# Dr. Chase's Old-Time Home Remedies

## INCLUDES TRADITIONAL ADVICE FOR ILLNESSES AND INJURIES, NURSING AND MIDWIFERY, MEALS AND DESSERTS, HOUSEHOLD MAINTENANCE, BEEKEEPING, AND MUCH MORE!

**Dr. Alvin Wood Chase**

CLYDESDALE

Originally published in 1903 by F. B. Dickerson Company

First Clydesdale Press Edition 2020

Clydesdale books may be purchased in bulk at special discounts for sales promotion, corporate gifts, fund-raising, or educational purposes. Special editions can also be created to specifications. For details, contact the Special Sales Department, Skyhorse Publishing, 307 West 36th Street, 11th Floor, New York, NY 10018 or info@skyhorsepublishing.com.

Clydesdale Press™ is a pending trademark of Skyhorse Publishing, Inc.˙, a Delaware corporation.

Visit our website at www.skyhorsepublishing.com.

10 9 8 7 6 5 4 3 2 1

Library of Congress Control Number: 2019912319

Cover design by Mona Lin

Print ISBN: 978-1-945186-60-8
eISBN: 978-1-945186-61-5

Printed in the United States of America

# DEDICATION.

THIS, MY THIRD AND LAST RECEIPT BOOK,

IS MOST RESPECTFULLY DEDICATED

To the Twelve Hundred Thousand Families, throughout the
United States and Dominion of Canada,

WHO HAVE PURCHASED

ONE OR BOTH OF MY FORMER BOOKS, AND TO THEIR CHILDREN

WHO HAVE THUS BECOME FAMILIAR WITH THEM, AND

WOULD, THEREFORE, DESIRE TO BENEFIT

THEMSELVES, AND PERPETUATE THE NAME OF THE "OLD DOCTOR,"

BY HANDING THIS, THE CROWNING WORK OF MY LIFE,

TO *THEIR* CHILDREN.

A. W. CHASE, M. D.

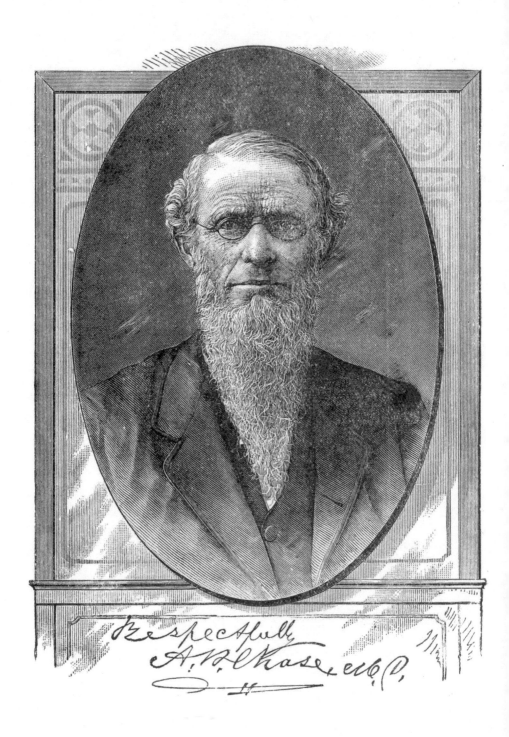

Respectfully,
A. B. Chase & Co.

# PUBLISHERS' PREFACE.

In presenting this book to the public, we make no apologies. There never was but one Doctor A. W. Chase. The immense sale of his former works is evidence that the public demand all that ever came from his prolific and philanthropic pen. There is no man now living, and none dead, whose writings have been so eagerly sought for, and no man, whose whole life was so devoted to the good of others. Through reverses in business, he left no pecuniary benefits to his family except the manuscript of this book, but died with the consciousness that his work had been appreciated and that he had been a benefactor to mankind. Dr. Chase's name is a household word in millions of homes; we trust this book will make it a familiar name in a million more, and, although this, his final work, is by him dedicated to the people whom he served so long and well, we, as publishers, think it befitting to such as he to inscribe it "The Memorial Edition" and dedicate it to HIS CHILDREN.

THE PUBLISHERS.

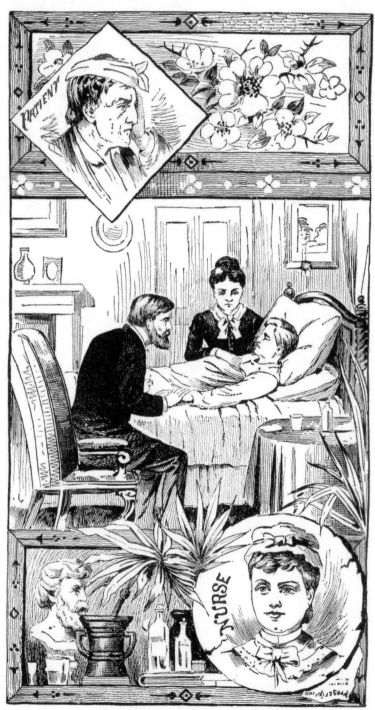

THE NURSE AND PATIENT.

# AUTHOR'S PREFACE.

The reason for the publication of this book is, that having given over fifty years of my life to the careful observation and test of Practical Receipes, as given in my first and second books, *i. e.,* "Dr. Chase's Receipts, or Information for Everybody;" and "Dr. Chase's Family Physician, Bee Keeper, and Second Receipt Book," by which it has become very natural for me to make notes of and preserve for future reference, items and receipts discovered by myself and those seen in the discourses of the Scientific, Medical, Agricultural, Mechanical and Household Publications of the day; and observing that as time advanced, every branch of Science and Art, by continued experience, became more and more perfect, practical and positive in its development, I continually selected and preserved the *very choicest* items until enough was accumulated for a THIRD BOOK. And fully believing that it would be appreciated by the people who had purchased over *twelve hundred thousand copies* of my former publications, within the thirty years they have been before them, I determined to prepare it before I could willingly and conscientiously lay down my life work. I have, therefore, labored over four years faithfully and diligently in experimenting, compiling and arranging this, my third and last book, as I knew it would do good in every home it entered. I am now willing and shall forever rest from this character of labor, that I may partake, a little at least, of the benefits and pleasures that I have done my best to prepare for others, feeling more than satisfied that if the people will give the time and earnestness in using this book that the author has in preparing it, the benefits and pleasures will not only be mutual, but more lasting than our lives, benefitting even our children's children.

As to the reliability of the information given in this volume, the unprecedentedly large sales of my two former works will testify. It is only necessary to say that the longer one labors in a practice or profession, or in the mechanical arts, the more mature is his mind and judgment and the better qualified he is to carry on his work. This being universally conceded, it need only be said, then, that one who has lived nearly seventy years, doing all the good possible to his fellow creatures, as I have done, if judged by the above evidence, would certainly make his last the crowning effort of his life, and that it shall be so found I feel assured. This work is the result of nearly thirty years practice and experience since the publication of my first book, and is not a "revised edition" of the former ones, but is made up wholly of new matter and new discoveries. I, therefore, believe that it will prove of infinite value to its purchasers, and although they may have both the former ones in their possession, they cannot, if they value my first and second book, afford to be without this, my third and last one. My mature years, numbering nearly three score and ten, will not allow me to ever undertake that great labor which, in this case, covers a period of nearly five years.

A Receipt Book, not being calculated for general reading, can very properly be set in closer type than an ordinary book, and as it is my aim to give the greatest possible amount of information for the money invested, I have instructed the type-setters to use the smallest type that can, with ease, be read; yet the following will serve to illustrate the fact that even a receipt book is, by some, read to a considerable extent. As I was once traveling through Illinois, a gentleman, just before we reached the crossing of the Mississippi at Burlington, approached me, and said, " Isn't this Dr. Chase, the author of Chase's Receipt Book?" (referring to my first) to which I replied, "Yes, sir," when he remarked: " I thought I recognized you from the frontispiece in your book;" and added, "We read it more than the Bible," etc. To which I remonstrated and begged to suggest that he instruct his family from that time forward to read the Bible most, inasmuch as eternity was of infinitely more importance than this life. His name I have forgotten, but I take the liberty of giving the name and address of a lady in Wisconsin, whose letter I received while preparing this last work, presuming she will take no offense, as I give her name and letter only to prove to the public in what esteem my former books are held by those who have them. The following is from Mrs. O. N. Alden, and dated at Neenah, Wisconsin:

DR. A. W. CHASE,
    DEAR SIR:
                It is not the author or compiler of every book who himself so permeates the contents that the reader feels in the author a personal acquaintance, but when I am consulting Dr. Chase's Books, it seems as though I was personally consulting him, and that he is a friend, he makes what is therein so individual. But, by so doing, he exposes himself to, perhaps, annoyance, as in this instance, by being personally addressed. * * *

The writer closes by relating her own condition of health, and making inquiry as to the character of goods made by another gentleman. I mention these circumstances among hundreds of others only to illustrate to those having neither of my former books what those who do have them think of them, hoping thus to convince the million that my third and last book shall, at least, be equally valuable. I have, however, done my best to produce a work in every respect superior to my former ones, and with the aid of thirty years' experience since my first book was published, during which time many new theories have come into vogue and many valuable discoveries have been made, I am confident that I have succeeded, and can only hope that my former works have opened the door to this, my Crowning Life Work, and that it will be a welcome visitor at every home, where either or both the first and second books have found their way and prove to be worth many times more than the sum paid for it.

                                THE AUTHOR.

Just two months after completing this work, and writing the foregoing preface, the "Old Doctor" passed away and his spirit took its flight to God who gave it.

                                PUBLISHERS.

# In Memoriam.

———✠———

DR. ALVIN WOOD CHASE, physician, and author of the celebrated Dr. Chase's Receipt Book, was born in Cayuga County, New York, in 1817. He was a son of Benjamin Chase, a native of the State of Massachusetts. When Alvin was eleven years of age his parents located near Buffalo, N. Y., where he grew to manhood, receiving a very limited education, in a log school-house. His desire for knowledge was so strong, coupled with an ambition peculiar to his naturally energetic disposition, that he far outstripped his more dilatory companions of that humble institute of learning. When seventeen years old he left New York and found employment on the Maumee River, in the meantime devoting his spare moments to study. In 1840 he located at Dresden, Ohio, where in the spring of 1841 he married Martha Shutts, daughter of Henry and Martha Shutts, natives of New York. To this noble and gifted wife, and mother of his children, may be justly attributed much of the success that followed the doctor during his long and eventful career. From the days of his boyhood he entertained a wish to study medicine, and awaited with impatience the time when he might become a member of the fraternity. After many wanderings he settled in Ann Arbor, Mich., in 1856, where, to his intense delight, he was enabled vigorously to prosecute his studies in what was to be his future life-work.

He attended lectures in the medical department of the State University during 1857 and 1858, and graduated from the Eclectic Institute of Cincinnati, Ohio, in the meantime. Prior to 1869 he traveled over a large part of the United States, acquiring valuable knowledge, only gained by practical experience, which proved a good foundation for the wonderful book which afterward gained such great celebrity. The first edition of the work, like all subsequent ones, proved a great success, and soon placed the author on the high road to fortune. In 1864 he built the first part of that magnificent structure that still bears his name. It stands on the corner of Main Street and Miller Avenue, and is an ornament to our city. The building was completed in 1868. The business had so increased that at this time fifty persons found constant and remunerative employment within the walls of the building; and the hospitality and liberality of the Doctor to the employes of the institution, as well as to the needy ones of the city, were always subjects of admiring comment.

In 1873 he published his second book, of which many thousand copies were sold, and it is safe to say that fully one million and a half have found their way into the homes of this and foreign countries.

A few years only have elapsed since Dr. Chase was considered one of the most prosperous and well-to-do citizens of Ann Arbor; losses by thousands and tens of thousands dollars greatly reduced his accumulations so honestly acquired. It is seldom the case that so much wealth is secured in so short a time by honest endeavor. He entered into no speculating schemes, but industriously pursued a very useful calling, bringing large profits without detriment to any, but, on the contrary, of great value to all. But, notwithstanding his losses, he did not lose his native energy and manliness of purpose, and stood before the community a conspicuous example of what energy, perseverance, and an indomitable will may accomplish. His liberality was remarkable, considering his income, though large. Many men, whose means were quadruple those of the Doctor, did not give one quarter as much for the advancement of education and benevolent enterprises.

He was once nominated for mayor of the city, but his business compelled him to decline the proffered honor. But the storms of life finally overtook him and swept with almost resistless fury around the now aged physician, and a few of the prejudices that characterize the human family found a resting place in the heart of this noble man; yet, when the last chapter shall have been entered in the book of life, the account will probably be balanced. The last earthly rites have been performed, and the aged veteran laid peacefully away beneath the shadow of the silent tomb. It may truthfully be said that he lived with malice toward none and charity to all. A beautiful monument marks the place where his earthly remains are laid away, but his real and ever-enduring monument is seen in his life, devotion and usefulness to his fellow man.

L. DAVIS,
*Secretary of the Washtenaw County
Pioneer Society.*

ANN ARBOR, Mich.

# CONTENTS.

# PHRENOLOGY DEFINED.

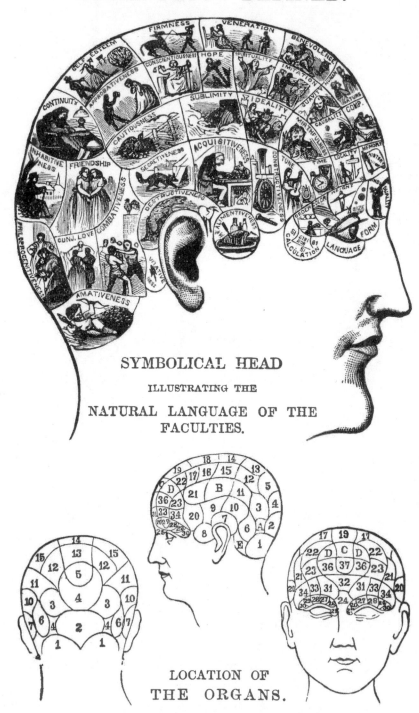

SYMBOLICAL HEAD

ILLUSTRATING THE

NATURAL LANGUAGE OF THE
FACULTIES.

LOCATION OF
THE ORGANS.

NAMES AND NUMBERS OF THE ORGANS.

# MEDICAL DEPARTMENT.

## SYMPTOMS OF DISEASES.

*Remarks.*—In preparing "Symptoms" I have carefully given all diseases that any person is liable not to be familiar with. There are some few common complaints, that "tackle" us without giving symptoms or warning, that I have omitted. A man would not need to be told that he had the *toothache* or *earache*, or what the symptoms are. He would be liable to find it out very suddenly without consulting any book or doctor. Some such simple diseases I have omitted in "*Symptoms.*"

**ABORTION OR MISCARRIAGE.**—When a woman in the family way throws off the contents of her womb, or loses her child, during the first six months, the accident is a *miscarriage*, or *abortion;* when the same thing happens during the last three months of her term, it is a premature labor.

*Symptoms.*—If abortion occur during the first month after conception, the symptoms may not attract much attention, or may be regarded only as an irregularity of menstruation. Occurring at later periods, it is frequently indicated by some feverishness, coldness of the feet and legs, a puffed-up condition of the eye-lids with purplish discolorations, shooting pains in the breasts, which become soft, pains in the back, bearing-down pains in the lower part of the bowels, which come and go, and at length take the character of real labor pains. As these pains increase, blood begins to appear, and, sooner or later, the bag of water breaks, and the fetus is thrown off.

*Causes.*—These are very numerous. Some of the principal are, displacement of the womb; ulceration of its neck; syphilitic disease of the fetus received from the parent; too much exercise; heavy lifting; falls, particularly when the woman comes down upon the feet, and is heavily jarred; emetics; powerful purges; and too much nuptial indulgence. REMEDY, pages **258, 259, 260, 261.**

**AGUE.**—The popular English name for *Intermittent Fever. Ague* is principally applied to the cold stage. The whole disease is commonly called *Fever and Ague.*

*Symptoms.*—This fever consists of various fits or paroxysms, each of which is made up of three stages or successions of symptoms. These stages are the cold, the hot, and the sweating stages. When the sweating stage is finished, the patient is free of complaint, or the disease intermits till a future period, when the same stages as before succeed each other. The time during which the patient is free of the disease varies in different kinds of intermittent fever, and gives its name and character to the disease. If the stages run through their course every day, it is called a quotidian ague; if they begin again every

1

third day, including that on which the former paroxysm occurred, it is called a tertian; if every fourth day, a quartan. Several minuter varieties occur, with which it is unnecessary to trouble the general reader. REMEDY, pages **86, 87, 88, 89, 90, 91, 123.**

APOPLEXY.— A disease in which the patient suddenly falls down, deprived of sense and motion; and which, in all languages, derives its name from the sudden manner of its attack, as if the patient were struck down by some invisible hand, by lightning, or some other agent equally sudden and violent.

*Symptoms.*—A person seized with apoplexy in its most perfect form, suddenly falls down, deprived of sense and motion, breathes heavily, and with a snoring sound; sometimes convulsions occur, and foam issues from the mouth. The pulse is full and strong, a cold clammy sweat breaks out over all the body; and the accumulating saliva, the bloated countenance, and the noisy laborious breathing, combine to form a distressing spectacle. The disease is not always so complete and violent, but varies in its symptoms, as is well described by Dr. Abercrombie:—"Sometimes the disease begins with a sudden attack of violent pain in the head, the patient becomes pale, sick and faint, generally vomits; and frequently, though not always, falls down in a state resembling fainting, the face very pale, the pulse very small. This is sometimes accompanied by slight convulsion. In other cases he does not fall down, the sudden attack of pain being only accompanied by slight and transient loss of recollection. In both cases he recovers in a few minutes, is quite sensible, and able to walk; continues to complain of intense headache; after a considerable time, perhaps some hours, becomes oppressed, forgetful, and incoherent, and thus gradually sinks into deep sleep, from which he never recovers. In some cases, palsy of one side occurs, but in others, there is no palsy. There is another form of the disease, in which the patient is suddenly deprived of the power of one side of the body, and of speech without stupor; or if the first attack is accompanied with stupor, this soon goes off; he appears sensible of his situation, and endeavors to express his feelings by signs. In some cases the attack passes gradually into apoplexy. perhaps after a few hours; in others, under the proper treatment, the patient recovers perfectly in a few days. In many cases the recovery is gradual, and it is only at the end of several weeks or months that the complaint is removed."

It is a matter of very great difficulty to determine what is the particular state of the brain which gives rise to the symptoms of apoplexy. Sometimes, after a fatal case, when the head is opened, we find a large quantity of coagulated blood, and we consider the pressure of this effused blood as completely explaining what has happened. But in other cases which have ended fatally, there is only a small quantity of fluid in some part of the brain; and in others, even after very marked symptoms, no injury whatever, or deviation from the healthy appearance, can be perceived in the brain.

There are certain habits of body that seem more peculiarly disposed to this disease. Men with short thick necks, large heads, and corpulent bellies, especially after their thirty-fifth or fortieth year, are very frequently the subjects of this disease; but very many examples occur of a make directly the reverse of this, viz., tall and slender, being also attacked with apoplexy. REMEDY, page **131.**

**ASTHMA.**—*Symptoms.*—A painful difficulty of breathing, recurring at intervals, with a sense of tightness across the breast; a wheezing cough, hard at first, but towards the end of each paroxysm more free, and followed by the discharge of a little mucus. The attacks of asthma are generally in the night-time, though they sometimes come on in the course of the day; and at whatever time they come on, it is for the most part suddenly, with a sense of tightness across the breast, impeding respiration. The person, if in bed, is obliged immediately to get up, and he requires the free admission of air. The difficulty of breathing increases, and is performed slowly, and with a wheezing noise. These symptoms sometimes continue for hours together; and a remission takes place by degrees; the breathing becomes less laborious, and the patient speaks and coughs more easily; and if there is something expectorated, the remission is greater, and sleep comes on. In the morning, and through the day, though the breathing is better than during the fit, it is not yet free from difficulty; a degree of tightness is still felt, and a very slight motion of the body is apt to bring back the paroxysm. In the evening the breathing is worse, and about the same hour as on the former night, generally between midnight and two o'clock, the same train of symptoms is renewed. After the fits have recurred for several nights in this manner, they suffer more considerable remissions; and, for some time, asthmatics may be free from complaint; but through the whole of life the paroxysms are ready to return, though in different circumstances in different patients.

Asthma seldom appears before the age of puberty, and seems to attack men more frequently than women; and in persons of a full habit whom it continues to attack, it commonly causes a great degree of emaciation. Though it does not often destroy life in the paroxysms, it may become fatal by passing into other diseases, as into consumption of the lungs, or by occasioning dropsy; and many cases, which have appeared a common spasmodic asthma, have been found at last to depend on organic diseases of the heart and great vessels.

*Causes.*—Some have the fits of spasmodic asthma brought on by heat, whether of the weather or of warm apartments; and frequently by warm bathing. Some are hurt by cold and moist air, or by anything worn tight about the breast, or by distension of the stomach from a full meal, or windy diet; or from exercise hurrying the circulation of the blood. Sometimes the disease is brought on by causes affecting the nervous system, as passions of the mind; or by particular smells, or irritations of the lungs from smoke or dust. REMEDY, pages **200, 201.**

**ATROPHY.**—*Symptoms.*—A disease, of which a very prominent symptom is wasting of the body, from deficiency of nourishment. It is well known to the nurses in Scotland by the term *Dwining.* It is very common in children, and proceeds in them from various causes; from teething; from acidity of the stomach, and disorder of the bowels; from rickets, from diseases of the glands of the mesentery; and this last cause is by far the most common. The patient is at first languid and inactive; has a bad appetite, a disagreeable breath, a pale complexion, a large belly; the bowels are not regular, sometimes costive, at other times loose; the stools smell badly, and are of a whiter color than natural. When the disease has continued for some time, the body becomes greatly emaciated, the belly still more swelled, and the digestive functions more disordered. REMEDY, page **190.**

**BARBERS' ITCH.**—*Symptoms.*—This is contagious and due to a fungus growth that invades the hair and hair follicles. It appears chiefly on the hairy parts of the face—the chin, the upper lip, the region of the whiskers, the eyebrows, and the nape of the neck. It consists in little conical elevations, which maturate at the top, and have the shaft of a hair passing through them. These pimples are of a pale yellowish color. REMEDY, page **102.**

**BLADDER—INFLAMMATION.**—*Symptoms.*—The bladder is also liable to inflammation without rupture. The symptoms of this formidable complaint are a burning pain at the lower part of the belly, increased by pressure; constant desire to pass water, which is done in very small quantities, and with intense pain; and more or less general fever. REMEDY, page **253.**

**BLOODY FLUX.—DYSENTERY.**—*Symptoms.*—The disease comes on with loss of appetite, costiveness, lassitude, shivering, heat of skin, and quick pulse. These are followed by griping pain in the bowels, and a constant desire to pass their contents. In general the passages are small, composed of mucus mixed with blood. These passages are attended and followed by severe gripings and inclination to strain, learnedly called *tormina*, and *tenesmus*. They are sometimes, in the early stages, attended by nausea and vomiting. The natural feces, which do not pass off much, are small in quantity, and formed into round, compact balls, or irregular, hardened lumps. This tenesmus, or great desire to strain, will continue, perhaps increase, for several days,—the discharges being mostly blood in some cases, and chiefly mucus in others. Having, generally, but little odor, at first, these discharges become, as the disease advances, exceedingly offensive.

*Causes.*—Dysentery is very frequently caused by sudden changes from hot to cold, by which sweating is suddenly checked, and the blood repelled from the surface. Hot climates, and dry, hot weather, are predisposing causes. All green, unripe, and unwholesome food; and all indigestible food of every sort, may induce it. REMEDY, pages **60, 139, 195, 234.**

**BOIL.**—*Symptoms.*—A circumscribed inflammation in the external parts, which terminates in a pointed swelling, sometimes as large as a pigeon's egg, attended with redness and pain, and sometimes with a violent burning heat, These inflammations generally suppurate, but they do so very slowly. They break at first on the upper part, and some drops of matter ooze out. What is commonly called the *core* is next seen; it is a purulent substance, but thick and tenacious, almost like a solid body, and may be drawn out of the abscess. Its discharge is followed by a flow of thinner matter, after which the pain ceases, and the part heals. REMEDY, pages **58, 59, 60, 97, 137.**

**BOWELS, INFLAMMATION OF.**—*Symptoms.*—This disease is characterized by the symptoms of general fever, heat of skin, thirst, restlessness, quick and hard small pulse; and by sharp pain in the belly, increased on pressure, and accompanied by vomiting and costiveness.

*Causes.*—Inflammation of the bowels is occasioned by acrid and irritating substances swallowed by the mouth, by hardened fœces, by vitiated bile, by long continued costiveness, and by constriction of some part of the canal in cases of rupture; a very frequent cause of it is cold, especially when applied with damp to the feet.

*Diagnosis.*—Inflammation of the bowels is distinguished from colic by the absence of fever in this last, and by the pain in colic not being increased on pressure, and in every case of severe pain of the bowels, with vomiting and costiveness, the practitioner should make very strict inquiries, lest a rupture should be the cause of them. REMEDY, pages **137, 252.**

**BRAIN — INFLAMMATION — CONCUSSION.**—Acute and general inflammation of the brain and its membranes has two stages.

*Symptoms.*— *The Stage of Excitement*, in which there is intense and deep-seated pain in the head, extending over a large part of it, a feeling of tightness across the forehead, throbbing of the temporal arteries, a flushed face, injected eyes, looking wild and brilliant, contraction of the pupils, great shrinking from light and sound, violent delirium, want of sleep, general convulsions, a parched and dry skin, a quick and hard pulse, a white tongue, thirst, nausea and vomiting, and constipation of the bowels.

*The Stage of Collapse*, in which there are indistinct mutterings, dull and perverted hearing and vision, double vision, the pupil from being contracted expands largely and becomes motionless, twitchings of the muscles, tremors and palsy of some of the limbs, a ghastly and cadaverous countenance, cold sweats, profound coma, and death

The disease will not show all these symptoms in any one case, It runs a rapid course, causing death, sometimes, in twelve or twenty-four hours; or it may run two or three weeks. REMEDY, pages **246, 247.**

**BRONCHITIS.**—*Symptoms.*—This disease is an inflammation of the membrane lining the air passages, or bronchi, is a very common, and a very serious disease. It is of two kinds, the *acute* and the *chronic* or "winter cough." The acute form, or severe cough, begins with the symptoms of common cold, or catarrh (see Catarrh); but difficulty of breathing, attended with a wheezing sound, and pain and cough, soon come on with great severity. There is also a degree of fever, generally much increased in the evening. With the cough, there is a tenacious and glary expectoration, sometimes purulent, and even mixed with blood. REMEDY, pages **123, 254, 255, 256.**

**BRONCHOCELE.**—*Symptoms.*—The goître, or swelled neck, which so frequently occurs among the inhabitants of mountainous regions. It is a common disorder in Derbyshire, and among the inhabitants of the Alps, and other hilly countries in their neighborhood; also in the valleys of Savoy, and at Milan, and among the Pyrennes, and Cevennes, in France. The swelling in bronchocele is at first without pain or any evident fluctuation, and the skin retains its natural appearance; but as the swelling advances, it grows hard and irregular; the skin becomes yellowish, and the veins of the neck put on a distended and winding appearance; then the patient complains of frequent flushing of the face with headache, and pains darting through the tumor. REMEDY, pages **44, 45.**

CANCER.— *Symptoms.*— By occult cancer or scirrhus, is meant a hard tumor, for the most part accompanied by sharp darting pains, which recur more or less frequently. This tumor, in course of time, breaks and ulcerates; and then is more strictly denominated cancer. The parts of the body subject to cancer are the following: The female breast and uterus (see Womb and its Diseases), the lips, especially the lower one, the tongue, the skin, the tonsils, the lower opening of the stomach, and some other parts chiefly glandular Chimney-sweepers are subject to a cancerous affection of the scrotum. REMEDY, pages **33, 34, 35, 99, 271.**

CARBUNCLE.— *Symptoms.*— An abscess or collection of matter, of a peculiarly gangrenous-looking nature. The first symptoms are great heat and violent pain in some part of the body, on which there arises a pimple with great itching; under this, there is a circumscribed tumor, seeming to penetrate deep into the parts below. This tumor soon puts on a dark red or purple color. A little blister frequently appears on the top of the tumor, which being broken. a dark-looking matter is discharged, and a slough makes its appearance. Sometimes a little slough of a black color is seen in the middle of the tumor. The progress of a carbuncle of the gangrenous state is generally rapid. The size of carbuncles is various; sometimes they are eight or ten inches in diameter. Considerable hardness and pain generally attend the disease. As it advances, several detached openings form in the tumor; and through these, a greenish, fetid, and irritating matter is discharged. Carbuncle most commonly occurs in constitutions that have been injured by luxurious living; and from this circumstance, and from its occurring not unfrequently in people advanced in life, carbuncle is commonly to be considered as accompanied with great danger; and this danger is to be estimated by the size and situations of the swellings, whether there be few or many of them, and by considering the age of the the patient, and the state of his constitution. REMEDY, pages **58, 59.**

CATARRH.— *Symptoms.*— The disease commonly called a *Cold*, of which the following are the ordinary symptoms:—The patient is seized with a coldness and shivering; and shortly after, there is a degree of difficulty in breathing through the nose, and a sensation as if something were stopping that passage; a symptom well known under the term of a stuffing of the nose or head. There is a dull pain and heaviness in the forehead, and the motion of the eyes is stiff and obstructed. There soon takes place from the nose, a plentiful discharge of thin watery matter, so sharp as to inflame and excoriate the skin of the nose and lips. There is a sense of weariness over the whole body; and the patient is usually sensible to the coldness of the air; and the pulse, especially toward evening, is more frequent than ordinary. These symptoms are very soon accompanied with hoarseness, and a sense of roughness and soreness in the course of the wind-pipe, with a difficulty of breathing, and tightness across the chest, and a cough, seemingly occasioned by something tickling or irritating the upper part of the wind-pipe. The cough is at first dry, and causes a good deal of pain in the chest, and about the head; and at times there are other pains resembling rheumatism, in various parts of the body. Gradually the cough becomes looser; that is to say, is accompanied by the discharge of mucus, which is brought up with more ease. The discharge from the nose becomes more mild, and also thicker; the pain of the head diminishes, but there is still a disagreeable sense of fullness about the nose, with a degree of deafness, ringing in the ears, and a wheezing sound when a full breath is drawn. There is also a bad taste in the mouth, with a foul tongue, although the appetite is good. REMEDY, pages **57, 155, 164, 183.**

**CHICKEN-POX.**—*Symptoms.*—A disease of the eruptive kind, in various particulars resembling small-pox, and apt to be confounded with it. Chicken-pox arises from a peculiar contagion, and attacks persons only once in their lives. It is preceded by chilliness by sickness or vomiting, headache, thirst, restlessness and a quickened pulse. After these feverish symptoms, which are generally slight, have lasted one or two days, pimples appear on different parts of the skin, in the form of small red eminences, not exactly circular; having a furface shining, and nearly flat, in the middle of which a small clear vesicle soon forms. On the second day, this is filled with a whitish lymph; on the third day, the fluid is straw-colored; and on the fourth day, the vesicles which have not broken begin to subside. Few of them remain entire on the fifth day; and on the sixth, small brown scabs appear in the place of the vesicles. On the ninth and tenth days, they fall off, without leaving any pits. REMEDY, page **224.**

**CHILBLAINS.**—*Symptoms.*—A painful inflammatory swelling on the extreme parts of the body, as the fingers, toes, and heels, occasioned by cold. A very common way of getting chilblains, is by bringing the hands and feet near the fire in cold, frosty weather. The color of chilblains is a deep purple or leaden hue, the pain is pungent and shooting, and a very disagreeable itching attends. In some instances, the skin remains entire; in others, it breaks, and a thin fluid is discharged. When the cold has been great or long continued, the parts affected are apt to mortify and slough off, leaving a foul ulcer behind. REMEDY, pages **142, 143.**

**CHILLS AND FEVER.**—See AGUE.

**CHLOROFORM.**—The formidable symptoms which sometimes arise from an overdose of chloroform are best met by opening the patient's mouth, and forcibly making the tongue protrude, allowing the free access of air, and applying ammonia to the nostrils. Chloroform should be administered only by a medical man. REMEDY, page **95.**

**CHOLERA.**—This disease is often attended by vomiting and purging, with cramps in various parts of the body. It first attracted notice as a wide-spreading and fatal epidemic, in the year 1817, when it appeared at at Jessore, in Bengal; and after ravaging the Continent and Isles of Asia, and spreading to China, it continued its destructive course westward through Germany and the Russian Empire, till it at length reached the British Islands in 1831. After committing frightful ravages, the disease disappeared from England in the end of 1832; but it reappeared in 1849, and carried off 15,000 people in London alone, and about 80,000 in the whole kingdom. In 1853 and 1854 the disease again caused a terrible mortality, upwards of 6,000 deaths having occurred in London alone during the first ten weeks of the epidemic which occurred in the latter year.

*Symptoms.*—The attack of the disease is sometimes quite sudden; at other times, there are precursory symptoms, of which the duration varies from a few hours to three or four days. There is a sense of general uneasiness and oppression, increased sensibility, not unlike a delusive feeling of high health and animation; pains about the navel; sometimes tremors and debility. The person is affected with derangement of the alimentary canal, more or less severe, indicated by sickness and vomiting, flatulent noises in the bowels, and frequent loose, but natural stools; these symptoms being accompanied or succeeded by thirst, headache, languors, and cramps or twitches in the limbs, breast, and other parts of the body. Such derangements often occur after some irregularity to which the patient has not been accustomed, as a luxurious meal, an indulgence in wine, spirits, beer, or porter, the eating of pastry, or other indigestible food; or after being exposed to the night-air, or to cold and damp. In ordinary seasons, these ailments might be left to nature, or carried off by a gentle laxative. But in seasons and districts where cholera prevails or is expected, no person, through fear of being thought whimsical, should neglect even very slight uneasiness; if the alarm be a false one, little harm is done; but if there be real danger to follow, it is of unspeakable consequence to have a medical man on the watch, to apply the remedies before the strength fails, and before the second stage, or that of collapse, comes on. REMEDY, pages **60, 127, 128, 139, 141, 236.**

**CHOLERA INFANTUM.**—See *Symptoms*, page **226.** REMEDY, page **226.**

**CHOLERA MORBUS.**—See *Symptoms*, page **225.** REMEDY, page **226.**

**COLIC.**—*Symptoms:*—A painful sensation spreading over the belly, and accompanied by a feeling of twisting or wringing at the navel. It is owing to spasms acting on the intestines themselves; and very frequently the skin and muscles of the belly are also drawn inwards and spasmodically contracted. These pains are very violent, unlike the transient gripings that occur in other affections of the bowels; and costiveness is a general attendant. Vomiting is also present; any thing taken in the mouth is apt to be rejected, and bile is thrown up.

*Causes.*—The causes of colic are various. It may arise from cold, from flatulence, from mechanical obstruction, from acrid matters taken into the stomach, from accumulation of fæces after long costiveness; it may also arise from passions of the mind. It is distinguished from inflammation of the bowels by the pain at times disappearing, by the absence of fever, and by pressure relieving the pain. Sometimes, however, long continued spasms induce inflammation. REMEDY, pages **41, 46, 127, 129, 197, 230, 277.**

**CONSTIPATION OR COSTIVENESS.**—The usual frequency of evacuating the bowels for persons in good health is once in twenty-four hours. The constitutions of different people vary in this respect; some having two or three motions in a day without any inconvenience or ill health; others not having above one or two in a week. When a person has habitually fewer motions than the generality of healthy people, he is said to be of a costive habit or constipated; and when he has at any time fewer than his ordinary rate, and when the fæces are hard, dry, and voided with difficulty, he said to be costive or constipated.

*Causes.*—Independently of medicine, it is not very easy to specify any diet or mode of living that universally predisposes to costiveness. Many articles have been blamed, and yet have been used by thousands without producing that effect. Rice in various modes of cookery; the finer kinds of bread; roast meat, eaten without a due proportion of vegetables; cheese; port and other dry wines; and indolent and sedentary life; and a sea voyage, are all known to occasion costiveness in certain individuals. In some infants this state is constitutional; and for some time, at least, appears to do them little harm. It is very apt to occur in children, as their volatility and playfulness cause them often to disregard the calls of nature, till a great and dangerous mass of feculent matter is accumulated in their bowels. The indolent and sedentary lives of females predisposes them much to costiveness. The structure of their pelvis also allows a larger mass to accumulate without inconvenience, from which circumstance the fæces are deprived of almost all their fluid parts, and the remainder becomes dry, hard, and difficult to be voided. Persons of the melancholic temperament; also those who are advanced in life, and those who take little exercise, are liable to become costive. REMEDY, pages **46, 47, 135, 136, 280.**

**CONSUMPTION.**—This disease is probably the greatest existing scourge of the human race, at least in the northern and middle latitudes. It is not deviating far from the truth to say that it causes about one-sixth or one-seventh of all the deaths north of the tropics. The duration of the disease is exceedingly variable. While some cases run their course to a fatal termination in less than a month, others have been known to continue thirty or forty years. The greater number of cases, as a rule, terminate in from one to two years. It is pre-eminently a hereditary disease.

*Symptoms.*—The earliest symptom of consumption that usually manifests itself is a short, dry cough, exciting no particular attention, being attributed to a slight cold. It, however, continues, and after a time increases in frequency. The breathing is more easily hurried by bodily motion, and the pulse becomes more frequent, particularly after meals and towards evening. Towards evening there is also frequently experienced a slight degree of chilliness, followed by heat and nocturnal perspirations. The patient becomes languid and indolent, and gradually loses strength. After a time the cough becomes more frequent, and is particularly troublesome during the night, accompanied by an expectoration of a clear, frothy substance, which afterwards becomes more copious, viscid, and opaque, and is most considerable in the morning; the *sputa* are often tinged with blood; or hæmoptysis occurs in a more marked form, and to a greater extent As the disease advances, the breathing and pulse become more hurried; the fever is greater, and the perspirations more regular and profuse. The emaciation and weakness go on increasing; a pain is felt in some part of the thorax, which is increased by coughing, and sometimes becomes so acute as to prevent the patient from lying on the affected side. All the symptoms increase towards evening; the face is flushed; the palms of the hands and the soles of the feet are affected with a burning heat; the feet and ankles begin to swell, and in the last stage of consumption there is nearly always profuse diarrhœa. The emaciation is extreme; the countenance assumes a cadaverous appearance, the cheeks are prominent, the eyes hollow and languid. Usually the appetite remains entire to the end, and the patient flatters himself with the hope of a speedy recovery, often vainly forming distant projects of interest or amusement, when death puts a period to his existence. Tubercular deposits are also usually found in other organs of the body; the liver is enlarged and changes in appearance, and ulcerations occur in the intestines, the larynx, and trachea. These are so frequent and uniform as to lead to the belief that they form part of the disease.

*Causes.*—The causes of this disease are divided into remote and exciting. Of the former, the most important is hereditary predisposition. It is not, however, an actual cause of the disease; and hence there are many cases in which the children of consumptive parents do not fall a prey to this disease; but it renders those who are in that condition much more liable to be affected by the exciting causes. Whatever weakens the strength of the system, or interferes with the oxygenation of the blood, tends to the production of this disease. Hence living in bad air, insufficient and unwholesome food, and sedentary pursuits, tend to it. Among the more exciting causes are exposure to cold or damp, especially after the body has been heated, intemperance of any kind, profuse evacuations, and exposure to the reception of dust into the lungs, as in the case of certain artificers, needle-pointers, stonecutters, and the like. REMEDY, pages 101, 109, 110, 112, 113, 117, 118, 125, 184.

**CONVULSION FITS OF CHILDREN.**—When we speak of convulsions, or convulsion fits, we most commonly mean epilepsy; and principally that species of it which occurs in very young children.

*Symptoms.*—In some cases convulsions come on suddenly, at other times the attack is gradual, and the first symptoms elude the observation of the attendants. In the sudden attack, the child, previously quite well, becomes livid in a moment; his eyes and features are contorted, and the limbs and whole body are violently agitated. These symptoms end by the patient falling into a state of insensibility, which in some cases proves fatal, and in others goes gradually off. In those cases where the attack is milder and more gradual, the child shows some degree of uneasiness; he suddenly changes color, his lips quiver, his eyes are turned upwards, and he stretches himself out, or his hands become clenched. Sometimes there is a rapid succession of fits; sometimes the intervals between them are long. Convulsions vary also in their degree of violence. Before the fatal termination of many of the diseases of infancy, convulsions occur, and appear to be the cause of death. Hence, their taking place after long or serious illness, may be considered as an indication of approaching death. But a single fit may destroy an infant. When the return of the convulsions is not suspended within forty-eight hours after active treatment has been adopted, there is reason to dread either a sudden fatal termination, or a long protraction of the disease. In this latter case, if the infant does not become emaciated, there is a probability of his eventual recovery, even although he had been blind and insensible for days or weeks. In some rare cases, though the health be restored, imbecility of mind remains. If emaciation attend the protraction of fits, the living powers at last give way.

*Causes.* — Convulsions arise from any thing capable of strongly irritating the nervous system; hence infants and young children, whose nervous system is so very delicate, and who are exposed to so many causes of irritation, are by far the most frequently affected with convulsions. These may arise from worms in the intestines, from certain kinds of food disagreeing with the child, from acidity, from wind; and, with remarkable frequency, from teething. Another cause of convulsions in children is the too sudden disappearance or going in of a rash or eruptive disorder. Children very frequently are seized with convulsions just before the appearance of small-pox; and in some cases, though very rarely, they occur before the appearance of measles. The general irritation arising from want of cleanliness, living in foul air, etc., may give rise to convulsions. Sometimes they are only the symptoms of a more deep and violent disease, as of water in the head, or growth of bone within the skull. In this case our attention is to be directed to the original disease; the symptoms and treatment of water in the head will be detailed in their proper place. REMEDY, page 232.

CROUP.—*Symptoms:*—In what is known as *false* croup the child coughs for two or three days, running at the nose, slight cold at first; or these symptoms may be absent. Between 10 and 12 o'clock at night may occur a sudden, loud, barking cough, whistling breathing, breathing hard, face flushed, great restlessness, skin hot and dry, pulse fast, lasts from 1 to 3 hours; patient generally gets well,—subject to return of disease.

*In true croup the symptoms are:* cold in head; hoarse, dry cough; voice hoarse, spittle frothy, membrane comes off when child vomits, breathing rapid, and the chest is quiet, the breathing being done by the bowel muscles; nostrils dilated, spasms of throat, and child throws itself from side to side; eyes wild; face anxious, fingers and lips blue, between spasms of throat, child is quite pulse, 110 to 190. If symptoms lull, do not think child is better, for usually they will recommence. Disease lasts from 2 to 14 days, and 19 out of 20 *die*. REMEDY, pages **105, 106, 107, 210.**

**DELIRIUM TREMENS.**—*Symptoms.*—This is a disease consisting essentially of excessive irritability and exhaustion of the nervine functions. Physicians term it *Delirium Tremens*, from the abberation of mind and the universal shaking of the body which characterise it. It is generally caused by excessive and long continued abuse of ardent spirits; or by their sudden withdrawal; but it may arise from any cause which exhausts the brain, or excites the nervous system for a length of time.

*Symptoms.*—The attack of this complaint is more or less sudden in different instances. For a few days at its commencement, the patient is merely incapable of his ordinary duties and exertion; a constant restlessness, debility, and inappetency, and occasional vomiting take place, with dullness and dejection of spirits, and headache. Vague suspicions are entertained of approaching danger, and he is haunted by visions and figures. Delirium generally accompanies these hallucinations, and the patient is always looking about, apprehensive of being seized, and distrusting every one who approaches. He is sensible for a moment when reasoned with, but soon reverts to his delusions. The pulse is quick, but soft, the skin cool or perspiring, and the pupil dilated. REMEDY, page **190.**

**DIABETES.**—*Symptoms.*—The name of a disease in which the urine is exceedingly increased in quantity. The normal amount of urine passed every twenty-four hours is about fifty fluid ounces, while in diabetes the patient will often pass from three to five gallons of pale colored urine within that time, and contains a great portion of sugar. There is great thirst and a voracious appetite, with wasting of the body; and the quantity of the urine far exceeds the food and drink taken in. Young persons are rarely attacked with this disorder. The most frequent subjects of it are those in middle age or in the decline of life, or who have made a free use of wine in their earlier years. It happens to persons of both sexes, and it is not easy to point out any particular constitution that is subject to it, or to say that any other disease is a forerunner of it. Dissection throws little light on the nature of this complaint; but it is now believed to be owing to a distinct lesion of the nervous system. Diabetes comes on insidiously without any previous disorder; it may continue for a long time without much emaciation, and it is commonly the great thirst and voracious appetite that first call attention to the disorder that is going on in the system. Severe headache is also a symptom of some importance. The emaciation is probably connected with increased metamorphosis, as indicated by the increased secretion of urea and phosphates. Sometimes, in the progress of the disease, the stomach is considerably deranged, the skin becomes dry, parched and scaly, and there is a sense of weight and pain in the urinary passages. When the disease has continued long, there is extreme emaciation, debility, and the usual symptoms of hectic fever. REMEDY, pages **176, 177, 184, 178-180.**

**DIARRHŒA, OR LOOSENESS OF THE BOWELS.**—A dis-ease consisting of more frequent and liquid evacuations by stool than usual, with griping and occasional vomiting. It is distinguished from dysentery by the absence of painful and ineffectual straining, and by the stools not consisting of blood and mucus.

*Causes.*—The causes of diarrhœa are many and various. 1. Cold applied to the whole body is not an unfrequent cause, and cold applied to the feet alone, in very many cases, produces diarrhœa. 2. Diseases of other parts of the body give rise to diarrhœa, as happens to infants while teething, and to persons who have a paroxysm of gout. 3. Certain emotions of the mind, particularly fear, are known to cause diarrhœa. 4. Certain articles of food taken into the stomach produce looseness. 5. Certain secretions of the body itself poured into the intestines, cause a laxity of them. In this way, heat is probably a cause of diarrhœa by first stimulating the liver; the increased secretion from which excites that from the small intestines, and looseness is the result.

Looseness *should not be rashly checked.* From the great variety of causes inducing diarrhœa, it must be obvious that it would be impossible to lay down any plan of cure that would apply to all cases, and it is often a matter of doubt whether it should be meddled with at all; thus, when from a surfeit, either in quantity, or from taking improper articles of food, a diarrhœa is produced, a wise physician will consider it as a salutary effort of nature to get rid of what would be noxious if retained; and he will allow it to go on for a time. taking care to watch that it does not come to excess. REMEDY, pages **60. 127, 128, 138, 139, 277.**

**DIPHTHERIA.**—The disease begins in the form of a whitish spot on one or both tonsils, unaccompanied at first by fever, and attended with only a trifling degree of uneasiness in swallowing. By and by this spot enlarges; its edges become of a florid color, fever steals on, and the act of swallowing becomes painful. A slough gradually forms, with evident ulceration at its edges; the fever increases, and headache and restlessness supervene. The partial separation of the slough, together with the rosy color of the edges of the ulcer with the moderate degree of fever for some days, promise a favorable issue But very unexpectedly, slowness of breathing, without either difficulty of wheezing takes place, with excessive and sudden sinking of the living powers; and it generally happens that within a day from this change the fatal event occurs; the breathing at first falls to eighteen respirations in the minute, then to sixteen, to twelve, and finally to ten or eight. Two other symptoms occasionally attend the disease; the one is a most offensive smell of the breath, and the other is the sudden appearance of croup. The disease attacks people of various ages. REMEDY, pages **50, 51, 52, 53, 54, 55, 56, 107.**

**DROPSY.**—*Symptoms.*—A disease, of which a very conspicuous symptom is the effusion of a watery fluid in certain cavities and cells, where it is not perceptible in the healthy state. Thus water may be accumulated in the ventricles of the brain, in the chest, in the belly, and the cellular texture generally, giving rise to a train of symptoms, different in each particular case, and requiring particular modes of cure. Water effused in the ventricles of the brain is commonly the consequence of previous inflammation; and gives rise to a variety of distressing symptoms, which generally prove fatal.  REMEDY, pages **45, 46, 161.**

**DYSENTERY, OR BLOODY FLUX.**—This is an inflammation of the mucous or lining membrane of the large intestine, of which the symptoms are frequent calls to stool, with a scanty discharge of mucus, alone or mixed with blood.  The stools are accompanied with copious discharges of wind, they generally exhibit a frothy appearance, and are often attended with a sense of scalding about the anus; the patient, after each evacuation, feels considerably relieved, and hopes, but in vain, to enjoy an interval of ease.  Along with this affection of the bowels, there is great dejection of spirits, prostration of strength, thirst, griping pains, and loss of appetite, with fever in very acute cases.  The disease varies in its duration; sometimes the patient sinks very rapidly, at other times lingers on for a long period, the slimy stools continuing, and being mixed with purulent and bloody matter from the ulceration of the bowels.

*Causes.*—It is a disease very common in warm climates, and is to be ascribed to exposure to heat, alternated with cold and moisture, especially in swampy localities, or the banks of rivers.  Whatever tends to congestion of the liver, such as intemperance, exposure, etc., in hot climates, will predispose to dysentery, by obstructing the return of the blood from the large intestines to the liver.  Sometimes dysentery attacks soldiers epidemically, when they are encamped on marshy ground, with a burning sun over-head, and having hard night duty to perform; and the disease may prevail with such virulence that there is good reason for supposing it infectious under these circumstances.  In ordinary cases it is not so.  At the same time, every precaution should be taken to promote cleanliness, to remove from the sick every thing putrid and offensive, and to give as little unnecessary disturbance as possible.  REMEDY, pages **60, 139, 195, 234.**

**DYSPEPSIA OR INDIGESTION.**—*Symptoms.*—These vary very much in different stages of the disease, and in different persons.  In general the complaint begins with a sense of fullness, tightness, and weight in the stomach, sooner or later, after meals, and a changeable, diminished, or lost appetite.  Occasionally, the appetite is craving, and when, in obedience to its promptings, a large meal is taken, there is pain in the stomach, with general distress and nervousness, and sometimes vomiting.  Flatulency and acidity are common, with sour and offensive belching of wind; and very often there is a water-brash, or vomiting of a clear, glairy fluid when the stomach is empty.  Dizziness is a prominent symptom.  There is a great deal of what patients call an "all-gone" feeling at the pit of the stomach,—a weakness so great at that particular spot that it is very hard to sit up straight.  There is a bad taste in the mouth; the tongue is covered with a whitish fur; there is headache, heartburn, palpitation at times, high-colored urine, and tenderness, now and then, at the pit of the stomach.  The bowels are generally irregular, sometimes very costive, at other times loose, when portions of food are passed off undigested.

Such are the symptoms in a case of simple disorder of the stomach, when no other part of the system is materially involved. This is *indigestion*, well marked, and distressing enough; but it is only a part of what is understood by a case of modern *dyspepsia.* In *this,* either the indigestion, in its course, disturbs and involves the nervous system, or the nerves become themselves disordered, and produce the indigestion. Sometimes one happens, sometimes the other, it matters not which; both are present,—the affection of the stomach and of the nerves, in a case of thorough dyspepsia. To make out a full-case, in its tormenting completeness, we must add to the above symptoms, great depression of spirits, amounting at times to complete hopelessness and despondency; a dread and fear of some impending evil; a lack of interest in passing events; unwillingness to see company or to move about; an irritable and fretful temper; a desire to talk of one's troubles, and nothing else; a sallow, haggard, sunken, and sometimes wild expression of countenance; a dry, wrinkled, and harsh skin, with unrefreshing sleep, disturbed by all sorts of annoyances and difficulties, such as shipwrecks, falls down precipices, and nightmare.

The man who has all these symptoms, or any considerable portion of them, has *dyspepsia,* and is about as miserable as if all the sorrows of life were electrical currents, and were running through him continually.

*Causes.* —Accidental fits of indigestion are of frequent occurrence, and arise for the most part from overloading the stomach with food, and indulging freely in wines, spirits, or other intoxicating liquors. Confirmed or chronic indigestion may depend on debility or want of tone of the stomach, or it may be caused by the lining or mucous membrane of this organ being in a state of irritation or chronic inflammation. Drinking large quantities of cold water while eating is a prevalent cause. Over indulgence of the sexual act is a predisposing cause. One of the most frequent causes of indigestion is not masticating the food we eat properly, by which such food is bolted, instead of being reduced to a natural pulp, thereby presenting to the digestive organs a hardened mass, which it has the greatest difficulty to operate upon. Another cause is habitual inattention to diet, both as regards the quality and quantity of food, irregularity in the times of eating, drinking large quantities of warm, relaxing fluids, and using malt liquors too freely. A third cause is insufficient exercise; a fourth cause, impure air; and, beside these, there are numberless other causes, which in a greater or less degree exercise their baneful influence upon this vital and all-important function of our natures. REMEDY, pages **59, 61, 135, 147, 148, 149.**

**ECZEMA, OR HUMID TETTER.** — This is a cutaneous disease, which is characterized by an eruption of small vesicles on various parts of the skin. These arise principally from some irritation, as from the heat of the sun or air in the summer season and in warm climates, as we see on the back of the hands and on the face; also on the neck and forearms in women. The eruption continues for two or three weeks, and there is not much internal disorder. Little can be done by medicine; much washing and rubbing is hurtful, and ointments and stimulants are to be avoided. Simple washing with tepid water relieves the smarting and tingling. Some persons have an eruption of this kind and even more severe, by the application of acrid substances; thus it occurs sometimes in grocers from handling sugar, and is then called the grocers' itch:

and masons and bricklayers may have it from the touching of lime. Similar
eruptions are also produced by the irritation of blistering ointment, not only
where the blister has been applied, but at some distance from it, and the eruption has a number of hard swellings and boils intermixed with it.  The
irritating cause must be removed, and emollient poultices applied to diminish
the heat and uneasiness, and to bring the boils to a suppuration.  Even a common bread and milk poultice often or long applied to a place, has sometimes a
similar effect.  In this case, the poultice must be left off, and simple dressing
applied.  A course of alteratives and gentle laxatives will do much good, and
the diet should generally be good and nourishing.  REMEDY, pages **97, 227.**

### EPILEPSY, CONVULSIONS, OR FALLING SICKNESS.—

A disease of frequent occurrence, and arising from many various causes, consisting of convulsions of more or fewer of the muscles of voluntary motion,
accompanied with a loss of sense, and ending in a state resembling deep sleep.
Epilepsy suddenly attacks persons seemingly in perfect health; and going off
after a certain time, the patients are left in their usual state.  In some patients
there is a very curious warning of the approach of an epileptic fit.  From some
point on the surface of the body, perhaps one of the fingers or toes, a sensation
begins, as of a cold wind, or the creeping of an insect; which appears to proceed to the head, and when it reaches that part, the patient is convulsed.  This
is called the *aura epileptica.*  In other cases, the patient fancies he sees a spectre
approaching him, and the contact of this figure is the commencement of the
convulsions.  Whether there be any warning or not, a person thus attacked
loses all power of sense and motion, and either falls or is thrown with convulsions to the ground.  In that situation, violent convulsions variously move the
limbs and the trunk of the body, and frequently with more violence on one
side than the other.  In almost all cases, the muscles of the face and eyes are
much affected, giving a very distressing and alarming distortion to the countenance.  The tongue is often affected, and thrust out of the mouth; and by the
convulsive action of the muscles which shut the jaw, the tongue is not unfrequently severely wounded, and has been known to be almost bitten through.
During the continuance of the convulsions, as the patient has not the power of
swallowing, the spittle issues from the mouth, worked into a frothy state by the
action of respiration.  This is always an unseemly appearance, though by itself
it is not to be greatly regarded.  The convulsions remit for a few minutes, and
are then renewed, perhaps with increased violence.  In a little time, the convulsions cease altogether, and the person is in a state of complete insensibility,
which remains for a considerable time.  Gradually he recovers his senses, but
has no distinct remembrance of what has passed from the first attack of the
paroxysm.  The pulse and breathing are somewhat irregular and hurried during the fit, but soon return to their natural state.

*Causes.*—In this, as in all nervous diseases, the explanation of causes is
very difficult.  The opposite causes of over-excitement and of debility are both
known to produce epilepsy.  Every thing that irritates the brain, or the mental
faculties, which we, in our imperfect knowledge, believe to be dependent on

the actions of the brain, has been known to produce epilepsy; thus an injury done to the skull, the growth of tumors in the internal parts of that cavity, splinters of bone scaling off in consequence of disease, and various alterations of structure which have been discovered after death in patients afflicted with epilepsy, give us just grounds for reckoning mechanical irritation among the causes of epilepsy.

*Remarks* —Persons subject to epileptic fits should be very careful to avoid excitement. REMEDY, pages **165, 212.**

**ERYSIPELAS, ROSE, OR ST. ANTHONY'S FIRE.**— An inflammation of the skin, often spreading rapidly, and extending to the *cellular tissue* below the skin. The disease comes on with shivering, thirst, and other feverish symptoms, and soon affects some part of the skin with swelling, and redness of an uncertain extent, on which blisters very commonly rise. It attacks various parts of the body, and very frequently the face. At the beginning of the disease, there is confusion of head, and some degree of delirium; and there is not unfrequently considerable drowsiness. About the second or third day, a slight redness appears, which gradually spreads till it has occupied the whole of the face, and from the face it extends to the scalp, and down the neck. The redness does not continue equally bright on all the parts affected, but fades a little on those where it began. The swelling is considerable, and sometimes so great as to disfigure the countenance, and to shut up the eyes. Blisters of various sizes, containing a thin yellowish liquor, rise on several parts of the face. Where blisters do not rise, the skin scales off at the conclusion of the disease. The fever and inflammation usually continue from eight to ten days. The severity and danger of the disease is to be judged from its effects on the brain. If there is much delirium and drowsiness, it portends great danger, especially when they appear early in the disease; but the absence of these symptoms is to be accounted favorable. REMEDY, pages **58, 175, 176, 183.**

**FELON.**—This is an abscess of the fingers, of which there are three kinds,—the first situated upon the surface of the skin, the second under the skin, the third within the sheath which contains the tendons of the fingers, and sometimes involving the covering of the bone.

The latter form of the disease is the most terrible, and begins with redness, swelling, and a deep-seated and throbbing pain, which gradually becomes so excruciating as to banish all sleep, and nearly drive the patient to distraction. Finally, matter forms and burrows in the deeper parts of the finger, and at length finds an opening which brings relief. REMEDY, pages **130, 164.**

**GALL-STONES.**—Concretions which form in the gall-bladder, and by their obstructing the passage leading from it to the intestines, prevent the bile from getting into them; hence jaundice is frequently produced. These gall-stones, when the obstruction is overcome, get down into the bowels, and are discharged by stool; then the disease abates, provided there is no other cause for it. The pain which gall-stones cause during their passage through the gall-duct into the bowels is very intense, and is felt in the region of the liver, sometimes also extending to the right shoulder. The pain is generally sharp, but it may be dull and aching; it comes on in paroxysms, is relieved by pressure, and is unaccompanied by fever. There is often vomiting of sour matter, and if the flow of bile is completely obstructed by the stone, jaundice comes on, and the urine becomes very highly-colored. The best way to relieve these symptoms, which often appear very suddenly, is to apply hot bran poultices assiduously, and to give a pill containing a grain of opium and ¼ of a grain of tartar emetic, every 3 hours until relief is obtained. If there is much retching or vomiting, the tartar emetic may be omitted. REMEDY, page **191.**

**GANGRENE (Mortification.)**—Gangrene is the first stage of mortification, so-called from its eating away the flesh. Gangrene may be considered as a partial death—the death of one part of the body while the other parts are alive.

*Causes.*—The causes are excessive inflammation, sometimes from hurts or injuries.

*Symptoms.*—All pain and sensation ceases in the part; and, if extensive, it turns from red to purple, livid, or black, with a quick low pulse and clammy sweats. If internal, there is a cessation of pain, but the body sinks and changes to a livid color, and often hiccoughs and other distressing symptoms attend. The face is pinched with cold, and the tongue brown. REMEDY, page **234.**

**GOITRE, OR BIG NECK.**-*Symptoms.*-A prominent, soft, elastic tumor, occupying the front of the throat, in the situation of the thyroid gland, and like it in shape. It is not tender, and the skin is not discolored. In old cases, the tumor becomes hard. In some instances the tumor is so large as to push the gullet to one side. REMEDY, pages **44, 45.**

**GONORRHŒA.**—See GLEET.

**GOUT.**—*Symptoms.*—The symptoms considered as characterizing gout are the following: The patient has a peculiar uneasiness about the stomach; there is a degree of fever; pain and inflammation attack the joints of the hands and feet, and principally the ball of the great toe; the feverish symptoms abate after some days; and at distant and uncertain intervals, the same series of symptoms again occur. The paroxysms of gout generally come on in spring, when the vernal heat succeeds to the winter's cold; and according as this takes place sooner or later, and according as the patient is exposed to the changes of temperature, so the period of attack will vary. The patient is affected with a degree of languor or heaviness, the functions of the stomach are disturbed; there is loss of appetite, flatulence or indigestion; the bowels are costive, the tongue loaded, and the urine high-colored and turbid. REMEDY, page **136.**

**GLEET, GONORRHŒA.**—*Symptoms.*—A continued running or discharge, after the inflammatory symptoms of a clap have ceased. The discharge is commonly thin and clear, and is not accompanied with pain or scalding in making water. It proceeds from relaxation or debility of the parts, and is best cured by some astringent or stimulant application to them; and at the same time, the general health is to be promoted by the use of bark, iron, and cold bathing  The best local applications are those made of the sulphate of zinc in the proportion of 2 grs to the oz., or 1 gr. of corrosive sublimate to 6 ozs. of water, and they require to be pretty frequently thrown up. They ought to excite a little pain on first being used.  If we do not succeed by astringent injections, we may be obliged to use bougies, either clean, or lightly touched with a little basilicon ointment.  Balsam of Copaiba in the dose of 1 dr. 3 or 4 times a-day, or the tincture of cantharides, 10 drops as often, may be given internally, or the following combination may be used: Take of citrate of iron and quinine, 1 scruple; tincture of cantharides, 1 dr.; water, 3 ozs.  Mix.  A dessert-spoonful 3 times a day in a wine-glass of water.  If we find no benefit from the above recommendation, we judge that the gleet does not arise from mere relaxation of the parts or from habit, but from unhealthy action of the glands in the urinary passage, and we attempt the cure of this by bougies, and by blisters to the perineum.  If the constitution is scrofulous, the remedies for that disease must be conjoined with our local applications.  Another cause of gleet is strictures in the urethra.  In such cases our attention is to be directed to the cure of the strictures, for which we refer to that article.  Sometimes a gleet is complicated with discharges of the seminal fluid; where this occurs in an originally bad constitution, which has been weakened by excesses, the sexual powers of the patient are much impaired, and may even be altogether destroyed.  REMEDY, pages **205, 206, 207, 208, 209.**

GRAVEL, OR STONE are the names applied to the diseases which are occasioned by concretions in the urinary passages.  *Gravel* signifies small stones that pass from the kidneys through the urethra into the bladder causing severe pain, hence the disorder induced in such cases is called a *fit* of gravel.  *Stone* is a calculous concretion in the kidneys or in the urinary bladder, which is too large to pass, or at least without great difficulty.  The symptoms to which such concretions give rise are of the most painful kind, and occur so frequently, as to become objects of very considerable interest.  There are so many different salts contained in the urine, that it does not appear wonderful that occasionally they should fail to be kept in complete solution  When this is the case, and when a nucleus is formed, they concrete around it, and by their getting into narrow passages, or pressing upon delicate organs, they occasion the severe symptoms of stone or gravel.  A *Fit of the Gravel* is accompanied by a fixed pain in the loins, a numbness of the thigh on the side affected, sickness and vomiting, and sometimes slight diminution of the quantity of urine.  Sometimes the acuteness of the pain occasions faintings and convulsion fits.  These violent and painful affections are generally terminated by the passage of small stones through the urethra; and the patient is for the time easy.  In those who are much disposed to gravel, these attacks may be expected again, at uncertain intervals.

When there is *Stone in the Bladder*, the symptoms are, a frequent inclination to make water, which flows in small quantity, and is often interrupted; and there is generally pain at the extremity of the passage, especially as the last drop  are expelled, and for some time afterwards.  REMEDY, page **48.**

**HAY-FEVER.**—Hay-asthma, and summer bronchitis, is a disease which occurs about the time of the hay harvest, and appears to be caused by the pol len of some wild plants getting into and inflaming the bronchial passages This theory is supported by the fact that those who live in situations where there is little or no vegetation do not suffer from it.

*Symptoms.*—A difficulty of breathing, and a burning sensation in the throat, are the chief characteristics of this affection. REMEDY, page 235.

**HEADACHE.**—Pain, heaviness, or oppression about the head is a very frequent occurrence, and arises from a great variety of causes. It is symptomatic of disorders of the stomach and bowels; and in such cases it often. proceeds to a very distressing height. We judge headache to arise from disorders of the stomach when the tongue is whitish, and slightly coated, with the edges of a pale red color. The patient has a dimness and indistinctness of sight; he has a dull pain or weight in the head, with some confusion, and he is somewhat giddy. The pulse is languid and feeble, but not very frequent. There is a degree of sickness and irritation about the stomach. There is a coldness and numbness about the fingers; and the patient becomes, what, in common language, is called *nervous.* This kind of headache commonly occurs in the early stages of digestion. It is best relieved by an emetic, but this is a remedy which should not be employed very often. REMEDY, pages **44, 74, 107, 108, 139, 183.**

**HEARTBURN.**—*Symptoms.*—A disagreeable sensation proceeding from acidity in the stomach, from which there are frequent belchings of sour flatulence, or discharges of water with a burning heat at the pit of the stomach. It is a very pertinacious symptom, and is not easily removed; it has its chance of abatement or cure like the other symptoms of indigestion, by air, exercise, and proper diet; but it is also to be palliated by giving such substances as will combine with an acid in the stomach, and form a tasteless and innoxious salt. REMEDY, pages **108, 244.**

**HEART DISEASE.**—*Symptoms.*—Of all the diseases of the heart the general symptoms are nearly the same. Respiration habitually short and constrained; palpitations and stiflings invariably produced by the motion of ascent, by rapid walking, by mental emotions, and returning even without known. cause; frightful dreams, and interruption of the sleep by sudden startings; occasionally the symptoms described under the name of *angina pectoris;* and, lastly, a cachectic paleness, with tendency to leucophlegmatic effusion, which eventually appears, are all symptoms which, to a greater or less extent, occur in persons affected with disease of the heart. REMEDY, pages **85, 108, 244.**

**HEMORRHAGE.** —Hemorrhage from the lungs may easily be distinguished from that of the stomach, as in the latter case the blood is vomited up, usually in large quantities, of a much darker color and more or less mixed with the contents of the stomach, whereas the blood from the lungs is of a florid color, is thrown up in small quantities, by coughing or hawking, and is more or less mixed with a frothy mucus. If bleeding from the stomach be but slight, a few drops of common table salt and vinegar may be sufficient to suppress it;

alum water may also be given. If these fail give a strong tea of the beth root. The bugle weed is also good — a strong tea, made from its leaves, to be taken cold during the day. REMEDIES— Hemorrhage of lungs, pages **48, 50, 188, 189**; nose, pages **84, 85, 188, 189**; uterus, pages **48, 179, 281.**

**HERNIA, OR RUPTURE.**—This signifies the displacement of any of the internal organs from their natural situation, but it is more commonly applied to that disease which arises from the bowels getting through some of the apertures designed for the transmission of other organs. When the parts of the bowels or omentum which have protruded can be replaced by change of posture or by the hand, the hernia is said to be *reducible,* when it is not, it is called *irreducible hernia;* and when dangerous or painful symptoms are brought on by its being constricted, it is said to be *strangulated.*

Ruptures are inconvenient and dangerous in proportion to their bulk, to the place where they occur, and to the stricture or pressure they undergo. REMEDY, pages **197, 234.**

**HYDROPHOBIA.** — *Symptoms.* — The symptoms of hydrophobia are the following: The bitten part begins to be painful, then there ensue uneasiness, restlessness, heaviness, a desire to be alone, sudden starting, pain, spasms, disturbed sleep, and frightful dreams. These symptoms increase, pains dart from the wounded place to the throat, with a sensation of choking, and dread at the sight of liquids. The person can swallow solids, but anything in a fluid form causes him to start back with horror; and the most painful convulsions are excited by any application of it to his throat or lips. In the course of the disease, vomiting comes on, with great thirst, dryness and roughness of the tongue, hoarseness, and a continual discharge of saliva. This saliva is very thick and viscid, and the constant efforts to get rid of it are very distressing. There is great watchfulness, a dislike of light and air, difficult breathing; in some cases, delirium occurs, but in others the judgment is unimpaired. The pulse becomes tremulous and irregular, convulsions arise, and the patient sinks exhausted, about the third or fourth day from the first appearance of the symptoms. REMEDY, page **243.**

**HYSTERIA, HYSTERICS, OR FITS.**—A disease presenting many alarming appearances, though the danger to life is by no means in proportion to the violence of the symptoms. It is chiefly confined to the female sex; and of them it principally attacks the high fed, the luxurious and the idle; also those who are addicted to the use of malt liquor or distilled spirits. It chiefly occurs between the age of 15 and 40; though in those who are peculiarly disposed to it, it may continue beyond the latter period. Hysteria is far more frequent at the monthly period than at other seasons. In those who are subjected to hysteria, it is very readily brought on by emotions of the mind, and especially by any surprise; and by long continuance of the disease, persons are brought to so morbid a state of sensibility, that the slightest noise or external impression agitates and alarms them. REMEDY, page **233.**

**IMPOTENCY.**—Impotency means incapacity in the male to perform sexual intercourse. This may arise from physical or moral causes, some of which are remediable, while others are not so. The loss of both testicles, or organic disease in them to a great extent, will render a man impotent for life; fear, weakening diseases, excessive drinking and smoking, may again make him temporarily incompetent. A skillful and kind physician should always be consulted where real or fancied incapacity exists, and under no circumstances whatever should advice be sought from advertisers of cordials, balms, restoratives, etc. REMEDY, pages 180–183.

**INFANTILE ERYSIPELAS.**—See ERYSIPELAS.

**JAUNDICE.**—This is a symptom of a disease, and not a disease, and depends upon the absorption of bile into the system from various causes. It is characterised by a universal yellowness of the skin, and of the white of the eyes; itching of the surface of the body, a white or claylike appearance of the stools; while the urine tinges linen of a yellow color. The disease is attended by a sense of weariness and languor, a feeling of pain or uneasiness about the pit of the stomach, and there is sometimes a slight difficulty of breathing. There is also sickness, vomiting, sourness of stomach, and various other symptoms of indigestion. There is sometimes an acute pain on the right side, below the margins of the ribs. There is not, in general, much fever. It is a vulgar error to believe that patients in jaundice see objects of a yellow color. REMEDY, pages **161, 201, 202, 203.**

**KIDNEYS, INFLAMMATION OF.**—*Symptoms.*—A weakness in the small of the back, and a dull, heavy pain in the kidneys. The urine is passed often, and in small quantities. It is alkaline,—sometimes white and milky,—and has in it deposits of phosphate of lime, and triple phosphates. REMEDY, page **252.**

**LIVER, INFLAMMATION OF.**—*Symptoms.*—These are sympathetic fever, with pain, and a sense of tension in the right side, inability to lie on the left side, difficulty of breathing, a dry cough, vomiting, and hiccough.

The pain is acute and lancinating generally, though sometimes dull and tensive. When sharp, it is like the stitch of pleurisy, and it indicates that the peritoneum which covers the liver is inflamed. When dull, it is the body of the organ which is suffering. When the convex surface of the liver is the seat of the disease, the pain is apt to run up to the right collar-bone, and to the top of the right shoulder. Breathing, coughing, and lying on the left side, increase the pain. A soreness is felt by pressing over the liver. The pulse is full, hard, and strong, the bowels are costive, and the stools are clay colored, owing to not being tinged with bile,—this having stopped flowing. The tongue is covered with a yellow, dark brown, or even black coat, and there is a bitter taste in the mouth. REMEDY, page **245.**

**LUNGS, INFLAMMATION OF.**—When the substance of the lung itself is inflamed, the disease is termed *pneumonia;* and the word *pleurisy* or *pleuritis* is restricted to inflammation of the pleura, *i. e.*, the membrane which envelopes the lungs, and lines the inner surface of the ribs. Sometimes both parts are affected, and then the term *pleuro-pneumonia* is used. For all practical purposes, the inflammation of these various parts may be included under one common name.

*Symptoms.*—The disease comes on with coldness and shivering, and other symptoms of beginning fever, then the heat of the body is increased, the pulse becomes more frequent, full, and strong, and there is very marked difficulty of breathing, especially when the patient attempts to draw in a full breath. The pain is generally greater when the patient lies on the side affected, but sometimes the contrary is the case. The pain is felt most commonly on one side, and some have supposed that the left side is more frequently attacked than the right, but this does not appear to be correct. Sometimes the pain is felt at the lower part of the breast, sometimes in the back, between the shoulders; the pain is commonly fixed in one spot, but sometimes shoots from the side to the shoulder, back, or breast, and such shooting pains are called in common language *stitches*. The disease is always accompanied by cough; and this cough, in every case, is attended with very considerable pain at the beginning of the disease, it is dry, but soon becomes somewhat moist, and the matter spit up is streaked with a little blood. REMEDY, pages **249, 250.**

**MEASLES.**— See *Symptoms*, pages **219, 220**; REMEDY, pages **220, 221, 222.** **Malignant Measles, page 221.**

**MUMPS.**—See *Symptoms*, page **223**; REMEDY, page **223.**

**NEURALGIA.**—(Neuralgia, nervous headache sometimes called), means pain in a nerve, and is generally of an excruciating, darting kind, but without any heat or swelling in the part. Neuralgic pains affect various parts of the body, but are most common in the head. REMEDY, pages **73, 74, 75, 76.**

**PAINTERS' COLIC.**—See page **230.**

**PALSY.—PARALYSIS.**—*Symptoms.*— Sometimes there are no premonitory symptoms; but often before the attack there are flushed face, swelling of the veins about the head and neck, vertigo, a sense of fullness, weight, and sometimes pain in the head, ringing in the ears, drowsiness, indistinct articulation of words, or even loss of speech, confusion of mind, loss of memory, and change of disposition,—amiable persons being made sullen and peevish, and irritable ones mild and simpering. After the attack the countenance acquires a vague expression; the mouth is drawn to one side; the lower lip on the palsied side hangs down, and the spittle dribbles away. The speech is altered, and the mind is generally impaired.

In some instances the patient recovers in a longer or shorter time; in others little or no improvement takes place, and the patient, after remaining helpless, often for a long time, dies either from gradual exhaustion, or suddenly from apoplexy. REMEDY, pages **130, 239.**

**PILES.**—Painful tumors in the neighborhood of the anus. Sometimes they are situated externally, and are found in clusters, hard, painful, and giving great inconvenience by their preventing the person from sitting; at other times they are within the gut, and are forced outwards with great pain when the patient goes to stool. Sometimes they are situated so far up, that they do not appear externally at all, but indicate their presence by very great pain, or by the discharge of blood. Sometimes the pain attending piles is less, and the principal inconvenience attending them is the discharge of blood, either pretty constant, or when a person goes to stool. In some cases very large quantities of blood are lost in this way. Sometimes, instead of blood, a whitish fluid is discharged.

*Causes.*—Few persons who have attained middle age are totally free from piles, but in some they are more troublesome, and require more attention than in others. Those who are frequently in a standing posture, who are subject to costiveness, and those who are much in the habit of taking purgative medicines, especially of aloes, are very liable to have piles. Pregnant women are very often troubled with piles. Whatever tends to prevent the blood from circulating freely through the veins of the intestines will produce piles; hence affections of the liver are a common cause of the complaint, especially in hot countries where that organ is apt to be congested. REMEDY, pages **141, 161, 185, 186, 187, 188.**

**PLEURISY.**—*Symptoms.*—This disease is most frequently introduced by *shiverings,* which are soon succeeded by high fever, with a peculiarly hard, resisting pulse; sharp, *stabbing* pain in the side,—generally just below the nipple, but sometimes extending to the shoulder, arm-pit, and back; hurried and interrupted breathing; and a short, dry cough

The pain is greatly aggravated by motion, coughing, or an attempt to take a long breath. It holds the patient under constant and powerful restraint. We find him lying upon his back, or his well side; his countenance full of anxiety,—fearing to move, cough, or even breathe needlessly; and often crying out from the keen torture these necessary acts inflict in spite of all his caution.

At a more advanced stage, when the tenderness has somewhat abated, he will prefer to lie on the diseased side, as this leaves the healthy lung more at liberty. REMEDY, page **191.**

**POISONING ACCIDENTS.**—Accidents from poisons are of such common occurrence, that every person should know the proper remedies, and not be obliged to wait the arrival of a physician before the proper corrective is applied. The *symptoms* are different in different poisons, but as *prompt action* and not symptoms, are necessary, we give the most common remedies, with the methods of applying them, under the proper heads. REMEDY, pages **47, 62, 93, 94, 216.**

**QUINSY.—INFLAMMATION OF THE THROAT.**—This kind of inflammatory sore throat generally commences with cold chills, and other febrile symptoms. There is fullness, heat, and dryness of the throat, with a hoarse voice, difficulty of swallowing, and shooting pains towards the ear. When examined, the throat is found to be of a florid red color, deeper over the tonsils, which are swollen and covered with mucus. As the disease progresses the tonsils become more and more swollen, the swallowing becomes more painful and difficult, until liquids return through the nose, and the viscid saliva is discharged from the mouth. Very commonly the fever increases also, and there is acute pain of the back and limbs.

*Causes.*—Exposure to cold, wearing damp clothes, sitting in wet rooms, getting wet feet, coming suddenly out of a crowded and heated room into the open and cold air. It may also be brought on by violent exertion of the voice, and by suppressed evacuations. REMEDY, pages **99, 154.**

**RHEUMATISM.**—*Symptoms.*—A painful affection of fibrous and muscular tissues, affecting principally the larger joints, and places covered by muscles; thus it affects the wrists, the elbows, the knees and hip-joint, and the back and loins. The internal parts also, as the heart and diaphragm, are considered to be capable of being affected by rheumatism. When the joints about the back and loins are affected, the complaint is called *lumbago*; when the pain is in the hip joint, it is called *sciatica*; and *pleurodyne*, or pain in the side, when the muscles of the chest are affected. Rheumatism may occur either with fever or without it; in the first case it is termed *acute*, and in the second *chronic rheumatism*.

Not long after the application of the exciting cause, the patient feels pain and stiffness in one or more joints when he attempts to move them; this quickly increases, till motion becomes almost impossible, from the excessive pain attending it. Along with this local, and often very general pain, there occurs very strong fever, much thirst, heat, and dryness of skin, strength, fullness, and hardness of pulse. The tongue has a white coating, but is red at the tip and the sides, and there is often profuse perspiration with a very sour smell. The appetite is deficient, but the bowels are often in their natural condition. The feverish symptoms are somewhat increased towards evening; and when the patient gets warm in bed, the pains are more severe. In a short time some of the joints swell, and the pain is a little relieved, but by no means removed. The pain is apt to shift from one joint to another, or at least several joints in succession are attacked; and when the pain seemed to be going off, it sometimes unexpectedly recurs.

*Causes.*—Rheumatism is a disease of the constitution, and depends on a morbid state of the blood, or, to speak more accurately, it is caused by a poison which circulates in the blood, and is probably carried from one joint to another. The tendency to rheumatism is hereditary, and in some families this predisposition is very marked, and the disease is excited by the most trifling causes. Cold and damp are the most common causes of this disease, and hence the poor suffer much from it. Thus, too, it is not an unfrequent disease with sportsmen, who, when hot and perspiring, are too apt to throw themselves down on the wet grass; and with travellers who sleep in damp and ill-dried sheets. Persons who get their clothes wet, and neglect to change them, are often seized with rheumatism. Acute rheumatism is most common between the ages of fifteen and forty. It is not a dangerous disease as long as it is confined to the joints, but there is always the risk of the heart being attacked; a most dangerous complication, and most to be dreaded when the disease has long existed, and when there is a strong hereditary predisposition to it. REMEDY, pages **33, 36, 37, 38, 39, 41, 42, 141.**

**RICKETS.**—*Symptoms.*—This disease is an affection peculiar to childhood, and supposed to depend upon the action of the causes which favor the development of scrofula. The signs of rickets are, a softened gristly state of the bones, large joints, large head, prominent forehead, straightness of the ribs and flatness of the sides of the chest, prominent breast bone, looseness of texture in the bones, crooked legs and distorted spine; many other symptoms of scrofula are sometimes also present. This, like scrofula, disposes the system to other diseases; the treatment of rickets is nearly the same as that of scrofula, (which you will find in its proper place in another part of this work,)—rickets, however, is a more curable disease, and less apt to continue after adult age. REMEDY, page **192.**

**RINGWORM OR TETTER.**—*Symptoms.*—This disease consists of minute water blisters, arranged somewhat in rings; it begins with slight redness —small blisters form and are attended with a colorless fluid—these break in four or five days, and are covered with a thin brownish scab, which falls off about the eighth or ninth day, leaving a red surface, which gradually disappears. The eruption seldom lasts more than ten days, but it sometimes appears a second time, and continues for several weeks; it is always attended with itching smarting, and burning. It often appears on the face, neck and arms of children —and may be communicated by contact. REMEDY, pages **163, 229.**

**RUPTURE.**—*Symptoms* (when it is reducible and not strangulated. A swelling in some part of the belly; this diminishes a little on pressure, but returns when the pressure is withdrawn; it goes off when the patient lies down, and is increased by coughing. Patients with rupture are sometimes troubled with indigestion; but frequently, all the functions of the alimentary canal are quite regular. When we succeed in getting up the bowels, there is commonly what is called a guggling noise.

*Causes.*—There are some persons in whom rupture takes place more easily than in others, and in whom it is constant. The reason seems to be, that the parietes of the abdomen, or the neighborhood of the openings in it, are more lax and yielding in them than in others. It is common in warm climates, in old people after long illnesses or debilitating fevers, and in the poor who have labored hard and been ill fed. The circumstance which immediately occasions ruptures, is generally some violent exertion, requiring a strong action of many muscles, especially those of respiration; hence ruptures are brought on by lifting or carrying heavy weights, jumping, running, vomiting, straining at stool, the efforts of women in childbed; or by coughing, sneezing, crying, laughing. REMEDY, pages **197, 234.**

**SALT RHEUM.**—See ECZEMA.

**SCARLET FEVER.—SCARLATINA.**—*Symptoms.*—Either mild, or malignant with putrid sore throat, exhibits different forms of a disease which is propagated by a specific contagion, like small-pox or measles, and like them is believed by the best observers to attack a person only once during life; though the apparent exceptions to this remark are more numerous in scarlet fever, than in the other diseases above mentioned. On the third or fourth day after exposure to the contagion of scarlet fever, a feverish attack occurs, and about the second day of this fever, a bright scarlet rash appears on the surface of the body, and within the mouth and about the fauces. The scarlet fever varies much in its degree of malignity and danger, even during the same epidemic; in some cases being so slight as to go off without the aid of medicine; in others; being accompanied with symptoms of great and fatal putrescency. It will be proper to notice separately, the mild and fatal scarlet fever; and to describe some cases, in which the symptoms are irregularly combined, it being always remembered that "the malignant sore-throat may be caught from a patient who has mild scarlet fever; and mild scarlet fever may, in like manner be contracted from one who is laboring under malignant sore-throat. These forms graduate insensibly towards each other." REMEDY pages **52, 64, 256, 257, 258.**

**Mild Scarlet Fever.**—The milder form of scarlet fever is distinguished by the rash, with a moderate degree of fever, and with very little affection of the throat. The rash first appears in innumerable red points about the neck and face, and by the next day they are seen over the whole surface of the body. The skin is rough to the touch, and sometimes there are small vesicles. About the fourth day the eruption is at its height, and on the fifth it begins to decline. The surface of the mouth and fauces appears red, and little red points appear on the tongue rising up through the white crust which covers it, and when this crust comes off, the whole is red and sore, and the points are still prominent, giving an appearance like a strawberry. There is sometimes considerable swelling of the face and of the throat. REMEDY, same as above.

**SCROFULA.**—*Symptoms.*—Scrofula and King's Evil, are names for a tedious and multiform disease, of which one of the most characteristic marks is a tendency to a swelling of glandular parts, which, when they come on to inflammation and suppuration, discharge an unhealthy, curdy, mixed matter, and form ulcers very difficult to heal. REMEDY, pages **141, 142.**

**SHINGLES.**—*Symptoms.*—A disease characterized by a number of vesicles, most commonly round the waist, like half a sash; but sometimes like a sword-belt across the shoulder. It very rarely surrounds the body completely; hence, a popular, but groundless apprehension, that if the disease goes round, it will be fatal. The disease is usually preceded, for two or three days, by languor and loss of appetite, rigors, headache, sickness, and a frequent pulse; with a heat and tingling in the skin, and shooting pains through the chest, and at the pit of the stomach. After these symptoms, more or less severe, there appear, on some part of the trunk, red patches of an irregular form, at a little distance from each other; upon each of which numerous small elevations appear, clustered together. In the course of twenty-four hours, they enlarge to the size of small pearls, and are filled with a limpid fluid. The clusters are surrounded by a narrow red margin. During three or four days, other clusters continue to rise in succession, and with considerable regularity. About the fourth day, the vesicles acquire a milky or yellowish hue, which is soon followed by a bluish or livid color of the bases of the vesicles, and of the contained fluid. Several of them run together; and those which are broken discharge a small quantity of a serous fluid for three or four days; this concretes into thin dark scabs, which soon become hard, and fall off about the twelfth or fourteenth day. Where there has been considerable discharge, numerous pits are left. The feverish symptoms commonly subside when the eruption is completed; but sometimes continue much longer, probably from the itching and smarting of the vesicles. Though resembling some other eruptive diseases in its rise and decline, it is not contagious, and persons may have it more than once The disease, in general, is slight and free from danger. REMEDY, page **192.**

**SMALL-POX.**—*Symptoms.*—The patient is seized with coldness and shiverings, which soon abate, and are then followed by a hot stage, lasting for two or three days; during which, children are liable to sickness and vomiting, to starting in their sleep, or to epileptic fits; and adults are disposed to sweating. Towards the end of the third day, the eruption appears, and increases during the fourth day. It commonly appears first on the face, then on the lower parts, and is completed over the whole body on the fifth day. The fever generally abates about the coming out of the eruption; the sickness, vomiting, fits, and other oppressive symptoms go off; and the patient is, for the time, free from uneasiness. The eruption appears in small red spots, hardly rising above the skin, but which by degrees form pimples. On the fifth or sixth day a small vesicle, containing a colorless fluid, appears on top of each pimple These get broader on the seventh day; and about the eighth are raised into round pustules. These pustules are surrounded with a circular inflamed border; and as they increase in size, about the eighth day the face is considerably swelled, and the eye-lids are sometimes completely closed. The matter in the pustules now becomes thick and white, or yellowish, exactly resembling the matter of an abscess On the 11th day the swelling of the face subsides, and the pustules appear quite full. REMEDY, pages **64, 68, 70, 71, 72.**

**STOMACH, INFLAMMATION OF**—*Symptoms.*—The symptoms of inflammation of the stomach are, acute pain, heat, and tension in the region of that organ, great increase of pain when anything is swallowed, vomiting, great and sudden depression of strength, a small pulse, thirst, restlessness and anxiety. REMEDY, page **251.**

**ST. VITUS' DANCE.**—*Symptoms.*—This disease is chiefly confined to children and youth between the ages of eight and fourteen. But few cases occur after puberty. The complaint affects both the muscles and the limbs. It excites curious antics. A few of the muscles of the face or limbs begin their mischievous pranks by slight twitches, which, by degrees, become more energetic, and spread to other parts. The face is twisted into all kinds of ridiculous contortions, as if the patient were making mouths at somebody. The hands and arms do not remain in one position for a moment. In attempting to carry food to the mouth, the hand gets part way, and is jerked back, starts again, and darts to one side, then to the other, then mouthward again; and each movement is so quick, and nervous and darting, and diddling, that ten to one the food drops into the lap. If the attempt be made to run out the tongue, it is snatched back with the quickness of a serpent's, and the jaws snap together like a fly trap. The lower limbs are in a state of perpetual diddle; the feet shuffle with wonderful diligence upon the floor, as if inspired with a ceaseless desire to dance. REMEDY, page **130.**

**SUN STROKE.**—*Symptoms.*—This begins by thirst, dizziness, headache and sometimes there is vomiting or difficult breathing. The symptoms, in fact, are pretty much the same as apoplexy; the patient should at once be taken into a cool shady place, and the first thing have a bucket of cold water poured slowly over his head, and, in all respects treat the case the same as a case of apoplexy. REMEDY, page **131**.

**SYPHILIS.**—*Symptoms.*—This disease is owing to a poisonous matter introduced into the system by absorption, thus producing more poisonous matter which in time corrupts all the fluids, and occasions many disorders in various parts of the body, and is generally the consequence of impure sexual intercourse. REMEDY, page **204.**

**THRUSH.**—*Symptoms:*—Comes on in the mouth, may extend down the throat, never attacks the nose or lungs, child becomes fretful, mouth and throat, red, inflamed and tender, vomiting and diarrhœa. The thrush consists of white points at first, which soon run together and become patches, they are slightly elevated, and look like white mould, or curdled milk, after the disease has run on for a short time the patches have a yellowish color, it comes on in young children and is very dangerous unless properly treated. If the previous health of the child is good the case should be cured in three to six days. REMEDY, pages **228, 296.**

**TONSILITES — INFLAMMATION OF THE TONSILS.**— *Symptoms.*—There is more or less thickness of speech, caused by enlarged tonsils and liability to *sore throat*, or quinsy. The only symptoms are inflamed and enlarged tonsils. REMEDY, pages **53, 140.**

**TUMORS — SWELLINGS.** — Are of various kinds, either of the whole body, or of particular members, or local and circumscribed. Watery swellings of the whole body are seen in general dropsy, and the same disease in its commencement occasions partial swellings, as of the lower extremities, or of the arms or face, according to the position of the body. Circumscribed swellings occur in various glands, as those of the neck, arm-pit, or groins, chiefly in scrofulous constitutions; or they may arise from inflammation, the consequence of cold. The tonsils swell in sore throat, and occasion a fullness of the external parts of the throat; gum-boils form during toothache, and swell the cheeks; and the bronchocele, or goitre, is an instance of a still more permanent swelling. The face, head, and limbs often swell exceedingly from various causes.

**Wen** is the common popular name for an excrescence or tumor growing on any part of the body, and frequently applied to tumors about the throat and neck. Tumors are distinguished by surgeons according to the nature of their contents; and they require treatment varied according to circumstances. REMEDY, pages **33, 96, 140, 210, 270, 296.**

**TYPHOID, OR TYPHUS.**—*Symptoms.*—The disease often has cautionary symptoms. For several days before its actual beginning, the patient droops. He may attend to his various duties, but does not seem well; he is low-spirited and languid, is indisposed to any exertion of body or mind has pains in the head, back and extremities; loses his appetite; and although dull and perhaps drowsy in the day time, his sleep is interrupted and unrefreshing at night. The immediate harbinger of the fever is a *chill* often so marked as to cause violent shivering.

The history of the first week shows increased heat of the surface; frequent pulse, ranging from eighty to one hundred and twenty; furred tongue; restlessness and sleeplessness; headache and pain in the back; sometimes diarrhœa and swelling of the belly; and sometimes nausea and vomiting.

The second week is frequently distinguished by an eruption of small, rose-colored spots upon the belly, and by a crop of little watery pimples upon the neck and chest, having an appearance of minute drops of sweat standing on the skin, and hence called *sudamina*, or *sweat drops*; the tongue is dry and black, or red and sore; the teeth are foul; there may be delirium and dullness of hearing; and the symptoms generally are more serious than during the first week. Occasionally, at this period, the bowels are perforated or ate through by ulceration, and the patient suddenly sinks.

If the disease proceeds unfavorably into the third week, there is low muttering and delirium; great exhaustion; sliding down of the patient towards the foot of the bed; twitching of the muscles; bleeding from the bowels; and red or purple spots upon the skin.

If, on the other hand, recovery takes place, the countenance brightens; the pulse moderates; the tongue cleans, and the discharges assume the appearance they have in health. REMEDY, pages **61, 62, 63, 64, 65, 66, 67, 193.**

**TYPHOID PNEUMONIA, OR TYPHOID LUNG FEVER.** —This is an inflammation of the lungs, differing from the preceding only in the character of the fever attending it, which is of a low typhoid character. The disease, like typhoid fever, is characterized by great debility and prostration. There are a combination of the symptoms of pneumonia and of typhoid fever. The disease begins with great weariness, lassitude, dizziness, pain in the head, back, and limbs. Soon there is much difficulty of breathing, tightness across the chest, with a dry, short, hacking cough.

As the disease advances, the active symptoms pass away; there is a dull pain across the chest; drowsiness is very apt to come on, with the various symptoms of sinking peculiar to typhoid fever. The skin is harsh and dry, the temperature uneven, the tip and edge of the tongue red, and the middle covered with a yellow or brown fur. The bowels are tender, swollen, and drum-head-like; while there is often a diarrhœa,—the discharges having a dirty-yellow color. REMEDY, page **193.**

**ULCER—FEVER SORE.**—When the nutrition entirely ceases in any portion of the body, the absorbents devour all the skin, flesh and vessels of the part—leaving an open cavity, the process of taking away the flesh, &c., is *ulceration*; the cavity left is an ulcer. REMEDY, pages **99, 101, 236, 237, 238.**

**VARICOSE, ENLARGED OR KNOTTED VEINS.**—In different parts, especially of the lower extremities, there are sometimes seen a number of unequal knotty swellings, of a deep blue color, occasioned by portions of the veins being dilated. The cause of these swellings is the obstruction to the free passage of the blood through the veins; hence tumors in the groin may cause varicose veins of the legs; and the appearance of such veins is frequent in pregnant women, from the enlarged uterus and its contents pressing on the large trunks of the veins. Sometimes the complaint arises from general debility, and from a sedentary life. When the distention is great, there is considerable pain; and the veins may be eroded, and cause a great discharge of blood; or troublesome and obstinate ulcers may be produced. The pain and inconvenience of varicose veins are not great at first, and hence they are too often neglected till they become very difficult to cure.

The varicose veins of pregnant women go off when they are delivered, and require very little treatment, except attention to posture. In other cases a moderate pressure by bandages is requisite. An elastic stocking makes a good and equal pressure. REMEDY, pages **235, 279.**

WATER-BRASH.—*Symptoms.*—This disease signifies the discharge of a thin watery fluid from the stomach, with belchings, and a sense of heat at the region of the stomach. It is not unfrequently one of the symptoms attending indigestion or stomach complaints, but it sometimes occurs as an original disease. It comes on in paroxysms, usually when the stomach is empty. The patient perceives a pain at the pit of the stomach, with a sense of tightness, and is increased by the erect posture. When the pain has continued for some time, it is succeeded by belchings, and the discharge of a thin watery fluid, sometimes acid, but generally tasteless. The belchings are repeated for a time, and then the fit goes off. When the disease has once happened, it is apt to recur frequently for a long time afterwards. It is most incident to persons of middle age; and to females, sometimes during pregnancy, sometimes when they are afflicted with the whites. It is not always connected with any particular diet; but is excited often by cold applied to the feet, and by emotions of the mind. REMEDY, page **229.**

WHOOPING, OR HOOPING COUGH.—*Symptoms.*—A catching or contagious disease, generally caught in childhood, between the ages of one and two years; has three stages: first stage, sneezing, cough and mild bronchitis, eyes slightly red, no spittle; this stage may last from three days to six weeks. The second stage then sets in, child feels a tickling in throat, which brings on a spasm of coughing, with tight feeling across the chest; child will put its head on its mother's knees or take hold of some fixed thing to help it during the coughing; pulse and breathing during the spasm are slightly faster; the sound during the spasm of coughing is called the "hoop" or "whoop." The face becomes flushed during this period; as soon as the coughing is over the child's face, pulse and breathing become natural again; the child will spit out a little frothy mucus; anger, fright, or exertion will bring on the cough. This stage lasts until the thirty-fifth day of the disease, when the third stage sets in. Spittle turns yellow and is thicker, cough becomes less and is neither so frequent nor severe. REMEDY, pages **125, 126.**

WORMS.—*Symptoms.*—When a child is afflicted with round worms, the face will become flushed and then pale, at irregular intervals; color leaden or bluish, lower eyelids swollen, and blue circle around them; thirst, sick stomach, vomiting, appetite variable, breath foul, tongue red and covered with points, pulse fast and irregular, may have spasms, twitching of muscles, disturbed sleep, nightmare, headache, eyes dilated, cross eye, colic, grinding teeth in sleep, generally diarrhœa. The symptoms of thread worm are not so pronounced; there is less fever, colic and nervous symptoms; the itching of the rectum is the most marked and prominent symptoms; the thread worm does not kill the patient, the round worm may. Never give worm medicine till the child has passed worms, and you have seen them. REMEDY, pages **134, 143, 144, 145, 146, 147**.

*Remarks.*—There are 21 kinds of worms. We shall take up two only, as they are the ones usually found, The first, or round worm, is reddish or reddish-yellow in color, tapers at both ends, and looks like the common earth or "angle" worm; they are prone to move from one place to another in the intestines, and may be found in the stomach. Each female worm lays about 60 million eggs. The thread, maw, or pin worm is white, and looks like a piece of white sewing thread; they are found in the large intestine and the rectum, where they create intolerable itching. Tape worms inhabit the small intestines, and will not be treated of more fully, as *no one* should try to doctor themselves for their removal, but should go at once to their physician.

**YELLOW FEVER.**—A dangerous fever, of the remittent and typhoid kind, common in the West Indies and America; and, with some little variety, occurring. too, often in Spain and Gibraltar. The yellow fever, like many others, attacks with lassitude and chilly fits, faintness, giddiness, and flushing of the face, thirst, pain in the eye-balls or forehead, pain in the back, scanty and high-colored turbid urine; irregular and diminished perspiration; the tongue is covered with a dark fur; the bile is secreted in unusual quantity, and being forced up into the stomach, is vomited; the skin is hot and dry. As the disease advances, the eyes become of a deep yellow, and the face and breast are of the same color; there is an incessant vomiting of frothy bile; great costiveness prevails, and delirium comes on. The fever sometimes remits so much about the end of thirty-six hours, that the patient thinks himself comparatively well; but the symptoms soon return with great aggravation, and extreme debility. In the last stage of the disease the debility is very great, and symptoms of universal putrescency occur; large livid patches are observed, the tongue becomes dry and black, the teeth are incrusted with dark fur, the body exhibits a livid yellow, blood flows from the mouth, ears, and nostrils, dark and fetid stools are discharged, hiccoughs come on, the pulse sinks, and death soon follows. The order and severity of the symptoms vary in different cases; some are seized very suddenly, and fall down insensible; others, for a few days, have the warning signs of costiveness, defect of appetite, pain in the head, yellowness of the eyes, hoarseness and sore throat, lowness of spirits. In the great majority of cases there are evident remissions or intermissions. All kinds of persons are affected by it, but those principally who are in the prime of life; men more frequently than women. People of color have the disease milder than others. REMEDY, page **224.**

# INTERNAL LOCATION OF THE ORGANS.

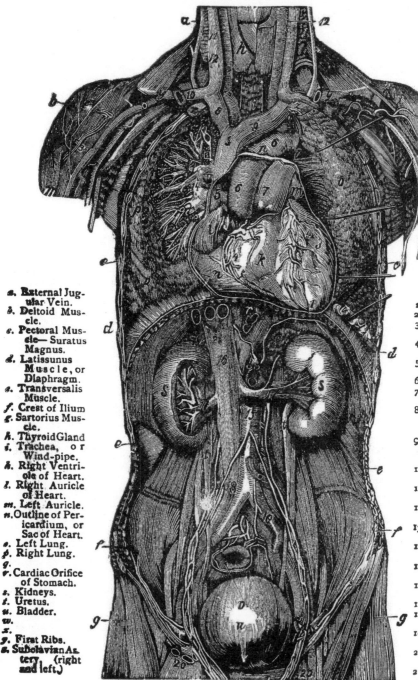

a. External Jug-
    ular Vein.
b. Deltoid Mus-
    cle.
c. Pectoral Mus-
    cle— Suratus
    Magnus.
d. Latissunus
    Muscle, or
    Diaphragm.
e. Transversalis
    Muscle.
f. Crest of Ilium
g. Sartorius Mus-
    cle.
h. Thyroid Gland
i. Trachea,  o r
    Wind-pipe.
k. Right Ventri-
    cle of Heart.
l. Right Auricle
    of Heart.
m. Left Auricle.
n. Outline of Per-
    icardium, or
    Sac of Heart.
o. Left Lung.
p. Right Lung.
q.
r. Cardiac Orifice
    of Stomach.
s. Kidneys.
t. Uretus.
u. Bladder.
w.
x.
y. First Ribs.
z. Subclavian Ar-
    tery  (right
    and left.)

1. Apex of Heart.
2. Lumbar Glands
3. Left Ventricle
    of Heart.
4. Coronary  Ar-
    teries.
5. Superior Vena
    Cava. (Vein.)
6. Arch of Aorta.
7. Left Pulmona-
    ry Artery.
8. Right — Vena
    Cava, or In-
    nomenata.
9. Left — Vena
    Cava, or In-
    nomenata.
10. Subclavian
    Vein.
11. Internal Jug-
    ular Vein.
12. Left Common
    Cartoid Artery.
13. Brachial Ar-
    tery.
14. Pulmonary
    Veins.
15. Descending
    Aorta.
16. Inferior Vena
    Cava.
17. Renal Vein.
18. Right—Com-
    mon Iliac Vein.
19. Left, Common
    Iliac Artery.
20. Femoral Ar-
    tery and Vein.
21. Hepatic Veins

# MEDICAL RECIPES.

**SWELLINGS TO REDUCE—Liniment for.**—Rum, spirits of camphor and laudanum, each 1 oz.; mix, shake well and keep corked. DIRECTIONS—Heat the mixture hot (when using) and bathe the swelling thoroughly, at least 3 times daily, by pouring into the hand and thorough rubbing in. For a pin-scratch, or small pimple, a finger application will be sufficient.

*Remark.*—This is claimed to reduce the worst swelling in a short time.

## RHEUMATISM, SPINAL AFFECTIONS, CANCERS, ETC.

**1. Dr. White's Remedy, or Liniment for.**—Strongest alcohol and spirits of turpentine. each 1 pt.; camphor gum and saltpeter, each 1 oz.; beef's brine, 2 qts. Dissolve the camphor gum and saltpeter in the alcohol; then add the turpentine. Scald and skim the beef's brine, and when cold, add it. To be shaken when used.

*Remarks.*—Dr. White, from whom this receipt was obtained, used it extensively, and with success, in weak backs and all other spinal affections, rheumatism, etc., and also claimed to have cured several cancers with it. I have no doubt of its value for general purposes, nor have I a doubt that, if taken or commenced early in the appearance of a cancerous growth, it may scatter it, and with an occasional active cathartic and the continued use of a good alterative, they may be cured.

**2.** Kerosene, ½ pt., and camphor-gum, 1 oz., cured a friend of mine, with whom I was acquainted for forty years; his fingers and hands were set nearly shut. Bathing his hands 3 or 4 times daily for 3 or 4 days made decided improvements, and finally cured them.

**CANCER—SUCCESSFUL REMEDIES.**—Persons suffering with cancers may expect to find the following beneficial:

**1.** Take a qt. bowl and fill half to two-thirds full of green sheep sorrel, then fill with water; let it stand one hour, then mash to get the strength; to be drank daily. Use dry sorrel same as green, only steep in hot water.

*For the Sore.*—Use a poultice, made by soaking the sorrel in warm water till soft; change often.

*To Make the Salve.*—Take a porcelain kettle holding a gallon; fill two-thirds full of the sorrel; then fill with water, and boil down to a strong ooze; take out the sorrel (pressing or straining, if necessary), and put in freshly made unsalted butter or lard; then let it simmer over a slow fire—do not burn it—and put in a lump of rosin the size of a hen's egg; when the water is simmered out, drain out the salve. Salve prepared in this way, will cure scrofula as well as cancers. I know whereof I affirm, as I have seen it tried successfully. It takes

33

perseverance, however, as it is in the blood; better that, than to be eaten up with either cancer or scrofula.

2.  Take equal parts of sweet fern and the bark off the north side of a black ash tree; burn both to ashes; leach and boil down thick; put a piece of sheet-lead upon the cancer, with a hole in it as large as the cancer, wet lint in the mixture; put on and place another piece of sheet-lead over that. Let it remain till it ceases to pain, when the cancer will be dead; then make a plas-ter of the white of an egg and white pine pitch; put on and cover with a warm Indian meal poultice; keep on till it comes out. In the case of the man from whom this receipt was obtained, the cancer came out in nine days. The poultice must be renewed when cold.

*Remarks.*—The idea of the piece of sheet-lead, with a hole in it the size of cancer, is to protect the sound flesh or skin from contact with the cancer salve. The sorrel water, as in No. 1, or some other good alterative, should be taken a reasonable length of time, in the treatment of any cancer, for the purpose of purifying the blood.

### 3.  Cancer—A New Remedy which Carbonizes the Cancer-ous Tumor with but Little or No Pain, and Not Poisonous.—

DIRECTIONS—Apply to the surface of the sore the chloride of chromium (a new salt of this rare metal), incorporated into stramonium ointment. This prepara-tion, in a few hours, converts the tumor into perfect carbon, and it crumples away. Specimens of cancers thus carbonized were inspected by a number of physicians at a recent meeting held at the N. Y. Medical University, where a paper was read on this new method of treating cancer, which had the appear-ance of charcoal, and were easily pulverized between the fingers. The remedy causes little or no pain, and is not poisonous.

*Remarks.*—In small places where this chloride-chromium is not obtainable, call in the assistance of a physician, and he will know where to get it; and as nothing is said as to how much of the chloride of chromium should be used, I would use 1 dr. to 1 oz. of the stramonium ointment, unless it was found by inquiry, when obtaining it, to need more or less—watch results. Poultic-ing, to remove the tumor, after it is carbonized, would be the proper way to do, then use any of the best healing salve.

### 4.  Cancer—Esmarch's or German Treatment.—I.  Fowler's

solution, 1 drop, 3 times daily, for three days, then increase the dose 1 drop every three days, till intolerance of the remedy follows. Apply the following locally, *i. e.*, upon the open sore:

*II.  Powder to Sprinkle Upon the Open Sore.*—Arsenious acid and muriate of morphia, of each 1 gr.; calomel, 1 dr.; powdered gum arabic. ½ oz.; mix. At first sprinkle only a little powder upon the open sore, gradually increasing the quantity to 1 teaspoonful. This overcomes the odor, and causes a hard eschar, or scab, to form, and healthy granulation takes place.

*Remarks.*—It will be understood that Fowler's solution contains arsenic, as well as the powder, and as injury might arise by their use, unless the symptoms from poisoning by arsenic are well understood, it would be well, when it is

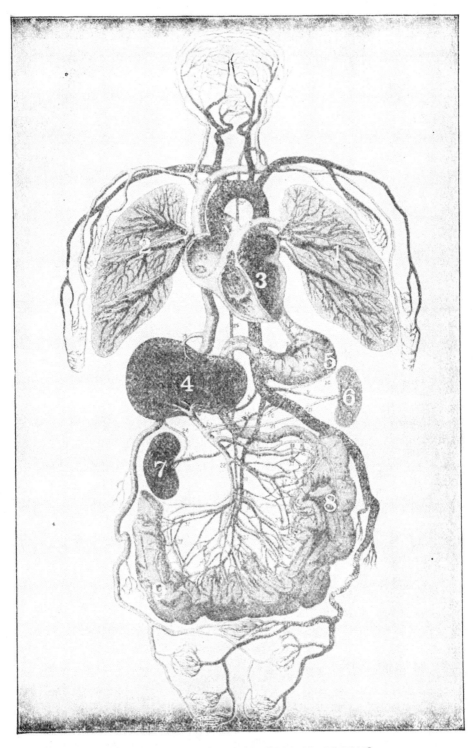

**SHOWING SYSTEM OF INTERNAL ORGANS.**
1 and 2, Lungs.   3, Heart.   4, Liver.   5, Stomach.   6 and 7, Kidneys.   8 and 9, Large Intestines.

used, to have it done by or under the care of a physician, so as to prevent any possible injury; although, if properly used, there is everything to encourage the hope of great benefit, rather than injury; but it is best, always, to be on the safe side, hence this caution.

**5. Cancer, Relief of Pain in.**—Dr. Brandini, of Florence, Italy, has recently discovered that citric acid will assuage (relieve) the violent pain of cancer. He applies to the part pledgets of lint soaked in a solution of citric acid, 4 grs.; dissolved in soft water, 350 grs. (about ¾ oz.), with the result of affording instantaneous relief in the most aggravated cases.

**6. Cancer, Chromic Acid Found Valuable in.**—Prof. John King, in his American Dispensatory, more than a dozen years ago, spoke of chromic acid being found advantageous in cancers, malignant tumors, ulcers, etc

*Remarks.*—The word "malignant," as applied to tumors, is generally understood to refer to those of a cancerous character, "tending," as Webster puts it, "to produce death, threatening a fatal issue," etc., and this fact gives me hopes, especially, that the chloride of chromium, No. 3, above, which is only another form of the chromium, will do what is there claimed for it, combined with the stramonium ointment. The acid, however, is being used more, of late, than formerly, as the following will show.

**7. Cancer, or Fungous Growth in the Ear—Removed Safely with Chromic Acid.**—Dr. Tangeman, Professor in the Medical College of Ohio, at Cincinnati, in Parke, Davis & Co.'s *Therapeutic Gazette*, reports the case of a young man of 18, with a running ear. The meatus, or opening into the ear, at the bottom was full of pus, or matter; the tympanum, or drum, of the ear wholly destroyed, and the inner ear filled with a fungus, or cancerlike growth; the boy wholly deaf on that side, the result of scarlet fever. The ear was packed with powdered boracic acid, which dissolved in 24 hours, and was repacked with the same, and repeated 4 weeks, but the fungus, or lacerous growth, had to be removed by a few applications of chromic acid, and the opening enlarged by it so they could get to the bones of the ear, which were necrosed (destroyed), it being the cause of the discharge. The case was cured.

Nitrate of silver was formerly used in such cases, but Dr. Tangeman thinks its use in ear cases is among the past, and that chromic acid will take its place; but, from its activity, must be used with care. It should not be put on too freely in any case, as to endanger, or extend to other parts.

Yet chromic acid will not continue, like other acids, to eat on indefinitely, but as a particle of it destroys a particle of flesh, or fungus, it is itself destroyed. This peculiarity shows its *great value over all other caustics or destroyers known.* See its value for warts, under that head. Best to be used under the care of a competent physician, or one accustomed to its use, especially in cancers where considerable tissue, or fleshy tumors, are to be destroyed.

**8.** M. Czartoryski, M. D., of Stockton, Cal., says in the *Medical Brief*, of June, 1884, under the head of "Cancer—California Cure":

"I accidentally discovered the secret process, by which an old man, living in this vicinity, has had remarkable success in removing cancers. He takes wild parsnip roots (the wild parsnip resembles our table vegetable, but the roots are poisonous), allowing them to simmer on the stove until they assume the the consistency of paste; then spread on chamois skin, and apply to the cancer At the beginning it will cause severe pain, and the cancer will contract and loosen, until it may easily be extracted with its roots. The resulting opening can be healed under any liniment or unguent (ointment) "

The best unguent, he thinks, is balsam of Peru.

*Remarks.*—The author rejoices in the hope that, with one or the other of these receipts, all cancer sufferers shall be materially benefited, if not abso lutely cured, adding many years to their lives.

**1. SCIATIC RHEUMATISM.—Successful Remedies.—I.** *In ternal and Alterative.* Fl. ex. of poke root, 1 oz.; fl. ex. of gelsemium, 1 dr.; mix. DOSE.—Take 20 drops, morning and evening, in a little water.

II. Fl. ex. of blue flag, 1 oz. DOSE.—Take 15 drops, at noon and bed time, in a little water.

III. Apply externally, along the back part of the thigh, as a liniment, tinct. of iodine and aqua ammonia, each 1 oz.; mix, and rub on thoroughly 3 times daily.

I cured a very bad case, with this treatment, for a fat, fleshy woman, in about a week's time, who could scarcely move when I took the case in hand.

**2. Sciatica Cured with Electricity.—A very Cheap, Simple Battery.—How to Make and Use.—**The following case of this disease —a bad case—was published in the *Physician and Surgeon*, of Ann Arbor, Mich., by Charles Ferhune, M. D., of that city, for Oct., 1880.

"An electric battery was constructed, consisting of a zinc and silver plate about two inches in diameter, connected by a coil of insulated copper wire long enough to allow the silver plate to rest on the front portion of the thigh, the zinc resting over the sciatic nerve, on the back part of the thigh.

"A thin slice of sponge was placed between the plates and the skin, and these were kept wet with a strong solution of salt in water. This apparatus was retained in its position by means of adhesive straps and rubber bandage. It was necessary to change its location every other day on account of the irritation caused by the formation of chloride of zinc and electric current.

"In a week's time the patient was so much better that a battery was placed on the left leg also, and these were kept on constantly, except when it was necessary to replace the zinc as it would become corroded. September 1st the battery was taken off from the right leg, as there was no more pain and felt perfectly natural. The battery is still kept on the left leg, which was always the worst, simply on account of a little numbness of the toes; other wise this leg also is free from any unnatural sensation.

"Whenever convenient, I applied the following preparation the whole length of nerve;

"Menthol, 12 grs.; alcohol, to dissolve the menthol, 7 minims (drops); oil of cloves, 1 oz.; mix. [Menthol is one of the newer remedies, sometimes also called Japanese camphor. It is made from a species of *mint* growing in Asia, Japan, and I think in China also. It is in the form of crystals, and smells much like peppermint.]

"This mixture I have known to be of almost immediate benefit in neu ralgic affections.

"Considering the long standing of the disease, that it was located in both legs, and the patient's habits (addicted to drink), and the great obstinacy and severity of Sciatica even under the most favorable circumstances, I feel it my duty to report a treatment so simple and easy and which has been of such signal service."

*Remarks.*—Having inquired into this case, and being well satisfied of the value of this treatment; also well acquainted with Dr. Ferhune, and as he speaks so favorably of the mixture, or liniment, for neuralgia, it would be well to try it for that purpose as well as in sciatica.

When Menthol is not kept by druggists, use one of the liniments given below.

Dr. Chase's Golden Oil (see recipe below), or strong Camphor Liniment, or some other—as preferred. The Golden Oil, however, made with capsicum, is very strong, and causes a glow of heat wherever it is freely applied.

3. The Author has several times cured Sciatica by the use of the simple Faradic current of the common Faradic "Family Battery," applying the *positive* pole along the sciatic nerve in the back part of the thigh, the *negative* pole at the feet, by means of a foot-plate, with very great satisfaction. Never use the current so strong as to cause additional pain, but simply to relieve it. Five to ten minutes to each limb, once or twice daily.

4. **External Remedy, or Liniment for Sciatica, Lumbago, Stiff Joints, Contracted Cords, Rheumatism, Etc.—Very Successful.— For External Use Only.—**Fl. ex. of aconite root (never of the leaf, for these purposes), 12 oz; oil of hemlock, 3 oz.; sulphate of zinc, 1 oz.; strongest alcohol, 1 qt.; soft or distilled water, 1 qt. DIRECTIONS.— Take at least a 3 qt. bottle and put in the alcohol, oil of hemlock, and extract of aconite root together; dissolve the sulphate of zinc in a little water and add lastly the water also, shake, always, before pouring out into a smaller bottle for use, and always shake before pouring out upon the parts, or into the hand for application. I have given it in these large quantities, because it is to be applied freely, at least twice daily, in any case, in very painful cases three times a day, pouring upon the parts and rubbing in several times at each application. Do not get into the eyes, *nor is it ever to be taken internally in any case.*

*Remarks.*—This is claimed by the person from whom I obtained the recipe to have cured stiff joints, as well as the other diseases named. For stiff joints I have had no opportunity of testing it, but in sciatica and rheumatism I have found it as valuable as he claimed.

3. **Rheumatism—Remedy for External Application.—** Cayenne pepper, 2 teaspoonfuls, steeped in 1 teacup of good vinegar, and the parts affected to be bathed with it, is claimed to be excellent. After steeping (not to boil), strain and bottle for use. It will cause considerable heat of the surface, and would, even, if a pint of vinegar were used. Apply 2 or 3 times daily, and if limb is very painful, wet cloths in the mixture and wrap around it, as long as it can be borne.

4. **Rheumatism—Golden Oil For.—**Linseed oil and spirits of turpentine, of each 8 ozs.; tinct. of iodine and aqua ammonia, of each 4 ozs.; mix, shake, and apply as often and as freely as needed.

**5. Inflammatory Rheumatism Remedy.**—A mixture of pulver-ized saltpeter, ½ oz.; and sweet oil, ½ pt., is a certain cure for inflammatory rheumatism. This mixture must be applied externally, to the part affected, and as it can do no harm and costs so little, we advise those afflicted with in-flammatory rheumatism to try it.

**6. Rheumatic Alterative.**—Colchicum seed, anise seed, black cohosh root, poke root, blue flag root, bitter root, gum guaiac, prickly ash bark and juniper berries, of each ½ oz.; mandrake root, 1 dr.; wintergreen leaves, spear-mint leaves, of each 1 oz.; iodide of potash, 3 drs.; good gin, 1 pt. DIREC-TIONS.—Bruise or grind coarsely all except the iodide, and put into the gin; keep corked, and shake daily for 10 or 12 days, strain and press out, put in the iodide, or if in a hurry, let it stand 3 or 4 days, then have a druggist to perco-late it (straining it drop by drop through a sponge pressed into the small end of a funnel-shaped percolator), adding sufficient gin to obtain 1 pt of the fluid. Good whiskey will do, but it is not so good, as gin is more diuretic; add the iodide of potash last, dissolved in a little of the liquor. DOSE—For a medium sized adult, 1 tea-spoonful 3 or 4 times daily in a little syrup, or molasses, with a small amount of water. While taking the above use a good liniment exter-nally, and the improvement will be more quickly realized.

**7. Rheumatism, Successful Alterative For—The Crutches Thrown Away by the Use of Half a Bottle.**—Tincts. of sarsapa-rilla and quassia, of each 3 ozs.; iodide of potash, 1 oz.; quinine, 20 grs.; water, 1 pt. DIRECTIONS—Put all into a quart bottle, and shake when taken, DOSE—1 table-spoonful just before each meal.

*Remarks.*—The person communicating this recipe, " W. W.," of Inde-pendence, Ohio, says: "I was 3 months on crutches, before I took half of it I threw the crutches away." It is probable that this amount of the iodide of potash may be more than some persons can take, as there are those who can not take it in large doses—this will be known by a stiffness of the nose, throat, etc., as though they had taken a bad cold. In such cases lessen the dose to a teaspoonful, and next time double the amount of tinctures, else use half the amount of the iodide.

**8. Rheumatism, an Alterative Tincture For.**—Tinct. of black cohosh, 2 parts; and tinct. of colchicum, 1 part (say the cohosh ½ oz.; colchi-cum, ¼ oz.) DOSE—Take 20 to 40 drops three times a day in a little syrup.—Mrs. E. L. Mills, of Romeo, Mich., in *Detroit Tribune.*

*Remarks.*—Twenty drops for a weak and feeble woman is plenty; 40 for a robust man, or even a tea-spoonful would be safe for him to take for a dose. While using this alterative internally, apply also any good liniment externally.

**9. Acute or Inflammatory Rheumatism — A New and Suc-cessful Remedy.**—After a fair trial of the salicylate of soda, in acute rheumatism, *i. e.*, in a rheumatism with pain and often swelling of joints, etc., from having taken a cold, the profession and doctors have come to a very favorable opinion of its use for rheumatism, as well as in tonsilitis and sick headaches, which see.

Dr. Clouston, in the June number of the *Practitioner*, thinks the action of the salicylate of soda on acute rheumatism is most marked, as in 63 per cent.— 63 in 100—the acute stage lasted only three days; the pain being relieved in a few hours, and the remainder of the disease having no serious symptoms; he thinks, however, its use should be commenced early in the disease, if benefit to any extent is to be experienced, and in doses not less than 10 grs. every hour, until the pain and severe symptoms are relieved, then less often, 2, 3, or 4 hours, and finally less amount. Dr. Clouston's recipe is as follows: Salicylic acid, 3 drs.; carbonate of soda, 1½ drs.; syrup of lemon, 1 oz.; cinnamon water to make 8 ozs.; mix. DOSE—A table-spoonful every two hours.—*Medical Digest.*

*Remarks.*—The *Medical Summary*, of New York, says: "The salicylate of potash has also been used with success: Salicylic acid, 2 drs.; bi-carbonate of potash, 3 drs.; water, 2 ozs.; mix. DOSE—A tea-spoonful every 2 or 3 hours."

**10. Confirmatory** of the use of salicylic acid; and also of the use of flannels, in inflammatory rheumatism, I will add Dr. Bell, of Canandaigua, N. Y., whom I met while at Eaton Rapids, Mich., in 1883, said, in speaking of inflammatory rheumatism, that his treatment, which had proved successful, was to put on flannel shirts and sheets and give salicylic acid, 120 grs.; acetate of potash, 320 grs.; simple elixir, or simple syrup, and glycerine, each 2 ozs.; well mixed and dissolved. DOSE—Take 1 tea-spoonful every 2 hours till relief is manifested, then 3 or 4 hours apart. John K. Owen, M. D., of Harrisville, Ind., confirms the above in the February number of the *Medical Brief* of 1883, but adds 1¼ ozs. of sweet spirits of nitre to the mixture, using the same dose.

**11. Rheumatism Internal.**—Try the following:

I. Salicylic acid, 3 drs.; acetate of potassa, 3 drs.; fl. ex. cimicifuga (black cohosh), 4 drs.; wine of colchicum seed, 4 drs.; elixir of ginger, or simple syrup, to make 4 ozs.; mix. DOSE—Take 1 tea-spoonful in a swallow of water, every 3 hours, until better, then 3 times a day till well.

II. EXTERNAL.—Alcohol, 95 per cent. (the best), 2 ozs.; gum camphor, 2 drs.; mix, and when the gum is dissolved add: oils of origanum and cajeput, tinct. of capsicum and tinct. of aconite root, each 2 drs.; mix and apply freely to the affected parts.—B. Frank Humphreys.

*Remarks.*—Here we have an excellent combination of the latest and best articles for internal use, and one for external, without going to different parts of the book for them. Remember, however, that in inflammatory rheumatism the flannel shirts and sheets are exceedingly valuable, and for wetting the blankets Miss McArthur's liniment next following is cheap and good.

**12. Liniment for Inflammatory Rheumatism.**—Miss Bell McArthur's recipe is as follows: Spirits of camphor and strong cider vinegar, each ½ pt.; muriate of ammonia, ½ oz.; soft water, 1 pt.; mix.

The gentleman, of whom Miss McArthur got the above receipt, said he had known it to cure one of the worst cases of inflammatory rheumatism he had ever seen, in a few days, the patient being wrapped in sheets kept wet with liniment. (The expense of this liniment is so trifling, it can be used freely.) Miss

McArthur's experience with it came in this way: she burnt her hand by accidentally putting it in a pail of boiling sugar, and it became very painful. She thought of this liniment, and as soon as it was applied the pain ceased. She tried it in many ways, and found it equally successful. It it is said to be a perfect preventive of sore breasts. Apply warm. Avoid using too near a flame.

*Remarks.*—This is undoubtedly an excellent liniment, especially where persons have to be wrapped in sheets wet with it, as it is inexpensive and will not cause smarting like the stronger alcohol liniments.

**1. LINIMENT—Mrs. Chase's—For Ladies.**—Best alcohol, 1 qt.; camphor gum, chloroform, laudanum, sulphuric ether, tinctures of myrrh and capsicum, and oil of red cedar, each 1 oz.; oil of peppermint, cloves, cajeput, and wormwood, each ¼ oz.; mix, and keep corked for use.

*Remarks.*—Mrs. Chase, during the latter years of her life, had occasion to use a liniment for rheumatism of the shoulder, and not liking the burning heat upon the surface, as experienced when using the stronger liniments containing capsicum, nor liking the oiliness of those known as "volatile," made with sweet oil, hartshorn, etc., asked me to get up something for her especially, avoiding both of these objections. This liniment is the result, and a very satisfactory one it proved, not only to her, but her sister who was visiting us, and who was afflicted in a similar manner. It has also given very great satisfaction in hundreds of cases since its origination. It has been used for all purposes for which liniments are applicable, and found very useful. It is applied night and morning for cold feet and limbs. For the severer cases of rheumatism in men, liniment for stock, etc., see next receipt.

**2. Dr. Chase's Golden Oil, or Strong Camphor Liniment.—** I. Gum camphor, 2 ozs.; oil of origanum, hemlock, sassafras, and tincture of cayenne, each 1 oz.; oil of cajeput, spirits of turpentine, chloroform, and sulphuric ether, each ½ oz.; best alcohol, 1 pt.; mix, and keep corked — as all liniments should be when not being used.

*Remarks.*—This I consider the best liniment for general purposes ever made, and it is a very strong one. This, with No. 1 (Mrs. Chase's) for the use of ladies to avoid the warmth or burning sensation of the skin as mentioned, I honestly think would fill the bill in all cases where liniments are needed. Still, I shall give a few others for special purposes, and some because cheaper than these; and I will further say, this liniment (the main features of it) I took from Dr. King's *Am. Dispensatory*, which I will give, as it is made with the capsicum itself in place of the tincture. I have found that for general purposes, on the flesh of persons, this is the best plan. I have also added the chloroform and ether, which materially help to allay pain externally as well as internally. These changes make it the best thing I know of as a "pain-killer" for internal as well as external use.

Dose—The dose may be from 15 drops to a tea-spoonful, according to the severity of the case, in sugar or in a little sweetened water or milk; to be repeated in 15 to 30 minutes, also according to the severity of pain, griping of bowels, etc.

Externally — For rheumatism, severe pains, etc., it should be poured upon the spot, or into the hand and applied, rubbing in well 3 or 4 times at each application; and, if the place allows it, hold the hand upon it till the heat and smarting subsides. Do this night and morning, and, if a severe case, at noon also. For exceedingly severe cases of painful rheumatism in men and for stock, make it as Dr. King did, by using the capsicum powder as follows:

II. Best alcohol, 1 qt.; camphor gum, 4 ozs.; oil of origanum and hemlock, each 2 ozs.; oils of sassafras and cajeput, each ½ oz.; capsicum in powder, 1 oz.; spirits of turpentine, ¼ oz.; mix, and let stand, shaking daily for two weeks, when it is ready for use. Keep it in the stable always, and apply for all bruises, swellings, lameness, etc. I have called this Dr. Chase's Golden Oil, to distinguish it from one or two other golden oils, which are not so strong, and consequently much cheaper.

**3. Liniment—Dr. A. B. Mason's—For Man or Beast.**—Best alcohol and sweet oil, of each 2 ozs.; aqua ammonia, spirits of turpentine, oils of origanum, spike and gum camphor, each 1 oz.; mix and keep corked for use.

*Remarks.*—Dr. Mason is a cousin of mine, and has used this liniment for 40 years, and knows its value for veterinary and general purposes.

**4. Liniment—Robinson's—For Sick Headache, Rheumatism, Colic, etc.**—Take a 2 quart bottle and put into it oil of origanum, 2 ozs.; chloroform and sulphuric ether, each 1 oz.; oils of sassafras, hemlock, wintergreen, anise, spirits of turpentine, and aqua ammonia, each ½ oz.; then add best alcohol, 1 qt. Keep well corked.

*Remarks.*—Mr. L. S. Robinson, of Jackson, Mich., formerly of Western New York, where, for many years, he made and sold this liniment, and various other medicines, cured several cases of sick headache with it, in Ann Arbor, Mich. He assured me that the person from whom he obtained the recipe offered to pay $50 for any case of rheumatism which he could not cure with it in 48 hours. It is also valuable for sore throat, to take a little on sugar, and apply freely upon the throat and holding the hand upon it while still wet with the liniment, till the heat and smarting subsides, or else wetting flannel in it, and laying upon the throat till quite red, and this mode of application should be adapted wherever necessary to use it. It is good for pains and aches of every description. Dose—From 15 drops to a teaspoonful, with sugar, according to age and the severity of the colic, or other pain. It has a pleasant flavor, is clear and does not soil the clothing. But bear this in mind, that to be successful with any liniment, it must be used or taken freely to get quick returns. In nervous headaches it must be applied to the back of the head and neck, as well as to the fore part, where the pain is located; snuff the fumes from the bottle also freely. A few drops put upon a pin scratch, small pimple, or slight burn frequently, will do very well. He recommended its use 3 to 5 times daily.

**5. Liniment, Nerve and Bone, Very Strong.**—Oil of spike, 6 ozs.; spirits of camphor, hartshorn, tincts. of anise and capsicum, oil of cedar and origanum, of each 2 ozs.; best alcohol, 8 ozs.; mix. DIRECTIONS—Shake well while using. Bathe the parts affected 2 or 3 times daily, and rub briskly with the hand 3 to 5 minutes at each application.

*Remarks.*—This recipe was obtained from Mr. Colman. It is recommended for deep difficulties, strains, sprains, sweeney, etc., as it is strong and penetrating

**6. Liniment, Mustang.**—Crude petroleum, or Seneca oil (so called because first gathered and sold by the Seneca Indians), 1 pt,; olive oil, or lard oil and spirits of hartshorn, each 4 ozs.; oil of origanum, 2 ozs. DIRECTIONS —Mix the olive oil with the hartshorn, then add the others.

**7. Oriental Balm, or Golden Oil Liniment.**—Linseed oil (raw, not boiled), 1 gal.; gum camphor, 4 ozs.; oils of thyme and cajeput, each 1 oz.; oils of wintergreen and anise, each ½ oz. DOSE AND DIRECTIONS—For an adult 1 tea-spoonful in 2 or 3 times as much water, and repeat as often as required. Use externally 3 or 4 times daily; put on frequently and as soon as possible after bee-stings.

*Remarks.*—This has been sold largely in South Western Michigan and Northern Indiana, and is liked very much.

**8. Another Golden Oil Liniment.**—Linseed oil (raw), 1 gal.; cam phor gum, 4 ozs.; oils of sassafras, hemlock, origanum, and cedar, each 2 ozs. DIRECTIONS, DOSE, ETC.—Mix all except the linseed oil, and when the gum camphor is dissolved, put in the linseed oil, shake well and bottle; if to be put up in small bottles, keep it well shaken while filling. It will be seen that this is the strongest liniment, as it contains more of the essential oils, still it may be taken in ½ to 1 tea-spoonful doses, with perfect safety. It has been extensively sold in the neighborhood of Marshall and Battle Creek, Mich., sometimes there called " Oil of Gladness." It will be found good, for a cheap liniment.

**9. Rheumatic Liniment, and for Pain in the Stomach, etc. —Donohue's.**—Oils of origanum, sassafras, cloves, and gum camphor, each ½ oz.; chloroform, ¼ oz. DIRECTIONS—Put all into a 3 oz. vial, and fill with alcohol; rub on the painful parts freely; take, for pain in the stomach, 5 to 20 drops on sugar, repeating in 15 to 30 minutes, if needed. This gentleman is an old friend of mine, living in Coshocton, O., where, he tells me, he has cured, or materially benefited 50 or 60 cases of common rheumatism. He thinks there is nothing equal to it.

**10. Liniments, Patent or Proprietary — Perry Davis' Pain-Killer.** — Some analysis recently made in the East, and published in the *Druggists' Circular*, gives the following as the articles composing the medicines named: Spirits of camphor, 2 ozs.; tinct. of capsicum, 1 oz.; gum myrrh, ¼ oz.; gum guaiac, ½ oz.; alcohol, 3 ozs.

**11. R. R. R. (Radway's Ready Relief).**—Soap liniment, 1½ ozs.; tinct. of capsicum ½ oz.; water of ammonia, ½ oz.; alcohol, ½ oz. This for a 50c. bottle.

**12. Hamlin's Wizard Oil.** — Spirits of camphor, ½ oz.; aqua ammonia, ¼ oz.; oil of sassafras, ¼ oz.; oil of cloves, 1 dr.; chloroform, 2 drs.; spirits of turpentine, 3 drs.; dilute alcohol, 3 drs.

**13. Giles' Liniment of Iodide of Ammonia.** — Iodine, 15 grs.;

camphor gum, ¼ oz.; oils of lavender and rosemary, each 1 dr.; alcohol, ½ pt.; strong aqua ammonia, 1 oz.

*Remarks.*—Any of these liniments, which have no directions accompanying them, would be used the same as the general run of liniments.

**14. Cure-All Liniment.**—Gum camphor, gum myrrh, opium, pulverized cayenne, and oil of sassafras, each 1 oz.; oils of hemlock, red cedar, wormwood, spirits of turpentine, and hartshorn, each ½ oz.; best alcohol, 1 qt. DIRECTIONS—Cut the opium finely; mix, and shake daily for a week or 10 days; then strain or filter.

*Remarks.*—It will be found a valuable liniment for all purposes for which liniments are used.

**15. Lightning Liniment.**—Chloroform and ether, each 1 oz.; laudanum, 2 oz.; spirits of turpentine, 4 ozs.; mix.

*Remarks.*—Mr. Johnson, of Grand Rapids, Mich., says: " Bathe legs, back, or any part of the body with it, and it will give immediate relief. Good for nervous affections, rheumatism, etc.

**16. Opodeldoc Liniment.** — Alcohol, ½ pt.; camphor gum, ½ oz.; almond or other good soap, and oil of cajeput, each 1 oz. DIRECTIONS—Shave the soap finely, and put it with the camphor gum into the alcohol and dissolve by gentle heat; when cool, add the cajeput oil, shake thoroughly before it sets, and pour into large-mouthed bottles, to allow the finger to reach it for application, else it has to be warmed, to pour into the hand for application.

*Remarks*—Some people prefer the Opodeldoc Liniment to others, especially for paralysis, enlarged joints, indolent tumors, rheumatism, lumbago, chilblains, etc., for which this is recommended, both to arouse the absorbents and to stimulate the nerves to action, by which a cure is effected when accomplished at all.

**17. Liniment—White's Nerve and Bone.** — Gum camphor, oils of sassafras, cedar, and origanum, each 2 ozs.; oil of cajeput, 1 oz.; aqua ammonia; 1 oz.; oil of tar, 2 drs.: sulphuric ether, 4 ozs.; best alcohol, 3 qts.; solution of analine (red), 10 or 15 drops—to improve the color; mix, and keep closely corked.

*Remarks.*—Mr. White is a druggist in Eaton Rapids, Mich., from whom I obtained this receipt. He kept this liniment on sale for a number of years. This is the liniment I refer to under the head of " Carbuncles." He speaks of it as a mild liniment, and the boys using it on their hands while playing ball, to prevent blistering, called it " Base Ball Liniment."

**18. Chloroform Liniment, Especially for Strains, Sprains, etc.**—Chloroform, 1 fluid oz.; camphor gum, ¾ oz.; shake together till dissolved, then add olive oil, 1 oz.; tinct. cantharides, 1 dr.; keep well corked, as chloroform is very evaporative.

*Remarks.*—A nephew of mine, from whom I received this recipe, found more benefit from it on a strained knee, with which he suffered for two years, than any other liniment. Let it be used freely, when used at all, and it must do good from the known nature of the ingredients.

**19. " The Best Liniment," for Strains, Bruises, Pains, Colic, Headache, Backache, and All Other Aches—Externally.—**A. Parsons, M. D., of Scottville, Ark., sends the following under the above title, to *Medical Brief*, page 508, of 1882. Chloroform, alcohol, aqua ammonia, spirits of camphor and tinct. of aconite root, each 2 ozs.; spirits of nitric ether, 6 ozs.; mix, keep corked. This is Thompson's chloroform liniment, improved, and is the best stimulating liniment that I ever met with. Any kind of ordinary colic may be relieved by saturating the bowels with it. Its application is very beneficial in all the above aches, and in nearly all cases removes them permanently.

*Remarks.*—I need only say from the nature of the articles composing it that it will prove an excellent liniment for external use; but do not take it internally, on account of the aconite it contains.

**Winter Itch—Certain Remedy.—**B. I. A. Cull, M. D., of Gamilla, Ga., page 330 of *Medical Brief* for 1880, under the head of "Eureka" (a Greek word, signifying I have found it), says: "After a fair trial, in several cases, to act as a specific (certain cure), in that disease. Blood root, pulverized and steeped in strong apple vinegar, to make as strong as can be made, applied 3 or 4 times a day, cures the disease."

**1. BRONCHOCELE—Goitre, or Swelled Neck, to Cure Without Coloring the Skin or Clothing.—**Compound tinct. of iodine, 4 ozs.; pure liquid carbolic acid, ½ dr.; glycerine, ¾ oz.; mix. DIRECTIONS—Have these articles put into a quinine bottle, having a good cork; put a small stick into the cork, suitable to tie a cloth swab upon it, with which to apply once or twice daily, as can be borne.

*Remarks.*—The carbolic acid prevents the iodine from coloring (aqua ammonia does the same thing), glycerine prevents speedy evaporation, and also keeps the skin soft and smooth. Constitutional, or alterative treatment, should also be made use of in connection with this local application. Electro-magnetism has also been found of great value, by hastening the reduction of the tumor. Dr. King, of Cincinnati, O., makes use of the following alterative pill

**2. Bronchocele, or Swelled Neck, Alterative Pill for—also Valuable in All Cases Needing an Alterative.** — Oleoresin of blue flag (irisin) 1 scru.; baptisin, 5 grs.; citrate of iron and strychnia, 80 grs.; alcoholic ex. of aletris farinosa, 80 grs. DIRECTIONS—Mix all thoroughly together and divide into 80 pills. DOSE—1 pill 1 hour after breakfast, dinner and at bed time.

*Remarks.*—If the treatment is begun soon after the commencement of the swelling, a cure may be expected quickly, but if of long standing and some hardening of the tumors already commenced, it will require a perseverance, perhaps, of several months, to effect a cure. The above tincture will be found valuable to apply to any node, or knotty tumors, from bruises or otherwise, upon man or beast.

**3. Goitre, Bronchocele, or Swelled Neck—Dr. Mason's Internal and External Remedy.**—-I. INTERNAL—Iodide of potash, 1 oz.; fl.

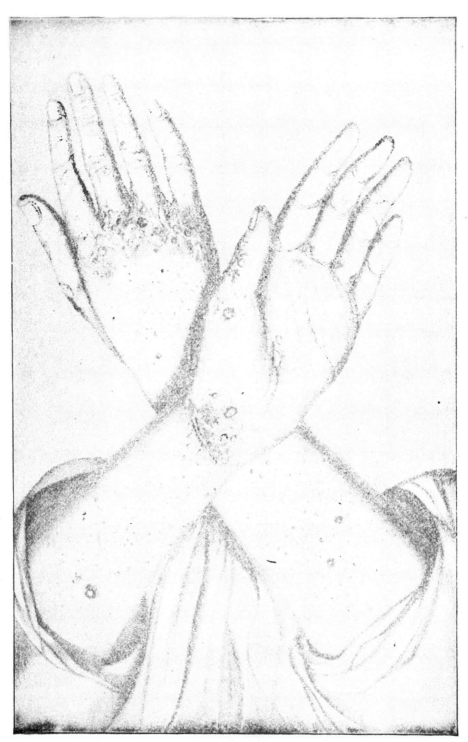

SCABIES, OR ITCH

ex. of sarsaparilla, 6 ozs.; fl. ex. of dandelion, 4 ozs.; dissolve the iodide in a tea-cup of soft water, then add to the extracts, in a bottle sufficiently large, 1 pint of simple syrup. DOSE—1 tea-spoonful ½ hour before each meal.

*Remarks.*—If in any case this causes a stuffing up of the nose, as is often said on taking cold, the dose must be lessened about one-half, or else as much more of the extracts and syrup must be added—with some people the iodide of potash causes this condition. Occasionally one cannot take it at all; the extracts, then, must be taken without it, but the cure will not be as rapid.

II. EXTERNAL—Take tinct. of iodine, 2 ozs.; soft water, ½ oz.; sulphite of soda, sufficient to remove the color of the iodine from the tincture before adding the water, which prevents the coloring of the skin or clothing. With a small brush, or swab, paint this tincture, once daily, upon the swelling, and so continue until cured.

*Remarks.*—The doctor says: " This remedy needs no recommendation, as it has been used by quite a number, and with good results. It was sent to my wife by a Mrs. P. M. Avery, of Pennsylvania, but the idea of discoloration," he says, " I got from the Boston *Medical and Surgical Journal.*"

**4. Goitre Alterative Syrup, and for All Purposes Requiring an Alterative.**—Fl. exs. of sarsaparilla and gentian, each 1 lb.; iodide of potash, ½ oz.; corrosive sublimate, 5 grs. DIRECTIONS—Rub the corrosive sublimate in a mortar, with a little of one of the fluid extracts to dissolve it, then mix all together. Shake occasionally, a day or so, to dissolve, and properly mix the iodide and sublimate. DOSE—1 to 2 tea-spoonfuls, according to the age and robustness of the adult, in a little water, sweetened. To be taken 4 times daily, a little before each meal and at bed-time.

*Remarks.*—This alterative has no superior for any general purpose. Some people, however, object to the corrosive sublimate, because it is a poison; but in the minute division of it into so many doses, it is a very valuable article, as an alterative, notwithstanding the objections. It can be left out if you wish, and still have a splendid alterative; but it will be better if put in. Having used it, and directed it for others, I know whereof I speak.

**1. DROPSY—Syrup For.**—Butternut bark, dwarf elder (bark of the root), and endives (chicory, also called succory), each 1 lb.; Indian hemp, ½ lb.; black root and dandelion root, juniper berries, yellow dock and burdock roots, each ¼ lb.; prickly ash berries, 2 ozs.; loaf sugar, 2 lbs.; pure whiskey, 3 pts. DIRECTIONS—The recently dried roots and barks are intended, and should be coarsely ground by the druggist; place all (except sugar and whiskey) in a four gallon jar and pour on sufficient boiling water to well cover the whole. Set the jar on the back part of the stove, cover with a cloth and plate, to keep in the heat, and let it stand 3 or 4 days, to sour; it is not to boil. When a little sour strain and simmer to one gallon, when the sugar is to be added, and when cool, the spirits· then bottle for use. DOSE—A wine-glass a little before meals.

*Remarks.*—This recipe was obtained from a Mr. Coleman, who spoke very highly of its success. It is diuretic. tonic and alterative, besides its action upon the liver by the black root (this is the *leptandra virginica*, from which the lep-tandrin is made), although it is not specially cathartic in its action, and must be found valuable. An ounce of essence of wintergreen would make it very pleasant to the taste.

**2. Dropsy and Anti-fat Medicine.**—M. Milton, M. D., of DuBois, Penn., in a report through the *Brief*, page 439, 1883, says:

"He cured a lady patient, having a dropsical tendency, of that difficulty, also reducing her weight from 247 to 198 lbs. in 15 days, by the following treat-ment: He obtained the juice of poke-berries, and evaporated it by means of sand-bath to the consistency of pill-mass, forming into 4-gr. pills, with a little powdered licorice-root."

Dose—Two pills half hour after each meal. In connection with these pills he gave ⅛ gr. of elaterium in solution at night. (If its action on the bowels should be so severe as to cause distress, skip a night or two.) By the continued use of these pills alone, for a few weeks, her flesh was reduced to 175 pounds, and she remained well up to the time of this report, 3 years after. See also "Fat People—Food to Reduce their Fleshiness."

**1. COLIC, OR OTHER INTERNAL PAIN—German Rem-edy or Liniment for.**—Alcohol, 1 qt.; oil of sassafras and hartshorn, each 2 ozs.; spirits of camphor and laudanum, each 1 oz.; spirits of turpentine, ½ oz.; tinct. of kino, ¼ oz.; mix. Dose—For colic, or any severe internal pain, from ½ to 1 tea-spoonful may be taken for a dose; to be repeated in ½ to 1 hr., according to the severity of the case.

*Remarks.*—This recipe was sent me by Mr. Frank Spurlock (a German), of Sedan, Kan. It certainly makes a good liniment for general use, and I give it a place, to meet the desire of my German readers; for they, like Americans, think their own prescriptions are the best.

**2. Colic—Cure by Quinine.**—Dr. N. R. Derby, of Bergen Point, N. J., says, in the *Medical Recorder*, that by accident he discovered that a dose of 8 or 10 grs. of sulphate of quinine will speedily put an end to an attack of colic. He had had such attacks from childhood, but cured himself and several others in this way. This dose is for an adult. I should try it if I had occa-sion to do so.

**1. CONSTIPATION OR COSTIVENESS—Valuable Pills for.**—I. Solid extracts of nux vomica and hyoscyamus, and pulverized capsi-cum, each 25 grs.; podophyllin, and ext. of belladonna, each 10 grs.; mix thoroughly and make into 100 pills. Dose—If very constipated when you com-mence taking them, take 2 each night for 1 or 2 nights, or until the bowels become easy; then 1 only at night till cured.

II. *Constipation — Hot Water as a Cure.*—A cup of hot water, a writer says, is a grand tonic and stomach cleanser, and a sure cure for constipation. It should be taken night and morning, just before retiring and after rising.

*Remarks.*—I have seen hot water recommended for this difficulty before, and think it worthy of trial. It is also recommended for dyspepsia, which often causes constipation. For the degree of heat and manner of taking, see " Hot Water for Dyspepsia."

## 2. Constipation or Costiveness—Newer Remedies.—For a few

years past the fl. ex. of cascara sagrada has been much extolled, and also found quite satisfactory in relieving the difficulty, and if properly combined with other remedies, has cured very many cases. I have been very successful with the fol-lowing combination:

I. Fl. ex. cascara sagrada, 1 oz.; tincts. nux vomica and belladonna, each 2 drs.; with syrup of Tolu, or syrup of wild cherry, 2½ ozs.; mix. DOSE—A tea-spoonful 3 times a day till the bowels become easy; then only at bed-time, till cured.

*Remarks.*—I have succeeded with this when other things, by other physi-cians, have failed.

II. I see that some physicians prefer the following prescription for consti-pation: Fl. ex. cascara sagrada, fl. ex. berberis aquifolium and simple syrup, each 1 oz.; tinct. nux vomica, 25 drops, and tinct. digitalis, 1 dr. DOSE—A tea-spoonful 3 times daily, till the bowels become easy, then drop off morning, then noon dose, and finally all, using only occasionally, for a while, till a healthy daily action is established. This would be the most valuable in female cases, as the berberis is claimed to be a " female regulator," uterine tonic, etc. But supposing there is no constipation, although the liver may be inactive in the secretion of bile, the stools, or passages, being light, or clay-colored, then I would use:

III. Fl. ex. of fringe tree, 1 oz.; fl. ex. of berberis, 1 oz.; adding also. as a stomach tonic, fl. ex. wahoo, ½ oz.; syrup of wild cherry, or Tolu, 1 oz.; and the tincts. of nux vomica and belladonna, each 2 drs., as in No. 1, above. DOSE and management the same as in No. 1, till the stools assume their healthy color again.

## 3. Constipation, More Recent Remedy.—My attention was re-

cently called to the following, and having a case of constipation on hand, and in which the liver did not give the usual amount of bile, giving a tendency to jaundice, I at once tried it with the happiest results—entire relief in both diffi-culties. The remedy was: Tinct. nux vomica, 1 oz.; podophyllin, 1 gr.; the podophyllin to be rubbed in a little of the tincture to insure it thorough mix-ing. DOSE—Take 5 drops only, before each meal, till the bowels become easy, then only 3 drops, or even 2, as required to keep them easy, for a few days; after which take occasionally, if needed, by the reappearance of the clay-col-ored stools.

*Remarks.*—The tincture of nux vomica in the small doses above given, is not only safe, but a very valuable medicine, still if left where children can get hold of it and drink the whole bottle, or considerable of it, it is poisonous; and hence I give in the next item the treatment for such a mishap, as follows:

## Poisoning by Nux Vomica or Strychnine—Remedy.—Should

ever poisoning occur by the careless taking of over-doses of tincture of nux, or strychnine (which is made from it), twitching of the muscles will be the first sign, then convulsions, no time should be lost in getting down oils of any character, sweet oil is considered best, but lard oil, or melted lard, in doses of from 1 cup to ½ pint for an adult answers very well, and strong coffee, and then producing vomiting in the quickest way, by mustard, or thrusting the finger down the throat after the oils or coffee has been given. A pint of strong coffee saved a dog, after it appeared he was nearly dead; four grains of camphor gum has done the same thing—then they are good for persons. It is better, however, to put such things out of the reach of children. See, also, "Poisons, Quick Emetics, Antidotes, etc."

**1. GRAVEL—Remedy.**—A strong decoction, made with a handful of smart-weed in ½ pt. of water, taken with a gill of gin, is said to have discharged a table-spoonful of gravel at a time in 12 hours from the time it was taken. Keep on taking it daily as long as any gravel is discharged.

**1. HEMORRHAGE OR BLEEDING FROM THE LUNGS, WOMB, RECTUM, ETC.**—Witchhazel and Other Specifics, or Positive Remedies for.—Hemorrhage, or bleeding from the uterus (womb) after child-birth, from the lungs and from the rectum, in some cases of piles, are of such frequent occurrence that I deem it of great importance to give the latest and most successful prescriptions for hemorrage in these cases.

Of late the homeopathists claim that the valuable properties of the witchhazel is a discovery of theirs, and they make ado over it in the form of "Pond's Extract of Hamamelis." If this is used, give it in doses of 10 to 15 drops, repeated every 3 or 4 hours.

Among eclectics, for many years past, the common witchhazel (hamamelis) has been considered a very valuable remedy for hemorrhages or bleeding from the internal organs. Prominent among these are Professors John M. Scudder and A. S. Howe, of the Eclectic Medical Institute of Cincinnati, who consider it a specific (positive cure) in all cases of debility of the nervous system—a weak and flabby condition that allows the blood to ooze through the membrane.

Prof. Howe has used this about 30 years, or long before homeopathy had become at all prominent in the United States.

Prof. John King, of the same institute named above, and also an extensive medical writer, thinks that in hemorrhages immediately following "delivery at full term" hamamelis is not equal to ergot, but in cases arising from debility, he agrees with the remarks above—that witchhazel is vastly superior.

A decoction or tea, made from the bark or from the dried leaves, will be as effectual as "Pond's Extract." which is kept by druggists.

The strength of a decoction will be 1 oz. of dried bark or leaves to 1 pt. of water. DOSE—A wine-glassful 3 or 4 times daily.

**2. Uterine Hemorrhage—Specifics in.**—C. J. Pitzer, M. D., of Detroit, Ill., a practitioner of over 16 years experience, in a communication to the *Eclectic Medical Journal*, asks for practical items from the experience of other physicians, and in giving his own, says: "Cinnamon and erigeron are specifics (positive cure) in uterine hemorrhage; I know it by actual experience. I don't tell you anything new, but recall your attention to the fact and confirm, as far as my evidence goes, what has been said of these articles by others. Let me say, while speaking of these invaluable remedies, that in uterine hemorrhage you can't have too much confidence in them. They are just what you want. Don't resort to ergot. Give oil of erigeron, 10 drops, every hour, and oftener, if needs be; and between each doze give 15 drops tinct. oil of cinnamon, made by adding oil of cinnamon, 1 fl. dr., to best alcohol, 95 % 1 fl. oz. I use both remedies in every case, alternating. Don't know which does the most good; neither do I care much, so I save my patient. Just had a bad case last week, caused by retained membranes. The case had been managed by other physicians, and 4 or 5 days after the delivery, the hemorrhage was very excessive and threatened the life of the patient in a short time. The doctor who sent for me had used ergot, opium, lead and tannin, and had resorted to the tampon. I suggested the above named remedies, and commenced the use of them at once. The hemorrhage ceased almost entirely in 4 hours, and we had no trouble in controlling it afterwards."

*Remarks.*—It is facts like these which have now well established the belief in the specific, or positive action, of medicines, and I trust that others may have sufficient confidence in them to use them when needed. This is one of the objects in writing this book, that these well established facts may reach the thousands, or hundreds of thousands, of the people, rather than stop with only a few physicians.

**3. Hemorrhage from the Womb, With High Pulse and Fever.**—Being called to a case where an abortion had been performed, in an early stage of pregnancy (not knowing for some time after, of the cause), finding the wasting, or hemorrhage, considerable, I gave:

I. Fl. ex. of ergot, ½ oz.; gallic acid, 40 grs.; mixed. Dose—½ teaspoonful every 2 hours, until pain and contraction of the womb was produced, then once in 4 or 5 hours only, until the wasting ceased.

II. *For the High Pulse*—I gave tinct. veratrum viride, 6 drops, with tinct. aconite, 3 drops, every 2 hours, alternating with the first, giving the second 1 hour after the ergot mixture had been given, dropping each into a tumbler, so as to get this number of drops, of each, in a tea-spoonful of water, when given. For instance, 36 drops of the veratrum and 18 drops of aconite, with 6 teaspoonfuls of water, gave the right dose each time.

*Remarks.*—Remember, however, that the veratrum and aconite mixture is only to reduce the pulse, which was about 120; when this comes down to 80, then give this only once in 4 or 6 hours, to keep the pulse at about this grade; if continued too long, it will reduce too much, and also distress and nauseate the stomach, which is not necessary, and should always be avoided if possible. The strength must be helped up with 2 or 3 grain doses of quinine, or "Dextro" quinine, in same doses three times daily.

The urine in such cases may need some attention, and call for acetate, or nitrate, of potash (I like the acetate best, some others prefer the nitrate-niter.

or the sweet spirits of nitre), to correct any disturbance of these organs, for which purpose. See " Diuretics" for directions.

**4. Hemorrhage, Slight, of the Lungs, with Cough—Regulator or Allopathic Treatment For.**—I. Give fl. ex. of ergot, 15 drops in a little water, putting in a little essence of wintergreen to lessen its bitter taste. (The author would say, in such a case, a few drops of essence of cinnamon, which will cover the bitter taste as well as the wintergreen, is of itself good for the hemorrhage.) Give the above every six hours.

II. Between these doses also give gallic acid, 4 grs., in a little syrup of lemon. This alternation brings the doses only three hours apart. A few doses of each will generally allay any slight hemorrhage. If the cough is pretty persistant, *i. e.*, continuous and irritating, give laudanum, 15 drops, once in 4 or 5 hours, and 25 drops at bed-time, to allay the cough and help in procuring sleep. Give also laxatives, if needed, to prevent costiveness.

*Remarks.*—I know this treatment to have proved eminently satisfactory when the hemorrhage was not very extensive.

**5. Hemorrhage, or Bleeding From Slight Cuts, etc.—Simple Remedy.**—To stop the flow of blood bind the cut with cobwebs and brown sugar, pressed on like lint. Wheat flour and salt, in equal parts, bound on with a cloth, for man or beast; mix well, without wetting, the blood will wet them enough.

**Treatment for Hemorrhage.**—Soon after the above was written we had the value of the cobweb treatment confirmed, by the Toledo *Post*, in a case of a lady of that city, who had a tooth drawn; hemorrhage from the cavity set in and continued, in spite of all common remedies, from Saturday noon until 3 o'clock Sunday morning, when the cobweb was procured and applied and the bleeding stopped by this move, leaving her very weak.

**7. Hemorrhage from Wounds—Styptic Colloid, to Prevent and Cure.**—The following will instantly coagulate blood, forming a consistent clot, under which wounds will readily heal: Collodion, 100 parts (grs.); carbolic acid, 10 parts; tannic and benzoic acids, of each 5 parts; mix the ingredients in the above order.

*Remarks.*—If the wound is so large that a slight application does not stop the hemorrhage or bleeding, wet lint with it and bind on if necessary, and leave on until the healing process is accomplished.

**1. DIPHTHERIA—Successful Remedies.**—My first remedy, although simple and easily obtained, is from a paper presented to the French Academy of Medicine by Dr. Revillout, who asserts from an experience of 18 years, that:

I. Lemon juice is one of the most efficacious medicines that can be applied in Diphtheria, and relates that when he was a dresser in the hospital, his own life was saved by this timely application. He got a quantity of lemons and gargled his throat with the juice, swallowing a little at a time in order to act on the more deep-seated parts.

It is also recommended for any inflammatory or irritable condition of the throat in their commencement.

II. Lemon juice in Diphtheria is endorsed by American physicians, as the following will show. Let it be tried by all means.

Dr. J. R. Page, of Baltimore, in the New York *Medical Record*, invites the attention of the profession to a topical use of fresh lemon juice as a most efficient means for the removal of the membrane from the throat, tonsils, etc., in diphtheria In his hands (he has heard several of his professional brethren say the same) it has proved by far the best agent he has yet tried for the purpose. He applied the juice of the lemon, by means of a camel's hair probang (a piece of cloth on a stick will do as well), to the affected parts every 2 or 3 hours, and in eighteen cases on which he has used it the effect has been all he could wish. A little remarkable—one has 18 years successful experience, the other 18 cases; either is enough.

**2. Diphtheria — Ice a Successful Remedy for.** — The French have also been very successful in the use of ice as a remedy in Diphtheria, which was introduced into this country by a Dr. Chapman, reported through the New York *Tribune*, by which means it was brought to the notice of the Oneida community in that state, where the disease was prevailing, and was successful in 60 cases. They aroused the mind of the patients, old enough to understand the necessity, to the greatest possible resistance to the advance of the disease. This determination of resistance is valuable against the advance of any disease. DIRECTIONS—The ice is broken into small pieces and given to the patient every ten minutes, night and day.

**3. Diphtheria, Cure For.**—A Mrs. R. S. K., of Toledo, Ohio., gives the following cure for diphtheria to the *Blade Household*: I. Syrup of squills, 1 oz.; gum camphor, ¼ oz.; laudanum, ½ dr.; cayenne pepper, ½ tea-spoonful; good whiskey, ½ pt. DIRECTIONS—Camphor to be dissolved in as small a quantity of alcohol as possible. Four large onions are to be cut in slices, put into a deep earthen plate (that will stand heat), sprinkle thickly with loaf sugar, cover with another plate, place a heated flat iron on the upper plate, leaving it set on the back of the stove. Heat and pressure will extract all the juices without losing any of its medical properties. All the juices thus extracted are to be mixed with the other ingredients; when all are mixed together and the camphor added, it will curdle; but when it stands awhile, it will become clear. DOSE—For an adult, 1 tea-spoonful every ½ hour; for a child, ½ tea-spoonful every ¼ hour; to be diluted for a child, as it is pretty strong.

II. Apply also the following: Salt pork, ½ lb , and 2 large onions; chop all together finely and put some upon the throat. For an infant place a thin piece of muslin on the poultice next the skin; change every 15 or 20 minutes

*Remarks* — A poultice of mashed onions to the arm-pits, stomach, soles of the feet and palms of the hands, in bad cases of fevers, has worked wonders. Why not good then for diphtheria?

**4. Diphtheria, Sulphur Treatment.**—Our attention was first called to the use of sulphur, in this disease, by a report from Dr. Fields, in England.

He found an advantage in its use, in some bad cases within ten minutes of its commencement. His manner of using it with those old enough, was in the form of a gargle, a tea-spoonful of the powder, or flour of sulphur, in a wine glass of water, gargling frequently. If the patient was unable to gargle, or too young, blow some of the dry sulphur through a quill upon the diseased parts of the throat, or burn some of the sulphur upon live coals near the patient, so that he will inhale the fumes. The patient should always be kept warm and the bowels open. In extreme cases, when Dr. Field was called, just in the nick of time, when the fungus was so near filling the throat, as not to allow the gargling, he first blew the sulphur through the quill into the throat, and after the fungus had shrunk to allow of it, then the frequent gargling. He never lost a patient from diphtheria under this treatment. He recommends after gargling a couple of times, to cleanse the throat, to swallow some of the sulphur water occasionally, so as to reach the fungus deeper in the throat, which also has a tendency to keep the bowels open, which is recommended a very important point to accomplish. This fungus is believed to be a living parasite, of plant-like growth, and that sulphur is absolutely destructive to them, as has been proved by its use, by applying upon the parasites of the grape vine. It has been proved that sulphur kills every fungus or parasite on man, beast, or plant. One Dr. Langautiers also found that one tea-spoonful doses every hour, of a mixture of sulphur, in 4 ozs. of water, taken every hour, is very beneficial in the treatment of croup.

**5. Diphtheria, Specific for—Also Scarlet Fever, and Preventive in Both.**—The best physicians of New York city, Brooklyn and Philadelphia are equally in favor of the sulpho-carbolate of soda.

[The sulpho-carbolate of soda is composed of soda combined with sulphur and carbolic acid, either of which alone is good in diphtheria, scarlet fever and any other inflammatory condition of the throat; and the combination is more decidedly beneficial than either would be alone; at least it seems so to me from my knowledge of their properties.]

Dr. May, of New York city, says the sulpho-carbolate of soda is a specific (positive cure) in diphtheria, also in scarlet fever, and claims that this article is a preventive to the development, even after exposure, as well as a cure for both these diseases. The writer of this report is very much impressed in favor of this article. He says:

"The use of sulpho-carbolate of soda in diphtheria has become a settled fact by the best physicians, as above named, to be the only certain specific (positive cure), for that dreaded disease which has taken off so many children in the United States during the past 8 years. He also says it is certain to destroy the parasitic fungus in the throat and glands in two hours.

"Ten grs. dissolved in a tumbler half full of cold water, and take from ½ to 1 tea-spoonful every hour, until the parasite is destroyed; then take 1 tea-spoonful every 2 or 3 hours, according to the circumstances of the case. There is no use in physicians fighting against this remedy, for they will have to use it if they have success in the treatment of scarlet fever and diphtheria. It is a specific in both diseases, as they are both zymotic (acting like a ferment, spreading quickly through the system) in their nature, and are produced by the parasite in the system. It will prevent both diseases, if given before an attack as well as a remedy. This remedy has been used for scarlet fever and diphtheria

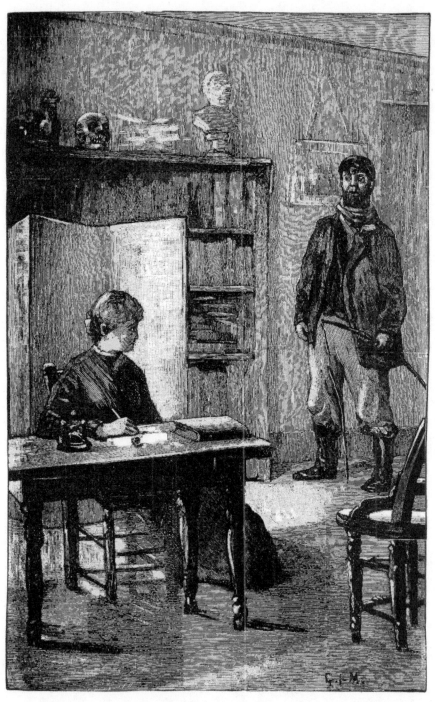

WHERE'S THE DOCTOR?  I AM THE DOCTOR, SIR.
WHEW!  I HADN'T CALCULATED ON A WOMAN DOCTOR;
BUT COME ON QUICK.

for over 3 years, and if given before gangrene (mortification) sets in, will work wonders in every case. It was discovered by an English physician, and has grown into favor as a specific ever since, particularly with children.

"The trichina parasite of pork, as soon as it enters the stomach, is absorbed by the blood, then into the muscles of the body. It is not so with the diphtheria parasite; it is generated in the stomach, and when it spreads up the œsophagus (comes from Greek words, signifying to bear, to carry and to eat; being the passage way of the food and drink to the stomach, commonly called the gullet), it produces such a high state of inflammation that gangrene sets in, which dissolves the parasite, and carries it all through the blood, which is always fatal. Gangrene always dissolves the parasite, but before that takes place the use of the sulpho-carbolate of soda will save every case. I have written these lines by special request of very many citizens and friends who desire it made public for the benefit of all."

*Remarks.*—I am only sorry that I have not had an opportunity to test this myself; but, as I have not, I can only say to physicians, and heads of families, try it, by all means. Whenever either of these diseases gives you an opportunity, have it on hand and lose no time in beginning its use.

**6. Diphtheria—Chlorine Water a Specific for.**—At a recent breaking out of Diphtheria in a considerable number of places, which was also alarming in its fatality, the *Springfield Republican*, in commenting upon the fact, called attention to some remedies which have entirely divested this fearful disease of its terrors, if applied in the early stages. Among these it claimed the most simple and effective to be chlorine water, diluted by adding 2 to 4 times the amount of water. A well known physician of that city, the *Republican* asserts, has used this specific conclusively for fifteen years with complete success, previous to its use having lost about half his cases. He repeatedly, by its use, eradicated the disease in different places, when all other remedies failed. Another medical writer claims that the chlorine water and sulphur treatments, as given above, are the only positive cures. DOSE—1 to 2 tea-spoonfuls, largely diluted with water, 2 or 3 times daily; also as a gargle in sore throat, even of a putrid character.

*Remarks.*—To give confidence to those who are not acquainted with the uses of chlorine water, I will say it is powerfully antiseptic (overcoming putrefaction), quickly destroying all bad odors arising from decay. It has been successfully used internally in chronic inflammation of the liver, typhus fever, malignant sore throat, scarlet fever, etc.

**7. Diphtheria — Successful Remedy in Forty Cases — Also Preventive.**—Dr. MacLean, of Norwalk, Ct., recommends the following as a preventive of diphtheria, remarking:

"During the past 4 years I have used it, and in 40 well marked cases of diphtheria, where 140 persons were exposed to a contagion, not a single case has been reported to me. I use 1 dr. of Monsel's salt in 8 ozs. cold water, adding plenty of sugar to overcome the taste of the iron. DOSE—2 to 8 tea-spoonfuls each day, according to the violence of the disease."

*Remarks.*—The dose would be 1 tea-spoonful, 2, 3 or 4 hours apart, as the case may require.

**8. Diphtheria, Sore Throat, Swollen Tonsils, Etc.—Homeopathic Remedy.**—Bin-iodide of mercury, 10 grs.; sugar of milk, 100 grs.;

triturate (rub) together 30 minutes in a wedgewood mortar. Then take 10 grs. of this triturated article and 100 grs. more of sugar of milk, and triturate again as before. DOSE—Give 1 gr. of this second trituration every hour in ordinary cases; if a bad case, give the same amount every 15 to 30 minutes, until relieved: then every hour or two, as needed. A few doses makes the cure.

*Remarks.*—Dr. Mason used this a number of years, and very successfully, on some very bad cases. The above is the Homeopathic treatment, except some of them use in addition to this a gargle, every hour, of ½ alcohol and ½ water.

**9. Diphtheria, Dr. Scott's Treatment for.**—After the foregoing recipes had been prepared I noticed Dr. W. A. Scott, of Sandyville, Iowa, reported through the Chicago *Inter-Ocean* his success with the following treatment:

I. Dissolve 20 grs. of pure permanganate of potassa (permanganate of potassa is a powerful disinfectant, also a great purifier of sick rooms, clothing, etc.) in 1 oz. of water, and apply it to the affected parts with a swab, gently, but thoroughly, every 3 hours, until better; then not so often. (Better get 80 grs. in a 4 oz. vial of water.) After the patient gets better weaken the solution by adding an equal quantity of water. This solution does not give any pain, nor is there any danger in its use, but it has a nasty taste, which is its only objection. (Its staining clothing is another objection.)

Prof. King, in his American Dispensatory, says:

"One dr. of permanganate dissolved in ½ oz. of water, in a saucer, and placed under the table, bed or other convenvient place destroys all odors. Another writer in speaking ot permanganate of potash to purify the air of sick rooms says: ½ oz. of it, in water, 1 qt., and cloths wet in it and hung up, is a quick and certain disinfectant. For disinfecting or cleansing clothing of diphtheritic, scarlet fever or small pox patients, bedding, etc., 1 oz. of the permanganate to 2 gals. of water is sufficient to soak them in, an hour or two, before the boiling and washing in the regular way.

II. "Apply a good liniment to the throat outside, 3 or 4 times a day. (Dr. Chase's golden oil or liniment, or Mrs. Chase's, will be found good for this purpose.) Keep a cotton cloth, not woolen, around the throat till well. The above is all I use in simple cases, and all that is needed.

III. "If there is much fever I mix 5 drops of fl. ex. of aconite root with 4 ozs. of water, and give to a small child ¼ tea-spoonful; a child 5 to 10 years, ½ tea-spoonful; 10 to 15 years, 1 tea-spoonful; over that age, 2 tea-spoonfuls. Give every 1 or 2 hours, as may seem needed, to lessen the fever.

IV. "If there is blood poisoning, which may be known by the bad smelling breath and quick beating of the heart, give: Chloroform, 1 fl. dr.; comp. spts. lav., 1 dr.; alcohol, 1 oz.; mix. DOSE—Five to 20 drops, according to the age, mixed in cold water, every ½ to 2 hours, as may seem necessary. This will quickly quiet the heart's tumultuous action and aid it to throw off the poison.

V. "Do not give harsh physics. If needed, give castor oil or purgative magnesia. Keep the patient from exposure to chilly air or cold baths. This treatment, which I have published in several medical journals, will rob this disease of its terror and save from the grave many a loved one."

*Remarks.*—Let the medicine be obtained where there are families of children, so as to have it in the house as soon as needed, on the approach of the disease into a neighborhood. Then when it begins, lose no time in applying the remedy, and the different aids he recommends, if needed.

**10. Diphtheria—Latest Allopathic Treatment For.**—In a recent conversation with Dr. Haney, of Toledo, Ohio, he claimed to cure every case of diphtheria, even in small children, by swabbing the throat with calomel; for quite a young child he gets 10 grs. into the throat, by a swab, and a child 5 to 8 years, 20 to 30 grs., so it will be swallowed. He says it stops the change in the blood, by which the fibrinous portions form the membrane in the throat. He follows 3 or 4 hours after with the liquid physic (see "Liquid Physic"), to help carry off the accumulation of the intestines; and then supports the strength with liquid food of a nourishing character. He is a successful physician, and claims not to have lost an average of one child a year for the eleven years, practice there; and I know he has a good share of practice among the children. I have also seen accounts in a recent medical journal, by some allopathic physicians, that they have been using calomel very similar to Dr. Haney, in this disease. Therefore I have not dared to pass it by without mention, as it may save many lives for future usefulness.

**11. Diphtheria—Remedy by the French Academy of Medicine.**—"The vapor from the burning of a mixture of tar and spirits of turpentine, near the bed, it is said, will dissolve the false membrane which is so often fatal in this dreadful disease. If this simple remedy is complete, as the French Academy of Medicine is said to have declared, it should be widely published." *American Messenger, October, 1884.*

*Remarks.*—Notwithstanding there are two "is saids" in this, yet, as it is simple, and would not interfere with any other treatment, and obtaining it from a purely religious paper, which seldom touches anything of this kind, I have felt, from the knowledge of love of the effects of these articles, it should have my help on its way to a wider publication. Equal parts should be used, although they do not so state, thoroughly mixed, and pour a few drops from a tea-spoon upon hot coals, to keep up the fumes, is all that is needed.

**Blistering in Diphtheria—History of a Case at Black Rock, N. Y., Saved by It.**—In the December number, 1884, of the *Therapeutic Gazette*, of Detroit, Mich., F. W. Bartlett, M. D., of Buffalo, reports the case of a man about 45 years old, to whom he was called, and who was very sick at the time, and continued to get worse for four days, when he considered it hopeless from the condition of the throat, and so informed his patient, who took it calmly, but asked to have something done to relieve the suffering of the stomach, for which he directed his wife to dip cloths in hot water, and wring out, then put on a few drops of turpentine, to be applied over the bowels; but in the confusion of such a case, expecting to lose her husband, she heated the turpentine, and saturated flannel with it, and laid it on, which he bore as long as he could, then violently flung it across the room, saying he "would rather die than suffer such agony." And when the wife saw what an inflammation she had caused, covered it with fresh lard, and waited the doctor's morning call; who found a blister (*vesication*, as M. D's most call it) a foot square, covered with a diphtheritic exudation, the throat better, and the patient saved. All I have to say further is, let others make similar mistakes in bad cases, and save their patients too. In other words, draw a blister in the regular way, in time, not to let the throat get beyond control. I would put a blister on both arms, breast and bowels too, if I thought it necessary to save my patient's life.

**12. Diphtheria, to Avoid by Diet — Pork Believed to be the Exciting Cause.**—With an explanation as to this exciting cause of diphtheria, I will close the subject, having given a large number of the most popularly known remedies, although there are many writers who think that the abundant use of pork in our diet is a very fruitful source of this disease, I shall only quote from one. A recent medical correspondent of the Lancaster *New Era* argues at considerable length: " That eating of pork is an inciting (arousing, stirring up,) cause of this terrible disease." His idea is that an unhealthy appetite is created by the use of so much pork, in the every-day diet of the country, until the specific pork poison is manifested in the exudatious deposits from the blood into the throat, which is the characteristic symptom in this disease. He especially advises parents not to allow their children to diet on pork, nor sausage, but fruit and vegetables in greater abundance.

*Remarks.*—Although beef, veal, lamb, chicken, etc., may be allowed to children generally, yet it would be well for parents during the prevalence of diphtheria in a neighborhood, to put their children upon a bread and milk and vegetable diet exclusively, lest their loss might be charged home to their neglect, which would not be a pleasant thought for after-consideration.

**13. Diphtheria—Closing Remarks Upon.**—The author leaves the subject with his readers, believing that he has presented a larger number and more reliable remedies or recipes for the cure and prevention of diphtheria than are to be found in any other publication whatever; he also believes that if these recipes are well studied, and one or more of them adopted by the heads of households containing young children, and the articles obtained and kept on hand ready for use, night or day, nothing like the fatality will hereafter take place from diphtheria, as has heretofore been the case. I feel certain that there can be no drug store where some of the articles mentioned may not be obtained. Then the responsibility rests with each one who shall have this knowledge, and yet neglect to use it. The author has done his duty, which is a great consolation to him. The same will also hold good upon many other subjects in this work. See "Disinfectants," to prevent this disease from spreading.

**1. SORE THROAT—The Good Old Grandmother's Gargle for.**—Steep 1 medium-sized red pepper in ½ pt. of water, strain, and add ¼ pt. of good vinegar, and a heaping tea-spoonful, each, of salt and pulverized alum, and gargle with it as often as needed.

**2. Sore Throat, New Gargle for.**—In all recent inflammations, or colds, affecting the throat, a gargle made by putting a heaping tea-spoonful of the bi-carbonate of soda (common baking soda) into a glass of water, and garging with it frequently, will be found exceedingly valuable. A tea-spoonful, or a little more, of it swallowed, will quickly relieve a tickling cough; also neutralize the acidity of the stomach often arising after meals, water-brash, etc. But if it should irritate, weaken one-half or more.

**3. Sore Throat—Heat Strong Tea as a Gargle for Speedy Relief in.**—It is well to know that sore throat can be speedily relieved by using strong, hot tea as a gargle. It is a convenient remedy and rather a pleasant one.

*Remarks.*—Hot water has proved valuable in many diseases of late, as dyspepsia, consumption, etc., taken internally before meals, which see, for these diseases.

**4. Sore Throat and Catarrh—Gargle for.**—Comp. spirits of lavender. ½ oz., into a 4 oz. vial; put in also the carbonate of ammonia, 20 grs.; fill with distilled, or rain water.

DIRECTIONS.—Put 1 teaspoonful of this to ½ cup of warm, soft water and gargle with it two or three times daily; and if any catarrh, or nasal inflammation, put into the hand, what it will hold, and snuff into the nostrils at each time. After the gargling and snuffing, a little vaseline, or cosmoline, mutton tallow, or some sweet oil, or sweet almond oil, should be introduced into each nostril with the finger.

*Remarks.*—Follow this course faithfully, and for a considerable time, in catarrh, if any good is expected to result; also use occasionally some good cathartic to act freely, together with an alterative and tonic course of medicine.

**5. Sore Throat, Common Gargle for.**—For common case of sore throat, a valuable gargle can generally be made at almost any dinner table.

DIRECTIONS.—Take ½ pt. tumbler, or common goblet, and put into it a small salt cellar of salt (about 2 tea-spoonfuls), ¼ tea-spoonful of black pepper, and a little cayenne (3 or 4 little taps on the bottom of the cruet, or pepper-box containing it, will be sufficient; a tea-spoonful or two of pepper-sauce, if on the table, is better than the cayenne powder), then fill the tumbler with cider vinegar and water, equal parts, stir well, a few times, and gargle with it often.

*Remarks.*—If you have alum and borax in the house, about ¼ tea-spoonful of each, pulverized, may be put in, or if only one of them, ½ tea-spoonful will improve the gargle. (Other gargles will be found in connection with the subject of diphtheria.)

**6. Sore Throat, Several Simple Remedies for.**—The following are some of the most common, or simple, remedies for sore throat, easily obtained and often effectual:

I  Salt and water is used by many as a gargle; but a little alum and honey dissolved in sage tea is better.

II. Others, a few drops of camphor on loaf sugar, which very often affords immediate relief.

III. An application of cloths wrung out of hot water and applied to the neck, changed as often as it begins to cool, has great potency in removing inflammation in recent cases.

IV. Borax the size of a pea in the mouth relieves hoarseness quickly (See also hoarseness, bronchitis, etc., for other remedies.)

**SORE NOSE — Akin to Erysipelas — Certain Cure.**—I had a case of sore nose, a very bad case, which nothing in the ordinary line of treatment would benefit at all, except for a very short time. The sufferer would cry out: "Cannot something be done to relieve this intolerable suffering," etc. DIRECTIONS—I prepared a little stick, 3 or 4 inches in length, and wound it with 3 or 4 thicknesses of cotton cloth, wrapped with thread, and dipped this into the full strength muriated tincture of iron, and held it firmly, for ½ minute, or so, to each spot, and over the inflamed nose, and to the inner edges, where it was sorest. The first moment or two it smarted like fire, but I held it the more firmly and said never mind that, it won't be so bad next time. So night and morning, for 3 or 4 days, then once daily as much longer, made a perfect cure—now over 6 months, without the least return and no sign of soreness remaining. I should continue to apply for a month or more, if necessary, or until cured. I gave him also internally 5 drops of the same tincture 3 times daily in a little water. Of course he had an iron-colored nose, but a piece of lemon rubbed on a few times soon removed that ornamental shade and left him all right again, the same as it will remove recent iron rust spots from clothing.

**Sore Fingers of Printers, etc., to Cure and Blood Blisters to Prevent.**—I. Generally a compositor's (type-setter's) sore fingers result from lye, low cases, splinters, scratches in handling brass rule, paper cuts, type poison, etc., and often occasion loss of time, expensive doctoring and great pain. For these sores a correspondent writes: "I have never lost an hour from business, nor been put to more than a trifling expense. Plentiful and frequent application of laudanum has been my panacea (cure all). It also cleanses, removes the soreness and rapidly heals old sores."

II. Blood blisters may be prevented from forming by immediately rubbing the bruise briskly with any non-poisonous hard substance.—*London Phonetic Journal.*

*Remarks.*—The fact here given as to the curative action of laudanum upon sore fingers, and old sores, is that laudanum alone would be valuable upon all ordinary chaps, or cracks upon the hands, lips, etc., no matter from what cause they may have arisen, as the opium relieves the pain, and the alcohol in it stimulates the parts to heal.

**CARBUNCLE—Treatment Which Saves Pain and Soreness —Also Applicable to Boils.**—Having just passed through a three weeks, siege with a six hole carbuncle, I feel competent to tell others how I saved myself much pain, soreness and suffering, although it is bad enough when all has been done that can be done for relief.

What it might have proved without my mitigating treatment, I do not know; it was the agony that compelled me to adopt some plan of relief; hence I took:

I. A mild liniment, Mrs. Chase's, given in this book (any mild liniment will do), 2 ozs.; chloroform, 1 oz.; laudanum, 1 oz.; mixed. Shaken, when used, and applied every hour or two, night and day. There were only short satches of sleep for about two weeks; after which, an hour or two was occasionally obtained.

After applying the above mixture freely at each time, I then applied the following anodyne, emollient, or softening mixture:

II. Sweet oil, 7 drs.; laudanum, 1 dr.; mix. The application of the foregoing mixtures would relieve very much of the agonizing pain, even before I would be done applying the first; and the second kept the surface soft, as well as to help keep down the pain. (The same thing will be just as effectual for boils, I have not a doubt.) The situation was such that no poulticing could have been done, if desired, to hasten it; and even if it could, I have never known one under the poulticing process to subside in less than 5 or 6 weeks, while by the above process nearly all the pain and soreness subsided in 3 weeks.

At one time I thought it was going to repeat itself: but by the application of the permanganate of potash, 1 dr. to 1 oz. of water, applied by rolling up a strip of cotton cloth, and tieing a bit of cord around it in the centre, the size of the roll being just to fill the mouth of the vial, by which means I could wet one end of the roll of cloth without spilling it upon the clothing (permanganate colors the clothes), and apply to the swelling, it was driven back, or scattered, and by taking an active cathartic dose of crab-orchard salts (any active cathartic will do the same) it was carried out of the system.

**2. Carbuncle, Specific for.**— R. H. Johnson, in the *Medical Review*, says, he has found tannin a specific for carbuncle. He sprinkles the tannin upon the openings as long as it will dissolve; and 24 hours after washes off with castile soap, and sprinkles it again. He claims it to soon heal up with but little pain. It is worthy of trial, as it can do no harm.

**BOILS.—Remedy Against their Continuance.**— Prof. Scudder, in his work on Specific Medication, speaking of lime, says: Its specific use is in cases of furunculus (boil), and other inflammations of the cellular tissue (the cell-like tissue immediately under the skin) terminating in suppuration. Why it has this specific influence I do not propose to say, but I have proven it in scores of cases. Taken in a case in which boils are continually developed, the use of lime water will effect a radical cure. [The proper strength for lime water to be used in these cases, in fact, in all cases, is: stone lime, 4 ozs.; distilled water, 1 gal., or in these proportions. Slack the lime with a little of the water, then pour the rest of the water over it and stir; cover the bowl and set aside for three hours; then bottle and keep the liquor upon the lime, well corked, and use only the clear liquid as wanted.] See "Milk Diet for Infants and Adults.". Dose—It is given in doses of a wine-glassful, 3 or 4 times a day. If too alkaline use additional water.

This lime water is often very properly used with the milk fed to infants which have to be raised upon the bottle; a tea-spoonful to a bottle of milk, or sufficient to prevent acidity of the stomach, and it is also valuable in Dyspepsia in adults when there are acid eructations of gas, or, as commonly called, belching or rifting of wind from the stomach, after eating. Dose—For adults in these dyspepsia cases, 3 or 4 table-spoonfuls to a bowl of milk; sufficient only is needed to keep down the acidity. See "Dyspepsia, Milk and Lime Water, Cure for." Lime water can often be borne by patients who cannot take the salts of soda, or potash. This also proves its value and adaptation to the human system.

**2. Boils—To Relieve the Pain of and to Scatter.**—The pain of boils, it is said, can be relieved very much by frequently applying castor-oil on the parts.

Painting a boil with tincture of iodine, it is also claimed, scatters them; but I prefer to scatter them by frequently applying a strong liniment. I have recently scattered two from my own neck in this way. I used Dr. Chase's golden oil, or strong camphor liniment; I think I applied it at least fifteen different times in the day, rubbing over the boil hard and long at each application, which scattered it, and is doing so again, at this writing, so that I see they are in the system, and I have therefore made 1 qt. of the lime water (1 oz. stone lime to 1 qt.), and am going to use it, expecting I shall thus cleanse the blood and eradicate them—the boils from the system or blood. It did do it, as I have not had any more, or any indications of them, now over four months, after writing the above.

**3. Boils, Alterative Syrup for.**—Blue flag and black cohosh root, each 1 oz.; yellow dock root and the bark of the root of bitter-sweet, Peruvian bark, the bark of the root of sassafras and prickly ash berries, each ½ oz.; pyrophosphate of iron, 2½ drs.; whiskey, ½ pt.; glycerine, 6 ozs.; water, 12 ozs. DIRECTIONS.—The barks, roots and berries are to be coarsely ground, or bruised, then steeped in water in a covered dish, to leave, when strained, 1 pt.; then add the glycerine, whiskey and pyrophosphate of iron. DOSE—A teaspoonful 4 times daily, at meals and at bed-time.

*Remarks.*—This is not only a valuable alterative in boils, but to follow the treatment of inflammations, after the acute stages have been overcome by cooling purgatives, such as salts, seidlitz powder or cream of tartar, attention to the skin, etc., especially so if there is a scrofulous tendency, or considerable debility, shown by the loss of strength, flesh, etc.

**1. MILK IN DIARRHEA, DYSENTERY, INCIPIENT CHOLERA, TYPHOID FEVER, ETC.**—Considerable has lately been said in medical journals concerning the value of milk as a remedial agent in certain diseases. An interesting article upon this subject lately appeared in the London *Milk Journal*, in which it is stated, on the authority of Dr. Benjamin Clark, that in the East Indies warm milk is used to a great extent as a specific for Diarrhea.

I. *For Diarrhea.*—A pint every 4 hours will check the most violent diarrhea, stomach-ache, incipient cholera and dysentery. The milk should never be boiled, but only heated sufficient to be agreeably warm, not too hot to drink. [The author would say 140° Fah. is as hot as one can take it comfortably with a tea-spoon.] Milk which has been boiled is unfit for use. He continues: It has never failed in curing in from 6 to 12 hours, and I have tried it, I should think, fifty times. I have also given it to a dying man who had been subject to dysentery 8 months, latterly accompanied by one continual diarrhea, and it acted on him like a charm. In 2 days his diarrhea was gone, in 3 weeks he became a hale, fat man, and now nothing that may hereafter occur will ever shake his faith in hot milk.

II. *For Typhoid Fever.*—Another writer also communicates to the *Medical Times and Gazette* a statement of the value of milk in 26 cases of typhoid fever, in every one of which its great value was apparent, checking diarrhea, nourishing and cooling the body.

III. *For Debilitating Diseases.*—People suffering from disease require food quite as much as those in health, and much more so in certain diseases, where there is rapid waste of the system. Frequently all ordinary food, in some diseases, is rejected by the stomach, and even loathed by the patient; but nature, even in all disease, is beneficient, and has furnished a food that is beneficial—in some, directly curative. Such a food is milk. The writer, Dr. Alexander Yale, after giving particular observations upon the points above mentioned, viz.: Its action in checking diarrhea, its nourishing properties and its action in cooling the body says: " We believe that milk nourishes in fever, promotes sleep, wards off delirium, soothes the intestines, and in fine is the *sine qua non* (an indispensable—just the thing) in typhoid fever."

IV. *For Scarlet Fever.*—The writer goes on to say he has lately tested the value of milk in scarlet fever, and learns that it is now recommended by the medical faculty in all cases of this often very distressing disease of children. He says:

Give all the milk the patient will take, even during the period of greatest fever; it keeps up the strength of the patient, acts well upon the stomach, and is in every way a blessed thing in this sickness. Parents, remember it, and do not fear to give it if your dear ones are afflicted with this disease.

**2. Milk as a Medicine.**—Under the head of "Milk as a Medicine," the *American Journal of Medicine,* of St. Louis, says that this article, once looked upon with distrust, has now become a valuable agent in treatment of disease, and is, on all hands, recommended by practitioners of medicine as being a safe and reliable article in the list of curables. Given warm it is declared to be almost a specific (positive cure) in diarrhea, stomach-ache, incipient cholera and dysentery. It is also pronounced invaluable in typhoid fever.

II. The *Journal* then quotes the sentence of Dr. Yale. given in III above, and closes by saying that he also agrees with the opinion of Dr. Benjamin Clark, in the London *Milk Journal,* given in I.

*Remarks.*—I understand that the milk is not to be boiled, that it is to be heated only to allow its being drank without scalding the mouth or throat. There can be no doubt of its efficacy with such an amount of testimony from the medical profession in India, England and America. See also "Treatment of Scarlet Fever with Sulphur," wherein I have recommended the milk to be also used.

**3. Milk Diet, with Lime Water—For Infants and Adults who have Weak Digestive Powers.—Dr. H. N. Chapman says that**

milk and lime water is not only food and medicine at an early period of life, but also later, when, as in the case of infants, the functions of digestion and assimilation have been seriously impaired. A stomach taxed by gluttony, irritated by improper food, inflamed by alcohol, enfeebled by disease, or otherwise unfitted for its duties, as is shown by the various symptoms attendant upon indigestion, dyspepsia, diarrhea, dysentery and fever, will resume its work, and do it energetically, on an exclusive diet of lime water and milk. A goblet of cow's milk to which 4 table-spoonfuls of lime water has been added, will agree with any person, however objectionable the plain article may be, will be friendly to the stomach when other food is apprehensive, and will be digested when all else fails to afford nourishment. Of this statement I have had positive proof in very many cases. The blood being thin, the nerves weak, the nutrition poor, the secretions defective, the excretions insufficient, the physician has at hand a remedy as common as the air, and as common, almost as water. In it all the elements of nutrition are so prepared by nature as to be readily adapted to the infant or the adult stomach, and so freighted with healing virtues as to work a cure where drugs are worse than useless.

*Remarks.*—It certainly needs no further remarks to show the estimation that milk is now held in. Let it be used accordingly, with the lime water, and you will also be satisfied.

**4. Milk an Antidote and Preventive to Lead Poison.**—The *Journal de Medicine* states, upon authority, that milk has been found to be an antidote and preventive to lead poisoning by those working in its manufacture. (Why not, then, for painters?)

A quart a day was furnished to each man, after which no colic nor other harm to health occurred.

The remedy is simple, easily obtained, and no doubt effectual. Used as a drink during the day would be the manner of taking it. See also its use in "Accidental Poisoning."

**5. Milk as an Aliment or Food.** — So much has been said on the use of milk as a medicine in diseased conditions of the system, it is but proper to say it ought to enter into our daily food to a very much greater extent than it does. It is believed to be good for children; but I beg leave to say it is as good for adults as it is for children ; and if every family would adopt the old plan of corn-meal mush and milk for supper for everyone in the family, as we used to do in an earlier day, the general health of the people would be better than it is. If it produces costiveness, in any case, put in a little lime water, or a little baking soda; but with the mush there is no danger of this.

**6. Milk, Hot, as a Restorative after Fatigue.** — A glass of hot milk, when one is fatigued, is so refreshing and strengthening it will astonish the one who takes it. A supper, made with a couple slices of toasted bread in a bowl of hot milk, is very satisfactory in the absence of the mush mentioned above.

**1. SCARLET FEVER—Successful Treatment of.**—Dr. Henry Pigeon writes to the London *Lancet* as follows:

" The marvellous success which has attended my treatment of scarlet fever by sulphur induces me to let my medical brethren know of my plan, so that they may be able to supply the same remedy without delay. All the cases in which I used it, were very marked, and the epidermis (outer or scarfskin) on the arms, in each case, came away like the skin of a snake. The following was the exact treatment followed in each case.

" The patients were thoroughly anointed twice daily with sulphur ointment [the sulphur ointment used was made by the London Pharmacopœia as follows: sulphur, 4 ozs.; lard, ½ lb.; oil of bergamot, 20 minims (drops); mixed]; giving 5 to 10 grains of sulphur in a little jam, or jelly. 3 times a day, according to the age of the child and severity of the case. Sufficient sulphur was also burned, twice daily (on coals on a shovel), to fill the room with the fumes, and, of course, was thoroughly inhaled by the patient.

" Under this mode of treatment each case improved immediately, and none was over 8 days in making a complete recovery; and I firmly believe in each; it was prevented from spreading by the treatment adopted. Having had a large experience in scarlet fever last year and this, I feel some confidence in my own judgment, and I am of the opinion that the very mildest cases I ever saw do not do half as well as bad cases do by the sulphur treatment, and as far as I can judge sulphur is as near a specific (positive cure) for scarlet fever as possible."

*Remarks.*—I can see no reason why the milk, as indicated under the head of milk in diarrhea, dysentery, etc., may not be given with the sulphur treatment; I believe both to be good; and as I see the medical journals speak with such confidence of Dr. Pigeon's sulphur treatment, I place also great confidence in it, and recommend it most heartily.

**2. Scarlet Fever, Sulphurous Acid Treatment of.**—Dr. L. Waterman, of Indianapolis, Ind., in an epidemic there, in 1876, gives his experience in the use of sulphurous acid. He says:

" I early adopted an anti-zymotic (anti-poisoning) principle, the administration of 10 to 30 drops, every 2, 3, or 4 hours, of sulphurous acid, diluted, in a little water. I treated eleven severe cases. The ten treated after its adoption recovered."

**3. Scarlet Fever, Simple Remedy, or Warm Lemonade for.**—An eminent physician says he cures 99 out of every 100 cases of scarlet fever by giving the patient warm lemonade with gum arabic dissolved in it. A cloth wrung out in hot water and laid upon the stomach should be removed as rapidly as it becomes cool

*Remarks.* A writer in *Good Health* gives the philosophy of the above treatment, with the warm lemonade, with an addition (which I know to be valuable), the wet hot sheet, or pack, over or around the whole body, guaranteeing that not one in one hundred will die of scarlet fever, if this treatment is properly carried out. He says,

**4. Scarlet Fever, Unnecessary for a Child to die with it.**— " It is as unnecessary for a child to die of scarlet fever, as it is that it should be blind with cataract. Let us see: At any time before the body has finished its ineffectual struggle we are able to help it, not by wonderful medicines, but by the knowledge of anatomy, and the application of common sense. * * * * Undress the child and place it in bed at the very first sign of sickness. Give it, if it has already fever, sourish warm lemonade, with some gum arabic in it,

Then cover its abdomen with some dry flannel.   Take a well folded bed sheet and put it in boiling water; wring it out and put this over the whole body and wait.   The hot  cloth will perhaps require repeated heating; according to the severity of the case and its stage of progress.   Perspiration will commence in the child in from 10 minutes to 2 hours.   The child then is saved; it soon falls asleep.   The hot, wet sheet must be continued, however, till perspiration takes place.   Soon after the child awakes it shows slight symptoms of returning in-clinations for food; help its bowels, if necessary, with injections of oil, soap and water, and its recovery will be as steady as the growth of a green-house plant, if well treated.   Of course if the child is already dying nothing can save it.   With this treatment I will guarantee that not one in a hundred chil-dren with scarlet fever will die."

*Remarks.*—I once succeeded in curing scarlet fever in one of my own chil-dren, before I had read medicine, by the cold pack, or sheet, but I should not try it again—I know the hot is better—the strain or struggle of the system being much less, and consequently the most safe and satisfactory.   There is no doubt of the value of the foregoing treatment, but any of the others may be tried, according to the conveniences to be obtained in different places.

### 5. Scarlet Fever and Small Pox—Successful Treatment.—

Dr. W. Fields, of Wilmington, Delaware, says to one of the medical journals:

"Having had much experience in the cure of scarlet fever and small pox of the most malignant type, I would thank you, for the sake of humanity, to publish a recipe, which, if faithfully carried out, will cure 45 cases out of every 50, without calling on a physician.

I.   *Scarlet Fever.*—"For adults give 1 table-spoonful of brewers' yeast in 3 table-spoonfuls of water, 3 times a day; and if the throat is much swollen gar-gle with the yeast, and apply the yeast to the throat as a poultice; mix with Indian meal.   Use plenty of catnip tea to keep the eruption out on the skin for several days.

II.   *Small Pox.*—"Use the above doses of yeast 3 times a day, and milk diet throughout the disease.   Nearly every case can be cured without leaving a pock mark."

*Remarks.*—I have had this used, in scarlet fever, with very great satisfaction.

### 6.  Scarlet Fever—Length of Time Dangerous to Others.—

In this disease the parent and the school teacher are often concerned to know how long a time must elapse before it is safe to admit those who have had the disease to mingle with other children, or with the family, and go to school.

For a month, at least, the body of a scarlet fever patient is casting off scales, or particles, from the skin.   The nose, throat, bowels and kidneys are also throwing off poisonous matter for this length of time, which will commu-nicate the disease to others.   The chief danger, however, is from the skin, as this is the main outlet for the blood poison to escape, and every scale or parti-cle of dry dust from the skin carries the infection.

Therefore greasing the patient, by rubbing a bacon rind over them, which, by some, has been recommended as beneficial to the patient, will certainty do this good, *i. e.* it will keep these minute scales from rising into the air, and thus prevent the communication of the disease to others from this source.   But *t.* Dr. Chapin, in a communication to the *Brief,* of St. Louis, informs its readers that he has used the ham fat (as he calls the bacon rind) in every case for 20 years, and has lost but few patients since using it, and must have treated some hundreds, and gives the following as his plan; "As soon as I diagnose (*i. e.,* determine it to be) a case of scarlet fever, I have the patient put on Canton flannel, or better, if in winter, fine all wool underclothing; then cut a piece of rind from a pretty fat, fresh smoked ham, with a half inch of the fat upon it; then warm the hand, also the slice of ham, rub the hand on the fat, and then on the patient, till they are well covered, except the face. (The author cannot see why the fat may not be rubbed directly upon the surface, rather think it is the best plan, then rub it in with the hand.) Do this night and morning as long as the eruptions and fever continue; put them in bed, cover up warm and give as much cold water as they like. (I prefer the warm lemonade if agreeable to the child, as named above in No. 3.) The greasing is very satisfactory, allaying the burning and itching, which are so annoying." (See also the sulphur ointment in No. 1 of scarlet fever; note for making it.)

7. **Scarlet Fever—To Prevent its Spread.**—Scarlet fever has been so prevalent and so fatal, for several years past, it has become of the utmost importance to prevent its spreading in schools as well as in families, and the above thoughts and statements being so fully corroborated by the following circular, prepared by the Boston Board of Health, and sent to every house in that city, I have deemed it best to give it in full. It says:

I. "Scarlet fever is like small pox in its power to spread rapidly from person to person. It is highly contagious (catching). The disease shows its first signs in about one week after exposure, as a general rule, and persons who escape the illness during a fortnight after exposure may feel themselves safe from attack. Scarlet fever, scarlatina, canker, rash and rash fever, are names of one and the same dangerous disease.

II. "When a case of scarlet fever occurs in any family, the sick person should be placed in a room apart from the other inmates of the house (an upper room is best), and should be nursed as far as possible by one person only. The sick chamber should be well ventilated and well warmed; its furniture should be such as will permit of cleansing without injury, and all extra articles, such as window drapery and woolen carpets, should be removed from the room. The family should not mingle with other people. Visitors to an infected house should be warned of the presence of a dangerous disease therein, and children especially should not be admitted.

III. "On recovery the sick person should not mingle with the well until the roughness of the skin, due to the disease, shall have disappeared. A month is considered an average period during which isolation is needed. The clothing before being worn or used by the patient or the nurse, should be cleansed by boiling for at least one hour, or if that cannot be done, by free and prolonged exposure to out door air and sunlight. The walls of the room should be dry rubbed, and the cloths used for that purpose should be burned without previous shaking. The ceiling should be scraped and whitewashed, the floor should be washed with soap and water, and carbolic acid may be added to the water, 1 pt. to 3 or 4 gals. The infected clothing should be cleansed by itself, and not sent to the laundry.

IV. "In cases of death from scarlet fever, the funeral services should be strictly private, and the corpse should not be exposed to view. Because children are especially liable to take and to spread scarlet fever, and because schools afford a free opportunity for this, the Board of Health has excluded from school every child from any family in which a case of the disease has occurred, and has decreed that the absence shall continue four weeks from the beginning of the attack, except in cases subject to the discretion of the Board, and that the scholar to be re-admitted to his school-room must have the certificate of a physician that the required time has passed."

*Remarks.*—I think the above directions are so plainly given that they will be readily understood, and if properly followed out, the spread of this disease will be almost, if not wholly prevented. I will say, however, that the use of the carbolic acid is not as much used as a disinfectant as formerly. See "Copperas Solution of the National Board." This and zinc solution will answer for all purposes, and are not only cheap, but absolutely reliable.

**1. TYPHOID FEVER — Treatment in Its More Malignant Character.**—The malignant character of this disease not being as prevalent in the North as in the South, I will first give the treatment used by Dr. J. J. Jones, of Conway Station, Ark., reported through the *Medical Brief*, of St. Louis, who has treated this disease in all its grades for over 25 years. When it takes on its malignant character of dysentery or pneumonia, which are inflammatory and dangerous if not properly met or treated in their commencement, he said that after testing various modes of treatment, he adopted the following:

I. First cleanse the alimentary canal with syrup of rhubarb and bi-carbonate of soda.

II. Follow this with spirits of turpentine, 30 drops; oil of sassafras, 6 drops; tinct. opium (laudanum) 25 drops; mix into well beaten whites of two eggs well sweetened with loaf sugar. Dose—Give an adult 1 table-spoonful of this emulsion every 3 hours.

III. If the pulse is full and firm, and over 100 per minute, give the following: Tincture of gelseminum, 1 oz.; fluid extract of aconite (of the root is best), 1/2 dr.; spirits of niter, 2 1/2 drs.; mix. Dose—Give 10 to 15 drops, for an adult, every 3 hours, until the pulse drops below 100. [The author would say, keep the pulse under 100, giving this alternately with the emulsion—first one, then, 1 1/2 hours after, the other; but these drops must not be continued to reduce the pulse much below 100 at the first. If it does this, lessen the dose, or make it 4 or 5 hours apart.]

IV. To control the temperature (heat of the surface), if it runs very high, which it frequently does, we resort to the wet sheet pack, as it is an important agent in the successful treatment of typhus and typhoid fevers. Use vinegar and spirits of camphor in place of water to wet the sheet, as it is much more sedative (calming, allaying irritation and pain), and less dangerous than water. After the pulse and temperature is brought below 100, we give large doses of tinct. of iron (muriated tinct. of iron is meant, and 15 to 20 drops would be large enough, once in 3 or 4 hours), checking the diarrhea, which is so common in typhoid fever. Alternate this (the iron tincture) with pure hard cider or lemonade. Diet: dried-beef tea, and milk gruel seasoned with pepper; give egg-nog if there are pneumonic symptoms.

*Remarks.* — It would be well to say here, see "Use of Milk in Diarrhea,

Dysentery, etc." I also say that my own plan has been to sponge the whole surface with bay rum and water (equal parts), sufficiently often to keep down the excessive heat; and if bay rum is too expensive, use whiskey and water—warm, if preferred by the patient; or vinegar and spirits of camphor will be good, if the heat is not too excessive. The bay rum, however, is more agreeable in flavor, especially for use about the face and hands. The patient can do this face sponging as often as the heat demands it, keeping a dish of the mixture and a small sponge near for the purpose. If the sponging, in place of the wet sheet, is resorted to, let it be done as often as the comfort of the patient demands it—doing it under the bed clothes, to avoid any exposure to cold air.

The lemonade recommended by Dr. Jones, or some of the drinks for fever patients in other parts of this work, would be very desirable; but what he calls "pure hard cider," unless reduced with cold water, would generally, I think, be a little too "hard;" however, it can soon be ascertained by trial. Whatever the patient craves in the line of drink or food, I believe in allowing moderately; and never to refuse even cold water right from the well or spring, as old allopathy used to do in the years "auld lang syne," by which, I have not a doubt, thousands of persons, burning up with fever, have lost their lives, where, if water had been allowed, they might just as well have been saved to their friends and usefulness. So well satisfied am I of this, that I cannot but give an incident reported recently by a Dr. Fairchild while lecturing in New York. Touching upon the old plan of the doctors not allowing water to fever patients, he gives the case of his uncle in the South, while slavery was in force, as follows:

"My own uncle, for one, lay, as we supposed, at the point of death.

"A trusty old colored man, his watchman, was called to his bed about midnight. Speaking just above a whisper, he said:

"'Abe, I am going to ask of you just one last request. Will you grant it?'

"'Yes, massa, anything you ask, I do.'

"'Take the old wooden jug; go to the spring back of the barn, fill it with cold water and bring it to me quick.'

"'Oh, massa, massa, anything else you ask, I'll do. Do you know what missus and doctor said?—'no water, no water.''

"'Abe, you go; if you don't and I live, I'll shoot you dead.'

"After deliberating for a moment, he said, 'Massa, I go.'

"It was brought to him. He drank his fill. By morning every drop was gone. The fever broke. He fell into a quiet, peaceful sleep, and was soon restored to health. And not until then, was any one told what cured him.

"Such examples as these finally changed the system of treating fevers. In this specific disease common sense is, at last, master of the situation."

It is to be hoped that such a condition of suffering and final death, as above spoken of, may never be allowed to gain the ascendency with any class of physicians again.

2. **Typhoid Fever, the Value of Coffee in.**—Dr. Guillasse, of the French Navy, on typhoid fever, says: "Coffee has given us unhoped for satisfaction; after having dispensed it, we find, to our great surprise, that its action is as prompt as it is decisive. No sooner have our patients taken a few table-spoonfuls of it than their features become relaxed, and they come to their senses. The next day the improvement is such that we are tempted to look upon coffee as a specific (positive cure) for typhoid fever. Under its influence

the stupor is dispelled, and the patient rouses from the state of somnolency in which he has been since the invasion of the disease. Soon all the functions take their natural course, and he enters upon convalescence." Dose—Dr. Guillasse gives to an adult 2 or 3 table-spoonfuls of strong, black coffee every two hours, alternated with 1 or 2 tea-spoonfuls of claret or Burgundy wine. A little lemonade or citrate of magnesia should be taken daily, and after awhile quinine. From the fact that malaria and cerebral fever appear first, *i. e.*, a general prostration, with head, or brain fever, accompanied with stupor, or great tendency to sleep, somnolency, from the Latin *somnus*, to sleep. The doctor regards typhoid fever as a nervous disease, and the coffee acting on the nerves is peculiarly indicated in the early stages before local complications arise.

## DISINFECTANTS FOR ALL CONTAGIOUS DISEASES—FOR THE SICK-ROOM, BODY AND BED-CLOTHING, WATER-CLOSETS, SEWERS, ETC.

The following instructions were published in the *Hospital Gazette* by the National Board of Health, which was composed of some of the most prominent men in the medical profession, as will be seen by the names accompanying the instructions.

"Disinfection is the destruction of the poisons of infectious and contagious diseases.

"Deodorizers, or substances which destroy smells, are not necessarily disinfectants, and disinfectants do not necessarily have an odor.

"Disinfection cannot compensate for want of cleanliness nor of ventilation.

**1. Disinfectants to be Employed.—**I. "Roll sulphur (brimstone) for fumigation.

II. *Copperas Solution.—*"Sulphate of iron (copperas) dissolved in water in the proportion of 1½ lbs. to 1 gal.; for soil, sewers, etc.

[The author, during the present summer, (in the month of August, 1882,) dissolved 3 lbs. of common copperas in a common wooden pail, holding about 2½ or 3 gals , by pouring on hot water, and with an old dipper threw it all about on the privy used by about 15 persons, which so completely deodorized and disinfected it that it required no more until late in the season.]

III. *Zinc Solution.—*Sulphate of zinc and common salt, dissolved together in water in the proportions of 4 ozs. sulphate and 2 ozs. of salt to 1 gal.; for clothing, bed linen, etc.

"Note.—Carbolic acid is not included in the above list for the following reasons: It is very difficult to determine the quality of the commercial article, and the purchaser can never be certain of securing it of proper strength; it is expensive, when of good quality, and experience has shown that it must be employed in comparatively large quantities to be of any use; besides it is liable, by its strong odor, to give a false sense of security.

**2. How to Use Disinfectants.—**I. "*In the Sick Room.*—The most valuable agents are fresh air and cleanliness. The clothing, towels, bed linen, etc., should, on removal from the patient, and before they are taken from the room, be placed in a pail or tub of the zinc solution, boiling hot if possible. All discharges should either be received in vessels containing the copperas solution, or, when this is impracticable, should be immediately covered with the solution. All vessels used about the patient should be cleansed or rinsed with the same. Unnecessary furniture—especially that which is stuffed—carpets and hangings, should, when possible, be removed from the room at the outset; otherwise they should remain for subsequent fumigation, as next explained.

II. *"Fumigation.*—Fumigation with sulphur is the only practical method for disinfecting the house. For this reason the rooms to be disinfected must be vacated. Heavy clothing, blankets, bedding, and other articles which can-not be treated with the zinc solution, should be opened and exposed during fumigation, as next directed. Close the rooms tightly as possible, place the sulphur in iron pans supported upon bricks placed in wash-tubs containing a little water, set it on fire by hot coals or with the aid of a spoonful of alcohol, and allow the room to remain closed 24 hours. For a room about 10 feet square at least 2 lbs. of sulphur should be used; for larger rooms, proportionally in-creased quantities.

III. *"Premises.*—Cellars, yards, stables, gutters, privies, cesspools, water-closets, drains, sewers, etc., should be frequently and liberally treated with the copperas solution, No. 2. The copperas solution is easily prepared by hanging a basket containing about 60 lbs. of copperas, in a barrel of water. [This would be 1½ lbs. to the gallon, or about that. It should all be dissolved.]

IV. *"Body and Bed-Clothing, etc.*—It is best to burn all articles which have been in contact with persons sick with contagious or infectious diseases. Articles too valuable to be destroyed should be treated as follows:

"(a.) Cotton, linen, flannels, blankets. etc., should be treated with the boiling hot zinc solution; introduce piece by piece; secure thorough wetting, and boil for at least half an hour.

"(b.) Heavy woolen clothing, silks, furs, stuffed bed-covers, beds, and other articles which cannot be treated with the zinc solution, should be hung in the room during the fumigation, their surfaces thoroughly exposed, and the pockets turned inside out. Afterward they should be hung in the open air, beaten and shaken. Pillows, beds, stuffed mattrasses, upholstered furniture, etc., should be cut open, the contents spread out and thoroughly fumigated. Carpets are best fumigated on the floor, but should afterward be removed to the open air and thoroughly beaten.

V. *"Corpses.*—Corpses should be thoroughly washed with a zinc solution of double strength; should then be wrapped in a sheet wet with zinc solution, and buried at once. Metallic, metal-lined, or air-tight coffins should be used when possible, certainly when the body is to be transported for any considera-ble distance. The following named gentlemen composed the board: George F. Barker, M. D., University of Pennsylvania, Philadelphia; C. F. Chandler, M. D., College of Physicians and Surgeons, Health Department, New York; Henry Draper, M. D., University of the city of New York; Edward G. Janeway, M. D., Bellevue Medical College, Health Department, New York; Ira Remson, M. D., Johns Hopkins University, Baltimore, Md.; S. O. Vanderpoel, M. D., Albany Medical College, Albany, N. Y.; Health Department, New York, Health Officer of the Port of New York."

*Remarks.*—Certainly no commendation of mine is needed to give strength to these instructions, as the most implicit confidence should be placed in them, coming, as they do, from the highest authority in the United States upon mat-ters of this kind. I will add, however, that no time should be lost in using them as soon as an occasion calls for them. The copperas solution I have found entirely satisfactory. See also "Note," following Dr. Scott's treatment of diphtheria, upon the permanganate of potash as a disinfectant; also see the "Nitrate of Lead as a Disinfectant in Small-pox," and also the "Use of Yeast and a Milk Diet in Scarlet Fever and Small-pox." It is well to keep all these valuable things before the mind, to be able to save pain and suffering of our fellow creatures.

**1. SMALL-POX— A Certain Cure.**—Wm. Grandy, of Detroit, communicated the following item of Mr. Hines' to the Detroit *Tribune*, which he had seen in the Toronto *Weekly Globe*, with these remarks:

"Small-pox being so fatal and so much feared, an unfailing remedy like the following, so simple and so safe, once discovered, ought to be brought to the knowledge of the masses without hesitation or delay."

"I am willing," says Edward Hines, "to risk my reputation as a public man if the worst case of small-pox cannot be cured in three days simply by cream of tartar. This is the sure and never-failing remedy· Cream of tartar, 1 oz., dissolved in boiling water, 1 pt.; to be drank when cold, at short intervals. It can be taken at any time and is a preventative as well as a curative. It is known to have cured thousands of cases without fail. I have myself restored hundreds by this means. It never leaves a mark, never causes blindness, and always prevents tedious lingering."

*Remarks.*—Although this seems to be very strong language, yet I have never seen it disputed, nor have I seen by any reports of cases that it has been adopted in this country; but, as it is deemed very important to keep the bowels in a solvent condition in this disease, no better and no safer medicine can be adopted for this purpose. Let it be used, by all means.

**2. Small-Pox—A Cure for, or Relief in.**—As the prevention or cure of this disease is a question that concerns every person, we take the following from the New York *Journal of Commerce*, one of the most conservative and reliable dailies published in this country·

"A lady, the mother of six children, had often sought relief for a pain in the back by taking saltpeter and brandy. She was exposed to the small-pox and contracted the disease. The premonitory symptoms were violent fever, severe pain in the head and excruciating pain in the region of the kidneys. A physician was called during the night, but in doubt as to the nature of the disease, though suspecting it to be a case of small-pox, he made no prescription, promising to return early next morning. The fever and pain increasing, she begged her husband to prepare for her the old prescription of saltpeter and brandy. The brandy was not to be had, but he crushed a piece of saltpeter as large as a common white bean. This she took in a tea-spoonful of cold water. Feeling better, the dose was once or twice repeated. Pain soon subsided and she slept well during the remainder of the night and awakened feeling perfectly well. She had 60 well defined pustules in her face, but they were but slightly inflamed and not at all painful. The developments of small-pox on her entire person were in number and appearance in keeping with those on her face. In due time all her children and her husband were affected, as she had been, by fever and pain in the head and back. They received the same treatment with the same favorable result. Several families caught the disease, used the same remedy, and in every case the result was favorable."

*Remarks.*—Not long after preparing the above given, I saw a report that "Mexican doctors were curing small-pox in 3 days, and no marks left," by the use of cream of tartar and water, which would go to strengthen the idea that Mr Hines' treatment above given is reliable.

**3. Small-Pox Pitting, to Prevent.**—It is well known that patients in rooms that are well lighted, pit very much more than in darkened rooms. I should, then, have the room as dark as possible for small pox patients; and not only this, but should cover the face, neck and hands with black cambric, or muslin, cut and made into suitable shape to keep off, or out, all possible rays of light. (The rays that make the chemical changes in photographing are absorbed into the pus, so changing it as to produce the deep pitting.) Certainly, then, no trouble, nor inconvenience, necessary to avoid this should be considered for a moment, to save a life-long annoyance, that none of us would like to have placed upon us by the terrible pitting we often see. Then take all these precautions and avoid it, certainly not overlooking the yeast and milk diet, before named; or pursue the following plan, as practiced in China:

**4. Small-Pox, to Prevent Pitting, Practiced in the English Army in China.**—It is very simple and easily followed, and if a blister on the arm of a diptheritic patient will draw off the irritation from the throat, as it has done, why should not this cause the small-pox eruption to come out on such parts ? It is done in this way: When the fever, which always precedes the eruption, is at its highest, and before the eruption appears, rub the chest with croton oil and tartar emetic ointment, which causes the whole eruption to appear on that part of the body, to the relief of the face; and as it is claimed also to cause a full eruption to appear, it prevents its attack upon internal organs, which is usually fatal. It is claimed by the *German Reformed Messenger* to be done in the English army in China by general order. It was reported through the *Medical Brief*, 1883, page 550, by J. A. Proctor, M. D., of Union City, Ind. It is worthy of trial.

**5. Small-Pox, the Nitrate, or Chloride, of Lead as a Disinfectant in.**—The mode of preparing and using the nitrate, or chloride, of lead, as a disinfectant, is from the *Physician and Pharmacist*, as follows: Chloride of lead is said to be the most powerful, safe and economical deodorizer and disinfectant known. To prepare it for use, on a small scale, for ordinary purposes, take nitrate of lead, ½ dr. and dissolve it in hot water, 1 pt.; dissolve also ½ oz of common salt in water, 2 galls., and mix the two solutions, which makes the chloride of lead, in solution, ready for use. A cloth wet with this and hung up in a room filled with a fetid atmosphere, will sweeten it instantly, and the solution thrown into a water-closet, sink or drain, will produce the same effect. It is not carbonic acid, but the sulphite of hydrogen and ammonium, which are eliminated with the breath and through the pores of the skin of the living body, that makes people who are exposed to such an atmosphere so depressed, and which, when highly concentrated, develops typhus poison, which causes, or at least aids, in developing fevers of a low grade, or typhoid character. Nitrate of lead is in dry crystals, and is sold according to its quality at 18 to 25 cts. per pound, which would make several hundred gallons of solution of chloride of lead.

*Remarks.*—Then let this, or those of the National Board of Health above, be used as freely as necessity insures the purification of the sick room, in all contagious diseases, cess-pools, water-closets, etc., and thus not only avoid the spreading of contagion, but prevent the development of the disease by the poisonous effluvia arising from these places.

**6. Small-Pox, Prevented by Vaccination.**—Dr. Woolsey reported the case in the *Pacific Medical and Surgical Journal* as follows: "Small-pox occurred in a Chinese boarding house, at a jute factory, containing seven hundred and ten persons, under the same roof. Seven were sick, one of whom died, when all were vaccinated, and no other case occurred, thus exemplifying the protective power of vaccination, or of some very remarkable coincident."

*Remarks.*—Webster says "coincident" is having coincidence (*i. e.. some circumstance*), agreeing, corresponding, *consistent.* I have italicised the word consistent merely to show how inconsistent it would be to suppose that any other circumstance could have given such protective power, except the vaccination. Then I think I have said enough when I say there cannot be a reasonable doubt but that vaccination is not only a protection, but that it is also safe; and therefore it ought to be adopted and insisted upon by boards of health, and also by parents and guardians.

**7. Small-Pox, the Origin of Vaccination for.**—Upon the question of vaccination, I will give an item from *Leonard's Medical Journal,* of Detroit, Mich., Oct., 1882, as to the origin of this practice; which, by this item, it seems must now be given to woman—the milkmaid instead of Dr. Jenner, as heretofore accredited. That is, his mind was capable of grasping or comprehending the philosophy of the fact communicated by the maid, and out of that he, Dr. Jenner, worked out the practice of vaccination which has saved millions of lives, no doubt; but it should also teach us, what some physicians have already claimed to be important, the fact that virus from the cow or some young and healthy animal should be used to vaccinate with, and not the virus from the human subject, which, it has been claimed, has communicated the disease to those vaccinated with it. Jenner, no doubt, used the virus from the cow of the "maid." Let others do the same from other cows. The poetry, it is claimed by the above named journal, is founded upon fact; but if it is not, it shows the greater power of the rhymer's imagination. It is as follows:

"Where are you going, my pretty milkmaid?"
"To see Doctor Jenner," the milkmaid said,
"I have such a cough, and it bothers me so,
I promised Jack Robin for sure that I'd go
    For a draught from the Doctor to-day."
And she nodded her head with so saucy a smile,
That no one would think, who was looking the while,
That she needed the Doctor, his pills or his plaster,
I doubt she could swear that she did, if you asked her;
    That sunny, bright morning in May.

Ah! how little she thought, that unthinking young lass,
While her little pink feet went atrip o'er the grass,
If Jack Robin had not been so true to his fancy,
As to fear the least whisper of harm to his Nancy,
    The great loss 'twould have been to us all.
But so it has proved such a number of times,
As I have not the space to recount in rhymes,
    Great events have beginnings so small.

Well! to keep by my milkmaid (as long as I can),
When she'd courtesied her best to the medical man,
And had told (heaven bless her) how badly she felt,
With such pouting red lips, and such ruddy good health,
  As no doctor could hope to improve,
She sat down to await his compounding her pill,
And their chat led along to the terrible ill
  That the small pox was threatening to prove.

Doctor Jenner looked grave when she mentioned the matter;
He thought it too bad for so careless a chatter:
But saucy young Nancy had nothing to dread,
"But few of the milkmaids would get it," she said,
  " For their hands had been sore from the cows,
And altho' it was horrid to milk when the beast
Had her bag all broken out, it was certain, at least,
  To keep the small-pox from the house."

I hope Doctor Jenner, that morning in May,
When he finished her pills and then sent her away,
Remembered enough of the lass and the stuff
  Not to give her a dose for a cow;
For his mind went far off
From the girl and the cough;
  But what does it matter, just now?
For her few simple words, while she waited,
Oh! think with how much they were freighted,
When Jenner's quick mind they awakened, to find
How science could conquer the foe.
And gave every nation that blessed VACCINATION
  That takes out the *sting* from the blow."

**1. NEURALGIA—German Cure of a Very Bad Case.—A** tea and poultice, made from the leaves of our common field-thistle, is reported to have cured a person who had suffered horrible pains from neuralgia. Failing to obtain relief in this country, and hearing of a noted physician in Germany who invariably cured the disease, he crossed the ocean and visited Germany for treatment. He was permanently cured after a short sojourn, and the doctor freely gave him the remedy as above given. DIRECTIONS AND DOSE — The leaves are macerated (soaked or steeped in water to become very soft) and used on the parts afflicted, as a poultice, while a small quantity of the leaves are boiled down to the proportion of a quart to a pint, and a small wine-glassful of the decoction drank before each meal.

*Remarks.*—The gentleman says: "I have never known it to fail of giving relief, while in almost every case it has effected a cure." It is certainly simple, and easy of trial, and no doubt will prove effectual in many cases.

There must be something in this thistle-cure, for a Mr. F. K. Ford, of Shellsburgh, Iowa, who was an agent of the Chase Publishing Co., wrote to the company desiring to get the same recipe into their Receipt Book. He also sent the onion and tobacco cure for earache, which will be found under that head. As Mr. Ford gives a more definite mode for preparing the thistle tea, I will give it. It is as follows:

I. *For the Tea.* — Take the leaves of the large field-thistle (not Canada). [The technical or botanical name of this species of indigenous (native) American thistle is *cirsium lanceolatum.* (Certainly it has many lances, or prickers, as sharp as a lance.) In western New York, where the author was raised, to distinguish it from the Canada, it was always called the "bull-thistle."] Press a gallon measure full of them; then put in all the water it will hold; boil down to ½ gal.: strain, and let cool (I should say, let cool and strain). DOSE—Of this take a wine-glassful every morning before breakfast; the same before tea.

II. *For the Poultice.*—Take the leaves of the same kind of thistle, put them into a clean cloth and pound to a jelly; put a layer of this on the afflicted part, bind on with cloth, every night. Be sure to get fresh leaves.

**2. Neuralgia, Headache, etc., English Remedy for.**—The intimate mixture of equal parts of chloral hydrate and camphor will produce a clear fluid, which is of the greatest value as a local application in neuralgia. Dr. Lenox Brown states, in one of the English medical journals, he has employed it in his practice, and induced others to do so, and that in every case it has afforded great and, in some instances, instantaneous relief. Its success does not appear to be at all dependent on the nerve affected, it being equally efficacious in neuralgia of the larynx, and in relieving spasmodic cough of a nervous or hysterical character. It is only necessary to paint the mixture lightly over the painful part, and to allow it to dry. It never blisters, though it may occasion a tingling sensation of the skin. For headache it is also found an excellent application. DIRECTIONS—Rub the two together in a mortar, which liquifies them, then bottle, and paint over the parts, lightly, as above. For toothache apply with lint, and rub upon the gums. I called upon one of the principal druggists of Ann Arbor, Mich., where I was then living, to see if they would mix, and also to see if they would make a clear fluid, as mentioned in the recipe; but I found he had mixed them several times for the last two years, and the result had been satisfactory. He had used the mixture personally, by wetting cotton in it and putting it into a decayed tooth, but the tooth was so extensively ulcerated at the roots, although it kept down the pain, yet it had to be extracted some two months after. But for common neuralgic pains the relief was generally instantaneous.

**3. Neuralgia and Sciatica, Simple Home Remedy.**—Dr. Ebrard, of Nines, France, states that he has for many years treated all his cases of neuralgic and sciatic pains with an approved apparatus, consisting merely of a flat-iron and vinegar, two things that will be found in every house. The iron is heated until sufficiently hot to vaporize the vinegar, and is then covered with some woolen fabric, which is moistened with the vinegar, and the apparatus is applied at once to the painful part. The application may be repeated two or three times a day. Dr. Ebrard states that as a rule pain disappears in twenty-four hours, and recovery ensues at once.

**4. Neuralgia, Facial—Quick and Permanent Cure.**—A quick and permanent cure of this disease, says a prominent physician, can be effected by using a spray-shower of sulphuric ether upon it. The intense cold is supposed to act upon the diseased nerves, so as to produce a complete change in their nutrition and action.

*Remarks* —I trust it will so prove. To do it properly a spray instrument kept by druggists would have to be used, continuing its use until relieved, and if to be permanent, I should say occasionally for a few days. I know its efficiency in ordinary pain—why not in neuralgia? But I cannot see why applying it as a liniment may not do as well.

**5. Neuralgia Pill, Tonic Alterative and Stimulant for.—** Quinine, 1 dr.; morphine, 1½ grs , strychnine, 1 gr.; arsenious acid, 1½ grs.; solid ex. of aconite, 10 grs.; mix very thoroughly and divide into 30 pills. DOSE—Take 1 pill only, 2 hours after each meal; never more than 3 daily, and never more than 1 at a time

*Remarks.*—This will be found a very valuable pill for neuralgia and all cases requiring tonic, alterative, anodyne or stimulating treatment, and especially so far as females of a weak and feeble habit, or condition generally. Valuable in ague, or chills and fever particularly. Some will say they contain some poisonous articles, so they do, and so does most medicines; but if they are made carefully and taken only as directed they will hurt none, but benefit many. (See also remarks after next recipe; see also tonic elixir, etc.)

**6. Neuralgia of the Head, Toothache, etc., Immediate Cure.** J. W. M Czartoryski, M. D., of Stockton, Cal., writes to the *Brief*, page 463, 1883, as follows: Dr. W. C. Frederick, of Lonoke, Ark., desires a remedy for the above diseases If he will moisten cotton well and introduce it into the previously cleaned ear of the patient, with the following lotion (mixture), he will be surprised with the miraculous effects: Fl. exs. of belladonna, viburnum opulus (high cranberry) and gelseminum sempervirens (yellow jasmine), each equal parts (say ¼ oz.); mix. By its local application on dental branches of the quintus trigemine, (fifth pair of nerves). It will relieve, in the same way, even toothache in the worst form in less than five minutes.

*Remarks.*—Druggists are now keeping all the prominent fluid extracts. If they have them not in any place, try tinctures, which will answer for most pur· poses. For toothache, wet cotton in the mixture and put into the tooth, if hol low, and rub a little on the gums and in front of the ears. (See also Ely's headache and toothache remedy, and the pain killer.)

**7. Neuralgia—Warning of a Poor State of Health.—**I cannot do better, in closing the subject of Neuralgia, than by giving the following sensible statement from the London (Eng.) *Lancet*, to show the importance of toning up the system of those afflicted with this terrible disease. (The Neuralgic Pills mentioned will do it nicely.)

" The great prevalence of neuralgia—or what commonly goes by that name —should be regarded as a warning indicative of a low condition of health, which must necessarily render those who are affected with this painful malady especially susceptible to the invasion of other diseases of an aggressive kind This is the season (autumn) at which it is particularly desirable to be strong and well furnished with the sort of strength that affords a natural protection against disease. There will presently be need of all the internal heat which the organism can command, and a good store of fat for use as fuel is not to be despised. It is no less essential that the vital forces should be vigorous, and the nerve power, especially, in full development. Neuralgia indicates a low or depressed state of vitality, and nothing so rapidly exhausts the system as pain that prevents sleep and agonizes both body and mind. It is, therefore, of the first moment that attacks of this affection, incidental to and indicative of a poor and weak state, should be promptly placed under treatment, and, as rapidly as may be, controlled. It is worth while to note this fact, because, while the spirit of manliness incites the 'strong minded' to patient endurance of suffering, it is not wise to suffer the distress caused by this malady, as many are now suffering it, without seeking relief, forgetful of the condition it bespeaks, and the con-·| stitutional danger of which it is a warning sign."

*Remarks.* — If the system is to be toned up, the first question is, how? Start out with a brisk cathartic; then follow with an alterative, as for rheumatism (which see), and also a good tonic bitters, or the Neuralgic Pills, as you choose; the pills are both tonic and alterative, and may cover both points with entire satisfaction, and especially so with females in a debilitated condition.

**8. Neuralgia—The Ladies' Cure.**—A lady writing upon this subject says: "If the lady that has neuralgia will make a strong tea of wild lady-slipper root—also called nervine (nerve-root is one of its common names, yellow moccasin flower, Noah's Ark, umbel, etc.)— and drink it, it will cure her; at least, it did me."

*Remarks.*—It is safe to try it, as it is tonic, stimulant, diaphoretic and antispasmodic. It is, in fact, valuable in most nervous and uterine difficulties. Take lady-slipper, with catnip and scullcap, equal quantities of each, powder and evenly mixed, and divided into powders of 1½ ozs.; then 1 pt. of boiling water poured over one of the powders, and steeped 15 or 20 minutes, taking at first 1 oz. or about 2 table-spoonfuls of the warm infusion, after which 1 table-spoonful every ½ hour for 3 or 4 hours, or until relieved, for sick or nervous headache, says Dr. King in his "Dispensatory," and repeating thus for 3 or 4 attacks, has permanently and invariably cured these neuralgic headaches.

**9. Neuralgia of the Face.**—The latest cure for neuralgia of the face is from a Dr. Nussbaum, which he reported in the Munich *Ærztliche Intelligence,* consisting of salicylic acid, 3½ grs., and salicylate of soda, 32 grs. To be pulverized and mixed for 1 powder, taking 4 to 6 such powders in the 24 hours.

*Remarks.*—Dr. Nussbaum considers this as a specific, or positive cure. It consist, of what has been recently brought out, as a cure for rheumatism. Neuralgia being, in fact, a species of rheumatism, why should it not cure it?

**1. EARACHE—Cure for.**—Take a large onion and cut it into slices; put a slice of onion, then a slice (the author would say a piece of leaf the size of the onion) of strong tobacco, then a slice of onion again, then tobacco, till the onion is all laid up, then wrap in a wet cloth and cover in hot embers, till the onion is cooked; press out the juice with heavy pressure, and drop into the ear. It gives instant relief. Solution of morphine will have a good effect also.

*Remarks.*—I should drop in only 3 or 4 drops of the onion and tobacco juice, at first, lest the influence of the tobacco might be too great, and repeat, if it was necessary. What is called a solution of sulphate of morphia, or *liquor morphia sulphatis*, kept by druggists, is of the strength of 1 grain of sulphate of morphia to 1 ounce of water only. Each tea-spoonful of it would contain ⅛ grain and would be a full dose, by mouth, which could be repeated, on an adult, in from 30 minutes to 2 hours, according to the severity of the pain for which it was given. To drop into the ear it might be, probably, twice as strong, without danger of injury. A few drops, say 4 or 5, of laudanum ought to have the same effect. The laudanum may be put with an equal amount of sweet oil, and the amount doubled, which would have a good effect in softening the wax of the ear. The onion cure is from Mr. Ford, of Iowa, who was referred to in the neuralgia (German cure, which see).

2. **Earache and Deafness, Valuable Remedy for.** — Wine of opium (not laudanum), 1 dr.; oil of anise, 10 drops; put into an ounce bottle, and fill with oil of sweet almonds (sweet oil will do very well). DIRECTIONS—Shake well, and drop from 3 to 5 drops into the ear, or ears, if both are affected. If no relief in 5 or 10 minutes, repeat; and follow along to relieve the sound or roaring in the ears.

*Remarks.*—"Old" Dr. King thinks this one of the most valuable combinations for earache or deafness which can be tried, having tested it several times. His remark was: "I think it will not fail once in 7000 cases, as it has not failed me in dozens of cases." He has been in practice fifty years. The one for "Ulceration" below is also from him.

3. **Earache, Remedy for.** — A writer says: "There is scarcely any ache to which children are subject, so bad to bear and difficult to cure, as the earache. But there is a remedy, never known to fail. Take a bit of cotton batting, put upon it a pinch of black pepper, gather it up and tie it, dip in sweet oil, and insert into the ear. Put a flannel bandage over the head to keep it warm. It will give immediate relief."

*Remarks.*—These simple remedies are easily tried, and will often prove successful.

4. **Ear, Ulcerations in — Very Certain Remedy.** — Pulverized sanguinaria canadensis (blood root), 1 dr., in soft water, 1 pt.; steep and strain. DIRECTIONS—Pour into the ear, or, what is better, syringe out the ear 2 or 3 times daily with it—a little warm.

1. **TOOTHACHE—Common Cures for.**—The following are common things recommended for the cure of toothache, outside of the profession, and are good remedies:

I. Alum, in very fine powder, ¼ oz.; spirits of nitrous ether, 7 drs.; mix, and apply with lint if the nerve is exposed, and also around the tooth. This is claimed to never fail, unless it is of a rheumatic character.

II. Equal parts of powdered alum and salt, mixed; then wet a bit of cotton, to make the powder adhere, and apply to the hollow of the tooth.

III. Saltpeter, pulverized and applied by cotton, cures nervous toothache at once.

**2. Toothache, to Cure so It Will Never Ache Again.—** If the following is the fact, it is the best of all the cures: Dissolve a piece of opium, the size of a small pea, in spirits of turpentine, ½ tea-spoonful. Put in the hollow of the tooth upon cotton. It does not stop the pain at once, says the writer, but, if well applied,—the cotton saturated and frequently changed—will soon cause it to never trouble again.

**3. Toothache Drops, Dr. Chase's.—** Best alcohol, 2 ozs.; chloroform, 1 oz.; sulphuric ether, 1½ ozs.; laudanum, oil of cloves, and oil of sassafras, of each ½ oz.; oil of lavender, 1 dr.; gum camphor, 1 oz.; mix all, and keep well corked.

*Remarks.*—I have used this very successfully for a long time; have manufactured and sold it, and have put others into the same business. I put it up in 2 dr. bottles, retailing it at 25 cts., and have yet to find anything better. Apply to the exposed nerve by means of cotton, and put freely around the gums.

**4. Toothache from Decaying Teeth—Solidified Creosote for the Pain of.—**Creosote has been for a long time used in its fluid state, to wet cotton in, and put into the tooth; but it has been found that 10 drops of collodion added to 15 drops of creosote makes a gelatinous mass that can be put upon the nerve, closing up the orifice and preventing the air from reaching the nerve, and it does not flow out into the mouth to irritate and make it sore.

*Remarks.*—This will prove a blessing to those preferring the use of creosote.

**1. POLYPUS IN THE NOSE—Very Effectual Remedy.—**Dr. King is very sanguine in the belief, or knowledge, that it is not necessary to twist off, nor to ligate (tie a cord around) them, but that the powdered blood root, snuffed into the nostril, will destroy and cure every case, unless the nostril is entirely filled with it, in which case it may have to be twisted off, and the powder applied to the base by wetting a piece of cloth tied on the end of a probe, or stick, dipping it in the powder, and touching it upon the base, or neck, from which the polypus was removed, to prevent a return.

*Remarks.*—The celebrated Dr. Wooster Beach, of New York, uses the powder of blood root and bayberry bark, in equal parts, for the same purpose. He, if the polypus was large, used the powdered poke root, introduced by the stick, or probe, as above, to cause them to slough off, often repeating, either medicine.

**2. Polypus of the Nose** has been cured by mixing the powdered blood root, 4 grs., with vaseline, 1 oz., and putting this upon cotton and pressing it up against the tumor. One month's application removed it. This was done by Dr. W. W. Carpenter, of Petaluma, Cal., and reported in the *Medical Brief.*

**3. Polypus, Another Cure for.—**A polypus, so large that it filled the whole nasal cavity, was cured by the use of carbolic acid, 1 part, and glycerine, 4 parts, and injecting 20 drops of this mixture by the hypodermis syringe (a syringe made to inject under the skin), into the base of the tumor. This, says Dr. Henning, of Redkey, Ind., who reported the case, is all I did. In one month it was gone, and it is still well, five months after the operation.

*Remarks.*—Certainly one of the plans ought to cure every case without twisting off or tearing out. Of course a physician would have to be called upon if this latter, or hypodermic, plan is adopted.

1. **BURNS—From Gunpowder, Prof. Gunn's Treatment.**— While Prof. Gunn was in the medical college, in Chicago, he gave the following item, through one of the journals of that city. It seems almost superfluous to add a word of endorsement, for, from several years acquaintance with him, as professor of surgery in the University of Michigan, it is well known that his recommendations could be relied upon. It is only for the benefit of those who are not acquainted with this fact that I have mentioned it. He says: "In burns from gunpowder, where the powder has been deeply imbedded in the skin, a large poultice made of common molasses and wheat flour, applied over the burnt surface, is the very best thing that can be used, as it seems to draw the powder to the surface, and keep the parts so soft that the formation of scars does not occur. It should be removed twice a day, and the part washed with a shaving brush and warm water before applying the fresh poultice. The poultice should be made sufficiently soft to admit of its being readily spread on a piece of cotton. In cases in which the skin and muscles have been completely filled with the burnt powder, we have seen the parts heal perfectly, without leaving the slightest mark to indicate the position or nature of the injury."

2. **Burns and Scalds, Instantaneous Relief for.**—The bi-carbonate of soda (the common cooking soda, found in almost every kitchen) has been found an exceedingly valuable remedy in the treatment of burns and scalds, giving almost, if not absolutely, instantaneous relief from pain, as well as a cure for the wound, by continuing its use. MODE OF APPLICATION—The injured part is to be moistened, then the dry soda, finely powdered, is to be sprinkled carefully upon it, to entirely cover the injury, and the whole wrapped with a wet cloth—linen is best. The relief is often instantaneous.

*Remarks.*—*Harper's Weekly* informs us that a Dr. Waters, of Salem, Mass., in speaking of the new remedy for burns and scalds, before the Massachusetts Dental Society, deliberately dipped a sponge into boiling water and sqeezed it over his wrist, producing a severe scald around his arm some two inches wide, and continued the application, despite the suffering, for half a minute. Then he at once sprinkled on the bi-carbonate of soda, and applied the wet cloth, which almost instantly deadened the pain; and on the next day after this single application of the soda, the less injured parts, were practically well, only a slight discoloration being perceptible, the severe portions being healed in a few days, by simply continuing the wet cloth bandage.

*Remarks.*—When I wrote this out some two or three years ago, I added to the above: I should have wet the cloth in a solution of the soda, for the continued wrappings, in every case. My idea above mentioned of wetting the cloths in a solution of soda, I have since seen, has been practiced by a Dr.

Froizke, of Russia, who reports its use, in this form, upon 25 cases of severe burns, caused by fire, in a conflagration, which shows that it is good for burns from fire, as well as scalds from hot water. In cases where the wounds were deep, and where there was considerable matter, the clothes were carefully removed and the wounds were cleansed to prevent the absorption of the matter into the blood before replacing the wet cloths.

**1  DROWNED PERSONS—Rules for Resuscitating—By the Michigan State Board of Health, and the Humane Society of Massachusetts.**—The following directions, or rules, for resuscitating, or bringing to life again, the apparently dead from drowning, are made up from a recent circular of the Committee on Accidents of the Michigan State Board of Health, and distributed throughout the State, and also from directions published at the request of the Humane Society of the Commonwealth of Massachusetts.

The general public should be well informed upon this subject; for, if life is to be saved, there must be no loss of time when one is taken from the water, and life apparently gone.

I.  Lose no time.  Carry out these directions on the spot:

II.  Remove the froth and mucus from the mouth and nostrils.

III.  Instantly loosen all neckwear, lacings, or waistbands.

IV.  Hold the body, for a few seconds only, so that the water may run out of the lungs and windpipe.

V.  If the ground is sloping, turn the patient upon the face, the head down hill; step astride the hips, your face towards the head, lock your fingers together under the belly, raise the body as high as you can without lifting the forehead from the ground, give the body a smart jerk, to remove the accumulating mucus from the throat, and water from the windpipe; hold the body suspended long enough to slowly count five; then repeat the jerks two or three times.

VI.  The patient being still upon the ground, face down, and maintaining all the while your position astride the body, grasp the points of the shoulders by the clothing, or, if the body is naked, thrust your fingers into the armpits, clasping your thumbs over the points of the shoulders, and raise the chest as high as you can without lifting the head quite off the ground. and hold it long enough to slowly count three.

VII.  Replace the patient upon the ground, with the forehead upon the flexed (bent) arm, the neck straightened out, and the mouth and nose free. Place your elbows against your knees and your hands upon the sides of his chest over the lower ribs and press downward and inward with increasing force long enough to slowly count two.  Then suddenly let go, grasp the shoulders as before and raise the chest; then press upon the ribs, etc.  These alternate movements should be repeated 10 to 15 times a minute for an hour at least, unless breathing is restored sooner.  Use the same regularity as in natural breathing.

VIII.  After breathing has commenced (and not before, unless there is a house very close), get the patient where covering may be obtained, to restore the animal heat. Wrap in warm blankets, apply bottles of hot water, hot bricks, etc., to aid the restoration of heat. Warm the head nearly as fast as the body, lest convulsions come on. Rubbing the body with warm cloths or the hand, and gently slapping the fleshy parts, may assist to restore warmth, and the breathing also.

IX. When the patient can swallow, give hot coffee, tea, milk, or a little hot sling. Give spirits sparingly, lest they produce depression. Place the patient in a warm bed, give him plenty of fresh air, and keep him quiet.

X. Let all the work be done deliberately and patiently, and do not give up too quickly,"for success,"says the Massachusetts society, "has rewarded the efforts of hours."

*Remarks.*—These rules cannot be too well understood (where it is possible for such accidents to occur), and no delicacy of mind or circumstances should prevent anyone from taking right hold of any case that may occur, because they have not done it before. No time to await the arrival of a physician— immediate action will insure success.

Let good judgment and great carefulness be exercised by everyone who finds himself called upon to act in any accident of this kind, and let no one hesitate a moment to do the best he can till some one more acquainted with the work, or a physician, may arrive, as life is too precious to allow of anyone neglecting to do what he can to save it.

**2. Drowned Persons—A Case in Hand.**—I will make a condensed statement here of a case reported in the New York *Mail and Express*, in 1882, to show what perseverance did in resuscitating a boy, by one of the officers of one of the life saving stations, who, with the reporter, happened to be passing along one of the wharves of that city, where a number of fishing vessels were tied, upon one of which was a boy who had been under water for 10 minutes, or more, and had lain as much longer upon the deck without an effort to restore him to life, and the bystanders, and even the police present, thought he was really dead; but the life-saving man took a different view of it, and went to work with a will; first opening the boy's mouth and removing the mud from it, he turned him over, on his face, and placed his coat, done up as a pillow, under the boys stomach, then took hold of the boy's ankles and raised them several feet above the boy's head, and put them into the hands of some of the bystanders, to keep them thus, he pressed gently, but firmly, upon the small of the boy's back, when immediately a stream of water gushed out of his mouth, which had all this time been in the lungs, waiting only for this treatment to help it out. This was continued a minute or two, to get out all the water he could, when he was turned upon his back, and the officer, kneeling over him, put one hand upon the boy's right side, the other on the left, just against the short ribs, he gave them a powerful compression, and then suddenly let go, the ribs springing back to their natural position, and the air rushed into the lungs; this was done a dozen or more times, but still no appearance of life, and the bystanders said to him: " Can't you let a drowned boy alone;" "why," says the officer, " I haven't begun yet, stand back and give more air here; " then he began slapping one of the boys hands, and put a man to the other, and one to each foot, they continued the slapping vigorously thus, upon each limb, and the reporter taking the officers place at that hand, the officer returned to the rib squeezing process, when after about five minutes of this vigorous work the boy gave a slight gasp for breath, to the great surprise of the bystanders and the delight of the life-saving officer. He then redoubled his efforts at the artificial breathing process, of pressing the ribs, etc., and called for brandy and warm blankets, the boy meanwhile gasping again and began to twitch in the legs, and as the boy began to breathe the brandy was given and the warm blankets were applied, and the boy was saved. (See hot sling in the rules above which, if it can be provided, is better than the raw brandy.) Thus you see what perseverance will sometimes do. Go then, in all such cases, and do likewise, and valuable lives may be saved.

1. **THE TRUE WAY TO HEALTH**—Simmered Down to a Few Short Rules.—A recent writer, whose name I do not know, has given us the most facts, in the fewest words, of anything I have seen. He says: The only true way to health is that which common sense dictates to man. Live within the bounds of reason; eat moderately; drink temperately; sleep regularly; avoid excess in everything, and preserve a conscience void of offence. Some men eat themselves to death; some drink themselves to death; some wear out their lives by indolence; and some by over-exertion; others are killed by the doctors, while not a few sink into the grave under the effects of vicious and beastly practices. All the medicines in creation are not worth a farthing to a man who is constantly and habitually violating the laws of his own nature.

**BANDAGING**—In Broken Limbs and Ulcers.—In broken limbs, it is necessary to use the bandage, and it has become quite common also, in the treatment of ulcers. They are more generally made of cotton sheeting, being torn off in strips of 3 to 4 inches in width, and sewed together until the required length is obtained, after which they are to be rolled into solid rollers for tne convenience of passing them around the limb, and to enable the one who applies them to draw them evenly at all stages of their application. In applying the bandage one can get a better idea from the illustrations than any other way. All parts should be covered evenly, lapping about one-half of the bandage upon the previous round, and in order to keep it smooth and not run up or down on the limb, it will be necessary to turn the bandage upon itself, as the cross lines in the cut will show, wherever the form of the limb causes the bandage to pass either way upon the limb from the center of the previous round. In this way the pressure is even, leaving no loose, or unbound place for an accumulation of blood, which would cause pain, and finally mortification. And it must not be applied so tight as to stop the circulation, for this would cause the same difficulty ; the object is to *lessen* the circulation, but *not* to stop it entirely.

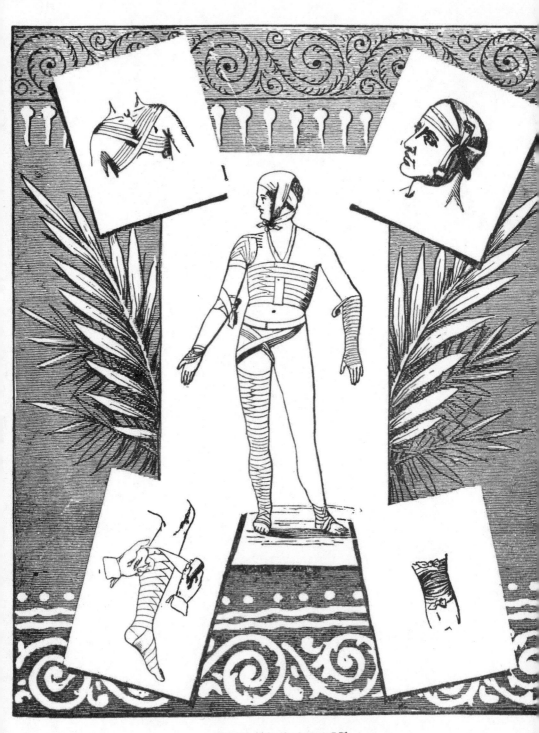

HOW TO BANDAGE.

**Ulcers.**—Most ulcers, in their early stage, upon the legs or arms, may be cured by judicious bandaging, and keeping the ulcer and the bandage wet with cold water, or perhaps cold water ¾ and whisky ¼ as much, merely to stimulate a little. This mixture I have found better than water alone in dressings. Our homeopathic friends are very much in favor of the arnica lotion in place of the cold water. It is certainly a valuable remedy if used in sufficient quantities to have its legitimate, or specific effects, say 1½ drs. of the *tincture* to a teacupful of cold water. A common teaspoon holds about 1 dr. Mix by pouring back and forth from one cup to another, then keep the bandage wet with it. Of this strength it does seem to have a specific effect upon fresh bruises, fresh cuts, etc. Two drs. of the tincture to alcohol, ½ pt., is highly recommended in rheumatism of the joints, pains of the feet or limbs from walking, etc., to be used freely as a liniment.

1. **PUNCTURED WOUNDS—New Cures to Avoid Lock-jaw.**—Mr. S. W. Hemenway writes to the *Scientific American* that he wishes to publish the following cure for punctured wounds for the benefit of all who may need it: As soon as such a wound is inflicted, get a light stick (a knife or file handle will do) and commence to tap gently on the wound. Do not stop for the hurt, but continue until it bleeds freely and becomes perfectly numb. When this point is reached, you are safe; all that is then necessary is, to protect it from dirt. Do not stop short of the bleeding and the numbness, and do not on any account close the opening with plaster. Nothing more than a little simple cerate on a clean cloth is necessary. I have used, and seen this used, on all kinds of simple punctures for thirty years, and never knew a single instance where a wound becoming inflamed or sore after the treatment as above. Among other cases, a coal rake tooth going entirely through the foot, a rusty darning needle through the foot, a bad bite by a sucking pig, several instances of file shanks through the hand, and numberless cases of rusty nails, etc., but never knew a failure of this treatment.

*Remarks.*—This being the class of wounds from which lock-jaw arises, let no one fail to adopt it or one of the following plans as soon as a small, deep wound is received.

2. **Punctured and Other Wounds and Bruises—To Relieve and Prevent Lock-jaw.**—The following remedy, simple as it is, is said to have saved thousands from death by lock-jaw: Smoke the wound or bruise with the smoke of wool. Twenty minutes in the smoke of wool will take the pain out of the worst wound, and repeated once or twice, will allay the worst case of inflammation arising from a wound.

3. **Lock-jaw or Tetanus Remedy and Preventive.**—A medical authority says: "Let anyone who has an attack of lock-jaw take a small quantity of spirits of turpentine; warm it and pour it into the wound—no matter what the wound is, or what its nature is—and relief will follow in less than one minute. Nothing better can be applied to a severe cut or bruise than cold turpentine: it will give certain relief almost instantly."

4. **Lock-jaw, or Tetanus, Quickly Relieved.**— A Dr. Bigelow reports, in the *Practitioner*, a case of lock-jaw, or tetanus, caused by a rusty

nail penetrating the foot, which was relieved in less than 20 minutes by introducing 1 dr. of the hydrate of chloral into the wound after it had been enlarged
by incision.

**5. Flesh Wounds and Fresh Cuts—To Prevent Bleeding,
Relieve Pain, Etc.**—Everybody is liable to be cut or to receive other flesh
wounds, away from surgical or veterinary aid; hence, they ought to know how
to proceed to save their own, or the life of a friend, or beast, by exercise of
common judgment.

I. If there is a flow of blood, close the wound with the hand and hold it
firmly together, so as to check the flow, and keep it thus until a bandage can be
obtained or stitches can be taken, if necessary, and the final bandaging is
applied. Bathing well with cold water, and keeping bandages wet with it, is
the latest method of treatment. I have known, however, one-half whiskey to
be used for this purpose, and believe it to be the best.

II. If the wound is painful, take a pan of burning coals and sprinkle upon
them common brown sugar, and hold the wounded part in the smoke. In a
minute or two the pain will be allayed, and the recovery proceed rapidly.

*Remarks.*—If the burning of wool will relieve pain and prevent lock-jaw
from punctured wounds, why should not sugar do the same? Although I cannot understand the why nor the wherefore, yet I still believe that both the
smoke of wool and sugar have cured many cases, otherwise these items would
never have been reported.

**6. Wounds, Hemorrhage or Bleeding from.**—It is also claimed
that bleeding may be stopped, on man or beast, by binding on a mixture of
equal parts of wheat flour and salt; of course they are not to be wet, but evenly
mixed, before binding on—the blood does the wetting.

**1. NOSE BLEED AND HICCOUGHS—Novel, but Certain
Remedy.**—The *Scientific American* reports the following novel plan for checking bleeding at the nose: The best remedy for bleeding at the nose, as given by
Dr. Gleason in one of his lectures, is in the vigorous motion of the jaws as if
in the act of mastication (chewing). In the case of a child a wad of paper
should be placed in its mouth, and the child should be instructed to chew it
hard. It is the motion of the jaws that stops the flow of blood. This remedy
is so very simple that many will feel inclined to laugh at it, but it has never
been known to fail in a single instance, even in very severe cases.

*Remarks.*—About the time of writing upon the subject I received a letter
from a Mrs. Harlan, of Hutton, Coles Co., Ill., wherein she confirmed the
above as to bleeding from the nose; and by the additional point of pressing the
fingers into the ears, with the motion as if chewing, it also cures hiccough.
And now I have an endorsement of my own as to its value in hiccough, for I,
at that time, had a little granddaughter living in the family who had been often
troubled with hiccoughs, and only a day or two after the receipt of Mrs. Harlan's letter the child again had an attack of them, and in two minutes, at most,
from the time I directed her and showed her how to do it, according to Mrs.

Harlan's plan of putting the fingers into the ears, and then "chew," the child was cured. She has had no further attack as yet, a little over three years, while before they had held her an hour or two, and sometimes longer, and it occurred quite frequently. It seems to have been an absolute cure. Mrs. Harlan included in her letter what she calls a simple cure for nose-bleed, hiccough and palpitation of the heart. I will give them in her own words, as follows:

**2. Nose-Bleed, Hiccough, and Palpitation of the Heart— Mrs. Harlan's Cure for.**—I. A simple cure for nose-bleed is to crowd the fingers tight into the ears and chew, pressing the teeth well together, as if chew-ing food.

II. It is said to be a cure also for a persistent hiccough. [This is what I tried with the grandchild.]

III. *Palpitation of the Heart.*—Hold the breath as long as possible and repeatedly. I have found it an almost certain remedy. And when it failed to stop the paroxysm at first it was relieved by it, and, after a time, stopped.

*Remarks.*—Mrs. Harlan is undoubtedly correct in the matter of relief, or cure, of "Palpitation;" for, in holding the breath, the blood is not invigorated by the absorption of oxygen in the air by its passage through the lungs, and hence the blood does not pass so freely nor quickly to the heart, and, therefore, its excessive action soon diminishes, and is finally quieted altogether. There is certainly philosophy in this. Mrs. H. had used these plans in her own family and among her friends, and sent them to me, as she expressed it, "for the good of the world."

**3. Hiccough, French Remedy for Children—Instantaneous Relief.**—According to the Lyons (France) *Medicale*, Dr. Grellety says:

"I have observed that hiccoughs in children are immediately stopped by giv-ing them a lump of sugar saturated with table vinegar. The same remedy was tried on adults with similar instantaneous success."

The sugar plan is confirmed by the following from Henry Tucker, M. D. in the *South Medical Record*, under the heading of "A Specific for Singulturs" (the physicians', or the Latin, name for hiccough):

"This very common affection, of infants and children especially, has a spe-cific remedy, at least one which I have never known to fail. Moisten granu-lated sugar with cider vinegar; give to an infant from a few grains to a tea-spoonful. The effect is almost instantaneous, and the dose seldom needs to be repeated. I have used it for all ages, from infants of a few months old to peo-ple on the down-hill side of life."

**4.** Another writer puts it in the following manner: "Take 3 or 4 swal-lows of sweetened vinegar."

*Remarks.*—Not much different, except in quantity. I should try this if Dr. Grellety's or Dr. Tucker's lump of sugar did not succeed.

**5. Hiccough, a Cure for by Pressure — French.** — The latest French discovery as to the cure of hiccoughs is given in *La Scalpel*, as follows: A very easy cure for a continued hiccough, sometimes complicated with spasms of the air-passage to the lungs, is introduced by Rostau, and highly recom-mended by Deghillaye, of Mons, France. It consists in placing the hand flat upon the pit of the stomach, immediately below the cartilage forming the end of the breast-bone, and making firm pressure. Should this prove unsuccessful, place a firm roll of muslin on the same place, securing it by a bandage bound tightly around the body. In an hour this may be removed, and it will be found that the hiccough has entirely disappeared.

*Remarks.*—The cure in this case is by the pressure, preventing the spasmodic action of the diaphragm, which is the cause of hiccoughs.

## BILIOUSNESS, BILIOUS FEVER, FEVER AND AGUE, CHILLS AND FEVER, INTERMITTENT FEVER, PERIODIC FEVER, ETC.

**BILIOUSNESS.**—The symptoms are too well known to need describ_ing. If your bones ache, and you feel languid, your mouth tastes unpleasant, etc., you are bilious, and if you don't remedy it soon your complexion will be sallow.

**Cholagogue or Bilious Tonic.**—Quinine, 1 dr.; oil of wintergreen, 1 teaspoonful; oil of peppermint, 5 drops; oil of lemon, 15 drops; alcohol, ½ pt.; water, ½ pt.; sulphuric acid, 30 drops. Mix well, then add red Peruvian bark, finely pulverized, 2 ozs.; rheubarb root, also finely pulverized, 2 ozs.; simple syrup, or molasses, to make all 1 qt. Those who are acted upon easily by cathartics can not bear more than half of this quantity of rheubarb. Let such have it made accordingly—the object of its use is to just keep the bowels solvent, not loose like diarrhœa.

The quinine, oils and acid should be put into the alcohol first, then the water, and afterwards the bark and rheubarb, and then the syrup; or what would be a little more palatable, would be to steep the Peruvian bark and rheubarb root in as little water as will answer, then strain off into the mixture and steep again, to get all the strength, by pressing out the second time; then make up the quart with syrup, as this avoids the sediment of the bark and root in taking off the medicine, as some people object to taking the medicine with the powders in it. It may be taken at once, if well shaken; or, if shaken 2 or 3 times daily for a week, after that it may be taken without shaking, as the strength of the Peruvian bark and rheubarb will by that time be extracted. DOSE—For an adult, 1 or 2 tea-spoonfuls 4 times daily, at meals and bed-time; for a child of 12 years, half dose. If very bilious take a full cathartic dose of rheubarb or such other cathartic medicine as you are in the habit of using, or prefer, to move the bowels freely.

*Remarks.*—This will be fonnd a very valuable *tonic* in all cases requiring one, and is absolutely the best known remedy for biliousness. If a person inclined to be bilious will take this every spring and fall, they will not be troubled. It will break up 99-100 of all the agues and remittent fevers in a few days; if not, repeat the cathartic, and continue the Cholagogue until the work is accomplished—never try to "*wear* out the ague"; it will either wear *you* out, or leave you the *worse* for wear." *Repeat* at intervals of a week, 2 or 3 times; and in nearly every case a permanent cure will be effected, if the medicine is taken for 3 or 4 days at each repetition.

[NOTE.—This is not an easy remedy to prepare. For a good many it will be cheaper to send $1.00 to the Chase Medicine Co., Detroit, Mich., and get a bottle already prepared.]

**Bilious Remittent Fever—Symptoms.**—The attack is generally sudden and well marked. Some writers say it has no premonitory symptoms; others, that it has. The more general understanding is, that for a day or two, or even longer, before the onset, there is a sense of languor and debility, slight headache, lack of appetite, furred tongue, bitter taste in the mouth in the morning, pains in the joints and general uneasiness.

The formal onset is nearly always marked by a distinct chill or rigor,— sometimes slight and brief; at other times severe and prolonged. The chill may begin at the feet, or about the shoulder blades, or in the back, and thence run like small streams of cold water poured in every direction through the whole body. There is *generally* but one well-marked chill, the returns of the paryoxysms of fever being seldom, after the first, preceded by the cold stage.

During the hot stage the pulse is up to one hundred and twenty, or one hundred and thirty. There are pains in the head, back and limbs, of a most distressing kind.

The tongue is generally covered with a yellowish, or dirty white fur; and in bad cases, in the advanced stage, is frequently parched brown or nearly black in the center, and red at the edges. There is no appetite for food, and generally nausea and vomiting; and usually there is pain and tenderness in the epigastrium. The bowels are at first costive, but afterwards become loose, and there are frequent evacuations of dark, offensive matter.

*Causes.*—This disease is produced by malarial exhalations from the decomposition of vegetable matter. It is most prevalent in hot climates, and in the summer and autumn.

*Treatment.*—If the fever be in the formative stage, and has not fully developed itself, give an emetic (see page 180), and follow it with a mild cathartic—rochelle salts, 2 drs.; bi-carbonate of soda, 2 scruples; water, ½ pt. Mix. To this mixture add 35 grains of tartaric acid, and take the whole foaming. This is the recipe for Seidlitz powders.

If the disease be already developed, sponge the body all over several times a day with cold or tepid water, according to the feelings of the patient, and give cooling drinks. To moderate the fever give 3 to 10-drop doses of tincture or fluid extract of veratrum viride. The compound powder of ipecac and opium is a valuable preparation for the same purpose. Give cold water as drink, if desired by the patient, or let him eat ice.

When the headache is very severe, let wet cups be applied upon the temples, or behind the ears; and the same remedy to the pit of the stomach, when there is great tenderness, is often desirable; though a mustard plaster will sometimes do better.

During the remissions of the fever, quinine and other tonics are to be given, as in fever and ague.

**AGUE.**—What is generally called ague is also known by all these names, which mean one and the same thing. Doctors generally say "intermittent fever," and what will cure it are also known as "anti-periodics." The two following recipes for ague originated with Dr. B. F. Humphreys, of Tyler, Texas, as substitutes, or to be used instead of quinine. He published them in the *Eclectic Medical Journal,* more especially for the benefit of other physicians; but if they are good for physicians, and I know they are, to use upon their patients and save the expense of quinine, they are as certainly good for the people to have them prepared by druggists for their own use. I have confidence in them, hence I give them. Dr. Humphreys gave the recipe for the "solution" to make 16 pts. (2 gals.), so that physicians could make up enough for a whole neighborhood; but I have reduced it by 16, so that families will make only 1 pt. If desired to make in larger quantities, simply keep the same proportions. The pills I will give for 240, as he gave them; if less are needed, to keep the proportions is all that is necessary. They are as follows:

**1. Ague Solution, Pills and Liniment for—Without Quinine.**—I. *Solution, or Dr. Humphreys' " Tip-Top Tonic."*—Sulphate of cinchonia, 1 dr.; sulphate of strychnia, 2 grs.; tinct. of stillingia, ½ pt.; tinct. of enonymus (wahoo), 4 ozs.; tincts. of leptandra (Culver's physic) and of podophyllum (mandrake), each 2 ozs.; oil of wintergreen, to flavor, (15 or 20 drops, only, in a little alcohol), and elixir of vitriol (aromatic sulphuric acid), to dissolve the sulphates. DIRECTIONS.—Rub the sulphate of strychnia, first, in a mortar; then put in the sulphate of cinchonia, and rub together, and add to them as much aromatic sulphuric acid as necessary to dissolve them; then put into the bottle with the other articles, shake well, and it is ready for use. DOSE.—For adults, 1 tea-spoonful 4 or 5 times daily. For a child, 3 times as many drops as it is years old, same number of times daily as for adults.

*Remarks*—Dr. Humphreys called this his "Calisaya Anti-Periodic: or, Tip-Top Tonic," and considered it as cheap and efficient as anything that can be got up. "Calisaya" is the name which the Indians of South America applied to what we know as Peruvian bark; hence the Doctor applies it here, as he knew all physicans, for whom he was writing, would know what he meant, *i. e.*, that the sulphate of cinchonia and calisaya was made from the Peruvian bark.

**2. Ague, or Chills and Fever — Simple Cure Without Quinine.**—H. G. D. Brown, of Copiah Co., Miss., gives the following as a certain and thoroughly tried cure for fever and ague: "Take 1 pt. of cotton-seed; 2 pts. of water boiled to 1; strain and take warm 1 hour before the attack. Many persons will doubtless laugh at this simple remedy; but I have tried it effectually, and unhesitatingly say it is better than quinine, and could I obtain the latter article at a dime a bottle, I would infinitely prefer the cotton-seed tea. It will not only cure invariably, but permanently, and is not at all unpleasant to the taste."

**3. Ague or "Chills"—Positive Cure, with Quinine.**—This receipt is from Dr. Joseph Spaulding, of Lafayette, Ind., in answer to an inquiry from a lady through the *Blade Household*, which explains itself. He says:

"DEAR MADAM:—You say 'don't prescribe *whiskey* nor *quinine*,' but I *will*, and I know whereof I speak, as I was a sufferer with the ague for three years, in the malarial district of Indiana, and this cured me, and I have not had a chill for five years; and I am sure it will do as much for others. The toper who takes his morning bitters out of this, will not want them a second time from the same bottle.

I. "A thorough cathartic. Now, I mean *thorough* when I say it.

II. "Two days after take quinine in 6 gr. doses every 4 to 6 hours, just as you can stand it, till you have missed a chill; then take the following:

III. *Tonic Bitters, to Strengthen and Tone up the System after Ague, or Chills and Fever have been broken, or for General Use.*—"Tinct. capsicum, 1 dr.; citrate of iron and quinine, 1 oz.; comp. tinct. of gentian, 1 oz.; elixir cinchonia, 2 ozs.; whiskey, 5 ozs. DOSE—Take 1 tablespoonful 3 times daily, just after meals."

The elixir of cinchonia is also known as "elixir of calisaya," or "elixir of bark," meaning, of Peruvian bark. It is made as follows: Peruvian bark, 1 oz.; fresh orange peel, ½ oz.; cinnamon bark, coriander seeds and angelica seeds, each 3 drs.; caraway and anise seeds, each 1 dr.; brandy and water, as given below; simple syrup, 10 ozs. Bruise or coarsely grind the bark and aromatics, and treat them with brandy until 10 ozs. are obtained; then continue the percolation with equal parts of brandy and water, until 22 ozs. have been obtained; then add the syrup to make 2 pts. tonic and cordial.

*Remarks.*—I know that some people object to using quinine, believing that it causes rheumatic or other pains, etc., but I am well satisfied that the pains, or other difficulties supposed to come from the quinine, came from the disease, or the climate, and not from the use of the quinine. It is not only a perfectly safe remedy, but is indeed a valuable *antiperiodic* and strengthening medicine. It can be obtained anywhere, and will cure ague everywhere, with only an occasional exception. The position I have taken above, that it is the disease, or *malaria* in the system, that causes the pain in the bones, etc., and *not* the quinine that does it, I have since seen, is also claimed to be the fact by some of our most eminent pysicians.

**4. Ague, or Chills and Fever—Certain Cure for.**—Quinine, 31 grs.; aromatic sulphuric acid and laudanum, each, 31 drops; water, 3 ozs. DOSE—A teaspoonful 3 times a day, before meals.

*Remarks.*—This was given me by Mrs. Catharine Baldwin, of Toledo, O., formerly of Put-in-Bay, where she obtained it, and knew of its curing several of the *most obstinate* or long standing chronic cases, which "nothing," as the saying goes, "would cure." I have used it with success, making only this difference with the receipt: Using 40 grs. of the quinine and 40 drops of the oil of vitriol and laudanum, in 4 ozs. of water (to make the quantity a little more); then, for an adult, directing a tablespoonful three hours, two hours and one hour, before the chill should commence—which will break it. After that, 1 tea-spoonful 3 times daily, just after meals, till all is taken, will cure most cases.

**5. Ague Pills, Very Cheap and Very Effective, Without Quinine.**—Chinoidine, 1 oz.; dovers powders, 3 drs.; piperine, 40 grs.; sub carbonate of iron, 2½ drs.; stiff mucilage of gum arabic sufficient to work into pills, and mix very intimately and make into usual sized pills. [The author would say to make into 440 pills, to be sure to have 1 gr. of chinoidine in each pill.] Dose.—Take 2 pills every 2 hours until 6 or 8 are taken, in the absence of fever. After the first day 2 pills 3 times a day, just before meals, in the absence of chills or fever.

*Remarks.*—This recipe is decidedly a good one, either as an ague cure or as a general tonic. Chinoidine pills, however, in warm weather get soft and should, therefore, have plenty of powdered liquorice root among them to prevent their sticking together; but from this tendency the following, in liquid form, may be preferable:

**6. Chinoidine for Ague—How to Give It.**—C. E. Ellis, M. D., of Gooch's Mill, Mo., in answer to an inquiry of Dr. A. Barry, of Dresden, Tex., in *The Brief*, page 505, 1883, for "a convenient mode of administering chinoidine," made the following answer: "The following is a prescription used by my father and myself with no dissatisfaction from any patient, except one colored woman, who complained of nausea after taking: Chinoidine, 2 ozs.; alcohol, 1 pt.; nitric acid, dilute (a formula druggists understand), 1 oz.; aromatic syrup of rhei. (rhubarb), 8 ozs.; water, 8 ozs. Mix. Dose.—When dissolved, take 1 tea-spoonful before meals and bedtime. If Dr. Barry will try this mode of giving the chinoidine he will find it all I recommend it to be. I have used it a great deal, and I hope he may have as good success with it as I have had."

*Remarks.*—Being so much cheaper than quinine is the main reason for its use. For those who oppose the use of quinine, and all similar ingredients, as cinchonidia or chinoidine, and would like to try a novel, yet a simple, cure, I give the following:

**7. Ague and Fever, Novel but Simple Cure.**—Take a medium-sized nutmeg and char it by holding it to a flame by sticking a piece of wire inside, permitting it to burn by itself without disturbance; when charred, pulverize it and combine with it an equal quantity of burned alum and divide into three powders. On the commencement of the chill give a powder. If this does not break it, give the second powder on the appearance of the next chill; and if not cured the third powder must be given as the succeeding chill comes on. Usually the first powder effects a cure, and it is seldom that the third powder will be required. The bowels should always be acted upon by a purgative previous to their administration. It is certainly deserving attention, though I do not pretend to account for its action.—*Prof. King.*

*Remarks.*—Prof. King says he has "known it to have cured several cases of intermittent fever" (fever and ague), and also says he has "been assured of its almost universal success in this disease;" and also adds that "it is recommended for the cure of other forms of fever." I am, like himself, unable to give a reason why or how it should so act; but that it has so acted I have not a doubt.

**8. Ague Pills for Obstinate Cases.**—Alcoholic ex. of nux vomica, 10 grs.; quinine, 30 grs.; pulverized capsicum, 20 grs. DIRECTIONS—Mix very thoroughly and divide into 30 pills. First give an active cathartic to get a good action upon the bowels; then give 2 of the pills an hour before eating, 3 times daily, until cured, then 1 pill for a dose the same way until all are taken.

*Remarks.*—This was from an old physician in Tennessee to a Baptist minister who had had ague a long time, not being able to get it cured. This did the work. He gave it to my cousin, Dr. A. B. Moon, of Toledo, O., who says he failed only in a single case for the many years he had used it.

**9. Ague, Tonic Elixir for.**—Tinct. of capsicum, 1 dr.; citrate of iron and quinine and compound tincture of gentian (the first is in crystals, the latter a fluid), each, 1 oz.; elixir of cinchonia, 7 ozs. Mix. DOSE—From 1 to 2 tea-spoonsful 3 times daily, just after meals; for a general tonic, once in 1 to 2 hours; if to break up an ague, 4 doses at least, the last to be taken one hour before the chill returns.

*Remarks.*—I know this to be a valuable tonic whenever one is needed.

**10. Ague, Tonic Pills for.**—Sulphate of cinchonia (made from the Peruvian bark), 40 grs.; arsenious acid, 1 gr.; iron reduced (ferri pulvis, or iron in a pulverized state) and solid ex. of gentian, each, 1 dr. Mix thoroughly and make into 40 pills. DOSE—As a general tonic, 1 pill 1 hour after each meal and at bedtime; or, if handier, half an hour before meals and at bedtime; to break up an ague, 2 pills, 4, 3, 2, and 1 hour before the chill should begin; then 4 daily for a few days as above.

**11. Ague, Elixir, or German Cure for.**—Quinine, 16 grs.; quinidia and cinchonidia, each, 20 grs.; comp. tinct. of Peruvian bark and tinct. of columbo, each, 2 ozs.; tinct. of rhubarb, 1 oz.; aromatic sulphuric acid, to cut the sulphates, and "Simple Elixir," to fill an 8 oz. bottle. [Lest some persons may want to have druggists fill this recipe, in small places where they may not have the simple elixir, I give the formula, it is as follows: Spirits, or essence of orange, ¼ oz.; essence of cinnamon, 10 drops; alcohol, 4 ozs.; simple syrup and water, each 6 ozs.; mix.] DOSE—1 teaspoonful every 3 hours, till the ague is broken; then 3 times daily, etc., as with other tonics.

*Remarks.*—I obtained this recipe of G. M. Nill, a druggist and pharmacist, of Broadway, Toledo, O.; and I had it filled by him several times, finding it very valuable. In one family the lady used it first, for herself, then for a child and finally for her father, successfully in each case, and I have used it in several other cases with equal success. Notice this, in this prescription, it contains three of the best anti-periodic and tonic preparations made from the Peruvian bark, and besides the compound tincture of bark itself, which will account for the great success I have had, and which I believe others will have, with its use, either as a cure for the ague or to prevent its return, and also as a general tonic.

**12. Ague, Tonic Febrifuge for — Not Needing a Cathartic Before Commencing its Use.** — Quinine, 40 grs.; elixir of taraxacum (dandelion), 2 ozs.; simple syrup to fill an 8 oz. bottle. Shake when taking.

Dose.—For an adult, 1 table-spoonful, or a small swallow, 3 or 4 times daily; for a child of 6 to 12 years, a dessert-spoonful; 3 to 6 years, 1 tea-spoonful; if very young, ½ tea-spoonful.

*Remarks.*—The beauty of this is, the elixir of dandelion acts on the liver and bowels, so you do not have to wait to take cathartics before you begin with the febrifuge. It is best, however, with this, as before remarked in several places, to begin with the doses 4, 3, 2 and 1 hour before the chill would come on. I obtained this from a friend of mine in Toledo—M. O. Waggoner—who has been familiar with its use for several years, and says "there is no equal to it." I have taken it, and given it to others, with entire satisfaction. It is indeed a febrifuge (opposed to fever) worthy of the name.

**13. Fevers in Low, Wet Country—Dr. Buchan's Preventive and Cure.**—Best red, unground Peruvian bark, 2 ozs.; Virginia snake root, root, 2 ozs.; gentian root and orange peel, each 1 oz.; brandy or good whiskey, 1 qt.; or whiskey and good worked cider, each 1 pt., will do nicely. Direc- tions—Grind coarsely, or bruise, and put into the spirit, and shake daily for 10 or 12 days, before using. Dose — Two table-spoonfuls immediately after each meal, either as a preventive or a cure.

*Remarks.*—Dr. Buchan, of the Royal College of Physicians of Edinburg, Scotland, in his *Domestic Medicine*, claims this to be the remedy for fluxes, putrid intermittents, and all other fevers in low, wet countries of an unhealthy climate. It is certainly valuable, as the gentian improves the appetite and the snake root benefits the kidneys and skin.

**14. Ague and Fever, How to Avoid.** — The foregoing remedies will cure ague, or chills and fever; but an important question is, how to avoid or prevent having them. To do this successfully, avoid exposure to the damp air of the early morning, except when exercising; and then do not remain in the open air to cool off. Avoid great fatigue; sleep eight hours of the twenty- four. Be sure that the water used for drinking and cooking is perfectly pure. Wear flannel underclothing at all seasons. Keep the feet dry and warm. And, after being careful in all these particulars, if you get the ague, take your choice in the foregoing list of remedies to cure it, until you can leave the ague district for a more healthy location.

**1. CINDERS OR DUST IN THE EYES — To Remove. —** A correspondent writes to the *Scientific American* this remedy for cinders in the eye: "A small camel's-hair brush dipped in water and passed over the ball of the eye on raising the lid. The operation requires no skill, takes but a moment, and instantly removes any cinder or particle of dust or dirt without inflaming the eye."

**2.** Another writer says: " Persons traveling much by railway are subject to continual annoyance from the flying cinders. On getting into the eyes they are not only painful for the moment, but are often the cause of long suffering that ends in a total loss of sight. A very simple and effective cure is within the reach of every one, and would prevent much suffering and expense were it more generally known. It is simply one or two grains of flax seed. It is said they may be placed in the eye without injury or pain to that delicate organ, and shortly they begin to swell and dissolve a glutinous substance that covers the ball of the eye, enveloping any foreign substance that may be in it. The irritation or cutting of the membrane is thus prevented, and the annoyance may soon be washed out. A dozen of these grains stowed away in the vest pocket may prove, in an emergency, worth their number in gold dollars.''

1. ACCIDENTS, POISONING, ETC.—Short Rules for Management. — Prof. Wilder, of New York, gives the following short rules to govern the action in such cases:

I. For dust in the eyes, avoid rubbing, and dash water into them; remove cinders, etc., with the rounded end of a lead-pencil.

II. Remove insects from the ear by tepid water; never put a hard instrument into the ear.

III. If an artery is cut, compress above the wound; if a vein is cut, compress below.

IV. If choked, get upon all fours and cough.

V. For light burns, dip the part in cold water; if the skin is destroyed, cover with varnish.

VI. Smother a fire with carpets, etc.; water will often spread burning oil, and increase the danger.

VII. Before passing through smoke take a full breath, and then stoop low; but if carbonic acid is suspected, then walk erect.

VIII. Suck poisoned wounds, unless your mouth is sore. Enlarge the wound, or better, cut out the part without delay. Hold the wounded part as long as can be borne to a hot coal or end of a cigar.

IX. In case of poisoning, excite vomiting by tickling the throat, or by warm water, or mustard and water, or salt and water, always warm, if possible.

X. For acid poisons give alkalies.

XI. For opium poisoning give strong coffee and keep moving.

XII. If you fall in water float on the back, with the nose and mouth projecting. (See falling into the river, etc.)

XIII. For apoplexy raise the head and body; for fainting lay the person flat.

2. Quick Emetics for Accidental Poisoning.—Another writer gives the following instructions for the management in accidents, poisoning, etc. He says: "Quickly mix a couple of ounces of powdered chalk or magnesia with a pint of milk and swallow the whole at one draught. Then run the finger down the throat and move it gently from side to side. This will induce vomiting; after which drink freely of warm milk and water and repeat the vomiting. Milk is an antidote for almost all poisons, narcotics excepted, especially if used promptly, and followed by vomiting. In narcotic poisoning, as by laudanum, opium or morphine, promptly give an emetic of mustard and water, followed by copious draughts of warm water and salt, until vomiting is induced. Keep the patient moving, and do not allow him to sleep. Send in haste for your family physician."

**3. Poisoning by Accident or Intention, What to do.**—Another medical writer on the subject of accidental or intentional poisoning, says: "To neutralize any poisonous mineral or vegetable, taken intentionally or by accident swallow 2 gills (½ pt.) of sweet oil; for a strong constitution, more oil."

*Remarks* —The sweet oil is good and a bottle of it ought to be kept in every house, to meet, immediately, any emergency of this kind; but lard oil or even melted lard will do. Vomiting is also very important.

**4. Poisoning by Poison Ivy—Remedy.**—Bromine, 15 grs., rubbed in 1 oz. of olive oil, or glycerine, and apply 3 or 4 times daily; one application at bed-time has been found effectual; a poultice of clay-mud has also cured many cases.

**5. Poison Ivy—Poisoning Cured by an Old Fox Hunter.**—The following was sent to *Forest and Stream*, which explains itself The writer says: "I have probably suffered more from poison ivy than any other man. Three times in one summer I have been blind from its effects. I have tried every remedy without success, until last summer. I was out shooting, and, with my usual luck, I got another dose that confined me to the house. I could not walk. An old fox hunter living in the neighborhood, hearing of my condition, came to see me, and brought me a remedy that acted like magic. In 3 days time I was up and enjoying what I love better than anything else in this world, the best of all field sports—fall woodcock shooting. I give you the recipe: Take 1 pt. of the bark of black spotted alder and 1 qt. of water, and boil down to 1 pt Wash the poisoned parts a dozen times a day, if convenient; it will not injure you."

*Remarks.*—Perhaps the better plan is to learn that the poison ivy has its leaves in clusters of three, while the non-poisonous has its leaves in clusters of five; knowing this, keep clear of the poisonous.

**6. Poisoning by the Poison Oak, Remedy.**—J. B. Murfree, M. D., of Murfreesboro, Tenn., says he has found the black wash made of calomel and lime-water (calomel, 1 dr. to lime-water, 1 pt.), an invariable success for several years.—*Medical Brief*. This is supported by the following, also from the *Brief*. by Dr. James A Douglass, of Poland, O., under the head of:

**7. Poisoning by Rhus,** wherein he says: "Since the discovery by Professor Maisch, that the toxic (poisoning) quality was due to an acid, which he denominated *toxicodendric* acid, the treatment has been based upon a true scientific basis (*i. e.*, that alkalies neutralize acids, and *vice versa*, that acids neutralize alkalies), I therefore," he continues, "apply alkalies to neutralize the acid. I prefer," he also says, "the liquor calcis (lime-water) applied locally; in severe cases use internally also. I sometimes combine it (the lime-water) with soda bi-carbonate, or hydrate of chloral, 1 oz. to 1 pt." This he closes by saying is as near a specific (positive cure) as any one could wish. (See tumor, poison wound, and wild vine poisoning, earth cure for.)

**8. Poisoning by Henbane, Tobacco, or Stramonium, and Bites of Snakes—Remedy.**—The oil of sassafras has been found a remedy against the poison of these articles. Given in 15 drop doses, 30 minutes apart, for six doses, restored consciousness when the flowers of stramonium had been eaten by a boy 4 years old; after which a dose of castor-oil was given to work it off by the bowels.

*Remarks.*—This is from a Dr. A. W. Lyle, of Castleton, Ind., in *Medical Brief*, in which he also gives Dr. Thompson's account of the value of oil of sassafras for henbane and tobacco poisoning, and also says: "It will destroy all insect life, and is an effectual antidote for the bite of venomous copperhead snakes." He recommends all physicians to try it, and, the author thinks, it is equally good for the people. He does not give the dose in these last cases; but if a boy of four years can take 15 drops, an adult may take at least 40. And in the snake-bites, I would rub it on the wounds also, and repeat as he directs.

**1. ACCIDENT FROM CHLOROFORM — To Prevent, by Mixing Spirits of Turpentine with it.**—"A preventive for those accidents which so frequently occur in the administration of chloroform to produce anæsthesia (insensibility to pain) has been suggested by Dr. Wachsmuth, of Berlin, Germany: the method consisting simply in the addition of one part of the rectified oil of turpentine (spirits of turpentine) to five parts of chloroform. The oil of turpentine in vapor appears to exert a stimulating or life-giving effect on the lungs, and protects those organs from passing into that paralyzed state which seems to be produced by chloroform narcosis (to benumb, or to become unconscious). It appears that Dr. Wachsmuth, while lying on a sick-bed, accidentally breathed the vapor of turpentine, and he experienced from this a strongly refreshing feeling—a fact which induced him to try the plan of adding oil of turpentine to chloroform when using the latter for anæsthetic purposes."

*Remarks.*—People, even physicians, speak unadvisedly when they say oil of turpentine, meaning the spirits, as it should be called; there is no oil of turpentine proper. The sticky mass, as it runs from the trees, is distilled, when it becomes very limpid, *i. e.*, pure and clear, having scarcely an appearance of oil—clear as water, as the common saying is. The only object of this explanation is, that no one shall suppose that there is an oil, and a spirit, too; they are both one and the same thing.

**2. Accident from Chloroform—To Prevent by Management.**—It is believed that many of the deaths from the administration of chloroform have arisen by the patient lying upon the back, and the tongue, from loss of muscular power or contractility, has fallen back into the throat and thus suffocated the patient. This should certainly be looked to by everyone who administers it. The tongue can be held with a cloth, if need be.

I see also by a recent statement in the Ann Arbor *Register* that Dr. McLean, of the University of Michigan, in his surgical practice of 25 years, prefers chloroform to any other anæsthetic, and has never had a death occur from it, nor seen a death by its use. He has always used it when necessary, and is a strong advocate for its use, and, all things considered, prefers it to ether. With the foregoing cautions as to the breathing, to prevent suffocation from the tongue falling over the glottis while the muscles are all relaxed by the chloroform, there need be no apprehension of danger from it; still, I can see no objection to mixing the turpentine with it.

The London *Lancet* confirms the idea advanced above, about the attention to the tongue, in the following words: "Death from chloroform need never occur, according to the doctrine of Syme, Lister and Hughes (all celebrated surgeons) if this simple rule is observed: Never mind the pulse, never mind the heart, leave the pupil (of the eye) to itself. But keep your eye on the breathing, and if it becomes embarrassed to a grave extent, take an artery forceps and pull the tongue well out. (A piece of cloth in the fingers will hold the tongue with but little difficulty.) Syme never lost a case from chloroform, although he gave it five thousand times "

**FALLING INTO DEEP WATER — What to do for Those Who Cannot Swim.**—For those who may fall into deep water, and cannot swim, it is thought best that a little fuller instructions ought to be given·

I.  When one falls into deep water let it always be remembered that he will rise to the surface at once; and now is the time to remember, also, that he must not raise the arms nor hands above the water, except there be something to take hold of; if he does it will sink the head so low he cannot breathe. But:

II.  Any motion of the hands may be made under the water, as you please, without endangering the life, for if the water is quiet, the head being thrown a little back, the face will float above the surface, unless heavy boots or clothing bear one down.

III.  And a motion of the legs as if walking up stairs, while it can be borne, keeping the perpendicular as nearly as possible, will greatly aid in keeping one afloat until help arrives; and even good swimmers had better not ex· haust themselves, if a boat is coming, only to keep afloat. (See also drowned persons, rules for resuscitation, etc.)

## SALVES, PLASTERS, OINTMENTS, POULTICES, ETC.

1.  **Salve or Plaster for Chaps, Cracks, etc.** — Rosin, 10 ozs.; mutton tallow, 2 ozs.; beeswax, 1 oz.  DIRECTIONS — Simmer together and work as shoemakers do their wax, and make it into convenient rolls.  Spread on slips of cloth to suit the place, and apply as hot as the flesh will bear it— It will need no tying.  If too stiff in very cold weather use a little more tallow and beeswax, or a little less rosin.

2.  **Ointment of St. John's Wort and Stramonium, for Tumors, Bruised and Blackened Spots, etc.**— Tops and flowers, recently picked, of St. John's wort (*hypericum perforatum*), fresh *stramonium* leaves, each ½ lb.; lard, 1 lb.  DIRECTIONS—Bruise the herbs and put into the lard and gently heat for an hour, then strain.  Rub and heat into the swellings, caked breasts, hard tumors and ecchymosed spots (spots which have been bruised and the blood settled under the skin) thoroughly.

*Remarks.*—Prof. King also says the saturated (as strong as can be made) tincture of the St. John's wort is nearly as valuable as that of arnica, for bruises, and may be substituted for it in many cases.  (See also the recipe for coughs, colds, hoarseness, etc., for the further value of St. John's wort.)

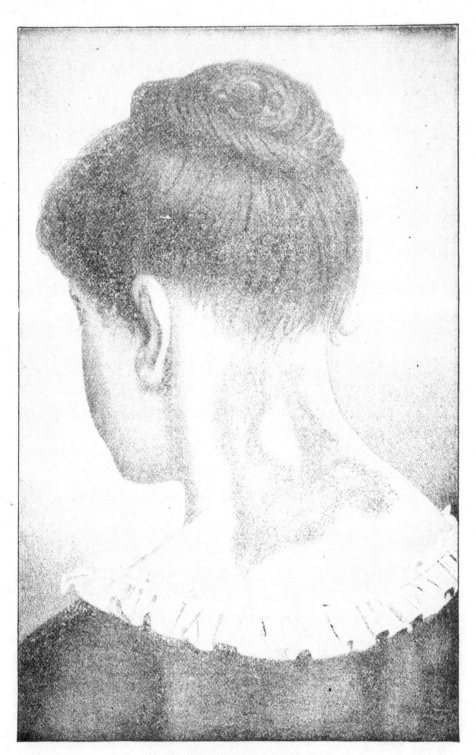

ECZEMA, OR SALT RHEUM.

**3. Salve or Ointment for Cuts, Sores and Cracks made in Husking, Salt-Rheum, Scurvey, Head Boils, etc.**—Mutton tallow, 3 lbs.; rosin, 1½ lbs.; sal-ammoniac (crystals),2 ozs.; sweet oil, 1 pt. DIRECTIONS —Melt the rosin and tallow together; dissolve sal-ammoniac in a little water, after having powdered it fine, then stir it into the mixture; put in the oil, or enough of it to reduce to a paste, or ointment, then place in boxes, or a jar that can be covered. To apply, it is best to keep a little of the sal-ammoniac dissolved in a little water, sufficient to give the water rather a sharp taste, and first wet the part to which the ointment is to be applied, with the sal-ammoniac water. The healing will be quick and satisfactory.

*Remarks.*—I obtained this from a Welsh blacksmith at Moawequa, Ill., who thought it had no equal in the world as a healing ointment, or salve, as he called it. It will be found valuable for cracked fingers in husking, as well as for general purposes.

**4. Itch Ointment, or Wash, Preferable to the Old Method.**— Quicklime (good stone lime, just slacked), 1 part; sulphur, 2 parts; water, 10 parts; by weight say ½ oz. of the lime, 1 oz. of the sulphur, and 5 ozs. of water, make the right proportions. DIRECTIONS—Boil together in a porcelain dish, stirring constantly with a stick, till it is the shade of cinnamon essence. When cool, bottle and keep corked. Apply a small quantity to the parts affected.

*Remarks.*—This is from Dr. A. B. Mason, who says of it: " It is much nicer to use than the old sulphur ointment: and will effect a cure with fewer applications." It can be relied upon.

**5. Ointment and Salve for General Purposes, Norton's.**— I. For the ointment, lard, 1 lb.; rosin, 5 ozs.; beeswax and gum camphor, each 2 ozs.; oil of origanum and spirits of turpentine, each 1 oz. DIRECTIONS —Melt the lard, rosin and beeswax together; break up the camphor gum as fine as you can, and when you remove the first from the fire, after all are melted, stir in the gum and continue to stir till the camphor gum is melted and all is quite cool; then put in the origanum and turpentine, and keep stirring until it sets, or stiffens; box, or put in a fruit can, and cover to exclude air.

*Remarks.*—" It is good, very good, for all general purposes," says my sister, Mrs. Norton, from whom I obtained it.

II. *For the Salve.*—Use 5 lbs. of rosin; and in place of the lard use 6 ozs. of mutton tallow; all the other ingredients as for the ointment, and melt; but as soon as the gum camphor is melted, and after having removed it from the fire, put in the oil and turpentine, and stir well for a minute or two; then pour into cold water, and pull and work the same as shoemaker's wax; then roll into sticks, and wrap each stick by itself.

*Remarks.*—Valuable as a strengthening salve or plaster to apply over all weaknesses, rheumatic and other pains, anywhere on body or limbs.

**6. Glycerine Ointment for Chapped Hands, Lips or Face, Chafes, Hemorrhoids, etc.**—Oil of sweet almond, 2 ozs.; spermaceti and white wax, each ½ oz.; best glycerine, 1 oz.; oil of rose, a little. DIRECTIONS —Melt the spermaceti and wax in the oil of almond by gentle heat; then stir in the glycerine and oil of rose, and put up in small jars or wide-mouthed bottles. In cold weather it must be warmed to apply. Keep covered or corked.

**6½. Balm of Gilead Ointment or Oil.**—Take any quantity of Balm of Gilead Buds, place them in a suitable dish for stewing, pour over them sufficient melted lard to cover them—or to make the Balm of Gilead Oil, pour the same quantity of sweet oil—stew thoroughly, then press out all of the oil from the buds, and bottle ready for use.

This will be found to be a very excellent ointment for cuts, bruises, etc., and the oil will also be found to be very healing.

**7. Salve, or Balsam, for Wounds, Cracks, or Internal Pains.** —Rosin, 2½ lbs.; spirits of turpentine, 1 qt.; balsam of fir, 4 ozs.; oil of hemlock, 2 ozs. DIRECTIONS—Melt the rosin, and remove from the fire; then, when a little cool, stir in the fir, turpentine, and last, the oil of hemlock, continuing to stir until cool enough to remain permanently mixed.

*Remarks.*—I saw this salve on the hands of a Mr. E. B. Mason, a farmer of Ann Arbor, Mich., upon cracks and a wound of considerable extent. Noticing its white appearance and adhesiveness, I inquired about it; he told me he had used it for several years, and thought it had no equal for wounds, sores, cracks from husking, etc., and also as a "plaster" over any internal pains whatever. He spoke of it so highly that I was induced to obtain it for my Third Book. I know it must be valuable; but I think it will prove too soft for hot weather. Then to use only half of the spirits of turpentine and possibly ½ lb. more rosin is all the modification needed to adapt it as a plaster to be applied to other parts of the body. It would be very valuable to wear over a sore breast, whether from strain or soreness of the lungs. See also the Centennial Recipes from "Poor Will's" Almanac, at the close of this department, for an ointment for these purposes.

**8. Salve for Inflamed Wounds, From Taking Cold in Them.** —Lard, 8 ozs., melted 3 or 4 times, and cooled each time in cold water (vaseline or cosmoline is now used without the purification, and will do as well, and possibly better,); then stew in it 2 fair sized onions sliced, and strain. This is an excellent salve for inflamed wounds. Apply twice or thrice daily, as needed. Twice is enough unless excessive ulceration, or running of considerable matter

**9. Salve, Carbolic, for Burns, Sores, etc.**—Lard, 10 ozs.; white wax, 5 ozs.; balsam of fir and carbolic acid, each 1 oz. DIRECTIONS—Melt the lard and wax together, then add the fir, and when it begins to thicken, by cooling, stir in the carbolic acid, and put up in tin boxes, or a suitable jar, covered tightly for use.

*Remarks.*—The balsam of fir is very soothing and healing, and makes the salve stick better to burns or other open sores, at the same time it hides the disagreeable odor of the carbolic acid  Many persons think there is no salve equal to those made with the carbolic acid.  I think vaseline, 10 ozs., would be better than the lard as above given.

**10. Salve, or Ointment, Green, for Old Sores, Ulcers, Cancers, etc.**—Rosin and beeswax, each 1 oz.; mutton tallow or lard, 4 ozs.; pulverized verdigris, 1 dr. DIRECTIONS—Melt the two first together and stir in the verdigris, stirring till cold. Dress the sores, ulcers or wounds, above named, morning and evening, after cleaning them properly with castile soap, if necessary, and apply a mixture of equal parts of tinctures of myrrh, aloes and blood-root. And if any fungus (proud flesh), sprinkle on powdered blood-root or finely pulverized burned alum, then the salve, or more properly, the ointment.

*Remarks.*—Dr. Gunn thinks this a very valuable treatment, especially for old or long standing ulcers.

**11. Salve or Poultice, Robinson's, for Sores, Inflammation, etc.**—Scrape plenty of raw potatoes and thicken it with finely pulverized charcoal. Apply freely to the sore, or inflamed part, and renew as often as it becomes dry, or once in 3 or 4 hours.

*Remarks.*—It cured a boy's leg which had been injured in such a way as to cause a large sore and extensive swelling, becoming so bad the doctors expected amputation would be necessary; but a neighbor recommended this salve, or poultice, which cured and saved the leg. Then it will do it for others too.

II. A flaxseed poultice thickened with pulverized charcoal will prevent the spreading, or extension, of mortification, separating the mortified parts from the healthy, at least it did this once on my own person, when only a boy, where one of my feet, and some of the toes, had been badly crushed by a threshing machine and mortification set in. Fail not to try one or the other, as occasion may demand.

**12. Pumpkin Poultice for Painful Inflammations, Swellings, etc.**—A correspondent of the New York Farmers' Club, published in the *American Agriculturist,* gives an instance in which a woman's arm was swollen to an enormous size and painfully inflamed. A poultice was made of stewed pumpkins, which was renewed every 15 minutes, and in a short time produced a perfect cure. The fever drawn out by the poultices made them extremely offensive as they were taken off.

*Remarks.*—In such cases after the inflammation is reduced by the poultices some good, mild liniment, like Mrs. Chase's, should be applied from time to time, for the purpose of strengthening, healing, etc.

**13. Salve and Other Treatment—For Quinsy and Gathered Breast.**—I. Obtain oil of spike, sweet-oil, British oil and spirits of turpentine, each 1 oz. Put lard, 1 pt., over the fire in a suitable dish, and burn or heat it till it is a brown color, then remove from the fire, and, when cool enough to allow the finger in it, add the oils and mix well.

II Take oats, 1 gal., and put in a kettle, with vinegar to cover, and boil; then fill two woolen stockings with the boiled oats, and sew up, and keep steaming hot, or as hot as can be borne, upon the neck; now grease the throat thoroughly with the salve, and apply one of the stockings to drive in the salve, changing every 10 minutes, greasing well each change until the sweating is kept up 2 or 2½ hours; then wash off with soda in warm water, change all damp clothing, and allow a good rest. It may be repeated next day, if needed, but seldom will be. It is equally good for gathered breasts; but in either case be careful not to take cold.

**14. Weak Back, Valuable Plaster for.**—Burgundy pitch and camphor gum, each 1 oz.; opium, 1 dr. DIRECTIONS—Melt the pitch, and having broken up the camphor, and made the opium gum into as fine bits as you can, stir them in and see that they are dissolved and evenly mixed. Spread the plaster very thinly on soft leather; wash the back with vinegar as hot as it can be borne; then rub the parts with dry flannel to make it red, and apply the plaster hot, and wear it as long as needed, renewing, if necessary. Remember this, in applying a plaster to any place, if there is any hair where it is to be applied, always clip it off as close as possible, or shave it off, as thought best. A bandage will have to be worn with this, as it will work out and soil the clothing without it.

*Remarks.*—I obtained this recipe from Mr. Moross, of this city (Toledo), a grocer, who said he was cured by it, after he had tried all the doctors, been to Saratoga for a season, etc., without benefit. And he also assured me that he had given it to others who were very bad (the doctor claiming disease of the the kidneys); one who had tried everything and was going home to die, by using this plaster became a well man. I have tried it personally and find it valuable, and deem it worthy of great confidence. I would suggest, however, that the addition of 1 oz. of rosin to this salve would prevent its running, without injuring its value.

**15. Counter-Irritation, Croton Oil for.**—In cases of chronic sore throat, lung coughs, asthma, bronchitis, consumption, inflammation of the liver, spleen, etc., as a counter-irritant, the following will be found very satisfactory: Croton oil, 1 dr.; spirits of turpentine, 2 drs.; mix. DIRECTIONS—Which be careful to follow: With the finger rub on the mixture thoroughly, covering a space about the size of a silver dollar, or larger, as deemed best, from the amount of cough, or soreness over the part affected, 4 to 6 times; the finger should carry enough for the size of the dollar. In about 12 to 24 hours, the skin becomes red, and slight pimples arise, but if they do not rise in 36 hours rub on again in the same manner, but not quite so freely. These pimples will ripen into pustules, and fill with water, or a thick yellow matter, according to the condition of the system, and must be opened with a needle, and the matter pressed out and carefully wiped off with a soft cloth, then washed with soap suds (castile is best), and this filling and refilling ought to go on for 3 to 6 days. Wash every night and morning, or at least once daily, according to the amount of matter, or itching which may occur. As this crop discontinues to run make another application as near to the first as you can, and continue this as long as needed.

*Remarks.*—The above mixture makes a mild and bearable sore; while the croton-oil alone, as formerly used, makes ugly sores and causes terrible itching or sharp burning pain, and so does the old Irritating Plaster, which is not necessary to produce the desired effect. This raises only in pimples, while the old Irritating plaster ulcerates the whole surface, and is very tedious and troublesome to be borne. Dr. Sykes, of Chicago, makes great use of this mixture, wherever and whenever needed, and I have used it with much satisfaction.

**16. Spiced Plaster or Poultice, to Remove and Prevent Nausea and Vomiting.** — Ginger, cloves, cinnamon, and black pepper, each ½ oz.; cayenne pepper, ½ dr.; all these in fine powder; tinct. of ginger, ½oz.; sufficient strained honey or molasses to make it to the consistency of a poultice—rather stiff; apply over the stomach.

**17. Itch, Valuable Ointment for.** — Lard, ¼ lb.; sulphur. ½ oz.; white precipitate and benzoic acid, each ½ dr.; sulphuric acid and oil of bergamot, each ½ fl. dr.; saltpeter, 1 dr. DIRECTIONS — Have the saltpeter in powder; melt the lard, remove from the fire, and pour into an earthen dish; then put in the other ingredients, stirring till cold. Anoint well, night and morning, until cured, which it is sure to do, as it kills the itch-mite, which burrows in the skin and causes the itch.

**18. Healing Ointment or Black Salve for Inflammations, Wounds, Ulcers, Burns, Etc.** — Olive-oil, 1¼ lbs.; bees-wax and unsalted butter, each 2 ozs.; white pine pitch, called also white turpentine, 4 ozs.; red lead, ½ lb.; honey, 6 ozs.; powdered camphor gum, 4 ozs. DIRECTIONS— Put the olive-oil into a suitable kettle, place on a stove, and bring it to a boiling heat (remembering that it takes nearly 3 times the heat to boil oil that it does to boil water); then, the lead being in fine powder, stir it in, as you would make "mush," and continue the heat, and stirring till it becomes a shining black or deep brown. Remove from the fire, the bees-wax being shaved finely, stir it in; then the other ingredients, the powdered camphor last. Spread on a cloth and apply.

**19. Stimulating Ointment for Cold Feet, caused by Sweating in Consumption and other Exhausting Diseases.**—Oil of butter, 1 pt.; oil of bergamot and strong tinct. of capsicum, each 1 oz. DIRECTIONS—To make the oil of butter, take sufficient butter and put into a kettle of water, boil well and stir; then set off till next day, and take the oily butter off the water, put in the tincture of capsicum and simmer, to evaporate what water is in it; when cool stir in the oil of bergamot. Box tightly, or put into a large mouthed bottle, for use. Rub on a tea-spoonful of this, night and morning, and heat into the bottoms of the feet and palms of the hands, which will soften them, remove all hardened skin, etc. By its stimulation it helps to relieve their tendencies to sweating and also of a sense of heat, or burning, which is sometimes very annoying.

**20. Magnetic Ointment, for Burns, Cuts, Sores, etc.**—Make the same as the above, except by using the oil of origanum in place of the tincture of capsicum.

*Remarks.*—This and the stimulating ointment will be found very reliable for what they are recommended; this last for all purposes of healing and soft-ening old sores as well as fresh cuts, bruises, burns, etc.

**21. Salve or Ointment, for Barber's Itch and Other Sores of a Chronic and Malignant Character.**—A Mrs. H. J. Merrill, of Toledo, O., gives me the following, which she had used many years, with great success, on all bad sores of long standing, and of an irritable character: Cleanse the sore well with warm castile soap suds, dry carefully with soft cloths and apply sparingly at first, as it will "bite," to show its power over the disease. Gunpowder, sulphur and alum, each, powdered, 2 table-spoonfuls; unsalted lard, or fresh made unsalted butter, ½ pt. DIRECTIONS—Put into an earthen dish and stew on the back of the stove for 24 hours, strain and box for use.

**1. ITCHING (Prurigo), TO CURE — Magical.**—Dilute (the medici-nal) hydrocyanic acid and sugar of lead, each 2 drs.; alcohol, 3 ozs.; distilled or soft water, 1 pt. DIRECTIONS—Dissolve the lead in the water, then add the acid and shake well, then the alcohol. Wet cloths and lay upon the itching parts, or apply with the finger, as the case will allow, frequently.

*Remarks.*—The acid is poisonous, hence keep it out of the way of children. It is claimed to be magical in its quick relief of itching of any part, but not upon open sores nor where the skin is broken. It is perfectly safe to use, when so extensively diluted as this is.

**2. Itching in Leucorrhœal Cases, etc.**-More recently in these cases of prurigo, or itching of the external parts, the following has been used con-siderably, and, it it claimed, successfully: Bi-sulphide, or bi-sulphite, of soda and soft water, each 2 ozs.; glycerine, 3 ozs.; mix and apply frequently, with cloths, if the patient is confined to bed, to be laid upon the parts.

**3. Itching, or Prurigo, Ointment for.**—My old friend, Dr. T. B. King, of Toledo, O., takes: Oxide of zinc ointment, 1 oz.; camphor gum, 20 grs., grind to a fine powder, with a few drops of alcohol, and mixed in, then 12 to 15 grs. of red precipitate, also rubbed into the zinc ointment. Rub a little upon the parts, and if a fold of the skin or flesh comes together and chafes, a little of the ointment upon a soft cloth and put between, soon relieves.

**4. Ointment for Chafing, Itching or Prurigo.**—Camphor gum and white wax, each 1 oz.; mutton tallow, 2 ozs.; red precipitate and oxide of zinc, each 3 drs.; tannic acid, 1 dr. DIRECTIONS—Triturate the camphor gum with a little alcohol, melt the tallow and wax by gentle heat, and stir, and rub all together thoroughly till cool. Used as above, or as for regular itch.

*Remarks.*—When it can be obtained, the oil from 4 ounces of freshly made unsalted butter in place of the mutton tallow is preferable. (To make oil of butter see stimulating ointment, etc.)

**1. CHAPPED HANDS, LIPS, CHAFES, ETC.**—Cold Cream of Glycerine and Rose for.—A cream, or liquid, for the above purposes is made by using 1 oz. of white melted wax; 4 ozs. of glycerine, with oil of rose or other flavor to suit, 4 or 5 drops, to flavor.

**2. Hands, to Soften, Remove Tan, Freckles, etc.**—Lemon juice and glycerine, equal parts, say 1 oz. of each, will not only soften the hands, but will remove tan, or sun-burn, and also freckles, by frequent applications. For freckles, however, I should add ½ to 1 dr. of powdered borax, which will not injure it for the other purposes. (See moles, freckles, pimples, etc.)

**1. AUSTRALIAN TREATMENT OF RUNNING OR OLD SORES.**—Wash them in brandy and apply elder leaves, changing twice a day. This will dry up all the sores, though the legs were like a honey-comb. Or, poultice them with rotten apples, but take also a purge once or twice every week.

**1. WHITLOW.—New Zealand Remedy for.**—The severity of the inflammation in whitlow varies considerably; there is the mild form, which generally yields to fomentation with hot water cloths or poultices; and if matter forms, if relieved by the lancet, it speedily heals; but there is a much more formidable affection, in which the deep textures of the finger are involved accompanied by severe pain, throbbing, and much redness, heat and swelling. This form is only to be relieved by free and early incisions with the lancet; for if this be neglected, the bones will become affected and will be destroyed. It would therefore be advisable to submit the finger to the inspection of a surgeon when it does not easily yield to fomentations or a poultice. (NOTE—The above most excellent remedies were sent the publishers in March, 1901.)

**1. NERVOUSNESS AND SLEEPLESSNESS.—New and Successful Remedy.**—Wm. A. Hammond, M. D., states that he has recently used the bromide of calcium (lime, from the Latin calx, lime), in a number of cases in which the bromides were indicated, and is satisfied of its great efficacy. He says:

"The dose is from 15 to 30 grs. or more for an adult. It is especially useful in those cases in which speedy action is desirable, as, owing to its instability, the bromine is readily set free, and its peculiar action on the organism obtained more promptly than when either of the other bromides is administered. Chief among these effects is its hypnotic (sleep producing) influence, and hence the bromide of calcium is particularly beneficial in cases of delirium tremens, or in the insomnia (inability to sleep) resulting from intense mental labor or excitement.

"I gave a single dose of 30 grains of this to a gentleman, who, owing to business anxieties, had not slept for several nights, and who was in a state of great excitement. He soon fell into a sound sleep, which lasted for 7 hours. The next night, as he was wakeful, I gave him a like dose of bromide of potassium, but it was without effect, and he remained awake the whole night. The subsequent night he was as indisposed to sleep as he had ever been, but a dose of 30 grains of bromide of calcium gave him 8 hours sound sleep, and he awoke refreshed with all unpleasant cerebral (head) symptoms—pain, vertigo, and confusion of ideas—entirely gone.

"In a number of other instances a single dose has sufficed to induce sleep —a result which very rarely follows the administration of one dose of any of the other bromides. [Then, of course, it is better than the others, as formerly used.]

"In those exhausted conditions of the nervous system attended with great irritability, such as are frequently met with in hysterical women, and which are indicated by headache, vertigo, insomnia and a mental condition of extreme excitement, bromide of calcium has proved in my hands of decided service. Combined with the syrup of the lacto-phosphate (milky phosphate) of lime, it scarcely leaves anything to be desired. An eligible formula is: Bromide of calcium (lime), 1 oz.; syrup of lacto-phosphate of lime, 4 ozs.; mix. DOSE—A tea-spoonful 3 times a day in a little water.

" In epilepsy I have thus far seen no reason for preferring it to the bromide of potassium or sodium, except in those cases in which the paroxysms are very frequent, or in cases occurring in very young infants; of these latter, several which had previously resisted the bromide of potassium, have yielded to the bromide of calcium. It does not appear to cause acne (a pustular affection of the skin) to anything like the extent of the bromide of potassium or sodium." *New York Medical Journal.*

**2. Sleeplessness, Simple Remedy, but Successful With Many.**—For those troubled with sleeplessness from literary labor, or other disturbances of the nervous system, a writer of experience says, " Just before retiring eat 2 or 3 small raw onions, with a little bread, lightly spread with fresh butter, which will produce the desired effect, saving the stupefying action of drugs."

*Remarks.*—This plan of eating raw onions has not only been satisfactorily tried to obtain sleep, but eating them once or twice daily with the meals has also proved valuable to those troubled with dyspepsia.

**3. Wooing Morpheus—The God of Sleep or Dreams.**—Wet half a towel, apply it to the back of the neck, pressing it upward to the base of the brain, and fasten the dry half of the towel over so as to prevent the too rapid evaporation. The effect is prompt and charming, cooling the brain and inducing calmer, sweeter sleep than any narcotic. Warm water may be used, though most persons prefer cold. To those suffering from over excitement of the brain, whether the result of brain work or pressing anxiety, this simple remedy is an especial boon.

**4. Sleep, Amount Needed by Different Persons.**—It has been found that tall and corpulent persons require more sleep than those of thin and spare habit of body. In health, generally, from 6 to 8 hours of sleep are required to restore the nervous energy exhausted by the labors of the day. At first, upon retiring, always lie upon the right side, to allow the easier and more ready passage of the food, as digested, from the stomach; and especially eat nothing heavy and hard to digest at supper—a light supper is far preferable and absolutely necessary to enjoy good health. If half sick, or debilitated persons can take 9 hours sleep it will be all the better for them.

**5. Sleep as a Medicine.**—A physician says: The cry for rest (sleep) has always been louder than the cry for food. Not that it is more important, but that it is often harder to obtain. The best rest comes from sound sleep. Of two men and women, otherwise equal, the one who sleeps the best will be the most moral, healthy, and efficient. Sleep will do much to cure irritability of temper, peevishness and uneasiness. It will restore to vigor an over-worked brain. It will build up and make strong a weary body. It will cure a head ache. It will cure a broken spirit. It will cure sorrow. Indeed, we might make a long list of nervous and other maladies that sleep will cure. The cure of sleeplessness requires a clean, good bed, sufficient exercise to produce weariness, pleasant occupation, good air, and avoidance of stimulants and narcotics. For those who are over worked, haggard, nervous, who pass sleepless nights, we recommend the adoption of such habits as shall secure sleep, otherwise life will be short, and what there is of it sadly imperfect.

*Remarks.*—It is claimed by many scientific men that it is best to always lie with the head to the north, on account of the fact—a supposed fact, at least,—that there is an electric current passing through the system when one is lying down, whether awake or asleep, and that its influence is best with the head to the north. Invalids, at least, had better do it, if the situation of their room will allow it. Lying with the head a little the highest prevents considerably the flow of blood to the head, and, therefore, induces sleep. A hot foot-bath, with mustard in it, on retiring, draws the blood from the head and aids in getting sleep; and sponging the whole length of the spine with hot water for 15 minutes just before going to bed often ensures a good night's sleep; active exercise in the open air, or a brisk walk, are great helps to this end—procuring a good night's sleep; but opium, chloral, or spirits of any kind, only tend to sleeplessness, rather than sleep, hence should never be resorted to, from the danger of establishing a habit which can not be overcome. It has been generally believed that fish furnished a large amount of brain food, or phosphorus; but this, of late, is considered to be an error, as it is now believed they do not have any excess of phosphorus over other animals. From the length this subject has reached, I trust I may be excused for closing it with an item to amuse rather than for any particular benefit which may be derived from it; yet, in one sense, it may do good to that class of persons who consider fun better than physic, and hence I trust that the subject of "brain tissue," as put forth by the *Springfield Republican* below, under the head of "Fun better than Physic," will be read with satisfaction. It says:

"There is a party, fat and stout
　　As any Turk on Bosphorus,
Who at our dinner table sits,
And ne'er his babble intermits,
But prates of mush and wheaten grits,
　　And ' mean amount of phosphorus.'

"He always airs his favorite theme,
　　Nor cares a penny's toss for us,
But rails at beef with ' Pooh!' and ' Pish!'
And calls for cod and other fish,
Hoping to gain—his dearest wish—
　　' The mean amount of phosphorus.'

"Oh! that he'd change his boarding place—
　　'Twould surely be no loss for us—
But there's one consolation yet,
His star, ascendant, soon will set,
Some time he'll die, and then he'll get
　　' His full amount of phosphorus.' "

**1. CROUP.—Instantaneous Relief—Internal Remedy.**—It is claimed that alum and sugar will cure croup in one minute, by shaving or grating off 1 tea-spoonful of the alum and mixing it with twice as much sugar, and giving it at once, the relief being almost instantaneous. Half these amounts may be repeated once or twice, ½ hour apart, if the relief is not permanent.

**2. Croup, External Remedy.**—Saturating (thoroughly wetting) flannel with spirits of turpentine, and placing upon the throat and chest, has the credit of being a sovereign remedy, *i. e.*, effectual in controlling the disease. If considerable distress is manifested when the child wakes up, and after the flannel has been applied a few minutes, 3 to 5 drops of turpentine may be given on a lump of sugar. Every family should keep turpentine in the house.

**3. Croup, Emetic for.**—If the foregoing fail in any case, an emetic may be given, of fl. ex. of ipecac, 5 or 6 drops, every 5 or 6 minutes, for a child of 4 years, giving warm water after 2 or 3 doses have been given, continuing the fluid extract as at first, until vomiting takes place, which will occur generally by the time 5 or 6 doses have been taken; a little more, or a little less, for older or younger children.

**4. Croup, Instantaneous Emetic for.**—Two tea-spoonfuls of mustard mixed in 3 or 4 table-spoonfuls of warm water, for a child with croup, relieves at once by causing vomiting. A tea-spoonful of lard warmed and given is also said to be an instantaneous emetic. Either may be repeated if necessary.

**5. Croup, Onions a Sure Cure for.**—A lady who speaks from experience, says: That probably 9 children out of 10 who die of croup might be saved by the timely application of roasted onions, mashed and laid upon a napkin, and a small quantity of goose oil, sweet oil, or even lard, put on and applied as hot as can be borne comfortably to the throat and upper part of the chest, and to the feet and hands.

*Remarks.*—The application of the roasted onions, with only a little oil upon them, to the throat and upper part of the breast will be very good; but, upon the feet and hands I should not apply any oil, as the object there is to draw the blood to these extremities, and hence it will be more drawing without the oil. Use such internal remedies also as the case seems to demand, and as are at hand. See the use of the juice of onions with sugar (making an onion syrup), for internal use in children's colds. I have no doubt of its value for croup, as well as colds and coughs.

**6. Croup, Instant Relief for.**—Dr. Bachelder, in the *Journal of Chemistry*, says: "Croup is relieved instantly with a solution of hydrochloric (muriatic) acid, about the strength of cider vinegar." This would be about ¼ oz. of the muriatic acid, as now more generally called, to 4 ozs. of water. It is often used as a gargle of this strength for elongated palate, sore mouth and sore throat in scarlet fever, etc. The doctor adds: "As far as my experience goes, this acid solution stops all morbid development in the throat as surely as the hoe will stop pig-weeds on a hot, sunny day. Apply it to the throat with a brush or sponge, or use as a gargle, if the child is old enough."

**7. Croup, Preventive of.**—For children who have a tendency to croup, or throat difficulties, get a piece of chamois skin, make it like a little bib, cut out the neck and sew on tapes to tie it on; then melt together some tallow and pine pitch, rub some of this in the chamois, and let the child wear it all the time. Renew with the mixture occasionally.

*Remarks.*—This will be found very valuable, as it will prevent the penetration of wind to the breast, keep the parts warm, and also impart the medical properties of the pitch, by absorption, to the system. About equal parts of tallow and pitch will be proper, or tallow enough to prevent it from sticking to the skin, as common plasters do.

**8. Croup, Diphtheria and Sore Throat, to Avert.**—The New York *Evening Post* recently made the following sensible remarks upon the necessity of watching the childrens feet. It says:

"A life-long discomfort or a sudden death, often come to children through the inattention or carelessness of the parents. A child should never be allowed to go to sleep with cold feet; the thing to be last attended to is to see that the feet are dry and warm. Neglect of this has often resulted in dangerous attacks of croup, diphtheria or a fatal sore throat. Always on coming from school, on entering the house from a visit or errand in rainy, muddy or thawy weather, the child should remove its shoes, and the mother should herself ascertain whether the stockings are the least damp. If they are, they should be taken off, the feet held before the fire and rubbed with the hands till perfectly dry, and another pair of stockings and another pair of shoes put on. The reserve shoes and stockings should be kept where they are dry, so as to be ready for use on a minute's notice."

**1. HEADACHE, TO CURE.**—Take a quart bottle and nearly fill it with water, then put in spirits of hartshorn and spirits of camphor, each 1 oz., and 1 table-spoonful of salt; shake well to dissolve the salt; then wet cloths with this and apply to the head, and renew as often as they become hot until relieved. If the stomach is sour, causing the headache, taking a little bi-carbonate of soda (baking soda) in water, may help in its cure.

**2. Sick Headache, Tea and Coffee Often the Cause.**—A distinguished doctor of New York, a man of wide experience, says of sick headache:

"Not a case of this disease has ever occurred within my knowledge, except with the drinkers of narcotic drinks (referring to tea and coffee), and not a case has failed of being cured on the entire renunciation of those drinks. Whatever may be said of the violations of physical law in other respects, tea and coffee may claim sick headache as their highly-favored representative."

Dr. Alcott, in writing on this subject, says: "We are driven to the conclusion that no person can use the smallest quantity of tea or coffee, or, in fact, of any drink but pure water, without more or less deranging the action of the stomach and liver, and ultimately, through these, the nerves and brain, of the whole system. Nay, we are driven to a position stronger still, which is, that no person can take these poisons at all, without, in a greater or less degree, abridging human happiness and human life."—*Christian Advocate.*

*Remarks.*—That the above is the general opinion of our best physicians and other scientific men, there is not a doubt. For my own part I know that the giving up of tea and coffee, and substituting half milk, and half water, for a few weeks at one time, did me much good. For great lovers of tea and coffee, among my patients, I have insisted that they take them of only half the usual strength, especially with those who have frequent headaches, and I claim it would be better for all; but I do believe that some warm drink, for general use, and taking tea or coffee of half the usual strength, as I now do, may be allowed, if not more than one cup is taken at a meal.

**3. Headache and Toothache, Ely's Magic Remedy for.—** Alcohol, the best, 8 ozs.: aqua ammonia, 2 ozs.; English oil of lavender,1 dr.; camphor gum, ½ oz.; chloroform, 1 oz.; sulphuric ether, ½ oz.; spirits of turpentine, 1 dr.; mix. DIRECTIONS—Smell it, changing from nostril to nostril, for a few minutes, and also bathe the head with it. Keep this up a short time, or until relieved, which must be quickly.

*For Toothache.*—Put cotton wet with it into the tooth, and also apply around the gums and front of ears, where the nerves pass near the surface. It is really magical in its action. Keep the finger over the bottle when not inhaling, as it is quite evaporative.

**4. Headache, Heartburn, etc., Remedy.—**A tea-spoonful of bi-carbonate of soda (baking soda) in 3 or 4 table-spoonfuls of peppermint, or cinnamon water, with ½ tea-spoonful of powdered ginger, or a little essence of Jamaica ginger added, and taken immediately after each meal, will generally remedy this in a few days. A dose of this, and repeated in an hour, will be good in headache arising from acidity of the stomach. If the regularly prepared water (cinnamon or peppermint) are not on hand, put ½ tea-spoonful of either of the essences in water, with the powdered ginger, or essence of ginger and the soda; or plain water will do, only not quite so pleasant.

**5. Heart Burn, Remedy for.—**Magnesia, ¾ oz.; pulverized Turkish rhubarb, 1 dr.; cinnamon water, 1 oz.; distilled, or soft water, 4 ozs.; spirits of lavender, 1 dr. DOSE—A tablespoonful half an hour after each meal.

**Heart, Palpitation of, Fluttering, etc., Remedies.—**When persons become weak and feeble, from whatever cause, there is often a palpitation or fluttering of the heart, as many call it, from this weakness. In such cases take any of our good alteratives and tonics to improve the condition of the system, as per directions; and besides this obtain fl. ex. of *cereus bonplandi* (a species of the cactus), ½ oz. DOSE—Take 10 drops, at bed-time only, in a little water, and generally relief will be realized soon and the cure permanent. At least, I have so proved it. Continue to use the tonic remedies as long as needed.

**7. Heart Disease, the Value of Buttermilk.—**In diseases of the heart the French claim that buttermilk is invaluable; as the lactic acid in it dissolves and prevents ossification (bone-like condition) of the valves, arteries, cartilages, etc.

*Remarks.*—It is worthy of a trial, and no doubt will prove valuable if continued faithfully for several months.

**1. CASTOR OIL—Its Nauseous and Disgusting Taste Overcome.—**I. A little glycerine (half the amount of the castor oil) mixed with castor oil, and 5 to 10 drops of any of the aromatic oils, as sassafrass, wintergreen, etc., put into the dose, the natural taste of the oil will scarcely be perceived; or,

II. Take the juice of a lemon or two, put a few drops of essence of cinnamon into it. Heat the oil and stir into the lemon juice, which forms an emulsion, and almost wholly covers the taste of the oil.

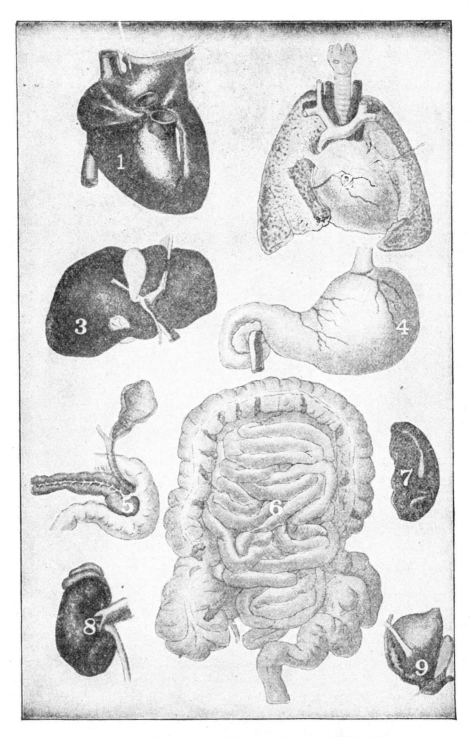

1, Heart.   2, Showing Trachea, Lungs and Heart.   3, Liver and Gall Bladder.   4, Stomach.
5, Pancreas and Gall Bladder.   6, Large and Small Intestines.   7, Spleen.
8, Kidney.   9, Bladder.

**2. Castor Oil Custard.**—Prof. King says: "I find it a very pleasant mode of administration, to boil the dose of oil with about a gill of sweet milk for a few minutes, sweeten with loaf sugar, and flavor with essence of cinnamon or other favorite aromatic; it somewhat resembles custard in its taste and appearance, and is readily taken by even the most delicate stomach."

*Remarks.*—This is certainly very desirable with children and delicate females, for whom it is often the best cathartic which can be given.

**1. CONSUMPTION, TROUBLESOME COUGH IN—Syrup and Tincture as Used in Charity Hospital, New York.**—I. Cough syrup: Bromide of potassium, chlorate of potassium, muriate of ammonia, each, 1¼ drs.; syrup of tolu, 4 oz.; mix. DOSE — One table-spoonful every 2 or 3 hours.

II. Cough Tincture: Paregoric, 1 oz.; tincture belladonna, 1 dr.; tincture of *hyoscyamus*, 2 drs.; compound spirits lavender, 1 dr.; mix. DOSE—Ten drops on a lump of loaf sugar every hour until cough is relieved.

*Remarks.*—For the hacking, or continuous coughing of patients far gone with consumption, either of these will be found satisfactory. But as prevention is better than cure for those who are liable to have consumption, but have not got it fastened upon them yet, I will give the rules of the celebrated Dr. S. S. Fitch, of New York, for its prevention, as they are certainly valuable and ought to be heeded by every one. He claims an absolute preventive in all cases and all persons, but as his rules are so very strict, if they are lived up to, they will certainly do much to prevent the establishment of this disease. They are as follows:

**2. Pulmonary Consumption—Absolute Prevention of—Dr. S. S. Fitch's Rules for.**—He says: "There is no disease to which we are liable that is so preventable as consumption. It is absolutely preventable in all cases and all persons.

I. "From earliest childhood stand erect, walk erect, sit erect, never stoop, always let the weight of the shoulders fall behind you.

II. "Keep your chest fully expanded by taking constantly, all your life long, full breaths so as to fully expand your chest. Do this at all times. Remember you can not have consumption until your chest shrinks in size, either wholly or partially; so if you keep your chest flexible and constantly expanded you will be safe from consumption.

III. "Never let a cold run on you. Break it at once by taking active physic and cough medicines, and putting your feet at bedtime in hot water; keep them in until you get in a perspiration, and then go to bed and keep up the perspiration with hot drinks (Thompson's old " Composition Tea " is one of the best to use to start perspiration; hot lemonade is good, too); then take a portion of physic, and the next day your cold will be well. By pursuing this course for a length of time you get out of the habit of taking cold, and will rarely take one. Always continue your treatment until your cold is well.

IV. "Avoid all debauching courses that weaken and reduce your constitution, such as soaking with liquor and actual drunkenness and dissipation of all kinds and gluttony and late night exposures.   In fact, lead an honest, orderly life, free from vice and every dissipation, your health will then be equal, regular and constant, and your life a long and happy one.

V.  "Keep your bowels always free by habit, diet or purgatives."

*Remarks.*—If these rules are strictly enforced, by parents, with their children, when small, and by themselves, as soon as they can be made to understand their importance, very much will be done to improve the general health, as well as to prevent consumption.   None are too old to take counsel from Rules IV. and V., and I might say also from Rule III.

**3.   Consumption Cured After Twelve Years' Suffering, Living About Sixty Years After the Cure.**—The transactions of the Connecticut State Medical Society contains the following paper from Professor S. G. Hubbard, of New Haven, in relation to the cure of the late Rev. Jeremiah Day, former President of Yale College, of tubercular consumption.   He says: "President Day, during early life, gave little promise of long life, and when, in 1789, in his 17th year, he entered Yale College, he was soon compelled to leave by pulmonary difficulty.   He rallied, however, and was able to finish the course and graduate in 1795.   He was very feeble, however, for many years. He became a clergyman, and in 1801 was elected Professor of Mathematics and Natural History in the college.   But he could not undertake the duties.   An alarming hemorrhage of the lungs prostrated him, which was treated learnedly by bleedings copious enough to have charmed even Dr. Sangrado.   He went to Bermuda, where he was plied with digitalis to such an extent as almost to take what little life he had left.   He came back to his native town, Washington, Conn., to die.

"He suffered from continued hemorrhage and repeated venesections (bleedings), which was 'all the go' at that time with the allopaths, for almost every disease.   He met Dr. Sheldon, of Litchfield, who had made the treatment with iron a hobby, and who expressed a belief that Mr. Day could be helped. Though the case was regarded as hopeless, the patient was placed under the care of Dr. Sheldon, who treated him with iron and calisaya (Peruvian) bark, feeding him carefully with wholesome food.   Under this regimen he soon exhibited symptoms of improvement and finally, in 1803, returned home as one restored from the dead, in sufficient vigor to be inaugurated in the Professorship.   He never afterwards exhibited symptoms of pulmonary disease, although he had been affected by it for more than twelve years.   He lived till August, 1867, and was 95 years old at the time of his death.   The cavity of the thorax was examined to ascertain the traces of his former malady   The lungs were everywhere free from tubercles and were apparently healthy.   In the apex (top) of each lung was found a dense corrugated (wrinkled) circular cicatrix (hardened scar) an inch and a half or more in diameter; also a third circular cicatrix (a scar as if remaining from a wound) on the left side of the left lung, a few inches below the apex (top), each involving such a depth of tissue as to indicate that the *vomicæ* (abscess, or hole from ulceration), of which they were the remains, had been large and of long duration.   Both lungs were slightly adherent at the apex.

" Here, then," remarks Prof. Hubbard, "was all that remained to mark the beginning, progress and cure of a case of tubercular consumption, occupying twelve years in its period of activity. A legible record surpassing in interest and importance, to the human race, those of the slabs of Nineveh or the Punic inscriptions."—*Peninsular Courier* (Ann Arbor, Mich., Oct. 1st, 1885.)

*Remarks.*—This publication in the *Courier* was within about a year of the death of President Day. The paper having been prepared by Prof. Hubbard soon after the president's death, and published in one of the New Haven papers, from which I obtained it, as I, at that time, published the *Courier*. And in looking over the bound volume of that year, after commencing to write this book, I was so forcibly struck with the "Medical Incident," as the paper was originally headed, I wrote to Prof. Hubbard to see if I could ascertain anything more definite as to Dr. Sheldon's treatment of the case. The professor answered my letter by saying, so far as he knew, "there was no record of the prescription or any part of the treatment." But, thinking it possible that there might be some one in Litchfield—Dr. Sheldon's home—who might have some knowledge of it, I wrote to the postmaster there, and found a Mrs. Lucy Beach, a daughter of Dr. Sheldon—the doctor having also passed away,—but there was no further knowledge to be obtained, no record having been made of the treatment. And all I can say further is, if iron and Peruvian bark would and did (of which I have not a doubt) cure President Day, it—the combination, properly made—will cure others. The compound tinct. of Peruvian bark, 1 pt., into which put pyrophosphate of iron, 2 drs., taken in 1 to 2 table-spoonful doses, just before or just after meals and at bed-time, will fill the bill, and I have not a doubt will cure very many cases, especially if the careful feeding with wholesome food is properly attended to, as Dr. Sheldon above indicates he did with President Day, to which I should add plenty of out-door exercise, with every other needed care of the general system. But remember that in President Day's case it took two years to accomplish the cure. So don't get discouraged and give it up for one year, at least. There is now a proprietary, or patent medicine kept by druggists, known as Elixir of Calisaya (which is Peruvian bark) and Iron, that may answer all purposes. It was not made in Dr. Sheldon's time. I have often recommended its use for frail and weakly females, and always with success. Still, I should prefer the compound tinct. of the bark and iron above directed, if the tincture has 2 ozs. of the unground red Peruvian bark used in making each pint. The bark should be coarsely ground or bruised when made. What I mean is that the powdered or ground bark kept by druggists must not be used, as it is generally made of inferior kinds of bark, and is also often adulterated by mixing other cheap things with it, so much so, at least, that it can not be depended upon.

**4. Consumption, New French Remedy for.**—M. J. Guyot informs the profession that the phosphate of lime, in the colliquative (rapidly exhausting) night sweats of consumptives, is not only almost a specific (positive cure), but tends also to improve the general health. DOSE—From 30 to 40 grs. in a little sweetened water, at night.

**5. Consumption, a New Discovery and Cure, by Crude Petroleum.**—Dr. M. M. Griffith, of Bradford, Pa., claims that out of 25 cases of well-marked consumption, treated by small doses of the crude petroleum, 20 are, to all means of diagnosis, cured; the rest have been materially benefited, and none have been under treatment more than 4 months. The nausea attending the use of ordinary crude petroleum led him to adopt the semi-solid oil that forms on the tubing of wells. METHOD OF USING—This made into from 3 to 5 gr. pills by incorporating an inert vegetable powder, was administered from 3 to 5 times a day in 1 pill doses. The first effect, he says, is the disappearance of the cough; night sweats are relieved, appetite improves, and weight is rapidly gained. These favorable symptoms continue until the patient is entirely recovered.

*Remarks.*—If half of what Dr. Griffith claims shall prove true, generally, he has indeed made a valuable discovery. I hope, as the *Scientific American* remarks, that Dr. Griffith has not mistaken some self-limiting phase of throat or bronchial disease for true consumption of the lungs; also, that continued trial of the alleged remedy will justify the high opinion he has formed in regard to its efficacy

**6. Consumption, a Substitute for Cod Liver Oil.**—According to the New York *Medical Journal* Dr. Thomas A. Emmet, in his recent work on the "Principles and Practice of Gynecology," (of the nature and diseases of women) recommends the fat of pork, properly prepared, as a substitute for cod liver oil, in consumption. To prepare it, he says: A portion from the rib, free of lean, is to be boiled slowly (the water being often changed) until the meat is thoroughly cooked. To be eaten cold, in the form of sandwiches.

*Remarks.*—He does not inform us whether mustard may be used to give them a relish or not, but certainly a very small amount can do no harm; and for my life, I cannot see why fat pork, so cooked, and thinly sliced, may not be as good, I really believe better, than the nasty, disagreeable, sickening cod liver oil. My substitute is ⅓ pt. of fresh cream, with 1 table-spoonful of brandy, or good whiskey in it, in place of cod liver oil. I direct this amount just before each meal. Make a part of the meal of the fat pork sandwiches too, if you like, or take the following, as you judge best; as some would not, and others could not eat fat pork.

**7. Consumption, a More Recent Substitute for Cod Liver Oil.**—It has been long known that whiskey has not only appeared, at least, to have lengthened the life of many consumptive patients, but also to have cured many. Then why is not the following combination an excellent substitute for codliver oil? I think it is a hundred per cent. better. Pure olive oil, 6 ozs.; strained honey, 4 ozs.; good (that is, not poor rot-gut) whiskey, 1 pt.; Shake when taken. DOSE—Take 1 to 2 table-spoonfuls just as you sit down to each meal.

*Remarks.*—I have used this personally in a continuous cough arising from having taken a very bad cold, and have also given it to others, consumptives, with very satisfactory results. It may not be an absolute cure, but with other proper tonics and supportive treatment, it will surprise those who try it, if not already past the reach of benefit from any medical treatment. (See Chronic Diarrhea, "Muscovite," or Raw-Beef Cure for, to obtain nourishment in very feeble and debilitated cases.)

**8. Consumption Cure, by Simple Home Means, if Taken in the Beginning.**—Mary Maybee, of Farmington, Conn., says: "Take 1 pt. of vinegar, 1 table-spoonful of tar, boil 15 minutes, Dose—Take 2 table-spoonfuls every time you cough."

*Remarks.* — "Maybe" it will cure the difficulty. Certainly it will be found good for common coughs; and some of these "simple means" are astonishing in their effects, if persevered with. Our American people change too quickly, hoping for something better. Stick to a good thing as long as there is a perceptible benefit.

**9. Consumption—Climatic Changes are Believed to Have Much to do in its Cure.**—Dr. Talbot Jones, in a communication to the New York *Medical Journal*, says there are 3,000,000 of persons who die annually of consumption; and also says that the medical resources are baffled by this disease and confesses "that climate is the physician's only dependence for the cure of his consumptive patient." He makes the following statements in relation to the disease:

I.   "No zone enjoys entire immunity from pulmonary consumption.

II.   "The popular belief that phthisis (consumption) is common in cold climates is fallacious, and the idea, now so prevalent, that phthisis is rare in warm climates is as untrue as dangerous.

III.   "The disease causes a large proportion of deaths on the sea-shore, the mortality diminishing with elevation up to a certain point.

IV.   "Altitude is inimical (opposed) to the development of consumption, owing chiefly to the greater purity of the atmosphere in elevated situations, its freedom from organic matter, and its richness in ozone. [This agrees with my own opinion, that high and dry situations, especially rolling and, consequently, dry pine lands, are the best places to take up a residence in if one has to change at all.]

V.   "Moisture arising from a clay soil, due to evaporation, is one of the most influential factors in its production.

VI.   "Dampness of the atmosphere, from whatever cause, or in any altitude, predisposes to the development of the disease, and is hurtful to those already attacked.

VII.   "Dryness is a quality of the atmosphere of decided value.

VIII.   "The most unfavorable climate possible for a consumptive is one of uniform high temperature and a high dew point (warm and moist).

IX.   "The effects, due to change in the atmosphere, are by no means so pernicious as are generally supposed, and on this subject present views require modification."

*Remarks.*—Dr. Jones commends the climate of Minnesota for those predisposed to consumption, or laboring under its first stages, and thinks "that a residence there would be very likely to cure or materially benefit them," and adds: "Between the pleasant rolling prairie, the wooded lake region, and the dense pine forests of the northern section of the state, they can choose what seems most agreeable and best adapted to them, while the dry, bracing atmosphere will enable them to live much of their time out of doors without fear of taking cold." He insists, however, as I have always done, that "'tis no use to send patients thither who are in the advanced stages of the disease." And this I know to be a fact. Some physicians think Colorado or Florida, New Mexico or Texas or Aiken, S. C., or Ashville, N. C., to be preferable places, whether it be consumption or bronchitis, with loss of voice, etc.

The following items by E. R. Ellis, M. D., in the Detroit *News*, in November, 1880, are so sensible and so pertinent to the subject, as to the climate of Michigan or Texas for consumptives, I give it in full. He says:

**10. Texas for Invalids or Consumptives.**—"The cold and bleak winds of winter, now so fast approaching, impel me to say a few words to a class of invalids now quite numerous in our state, which your paper may reach. The list of deaths from consumption and other debilitating diseases, while not large in Michigan, does every year include a few in every community.

"While there is no way known to remedy all this mortality, yet a large share of it is avoidable. This last consists in a change of climate. For some years I have given this matter considerable attention, and am satisfied that there is no locality in the United States, and perhaps not on the western hemisphere, equal to the highlands of central and southwestern Texas.

"The climate there is dry, mild and salubrious. The elevation takes one above the damps and fog which are so fatal in Florida and on the sea coasts generally. Incidentally I might say that there is nothing more fatal to human life in any country than the near presence of marshes or lowlands, where fog settles, or where dampness collects, as it does in many habitations which are too much shaded with trees and shrubbery. In such houses the physician encounters an odor of mildew, and its intensity determines the activity of his business at that place. I should estimate that there are two or three thousand invalids now in this state who would be cured or greatly benefited by a temporary or permanent residence in Texas. If we have a severe winter and they attempt to remain here, by the end of March next, three-fourths of them will be 'chirping with the angels;' and while they make rich harvest for doctors with their tonics, syrups, elixirs, inhalations, etc., one-fourth of them only will survive, and not many of these fully cured. A removal to Texas will cure or greatly benefit three-fourths, which makes an amazing difference in mortuary results.

"It is lamentable that the pecuniary condition of many will not permit their removal, but many others are blessed with wealth and will gladly do whatever will prolong their life or that of their dear ones. Consider well the matter before it is too late, and act promptly.

"Physicians are usually, and sometimes excusably, reluctant to advise invalids to go away from home and friends, and thus the matter is delayed until a fatal result is inevitable.

"But every consumptive patient of mature years may know this for himself. If, in spite of the favorable weather of summer and autumn, he is declining with increased cough and shortness of breath, and occasional spitting of blood, his condition is alarming. He should change his physician or climate, or both, immediately.

"If, with the above, his pulse is habitually up to or over 100 in a minute, a destructive process is going on, which, in this climate, the most skillful physician can arrest in not more than one case in four.

"In all such cases go south at once, if not too far gone already. The quack here will encourage you to stay and make you brilliant promises up to the time of your death, but it is your own loss and folly if you believe him."

**11. Where to go to in Texas.**—As to the best place to go to in Texas, A. G. Hayson, M. D., of Minden, La., in *Medical Brief*, '83, page 508, says to the editor:

"If 'F. H. G.' (a man who previously inquired through the *Journal*) will go 80 miles west of San Antonio, Tex., he will find a beautiful valley lying in the gap of the mountains, with an average width of 4 miles by 18 long. This valley, or 'Sabinal Canyon,' as it is called there, has gushing mountain springs and bright, clear running streams that never go dry. I met there, in 1875, two gentlemen who had, previous to going there, pulmonary hemorrhage. Both seemed to be in perfect health, and so expressed themselves.

"This canyon, with its pure-aired atmosphere, its mountain scenery, with beautiful stretches of prairie and timber, and here and there, standing alone in the distance, knots of live oak and pecan, make it one of the most beautiful as well as romantic places I have ever seen. I do not think a better place for consumptives can be found." Another physician, B. F. Rowls, M. D., writes to the same journal, from Union, S. C., and directs attention of physicians to western North Carolina, "known," he says, "as the land of the sky, Ashville being the principal town in the vicinity, which is 2,250 feet above the level of the sea. This climate is one of inestimable value in the disease, consumption. Very dry, and neither the heat of summer nor the cold of winter is at all unbeneficial to the patient." Just such a place is wanted by invalids with any disease; then, persons in the eastern or northeastern States can take this place, Aiken, S. C., or Florida; while those of Michigan and the northwest or western States can take the San Antonio section of Texas, or go on to Los Angeles, or San Antonio, in the southwestern part of California, if they choose, and enter into the culture of oranges, lemons, etc., as a friend of mine did, and regained his health. Let there be no confusion about the two San Antonios spoken of; that in Calfornia is in Monterey county, and the other is the county seat of Bexar county, Texas.

**12. An Alabama Physician's Idea of the Best Place for Consumptives to go to.**—I learn from O. F. Harrell, M. D., also given in the *Brief*, that he considers Healing Springs, Ala., where he now lives, or in that neighborhood, which is a ridge of considerable extent, and heavily timbered with pine, to be the best place for those to go who have a tendency to, or actual consumption. The land, being unsuited to farming is now an almost unbroken turpentine orchard, giving employment to many hundred people engaged in this industry. "Along this elevation," he says, "commencing at Citronville, Ala., and going northward 40 or 50 miles, I believe to be the best location for consumptives, or for persons predisposed thereto, in the United

States." Dr. Harrell then went on and gave a history of his own case and the reason for the faith that was in him, *i. e.*, as to the region of Healing Springs being the best place for consumptives to go, as he was predisposed to it from his mother, who died with this disease. While the doctor was engaged in active practice in 1863 he had to give up, was confined to his room, and all his professional brethern pronounced his case to be a clearly-defined, well-developed case of tuberculosis—consumption. From this on it was a struggle with him for life. In his efforts to find a location—after rallying in 1864—suited to his condition, he says:

"I have been made familiar, I believe, with all the states embraced in the area of New York on the north and east, Missouri on the west and Florida on the south. In the winter of '79 I went to Florida, where, after a stay of two years, I was much worse than when I went there." [The author will state here, what he afterward learned by letter, that he spent these two years on Pensacola bay, which is a low section of the state like St. Johns river, Fla., neither of which sections, nor any other low places along any of the rivers, should any one allow himself to remain in, but get to the highest and dryest pine sections he can find, as mentioned further on.] "In the winter of '81-'82, with a distressing and uncontrollable cough, profuse, purulent expectoration and frequent (sometimes daily) hemorrhages from the lungs, I was finally brought to my bed again, upon which I was brought to this country in February, '82. Since I arrived here I have steadily improved in health, and gained in flesh from 125 to 160 pounds.

"I have never had a hemorrhage since I came here, and with almost a complete absence of the cough and expectoration, I think I can claim that the country has restored me; relieved me not only of my lung trouble, but also cured me of an obstinate vesical catarrh (catarrh or chronic inflammation of the bladder), from which I have greatly suffered for more than 20 years. For the relief of the latter disease, however, it is perhaps proper that I should give credit, in part, at least, to the waters, of which I have drank here."

*Remarks.*—He says there is no malaria there, referring to an inquiry as to a "place that was free from it." In conclusion he says: "I do think that a large majority of persons suffering with this disease (consumption)," or in whom there may be a predisposition to it, would find relief here." So it seems to the author; and possibly some persons who are not very bad, and yet have not large means, might find employment in the turpentine orchards of that section, or start it up for themselves, so as to stay among the pine hills, at all events. Dr. Harrell's town, Healing Springs, has a charm in its name that leads me to hope that every one who may go into this region of country will derive a great advantage from it. I will only add here, let whoever goes into this, or any other section, ramble as much as possible among the pine forests, for they certainly have an advantage over those places where there is no pine, as I fully believe.

**13. Places in Florida Where Consumptives May Visit.—** Any place in Pensacola bay, or upon the streams emptying into that bay, or any of the towns along the St. Johns river, are but very little above the sea level, and, consequently, must be damp and foggy, and not the sections that consumptives should locate in; but there are sections which, although hilly, like some other states, are sufficiently rolling and timbered with pine, which makes them far better to locate in for those seeking health.

I.   Such a place is Brockville, the county seat of Hernando county, which I see spoken of by a lady who has been there, and reported through the *Free Press,* of Detroit.   She says of this section: "It is said to be a splendid country to cure even bad tempers.   Chronic grumblers (referring to those who had complained of Jacksonville and the low country along the St. Johns river) have been here, to succumb under the combined influences of balmy air, moonlight and orange flowers."

*How to Reach Brockville.*—Take a boat at Jacksonville, up the St. Johns, to Astor, 134 miles.   Then the cars through the pine forests, via. Fort Mason, on Lake Eustice.

II.   Twin Lakes, Orange county, is also reported to the *Rural New Yorker* by another lady, who was there for her health, to be a very desirable place for consumptives.   She first spoke of the fact that the country along the St. Johns and all the other rivers of the State is damp and unhealthy.   She says to those who might be coming, "Come up to the hills, where there is no damp."   And I would add that those who do may really expect to be greatly benefited if they stay long enough to allow the climatic changes to take place in their systems.   For this lady closed by saying: "When we left home every breath seemed to rasp and last, but now 'tis all gone, and with it the weariness and languor."   Then, surely, if one stays long enough, the same "balmy air, full of the resinous aroma of the pine forests," as she expresses it, will accomplish a cure.   There may be many other places in Florida equally dry and salubrious, with pine forests, making them equally valuable as health resorts, but I leave every one to judge of this fact for himself, relying upon the statements of friends who know, or upon enquiry when they reach there: but do not stay in the low, marshy grounds of any section whatever, if health is to be regained, or even retained, in any country.   I will only add one thought further on the subject of going south, or to any point, for a change of climate; do not wait until nothing but a miracle can cure, for·I fully believe that God works by the use of means—medicines judiciously administered, change of climate, care of one's health, etc.   Where one lives may make a difference as to where they might or should go.   Living at Toledo, O., as I do, if I had to go south on account of consumption, I should go to the Healing Springs section of Alabama, as it is about south from here.   If I lived in the east, or New England States, I should go to the neighborhoods of Ashville, N. C., Aiken, S. C., or Florida; if in Illinois or the west, I should strike for San Antonio, Texas, or southwestern California, as before mentioned, as circumstances made it appear best.

I will give an item or two more for consumptives, hoping thereby to benefit, if not actually cure, many persons suffering from it.   The following I take from a report by Wm. H. Hull, M. D., in the June number of the *Medical Brief* of 1877, upon the use of gallic acid, with which he had been very successful, as you will see in the heading of the recipe, and I shall also mention a case where·

another physician has been equally successful with the same remedy in a very bad case. It is as follows:

**14. Gallic Acid in Consumption.**—Gallic acid, 1 dr.; pulverized Dover's powder, ½ dr.; pulverized cubebs and pulverized gum arabic, each, 1 dr., and pulverized licorice root, ½ oz. Mix thoroughly. Dose—Half a tea-spoonful, dry, every 3 or 4 hours.

*Remarks.*—Dr. Hull said of this: " Out of 200 cases treated during the past seven months, I found only 2 that this remedy would not relieve." Certainly a very marked proportion of cures. The corroboration I referred to above in the very bad case was reported also in the *Brief* by R. H. Holliday, M. D., of Guntley postoffice, N. C. His patient was a man who had been confined to his bed for 170 days, and upon whom he had exhausted his book knowledge without benefit, the man raising 2 quarts of thick, purulent matter daily that smelled terribly, so that he says " the ferryman was waiting to carry him over, etc., when, upon the appeal of the wife, if I could not do something more for him, I took up the *Brief*, and fell upon Dr. Hull's gallic acid treatment (above given) and saved my patient."

**15  Gallic Acid in Liquid Form.**—The editor of the *Brief*, in commenting upon the gallic acid in powders, gave the following formula as preferable. He said: Gallic acid, 1 dr.; glycerine, 3 ozs.; listerine, 5 ozs.; mix. Dose—Take 1 or 2 tea-spoonfuls 4 or 5 times a day.

*Remarks.*—This the editor found a better formula, from its fluid form no doubt, and from its containing the listerine, which is considered a valuable antiseptic, *i. e.*, as against the destructive tendency in cases where the matter raised, smells terribly, as in Dr. Halliday's case above. The listerine is manufactured at St. Louis, Mo., I think, and therefore can be obtained, if not found in the drug stores, by inquiring through the *Medical Brief*, of that city. See the next item, on the use of hot water, to know that the editor of the *Brief* is well qualified to judge of the nature of any article of medicine which he may recommend.

**16.  Consumption, Hot Water Cure for.**—The latest thing claimed to cure consumption was given in the St. Louis, Mo., *Medical Brief*, by the editor, J. J. Lawrence, A. M., M. D., page 561, 1883, and as it is more than probable that it will help very many sufferers, I shall give it, not to be tried as a last resort, but to be tried as early in the disease as any wasting of flesh and debility is manifested: and to be tried faithfully for two or three months, at least, remembering that the diet of tender beef and stale bread, (bread never less than one day old) must be attended to, as well as the hot water. Dr. Lawrence says: A young man who was compelled to resign his position in one of the public schools of New York because he was breaking down with consumption, and who had ever since been battling for life, although with little apparent prospect of recovery, was encountered several days ago in a Broadway restaurant. "I see," he said, "that you seem surprised at my improved appearance. No doubt you wonder what could have caused such a change. Well, it was a very simple remedy, nothing but hot water." Hot water!

"'That's all.'" You remember my telling you that I had used the usual remedies. I consulted some of the leading specialists in affections of the lungs, in the city, and paid them large fees. They went through the usual course of experimentation with me, under all resorts to medicine. I went to the Adirondacks (a range of mountains in northern New York) for the summer, and to Florida in winter, but none of these things did me any substantial good. I lost ground steadily, grew to be almost a skeleton, and had all the worst symptoms of a consumptive whose end is near at hand. At that juncture a friend told me that he had heard of a cure effected by drinking hot water. I consulted a physician who had paid special attention to this hot water cure, and was using it with many patients. He said: 'There is nothing, you know, that is more difficult than to introduce a new remedy into medical practice, particularly if it is a very simple one, and strikes at the root of erroneous views and prejudices that have long been entertained. The old practitioners have tried for years to cure consumption, but they are as far from doing it as ever. Now, the only rational explanation of consumption is that it results from defective nutrition. 'It is always accompanied by mal-assimilation of food.' [Mal, means bad and assimilation means, to make food.] 'In nearly every case the stomach is the seat of a fermentation that necessarily prevents proper digestion. The first thing to do is to remove that fermentation and put the stomach into a condition to receive food and dispose of it properly. This is effected by taking water into the stomach, as hot as it can be borne, an hour before each meal. This leaves the stomach clean and pure, like a boiler that has been washed out. Then put into the stomach, food that is in the highest degree nutritious and the least disposed to fermentation. No food answers this description better than tender beef. A little stale bread may be eaten with it. Drink nothing but pure water, and as little of that at meals as possible. Vegetables, pastry, sweets, coffee and alcoholic liquors should be avoided. Put tender beef alone into a clean and pure stomach, three times a day, and the system will be fortified and built up until the wasting away, which is the chief feature of consumption, ceases and recuperation sets in.

"'This reasoning impressed me. I began by taking one cup of hot water an hour before each meal, and gradually increased the dose to three cups, or nearly a pint. At first it was unpleasant to take, but now I drink it with a relish that I never experienced in drinking the choicest wine. I began to pick up immediately after I began the new treatment and gained fourteen pounds within two months.'"

The editor then closes in a way which you will see encourages the use of hot water in dyspepsia. He says:

"Combined with carefully selected foods, and some mild medicine to assist nature in eliminating (carrying out) poisons from the system, it is said by those who have tried it to be very efficient in dyspepsia and all forms of indigestion. If this be true (and of this the author has not a doubt), it will certainly be a blessing, as medicines almost universally fail to effect cures in these diseases. Many prominent New York physicians are abandoning medicines for simple, nutritious foods, and report more than ordinary success in the treatment of many forms of disease from want of nutrition. A prominent English physician, who has had much experience in India, says, cholera will not attack a person in whose stomach and bowels there is no ferment (gaseous condition from food that does not readily digest); or, if it does, the attack will be light and easily controlled." He regards good nutrition (healthy digestion) as the only real prophylactic (prevention) for disease.

**HIVES.**—This disease manifests itself in the form of an eruption, or red blotches upon the surface, or skin of children, mostly.

**Cause.**—Obstruction of the circulation, and the absorption into the blood of some poisonous vapors in the atmosphere, similar to that of the more simple fevers are the undoubted cause of the disease.

**Symptoms.**—Large red patches with a somewhat swollen center more white than the rest, with an almost intolerable itching, something like the irritation from nettles, make their appearance, and have also given another name to the disease—"nettle rash." This rash, or blotches may subside after a few hours, then re-appear for a day or two, causing considerable sickness of the little patient unless properly attended to.

**Treatment.**—Bathe the whole surface, but more thoroughly the affected parts, with spirits of camphor and soft water, equal parts of each, and give a dose of the cathartic tincture, to operate tolerably free ; and also a tea of saffron and spearmint, every hour or two to keep the disease to the surface, and but little danger need be feared. I am partial to the spearmint plant, in preference to the peppermint, because of its greater *diuretic* properties.

**CANKER AND NURSING SORE MOUTH—Remedy.**—Take epsom salts, gun-powder, borax, alum, copperas, and sulphur, of each 1 teaspoonful; soft water, 1 quart.

The alum and copperas will be burned, or heated on a shovel, and pulverized ; then all mixed and bottled for use. Shake when used. Hold a little of the wash in the mouth, for half a minute, and gargle the throat with it twice daily. And at the same time take a little sulphur and cream of tartar for 3 or 4 mornings, to correct the blood. It has cured bad cases after a failure of the "regular" remedies.

**SINGERS AND PUBLIC SPEAKERS—Loss of Voice,** **Hoarseness, etc.**—It has been found that borax has proved a most effective remedy in certain forms of colds. In sudden hoarseness or loss of voice from colds by public speakers or singers, relief for an hour or so, as by magic, may be often obtained by slowly dissolving and partially swallowing a lump of borax the size of a garden pea, or about 3 or 4 grains, held in the mouth for 10 minutes before speaking or singing. This produces a profuse secretion of saliva, or watering of the mouth or throat, probably restoring the voice or tone to the dried vocal cords, just as the wetting brings back the missing notes to a flute when it is too dry.

*Remarks.*—There need be no fear in using 2, 3 or 4 pieces of the size above named, within the hour before speaking or singing is to commence. Keep it handy, to use, as needed, during the evening.

**1. COUGH SYRUP—Effectual Remedy for Coughs, Colds, Hoarseness, etc.**—"E. J. R.," from an inquiry through the Detroit *Tribune*, sends for publication the following sure cure for cough, cold, hoarseness, etc., saying it has been tried repeatedly, and is a most invaluable remedy. It is always kept in our family. It cured a cough of three years standing to my knowledge. Syrup of squills, 2 ozs.; paregoric 1 oz. ; fl. ex. of licorice, 1 oz.; fl. ex. of ipecac, ½ oz.; antimonial wine, ½ oz.; ess. of wintergreen, or peppermint, 1 dr. DOSE—One tea-spoonful every 2 or 3 hours, but not on an empty stomach.

**2. Cough, Hoarseness, Incipient Consumption, etc.**—Take of horehound, boneset and lobelia (herbs), each 1 oz.; comfrey root, spikenard, St. John's wort (*hypericum perforatum*), and poppy capsules, each ½ oz; pour on 3 pts. of boiling water and let it stand covered over for 3 hours. Then strain through a fine cloth, add ½ lb. of loaf sugar, and let it just boil (no more), then add a full wine-glass of Jamaica rum, and cork tightly. DOSE—1 to 2 table-spoonfuls 3 or 4 times daily. This will be found invaluable in coughs, hoarseness, incipient consumption, etc.—*Hearth and Home.*

*Remarks.*—This is an excellent syrup. Dr. Beach, in his *Family Practice*, says of the St. John's Wort: "A syrup of this with sage is a specific (sure cure) for coughs." [The St. John's wort grows abundantly in this country and Europe, to the great annoyance of many persons, flowering from June to August. The stem is two-edged, and grows about 2 feet high, the flowers of a bright yellow color, the leaves being marked with clear transparent spots of a greenish shade, the whole herb being a dark green; the petals, or leaves of the flowers, are streaked and dotted with black or dark purple, and if bruised with the finger give a purple stain. This, I think, will enable any one to distinguish it from any other plant.] But this article, so far as I know, is but little known and little used. Its flowers are a bright yellow, although King says if they are infused in sweet-oil or bears-oil by means of exposure to the sun, they make a fine red balsamic ointment for wounds, ulcers, swellings, tumors, etc. See also "Ointment of St. John's Wort and Stramonium."

**3. Best Cough Syrup—To Break Up Bad Colds.**—I. *The Syrup.*—Horehound leaves and blossoms, spikenard root, comfrey root, elecampane root, and sun-flower seeds, each 1 oz.; water sufficient. DIRECTIONS.—Boil 1 hour, having 1 qt. when done; strain, add sugar, 1 lb.; dissolve by heat, and add a little brandy (½ pt. of spirits will be enough to prevent souring). DOSE.—One table-spoonful 3 times daily. Tested.—*Home Cook Book.*

*Remarks.*—This will be found good, as it contains most of the roots used in "lang syne" for coughs, when there were far less deaths from consumption than now, in proportion to the attacks.

II. *To Break Up Bad Colds.*—The same book recommends glycerine, 1 tea-spoonful with spirits, 1 or 2 table-spoonfuls to a pint bowl of hot lemonade, to break up bad colds at bed-time. This is also good if taken as hot as it can be drank after getting into bed; but don't take additional cold next day after the free perspiration which it produces.

III. *How to Cure Recent Colds.* — A writer gives the following sensible plan for quickly curing a recent cold. He says: "When you get chilly all over and begin to sniffle and almost struggle for breath, just begin at once and your tribulation need not last very long. Get some powdered borax (it should be kept in every house), and snuff it freely up the nostrils frequently. Smell freely and frequently also from the camphor bottle (which also ought to be kept in every house), and pour a little of the camphor upon the handkerchief to wipe the nose with as often as is needful, which will be quite often as the cold begins to break. The nose will not become sore with this treatment, and if begun quickly and followed faithfully at intervals, by bed-time you will wonder what has become of your cold, and your sleep will seldom be disturbed."— *Experience.*

*Remarks.*—If a cold is not broken up within two or three days at most, it will run about two weeks in spite of all known remedies. Take note, then, of the very first symptoms, and besides the snuffing of the powdered borax, and the hot lemonade on getting into bed, heat the feet by the fire, or put them for 15 or 20 minutes into hot water, before getting into bed, and then take the hot lemonade and put a bottle of hot water or a hot flat-iron to the feet, cover up with an extra amount of clothing, and your chances are as good to break up the cold as it is possible to make them. Avoid exposure again for a day or two, if possible, and you will be safe; at any rate, nothing better can be advised.

**4. Coughs, Indian Vegetable Syrup for.**—Soft water, 2 qts.; boneset, 2 ozs.; cinnamon bark, ginseng root, spikenard and comfrey roots, each, 1 oz.; blood root, ¼ oz.; loaf sugar, 1 lb.; gin, 6 ozs.; water sufficient. DIRECTIONS.—Bruise the roots and bark, and steep (not boil) to 1 qt.; strain and add the sugar, and when cool add the gin and bottle. DOSE.—One table-spoonful half an hour before meals and at bed-time.

*Remarks.*—This has proved valuable in coughs and in incipient consumption, *i. e.,* in the commencement of the disease. It was obtained of an Indian, at an early day, by an uncle of mine, in whose family it was held in high estimation for the good it had done them.

**5. Colds with Cough, Simple and Easily Taken Remedy.**—Roast a lemon, avoiding to burn it; when thoroughly roasted, cut into halves and squeeze the juice upon 3 table-spoonfuls of powdered sugar. Mix, and take a tea-spoonful whenever the cough or tickling of the throat troubles you. It is good as well as pleasant, even for children.

**6. Irritable, Dry or Hacking Coughs, Flaxseed Lemonade for.**—Put 2 or 3 table-spoonfuls of flaxseed and the juice of 2 good sized lemons and 2 or 3 table-spoonfuls of sugar into a dish which can be covered, and pour on boiling water, 1 qt.; cover and let steep until the mucilage has been drawn out of the seed. DOSE—A table-spoonful of it may be taken every hour or two to relieve the hacking, but sipping a little often is better than larger doses at longer intervals.

**7. "Winter Cough," or Chronic Bronchitis, Remedy for.—** Dr. Fletcher, of Washington, strongly recommends the employment of the spray of chloral in the treatment of the form of chronic bronchitis known as "winter cough," which often offers a very obstinate resistance to remedies. He says: "A solution of 10 grs. of chloral to an ounce of water may be inhaled through a steam atomizer morning and evening."

**8. Bronchitis, Valuable Remedy for.—**A simple, but oftentimes efficacious, remedy for bronchitis in its early stages, is: Syrup of tolu, 1 oz.; syrup of squills, ½ oz.; wine of ipecac, 2 drs.; paregoric, 3 drs.; mucilage of gum arabic, 1½ozs. Dose.—A tea-spoonful 3 to 5 times daily, as needed.

**9. Indian Cough Syrup.—**Elecampane root and Indian turnip (known also as wake-robin, Jack-in-the-pulpit, etc.), bruised, each, 1 oz.; honey, 1 pt. Steep thoroughly and strain. Dose.—A tea-spoonful to a table-spoonful as often as the cough or tickling requires it, at least 3 or 4 times daily.—*Reliable.*

**10. Recent Colds, Simple, but Sensible, Remedy.—**A medical writer says: "Hot lemonade is one of the best remedies in the world for a cold." Directions.—Roll a good sized lemon, squeeze out the juice, cut the rind in slices, put in 2 or 3 table-spoonsfuls of sugar, and pour on ⅔ of a pt. of boiling water, stir well and cover up while the patient is getting into bed; then drink it all, cover up warm, and the result will be almost magical.

**11. Chills or Ague, to Ward off.—**It is said, also, that the same thing, only doubled in quantity, and taking half of it as hot as can be drank, an hour before the chill would set in, (being covered warm in bed) and the balance in 15 or 20 minutes after, also hot, will ward off "the chills," as ague is often called. Certainly it is a pleasant remedy to take.

**12. Colds—General Washington's Cure.—**The *Baltimore American* informs us that Gen. George Washington gave the following recipe for a cold, to an old lady now living in Newport, when she was a very young girl, 1781—103 years before this writing. He was lodged in her father's house, the old Vernon mansion. As she was being sent to bed early with a very bad cold he remarked to Mrs. Vernon, the mother of this lady: "My own remedy, my dear madam, is always to eat, just before I step into bed, a hot roasted onion if I have a cold."

*Remarks.*—It may be taken for granted that this simple remedy will be found very efficacious, and, if the cold is of recent taking, with the help of either toasting the feet before the fire or stove through the evening, otherwise soaking them in hot water for 15 to 20 minutes before going to bed, it will be the more likely to succeed. If necessary, however, to effect a complete cure, repeat it for one or two evenings. And if a hot roasted onion was eaten two or three times during the day it would also help the cure.

**13. Colds and Inflammation—Health Rules for Winter.—**I. "Never lean with the back upon anything that is cold.

II. "Never begin a journey until the breakfast has been eaten.

III. "Never take warm drinks and then immediately go out in the cold air.

IV. "Keep the back, especially between the shoulders, well covered; also the chest well protected.

V. "In sleeping in a cold room, establish the habit of breathing through the nose, and never with the mouth open.

VI. "Never go to bed with cold or damp feet; always toast them by a fire 10 or 15 minutes before going to bed.

VII. "Never omit weekly bathing, for, unless the skin is in active condition, the cold will close the pores and favor congestion or other diseases.

VIII. "After exercise of any kind, never ride in an open carriage or near the window of a car for a moment; it is dangerous to health and even to life.

IX. "When hoarse, speak as little as possible until it is recovered from, else the voice may be permanently lost or difficulties of the throat be produced.

X. "Warm the back by a fire, and never continue keeping the back exposed to heat after it has become comfortably warm; to do otherwise is debilitating.

XI. "When going from a warm atmosphere into a colder one, keep the mouth closed so that the air may be warmed by its passage through the nose ere it reaches the lungs.

XII. "Never stand still in cold weather, especially after having taken a slight degree of exercise; and always avoid standing on ice or snow, or where the person is exposed to cold wind; in short, keep your feet warm, your head cool, and your mouth shut and you will seldom 'catch cold.'"—*Common Sense.*

XIII. To the foregoing rules from "Common Sense" allow the Old Doctor to make a "baker's dozen" of them, by saying that the most fruitful seed from which colds, and often consumption arise, is the pernicious habit of young people loitering at the gate. Never do it.

**14. Deep-Seated, or Heavy Cold that Has Settled in the Breast.**—"J. P. S.," of Holmdel, N. J., writes to the Toledo *Blade* on this subject and says:

"For a heavy cold that has settled in the breast, take 4 table-spoonfuls of molasses, 3 of paragoric, 2 of castor-oil, and 1 of turpentine. Mix it well together. Take a tea-spoonful before each meal. It is considered one of the best remedies known in the New England states, and I know no equal."

**15. Colds of Young Children—Onion Syrup for—Very Valuable.**—Slice up thinly a few mild onions and sprinkle sugar over them, set in the oven in a suitable dish to simmer until the juice may be all squeezed out, then thoroughly mix with the sugar, forming a very nice thick syrup, or sugar, according to the amount of each used. DOSE — A tea-spoonful, or less, according to the age of the child, 4 or 5 times daily, as needed. It is perfectly safe and reliable for the smallest child; also valuable for adults.

*Remarks.*—This might claim to be a half-brother to General Washington's cure for colds.

**16. Coughs, Colds, etc., Recent Remedy for—Very Satisfactory.**—I have recently tried the following with a good deal of satisfaction. I obtained it of a Dr. A. Galloway, formerly of Rochester, N. Y.: Solid extract of licorice, ½ dr., rubbed with muriate of ammonia, 3 drs, and added to syrup of senega and ipecac, each, ½ oz.; syrup of tolu, 2 ozs; syrup of wild cherry,. 6 ozs; tincture of lobelia, ¼ oz. Mix. Dose—Shaken when used; 1 tea-spoonful 3 or 4 times daily for adults. I have sipped it oftener than this without sickening at the stomach. That is all that needs guarding against. Children 5 to 20 drops, according to age. I believe I would sooner risk it than Ayer's, which follows:

**17. Ayer's Cherry Pectoral, for Coughs, Colds, Consumption, etc.**—Tinct. of blood root, 2 ozs.; antimonial wine and wine of ipecac, of each 3 drs.; syrup of wild cherry, 2 ozs.; acetate of morphia, 4 grs.; mix. Dose—Take 1 tea-spoonful 3 or 4 times daily; or sip a little, as the cough is troublesome; and if nausea is felt take less, or stop until the nausea passes off. —*Druggist Circular.*

*Remarks.*—And now allow me to say, with all the recipes here given, there need be but little suffering with coughs, colds and consumption in its commencement, as compared with what it must have continued to be without this knowledge. I will close this subject with a cough syrup given by Dr. Hildreths, of Zanesville, Ohio, as follows:

**18. Cough Syrup, Very Valuable in Recent Colds.**—Paregoric, 1½ ozs.; tinct. of capsicum, 1 dr.; tinct. of tolu, 3 ozs. Dose—A tea-spoonful every 3 hours, in a little water.

*Remarks.*—Dr. Hildreth has had a long experience in the practice of medicine, and this was his dependence in recent colds. I once heard a man say: "Paregoric is the best cough medicine I ever used," which showed his opinion, at least, of the value of one of the articles in this syrup. The combination will be found indeed valuable.

**1. WHOOPING COUGH—Remedy for.**—A paper recently read before the New York Academy of Science, by Dr. H. A. Mott, holds that much of the mortality among children from whooping cough is attributable to the prevalent faulty belief that it will be much worse for the child if the disease is broken up. He says: The disease is now known to be caused by a fungoid growth (in plants, growing quickly like mushrooms, coming up in a night; but in animal bodies being slower in growth and being much of the character of proud flesh, but below he calls them spores, which indicates them to be more of the nature of an animal parasite), which begins under the tongue, and spreads backward to the throat and lungs, the spores requiring from 9 to 15 days to develop. When the fungus enters the bronchial tubes, most alarming complications arise. It is, then, best to kill the fungus in its earliest stage; there would then seldom be any trouble from bronchitis, cholera infantum, or cerebral (head) difficulties. Quinine, just after a coughing spell, and before retiring for the night, is the best remedy.

*Remarks.*—I have had no opportunity to try this remedy, yet I do not doubt its value, for some physicians claim that even chills and fever are developed by spores. Then as quinine does cure ague may it not be by killing the spores? most likely. Then, by all means try the quinine immediately after it is known that a child, or anyone, has been exposed; and if it does not entirely abate it, I believe it will give it a mildness not otherwise attained. Probably as good a way, or the best way, to take the quinine for this purpose, is to dissolve it in one of the following ways:

I. *Quinine, to Dissolve, or Solution of Quinine.*—Put 20 grs. of sulphate of quinine into a 2 oz. vial, and add 1 dr. of aromatic sulphuric acid, then fill the vial with water. DOSE—For an adult, 20 drops once an hour, in a table-spoonful of water. The proper dose for a child will be 1 drop to each year of its age, in 1 tea-spoonful, only, of the water, or if it is a nursing child, in the mother's milk. And, in all cases, (if the spore theory is correct, which I have no reason to doubt) the longer the quinine solution is held in the mouth, the more certain it will be to kill them.

II. Rub 20 grs. each of quinine and tartaric acid together, put into the same sized vial and fill with water, as in the first case. Dose and manner of using, the same.

The following are a few of the more common remedies for this disease; the chestnut leaves, however, I believe are not, as yet, very common; but I can not see why they may not be as efficient as claimed to be.

**2. Whooping Cough, Efficient Remedy for.**—Somebody's friend gave a correspondent of one of the Detroit papers the following as a cer-tain cure for whooping cough, by simply "boiling chestnut leaves and sweet-ening with brown sugar," adding: "Whooping cough generally remains eighteen weeks, while by the use of this tea it can be cured in a few days."

*Remarks.*—I should gather the leaves before the nuts fall off.

**3. Whooping Cough Tincture.**—Tinct. of blood root, 1 oz.; syrup of garlic, 1 oz.; solid ex. of belladonna, 3 grs. Mix, and be sure the extract is dis-solved. DOSE.—Ten to 20 drops, according to age of the child, 3 times daily.

*Remarks.* —This is the favorite prescription of Dr. T. B. King, of this city— Toledo, O.,—an old English physician who practiced in the army of India a number of years, and then in the United States, with very great success. This is his dependence in bad cases.

**4. Whooping Cough Syrup.**—Make a syrup of prickly-pear (*Opuntia vulgaris*, a species of cactus,) and drink freely. Take about three moderate sized leaves of the prickly pear to a quart of cold water, cut up in pieces and boil slowly about half an hour, strain out all the prickles through close muslin or linen, sweeten with white sugar and boil, a little longer. A safe and sure cure, and so pleasant to the taste that infants will take it with a relish. It is also good for a cold that settles in the throat or lungs. This species of cactus grows in rocky and sandy places, and is grown in gardens.

*Remarks.*—There is nothing said by this writer as to a dose, but I should say from a tea-spoonful to a table-spoonful for a child, as needed, according to age. An adult 1 to 2 table-spoonfuls.

**5. Whooping Cough, Help for.**—I. Cut in small pieces a large red onion, put it in a bottle with a piece of asafœtida half the size of a nutmeg, cover with good whiskey, shake well, and it is ready for use; weaken, sweeten and give according to age, three or four times a day

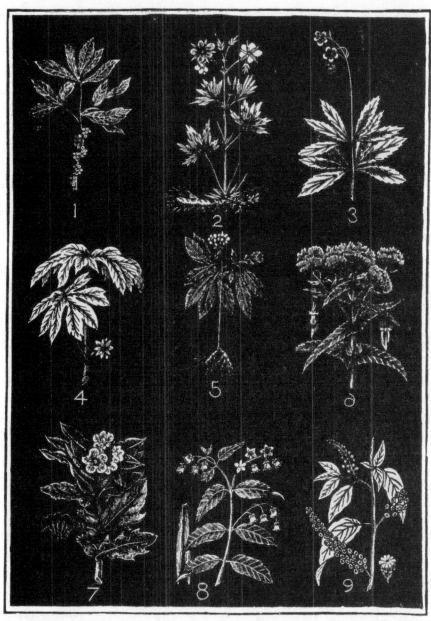

1—Bayberry, or Wax Myrtle.  2—Cranesbill, or Doves Foot.  3—Pipsissewa, or Princes Pine.  4—Mandrake, or May-Apple.  5—Ginseng.  6—Boneset, or Thoroughwort.  7—Henbane.  8—Bitter-Root, or Dog's Bane.  9—Poke, or Pigeon-Berry.

II. Also mix Radway's Relief with a little sweet-oil, bathe the chest, stomach, sides, and along the back-bone before going to bed, and take a drop or two inwardly, in a little syrup or honey.

*Remarks.*—This will be found valuable, but it would be better to allow it to stand 3 or 4 days before using.

**1. CHOLERA—Drops and Powder for, also Valuable for Colic, Diarrhea, etc.**—Alcohol, ½ pt.; gum myrrh, 1 oz.; gum guaiac, ¼ oz.; gum camphor, capsicum, and opium, each, 1 dr DIRECTIONS. — Mix, and keep in a well-stoppered bottle, shaking often for 10 or 12 days, when it will be ready for use. DOSE.—A tea-spoonful in well sweetened water; or, what is better, use sugar alone, just enough to absorb all the drops, and not use any water.

II. *For the Powder.*—By omitting the alcohol in the above, and pulverizing each article, the medicine can be used as a powder, 10 grs. being a dose; or the same may be made into pills of 4 grs., 3 pills for a dose.

*Remarks.*—Dr A. B. Mason, of Toledo, O., of whom I obtained this recipe, says: The above has twice saved my life when attacked by cholera. I have never known it to fail in giving almost immediate relief in all cases of colic, diarrhea, dysentery, cholera-morbus and cholera. In the summer of '77 I cured a lady of the regular dysentery, who had been doctored for four weeks by one of the best doctors in a city of 20,000 inhabitants, and then lived along for four weeks more without a doctor, every one saying she could not live long. The night I gave her this medicine was the first good night's rest she had had for weeks. In two days all discharges were stopped, and I gave a small dose of podophyllin, and in eight days she was well, and was soon in better health than for years before. In this case I used the medicine in the form of a powder. In severe cases, he says, repeat the dose often, and even give two times the above dose. If vomited up as soon as taken, repeat the dose. The utmost confidence may be put in this treatment.

**2. Cholera, Infallible Cure for.**—Gen. Jordan, of the *Mining Record*, makes the following statement in relation to the infallible cure of cholera by the use of chloroform only. It is somewhat strange that such facts as here stated should not become generally known quicker than they do; still I can not doubt their being facts, and as I know that a dozen drops of chloroform, in a little water, will at once correct a gaseous condition of a dyspeptic stomach (which see), why should it not correct a much more disturbed condition, by using larger quantities? I would certainly "go for it," on the "double quick" if occasion called for it. He says:

" A ½ tea-spoonful of chloroform in about eight times as much water is an infallible cure for cholera. A doctor who had lived in Mobile, Ala., and had great success in curing people during a cholera epidemic there, told me about it. When, in the Cuban revolution, I went to Cuba to help organize the insurgent army, I had a chance to try the remedy, for a cholera epidemic broke out among the troops. My first experiment was on a negro who was in the last stages. It cured him and hundreds after him. When we marched, the officers carried bottles of chloroform, and if a man fell out, sick with cholera, the remedy was given and he was able to resume his place. I have seen men lying by the roadside in a state of collapse, almost dead. An officer would ride up, dismount and give the remedy, and before the column had passed the man would be in the ranks again."

**3. Chronic Diarrhea, Muscovite, or Raw Beef Cure for.**—About the year 1852 Dr. Weisse, director of the Hospital for Foundlings at St. Petersburg, Russia, called the attention of the medical world to the use of raw beef in the treatment of chronic diarrhea. His method, to which was applied the title of the "Muscovite method," was adopted in England, Germany, Italy and France. In the last named country Drs. Trousseau and Bouchut were the first to test it, and reported it to have good results in cases of children severely afflicted. A little later, Dr. Labadie, of Bordeaux, communicated to the profession some facts in regard to three children afflicted with tubercles, whom he had treated and cured by the Russian "Muscovite" method. We give below Dr. Trousseau's formula for preparing the meat: Take 100 grammes (1 gramme is about 15½ grs., and 100 are equal to about 3½ ozs.) of fillet of beef, from which the gristle and fat should be carefully removed; mince it fine and bray (pound) it in a wooden mortar; 20 grammes (¾ oz.) of powdered sugar, 1½ grammes of chloride of sodium (common salt, 23 grs.,); ½ gramme chloride of potassium (7½ grs.); 1½ grammes (23 grs.) powdered black pepper. Take by the table-spoonful during the day.

*Remarks.*—As but few would understand these French technicalities, I have put their "grammes" into grains, to be easily understood. I have used the above with satisfaction in consumption, although there is no doubt that Dr. Labadie, by "tubercles," refers to a tuberculous deposit in the mesenteric glands of the bowels, as children are frequently troubled with them, and they are very wasting in their effect upon their tender constitution. It is undoubtedly a valuable diet in either of these exhaustive diseases, whether of children or adults, and may be used in any disease of a debilitating character, where some physicians have recently adopted the plan of giving what they call "powdered beef," that is grated, or pounded fine, then dried. I should prefer this "Muscovite" plan of using it. It will prove exceedingly valuable in consumption.

**4. Chronic Diarrhea, a Well Tried Remedy.**—Powdered opium and tannin, each 10 grs.; mix thoroughly and divide into 20 powders. DOSE—Take 1 powder in a little syrup every 4 hours, till improved, then 1 or 2 powders daily, as occasion requires, until the cure is complete.

*Remarks.*—It is not best to check too suddenly, lest fever or other disturbance of the system arise. Watch carefully, with this, and it will generally be found effectual.

**1. PAIN KILLER, INTERNAL—For Cholera, Diarrhea, etc.**—Oil of cloves, cinnamon, anise and peppermint, each 45 drops; laudanum and ether, each 1 oz.; alcohol, 3 ozs. DOSE—A tea-spoonful in 2 table-spoonfuls of sweetened water, and for an adult it may be repeated in from 5 minutes to ½ an hour, or 1 hour, according to the severity of the pain, or the frequency of the discharge. Children proportionately less, according to age. A teaspoon is considered to hold 60 drops; then at 14 years, ½; at 7 years, ⅓; at

4 years, 1-5; at 3 years, 1-6; at 2 years, ⅛; decreasing in like proportion for infants; at 21 years the full dose is to be given, up to 60 years, then diminish, in like proportion on each 5 to 10 years.

*Remarks.*—This prescription is from "Old" Dr. T. B. King, who used it in India with great success, curing internal aches and pains, diarrhea and bloody dysentery as well as cholera. I would now suggest the addition of half as much chloroform as ether, and also one-fourth as much tincture of cayenne. In the "Old" Doctor's day in India chloroform was not as much in use as since then, and the cayenne has, of late years, also been found a very valuable aid in curing internal pains, as well as the free discharges from the bowels. It is one of our best and purest stimulants. And with these additions it would be a valuable embrocation, or liniment, to use externally on the stomach and bowels in these painful diseases.

**2. Pain Killer, Truly Magical, for All Purpose and Places of Pain.**—Morphine, 10 grs.; chloral hydrate and camphor gum, each, ½ oz.; chloroform, 1 oz.; nitrite of amyl, 2 drs.; oils of cloves and cinnamon, each, ¼ oz.; alcohol (best), to fill a 4 oz. bottle. DIRECTIONS — Dissolve the morphine in a little of the alcohol; rub the chloral hydrate and the camphor gum together, which forms a liquid, and add the dissolved morphine and the others, the nitrite of amyl to be the last, as it is very evaporative; then add 3 or 4 drops of strong sulphuric acid, which keeps the morphine in solution. DOSE—It may be taken on sugar in doses of 5 to 20 drops, and repeated in 30 minutes to an hour, according to the severity of any internal pain. For headache inhale from the bottle, from nostril to nostril, and apply also over the pain.

*Remarks.*—This will stop any kind of pain almost immediately, and does seem, at least, to be magical by its quick action upon the nerves, relieving pain at once. I have applied it upon the eyeball (not in the eye, but with the eye closed) holding the finger wet with it for a minute or two, which causes a counter, or external, irritation, and would soon cause a blister, which proves its value as well as its strength and adaptation to the relief of pain in all situations. I cannot speak of it too highly, for slight pains or neuralgia of the eye. I shall use it upon painful teeth, neuralgic, and, in fact, in all pains anywhere, internally and externally It will be hard, very hard, to excel. The only objection against it, is its cost (about 25 cents an ounce), when made in small quantities. It would still be valuable as a liniment if an equal amount of alcohol was added, which would make it cheaper, but to retain its magical power it must be kept full strength.

**3. Pain Killer, or Rubefacient, in Place of Mustard Plaster, Immediate in its Action.**—When there is internal pain, as in pleurisy, inflammation of the lungs, etc., wherein it would be thought advisable to put on a mustard plaster, for quick relief take the following: Chloroform, spirits of camphor and sweet oil, equal parts, say 1 oz. each. Mix. DIRECTIONS— Fold a piece of muslin 3 or 4 thicknesses, shake the bottle and wet the cloth thoroughly with the mixture and apply, covering with a folded towel to prevent evaporation. Dr. T. B. King, of this city (Toledo), claims it will remove ordinary or rheumatic pain in one minute, and that it will blister in three minutes. So be careful when you do not desire to blister. If the pain moves to any other part, follow it up in the same manner.

**BLEEDING—A Styptic Which Will Stop Bleeding of the Largest Vessels.**—Brandy, or common whisky, 2 ozs.; castile soap, 2 drs.; carbonate of potash, 1 dr. DIRECTIONS—Scrape the soap fine and dissolve it in the spirits; then add the potash; mix well and keep corked. Warm it and wet pledgets of lint in it and apply to the wound. It immediately congeals the blood and coagulates it some distance within the vessel. It may need repeating for deep wounds and when limbs are cut off.

*Remarks.*—I am sorry I cannot give the name of the writer, or the paper in which this was published, having had it in my scrap-book for some time; but I am satisfied that it is reliable.

**ST. VITUS' DANCE, or Shaking Palsy, Cure for.**—Tincture of black cohosh, 6 ozs.; bromide of potassium, 1½ ozs.; mix. DOSE—For an adult, 1 tea-spoonful 3 times daily, an hour after meals.

*Remarks.*—W. W. Stimson, M. D., of Connersville, Miss., reports in the *Medical Brief*, the cure of a young lady of 15 years, who had had this annoying trouble so bad that she would not go into company for over a year, her speech even being affected. Two weeks cured this case. But in older persons and of longer standing it may require months. There is no danger in its use; but after taking the above amount I would wait a week before beginning on a new prescription of same amount. Look after general health in all cases. Younger persons will take less according to age.

**1. FELON—Remedy for.**—A small piece of calf's rennet soaked in milk and tied around the finger, renewing occasionally, will cure any case of felon.

*Remarks.*—I do not know who tried this, to make the assertion, nor have I had a chance to test it; yet I have no doubt of its value. But as the rennet may not always be at hand, I will give the following, the ingredients of which may always be obtained:

**2. Felon Salve—Successful Treatment.**—A salve made of soap and spirits of turpentine, a very small proportion of the latter, just enough to moisten the soap, which has been shaved from a bar. "I have known it," says "H. S. P.," of Byron, Wis., to one of the papers, "to cure the worst felons, and I never knew it to fail when applied." To which the editor added: "The above is a well-known remedy in the editor's family, and has always been considered infallible, if applied in the earlier stages."

**3. Felon—Warranted Cure for.**—F. F. Lewis, of Whitewater, Wis., says: "Wind a cloth loosely about the finger, leaving the end free. Pour in common gunpowder till the afflicted part is entirely covered; then keep the whole constantly wet with strong spirits of camphor. Warranted to remove all pain in two hours. Have seen it tried many times, and never without absolute cure and without pain or injury to the hand."

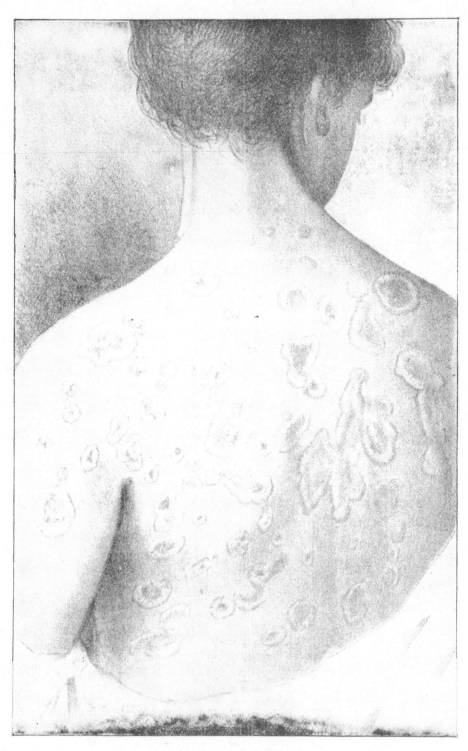

PSORASIS, OR DRY TETTER.

1. **HYDROPHOBIA; or, Mad Dog Bites—Hot Vapor Baths for.**—The following item comes from G. F. J. Colburn, of Washington, D. C., who says: " For God's sake, give the remedy a trial, should a case present itself.' The report was first published in the *Salut Public*, of Lyons, France, as follows·

" Dr. Buifson claims to have discovered a remedy for this terrible disease. In attending a female patient in the last stages of canine madness, the doctor imprudently wiped his hand with a handkerchief impregnated with her saliva. There happened to be a slight abrasion on the index finger of the left hand; but, confident of his own curative system, the doctor merely washed the parts with water. He was fully aware of the imprudence he had committed, and says: 'Believing that the malady would not declare itself until the fortieth day, and having various patients to visit, I put off from day to day the application of my remedy—that is to say, vapor baths. The ninth day, being in my cabinet, I felt all at once a pain in my eyes. My body felt so light that I felt as if I could jump a prodigious height, or, if thrown out of a window, I could sustain myself in the air. My hair was so sensitive that I appeared to be able to count it separately without looking at it. Saliva kept constantly forming in my mouth. Any movement in the air caused great pain to me and I was obliged to avoid the sight of brilliant objects. I had a continued desire to run and bite—not human beings, but animals, and all that was near me. I drank with difficulty, and I remarked that the sight of water distressed me more than the pain in my throat. I believe that by shutting the eyes, any one suffering from hydrophobia can always drink. The fits come on every five minutes, and I then felt the pain start from the index finger and run up the nerves to the shoulder. In this state, thinking that my course was preservative, not curative, I took a vapor bath, not with the intention of cure, but of suffocating myself. When the bath was at 52 centigrade (93 3-5 Fahrenheit), all the symptoms disappeared as if by magic, and since then I have never felt anything more of them. I have attended more than 80 persons bitten by mad animals, and I have not lost a single one. When a person is bitten by a mad dog he must for 7 successive days take a vapor bath, *à la Russe*, of 57 to 63 degrees. This is the preventive remedy. A vapor bath may be quickly made by putting 2 or three red-hot bricks in a bucket for 15 or 20 minutes. The person to be covered with a blanket. When the disease is declared, it only requires one vapor bath, rapidly increasing to 37 centigrade, then slowly to 53, and the patient must strictly confine himself to his chamber until the cure is complete."

2. **Hydrophobia, Portuguese Physician's Cure.**—A Portuguese physician claims to have cured several cases of hydrophobia by simply rubbing garlic into the wound, and giving the patient a decoction of garlic to drink for several days. This is the old Greek treatment, which, it is claimed, was practiced by them with success.—*Medical Brief.*

1. **SUN-STROKE AND APOPLEXY, How to Cure.**—Sunstroke and apoplexy, can be cured almost surely if taken in any kind of time. Dr. E. B. Babbitt says:

I. " Rub powerfully on the back of the head and neck, making horizontal and downward movements. This draws the blood away from the front of the brain and vitalizes the involuntary nerves.

II. " While rubbing call for cold water immediately, which apply to the face and to the hair on the top and the side of the head.

III. " Call for a bucket of water as hot as can be borne, and pour it by dipperfuls on the back of the head and neck for several minutes. The effect will be wonderful, for vitalizing the *medulla oblongata* (that part of the spinal column within the head); it vitalizes the whole body, and the patient will generally start up into full conscious life in a very short time.

"Last summer I was called in to see a man on Fourth avenue. I found him in a state of coma, and his wife greatly alarmed, supposing him to be dead. He had lain thus for about 3 hours. I had him brought out where he could get the air, jerked off his clothes, rubbed his back, head and neck powerfully, slapped his back, legs and feet briskly, and called for iced water, which I applied to his front and upper head. I then had a bucket of hot water brought, which I poured on his back, head and neck. Before doing this I had noticed some signs of life while applying the cold water in front, but after applying the hot water on the back of the head and neck a few minutes, he started up, vomited, and exclaimed "All right!" I occupied about 20 minutes in thus resuscitating him. He rose up, put on his clothes with a little help, and did not lose an hour more from his business. Persons of large and active brains and weak bodies are more liable to sun-stroke and should wear light-colored, cool hats in summer, wet the hair occasionally, and if they feel a brain pressure coming on, should rub briskly on the back of the neck and put cold water on the top and front of the head. These remarks, if heeded, will prevent great danger and great suffering. I have never known this method to fail."

*Remarks.*—Heretofore it has been customary to use only cold water upon the head in sun-stroke or apoplexy, but it seems by the above treatment of Dr. Babbitt, with the hot water upon the back of the head and neck, that consciousness is restored much more quickly, as well as more certainly, for without it, on the old plan of the cold water only, many have never been restored at all; hence the hot water should be provided as quickly as possible, and applied freely with a dipper, while the cold water, by wet cloths, may be kept on the front and top of the head. Small things, when you get the right thing, are often "wonderful," as the doctor puts it above. The colder the water on the front and top of the head, the better, and the hotter it can be borne on the back of the head and neck, the better, also. It would seem to me preferable, to dip cloths into the hot water and apply as hot as they can be borne, re-wetting often, than to pour it. For those who have a tendency to head troubles let them dampen a flat piece of sponge and put it in the hat before going out into a very hot sun. It may be well to know that what is good for sun-stroke is also good for apoplexy.

When one is stricken down in the sun, he should be placed in the shade as quick as possible, and cold water applied to his face, and the limbs kept warm by rubbing, etc., until he can be removed to the house, where the above plan can be carried out fully.

**1. MOLES, FRECKLES, PIMPLES, ETC.—To Remove.—** W. H. Riddle, of Crystal Lake, Cal., says to "Mary," of Zenia, Ind., through the *Blade Household:*

"Do not use nitric acid on your face. I would advise you to use the acid nitrate of mercury, in removing moles from the face. The acid should be applied with a splinter of wood, and gently rubbed in the part (with the splinter) for several seconds, according to the thickness of the growth. Great care should be taken to prevent the acid from reaching the surrounding skin. There is absolutely no pain attending the application, and the growth gradually shrivels away, and the slough falls off in about a week. I know a lady who had a very large mole removed in this way from the chin, leaving scarcely any depression in the skin. It is now some five years since the operation was performed, with no return of the growth."

*Remarks.*—It will be safe to use it for this purpose. Have it labeled, and keep it out of the way of children.

After writing the above, having a mole on one of my wrists, I tried it, and removed it successfully. At the first application it only took off about half the thickness of the mole; I then applied it again, using the end of a match-splint; I put on so much and rubbed it in so thoroughly that it killed the mole entirely, making a deep sore, although no larger than the mole; but putting on a liniment, followed with a little vaseline, 5 or 6 times daily, removed all soreness and healed it up in a few days, leaving the skin perfectly smooth and soft. I have since cured 3 or 4 others with the same, 2 of which were cancerous (open sore), and consequently, know the value of the acid nitrate of mercury for such cases.

**2. Pimples or Skin Diseases, Valuable Remedy for.** — Glycerine (English or Price's), 100 grs.; corrosive sublimate, 5 grs. DIRECTIONS— Rub the corrosive sublimate in a little of the glycerine; then mix all, and apply morning and evening.

*Remarks.*—M. Pierre Vigier, a French professor, finds, from experiments upon himself and upon his pupils, that substances incorporated with glycerine are not absorbed by the skin, therefore he advises this as a substitute for blue ointment, which stains the linen and is absorbed, while with a glycerine prepared as above, in spite of the causticity of the bichloride (corrosive sublimate is the bichloride of mercury), the skin is not irritated by this mixture, and after extensive applications to the skin, no mercury is found in the urine.

The fact that by this form of mixing the corrosive sublimate prevents its absorption into the system, it should be so prepared; as it thus cures these and other skin diseases, it becomes valuable for these purposes. It will also cure itch, as well as pimples, blotches, black-heads (worms in the skin of the face). See " Pimples, Tetter, etc.," where corrosive sublimate is also used.

**3. Freckles, Remedy for.** — The following remedy is said to have been found efficacious in Europe: Finely powdered sulpho-phenate of zinc (one of the newer remedies), 1 part; oil of lemon, 1 part; pure alcohol, 5 parts; collodion, 45 parts; drops, grs. or drs.— as you please — may be used. DIRECTIONS—Mix well; then apply to the freckles, twice daily, until the change is affected.

**4. To Remove Freckles.**—Rub them twice, daily, with a piece of saltpeter, moistened by touching it in water.

**5. Sunburn, to Remove.**—Water, 1 pt.; pulverized borax, 1 oz. DIRECTIONS—Put in a bottle and shake before using. Wet the parts, blackened by exposure to the sun, twice daily.

**6. Pimple, Tetter or Bad Skin Diseases, Remedy.**—Put corrosive sublimate, 30 grs., into a 4 oz. vial, with ½ oz. of oil of sassafras (these to be rubbed together), and fill the bottle with alcohol.

*Remarks.*—Upon pimples of an ulcerative character, or on eruptions, like tetter or salt-rheum, apply this corrosive mixture, once a day only, until some inflammation manifests itself, then discontinue, and apply simple glycerine, vaseline or some mild ointment, until healed.  If in any case the pimples or eruptions show again. do the same for 2 or 3 times, which will generally cure them, especially if a proper cathartic is first given, then an alterative course of medicine is given.  But should the above fail in any case, double the amount of corrosive sublimate and try it again.  It has been used as strong as here recommended; but if of less strength will do, so much the better.  Of course it will be understood that this is a poison, and children should not have access to it; although it is safe and valuable to use as above directed.

**7. Tetter, Simple Cure for.**—It is claimed also that to wet gun-powder and smear on the tetter twice a day, for 2 or 3 days, will effect a permanent cure.  It would undoubtedly be rather severe.  I should rub it up in water, or spirits of camphor, to use it, and make the strength bearable, as it is no use to kill it dead the first pop, but use it milder, and longer, will do as well.  If the gun-powder was rubbed fine, then rubbed into an ointment with lard, or vaseline, I think it would do just as well.  A tea-spoonful of the powder to 1 oz. will be strong enough.  But do not forget a laxative treatment with sulphur and cream of tartar, salts or magnesia, as may be preferred.

**8. Face Worms, to Remove.** — To remove worms in the face, place over the black spot the hollow end of a watch-key, and press firmly. This forces the foreign substance out, so that it may be brushed off, and is a cure.  A lady writer gives us the following, also:

**9. Face Worms, Pimples, etc.**—Wash your face night and morning in strong cologne water and rub dry with a coarse towel.  Also take a thimbleful of sulphur in a glass of milk 2 or 3 times a week, before breakfast. Continue the practice a couple of weeks.

*Remarks.*—It is a well known fact that sulphur is a valuable thing to take internally, from its alterative effect in all diseases of the skin; and one of the handiest ways to take it, is to mix it up quite thick, with a little syrup, or molasses; and when thus mixed, in place of stopping to measure out the lady's thimbleful, as above, take what you can in a tea-spoon, three mornings, and skip three, till nine doses are taken.  Some prefer to make it half-and-half, with cream of tartar, and to take it in the same way; but the cream of tartar is not as necessary in skin difficulties, as it is in more general inflammations, such as boils, swellings, etc.

**10. Pimples, Bad and of Long Standing.**—Prof. Scudder, of Cincinnati, Ohio, reports through the *Eclectic Medical Journal*, the case of a girl who had been troubled for years with pimples, which left large scars, cured in 10 days, by the simple use of bi-carbonate of soda (common baking soda).  He claimed, because of a broad, pallid or pale tongue, the soda was needed to neutralize an acid condition of the system.  The cure proved him correct.  DOSE—For a girl of 15 years, the age of the one cured, ½ tea-spoonful in a little water, 2 or 3 table-spoonfuls only, after each meal.

*Remarks.*—It will prove valuable in many cases, and in all cases with acidity of the stomach, "belching" wind, or passing large amounts of gas per rectum. In these cases, "belching" of the wind, or gas distending the stomach and bowels, mix ivory black (which is an animal charcoal), with equal parts of sugar and half a tea-spoonful of the mixture, taken before meals, by placing on the tongue dry, then taking a sip of water to swallow it. These two will soon correct this condition which arises from dyspepsia.

**1. PILLS, Compound Cathartic and Liver.**—Comp. ext. of colocynth, ext. of jalap and calomel, each, 100 grs.; gamboge and ext. of hyoscyamus, each, 25 grs.; castile soap in powder (in fact, all in powder except the extract of hyoscyamus, which is gummy). Mix and make into 100 pills. Dose—As an active cathartic, 2 or 3 pills, to act on the liver 1 pill at bedtime each night until the action is sufficient.

*Remarks.*—I have prescribed them and found them to have the desired effect with those persons who prefer calomel to podophyllin. But if there are those who think they would like this pill best if it was not for the calomel, they can leave it out, or put in only 25 grs. of it, so as to have one-fourth of a grain only in each pill. Either way it will be found efficient and satisfactory. I prefer it with only ¼ gr. of calomel to each pill. The old plan of giving large doses of calomel, I feel thankful, is among the things of the past.

**2. Butternut Pills.**—A very valuable cathartic is made by taking the inner bark of the butternut tree and roots (not old trees), strip it into strips and put in a clean boiler, with plenty of water, and keep moderately hot for 48 hours, then boil for a few hours longer, after which pour out and strain; then boil down to a consistency of thick molasses, adding at this point as much molasses as there is of the extract, and continue to boil down carefully until quite thick; then preserve in covered jars. Dose—A piece the size of a small hickory nut, or less, as may be found to be necessary to produce proper cathartic action. During the Revolution there was but little other physic used. This, however, was very satisfactory; and still in places where the tree abounds, it may be adopted with a like satisfaction. In case that it gripes or gives pain in its action, a little powdered ginger, or capsicum may be incorporated with the gummy mixture to overcome this tenesmus, as doctors call it. One-fourth as much bulk of the ginger or one-eighth of capsicum will be sufficient.

**3. Liver Regulator, or Liver Complaint, Dyspepsia, etc., Liquid Remedy for.**—Fluid exts. of dandelion, blue flag-root and rhubarb, each, 1 oz.; fl. ext. leptandra (Culver's physic) and simple syrup, each, 2 ozs. Mix. Dose—One-half tea-spoonful every 6 hours.

**4. Liver Syrup, or Liver Regulator, in Place of Pills for an Inactive Liver, Constipation, etc.**—The fl. exts. of wahoo, butternut and cascara sagrada, each ½ oz.; fl. exts. of fringe tree and white ash, each, ¼ oz.; fl. exts. of berberis aquafolium, prickly ash and bitter root (Culver's physic), each, 1 dr. Mix and add simple syrup to fill a 4 oz. bottle; shake when used. Dose—Take ½ tea-spoonful at bedtime only, and if it does not start the action of the liver in 3 or 4 days at most increase the dose to ¾, or even 1 tea-spoonful; then drop back to the ½, or it may be to 15 or 20 drops, to keep a little action on the liver until it will continue its secretion of bile, producing natural colored stools.

*Remarks.*—As there are persons who cannot take pills, and others also who prefer laxative medicines in liquid form, as well as many whose livers need a mild medicine so it can be continued for some time to overcome the inactivity of the liver, etc., such persons will find this recipe to "fill the bill" in all these cases. Hence, this will be found a very valuable substitute for pills. A little oil of wintergreen may be put in as a flavor and to hide the bitter taste, if desired.

**5. Liquid Physic for Constipated and Weakly Women and Children.**—Fl. ext. of butternut, 2 ozs.; tinct. of aloes, 5 drs.; comp. tinct. of cardamon, 1 oz.; simple syrup, 4 oz. Mix. DOSE—According to age of children, from 1 to 3 tea-spoonfuls in the morning is the best time to give to children, and repeat next morning, if no operation before. For weak constipated women, the physician whom I first knew to use this preparation was in the habit of triturating calomel, 10 grs., with 100 grs. of the sugar of milk, and dividing into 10 powders; then giving 1 powder at 10 in the evening, and at 2 in the morning, followed by 1 or 2 tea-spoonfuls of this liquid physic, which carries off all otherwise ill effects of the calomel, arouses the action of the liver and overcomes the tendency to constipation. Those in favor of using calomel will undoubtedly be satisfied to use it in this manner; the trituration, or thoroughly rubbing the calomel, or any other medicine, with sugar of milk, divides it into more minute particles and then it takes less to have the desired effect. Of course, this liquid physic can be taken without the calomel by doubling the dose. See the remarks closing the subject of "Jaundice," for the author's experience and opinion of calomel in small doses. Since writing this I have given the twentieth of a grain calomel pill with entire satisfaction, arousing the action of the liver.

**6. Pills for Constipation—Very Successful.**—Pulverized aloes, 40 grs.; solid ext. of nux vomica, 20 grs.; solid ext. belladonna, 15 grs. Mix thoroughly and divide into 50 pills. DOSE—One pill only; never more than 1 pill for a dose, at bedtime every night until cured or all taken.—*Dr. T. B. King.*

*Remarks.*—The doctor says this is the best thing he knows, and pretty sure to cure the difficulty. I have used it with success in one case of long standing constipation. It was a lady who was pretty well run down in strength, but with this pill at night, and a 2 gr. pill of quinine 3 times daily, for a month, she has enjoyed an excellent condition of health now for several months. If they fail to touch the spot, ¼ gr. of podophyllin, or calomel, as one prefers, may be added to each pill; neither will be required unless it may be for an occasional case of constipation which has withstood all other remedies.

**GOUT—Cured by Garlic**—The London *Truth* makes the following remarks upon the garlic as a specific (sure cure) for gout. It is amusing, and is, no doubt, valuable: "Many people would be overjoyed to pay large sums for a specific for gout. I will give them for nothing a sure but simple cure. A friend of mine had chalkstones on his fingers so bad that he might have marked half the trees in Windsor Park with them. After consulting almost all the specialists in Europe he was advised by an old woman (some old women know more than half of us doctors) to try a clove of garlic (a clove of garlic means one small bulb from a cluster) night and morning. He did so, and the chalkstones totally disappeared. No doubt such a cure involves the social duty of retiring to the summit of an exceedingly high mountain, or going to sea, alone, in a yacht; but it is worth even the penalty of absolute seclusion to get rid of chalkstones." (See next recipe.)

1. **PURIFYING THE BLOOD—Safest Way by the Use of Onions.**—Sherley Dare, in answering correspondents through the *Blade Household*, says to "A. E. W.," of Waterloo: "The safest and quickest prescription for clearing the blood is to eat a raw onion, finely minced, at breakfast; the whole of a common sized onion is enough, and a dose of charcoal or ground coffee, and brushing the teeth, will deodorize the breath. The onion can be taken with salt and vinegar as a salad. Consumptives find this of benefit."

*Remarks.*—I have much more faith in the onion as an alterative, than I have in the idea that the charcoal or powdered coffee, even with the brushing of the teeth, will remove the odor of onions from the breath; but what of that? let the " bref " smell of garlic; if onions will do what they are here credited with, they are certainly more valuable than is generally set down to their credit; but I remember of once being told by a gentleman that a moderate sized onion minced and eaten at each meal, with the salt and vinegar, as above mentioned, would cure dyspepsia. I have no doubt of their utility, both as an alterative upon the blood and as a tonic to the stomach; not one is eaten when ten ought to be.

2. **Roasted Onions—As a Poultice to Boils, Inflammation of the Bowels, etc.**—A poultice of roasted onions applied to boils, tumors, etc., hastens suppuration, and are often applied as "drafts" to the feet, and I have heard, from the old women, of their being applied in excessive fevers, by mashing or pounding onions and placing them under the arms and upon the bowels or other parts swollen from extensive inflammation (to be changed often), and they are very valuable indeed.

3. **Onions, Their Value as Food.**—Onions contain 25 to 30% (*i, e.,* 25 to 30 parts in 100) of solid substance, when dried; while potatoes, even, do not average 25%; but from some peculiarity of the onion its nourishing properties more than double those of the potato, and in some cases nearly treble it; hence its value as food may now be the better understood, and without regard to its peculiar flavor, the onion should be much more eaten than it is. If health is desirable, eat onions.

1. **STOMACH BITTERS, OR ALTERATIVE.** — Culver's physic, root, and wahoo, bark of the root, each, 1½ ozs.; prickly ash bark and poke root, each, ½ oz.; Peruvian bark, the best red unground, wild cherry bark and anise seed, each, 1 oz.; blue-flag, yellow-dock, dandelion and pleurisy roots, known also as white root (*asclepias tuberosa*), with our home yellow parilla

and Honduras sarsaparilla and golden seal roots, each, 1 oz.; water, 1 gal.; alcohol, 1 pt., or good whiskey (if there is good (?) whiskey), 1 qt. DIREC- TIONS—Have all the roots and barks ground coarsely if you buy the dry articles of the druggist, and if you use the green ones, gathered yourself, use half as much more, and even twice as much will do no harm; bruise them with a mallet or hammer, and steep all in the water 3 or 4 hours, covered; then strain and press out all the virtue, and when cool, strain again to get rid of the fine sediment; add the alcohol, or whiskey, and if it lacks any of 1 gal. make it up with wine- worked cider, or whiskey. Bottle and keep in a cool place. DOSE—According to the size and robustness of the person, take from 1 to 2 table-spoonfuls a short time before each meal. If costive, or considerable dyspeptic disturbances of the stomach, see remarks and further directions below.

II. *Remarks and Further Directions if at all Costive.*—In such cases take a quart of this bitters and add ½ dr. of the alcoholic ex. of mandrake, dissolved nicely in the bitters by rubbing in a cup with a tea-spoon; pour off into the bottle and put on more, as it is slow to dissolve. DOSE—This can only be taken in doses of from 1 to 2 tea-spoon fuls 3 times daily, more or less, to keep the bowels easy. The mandrake is very gentle in its cathartic and laxative proper- ties, but it is very certain.

III. If dyspeptic, take a pint bottle and pour into it fl. exs. of leptandra and blue-flag, each, 1 dr.; and fl. ex. of balmony, ½ oz., and also iodide of potash, 25 grs., and fill the bottle with the No. 1 Bitters, which has no man- drake in it. DOSE—Then take 1 table-spoonful for a dose, just before meals and at bed-time; and if the urine is scanty or high-colored, 2 drs. each of fl. exs. of buchu and uva ursi may also be put in. DOSE—The same, as with the above bitters as a base, almost any condition can be met.

**1. DIARRHEA COMPOUND.**—Compound spirits of lavender and tinct. of rhubarb, each, 1 oz.; laudanum, 3 drs.; oil of cinnamon, 10 drops; mix. DOSE—One tea-spoonful every hour or two, for an adult, as needed, until relieved; then 2 or 3 times a day only, for a day or two.

**2. Loose Bowels, Simple Remedy for.**—For loose bowels, not of long standing nor very severe, the following powder will prove effectual and satisfactory. I have used it many times. Powdered opium and tannin, each, 5 grs. Mix thoroughly and divide into 10 powders. DOSE—For an adult, 1 powder every 4 hours, or 3, or even every 2 hours, if needed to control the con- dition; children of 8 to 12 years, half a powder only, and of a less age—above 2 years—one-fourth only of a powder.

**3. For Infantile Diarrhea.**—That is, for children at the breast or less than 2 years old: Powdered rhubarb, 10 grs.; calomel, 1 gr.; morphine, ½ gr., and divide into 10 powders, 1 powder for a dose. No danger of saliva- ting a child at the breast.

**4. Diarrhea of an Exhaustive Character, Dr. T. B. King's Remedy for.**—Blue mass and pulverized ipecac, of each 3 grs.; prepared chalk and pulverized rhubarb, each 10 grs.; pulverized opium, 3 to 10 grs. Mix and make into 10 pills. DIRECTIONS, DOSE, ETC.—For adults, bad cases, use the 10 grs. of the opium and give 1 pill every 3 hours; for children and slight cases, only 3 to 5 grs. of opium should be used; small children, only half a pill cut up and dissolved in molasses will be sufficient for a dose, to be repeated in 3 or 4 hours, as needed.

**5. Diarrhea, Simple Home Remedy for.**—The journals of late have said considerable about the use of pure cider vinegar in diarrhea. It was started, so far as I know, by T. E. Stellwagen, in an edition of Coleman's "Dental Surgery." Dose—For an adult about 2 ozs., or 4 tablespoonfuls, without water; for a child of 1 year, a tablespoonful with a little water.

*Remarks.*—Its effect is said to be to check the colicky pains at once, to relieve the chills and cramps, if any present, and to give a feeling of warmth and comfort over the surface. I trust it will prove as reliable as reported. It is claimed to have been satisfactory even in long standing cases.

**1. DYSENTERY – Successful Remedy for.**—Laudanum and ipecac. Directions, Dose, etc.—For an adult first give laudanum, 20 drops, to prepare the stomach so it shall retain the ipecac, which is to be given half an hour after, in 20 gr. doses, repeated every 6 hours until cured. The first dose may be vomited, or partially so, as this article is well understood to possess this property—of vomiting—but it is also known that the stomach can be trained to tolerate (bear) it. It also acts as a mild laxative, tonic, and stimulant, to the coats of the stomach and intestines, producing slight sweating, moist and pliable skin, and thereby reducing the fever, controlling also the tenesmus (pain and griping) of the rectum at the time of the passage, almost if not wholly relieving this difficulty soon after its use is commenced.

**2. Dysentery, Diarrhea and Incipient Cholera—Milk a Specific for.**—It is reported through the *Milk Journal*, of London, Eng., that in the East Indies, 1 pt. of warm milk every 4 hours, will check the most violent of the above complaints. The milk must not be boiled, but just hot enough to drink comfortably. Boiled milk, contrary to our American custom, is not to be used.

**NERVOUS HEADACHE—Such as People Used to be Bled for.**—Iodide of potash, 2 drs.; tinct of gelsemium, 2 drs.; pure water, 2 ozs.; mix. Dose—1 tea-spoonful once in 2 to 4 hours until relieved.

*Remarks.*—This is a prescription of a physician of Grand Rapids Mich., for a lady who called upon him to be bled for the difficulty, according to what she had been accustomed to. But he made this prescription for her and it relieved her. The next season she called upon myself for the same purpose, at the same time showing me the prescription, which I changed to bromide of potassium, in the same quantity for the iodide, which she took with the same success. I prefer the bromide, as I think its action upon the nerves more satisfactory.

**2. Nervous Headache, New Remedy for.**—Salicylate of soda, 10 grs., every 3 hours for an adult, followed next day in 5 to 8 gr. doses. If of long standing, continue 1 or 2 doses daily for a few days longer. Taken by dissolving in water.

*Remarks.*—This was given in the *Scientific American* by a celebrated physician who gave a case of a boy of 16 years, who had had nervous headache several days each week from the time he was 6 years old, entirely cured by this remedy, and at the time of the report he had been free from the disease several months. See next item also for other uses of this new remedy.

**TONSILITIS — Salicylate of Soda for — Also as a Gargle in Ulcerated Cases.**—Given in 10 gr. doses, every 2 to 4 hours, internally, and is also used as a gargle in ulcerated cases. Strength of gargle is not given; but I should say, 5 to 10 grs. to the oz. of water, according to the degree of ulceration.

*Remarks.*—I certainly expect much from its use upon a fair trial, and say to all who need it, try it.

**ULCERATING TEETH OR SORE GUMS — Dr. Mason's Remedy.**—Take what the homeopaths call the "third decimal trituration of mercurius" (quick-silver). [Quicksilver was named mercurius after the god Mercury; it is also known as hydrargyrum, from another god or deity, worshiped by the ancients. These deities were held in higher estimation by them, as compared with other deities, from the fact that mercury or quicksilver was held, long ago, to be a very important article or medicine in the treatment of diseases, as compared with other remedies. But my school of medicine (eclectic) generally claims and believes that it has been proven not only of little value but to have been one of the greatest curses to humanity that ever found a place in the annals or history of medicine. Of late, however, I am led to believe the harm to have arisen from its over-doses and abuse in giving it for everything rather than in the article itself. See my remarks following "Jaundice, Liver Complaint, etc."] DOSE—The size of a wheat kernel, every half hour or hour, until cured, which will be in 2 or 3 days.

*Remarks.*—Dr. Mason, in writing to me, said: "Doctor you know that I am not a homeopath, but I know, after having used the above in my practice as a dentist for over fifteen years for ulcerating teeth, that it is a good remedy. In the winter of 1878-79 I extracted some teeth for my wife; and, in common parlance, she took cold in the jaw. Although it was nearly 2 days after it commenced aching before I prepared the remedy, the pain entirely ceased in less than 2 days from the time she began its use. But let no one put it off, as I did, through pressure of business—'a stitch in time,' etc."

In case no homeopath or druggist is near, who keeps this triturated preparation, see "Diphtheria, Sore Throat, etc.," (Dr. Mason's, or homeopathic remedy), for the manner of trituration, use the quicksilver instead of the biniodide of mercury, as given in that case.

**1. VOMITING — Ejects a Dime from the Trachea.**—Lorenzo Hubbard, M. D., reports a case to the *Pacific Med. and Surg. Journal* as follows:

"Carpenter Simes, a private in Company A, First U. S. Cavalry, while playing with a dime, by tossing it into his mouth, accidentally threw it far back into the pharynx, where, coming in contact with the posterior nasal orifices, it excited a strong disposition to sneeze. The spasmodic inspiration which followed drew the piece through the glottis (the opening into the windpipe) into the trachea (windpipe), and subsequent inspirations lodged it at the point of the bifurcation of the right bronchus. By inflating the lungs, and then making a strong effort at expiration, the 'piece' would rise into the trachea, but when it reached the glottis suffocation was so imminent he was forced to allow it to descend. When he first made his situation known to me, three hours after the occurrence of the accident, he said he could feel the 'bit' resting directly under the right nipple, and that the parts at this point had become quite sore.

"While the piece was yet movable, and had not yet found a lodgement, I determined to try the experiment of vomiting, with the hope that in the spasmodic effort of retching and coughing it might be ejected. In this I was not disappointed, for in the very first effort it was thrown out to the distance of several feet, with considerable force. I also send you the 'bit' with which this strange experiment was made, supposing that possibly the case might interest our society."

*Remarks.*—I have given this to show not only the danger of thus throwing pieces of money into the mouth, which I have often seen done, but also to say it is dangerous to allow small children to have small pieces of money to play with, for the mouth is about the first place they put it; but if a piece lodges in the throat, no time should be lost in trying one of the quick emetics found in "Accidental Poisoning."

### 2. Vomiting and Watery Discharges, to Check in Cholera.

—Black pepper, in powder, fine table salt, each 1 tea-spoonful; vinegar, 5 tea-spoonfuls; hot water, ½ tumbler. DOSE—A table-spoonful every 5, 10 or 15 minutes, as circumstances required, speedily checked vomiting, abated the watery discharges and removed the cramps. It succeeded in many cases where every other means had failed.

*Remarks.*—This was during the Cincinnati cholera in 1849-50-51, when the eclectics saved hundreds of their patients in this disease, while other branches of the profession lost most of theirs. This is no fancy statement, simply for effect, but is susceptible of proof, and it was by simple common sense remedies, like this, that it was done.

### 1. SCROFULA, PILES AND RHEUMATISM.—Cure for.

Sulphur, cream of tartar, and licorice root, equal parts of each, all finely pulverized, ¼ part nitre, and put into just honey enough to mix like mush. DOSE—One tea-spoonful ½ hour before eating, 3 times a day, for 3 days; then cease 3 days, continuing until a cure is effected. But after the first 3 days, ½ tea-spoonful doses will be as much as can be taken without making the bowels too loose. It may be made into pill form by using only honey enough to dampen. DOSE—In this way 3 good sized pills, before each meal, as the other.

*Remarks.*—This was communicated to me by a sister, at that time living in Mt. Pleasant, Iowa, from the fact that a young girl, a Miss Conner, had been cured by it, who had been under the doctor's care for over a year, without benefit. Her breast and throat were covered with ulcers, deep and penetrating, so when pressed up on one side of the neck, matter would ooze out of the other side. Under these circumstances, the girl's mother (the wife of a barber) paid $10 for this recipe, which cured the girl in a few weeks. At the time my sister sent me this recipe, six years after the cure, the girl had had no returning symptoms of the disease. But the scars, my sister said, she would always carry. A child had also been cured by the use of the same, whose head was a solid scab at the time the treatment was commenced. My sister had obtained the recipe for the purpose of curing bleeding piles upon herself, which had reduced her strength very greatly by the loss of blood. And it was as successful with the piles as in the other cures. I have had no opportunity of using it except for rheumatism, which I have cured with it. I believe much good will be derived by its use whenever needed, as an alterative, for the value of sulphur and cream of tartar have been long known as alteratives in rheumatism. Why should not the combination prove valuable in scrofula? I have no doubt it has, and that it will continue to do so, most effectually. The licorice I look upon as merely to improve the taste.

**2. Scrofula, White Swelling, etc., Salve for.**—Scrape sweet elder (inner bark), bitter-sweet (roots and twigs are used), and mullein leaves, each, a good handful; boil these, (the roots and twigs, being bruised,) in a little water; then put in half as much golden seal root, and stew all in two table-spoonfuls of freshly churned and unsalted butter, not level spoonfuls, but as you would take them up heaping, from rather soft butter, and an equal quantity of mutton tallow. Stew till the water is all out, and the mass crisped, or dry, but not burned; then strain, and put back into the skillet, and add half as much beeswax, as of tallow and half as much pine pitch as of the beeswax. DIRECTIONS—For white swelling spread on a cloth, and apply; for scrofulous sores put on cotton, and put into the sores, or openings, if any, otherwise the same as for white swellings.

*Remarks.*—I should apply this salve while taking No. 1, internally, as I think it will hasten recovery. It will be found valuable for all purposes, as an ointment, rather than a salve, if not made too stiff with the beeswax. As an ointment, use but very little beeswax.

**PLIABLE COLLODION—Or Artificial Skin—For Abrasions, Burns, Sores, etc.**—A French journal gives us the following plan of making collodion pliable, for all purposes where water may come in contact with the spot, as upon the face, hands, lips, etc.: Collodion, 30 grammes; castor-oil and soft turpentine (Venice turpentine or pine pitch), each 50 centigrammes, mix.

*Remarks.*—As a gramme is so nearly 15½ grains (being actually 15 and 834 of 1,000 parts of a grain, we call it 15½ grains,) and as a centigramme is the 1-100th of a gramme, in the 50 centigrammes we get nearly 8 grains, hence we say: Collodion, 1 oz.; and castor-oil and soft turpentine, each 8 grs. And thus we have the recipe Americanized, so that it can be filled understandingly by anyone, or druggist. Apply with a brush. It will be found quite satisfactory to apply upon any injured parts, scratch, bruise, etc., as by putting on two or three times, as the first coat dries, it forms an artificial skin over the sore.

**1. CHILBLAINS, FROST BITES, ETC.—Valuable Remedy for.**—Spirits of turpentine and sulphuric acid, each ¼ oz.; olive oil, 1¼ oz.; mix; shake and apply frequently.

**2. Spirits of Turpentine,** 1 oz.; ammonia, ½ oz., with as much camphor gum as this will dissolve, used as a liniment, will cure these hateful things.

**3. To Relieve** the intense itching; 2 or 3 bathings of the parts, warming in before the fire, or strong alum water, gives relief.

**4. An Ointment** made by rubbing as much tincture of cantharides into any simple "cerate," as it will take up (any druggist will prepare a small box of it, for about 15 cts.). Bathe the feet in warm water, wipe and rub this on at bed-time. I cured a bad case of 6 years standing, in 2 or 3 applications, and afterwards cured several other cases.

**5. Frost Bites, Remedies for.**—The Lansing (Mich.,) *Republican* recently gave the following, as to the management and cure of frost bites. It says: "Extract the frost by the application of ice-water till the part is pliable, but let no artificial heat touch it; then apply a salve made of equal parts of hog's lard and gunpowder, rubbed together until it forms a paste, and in less than 24 hours the frozen parts will be well."

**6. Chilblains, Warranted Cure for.**—Olive oil, spirits of turpentine, aqua ammonia, and oil of peppermint, each, ¼ oz. Mix, and anoint night and morning. Is warranted to cure every case. This was given me on "experience," also.

## WORMS—REMEDIES, VERMIFUGES.

There are seldom found but three varieties of worms in the human intestines.

I. The principal, or most common one, is the long, round worm, found in the small intestines.

II. The second variety is the small, round, or pin-worm, so called because scarcely ever longer or larger than a pin. These are chiefly found in the rectum, and known to be there from an intolerable itching.

III. The last, or third variety, is the tape-worm, called by physicians *tænia solium* (from *tænia*, tape, and *solus*, alone); for, as a general thing, there is only one of them found to annoy the patient. The remedies for them, I shall give in the order in which I have mentioned them. First:

**1. The Long, Round Worm.**—Pink and senna were the old "standby," for the common long worm, followed by a cathartic; but the following combination is better, as it has the cathartic in combination, and as the good old saying is, "kills two birds with one stone."

Pink root and senna, each ½ oz.; cream of tartar, 1 dr. (1 tea-spoonful); pulverized jalap, ½ dr.; cardamon seeds, 1 dr.; and ext. of licorice, or powdered licorice-root, ¼ oz. Mix, and pour on ½ pt. of boiling water and steep ½ to 1 hour; and, according to the age of the child, give 1 to 2 table-spoonfuls every hour until the worms are expelled, or a brisk action of the bowels is obtained. Repeat every day or two, until you are satisfied there are no more worms present, or see that they have been expelled, as it does not always, but generally, expels them on the first trial.

**2. The Eclectic Vermifuge — The Latest and Least Distasteful.**—Santonin, 30 grs.; white sugar, 50 grs. DIRECTIONS—Rub together evenly, and divide into 10 powders. DOSE—Give 1 powder an hour before supper and 1 at bed-time; next day 1 powder before each meal and at bed-time, and the following day the same, which uses up all the powders. Next morning take an active cathartic, to carry off the worms.

*Remarks.*—I recently took this remedy in just this way, realizing that I, at nearly 68 years of age, had them. For the cathartic I took 2 blue papers of seidlitz powders and 1 white paper, to be sure and get quick and thorough action. It did act quickly, and brought them away. I have enjoyed better health since.

**3. Worms, Allopathic Vermifuge for.**—Santonin and white sugar (or sugar of milk), each 10 grs.; calomel and ipecac, each 1 gr. DIRECTIONS—Rub the two first well together; then rub in the two last, and divide into 10 powders. DOSE—For child, 1 powder, night and morning, till all are taken; then an active cathartic, unless the worms pass off freely by this time. I should give a cathartic of cream of tartar, or some mild one, at any rate. This is the favorite, of an old friend of mine, of the allopathic school.

**4. Vermifuge or Vermicide—Extraordinary.**—Dr. A. S. Sweet, of Southhold, L. I., informs the readers of the *Brief* that he gave Mrs. C. the following mixture as a vermifuge: Santonin, 16 grs.; fl. ex. of pink, 160 drops; simple syrup, 2 ozs.; mix. DOSE—A tea-spoonful morning and night. She gave it about equally between 4 children of her own and 1 of a neighbor's. The result was the expulsion of 67 worms. As having a possible bearing upon the question whether worms cause any special symptoms by their presence in the intestines, Dr. Sweet says that the child for which the vermifuge was particularly desired had, previous to taking it, several attacks of convulsions. They ceased with the expulsion of the worms.

*Remarks.*—Any person of common sense would say the worms caused the convulsions, else their removal would not have stopped them. Dr. Sweet says nothing about giving any cathartic; but as the *Brief* is taken only by physicians, he leaves it to their judgment to direct it. I would say, give an active cathartic on the third or fourth day, whether any worms have passed or not. In all cases, after expulsion of worms, give a tonic to build up and strengthen the general system, which will also strengthen the bowels, and thereby make it less liable for another "crop" of worms. For, as a general thing, it is only the weakly children who are troubled with worms, although sometimes adults have them, as in my own case.

**5. Pin Worms, Remedy.**—A "Mrs. C." made inquiry in the Toledo, O., *Blade*, for a remedy for pin-worms, receiving the following answers: A Mrs. "A. P. A." (a pity that so many writers are ashamed of their names), says: If "Mrs. C." will give the child a tea made of common spearmint, both using it as a drink and as an injection, I am confident it will suffer no more from pin-worms, as I have known a very bad case, of long standing to be cured by this remedy, when many others had been tried without success. If one trial does not cure, repeat, as the remedy is harmless.

*Remarks.*—The spearmint is safe, and quite a diuretic, with its other valuable properties.

**6.** A "Subscriber, of Rochester, O., gave the following answer: Tell "Mrs. C." to use the following, which I have used, in a great many cases, without failure: Carolina pink root, senna, American worm seed and manna, each ½ oz.; steep for 1 hour in water, 1½ pts. Dose—1 gill (about 8 table-spoonfuls), once a day, in one-half as much new milk, well sweetened There is no "ifs" or "buts" about this, it will cure. I cured myself after having con-vulsions for over three years, and being given up by doctors; and since then it has cured many of my neighbors.

*Remarks.*—This writer says nothing about injecting it; but there would be no impropriety or danger in doing so, as it is for pin-worms, which mostly infest the rectum, and for which injections are the most effectual. The injec-tion should be kept in place as long as it can be borne, by holding a wad of cloth to prevent its voluntary escape, or discharge. This preparation, however, is very appropriate for the long round worm, and the author is of the opinion that it was for that, and not pin-worm, that this writer gave it.

**7. Pin-Worms.**—A solution made by soaking rasped quassia, ½ oz., in cold water, 1 pt., for 12 hours, then straining, for the purpose of injection, is very effectual to remove pin-worms. A solution of aloes, ½ oz., with carbon-ate of potash, 15 grs., in ½ pt. of decoction, or tea, of barley, dissolved by rubbing together, for an injection; or an injection of simple sweet oil, says Dr. Warren, of Boston, are very effectual in removing pin-worms. Lime water (which see how to make) is also frequently used as an injection for the removal of pin-worms.

**8. Tape Worm, Dr. Turnbull's Successful Remedy.**—Dr. R. J. Turnbull, of Duncansley, Miss., in a recent issue of the *Medical and Sur-gical Reporter*, says: I notice a request for a recipe for tape worm. The fol-lowing prescription proved most efficacious with me in the treatment of a patient who suffered for more than 3 years with tape worm. Bark of the pom-egranate root, ½ oz.; peeled pumpkin seed, ½ dr.; ethereal ex. of male-fern (an extract made with ether), 1 dr.; powdered ergot, ½ dr.; powdered gum arabic, 2 drs.; croton oil, 2 drops. Directions—The pomegranate root and pumpkin seed must be thoroughly bruised, and, with the ergot, boiled in 8 ozs. of water, for 15 minutes (the author would say not less than 30 minutes), then strain through coarse cloth. The croton oil must be rubbed up with the gum arabic and extract of male-fern, and then formed into an emulsion (by rubbing or thoroughly stirring), with the decoction. This is the prescription of Dr. A. J. Schafish, of Washington, D. C., who employs no preliminary provision, except forbidding the patient to take only breakfast the day on which it is intended to remove the worm, and give a large dose of Rochelle salts the night before. No unpleasant effects follow this remedy.—*Brief*

*Remarks.*—The author would say, if the croton oil does not cause a passage in 2 hours at most after taking the mixture, give 2 blue and 1 white paper of seidlitz powder to get thorough action from the bowels.

**9.** Dr. Currie, of Lebanon, N. H., gives an account in the *Brief* of removing a tape-worm from a girl 16 years old, by the simple articles of pumpkin seed, 1 oz.; white sugar, ½ oz.; the seed pounded fine, and mixed with the sugar. Dose—A tea-spoonful of the mixture every 2 hours, till all was taken: following the last dose with castor oil and spirits of turpentine. The next morning I was presented with the worm entire, 7 meters long.

*Remarks.*—A meter is a little less than 39¼ inches, or a total length of worm equal to 23 feet, at least. They have been expelled from 60 to 100 feet in length. The proper dose of castor oil for a girl of 16 would be 1 table-spoonful, with the spirits of turpentine, 1 tea-spoonful, mixed; and to avoid nausea or its disagreeable taste, add a few drops of oil of cinnamon. Repeat the dose in 2 or 3 hours, unless a free passage is obtained before this time. Unless the worm put in an appearance, I would repeat the whole on the third day, at farthest; the second, unless the stomach was considerably disturbed, would be better. More or less, according to the age and robustness of the person, may be given.

**10. Other Remedies.**—Dr. Bennett says: "Of all the vermifuge remedies proposed for the expulsion of tape-worms, I have found ethereal ex. of male-fern the most effectual." (See Dr. Turnbull's remedy above.)

Dr. Caldwell, Baltimore, Md., claims that the Dundas, Dick & Co.'s capsules of male-fern and kamala, produced with a patient of his, the happy result of expelling a monster of some 31 feet in length, after taking 6 capsules according to printed directions accompanying them; also relieving a cough, vomiting, and all other unpleasant symptoms attending its presence.

**11. Tape-Worm—The Latest, Most Easily Taken, and Most Successful Remedy for.**—There has been quite a stir made recently by two or three traveling physicians with the French chemist Tauret's "pellètierine," in removing tape-worms. I have seen several that have been removed here within a few months. I had known that one physician was using it here with success before, but not being of the talkative kind, very little was said about it. With this introduction, I will say: Tauret's "pellètierine" is put up in bottles containing *one dose* only, and retails at about $3 per bottle. Its action is to numb the worm, causing more or less giddiness, according to the nervousness of the patient. This soon passes off by the patient laying down and keeping quiet. It is perfectly safe, and but slight preparation is necessary to take it. Doze — One bottle being a full doze for a man, delicate females and youths of about 15 years would take only two-thirds; children of 10 or 12, one-half, and of 4 to 8 years, only one-third of a bottle. Directions — The day before it is to be taken, take a laxative or gentle cathartic, or a copious injection; and, for supper, eat only a milk diet. In the morning take half a glass of water on an empty stomach; then, five minutes after, take the pellètierine, and, immediately after, half a glass more of water, slightly sweetened. Three-fourths of an hour after take a dose of comp. tinct. of jalap; or infusion of senna (made by steeping ½ oz.), sweetened with syrup of orange-peel. If in a few hours there are no stools, take a purgative injection or repeat the purgative medicine. The giddiness will come on in about 15 minutes after taking the pellètierine, and the worms ought to be expelled in 2 to 4 hours. I have seen one passed in 1½ hrs. from the taking of the remedy. It is important to remember, say the instructions sent out, that the purgative must act rapidly. Don't stay in bed any

longer than the giddiness lasts; then move about, to help the action of the medicines. I have taken these instructions from a pamphlet sent out by E. Fougera
& Co., 30 North William st., New York, who supply the article if your druggist has not got it. This is not an advertisement for them, but to help any one
to obtain it who needs it. They do not know that I have mentioned them even;
but, knowing its value, I have given it, to save those needing it from paying
$10 to $50, as these tramping doctors charge for their removal. The pellètierine is made from pomegranate bark, which has been the main dependence for
removing tape worms; but as it had to be made in the form of an infusion and
taken in large doses of a ½ pt. or more, often causing sickness of the stomach,
this new preparation is as great a boone as quinine was over having to take the
Peruvian bark in powder, as formerly; and as the pellètierine has proved very
successful, it will, undoubtedly be but a short time till our druggists will keep
it, and it will enter into general use. Speaking of its success, I will mention a
few cases, only to show the estimation it is held in.

Professor Lahoulbène gives 19 successes in 19 trials. Dujardin-Beametz,
member of the Academy of Medicine, France, succeeded 37 times in 39 trials.
Dr. Ed. Mount, of Montreal, had 4 successes out of 4 trials; one of the cases
had been troubled with tape worm for 26 years. Dr. H. Wilfert, of the Cincinnati Academy succeeded also in every case.

I will mention only one case more, the worm I spoke of being removed
in one hour and a half, in the foregoing. The medicine was administered by a
boy of less than 20 years, who had been with a doctor for a short time only, and
learned what was used. The man was a butcher, and was well pleased to be
rid of his tormentor.

*Remarks.*—Certainly, with the foregoing list of remedies to select from, no
one should long be permitted to suffer the presence of either variety of worms,
unless it should be thought worth while to keep " His Majesty " (the tape worm)
in a bottle of alcohol, as a trophy of success in his removal.

1. **DYSPEPTICS—Bad Cases Put Upon the Right Tack.—**
A writer in the *Medical Journal*, discoursing upon dyspepsia, says: " We have
seen dyspeptics who suffered untold torments with almost every kind of food.
Bread became a burning acid. Meat and milk were solid and liquid fires. We
have seen these same sufferers trying to avoid food and drink, and even going
to the enema (syringe) for sustenance. And we have seen the torments pass
away and their hunger relieved by living upon the white of eggs, which have
been boiled in bubbling water for thirty minutes. At the end of a week, we
have given the hard yolk of the egg with the white, and upon this diet alone,
without fluid of any kind, we have seen them begin to gain flesh and strength,
and refreshing sleep. After weeks of this treatment they have been able, with
great care, to begin upon other food, and all this, the writer adds, without
taking medicine. He says that hard boiled eggs are not half so bad as half
boiled ones, and ten times as easy to digest as raw eggs, even in egg nog."

2. **Voltaire's Food for Indigestion, or Dyspepsia.—**In the
memoirs of Count de Segur (Vol. 1, page 168) there is the following anecdote:
My mother (the Countess de Segur) being asked by Voltaire respecting her

health, told him that the most painful feeling she had arose from the decay of her stomach, and the difficulty of finding any kind of aliment (food) that it could bear. Voltaire, by way of conversation, assured her that he was once nearly a year in the same state, and believed to be incurable; but that, nevertheless, a very simple remedy had restored him. It consisted in taking no other nourishment than the yolks of eggs, beaten up with flour of potatoes and water. Though this circumstance took place as far back as about 48 years ago, and respecting so extraordinary a personage as Voltaire, it is astonishing how little it is known, and how rarely the remedy is practiced. Its efficacy, however, in cases of debility, cannot be questioned; and the following is the mode of preparing this valuable article of food, as recommended by Sir John Sinclair. RECIPE—Beat up an egg in a bowl, and then add 6 table-spoonfuls of cold water, mixing the whole well together; then add 2 table-spoonfuls of the farina (flour of) potatoes, or mashed potatoes (I have used the mashed potatoes), mixing it with the liquor in the bowl; then pour in as much boiling water as will convert the whole into a jelly (like starch), and mix it well. [The author thinks it best to boil it a little, after pouring on the water.] It may be taken either alone, or with the addition of a little milk sweetened with sugar, not only for breakfast, but in cases of great debility of the stomach, or in consumptive disorders, at other meals. This dish, or food, is light, easily digested, and extremely wholesome and nourishing. Bread or biscuit should be taken with it, as the stomach gets stronger.—*Beach's Family Practice.*

*Remarks.*—I have recommended this food for several weak patients, with entire satisfaction; but I would say no bread, nor biscuit, should ever be eaten by a dyspeptic, or any person in a weak or debilitated condition of the system, from sickness, or naturally of feeble digestive powers, until at least the next day after the baking. I will only add, that in extremely weak patients, this, if relished, may constitute the entire nourishment taken for days, or weeks, according to the necessity of the case. But when one tires of this, some of the beef teas, essences, soups, porridges, as given under these heads in this work, or the oatmeal gruel for invalids, or delicate children, may be used to vary the food for the sick.

The two following dishes are given by Dr. Beach, in connection with the above food, as valuable for dyspepsia:

**3. Dyspepsia, Liquid Food for.**—Take fresh, lean beef, cut thin, 1 lb. Put it into a large-mouthed bottle or jar: add a little salt; place the bottle in a kettle of boiling water, and let it boil 1 hour; then strain through a woolen cloth. (It seems to the author that a stout piece of muslin is just as good.) There will be about 1 gill (4 ozs.) of clear, nutritious liquid. Begin by taking 1 tea-spoonful, and increase the quantity as the stomach will bear. This has been retained on the stomach when nothing else could. It cured an old captain when nearly gone with dyspepsia.

**4. Dyspeptics, Excellent Food for.**—Take a piece of stale wheat bread and a little white sugar, and cover with boiling water; then cover with a plate for a short time; add cream or good milk. This dish rests easy on the stomach, and is very pleasant.

*Remarks.*—This, of course, is not understood to be toasted, but in its simple state—to toast bread makes it much the nature of freshly baked, which is not good for the healthy, and especially bad for dyspeptics or the debilitated from any disease or cause whatever.

**5. Dyspepsia and Weak Stomach, The Value of Milk and Lime-Water for.**—Milk and lime-water are now frequently prescribed by physicians in cases of dyspepsia and weakness of the stomach, and in some cases are said to prove very beneficial. Many persons who think good bread and milk a luxury, frequently hesitate to eat it, for the reason that the milk will not digest readily; sourness of the stomach will often follow. But experience proves that lime-water and milk are not only food and medicine, at an early period of life, but also at a later, when, as in the case of infants, the functions of digestion and assimilation have been seriously impaired. A stomach taxed by gluttony, irritated by improper food, inflamed by alcohol, enfeebled by disease, or otherwise unfitted for its duties—as is shown by various symptoms attendant upon indigestion, dyspepsia, diarrhea, dysentery and fever—will resume its work, and do it energetically, on an exclusive diet of bread and milk and lime-water. A goblet of cow's milk may have 3 to, 4 table-spoonfuls of lime-water added to it with good effect.

These ideas are fully endorsed by Dr. E. N. Chapman, who presented the following valuable notes on the use of milk and lime-water for invalids, to the Medical Society of the State of New York. He says: " I have used milk and lime-water for years as a diet with my patients with great success, particularly in cases involving nerve centres, that are acknowledged to be little under the command of the accepted modes of treatment, such, for instance, as marasmus (a wasting of flesh), anemia (debility from poor blood), paralysis, indigestion, neuralgia, cholera, dementia (insanity), and alcoholism. Also in cases where the nutritive functions are at fault, milk with a pinch of salt, being rendered very acceptable to the stomach by the lime, is the most digestible and nourishing food that can be given. It allays gastric (stomach) and intestinal irritability, offers a duly prepared chyle to the absorbents, supplies the blood with all the elements of nutrition, institutes healthy tissue changes, stimulates the secreting and excreting glands, and, in a word, provides nature with the material to sustain herself in her contest with disease. * * * Milk, acted on with limewater, has a range of application almost as extensive as disease itself, whatever its character and whoever the patient."

*Remarks.*—I trust that enough has now been said to satisfy everybody of the value of milk in disease, and I will add that I know it to be equally valuable as a regular family diet.

**6. Dyspeptic Invalids or Weakly Children, Oatmeal Gruel for.**—A Mrs. " H. K.", of Evanston, Wyoming Territory, in writing to the *Blade,* upon what Mrs. Jane F. Hollingsworth said of strained oatmeal gruel for invalids, gives her own experience with it for children. She says:

"Nothing is better for either invalids or young children. Let me give my experience. Our baby was delicate; cow's milk did not agree with her while nursing; I began feeding her corn starch and oatmeal gruel, and now a heartier, happier and fatter baby than ours you will seldom see, and oatmeal gruel is her daily food.

"I take 2 table-spoonsful of oatmeal and pour on a pint, or a little more, of boiling water; let boil until thick enough for jelly, then I strain it through a little sieve, add 1 tea-spoonful of sugar and 2 of cream to a coffee cup of gruel, and it is a dish fit for a king.

"For very young children or very weak invalids of a dyspeptic character, make thinner with water while boiling, or with cold milk, after done boiling."

**7. Food for Dyspeptic, or Weakly Babes.**—Boil slowly, for 2½ hours, ½ cup of oatmeal, in 1 qt. of water, with a very little salt, the dish being covered to prevent evaporation; then strain. A double, or rice kettle (which see) is just the thing to avoid burning. When cold, to ½ pt. of this gruel, or food, add an equal quantity of thin cream, and 2 tea-spoonfuls of white sugar; then, to this mixture, add 1 pt. of boiling water, and when cool enough it is ready for use, and will set easy on the stomach, when milk and all other food cannot be digested by a feeble or weak babe, unless aided by the use of lime-water, as above.

**8. Drinks for Small Children Having Dyspeptic or Diarrheal Tendency.**—Rice-water, barley-water, oatmeal-water, made by boiling a single handful of either of these to 1 qt. of water, with lemon and sugar, should be ready in every house where there are children. These drinks are surely better than cold tea, which is often given. However, milk is considered better than anything, when it is sweet and pure, and given in only small quantities at any one time, with lime-water.

**9. Dyspeptics, Healthy Food for.**—It is a well known fact that meats are much more needed in winter than in the heat of summer, and the following, written by a well known physician (Dr. Hunt, of New Jersey), explains the whole matter so fully, I will give it a place. Dr. Hunt, the editor of the Newark (N. J.) *Advertiser*, wholly regardless of the loss of his fellow-practitioners, by "a fearful state of healthfulness" in that vicinity, and honest as he is skillful in his professional work, gives this advice for the summer season:

"Fruits and vegetables, with an abundance of good milk and bread, should be the main substantials and not the mere side dishes of the table. There are too many who simply add what the summer brings to their usual bill of fare. They still indulge in heavy meats and stimulating condiments, adding some badly cooked vegetables, and finishing with the usual flatulent pastry, or may-hap a few berries; but this is an injustice both to the system and to the Providence whose blessings are showered upon us in such prodigal profusion. Meat should now become the side dish; gravies, stews and condiments should be utterly abandoned; and the system should be toned and purified by the tonic of the field and garden. Milk is better than medicine, and the entire pharmacopœia contains nothing equal to what now comes to us from the true laboratory —comes to us not only with healing wing, but with a flavor for the palate which all the French cooks in Paris could not imitate. And the offerings arrive with such glorious progressiveness! First comes the strawberry, like a blush on the cheek of Mother Earth; then the berries and vegetables of more vigorous growth; then the stately, luscious melon, the charm and glory of the breakfast-table; then corn, which is meat in nutrition; with the juicy apple, the pride of prince and peasant. Then we come to the pear and to the orchard—

> Where peaches grow with sunny dyes,
> Like maiden's cheeks when blushes rise,
> Where huge figs the branches bend,
> Where clusters from the vine distend.

There is the feast which nature spreads. Let every man say grace in his heart, and partake of it thankfully."

**10. Gaseous Dyspepsia, Simple but Effectual Remedy.—** Where gas distends the stomach, or bloats the bowels, taking 15 to 20 drops of chloroform in a little syrup, after eating, will expel the gas, and stop the fermentation in a few minutes.

*Remarks.*—Chloroform is well known to be a very diffusive stimulant, and hence this action of it might be expected. It is easily tried and may prove as effectual as it is claimed to be. (See the closing remarks on pimples, bad and of long standing, etc., for the use of animal charcoal, with sugar, before meals, also of soda after meals, for this gaseous condition of the stomach.)

**11. Dyspepsia, or Indigestion, Very Valuable Treatment of.—** I am now using a very valuable medicine, or combination, on a case where the indigestion was very bad, so much so, it might be considered real dyspepsia; but the treatment allayed the distress so promptly, and helped, or enabled the food to digest, so effectually that I will give the recipe. First I used the following fluid preparation.

I. *Solution for Dyspepsia.*—Pepsin in crystals, 30 grs.; glycerine, 1 oz.; concentrated lactic acid, ½ oz.; distilled, or soft water, 4 ozs.; mix. Dose— A tea-spoonful in 3 or 4 tea-spoonfuls of water, immediately after each meal.

*Remarks.*—After a week or two, as the case may improve, less, and still less, may be used, say ½ tea-spoonful only, till finally cured. And in case there is a diarrheal tendency, or any inflammatory condition of any part of the system, in which the lactic acid is not good, take the following powder, in place of the solution, as above.

**12. Powder for Dyspepsia, Diarrhea, etc.—** Sub-carbonate of bismuth, 200 grs.; Scheffer's, or other good pepsin, 100 grs. Mix thoroughly, and make into 20 powders. Dose—Take 1 powder in a little molasses and water, half-and-half, immediately after each meal, the same as the solution; and after some time, or suitable improvement has been made, divide a powder for 2 doses, as long as needed

*Remarks.*—This will meet very bad cases of either disease, and prove, generally, all that can be desired. See the use of bismuth with Dover's powders, in looseness of the bowels, from teething—where it is effectual, although the cause, in the case of teething is continued for several months, or as long as the teething continues. It holds the fort, however, notwithstanding this continuance of the cause, so it will with the pepsin here as well as in the other case. But whether the solution or the powder is being used, if there is heat and an uneasy or distressed condition of the stomach, it is an evidence that the hot water, given next below, is called for, and will prove valuable.

**13. Hot Water for Dyspepsia.**—The following item is from the *Hartford Courant*, which I have since proven to be very valuable. By using the hot water an hour before each meal, instead of only at breakfast. The *Courant* says: "A gentleman who is in business in this city has cured himself of a chronic and ugly form of dyspepsia in a very simple way. He was given up to die; but he finally abandoned alike the doctors and the drugs, and resorted to a method of treatment which most doctors and most persons would laugh at as an 'old woman's remedy.' It was simply swallowing a tea-cupful of hot water before breakfast every morning. He took the water from the cook's tea-kettle, and so hot that he could only take it by the spoonful. For about three weeks this morning dose was repeated, the dyspepsia decreasing all the while. At the end of that time he could eat, he says, any breakfast or dinner that any well person could eat—had gained in weight, and has ever since been hearty and well. His weight is now between 30 and 40 pounds greater than it was during the dyspepsia sufferings; and for several years he has had no trouble with his stomach—unless it was some temporary inconvenience due to a late supper or dining out, and in such a case a single trial of his ante-breakfast remedy was sure to set all things right. He obtained his idea from a German doctor, and in turn recommended it to others—and in every case, according to this gentleman's account, a cure was effected."

*Remarks.*—After seeing the above item in the *Courant* I have had occasion to use the hot water personally, and to direct it for others; and I have found it satisfactory, if taken faithfully before each meal, instead of only at breakfast. I also find that heating it in summer to about 40 degrees and in winter to 145 degrees F., is about the right degree of heat. I heat it over a small coal-oil stove, in a pint tin cup, about ¾ full, which I find about the right amount to be taken at one time. It can be heated in a tea-kettle and poured into a cup or bowl; but it is well to have a thermometer to know just what the heat is. A tea-spoonful of sugar makes it pleasant for me, but a bit of lemon juice might suit some better. It must be followed for several months, in long standing cases, to prove of lasting benefit, eating only easily digested food, and nothing that disagrees with the stomach. The sipping of the hot water has this advantage also, it allays the great thirst of dyspeptic patients, as well as the heat and distress in the stomach, better than anything else I know of, contracting the lax and flabby condition of the muscular coating of the stomach, giving tone and strength to this organ, which immediately diffuses itself to the whole system. Take the hot water before each meal and at bed-time as long as you have any considerable thirst. Be careful, also, not to eat too much, and only at meal times, and a cure must be the result. (See also Hot Water Cure for Consumption.)

**APPETITE—To Increase or Restore.**—Obtain valerian root, ¼ or ½ lb. Have it ground coarsely, or well bruised. Make a tea of it by steeping a rounding table-spoonful of the powder in water 1 pt. DOSE—One to 2 table-spoonfuls just before meals, and half to a wine-glassful at bed-time.

*Remarks.*—This plant is known as the American Greek-valerian, abscess root, blue bells (from its blue flowers), sweat root, Jacob's ladder, etc. The Latin, or technical, name is *polemonium reptans*. It grows in the northern states, and was a great favorite with the Indians, the tea being given freely in fevers, pleurisy, and to produce copious perspiration. It is claimed also to cleanse the blood, and to have cured many cases of consumption.

**PECKHAM'S GENUINE BALSAM— For Coughs, Sore Throat, Sore Chest, Kidney Difficulties, Wounds, etc.**—Rosin, 10 lbs.; spirits of turpentine, 1 gal.; or, rosin, 2½ ozs.; turpentine, 2 ozs., is the same proportion. DIRECTIONS—Melt the rosin in a suitable kettle, or pan, over a stove, in the day time, so that it shall not be necessary to have a lamp, or candle, near; and when not too hot put in the turpentine, gradually. It must not be made over an open fire, as the gas arising from it as the turpentine is put in takes fire very readily, and would quickly fill a whole room with its blaze, and perhaps fire the house; hence I have given these necessary precautions. Bottle while moderately hot, else it will run too slowly. DOSE—For a grown person, take from 5 to 10 drops on sugar; children, 1 or 2, to 5 drops, night and morning.

*Remarks.*—I obtained this recipe of L. S. Robinson, of Jackson, Mich., who says he has made and sold thousands of dollars worth of it, claiming that it is the original Peckham's balsam, and that all additional articles put in and claimed to be an improvement, should not be used. With this balsam Mr. Robinson claims he has made some remarkable cures in the diseases mentioned, both internal and external, and mentions the following cases.

I. A mare of his own, being in a strange pasture with some cows, was badly hooked one night. The wound was long, deep and jagged, upon the side; but he put some of this balsam into every part of the wound, then sewed it up, except a little opening at the lowest point of the wound, to allow the matter in healing to drain off. Then drove home, 30 miles, the same day, and the wound made a very rapid healing.

II. A remarkable case, that of a lady who had had several miscarriages, and feared another, there being an inflammation of the parts, and also of the neck of the bladder; but 5 to 8 drop doses, night and morning, of this balsam, cured both difficulties; the lady, upon a subsequent trip he was making over that route, showing him the babe, healthy and well, and herself the same, telling him, "There, doctor, that is your child, you saved it; nothing else was used."

III. A gentleman who had recently buried a wife from consumption, and who considered himself past help, with the same disease, when Mr. Robinson first made his acquaintance. But with this balsam internally, and Cook's electro-magnetic liniment, externally, he was entirely cured, and is still alive, at this writing, hale and hearty, living with a second wife, some 30 years after the cure.

**BRIGHT'S DISEASE OF THE KIDNEYS.—A Novel Cure for..**—A correspondent of the New York *Evening Post* gives the following novel item to that journal. He says:

"About 20 years ago, a daughter of mine—then about 6 years old—was given up to die by the family physician, who said that she had Bright's Disease of the Kidneys, and that it was incurable, and never known to be cured either in Europe or America. The physician, on giving the case up, told my wife to give the child anything that she wanted, and to make her as comfortable as possible while she lived. The child constantly called for beans; so my wife cooked some as quickly as possible, not stopping to parboil them, as is usually done, but boiled beans, pork and potatoes together, in the first water, and when well cooked she gave them to the child to eat. The child then went to sleep and from that time began to improve. She is now the mother of two children. She is not troubled with the disease unless she takes a severe cold, and when that happens she at once uses her old remedy, and it is always effectual.

*Remarks.* There is nothing said here about continuing to eat the beans; but I take it for granted that this was, and should be done in all cases; and tell me, pray! why beans should not have this power as well as any drug? And it is admitted, as this writer says, that it is seldom, or never known to be cured. Let this remedy, therefore, have more than a fair trial by a long continued use. Beans are certainly a healthy and agreeable food for a general diet. But if used especially for kidney difficulties keep all their virtues by not changing the water. Beans over a year old are liable to become musty as well as doubly hard, and unfit for this, or any other use.

**2. Bright's Disease—Sixteen out of Nineteen Cases in a London Hospital Cured.**—Notwithstanding the statement in the item above, that Brights disease was never to be cured in Europe or America, still some years ago a London (Eng.) physician reported in the *London Lancet*, the cure of 16 out of 19 cases, in the Hospital, by the use of 15 gr. doses of powdered valerian, 3 or four times a day, with supporting diet. Now the fl. ex. would be used, in ½ to 1 teaspoon doses, with the same effect; but I am not aware of its having been used by others. But if one has the difficulty it had better be tried, and may, with the beans, as above, cure more than without them.

**QUINSY.—A New and Successful Remedy for.**—A Dr. Gine, Professor of Clinical Surgery, at Madrid, Spain, reports through the *La Presse Med. Belge*, July 17, 1881, the bicarbonate of soda (the common baking soda, the best, however is the English bicarbonate, kept by druggists) applied to the tonsils in fine powder in Quinsy, repeating frequently, is of inestimable efficacy, he having cured dozens of cases—in no case without benefit, and, usually a cure in 24 hours; and in no case when he had used it had he found it necessary to remove the tonsils.

DIRECTIONS FOR APPLICATION. It may be applied by rolling a bit of paper of suitable length into cylindrical form, then putting the end into a fine powder of the soda, to get a suitable amount into the hollow, the size of an ordinary goose quill and blowing it upon the tonsils; or applying it by wetting the finger, then putting the finger into the powder, then upon the tonsils.

*Remarks.* I have had no opportunity for trying it for this purpose, but I have proved its value as a gargle in "Sore Throat,—which see. See also its value in "Burns, Scalds, etc." See, also, "Inflammation of the Tonsils following Sick Headache," where the latter remedy—the salicylate of soda—is used as a satisfactory cure in both these diseases, as inflammation of the tonsils is only another name for quinsy.

1. **EYE-WATERS.**—Sulphate of zinc, and fine table salt, each 4 grs.; sugar of lead, 2 grs.; morphine, 5 grs.; loaf sugar, 10 grs.; distilled or rain water, 4 ozs.; mix and keep corked. DIRECTIONS—Drop 1 or 2 drops in the eye morning and evening, else apply with the finger between the lids which is the most common way. Best done when laying down. It can be done very well by holding the head back.

*Remarks.*— This will be found a very valuable eye-water in all cases of weakness, or slight inflammation of the eye. It may be applied three or four times a day, if needed so often. It is well to shake it two or three times a day at first, for a week or ten days, then allow to settle, and strain. If this causes too much smarting in bad cases, reduce some of it with more rain water, so it shall not smart more than five minutes at most.

2. **Eye-Water for very Sore Eyes or Catarrhal Ophthalmia.** —Tincts. of aconite, and veratrum viride, each 10 drops; acetate of lead, 5 grs.; morphine, 3 grs.; water, as in No. 1, 4 ozs. DIRECTIONS—Open the lids and put in freely.

*Remarks.*—I. It is claimed by physicians that this has cured very bad cases. These very bad cases are generally the result of an acute inflammation of the eyes which, instead of having been cured, have degenerated into a chronic or long standing condition, with considerable watering of the eyes, and also, especially in the mornings, a thick matter is found in them, all for the want of proper treatment, else a scrofulous condition of the system. In all these cases, bathing the feet in hot water evenings, and taking cream of tartar, 1 oz., dissolved in 1 pt. of boiling water, and drank of freely, when cold, to produce gentle cathartic action, will be found a valuable help in curing them; or, the old plan, taking cream of tartar and sulphur, equal parts, or of late, 2 ozs. of cream of tartar to 1 oz. of sulphur, mixed and stirred into syrup, and take 3 mornings and skip 3, until 9 doses are taken, was a good way, if enough is taken to act pretty freely on the bowels by the 3d day. Being also careful to avoid a greasy diet, and using only plain and nutritious food, avoiding also stimulating drinks, if a cure is hoped for or desired.

II. *If the Urine* is high colored or deficient in quantity, take acetate of potash, ½ oz., in water, 8 ozs. DOSE—1 to 2 tea-spoonfuls 3 or 4 times daily until free and clear, will aid much in bringing about a healthy condition of the system in most cases.

III. *Case in Hand.* Prof. Scudder, in the *Eclectic Medical Journal,* gives the case of a child 11 months old having this catarrhal ophthalmia, with the matter sticking the lids together in the mornings, cured by him with the above treatment after other physicians had failed to give any relief; with the addition only of the tinct. of *rhus toxicondendron* (poison oak) 4 drops in 4 ozs. of water.

Dose—One tea-spoonful 4 times daily.   His cure was effected in 5 weeks, and very satisfactory.

**3. Weak Eyes, Mild Remedy for.**—Put 1 dr., or a tea-spoonful, each of spirits of camphor and laudanum into a 4 oz. vial and fill with rose-water.   Shake and apply as often as needed.   Rain water will do.   Shaken when used, works very satisfactory.

**4. Another Mild Eye-Water — For Children.** — Take 1 oz. of elder flowers and steep in ½ pt. of soft water (steep in an earthen dish); strain, and add ½ tea-spoonful of laudanum.   Keep in a cool place, and use as needed.

*Remarks.*—If the eyes are painful, wet soft cloths with this, and bind on at night.   If of long standing or chronic, make a tea of the elder flowers and drink, or give to children in these cases, to cleanse the blood.

**5. Weak Eyes, Wash for.**—Some writer for weak eyes says: "Bathe your eyes night and morning in a tolerably strong solution of common table salt and water.   We have known some remarkable cures effected by this simple remedy.   After bathing the eyes daily for about a week, intermit a day or two; then resume the daily bathing, and so on till your eyes get strong again."

**6. Eyes, Acute Inflammation of—Valuable Remedy.**—For an acute inflammation of the eyes I know of nothing better than to take the white of an egg, in a tin cup, and beat into it thoroughly about ½ a teaspoon of powdered alum; set on the stove to heat, and stir constantly till it curdles; then strain off the whey, breaking up the curd and putting it upon a cloth, and lay upon the eye; and as it becomes dry, take it off and fold the cloth around it to keep the curd together; re-wet it, by putting it into the whey, drain off the surplus whey, and re-apply.   This may be done 2 or 3 times; then make more, if needed, and use the same way, until the inflammation subsides; after which any of the eye waters, reduced with water to be very mild, may be used to strengthen the eyes.   I have used this in just this way, upon my own eye, with entire success.   If the inflammation should continue long, take some salts or cream of tartar, or the sulphur mixture as in No. 2 for "Catarrhal Ophthalmia." I see this alum cure is recommended, in about the same way, for sprains. I have not used it upon them; yet, as a sprain produces an inflammation, I think it will prove valuable there also.

**7. Eyes, to Remove Iron and Steel from.** — Iodine, 2 grs.; iodide of potash, 12 grs.; soft water, 3 ozs.

*Remarks.*—Accidents are often occurring to millers, while picking the mill-stones, by a small bit of steel from the pick penetrating into the coating of the eye.   Dr. T. B. King, of Toledo, an old English physician, referred to several times in this work, informs me that he has cured several cases with this preparation.   I have had no opportunity to test it since I obtained it, but had one just before, which I was relating to the "Old Doctor," when he gave me this. He says, by putting one or two drops of it into the eye a few times, the steel or iron will be loosened in 24 hours.   Then let no one fail to try it, as soon as needed.

**8. Eyes, Granulation of.**—For granulations (small grain-like elevations inside of the lids) of the eye, Dr. King puts corroscive sublimate, ½ gr., into the reddish codliver oil, 1 oz., dissolves and applies 2 or 3 times daily, with great success.

**9. Films o.' the Eye — One Case of Five and One of Nineteen Years Blindness Cured.**—I. Dr. M. P. Greensword, of Poughkeepsie, N. Y., reporting through the *Medical Summary*, in Dec. No. for 1882, says: "I took a patient that had been blind five years from opacity (thickening of the cornea membrane covering the front of the eye, which prevents seeing through it) and gave him the nitrate of silver in doses as follows: Nitrate of silver, 5 grs.; tannin, 2 grs.; rain water, 6 ozs. DOSE—A tea-spoonful 15 minutes before each meal. In 10 days he began to receive sight, and in one year his sight was nearly perfect.

"After this I took a man aged 82, and blind nineteen years from opacity of the cornea: I gave him the same remedy, in the same way, and in 6 months his sight was restored nearly perfect. I have since cured a great many cases from opacity by the same remedy. It is far superior to mercury in any shape. Another advantage in using this remedy is that the patient continues to grow better for a year after discontinuing its use, if he lets all other medicines alone during that time."

*Remarks.*—The Doctor admits having failed to cure some cases of females, who were troubled with leucorrhœa, until he cured that difficulty by applying a sponge to the parts wet with a strong solution of cadmium, for 24 hours; then alternate with a sponge pessary, saturated with pure glycerine, for the same length of time. The words, "a strong solution," may do very well for a physician, but for the people it is not as well as to say how many grs. to 1 oz. of water—from ½ to 4 grs to the oz. are used as an eye-water, and double this strength is used in ulcerations of the ear; then 5 or 6 grs. to 1 oz of soft water would be as strong as I would recommend. It is much like the sulphate of zinc in its action. I trust the nitrate of silver, as above, will continue to give satisfaction in blindness.

If nitrate of silver is taken very long in any case, I should fear it might give a dark color to the skin and whites of the eyes, that could never be removed. Look out for that, by consulting with your physician, and stop its use if these conditions show at all, but even this is better than blindness.

II. The old plan of removing films from the eyes, by rubbing a piece of "blue stone" (blue vitrol—sulphate of copper), made very smooth, over them, once daily, which has been done also for granulations, is a quicker way, and no danger of discoloring the skin. But this would have to be done by a physician or some one a little skilled in turning up the lids out of the way, then simply passing it carefully over the film or granulations, as the case may be. It is pretty severe but effectual, if properly done. The eye-lid should be held open 2 or 3 minutes before allowing it to close.

III. Films are also removed with corrosive sublimate, ½ gr. dissolved in ½ oz. of sub. acetate of lead water, then ½ oz. of white cod liver oil, added

and shaken until thoroughly mixed, and shaken when used.   Put on a little
with a brush once daily.   Of course, in all cases, correct the blood and general
health.

**10.   Stye upon the Eye—Lid Remedy.**—Put a teaspoonful of black
tea in a small bag; pour on it enough boiling water to moisten it; then put it
on the eye pretty warm.   Keep it on all night and in the morning the stye will
most likely be gone; if not, a second application is certain to remove it."

*Remarks.*—The infusion or weak tea, made from black tea, has been for
some time considered good as an eye-water, then why not the grounds good as
a poultice?   I believe it may be worthy of trial.

As a beverage the black tea is preferable for invalids and for nervous
people—a weak infusion.   Should the above poultice of tea fail, try the following, which I know must be good in any kind of swelling, as styes, boils, etc.,
if followed up properly.   It is from the *Cricket on the Hearth,* a valuable paper.
It is headed:

**11.   A Stye, to Remove from the Eyelid.**—"The stye is strictly
only a little boil, which projects from the edge of the eye-lid.   It usually disappears of itself after a little time, especially if some purgative medicine be taken.
If the stye should be very painful and inflamed, a small warm poultice of linseed meal and bread or milk must be laid over it, (a poultice of powdered
slippery elm is also good for any inflammation), and renewed every 5 or 6 hours,
and the bowls freely acted upon by a purgative draught, such as the following:

I.   *Purgative Draught for Stye, or Other Purposes.*—"Take Epsom salts,
½ oz.; best manna, ¼ oz.; infusion of senna, ¾ oz.; tinct. senna, ¼ oz.; spearmint water, 1 oz.; distilled or soft water, 2 ozs.   Mix and take 3, 4 or 5 table-
spoonfuls.   When the stye appears ripe, an opening should be made into it with
the point of a large needle, and afterward a little of the following ointment may
be smeared over it once or twice a day.

II.   *Ointment for Stye, Chaps, etc.*—Take spermaceti, ¾ oz.; white wax,
1¼ ozs.; olive oil, 3 ozs.   Mix them together over a slow fire, and stir them
constantly until cold.

*Remarks.*—Box the ointment for use, as above indicated.   A faithful use
of these will soon tell.

**1.   CORNS—Hard and Soft, Warts, Bunions, etc.**—I.   *Corns.*—
Probably but few subjects of more universal interest could be found than the
very humble one of corns.   A writer in the *Christian Weekly* says: "They are
of two kinds—soft and hard—the result of pressure which stimulates the skin
so that an increased flow of blood to the excited part is caused, and the cells of
the cuticle (from the Latin *cutis,* skin,) are more rapidly produced than is
natural.   Soft corns occur between the toes, because of the pressure of the joints
of the smaller toes on the opposite skin, and the corn is constantly moist with
perspiration.   The first thing in the cure of corns is to remove the cause—wear
soft, broad-toed shoes and boots, and thus remove the irritating pressure.

I.   *Hard Corns.*—Soak hard corns in warm water, shave down, touch them
with a little acetic acid occasionally, and put a thin plaster over the corn to prevent chafing after the application of the acid.

II. *Soft Corns.*—In the case of soft corns great cleanliness must be observed, the suffering toes must be kept separate by a bit of cotton, and the dead skin, after touching lightly with the acid, must be removed as fast as its tenderness will allow. But no cure can be accomplished while an ill-fitting shoe is still doing its mischievous work. Too tight a shoe, especially one too narrow-toed, is an ill-fitting shoe.

*Remarks.*—I wish to say as confirming the idea above advanced, that if any one will not give up their "tight fits" they may rest assured that they will always have a crop of corn(s) on hand, or rather on foot. So suit yourself as to keeping a full supply.

## 2. Bunions, Corns, Warts, etc.—Brister's Spanish Destroyer.

—Concentrated ether, 1 lb.; gun cotton, 1 oz.; best alcohol, 8 ozs.; glycerine, 1 oz.; a trifle of red aniline to color.

I. *Directions to Make.*—Put the gun cotton on a plate and wet it with a little alcohol, and then put all into the ether. If a less amount is desired keep the same proportions. Keep corked. To color, if to put up for sale, put 5 cts. worth of aniline red into 1 oz. of alcohol, and 1 tea-spoonful of it will color all a nice red, more or less as you choose.

II. *Directions for Use.*—Soak the feet in warm water from 5 to 10 minutes; scrape the outside of the corns, or bunions, with a knife. Apply the destroyer to the afflicted parts with a brush, as thin as possible, about three times a week, 4 or 5 applications being sufficient to cure the affected parts. Should the corns be between the toes (soft corns), place a little piece of cotton between them, to keep them apart, and to keep the medicine from being rubbed off.

For warts keep covered with the remedy, or destroyer, till they are removed. Keep the vial corked tightly.

The destroyer, when applied to the afflicted parts, forms a thin plaster (artificial skin) over the same. Discontinue the use of the destroyer until the plaster disappears. When my wife used it upon her bunions she put some washing fluid (made of sal-soda and lime, which she always kept for washing purposes), into the water in which she soaked the bunions, then scraped off all the dead matter and softened skin, and applied the remedy. It did not take but a few days to reduce her bunions more than one-half in size, and to remove all soreness. This is really a valuable thing for bunions.

But sal-soda put in the water to soak the corn, or bunion in, making it pretty strong, will do as well as the washing 'fluid, referred to above; it softens the hard scaly surface, which is to be scraped off; then apply as above directed, with a brush.

*Remarks.*—I obtained this recipe of Wm. H. Brister, of Springfield, Ill., at the depot where he was selling the "Destroyer," as he calls it. He had a circular, calling himself "The Great Western Corn Doctor," and told me he had traveled 8 years in its sale, and had cleared his living for himself and family and built a house in Springfield worth $8,000 made out of the business. This remedy must certainly have been very valuable, or he could not have continued its sale for so many years; for he showed me certificates from prominent men, governors, senators, lawyers, doctors, etc., all over the country whom he had cured. I have made it and cured many bad bunions, and hence I know its value. It forms an artificial skin over the parts and hence it is good in slight bruises or abrasions, to put on for this purpose, to protect them from water, etc.

**3. Corns, Simple Remedy for.**—Having removed the friction and pressure causing corns, by the substitution of well constructed shoes and boots, the thickened cuticle may be removed by applying equal parts of carbonate of soda and common brown bar soap. Rub these substances together, with a spoon handle or knife blade on the surface of a plate, forming a strong alkaline ointment. DIRECTIONS—Spread a little of this on a piece of buck-skin or wash-leather and apply it to the surface of the corns at bed-time, after soaking them for 5 or 10 minutes in hot water, allowing it to remain until morning. When the soap plaster is removed in the morning, the corn to which it has been applied, will be found white and soft, and by scraping a little around its base with your finger nail, or a dull knife, it may be easily raised up and removed. Then apply the colodion or artifical skin, or a bit of court plaster, till it heals. This is all that is needed, except to wear easy shoes and boots.

**4. Corns, A Sure Cure for.**—Bathe in a strong solution of sal soda; pare off close, and touch the corn with carbolized iodine; repeat the application of iodine next day, and a cure will speedily follow.

*Remarks.*—A druggist will prepare this mixture, if desired, and either of the plans here given, with proper care not to wear tight boots or shoes, will cure corns.

**5. Corn Salve, Effectual.**—Pine pitch, or pine tar, as some call it, brown sugar and saltpeter, each, 1 tea-spoonful. Simmer together. Pare the corn as close as you can. Spread some of the salve on an old kid glove or other thin, soft leather, the size of the corn; bind it on for 2 or 3 days; when taken off the corn comes off with it. A lady who had used it gave me this.

**6. Warts, Simple Cure for.**— Cut a piece of wild turnip, from the woods, and rub several times upon the wart or warts. A writer says: "I removed nearly a hundred from hands, leaving no scar at all."

*Remarks.*—This is simple, and is, no doubt, as good as represented.

**7.** It is also claimed that our simple potato, cut and rubbed on, the same as the wild turnip, in the receipt above, 3 times a day for a few days, removed 20 warts from the writer's hands.

**9.** Another writer says: "Chromic acid, a drop or two to each wart at bed-time, I will warrant to cure in 3 days."

*Remarks.*—Be careful not to get it on the hands or clothing, nor leave it where children can get it. Carbolic acid, full strength, will do the same thing. The best way to apply any acids is to take the end of a match-stick and mash one end between the teeth, to make a broom-like end, to hold only a drop or two, and just touch the head of the wart, or corn with the acid 2 or 3 times. Remember this—if you get too much acid on, so it runs down into the flesh, soda will neutralize it. The chromic acid is considered the safest of the acids.

(See Cancer, Chromic Acid in, etc.) Don't use enough to spread upon other parts.

**9. Warts, Simple and Easy Cure.**—Rubbing warts night and morning with a moistened piece of muriate of ammonia (sal ammoniac), will cause their disappearance without pain or scar.

**10. Warts on Cows' Teats; or, The Hand's Remedy.**—E. Walcott asks the readers of the Detroit *Tribune* for a remedy for warts upon cows' teats, and "J. L.," of Maple, Mich., makes him the following answer: "Take a handful of green bean leaves and rub them in the hands until the hands are thoroughly wet with the juice; then proceed to milk. As often as the hands get dry while milking, moisten again with the bean leaf juice. Do this twice or three times a week, and in a few weeks there will be no warts on the cow's teats or the hands of the milker."

**1. SEASICKNESS, CURE FOR.**—Dr. Landener, of Athens, Greece, claims to have discovered that 10 to 12 drops of chloroform cures seasickness. One dose cured 18 out of 20; the second dose cured the others.

*Remarks.*—It is simple, easily obtained and not unpleasant to take in a little water. And a lady who has had considerable experience in crossing parts of Lake Erie informs me that the smelling of chloroform a few times has relieved much of the nausea attending seasickness. So, also, my judgment is that the taking and inhaling a little of it from the bottle will do great good.

**2. English Remedy.**—The bromide of sodium, for long voyages, has been found very effectual in doses of 10 grs., 3 times a day, in treating 200 cases of ocean seasickness.—*Dr. Kendall in British Medical Journal.*

*Remarks.*—The bromide of sodium was first used by the late Dr. Beard. The indiscriminate use of oranges, lemons, brandy and champagne, Dr. Kendall condemns, as making the case worse than without them.

**CALOMEL, a Substitute for, in Jaundice, Hepatic Dropsy, Hypochondriosis, Hemorrhoids, Throat and Bronchial Inflammations, etc.**—A medical writer says: "Sulphate of manganese is now being introduced as a substitute for mercury in various bilious troubles. In jaundice, hepatic dropsy (dropsy arising from liver difficulties, and most generally affecting the abdomen), hypochondriasis (a condition of melancholy, or low spirits) it is stated to have produced most remarkable results; and in hemorrhoids (piles) and in congestion (inflammation, or an unnatural accumulation of blood) of the throat and bronchial tubes it has proved no less efficacious. Anæmic patients (persons of a pale or bloodless appearance), who cannot take any of the preparations of iron, are enabled to take iron with benefit it combined with 2 to 5 grs. of sulphate of manganese. It is generally found preferable to administer the manganese in 10 to 20 grs. dose, in a glass of water. adding a little citrate of magnesia to cause effervescence. By these doses large bilious dejections (passages) are produced. Half a drachm (30 grs.) is said to be the utmost dose ever necessary, 10 grains being usually quite sufficient."

*Remarks.*—Prof. King, in his "American Dispensary," says: "It acts like a powerful *cholagogue*, (a Greek word signifying "to carry off bile"), causing a profuse secretion of bile, and has been used with efficacy in scrofula, chlorosis (whites), jaundice, torpid liver, diseases of the spleen and cachexia (*i. e.*, any depraved or bad condition of the system, as from cancer, syphilis, etc.). Dose—The dose is from 5 to 20 grs., 3 times a day. A dr. or two (60 to 120 grs.) dissolved in a ½ pt. or 1 pt. of water will act as a prompt purgative, with scarcely any depression of the system. "But," he continues, "large doses, or its long continued use in small doses, injures the tone of the stomach. One dr. of the sulphate of manganese mixed in 1 oz. of lard has been used externally as an ointment in buboes, chancres, indolent ulcers and some diseases of the skin." And the author thinks this ointment might prove valuable to rub in thoroughly over the liver. So it will be seen that this preparation of manganese, is a valuable article, and if it is made to take the place of calomel, it will be a grand thing for the people. Almost any cathartic, if very long continued, will depress and injure, more or less, the condition of the stomach; so this is not alone in thus injuring "the tone of the stomach," if long continued.

**ALTERATIVES, OR BLOOD PURIFIERS—By Food, Beers, etc.**—An inquiry through the *Blade* for a plan to improve the complexion by removing pimples, etc., was made in the following words: "My complexion is sallow and bad, my skin pimply all over. I am run down, and want to feel alive again. What is the matter, and what is to be done?" To this inquiry the editor of the "Household Department" made such a common-sense reply that I give it a place, hoping that every one needing such an alterative effect will adopt her suggestions, and save the necessity of taking something which is more of a medicinal character. She says:

I. The matter is that the blood is thoroughly vitiated, and improving it must be a matter of time. Spring diet should do the work of medicine, largely. And first in importance, are salads of all sorts. Every family should have its beds and boxes, its borders and hot-beds full of fresh sprouts, from the pepper-grass and the water-cress to the tender turnip, mustard, cabbage and beet shoots, the first leaves of dandelion and sorrel, cheril, mint and parsely, all good to mix for some of the most inviting salads.

II. But the vegetable which combines the most beneficial qualities, which ranks as a medicine and purifier of the finest sort, is one, which, though its stigma is now removed among gourmands and in polite society, is under the ban in ordinary circles. The virtues of the onion render it a pharmacopœia in itself. Eaten raw, with or without vinegar, it is the most effective purifier of the blood known. It has been known to leave consumptives plump and rosy. It cures dyspepsia, and is a thorough worm-medicine for children. As a toilet prescription, it will do as much to refine the complexion, renew the hair and remove spots as any one article known. More people like its piquant flavor, indispensable in all high-class cookery, than care to own a preference they suppose ungenteel. But there need be no hesitation in eating onions freely, since the use of a tooth-brush and a dose of charcoal, always good in itself, or the chewing of some roasted coffee or corn, will remove the odor. The only care to be

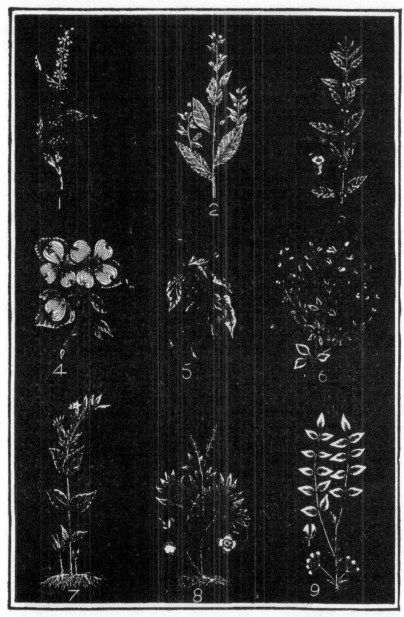

1—Yellow Dock.   2—Lobelia, or Indian Tobacco.   3—Bugleweed, or Water Horehound.   4—Dogwood, or Boxwood.   5—Deadly Nightshade, or Belladonna.   6—Wild Indigo, or Rattle Bush.   7—Pink Root, or Carolina Pink.   8—Black Cohosh, or Rattleroot.   9—Prickly Ash, or Yellow Wood.

observed is, that as onions absorb impurities very quickly, they should be kept in a dry place where there is pure air, not in musty cellars or closets, with decaying provisions and sour milk. To get their full benefit, raw onions and their young shoots should be eaten at breakfast, as a salad, with bread and butter. They banish worm complaints of the most aggravated type, and prevent throat and blood disease in a large degree, absorbing and removing impurities in the blood. * * * * I am going to give one or two old-fashioned recipes for spring bitters which, home-made, of fresh roots and simples, are better than expensive medicines, and the two following have especial virtues for the complexion.

III. *Alterative Bitters, Cheap and Good.*—Put 1 oz. of yellow dock root and a cup of grated horse-radish in 1 quart of hard cider, cold. It will be ready the next day and should be taken, a wine-glass full before each meal. This made by the gallon and taken through the season will affect the growth of the hair and improve the appearance in every way, provided the strength is kept up by well selected food.

IV. *Alterative Beer of Our Grandmother's Make.*—The next is a strictly temperance beer of the sort of our grandmothers used to administer in powerful doses. Take of best Jamaica ginger root, sassafras bark, from the root, and wild cherry bark, each 2 ozs.; burdock root and dandelion root, each 4 ozs.; bruise all, and add cream of tartar, 1 oz., and water, 2 gals. Boil 10 minutes, strain, and add white sugar, 1½ lbs.; the rind of a lemon in bits; heat, stir until the sugar dissolves, and pour into a stone jar with 3 ozs. of tartaric acid. When lukewarm, put in a tea-cupful of hop yeast, stirring well. In a few days it will be in high perfection and a very pleasant beer, with valuable alterative properties.

*Remarks.*—The author thinks that 1 oz. of tartaric acid will be plenty, because, with the above amount, 3 ozs., it will become hard and sour too quickly.

**Ring-Worm Remedies.**—The form that this eruption takes gives its name, as it is generally in a circle, itching considerably when the body is heated by exercise, or in hot weather; and also if rubbed or scratched. A saturated solution (all that will dissolve) of blue vitriol in water, touching the parts several times daily, will cure them.

**SPRAINS—Capital Remedy for.**—The white of an egg, into which a piece of alum about the size of a hickory-nut has been stirred, stirring constantly until it forms a jelly or curd, is a capital remedy for sprains. It should be laid over the sprain upon a piece of lint, and be changed or re-wet in the whey as often as it becomes dry.

*Remarks.*—I think it best to lay on a cloth, rather than lint, for convenience of re-wetting, as in for Inflammation of the Eye; full directions there how to make and use it. It allays inflammation and soreness quickly.

**1. CUTS AND BURNS Shorn of Their Terrors.**—A writer in the Stratford (Ont.) *Weekly Herald* gives the following remedy for slight cuts and small burns, which she claims to be so effectual as to remove the usual terror arising in a family upon such occasions. She says: " Our own remedy for cuts and burns is glue or mucilage. This closes up a cut nicely, and one will experience no inconvenience thereafter. Cuts and burns are shorn of their terrors when the glue or mucilage is handy and ready for use. Let our lady readers bear this in mind. The good right-hand which penned these lines was caught under a stick while replenishing the fire in the kitchen stove, and pressed closely against the hot iron plate so that one finger was quite roasted. We released it and almost fainted before we could reach the cool, thick mucilage on our writing-desk, when, lo! all pain, and smart, and annoyance were gone, and the hand was ready for duty just as soon as the transparent covering could dry. How many useful things there are, the value of which we know almost nothing of."

*Remarks..*—I was aware that carriage varnish was good for slight cuts, burns and bruises, when the skin is more or less abraded, or scraped (from the Latin *abradere*, to scrape off), and I have no doubt a good liquid glue or the common mucilage, made with gum arabic, 5 ozs., to water, ½ pt., will do just as well. I should prefer the mucilage in place of the glue.

**2. Cuts, An Excellent Remedy for.**—"It is not generally known," says a writer, "that the leaves of the common geranium are an excellent remedy for cuts, or where the skin is rubbed off, and other wounds of that kind. One or 2 leaves, bruised and applied to the parts, and the wounds will be cicatrized (healed) in a short time." (See Burns, Scalds, etc., for the use of the new remedy—bi-carbonate of soda.)

**3. Cuts, Wounds, Felons and Other Inflammations, Hot Water Poultice for.**—A paper called the *Home Health* says that a hot water poultice is the most healing application for cuts, bruises, wounds, sores, felons and other inflammations, that can be used. The poultice is made by dipping cotton in hot water and applying, changing often. A convenient way is, in case of felons or other painful abscess, to hold the hand for hours in water as hot as can be comfortably borne.

*Remarks.*—This is undoubtedly valuable. I have for some time past used hot applications to an inflamed eye, while most physicians apply cold. It is good for internal use, as seen by the use of the hot water cures for dyspepsia, consumption, etc., in this book, which see; why not good for external applications? I believe it will be found so, if a wound or other sore manifests the least tendency to inflame and become tedious in healing.

**1. CATARRH, NASAL—Common-Sense Treatment for.**—Notwithstanding Dr. Dio Lewis has sometimes appeared, at least, to run the "diet" question into the ground, as we often hear said, yet his remarks upon it in connection with nasal catarrh are perfectly sound. He says:

"For nasal catarrh, eat only a piece of beefsteak (broiled is best) half as large as your hand, one baked potato and one slice of bread for your breakfast; a piece of roast beef as large as your hand, with one boiled potato and one slice of bread, for dinner; take nothing for supper, and go to bed at 8:30 o'clock. Sleep, if possible, half an hour before dinner. Drink nothing with your meals, nor within two hours after. Drink as much cold water on rising and going to bed as you can. Live 4 to 6 hours daily in the open air, riding or walking. Bathe frequently, and every night on going to bed rub the skin all over with a hair glove. [There are two kinds of hair gloves, the English and American, usually kept by druggists. The English are the best, being more durable.] In less than a week you will get along with one handkerchief daily. To cure even bad cases you have only to make your stomach digest well—only to make yourself healthier—and your nose will quickly find it out and adapt itself to the better manners of its companions."

*Remarks.*—Dr. Lewis claims, and the above treatment indicates, this disease to be constitutional, and, therefore, he works upon the constitution alternatively through the digestion, which, not directly but impliedly, forbids tea, coffee and all pastry; but while he leaves the substantials, we may well allow him to cut off, as he does, all hurtful superfluities. It has only to be tried faithfully to satisfy the most incredulous of its value. It will prove equally valuable in consumption, salt-rheum, discharges from the ears, fever-sores, etc., etc., as he claims them all to be constitutional rather than simply local, as has been generally believed. Certainly this common-sense plan of eating and care of the person will do great good in these and all chronic diseases; and it would be wise for everybody to use much less of the superfluities and confine themselves to the simple necessaries in the line of food, if health and consequent long life is worthy of consideration. It will not be possible for those living in the country to always have fresh steak or roast beef, but they must confine themselves to the substantials, and let cake, pie and puddings alone, if they hope to get rid of long-standing disease. And I will only add here that in any chronic, *i. e.,* long-standing, disease, the salt-water washings (which see) should be resorted to, with the dry rubbings, as there directed.

**2. Catarrh Snuff.**—Pulverized borax, 1 oz.; loaf-sugar, pulverized, ½ dr. Mix thoroughly, and take 6 to 10 pinches daily.

*Remarks.*—It may be used in connection with any other treatment, and will be found especially valuable in all recent cases, and has cured many chronic, or long-standing cases, without other aids Still it is always best to use general treatment in connection with it. If the throat is at all sore at the same time you take a pinch of the snuff, it will be found valuable to take another pinch and drop it into the fauces, or back part of the throat. It helps the cure materially.

**3. Catarrh, Ointment for.**—Pure tar, ¼ oz.; freshly made, unsalted butter, 1 oz., or 1 oz. to 4 if it is thought that much will be needed. Simmer together and apply inside the nostrils from 3 to 6 times a day, as the case seems to require. This is claimed to be very valuable, keeping the membrane moist as well as being curative in itself.

**EPILEPSY—Of Long Standing—German Cure for.**—According to Kunze, we possess in Curare a remedy by which cases of epilepsy of very long standing can be cured. He uses a solution of ½ grs. of Curare in 1 dr. and 15 minims of water, to which 2 drops of hydrochloric acid have been added. At intervals of about a week he injects 8 drops of this solution subcutaneously (under the skin), and he has found that in some cases where con. vulsions had occurred for some years, a complete cure was effected after about 8 to 10 injections.—*Deutsche Zeitsch. f. prakt. Med. 1877, No. 9.*

*Remarks.*—The Curare is one of the newer remedies, and may not be generally kept by druggists; but as this would have to be done by a physician, having a suitable instrument to inject with, he can obtain the remedy without trouble to the patient. It will be a grand thing if we have a cure, at last, for this terrible disease. The following, however which came to me in the *Medical Summary,* of Landsdale, Pa., for December, 1882, long after the above was written, seems to hold out great hopes, with much less trouble, than the foregoing. It was first communicated to the *Medical and Surgical Reporter* by Edward Vanderpoel, M. D., who says:

"When I commenced practice, in 1833, nitrate of silver was the grand remedy for this complaint. After repeated failures, however, with it, I was told by Dr. Boyd, an octogenarian (one of 80 years, who might have seen 50 or 60 years of practice), of our city, that he had no trouble in its cure. He had treated a man successfully who had not earned a dollar in 20 years, and who afterwards supported his family by his labor. I gladly adopted his practice, and have been successful ever since. The remedy, oxide of zinc. DIRECTIONS— Begin ½ gr. dose, 3 times a day, for 24 doses (8 days). Then 1 gr. for 24 doses. Then 1½ grs. 3 times a day, rubbing the spine with stramonium ointment, morning and evening, and stimulating embrocations (liniments), which I have seen used. Since then I have been successful; never going beyond 5 gr. doses, except in one case of a hard drinker and opium eater who, at the time I com menced with him, had been treated for a year with bromide of potash; impairing his memory badly, which was restored with the use of the zinc."

*Remarks.*—I have great confidence in this treatment, from the age of the originator and the length of time Dr. Vanderpool had used it, he being in practice for 50 years. (See also " Chorea, or St. Vitus Dance," which is a species of nervous disease, much like epilepsy.)

**FAT PEOPLE—Food to Reduce Their Fleshiness.**—The *Medical Journal,* speaking of the plan to reduce fat people, to a reasonably stout and healthy condition, says: " If any reader is growing too fat for comfort, he may, possibly, find the following suggestions valuable: There are three classes of food, the oils, sweets and starches, the special office of which is to support the animal heat and produce fat, having little or no influence in promoting strength of muscle or endurance. If fat people, therefore, would use less fat and more of lean meats, fish and fowl, less of fine flour and more of the whole products of the grains—except the hulls—less of the sweets, particularly in warm weather, and more of the fruit acids, in a mild form, as in the apple, sleep less, be less indolent, and labor more in the open air, the fat would disap- pear, to a certain extent at least, with no loss of real health. In food we have almost a perfect control of this matter, far better than we can have in the use of drugs. If we have too much fat and too little muscle, we have simply to use less of the fat forming elements and more of the muscle food, such as lean meats, fish and fowl, and the darker portions of the grains, etc., with peas and beans."

*Remarks.*—The above principles are facts; then, if any person desires to be less fat, let them be governed by them, and they will obtain their desire; indolence and self-indulgence are the mothers of fatness. (See also "Dropsy and Anti-fat Medicine in One.")

**1. LIQUOR—A Cure for the Love of it.**—At a festival at a reformatory institution recently, a gentleman said, of the cure of the use of intoxicating liquors: "I overcame the appetite by a recipe given to me by old Dr. Hatfield, one of those good old physicians who do not have a percentage from a neighboring druggist. The prescription is simply an orange every morning a half hour before breakfast. 'Take that,' said the doctor, 'and you will neither want liquor nor medicine.' I have done so regularly, and find that liquor has become repulsive. The taste of the orange is in the saliva of my tongue, and it would be as well to mix water and oil, as rum, with my taste."

*Remarks.*—I will add to this, keep away from where it is sold, taking the orange as directed, and you will be safe. If you go into saloons, no matter how much you may try to avoid drinking while there, there will be pretended friends —real enemies—who will urge you to drink, and even attempt to pull you up to the bar, and try to force it into your mouth. I speak from knowledge. I once had two young men—I was then young myself—get a cup of brandy, and one of them behind me and the other in front, tried to force me to drink it; but I got a chance to get a foot against a bureau and pushed back enough to get room for a kick, and that cup and brandy went, as the saying is, "higher'n a kite,"—it went to the ceiling,—and then I said, " Boys, if you don't let me alone, I will kick you, too, but drink I will not." But I should have had to fight, if the boss for whom we all worked, had not stepped forward at this juncture, and said "Boys, you ought to be ashamed of yourselves. You know Chase told us this morning that he did not drink, and, hence, went and borrowed a rifle, and has spent all day to get a deer for us to eat; now, let him alone." At this they gave it up. The occasion being when a saw mill, in which we worked, had been sold — this was in 1834 or '35—and the giving possession had to be done with whiskey and a high day. The difficulty is, people—men or boys—do not say *no* with sufficient vim. When enticed to evil, let the *no* have a ring as though you meant just what you said; then, unless the enticers are drunk, as they were in the above case, you will generally have no trouble, especially if you do not put in your presence at their haunts of vice. In the above case, it was a boarding-house for the mill, and I had nowhere else to go. I will only add, if a man does not want to drink, he need not; if he wants to drink, nothing can save him. He is bound to destruction. He is, like Ephraim, " joined to his idols," —you may just as well—"let him alone."

**2. Liquor—The Use of It Leaves a Permanent Injury.**—An American physician, who has given attention to the study of alcoholism, said in the course of an address recently delivered before a learned society: " There are constantly crowding into our insane asylums persons, 50 to 80 years of age, who in early life were addicted to the use of alcoholic liquors, but who had reformed, and for 10, 20, or 30 years had never touched a drop. The injury which the liquor did to their bodies seemed to have all disappeared, being triumphed over by the full vigor of their manhood; but when their natural force began to decrease, then the concealed mischief showed itself in insanity, clearly demonstrating that the injury to their brain was of a permanent character."

*Remarks.*—Then is there not a double reason for not using it? The loss of time and money, and often the abuse of wife and children, or other friends, while using it, and the probability of the loss of one's reason in old age. It is greatly to be hoped that a word to the wise may be sufficient.

**1. LIFE LENGTHENED—Sensible Rules for.**—Dr. Hall, in his excellent *Journal of Health*, gives the following sensible and suggestive rules · under the above heading:

I.   Cultivate an equable temper; many have fallen dead in a fit of passion.

II.  Eat regularly, not over thrice a day, and nothing between meals.

III. Go to bed at regular hours. Get up as soon as you wake of yourself, and do not sleep in the day-time—at least, not longer than ten minutes before dinner.

IV.  Work in moderation, and not as though you were doing it by the job.

V.   Stop working before you are very much tired—before you are "fagged out."

VI.  Cultivate a generous and accommodating temper.

VII. Never cross a bridge before you come to it; this will save you half the troubles of life. (In other words, "don't borrow trouble.")

VIII. Never eat when you are not hungry, nor drink when you are not thirsty.

IX.  Let your appetite always come uninvited.

X.   Cool off in a place greatly warmer than the one in which you have been exercising. This simple rule would prevent incalculable sickness and save thousands of lives every year.

XI.  Never resist a call of nature, for a single moment.

XII. Never allow yourself to be chilled through and through; it is this which destroys so many every year, in a few days' sickness, from pneumonia—called by some, lung fever—or inflammation of the lungs.

XIII. Whoever drinks no liquids at meals will add years of pleasurable existence to his life. Of cold or warm drinks, the cold ones are the most pernicious. Drinking at meals induces persons to eat more than they otherwise would, as any one can verify by experiment; and it is excess in eating which devastates the land with sickness, suffering and death.

XIV. After fifty years of age, if not a day laborer, and sedentary persons at forty, should eat but twice a day—in the morning, and about four in the afternoon; for every organ without adequate rest will "give out" prematurely.

XV.  Begin early to live under the benign influence of Christian religion, for it "has the promise of the life that now is and of that which is to come."

*Remarks.*—These rules need no extended commendation—they are certainly sensible.

**2. How Long Have We to Live, as Shown by the Life Assurance Tables.**—The following is one of the authenticated tables, in use among insurance companies, showing the average length of life at the various ages. In the first column, we have persons of average health, and in the second column we are enabled to peep, as it were, behind the scenes, and gather from their table the number of years they will give us to live. This table is the result of careful calculation, and seldom proves misleading. Of course, sudden and premature deaths—from accidents, unusual severity of disease, etc.—as well as lives unusually extended, occasionally occur; but this is the average expectancy of life, of an ordinary man, who lives prudently and avoids all undue exposures, etc. In the earlier years of life, the female, from less exposure, has from 1 to 2 years more of life in expectation than the male; but as life advances, this over-average comes down gradually to nearly the same; but still there is a trifle, or small part of a year, always in favor of the woman. I will say, at the start, that the average life of all born into the world is, for males, about $39\frac{90}{100}$ years, and for females, $41\frac{85}{100}$ years. I shall only give the figures for every 10 years, up to 20 and after 60, for, so far as business is concerned, before 20 and after 60, it will not be of much account, yet interesting as a matter of curiosity. The table is given in years and hundredths of a year, by Dr. William Farr.

| Age. Those who reach. | More years to live. | Age. Those who reach. | More years to live. |
|---|---|---|---|
| 0 | 39.90 | 45 | 22.76 |
| 1 | 46.65 | 50 | 19.54 |
| 10 | 47.05 | 55 | 16.45 |
| 20 | 39.48 | 60 | 13.53 |
| 25 | 36.12 | 70 | 8.45 |
| 30 | 32.76 | 80 | 4.93 |
| 35 | 29.40 | 90 | 2.84 |
| 40 | 26.06 | 100 | 1.68 |

*Remarks.*—With this table before us, taking the present age of any person in ordinary good health, we see at a glance how much longer they may be expected to live. By considering these things, we can tell whether or not it would be best to enter into new business enterprises, marriage relations, etc. And, with the table, on "The Pulse in Health," we can tell pretty nearly whether we are in an average condition of health or not, as these figures do not lie; if they do not hold good in any particular case, it is from a want of average health.

Supposing the ladies will desire to know their chances or probabilities of marriage, I will append a table showing what their prospects are, between thirteen and forty, as follows:

**3. Chances of Women for Marriage.**—The following statement is drawn from the registered cases of 876 married women in France. It is the first ever constructed to show ladies their chances of marriage at various ages. Of the above number there were married:

| | | | | | | |
|---|---|---|---|---|---|---|
| 3 at 13 | 45 at 17 | 86 at 21 | 36 at 25 | 17 at 29 | 7 at 33 | 2 at 37 |
| 11 at 14 | 77 at 18 | 85 at 22 | 24 at 26 | 9 at 30 | 5 at 34 | 0 at 38 |
| 16 at 15 | 115 at 19 | 59 at 23 | 28 at 27 | 7 at 31 | 3 at 35 | 1 at 39 |
| 43 at 16 | 118 at 20 | 53 at 24 | 22 at 28 | 5 at 32 | 0 at 36 | 0 at 40 |

**4.  The Pulse in Health—Average Beats per Minute—From Physiologist Carpenter:**

| | | |
|---|---|---|
| New-born infants,        -        -        - | From 140 down to 130 |
| During 1st year,   -     -     -     = | "    130   "    115 |
| "      2d  year,     -     -     - | "    115   "    100 |
| "      3d  year,   -     -     -     ◦ | "    105   "    95 |
| From 7th to 14th year,        -     . | "    90   "    80 |
| "    14th to 21st year,   -     .     - | "    85   "    75 |
| "    21st to 60th year,        -     . | "    75   "    70 |
| In old age,        -     .     -     - | "    75   "    80 |

In inflammatory or acute diseases the pulse may rise to 120, or even to 160, in the adult, and becoming so frequent in the child that it cannot be counted. Muscular exertion, mental excitement, digestion, alcoholic drink, and elevation above the sea level, accelerate the pulse, and as a rule it is more frequent in the morning than in the evening.  It is slower in sleep, and from the effects of rest, diet, cold, or blood-letting.  The pulse of a grown woman exceeds that of a man of the same age, as much as 10 to 14 beats a minute, and, according to some authorities, is less frequent in the tall than in the short person, the variations being about 4 beats for each 6 inches of height.

*Remarks.*—With this tabulation, any person of average ability (we are now talking of averages) can form a fair opinion of how much disturbance there may be in one's system, to cause any variation from the general average, and hence, tell how sick a person may be and the probability of returning health, under favorable circumstances; also the general average of the length of life and probability of marriages, etc.  But it may not be amiss here, to state that while standing, a healthy man's pulse beats about 74 times in a minute; when sitting, only about 70; and when he lies down, only about 64.  Thus the heart takes its rest at night; and as the heart passes in its beats about 6 ozs. of blood, it is saved the lifting of about 30,000 ozs. of blood in 8 hours' sleep.  But now suppose he is a drinking man, and takes his wine or liquor day and night, the heart must not only get no rest, but is increased by at least 15,000 beats in this 8 hours and he rises more tired than when he retired, and wholly unfit for the day's work, and so strikes out again for the "ruddy bumper," as some call it, to "settle his nerves," and thus in a few years he settles, also, into a drunkard's grave, mourned for only by those who ought to have been helped by him yet, for many years, if he would have cast away his "cups."  O, why will men so far forget the object of their being?

**1.  THE TONGUE—WHAT IT TELLS.**—I am very sorry that I do not know who wrote the following soliloquy upon the tongue, as it is both sensible and sound in its teachings; hence, I say, let it be read with care and its teachings heeded.  He says:

"A man can never be happy if his stomach is out of order; and dyspepsia and hysteria imitate the symptoms of innumerable disorders.  But how, the reader may ask, can I tell the illness, from which I think I am suffering, to be real or imaginary?  At any rate, I should answer, look to your stomach first, and, pray, just take a glance at your tongue.  If ever I was so far left to myself as to meditate some rash act, I should, before going into the matter, have a look at my tongue. If it was not perfectly clean and moist I should not consider myself perfectly healthy, nor perfectly sane, and would postpone my proceedings in the hope that my worldly prospects would get brighter. What does a physician discover by looking at the tongue? Many things. The tongue sympathizes with every trifling ailment of body or mind, and more especially with the state of the stomach. That thin, whitish layer (fur) all over the surface, indicates indigestion. A patchy tongue (*i. e.*, the fur in patches) shows that the stomach is very much out of order indeed. A yellow tongue points to biliousness. A creamy, shivering, thick, indented tongue, tells of previous excesses; and I do not like my friends to wear such tongues, for I sincerely believe that real comfort can not be secured in this world by any one who does not keep his feet warm, his head cool, and his tongue clean."

*Remarks.*—That we may know what further the tongue may teach us we will give the "Synopsis of a Paper read before the Eclectic Medical Association of Ohio, by Prof. John M. Scudder, of the Eclectic Medical Institute of Cincinnati," and published by him in the *Eclectic Medical Journal*, of which he is the editor and proprietor. The paper was prepared to explain, and does fairly explain, the leading point, or basis upon which "Specific Medication" is established or founded, and that is, the indication for treatment as shown by the condition of the tongue, or "What the Tongue Tells Us," as shown in our first heading above. And although it is quite lengthy, yet as it contains so much valuable information for those who may desire to take care of themselves and their families, I think it best to give the full synopsis as he gave it in the *Journal*, Vol. XXXI., pages 425-8, under the head of "Specific Medication," but as it relates largely to what the tongue teaches or shows us, I will head it accordingly.

### 2. The Tongue, the Condition of the System Shown by it, and the Remedy their Conditions Call for.—After the preliminary business of the association was completed, he addressed them as follows:

GENTLEMEN:—At the last meeting of the State Society I was requested to prepare a paper on Specific Medication, which should serve as a basis for a discussion in this new departure (as it has been called) in medicine.

I do not propose, in doing this, to occupy much of your time in details, but rather to present the principles upon which specific or direct medication rests.

It will be well for us, first, to think for a moment (if it is possible for us to realize it) what an un-specific or indirect medication is. · It means that we never oppose remedies directly to processes of disease, but, on the contrary, influence diseased action in a roundabout, indirect, and uncertain manner.

As examples—We violently excite the intestinal canal with cathartics to arrest disease of the brain, the lungs, the kidneys, or other distant parts. Or it is possible that we confine our ministration first to the gastric sac (stomach), then follow with potent cathartics. In order, we excite the skin and the kidneys in the same manner. This not sufficing, we counter-irritate with rubefacients, blisters, etc., and so far as possible keep up an influence counter to the disease, by unpleasant, nauseating and irritant medicines.

Whatever may be said in favor of such a practice, and how fine-so-ever the theories in reference to it may be spun, it is based upon the idea that two diseases can not exist in the body at the same time, and if the medicines are sufficiently potent their action will surely be the strongest—and the disease will stop —leaving the patient to recover slowly from the influence of the medicines.

Did you ever know the patient to stop instead of the disease? I have, many a time, and have in this way, myself, been a wonderful dispensation of Providence. In the olden time men would not believe that the doctors aided large numbers of people out of the world. Oh no! The doctors, God bless them, pulled the sick through; they would all have died if it had not been for the faculty.

It is wonderful how statistics take the conceit out of some people and some things. When we find hundreds of cases of severe diseases tabulated—such as typhoid fever and pneumonia—with a mortality of but one to three per cent., with only good nursing and food, no medicine; and active, potent medication gives a mortality of five to fifty per cent.

Do Eclectic physicians kill people too? This brings the matter home, and one doesn't like to confess his own sins, as a rule. But in this matter I am like Artemus Ward in the last war—I am willing to shed the blood of all my relations—and I answer in the affirmative—they do kill—not so many as the old practice, it is true, but yet enough to cause us to look at home and rid ourselves of the evil.

Now, I am glad to know that you, and Eclectics as a rule, have a very much better practice than theory. Whilst they occasionally wander off after these phantasms, it is the exception and not the rule.

As a body of physicians, we recognize the fact that disease in all its forms is an impairment of life. And we recognize the necessity of conserving this life, and of employing such means as will increase it, and enable it to resist and throw off disease, and restore normal structure and function.

We recognize the importance of the functions of circulation, innervation (healthy action of the nerves giving strength), excretion, etc., and the necessity of obtaining as nearly a normal (healthy) performance of them as possible. And all experience shows that just in proportion as we get this normal performance disease is arrested.

From its inception (commencement) Eclecticism has been, to a very considerable extent, Specific Medication. The earliest writings point us to Dioscorea (wild yam or colic-root) as a remedy for bilious colic, Hydrastis (golden seal) for enfeebled mucous membranes, Aralia (dwarf elder) and Apocynum (Indian hemp) for dropsy, Baptisia (wild indigo) for putrid sore throat, and similar conditions of mucous membranes, Hamamelis (witch-hazel) for hemorrhoids, Macrotys (black cohosh) for rheumatism, etc.

In our Materia Medicas remedies were classed as emetics, cathartics, diaphoretics, tonics, alteratives, etc., but in reading the description of medical properties, some special use or curative action would be pointed out, and for this it would be commonly used.

In all acute, and most chronic diseases, our examination of the patient and our therapeutics will take this order: 1. With reference to the condition of the stomach and intestinal canal—bringing them to as nearly a normal condition as possible, that remedies may be kindly received and appropriated, and that sufficient food may be taken and digested. 2. With reference to the circulation of the blood and the temperature—obtaining a normal circulation as regards frequency and freedom, and a temperature as near 98° as possible. 3. With reference to the presence of a *zymotic* poison, or other cause of disease, which may be neutralized, antagonized or removed. 4. With reference to the condition of the nervous system—giving good innervation. 5. With reference to the processes of waste and excretion—that the worn-out or enfeebled material may be broken down and speedily removed from the body. 6. With reference to blood-making and repair—that proper material be furnished for the building of tissues, and that the processes of nutrition are normally conducted.

We may illustrate this further by calling attention to the tongue as a means of diagnosing (determining) the conditions of the stomach and intestinal canal, and of the blood.

You will bear in mind that diagnosis—or determining the real condition of disease is the most important part of specific medication. And that it is not that rough diagnosis which will enable us to guess off a name for the associated symptoms, at which name we will fire our Materia Medica promiscuously. Hence when we question the tongue, it is not with reference to a remittent or typhoid fever, an inflammation of lungs or rheumatism, but it is—I want you to tell me the condition of the stomach and intestinal canal, and especially the condition of the blood.

Now let us briefly see what it will tell us, with regard to the condition of the *primæ viæ* (first passages—stomach, intestines, and kidneys).

If the tongue is heavily coated with a yellowish-white fur, we know that there are morbid accumulations in the stomach; and we have to determine between the speedy removal by emesis (vomiting), and the slower removal by the alkaline sulphites (sulphite of soda is generally used), or the indirect removal by catharsis (cathartics).

If the tongue is uniformly coated, from base to tip, with a yellowish fur, rather full and moist, we have the history of atony (weakness) of the small intestine, and we give podophylin, leptandrin, and this class of remedies, with considerable certainty.

If the tongue is elongated and pointed, reddened at the tip and edges, papillæ elongated and red, we have evidence of irritation of the stomach with determination of blood. The therapeutics (application of the proper medicine) is plain: get rid of the irritation *first*, and be careful not to renew it by the application of harsh medication.

Again, we have a tongue that might be designated as "slick." It is variously colored, but it looks as if a fly should light upon it he would slip up. It is an evidence of a want of functional power, (general weakness), not only in the stomach and bowels, but of all parts supplied by sympathetic nerves. We treat such a case very carefully, avoid all irritants, and use means to restore innervation (strength) through the vegetative system of nerves.

The tongue tells us of the acidity and alkalinity of the blood, and in language so plain, that it can not be mistaken.

The pallid tongue (pale, or without color), with white fur, is the index of acidity, and we employ an alkali—usually a salt of soda—with a certainty that the patient will be benefited. Indeed, one who has never had his attention directed in this way, would be surprised at the improvement, in grave forms of disease, from one day's administration of simple bi-carbonate of soda.

The deep-red tongue indicates alkalinity, and we prescribe an acid with the positive asssurance that it will prove beneficial. Grave cases of typhoid fever and other zymotic (epidemic or contagious) diseases, presenting this symptom, have been treated with acids alone, and with a success not obtained by other means. But it makes no difference what the disease is, whether a recent diarrhea, or a grave typhoid dysentery, if there is the deep-red tongue, we give muriatic acid with the same assurance of success.

Impairment of the blood—sepsis (blood-poisoning)—is indicated by dirty coating, and by dark-colored fur—brownish to black. When we have either the one or the other we employ those remedies which antagonize the septic (poisoning) process.

The bitter tonics are indicated by fullness of tissue, with evident relaxation, impairment of circulation and muscular movement. The same condition will be an indication of iron. We give tincture of chloride of iron, if the tongue is red, iron by hydrogen if the tongue is pale.

The pale, trembling tongue, is a very good indication for the hypophosphites.

The pale blueish tongue, expressionless, is the indication for the administration of copper.

The dusky, swollen tongue demands baptisia (wild indigo).

You will notice that we have made this unruly member tell us a good deal, yet it might tell us more—it will tell us more when we thoroughly study it. My object, is not to point out all that we might learn from it, but to show that it is possible to arrive at positive conclusions, from symptoms that are always definite in their meaning.

In making our diagnosis, we question every function in the same way. We make the pulse tell us the condition of the circulation, and to some extent the nervous system that it supplies. We question the nervous system, the secretory organs—in fact every part.

One might suppose that diagnosis in this way would be a matter of great difficulty, as would the therapeutics based upon it, from the large number of remedies needed to meet these varying conditions of the several functions. But this is not so. On the contrary, the method is not only direct and certain, but it is easy.

We have but one life, though its manifestations are so varied. The control of this life is centered in a common nervous system—the ganglionic, and through this the various parts and functions are united. Disease is an aberration of this life—life in a wrong direction. Though it manifests itself in various ways, and though we study in detail, as I have named, it is to grasp it at last, as a unit, and oppose to it one or more remedies.

In some cases we have a first preparatory treatment, to fit the patient for the reception of remedies which directly oppose disease. As when we gave an emetic to remove morbid accumulations, or means to relieve irritation of the stomach, or give an acid or an alkali, or use veratrum and aconite to reduce frequency of pulse and temperature, to obtain the kindly action of quinine in intermittent or remittent fever.

In other cases there are certain prominent symptoms indicating pathological conditions which may be taken as the key notes of the treatment. As, when we have the full, open pulse, indicating veratrum; the hypochondriac fullness, umbilical pains, and sallowness of skin, indicating nux vomica; the bright eye, contracted pupil, and flushed face, calling for gelsemium; or the dull eye, immobile pupil, tendency to drowsiness, which calls for belladonna.

In some cases the indication for a special remedy, like one of these, is so marked, that we give it alone, and it quickly cures most severe and obstinate diseases.

I would like to continue this subject further, for it is one in which I am greatly interested, and I know it is one in which you are interested, but the shortness of our session will not permit further remarks. But when we come together another year, with another year's experience, we may discuss it again.

*Remarks.*—If the foregoing is studied well, "it will pay," by helping to understand the diseased conditions to which all are liable, as shown by the tongue; and, besides this, there are quite a number of things explained, which, if studied and heeded, will also prove of great value to those who are sick, or who have the care of the sick.

**LEMONS—Their Value in Sickness and in Health.**—One of the journals, speaking of the use of lemons, says: "For all people, either in sickness or in health, lemonade is a safe drink. It corrects biliousness. It is a specific (positive cure) against worms and skin complaints. Lemon juice is the best antiscorbutic remedy known. It not only cures the disease but prevents it. Sailors make a daily use of it for this purpose. A physician suggests rubbing of the gums daily with lemon juice, to keep them in health. The hands and the nails are also kept clean, white and soft by the daily use of lemon instead of soap. It also prevents chilblains. Lemon used in intermittent fever is mixed with strong, hot, black tea, or coffee, without sugar. Neuralgia may be cured by rubbing the part affected with a lemon. It is valuable, also, to cure warts and destroy dandruff on the head, by rubbing the roots of the hair with it. In fact, its uses are manifold, and the more we use of them the better we shall find ourselves."

*Remarks.*—See also their value for freckles, and the use of hot lemonade to cure colds, and also lemon juice a cure for small-pox, etc.

**Food as Medicine.**—Dr. Hall relates the case of a man who was cured of his biliousness by going without his supper, and drinking freely of lemonade. Every morning, says the doctor, this patient arose with a wonderful sense of rest and refreshment, and a feeling as though the blood had been literally washed, cleansed and cooled by the lemonade and the fast. His theory is, that food will be used as a remedy, for many diseases, successfully. For example he cures cases of spitting blood by the use of salt; epilepsy and yellow fever, by water-melons; kidney affections, by celery (water-melons are very valuable also for the kidneys); poison, olive or sweet oil; erysipelas, pounded cranberries applied to the parts affected; hydrophobia, onions, etc. So the way to keep in good health is really to *know what to eat* — not to know what *medicines* to take.

*Remarks.*—These are all good for what he recommends them; then use them freely, in their season.

**1. ERYSIPELAS—New and Successful Remedy.**—Dr. T. B. King of this city (Toledo, O.), an old physician, of the "Old School,"—Allopathic—tells me he has cured erysipelas upon a woman's leg (by the way do women have "legs"—I believe not so understood, but "limbs"), after ulcerated and swollen so bad that other doctors said it must be amputated. But by simply dusting upon it, freely, the per sulphate of iron (Monsel's salt), cleaning off twice daily, with warm suds, and re-applying, without other treatment, effectually cured her.

*Remarks.*—This salt, or preparation of iron, is a great favorite with Dr. King. He applies it, through a speculum (from the Latin *specere*, to look), to ulcers at the mouth of the womb, or upper part of the vagina, he says, with equal success. I have also used it, with success, in several of these ulcerations, so I have confidence in it, in erysipelas also. To avoid staining the clothing, in these cases, wear a suitable bandage to absorb any escaping fluid, as the iron in this leaves an iron-rust appearance upon the clothing.

**2. Erysipelss of the Face (Facial Erysipelas).**—Dr. J. B. Johnson communicated the following to the *Medical and Surgical Reporter*, which he has always found to arrest the disease at once and allay the heat and burning promptly. He says: "As the tongue is always more or less coated, I usually introduce my treatment by a dose of pills composed of blue mass, 10 grs.; calomel, 5 grs.; mix and make into 3 pills; to be taken at one dose; and to be followed in 3 hours by a dose of sulphate of magnesia (epsom salts, dose, ordinarily, a heaping table-spoonful); and without waiting for the action of the pills and salts, I immediately commence with iodide of potassium, 1 dr.; tinct. of hyoscyamus, 2 drs.; tinct. aconite leaves (tincture of aconite root is seldom given internally), 12 drops; distilled water (clear soft water will do) 8 ozs.: mix. Dose—A table-spoonful every hour, day and night, when awake; and I have the face bathed every 2 or 3 hours, and constantly covered with a linen cloth saturated (all it will hold) with the following solution:

"Hyposulphite of soda, 1 oz.; carbolic acid No. 1, 1 oz ; distilled water (soft water will do), 8 ozs. Mix.

"This allays, most promptly, the burning and itching of the skin and face, and is in no wise disagreeable.

"This treatment, I have always found, to arrest the erysipelas almost at once, and my patient to be about his room in 4 or 5 days. My cases have not only escaped complications of congestion and inflammation of the brain, but of the throat also, and without the use of either iron, quinine or wine; 5 gr. doses of iodide potassium (as above) every hour, has never disappointed me in their action; and long experience has enabled me to declare, in my opinion, the internal use of iodide of potassium, to be a specific (positive cure) for facial erysipelas."

*Remarks.*—This will please all who prefer calomel to the other treatment, and the author has confidence in this plan of treatment, as he is not afraid of a small dose of calomel, nor blue mass, if worked off directly as was done in this case.

**3. Facial Erysipelas, The Author's Treatment of.**— Having been recently called to a case of this kind, I will give my treatment of it, as it may help others. It was a young lady of about 18 years of age, in which there was an hereditary tendency to this disease, her grandmother having died of it. I found the left side of the face swollen and inflamed, and just below the eye the flesh was quite hard and very tender. I had it painted, or wet, at once, with muriated tincture of iron, full strength, and covered with a soft cloth, to protect it from the air. This was in the forenoon, and in the evening I instructed the same application, and then a poultice of stewed cranberries to be applied, always wetting with the tincture before applying the poultice. I gave her a seidlitz powder at once, to open the bowels, the next morning to be followed with a rounding table-spoonful of epsom salts, and after that, every other day a seidlitz powder and salts, alternately. I gave her 5 drop doses of the tincture of the iron 3 times a day from the first, by dropping it into a spoon and adding water, and telling her to put the spoon past the teeth, so the iron should not stain them, which it does without this precaution. After the first 24 hours, as the inflammation began to go down and the hardened spot below the eye to become more soft and natural, I weakened the tincture to be applied with one-third water, keeping up the cranberry poultice nights, until the inflammation was cured, reducing the strength of the tincture for application as the case improved, until it was only one-third tincture and two-thirds water; and thus, in one week, she was again able to resume her labors in a candy manufactory where she was engaged, no ulceration or open sore having occured; the scarf-skin only peeled off from the effect of the iron, poulticing, etc. Let each one, then, afflicted with this disease, suit himself as to which plan he will adopt, as circumstances seem to demand.

**1. DIABETES—Valuable Diet for, and Diet to be Avoided.**
—Experienee has shown that the only way to cure diabetes is to change from the ordinary to the following plan of diet:

I. *Food and Drinks which may be Used.*—The quickest way is to confine the patient to beef and bread made of gluten flour, which has all the starchy parts of the wheat removed from it in its manufacture; but mutton, tripe, tongue, ham, bacon, sausage, poultry, game, oysters, clams and eggs may be occasionally used for variety's sake (but liver never); so also salads, made with cabbage or lettuce; cucumbers, water-cress, cauliflower, spinach and string-beans in their season; so also peaches and strawberries with cream, but never with sugar; in fact, all tart fruit may be used, especially nice sour apples, 'peeled, quartered and cored, dipped in beaten eggs and rolled in fine or powdered crumbs of the gluten bread, then fried in very hot fat and drained while hot, make the best substitute there is for potatoes, which you will see below, must not be eaten. Milk in moderate quantities, cream, nice butter, buttermilk, and all freshly made cheese and Neuchatel (Swiss) cheese may be eaten. Nuts in moderation may be allowed, and eggs freely, cooked to suit the patient. Coffee or cocoa, in moderation, with cream, but never with sugar. If tea must be used, let it be weak, and only taken in small quantities. Sour wines, as claret, Burgundy, Rhine, etc., for those who will use them, may be taken in moderation at dinner time. For variety's sake, instead of being absolutely confined to the bread made of the gluten flour, it may be made into rolls, pancakes, fritters, mush, and baked puddings, but never with sugar or molasses, nor may these ever be used, even in pudding sauces. Eat slowly, *i. e.,* masticate (chew) very finely, and what drinks are used let them be taken at the close of the meal—as little as possible between meals, of such as have been named above.

II. *Food and Drinks which Should Never be Used.*—Potatoes, turnips, beets, carrots, parsnips, peas, beans (only string-beans above named), rice, celery, asparagus, or tomatoes; nor soups in which common flour has been put, as vermicelli, noodles, nor any of the vegetables above prohibited. No cake nor pastry of any kind, except it be made from the gluten flour; and nothing that contains sugar or starch in any form; and no spirits, malt beers, nor any of the sweet wines can ever be allowed. Take tepid or warm baths, according to the season, as often as necessary, followed with friction and exercise, as needed to bring a glow of warmth and heat to the surface. [I can not see why the Salt Water Washings, (which see) should not be used with the friction or rubbings, as there given; certainly diabetes is a chronic disease.] Also stick to the above directions as to diet, the year round, to avoid a relapse.

*Remarks.*—This plan was, I think, adopted by some eminent physician in Europe—I do not remember his name.—then by American physicians, by which it has been fairly tested, and found to be about the best thing that can be done; and it has heretofore been considered to be about all that could be done; but later, as shown below, a few remedies have been found also valuable, and the closer the confinement to the beef and gluten flour bread, for a few months, the better will it be for the patient, using the allowables only, as it may be absolutely necessary for variety's sake.

2. **Diabetes, Ammonia-Saline Treatment for.** — It has been found recently, by analysis of diabetic blood, that there is a great deficiency

of certain alkaline salts. These salts are absolutely necessary in order that the sugar which is formed in this disease, just as in health, should be burnt off at the lungs. M. Mialhe, who discovered the above fact, considers this deficiency the primary (first) cause of diabetes. Whether this is so or not, there is no doubt that such deficiency must re-act upon the disease. Accordingly, treatment directed to supply this deficiency is likely to prove of service, and in actual practice such is found to be the fact. The best saline mixture is composed of carbonate of ammonia, phosphate of ammonia, and carbonate of soda, each, 10 grs.; tinct. of ginger, a few drops; 3 times a day in an oz. (2 or 3 table-spoonfuls) of water.

This mixture is very gratifying to the patient, relieves thirst, and mitigates (lessens or relieves) the morbid (unhealthy or craving) appetite. The tongue generally becomes moist, the urine diminishes in quantity, and contains less sugar. In one case, which may be taken as an average one, the amount of sugar was reduced from 30 grs. to the oz. of urine, to 6 grs., and the amount of urine daily from 14 pts. to 4 pts,—*Dr. W. R. Basham.*

*Remarks.*—I have taken this from the *Eclectic Medical Journal* of 1872, page 327, and therefore, I have confidence in it, although I have had no opportunity to try it, as I did not see it until the writing of this department was nearly completed, and especially not till the subject of diabetes had been written; still, I shall try it at once if a case comes under my care.

**3. Ergot in Diabetes Insipidus.**—Dr. Saunders—*St. Louis Courier of Medicine*—reports a case of diabetes insipidus successfully treated, with dram (small tea-spoon) doses three times a day of fl. ex. of ergot. The use of ergot was suggested by an article from Dr. Do Costa.

*Remarks.*—These French physicians, are generally pretty certain of their facts, before they report their cases.

**4. Diabetes—Incontinence and Dribbling of Urine, Successful Remedy for.**—After the foregoing matter upon diabetes had all been prepared, I saw a report of the very remarkable success of J. T. McClanahan, M.D., of Brownville, Mo., in the " Newer Materia Medica" of Parke, Davis & Co., Detroit, Mich., especially upon diabetes, and incidentally upon the others above named, having been successful in both kinds of diabetes — *mellitus,* from *mel,* honey or sweet,—the kind that has sugar in the urine; and also in what is called *insipidus, i. e.,* no sugar in the urine, and hence insipid or tasteless. This latter kind, however, has been, heretofore, much more readily cured than that with the sugar in the urine, but Dr. McClanahan, even in a case of this almost incurable kind—diabetes mellitus—reports the following successful cure. He says:

I. " My case was that of a woman aged 37, mother of children, who was completely run down by large discharges of urine, general lassitude or weakness, (so that she had to give up housework,) pain in the back, considerable thirst, appetite variable, sometimes ravenous, and sometimes deficient, skin sallow and doughy, temperature 101½, slight cough, and occasional night sweats, loss of flesh, pulse little affected except when diarrhea was present for a few days, it would then present the usual feebleness and rapidity. I found the urine contained sugar; specific gravity, 1.032. I gave the saturated tinct. of rhus aromatica, in ½ tea-spoonful doses every 4 hours, until she was under the influence of the remedy, with a diminution of urine from the first day. The dose was lessened and the interval lengthened from week to week, and finally, in 3 months, the medicine was discontinued. In the meantime, strict dieting laws were observed, carefully avoiding such diet as favored the sugar forming process in the body. She being of a scrofulous diathesis (tending to scrofula), I gave cod liver oil with hypophosphite for some time after discontinuing the rhus aromatica. He continues by saying:

"I have had the same results with two cases of diabetes insipidus under the same treatment; and I am at present treating another case of diabetes mellitus, a very interesting case, which I will report in a future article."

II. *Incontinence.*—In incontinence of urine, whether from atony (weakness) of the muscular fiber, or irritation of the nervous fiber, which prevents normal (usual, healthy) distention of the bladder, it is applicable.

III. *Dribbling.*—I have relieved several cases in which the person was unable to prevent a constant dribbling of urine; also, those cases in which the patient has no control over the urine whatever, will be promptly met by the action of the rhus aromatica. DOSE—For adults in these cases of dribbling, or incontinence, he gave 10 drop doses only, 3 times daily. For children, strong tinct. rhus aromatica, ½ oz.; glycerine, 1½ ozs. DOSE—One-half tea-spoonful 3 times a day; and when allowable, drop the morning dose, then the noon, and when cured, stop all. But in all such cases have the child urinate, at once, when nature calls for it, even in the night, and especially before retiring in all cases.

IV. *For Summer Complaint of Children.*—Dr. McClanahan, above named, reports the case of a little boy, with chronic diarrhea and dysentery, stools pale and thin, running from him like water; no particular pain, or fever. Pale and emaciated; limbs, trembling, scarcely able to stand alone; skin cool and bowels flabby. Gave tinct. rhus aromatica, ½ oz. DOSE—Only 3 drops, in a little water, after each passage; with proper diet and care he recovered rapidly.

V. A laborer, with chronic dysentery for two months, he gave: Tinct. rhus aromatica in doses of 10 drops, together with a boiled milk diet; made a complete recovery. He gives an account of cases where almost wholly the passages were blood, equally successful in treatment; increasing to 15 drop doses, after each stool, with the boiled milk diet. And also many other cases of incontinence of urine, but these will suffice on this class of diseases. Then he comes to:

VI. *Uterine Hemorrhages, Menorrhagia (profuse flowing) Leucorrhea, etc.*
—He first cautions against the frauds of some persons putting out bad articles, etc. But he thinks, and so does the author, that Park, Davis & Co., of Detroit, will furnish a genuine article of fluid extracts of the rhus aromatica, and if I failed with that, I would get the crude article of them, and make the strong tincture, as Dr. McClanahan had always used, up to the time of the foregoing reports. He was then called to a bad case of uterine hemorrhage, after an abortion; at least two quarts of blood lost; first gave a stimulant, then gave doses of 10 drops of the strong tincture rhus aromatica, every 15 minutes, and

applied' to mouth of the womb, cloths wet in water with a fifth as much tinc ture of rhus, gently kneading over the uterus until it contracted, and after two hours the hemorrhage ceased, and patient comfortable. Then directed the tinc ture every hour, and left to call in 6 hours. Found her comfortable, removed the cotton without any more hemorrhage, improvemen* rapid, and recovery complete in 10 days; but there was a slight discharge during this time, for which he gave smaller doses, probably 5 or 6 drops, every 2 or 3 hours, as required.

VII. *Leucorrhea.*—He uses the same tincture when there is a relaxed con dition of the uterus, as in leucorrhea, and also hemorrhages from falls, blows, etc.

VIII. *Hemorrhage From the Kidneys.*—For blood passed in the urine, mak ing it dark, he prescribed: Tinct. rhus aromatica, ½ oz.; tinct. nux vomica, 15 drops; glycerine, 3 ozs.; mix. Dose—A tea-spoonful 3 times a day. Man able to be out in a week; good recovery.

*Remarks.*—These last clauses are condensed from the doctor's report, giv ing all that I deemed necessary to understand how, and when, and how much, to give of the remedy, not doubting that much good will arise from the further use and study of this article, of the " New Remedies." For, certainly, if it proves as successful in diabetes, which has been one of the incurables, in other hands, as it has in Dr. McClanahan's, and several other physicians whose reports were given in connection, it will be a great blessing to suffering humanity. The report was made in Vol. I, Parke, Davis & Co.'s " Newer Materia Medica," Detroit, Mich.

**TOBACCO CHEWERS' WEAK STOMACH—Antidote for— Which Also Weans One From its Use.**—A writer to the " Household" of the *Blade*, in answer to an inquirer for such an antidote, says: " I herewith send you my prescription, which has never failed yet. Take the inner bark of the root of poplar or whitewood, and when your friend wants a chew of tobacco let him take a chew of this bark. If he will follow this for 3 weeks, I will guarantee he will not be troubled with a weak stomach or have any more desire for the filthy weed."

*Remarks.*—This being just the thing desired by many, let it have a fair trial, twice as long as the writer claims to be necessary, rather than fail. Not being a " chewer," I have not tested it.

**EMETIC—The Best in Use.**—Lobelia and boneset (*eupatorium per foliatum,* also called thoroughwort). each ½ oz.; infused or steeped in water, 1 pt. Dose—Give one table-spoonful every 10 minutes until thorough *emesis* (vomiting) has taken place.

*Remarks.*—This is the best emetic in use, from the fact that it injures none, and will not continue its action any longer than you give it. It is necessary, therefore, to continue to give it until the contents of the stomach are thoroughly evacuated. This was the great favorite of Prof. I. G. Jones, one of the early Eclectics, who claimed it the best emetic in use.

1. **IMPOTENCY—Especial Tonic for.** — Strychnine, 1 gr.; sul phate of quinine (phosphate of quinine is the best, but it is not kept by drug

gists generally), 30 grs.; tinct. of muriate of iron, ½ oz.; glycerine, 4 ozs. DIRECTIONS—Put the strychnine into a mortar and rub first, then the quinine also, and rub together a little, then put in the tincture of iron, and rub till all are dissolved, then rub in the glycerine, and bottle for use. DOSE—Take ⅙ tea-spoonful in a little water, 4 times daily, just before each meal and at bed-time. Shake well before taking.

*Remarks.*—When the amount here given has been taken twice, take no more for two weeks, after which, should there be still further need for the tonic, do the same again as long as needed, whether it be a year, or more. It is much to be regretted that young persons, of both sexes, very frequently are led into evil habits by seeing others do the same, and too often by persuasion and instruction, which undermines their strength and vitality; and if long fol-lowed, destroys all happiness by what is called "loss of manhood"—the destruc-tion of the powers of nature, created for the wise purpose of continuing the existence of the human race; it is also to be regretted that men, not to say women, even after marriage, are so excessive in their indulgences, that they also become equally prostrated. And, allow me to say, that while these evil prac-tices are continued there need be *no* expectations of cure. Stop them, and take the medicines necessary as long as needed, and a cure may be expected, with this drawback, however,—I care not what the evil habit may be, nor what the disease may be, if it is very long continued the same degree of health will never afterwards be obtained as that before indulgence or the disease—it is not in the nature of the human system, any more than it is for a tree to heal without leaving a scar or dead spot, although the bark may heal over after a piece has been knocked off, but there will be found always the dead spot underneath it; and although the spot may not be easily found by the physician when called to these old cases, the persons themselves will generally realize it as long as they live. Then, let every family of children be instructed against these evil habits, and every married person avoid all excesses.

The tonic effects may be increased by taking the elixir of calisaya and iron after meals. This is kept by most druggists, and the directions as to dose, etc., found upon the bottle. Calisaya means Peruvian bark. The above treatment, with an occasional change to some of the following tonics, will be found valuable in spermatorrhea (loss of semen), as well as for all purposes of debility or disease needing a tonic. (See also, Female Debility, Tonics for, etc.)

**2. Tonic or Stimulant for Sexual Debility.**—Tincture of iodine, 80 drops; simple syrup, 4 ozs. DOSE—Take 1 tea-spoonful 4 times daily, one being at bed-time.

*Remarks.*—Even in these small doses, Prof. Scudder says, it stimulates and increases the power of the sexual organs

**3. Tonic Tincture, etc., for Sexual Debility.**—Geo. W. Hom-sher, M. D., of Fairfield, Ind., in answering several inquiries made through the *Brief,* gives the following plan, as being very satisfactory; and although I have not as yet tried this, I know it will be found valuable·

" Ferro-cyanuret of potash, ½ oz.; ay bul (boiling water) 3 ozs , dissolve, then add glycerine, 1½ ozs.; specific tinct. (fl. ex., I think, will do as well when the specific tinct. is not kept by druggists) of staphisagria, 1 dr.   DOSE— Take 1 tea-spoonful 3 times daily, and at bed-time have the patient take a sponge bath over the spine and hips, and give, on retiring, 10 grs. lupulin (I think B. Keith & Co., of New York city, prepare the best lupulin in use) in a little cold water.   Not only," he continues, "will this treatment relieve the dis- charge of semen, but will cure 9 cases out of ten of sexual debility, by prohib- iting sexual intercourse for 2 months, and giving these medicines that length of time; then suspending all drugs, with the exception of the lupulin at bed-time, and continuing the hip baths."

*Remarks.*—Should not a cure be perfected in two months, I should say, go over the same treatment again, after two weeks' discontinuance, until a cure is accomplished, avoiding absolutely all the causes which led to it in the first place.   In these cases there is always an inflammatory condition of the ureter and other parts of the organs of generation; hence I have found that a 10 to 15 drop dose of the fluid extract of gelsemium, in connection with the other treat- ment, at or near bed-time, will greatly aid in overcoming this inflammatory condition.

**4. Tonic Tincture for Impotency, Spermatorrhea, etc.**— Dr. R. M. Griswold, of North Manchester, Ct., reports through the *Brief*, that he has made several quick cures of the above diseases with the following: Tincts. of nux vomica and cantharides, each 1 dr.; tinct. ferri-mur (muriated tinct. of iron), 3 drs.; fl. ex. ergot, 1 oz.; acidi phos. dil. (dilute phoshoric acid), 3 drs.; mix.   [The author would say, double the amount, as it will be needed.] DOSE—Thirty drops (½ tea-spoonful) in a wine-glass of water, 3 times daily.

"Within the last six months," the doctor says, "I have treated several cases of the above diseases with uniform success, a radical cure being effected in each case.   Two cases occurred in young men of about 20 years of age, resulting from masturbation; one case, following gonorrhea; the fourth case, a married man, was the result of excessive indulgence; and three other cases, where the search for the direct cause was unsuccessful, yet the same treatment was successful."

*Remarks.*—He required abstinence from all stimulants (liquors) and condi- ments (high-seasoned food), using light but nourishing food, especially milk, eggs, fish; sleeping on a hard bed, and in a cold, well-ventilated room; total avoidance of all sexual excitement and all undue exertion of strength.   By ob- serving the foregoing, the success was satisfactory.

The only apology I have to offer for the introduction of this class of reme- dies, for the above diseases, is a positive knowledge that such conditions are found throughout the country—I mean the whole United States and Domin- ion of Canada, and, I have not a doubt, of all other countries—and also a knowledge that those who have need of such remedies have so great a delicacy in going to home physicians, they either put off treatment too long, or are so egregiously humbugged by advertising quacks that I have felt compelled to come to their relief, as well as those troubled only with the common, or ordinary, diseases affecting the health of the people.   Faithful attention in taking the medicines, and the avoidance of all the causes leading to these difficulties, with care also as to diet, etc., will ensure success, with but trifling expense as compared with the charges of those who can cure, at most, but few of the cases they succeed in obtaining through their advertisements. I will close this subject with the following:

5. **Tonic Pill for Sexual Debility.**—Dr. Benj. A. Penn, of Bryantsburg, Ind., gives a valuable pill for sexual debility, in the May number of the *Brief* of 1882. "Strychnine, 3 grs.; sulphate of quinine (phosphate is best, if it can be obtained) 120 grs.; iron by hydrogen, 120 grs.; mix thoroughly and make into 240 pills. Dose—Take 1 pill every 6 hours during the day; and after the system becomes used to them take 1 every 4 hours."

*Remarks.*—The only change I would suggest in this pill is that the quinine should be doubled in amount, or one grain to each pill, as I think this would greatly increase its tonic power.

**BORAX—Its Value in Catarrh, Throat Difficulties, Inflamed Eyes, Dandruff, etc.**—I. A solution of 1 dr. to soft water, ½ pt., snuffed up into the nostrils, is valuable in catarrhal difficulties; if recent, it will effect a cure. Use 3 times daily; though I must say I think it is easier taken in powder, as a snuff, and better too, taken 5 to 10 times daily. I combine sugar, ½ dr., with powdered borax, 1 oz.; and put in a few drops of white rose perfume, as a snuff; and if the throat is sore, drop a pinch of it into the throat at each time of snuffing. It soon benefits both difficulties.

II. The same strength makes a good wash for weak inflamed eyes.

III. Use as a gargle, in recent affections of the throat.

IV. It makes a valuable wash for the head if troubled with dandruff, leaving the hair soft and glossy.

V. In nervous headaches, wash the head with it two or three times as strong, then wash out with cool, clear water, rubbing well with the towel, and take a nap, and generally all headache will subside, and the patient be much refreshed. After washing the head in this way it will be very proper to use the magic headache cure, as there directed, which see.

VI. In erysipelas, a writer in the Philadelphia *Medical Times* says, from 8 years experience, he has found a solution of borax in glycerine, 1 dr. to 1 oz., to be a remarkably effective remedy, to be locally applied on linen. In connection with this borax solution upon the inflamed part, I would give 5 to 10 drops of muriated tincture of iron, every 4 or 5 hours, internally, when a cure may be expected in 2 or 3 to 6 days. If it irritates the stomach, or causes too much flow of urine, lessen the dose, or lengthen the time between them. (See also erysipelas, where the treatment may be preferable.)

VII. As a shampoo, once or twice a week, it will be valuable for everyone; but for students, clergymen and others who have considerable mental work, it will be found especially valuable, after the labors of the day, rubbing and drying the hair and head well, before retiring. The powdered borax is readily dissolved, and a small tea-spoonful to a tumbler of water makes all ready for general purposes. If there is any inflammation of the gums, rinse them with it 3 or 4 times daily.

VIII.  For clothes washing, in Holland, Belgium and France the washer-women and washer-men (for in some of these countries the men do a good share of the washing) use a large handful of refined (powdered) borax; being a neutral salt (having no excess of acid or alkali) it does not injure the clothing at all, but softens the hardest water, or at least materially improves it for washing purposes.  Many people use ammonia for most of the purposes here named, but the borax is generally preferable.

1.  NIGHT SWEATS—Remedy for.—Dr. Charles D. Carpenter reports a case through the *Medical Brief*, of St. Louis, wherein he was attending a "medical" friend, suffering with rheumatism, which continued 7 weeks (I have heard of a case wherein the celebrated Abernethy, of England, was asked what should be taken for rheumatism, and the answer was, "Take six weeks," —in other words, there was no cure, but it would get well in that time).  In this case, after the acute stage had passed, recovery was retarded by terribly prostrating night sweats, and after trying half a dozen or more of the common remedies for them, at the suggestion of the "medical" friend, he gave 2 full doses of chloral dydrate.  When the patient was fully under the influence of the chloral the sweating ceased and returned no more, the patient making a rapid recovery.  He afterwards tested it in a number of obstinate cases of night sweats, and with uniform success.  Dose—A full dose may be put down as 15 grs. for a large man; 8 to 10 grs. for a large woman; repeating or giving the second 2 hours after, dissolved in water, say a wine-glassful or $\frac{1}{4}$ of a common tumblerful.  I should not give beyond the 2 doses.  It has been given in much larger doses, but it is not best to run any risk, unless absolutely necessary in great and long-continued pain or nervousness arising from delirium tremens, etc.

*Remarks.*—If it is good for night sweats arising from rheumatism, it is good for them arising from consumption, or any other prostrating disease. Further, it is very probable that one of Dr. Carpenter's obstinate cases above mentioned was a consumptive; although he does not say what they were, it is enough to know it is good for this symptom.  It matters not, then, what the disease is in which they are present.

2.  Night Sweats, Consumption, Spitting Blood and Diabetes, Valuable Remedy for.—Bugle weed (*Lycopus Virginicus*), also known as Paul's betonia and water hoarhound; the tincture or fluid extract has been found valuable remedy in all the diseased conditions above named.  Prof. Scudder uses it in all chronic diseases when the pulse is too frequent and the debility considerable, for, as it lessens the pulse—which it does—so also it increases it in strength, acting, as he believes, through the sympathetic system of nerves, improving the circulation, the appetite, blood-making, nutrition, and the secretions. In consumption, he says: " We find it relieving the cough, checking the night sweats and the diarrhea, lessening the frequency of the pulse, improving the apppetite and giving better digestion.  It has been used more in hemoptysis (spitting of blood) than in any other disease, its action being slow but certain." —*Scudder's Specefic Medication.*

Prof. I. J. M. Goss, of Marietta, Ga., author of " Materia-Medica and Therapeutics," in his " New Medicines," says, among other things, that he has had it—the *lycopus*—to arrest hemoptysis (spitting blood) in a few hours, when it was profuse and alarming. It seems to control the vascular excitement (excitement of circulation) in a manner peculiar to itself.

This, however, I do not look upon as at all singular — all remedies have their own peculiar action, and none of us can tell why, and in but few circumstances can we tell how; but it is enough for it to be known, they do it.

Prof. Goss further says, that it is also a valuable remedy in the treatment of diabetes *insipidus* (when the urine is tasteless) and *sacharina* (the urine containing sugar), and in chronic coughs, with profuse expectoration.

The dose of the infusion is 1 to 2 ozs. (2 to 4 table-spoonfuls), and the dose of the fl. ext. is 1 to 2 drs. (tea-spoonful).

*Where It Grows, When to be Gathered, etc.*—It grows over large portions of the United States. Has a small purplish flower through July and August, when it should be gathered, dried in the shade and carefully kept in paper sacks, for each year's use, as age injures it. It yields its strength to boiling water, 1 oz. to the pint of river or rain water—giving 1 to 2 ozs., which would be 2 to 4 table-spoonfuls, as a dose. None of these writers say how often it should be given, hence I would say, 4 to 6 times within the day and evening, as found to agree with the stomach and the action desired. It is not poisonous nor dangerous. See "Diabetes" for diet, etc., in that disease.

Prof. King, of Cincinnati, in his "American Dispensatory," in his explanation of the uses of the bugle weed (*lycopus*), after corroborating its uses in the diseases above named, adds: "It acts somewhat like digitalis, in reducing the velocity of the pulse, but it is devoid of the dangerous effects resulting from the use of that drug, and hence has proved useful in some heart affections. It is decidedly beneficial in the treatment of diabetes, having cured when all other means were useless; and has been of service in chronic diarrhea and dysentery, inflammatory diseases of drunkards, diseases of the heart, and intermittents (agues)."

Dose of the powder, from 1 to 2 drs. (1 to 2 small tea-spoonfuls); of the infusion, 2 to 4 fl. ozs. (from 4 to 8 table-spoonfuls), and of the concentrated tinct. of the recent plant (tinct. made with 8 ozs. of the bruised plant to 1 pt. of diluted alcohol), from 5 to 60 minims (drops).

Thus it is seen, the bugle weed is a very valuable remedy. Especially is it worthy of a fair trial in the coughs and prostrating night sweats of consumption, as well as in all the other diseases mentioned.

**PILES (Hemorrhoids) — Bleeding or Only Tumors, Some Remarkable Remedies for.**—Stephen Adams, M. D., of West Newfield, Me., in answer to a call in the *Medical Brief*, of St. Louis, Mo., for hemorrhoids (piles), says: "I use a remedy which I have used a long time, and which has cured every case where it has been used. Mix citrine ointment and rosinous ointment (both kept by druggists), about equal parts; put a few grs. on a piece of paper, rub on and about the anus (rectum) 3 or 4 times a week, at night. It will stop the hemorrhage (bleeding), and soon discus (drive away or scatter) the tumor. You need no knife or caustic. Should the bowels incline to constipation, use, 2 or 3 times a week, ⅓ gr. solid ex. of belladonna, and some gentle laxative (as cream of tartar, sulphur, magnesia, etc., or the pile laxative below), or, if possible, a better plan is to keep the bowels regular by proper diet and exercise."

*Remarks.*—This would be considered a pretty good thing, without other testimony or corroboration; but in accordance with my general custom, although I have not had a bad case on which to try it, yet as others have, and are reported through the *Brief* above named, I will quote from one more of them. G. A. Graham, M. D., of White Hall, N. C., June 18, 1880, page 318 of that year, says: "Being a sufferer from hemorrhoids myself, I was especially interested in the many articles which appeared in the *Brief*, for the cure of this trouble without the knife. I concluded to try citrine and rosinous ointment, recommended by Dr. Stephen Adams; I only used it twice last November, and have not suffered once since. Four weeks since, an old man came to me for treatment, who had piles for forty years, in which time he tried any number of doctors and remedies, without any marked benefit. I did not care to treat his case with ointment alone, but, as he refused any more radical procedure (as the knife or ligature), I gave him, as an experiment, a little of Adams' ointment; he reports a wonderful relief. The tumor, which was two inches in length, and nearly as hard as a bone, almost entirely disappeared, causing no pain, no hemorrhage (bleeding), and leaving him like a new man. I write this hoping that others may be induced to try this remedy and report."

**2. Piles, Laxative for.**—The inquiry for the best medical treatment for the cure of hemorrhoids, or piles, which brought out the above and many others also, was made by Dr. Hendien, of Nicholasville, Ky., among which was the following, by Clarence H. Clark, M. D., of Haverhill, N. H. I give it, because I think it valuable as a laxative in these cases, rather than with an expectation of its making an absolute cure, although Dr. Clark says of it: "What I think to be the best remedy is the following recipe, which I have thoroughly tested. Jalap, confection of senna, bitartrate of potassa (cream of tartar) and sulphur, each 3 drs.; nitrate of potassa (purified saltpetre) 20 grs. (all in powder); syrup of tolu, sufficient to make a soft mass. DOSE—A pill the size of an ordinary bean or small chestnut, 3 times a day, before meals; or sufficient amount to produce a gentle movement of the bowels; continue till the bowels become regular and natural."

*Remarks.*—This will, however, be found quite efficient as a laxative; and also an alterative of considerable value. The fig remedy below is an excellent laxative also, for piles, and I think more curative in itself. (See "Bleeding Piles, Laxative for, etc.")

**3. Piles, Simple Remedy for Tumors in.**—E Parsons, M. D., of Savannah, Ga., gave the following. He says: "For many years I was very much troubled with piles, the tumors often being as large as a walnut and very painful. I tried many remedies with only temporary benefit; three years ago I prepared the following: Glycerine, 1 oz.; carbolic acid dissolved in the least water that will dissolve it, 20 drops; mix. At night, on going to bed, I washed the parts in cold water, and with my fingers I annointed the parts. In one week's time, six applications cured me, and I have had no return since of this very troublesome disease. I have recommended it to quite a number of my friends, who tell me it has cured them."

4. **Piles, Cured by a Simple Internal Remedy.**—Another writer claims to have cured piles of long standing by taking a tea-spoonful of glycerine, twice daily, only.

5. **Bleeding Piles, Valuable Laxative and Cure for.**—A nephew of mine, who had been troubled considerably with piles, gave me the following recipe which had done him much good. He said it was "going the rounds of the newspapers," as we often hear remarked. It was as follows: "Take nice soft figs, 1 lb.; best powdered senna, 2 ozs.; manna and fennel seed, each 1 oz. DIRECTIONS—Trim off the stems, flower end and other hard and dry spots, if any, from the figs; then chop them in a chopping-bowl, to a salvy consistency, and mix in the other ingredients with the hand, using a little molasses, if necessary, to work all in nicely and evenly. Then put into a tin box, and put a moistened cloth over the top, and cover tightly, for use. And if no fennel seed are to be had, anise seed or caraway seed may be used in their place. The seed, whichever may be used, are a carminative, to prevent griping from the action of the senna; whichever is preferred, as to taste, may be used. DOSE—Take a piece the size of a common hickory nut, at bed-time, to move the bowels next day; and continue to take such a sized piece every night, or every other night, as will keep the bowels easy, or soluble, until cured. If there is griping to any extent, use half as much more of whichever seed was used. Additional flavor might be used, if desired, a little oil of peppermint or wintergreen, as both are highly carminative."

*Remarks.*—This was claimed to have been very effectual in bleeding piles, as well as where only tumors were present.

6. **Piles, Simple Laxative for.**—Confection of senna, 2 ozs.; cream of tartar and sulphur, each 1 oz.; syrup of ginger, enough to make a thick paste; mix well. DOSE—Take a piece the size of a medium sized nutmeg, every bed-time, or sufficiently often to keep the bowels lax or loose. That is, in piles, the bowels must be kept easy, as the soreness of the parts do not admit of strain without causing great suffering to the patient. With this laxative, or the one before it, the tendency to costiveness can easily be avoided. Dr. Warren, in his "Household Physician," says this is one of the very best laxatives for piles.

7. **Piles, Lead Ointment for.**—Rub well together, lard, 2 drs.; sulphur, 1 dr. Then rub it between two plates of lead, or large flat pieces of lead, until the whole is well blackened. Dr. Warren says: "It is not only soothing but curative, both in bleeding and blind piles (where no tumors come down). The food should be of a laxative nature—corn bread, rye mush, bread of unbolted flour (Graham), mealy potatoes, ripe fruit, pudding and milk, buckwheat cakes, broths, and a little tender meat once a day."

*Remarks.*—When the digestion and circulation are good, there never are any piles. So keep the digestion and circulation good and have no piles, is the author's advice.  But as many persons will still have them, I will give a recipe for a suppository for intruducing into the rectum, which W. M. Bemus, of Jamestown, N. Y., tells us through the *Brief*, in answer to an inquiry, he has for some time used with marked success, and as it is also good for "enlarged prostrate," will be found doubly valuable.  It is as follows:

**8. Piles and Enlarged Prostate, Suppository for.—I.** *For the Piles.*—Iodoform, 30 grs.; solid ext. of hyoscyamus, 18 grs.; cocoa butter, or spermaceti, sufficient to make into suppositories—6 in number; and intro- duce one into the rectum night and morning.

II.  *For the Enlarged Prostate.* — This suppository, with the addition of solid ext. of belladonna, in the proportion of one-half gr. to each suppository, is a very satisfactory mode of treatment for enlarged prostrate.

*Remarks.*—Although the description is sufficient for physicians, for whom, as before remarked, the *Brief* is published, to understand the treatment of enlarged prostate, it is not so for the people for whom, especially, this work is published; therefore, the author will explain, by saying, the "prostate" is a gland in the male, lying immediately in front of and below the neck of the bladder, across, as it were, and upon the ureter just at the entrance into the bladder; hence its enlargement causes a pressure upon the urethra or water pas- sage from the bladder, making it difficult to pass the urine, and sometimes pre- venting it wholly, except by passing a catheter to evacuate the contents of the bladder.  Then, of course, it lies so near the rectum, into which the suppository is to be introduced for enlarged prostrate, the same as it would be for piles; and I have not a doubt that it will be found very satisfactory for this difficulty. Knowing the importance of understanding, as perfectly as possible, anything I desire to do myself, I try, at least, to make everything as plain as possible for the people, for whom I have given a life time of service, and, I trust, have done and may continue, through my books, to do a good many years after my tongue and pen have ceased their labors.  This, to me, is the grandest thought of my life—I have done what I could—to benefit mankind.

**9.  Piles, Common or Bleeding—Bleeding of the Nose, Womb, Wounds, etc, Remedy for.**—Samuel Wimpelberg, M. D., of Pough- keepsie, N. Y., writing to the *Medical Bulletin* on the subject of piles (of course called hemorrhoids by the doctors), says: " There are numerous remedies recom- mended for the cure of hemorrhoids, and I have tried many; but I can safely say that not one in the whole Pharmacopœia (whole range of medical books) has given me results half as favorable as the persulphate of iron.  [Monsel's salts is the common name, and I will use it in this connection.]

"In cases known ordinarily as bleeding piles it acts promptly and posi- tively, thus giving the best results.  In such cases the dose should be Monsel's salts, 1½ grs., *ter in die* (3 times daily), internally, and the following ointment, applied locally: Simple ointment, 1 oz.; Monsel's salts, 12 grs.; mix and apply night and morning.  I have known hemorrhoidal tumors, the result of preg- nancy, to disappear entirely in less than a week on the application of the inter- nal use of Monsel's salts, as directed above.

"Piles, the result of violent efforts at stool (to force a passage), disappear promptly by combining the internal use of the powder and the local use of the ointment. In this connection I would also mention that in *proctocele* (a species of piles in which the mucous membrane of the rectum, or intestine, comes down with every passage), a most satisfactory result can be obtained from the internal use of the per sulph of iron (Monsel's salt), in doses of 2 grs. 3 times daily, besides the local application of the ointment."

**10. Hemorrhage of the Lungs, Nose, Womb, etc.**—The Monsel's salts being so prompt and positive in closing piles, the author cannot see why it would not be equally prompt in bleeding from the organs above named; still, I know that the fluid extract of ergot and tannic acid combined, say, fl. ex. of ergot, 1 oz.; tannic acid, 180 grs.; mix. Dose—Take ½ tea-spoonful every 2 hours, if the hemorrhage is moderate, or if more free, repeat once or twice only, 1 hour apart, then once in 3 or 4 hours, according to the severity of the case. I have used this latter in hemorrhage from the womb, with success, and hence know its value for all these purposes, using friction over the womb, occasionally, until it contracts, and thus ends the hemorrhage.

*Remarks.*—In speaking of the uses of Monsel's salts, King, in his "Dispensatory," says: "The action of this salt on blood and albumen (albumen forms a part of the blood) is powerful; with the former it produces a voluminous clot, absolutely insoluble, which continues to enlarge for several hours after its application, and becomes quite hard and firm. Dr. H. H. Tolland, of San Francisco, Cal., who has successfully used this salt says: ' If applied to a superficial (surface) wound, as soon as made not a drop of blood escapes, and no pain results from the application. It acts by producing instantaneous coagulation (thickening) of the blood, and will be found invaluable in hemorrhages from the mouth, nose and throat, when it is impossible to ligate (tie) the vessel, and may be equally efficacious in alarming uterine (womb) hemorrhages, either active or passive. [That is profuse or slight hemorrhages from the womb.] In solution, it could be readily applied; it is very deliquescent (dissolves quickly in the air), and dissolves speedily in water.' "

*Remarks.*—Pill form is the easiest way to take this Monsel's salt, or per-sulphate of iron, as it has an unpleasant, astringent taste in solution; still the solution is the quickest to act, in case of profuse or active hemorrhages. In wounds or ulcerative sores the powder may be sprinkled into them, or in cuts with much hemorrhage. It is the same powder that Dr. T. B. King, of Toledo, O., used in curing an ulcerated erysipelatious sore leg, on a woman in Detroit, Mich., after the doctors said nothing could help her. As in that item remarked, he applies it, and so have I, to the mouth of the womb, when ulcerated, with great success. Mind, however, it is iron, and stains clothing; so protect them.

**ABSCESS.**—An abscess is the collection of pus or matter in the substance of some part of the body. When the matter is poured out from some part, the process is said to be suppuration; when it collects in a tissue, it is an abscess. When the matter collecting in some organ, comes toward the surface, and a place in the centre rises above the surrounding skin, and turns white, the abscess is said to point. Some abscesses point and break in a week; others of a more chronic character, will linger on for months.

TREATMENT.—When the abscess is completely formed, and there is no longer any doubt of the presence of matter, it should be opened at once. To let out the confined pus alleviates the pain and lessens the inflammation. If the matter lie close to the bone, the opening should be made without delay. The opening should be large enough to let the matter out freely. It is a rule to keep the incision open till the cavity of the abscess is so far filled up that another collection of pus is not likely to occur.

If the matter do not readily get to the surface through the opening, it may burrow itself in the flesh, in a long narrow channel called a sinus. To relieve this the opening must be extended in such a way as to give vent to the new collection.

An abscess is sometimes indisposed to heal at the bottom, and pus continues to be formed a long time, and is discharged through an opening smaller than the sack which contains it. This is a fistula; and the opening to it should be enlarged so as to let out the matter more freely. A little soft lint may then be gently pressed into the wound to prevent its healing before the cavity below.

An abscess from acute inflammation requires to be poulticed for a time after it has been opened. When the swelling and inflammation are gone, the poultices are to be laid aside, and a bandage put on. When the inflammation is gone, let the diet be improved; and if the discharge of matter be large, give wine and tonics.

**ATROPHY, OR SHRINKING OF THE HEART.**—The heart, like any other organ, is liable to defective nutrition, and in consequence of it, may become small; it shrinks in some cases to the size of an infant's heart.

The complaint is generally caused by whatever reduces the general flesh, as in consumption, diabetes, chronic dysentery, cancer, and excessive loss of blood.

It can hardly be called a disease. Persons who have it are less subject to inflammatory diseases than others, though they faint from slight causes, and have nervous affections.

TREATMENT.—If its causes can be discovered, treat them; if not, the treatment should be the same as for dilatation.

**DELIRIUM TREMENS.**—This is often mistaken for brain fever; but it is quite a different disease. It is not the result of inflammation of the brain, but of irritation. It is important to distinguish it from inflammation. because the remedies which are employed for that would be injurious if used for this.

TREATMENT.—Opium and its preparations are the sovereign remedies. Give ⅓ of a grain of morphia; if this does not quiet the patient, give 30 drops of laudanum every two hours, till sleep is produced. Sleep will cure him, and nothing else will. A draught or two of his accustomed drink, brandy, gin, or whatever it may be, will also generally dispose him to sleep.

Recently, a very effectual remedy has been found in the use of tepid baths, prolonged from four to ten hours, in connection with cold applications to the head. In connection with this, small doses of opium are required; but the treatment may yet prove to be very valuable by enabling us to dispense with excessive doses of opium.

**FAINTING.**—TREATMENT.—Lay the patient upon the back, with the head low; let fresh air into the room instantly, and apply gentle friction. Sprinkle a little cold water upon the face, and hold spirits of camphor, ether, hartshorn, or vinegar to the nose,—rubbing a little of the spirits of camphor upon the forehead, and about the nostrils. As soon as the patient can swallow, give a tea-spoonful of compound spirits of lavender, with 10 drops of water of ammonia in it.

Persons subject to fainting should not go into crowded assemblies where the air is bad; neither should they wear tight dresses, or allow themselves to get excited. Cold bathing, a well regulated diet, and vegetable tonics, will do much to break up the habit.

*Remarks.*—Whatever causes debility, particularly of the nervous system, will predispose to fainting. Persons much weakened by disease, faint easily— especially when they attempt to stand still. When on their feet, such persons should keep moving. Fainting is sometimes induced by sudden surprises and emotions, by violent pains, by the sight of human blood, and by irritation of the coats of the stomach by indigestible food.

**GALL STONES.**—TREATMENT.—To reduce the spasm, give Dover's powder in full doses, or chlorodine. Also apply mustard over the right hypochondrium and stomach, and follow it with hot fomentations with hops, or use wet cups.

If the stomach is irritable, give the neutralizing mixture until it moves the bowels. A warm infusion of thoroughwort, given to the extent of producing vomiting, will sometimes do well, and lobelia enough with it to relax the duct may be useful.

To relieve the acidity on which the formation of these stones so often depends, the following neutralizing preparation may be given for a long time, the diet, in the meantime, being well regulated: Rhubarb, pulverized, ½ oz.; spearmint herb., pulv., ½ oz.; pulv. cascarilla, ½ oz.; pulv. bicarbonate of potassa, ½ oz.; pulv. wild cherry bark, ½ oz. Mix. and pour on one quart of hot water. Let this stand till cold, and add ½ pint of brandy. DOSE— Half a wine-glassful. The sponge bath, with saleratus and water, should be taken daily, followed by brisk rubbing; and free exercise in the open air should on no account be omitted.

**PLEURISY.**—TREATMENT.—As a general thing I am opposed to bleeding, and am even reluctant to recommend it in pleurisy. Yet if there is a human ailment which will justify it, pleurisy is that one.

Sweating should be encouraged immediately. The compound tincture of Virginia snake root, given every half hour, in tea-spoonful doses, will generally produce a free perspiration, and give immediate relief. It may be given in infusion of catnip, balm, or pleurisy root. At the same time, the affected side should be fomented with hops, tansy, wormwood, etc., applied very hot.

If this does not afford relief, or only partial relief, give an emetic of the compound powder of lobelia, and follow it with the compound powder of jalap, or the compound powder of leptandrin, or prescription as physic: Pulverized gamboge, 12 grs.; pulverized scammony, 12 grs.; elaterium, 2 grs.; croton oil, 8 drops; ex. of stramonium, 3 grs. Mix. Make 12 pills. One pill is a dose, repeated every hour until it operates. At the same time keeping up the perspiration, with full doses of tincture of veratrum.

To produce sleep and perspiration at the same time, Dover's powder may be given in 6 grain doses.

For the fever, nothing is equal to the tincture of veratrum viride.

The diet must be of the very lightest kind.

When absorption of the fluid does not take place, a puncture is sometimes made through the walls of the chest, and the water drawn off. This operation is called paracentesis thoracis, and is generally, in uncomplicated cases, entirely successful. When this is not done, let the affected side be painted daily with tincture of iodine, keeping up considerable soreness, and giving iodide of potassium at the same time.

Fluid ex. of sarsaparilla, 4 ozs.; fluid ex. of pipsissewa, 1 oz.; water, 1 qt.; iodide of potassium 2 ozs. Mix. Take a table-spoonful 3 times a day.

**RICKETS.**—This is also a disease of scrofulous children. By some bad process of nutrition in such children, there does not enough phosphate of lime enter into the bones to harden them, and the weight of the body, or the pulling of the muscles, or the pressure of the clothing, bends and distorts them in all manner of ways. The heads of the thigh bones are pushed nearer together making the lower belly narrower, the backbone is so curved as to lessen the height; the shoulder blades stand up like wings when flying is contemplated; and the shoulders are so lifted up that the head seems only a little higher than the elevations on each side.

TREATMENT.—A good, generous, wholesome diet, properly regulated; out door exercise; the tepid or cold salt water sponge bath, with friction, and but little medicine. The hypophosphite of lime, in 2 gr. doses, given in a little sweetened water, 3 times a day, or the syrup of the hypophosphites, in ½ tea-spoonful doses, 3 times a day, may be given with advantage.

**SHINGLES.**—TREATMENT.—Light diet and gentle laxatives. If the patient be advanced in life, and feeble, the following tonic will be desirable:

1. Bicarbonate of soda, ½ oz.; compound infusion of gentian, 4 ozs.; tincture of colombo, 1 oz.; syrup of orange peel, ½ oz. Mix. Take a table-spoonful 3 times a day.

For external application·

2. White Vitriol, 1 dr.; rose water, 3 ozs. Mix. Apply outwardly.

Or the following ointments:

3. Sulphuret of lime, 1 dr.; camphor, in powder, 15 grs.; lard, 1 oz. Make an ointment.

4. Elder-flower ointment, 1 oz.; oxide of zinc, 1 dr. Make an ointment.

## SPASM OR CRAMPS IN THE STOMACH.—TREATMENT.

The following strong purgative injection will often bring immediate relief:

1. Castor oil, 2 ozs.; tinct. of prickly ash bark, ½ oz.; comp. tinct. of Virginia snake root, 2 drs.; infusion of boneset and senna, equal parts, ½ pt. Mix.

2. Sweet tinct. of rhubarb, 4 ozs.; bicarbonate of soda, 2 drs. Mix. From a tea-spoonful to a table-spoonful, as occasion may require. This, with a few drops of tincture of cayenne mixed with it, will often bring speedy relief. So will a mustard poultice laid upon the stomach. The mustard poultice is a remedy of great excellence in many cases. It deserves to be called the poor man's friend.

*Remarks.*—Though generally of shorter duration, this is more violent than heartburn. It is attended by a sense of fullness, by anxiety, and by great restlessness. In females hysterical symptoms are often coupled with it. Great quantities of air or a gas are generally expelled, and the pain shoots through to the back and shoulders.

## TYPHOID PNEUMONIA. — TREATMENT.

This should be like the treatment of pneumonia and typhoid fever united. Great care must be taken not to use reducing remedies. While active purging must not be used, yet if there are symptoms of an inactive state of the bowels, the following may be employed:

1. Leptandrin, 1 dr.; podophyllin, 1 scruple; scutillarine, 2 drs.; pulv. cayenne, 1 scruple; pulv. loaf sugar, 4 ozs. Rub together for some time in a mortar. DOSE—For an adult, $\frac{1}{8}$ of the above.

2. Leptandrin, 30 grs.; podophyllin, 10 grs.; pulv. cayenne, 10 grs.; ext. nux vomica, 6 grs.; quinine, 12 grs. Mix. Make 24 pills. One, two, or three times a day.

When there are symptoms of great depression, use the following tonics:

3. Podophyllin, 4 grs.; leptandrin, 8 grs.; quinine, 8 grs.; ext. nux vomica, 2 grs. Mix. Make 16 pills. One, two, or three pills, at bed-time.

4. Pulverized Peruvian bark, 1 oz.; pulv. rhubarb, ½ dr.; pulv. muriate of ammonia, 1 dr. Mix. Divide into eight powders. Take 1 three times a day.

5. Aromatic syrup of rhubarb, 1 oz.; tinct. of colombo, 1 oz. Mix. DOSE—Two tea-spoonfuls 3 times a day. Taking care to keep the cough loose by flaxseed, slippery elm, and marshmallow tea, and by some external irritant.

## CHILDREN, MANAGEMENT OF.—1. Diet.

Between the period of weaning and the seventh year the diet should consist very much of farinaceous food, and milk; with a moderate allowance of animal food once or twice a week.

2. **Bowels.**—To keep the bowels of children in a healthy and regular state, is a matter of the utmost consequence. They are too apt to neglect the calls of nature, not being aware of the importance of regularity in this respect.

**3. Sleep.**—Children generally take a great deal of rough and boisterous bodily exercise; and during their education, their minds too are pretty much employed; all which occasions considerable exhaustion, so that it seems quite proper to allow them a due share of sleep, from eight to nine or ten hours at least. But it should be at sleeping time; and they should not be allowed to doze and saunter during their waking hours.

**4. Clothing.**—Children should have their dress accommodated to the season; and a due degree of warmth should be kept up. It is wrong to expose them to cold in order to harden them; but a proper degree of exercise in the cold air should be taken. The great evils to be avoided are, cold accompanied with moisture, and any check to perspiration; which boys too often sustain, by throwing themselves down on the moist ground, when heated by their games. Flannel next the skin need not be ordered for healthy children; but where there is much tendency to catch cold, or to have loose bowels, or continual paleness of the skin, and weakness of the system, it will be prudent to make children wear flannel. Much care should be taken to have the feet always warm and dry; and to make them change their shoes as well as their clothes, whenever they get wet.

**5. Cleanliness.**—Children should very early be taught the necessity and importance of cleanliness. They should be made to keep their hair, their teeth, and nails in good order, as it not only promotes their own health and comfort, but renders them agreeable to all around them. It is of the utmost consequence to keep the skin very clean, as this tends to prevent many of the cutaneous diseases which are so common with children, but which are so disgusting. Washing with cold water about the chest will lessen the susceptibility to cold; and about the feet, will strengthen them, and render them less liable to chilblains. Sea-bathing and swimming in safe places, are excellent both for health and cleanliness. Cleanliness is not without a degree of moral influence, and has been very properly styled one of the minor virtues.

**6. Exercise.**—Children when in tolerable health, and not of an indolent disposition, seldom require to be urged to take exercise; they are rather inclined to take it too much, and too violently, and need a little regulation and superintendance in this respect. The practice of gymnastics or dancing is a good exercise; and girls should use the skipping ropes. When out of doors, children should be allowed to choose their own amusements, and interfered with only when they are in danger of doing anything unbecoming, or hurtful to themselves or their companions. Even girls should have ample scope in their playtime, and their own sense of propriety, will soon enough correct any tendency to improper romping; their health will be promoted, and their figure expand; and it is better to posses a sound constitution and an active frame, than to be celebrated for proficiency in drawing or music, before the age of twelve or thirteen.

**Moral Treatment.**—We charge upon nature many of the bad passions which we ourselves implant in children. The moral treatment of children is generally bad. We are apt to begin by either making them our masters or our slaves. Sometimes we do both,—allowing them to govern us for a time, and

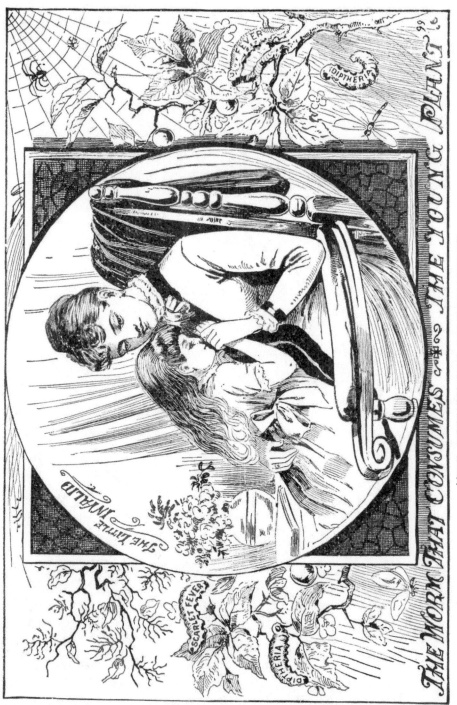

THE AFFLICTIONS OF CHILDHOOD.

then, getting into a passion, or a mood for playing the tyrant, we turn upon, and govern them as if we were autocrats. We submit to their whims until we grow irritable, and then, by way of retaliation, we compel them to submit to ours. This is all wrong. Children should be *governed always*, but with an even, a gentle, and a loving hand. They should early be subjected to habits of self-control, and of regularity in eating, and sleeping; and should be taught absolute and continued obedience. All this can be brought about only by firmness, self-control, and great gentleness on the part of parents. If they would make a child cheerful and happy in its disposition, they must themselves be cheerful, and never let it see anger, passion, and fretfulness, marring their conduct. Nothing is more injurious to the health of a child than a peevish, complaining, and soured disposition; and these vices are seldom acquired, unless seen in the lives of parents.

**1. DISEASES OF CHILDREN — Prickly Heat, Dysentery, Diarrhea, etc.—Remedies.**—Mrs. Jay, of Fern Grove, Ill., reports through the *Blade*, that an experienced physician taught her the following, in caring for children broken out with prickly heat:

I. Keep them as cool as possible.

II. For a child of 2 years, give ½ tea-spoonful of cream tartar in the morning, for a few mornings.

III. Bathe them in tepid (a little warm) water, with a little soda in it, every night. It is also good to have a tubful of water (the chill off, of course), and let the child splatter in it for about fifteen minutes.

IV. When the heat breaks out in little pimples, which are all sore, grease them over with fresh (unsalted) grease of any kind; then dust over with pulverized starch, at least once a day, to keep them from smarting.

**2. Dysentery, Diarrhea, etc., of Children, Cordial for.**—This lady continues: I. These little ones require much care during warm weather, with their dysenteries, diarrheas, etc., from teething. I have found the blackberry balsam, as I call it, a most excellent remedy, but when the disease is of long standing, and there seems to be pain and soreness of the bowels, it is best to keep them very quiet, scarcely rocking them (so the doctor told me) and apply spirits of turpentine over the bowels. Take a cloth dampened with the turpentine, large enough to extend up over the stomach, as well as to cover the bowels, and leave it on long enough to cause redness, but not to blister. Then take it off, and when the redness goes away, apply again, until it seems to be out of pain, or easier, or:--

II. *Onion Poultices*—Applied in the same way, are very good; but the turpentine, if at hand, acts quicker. Onion poultice is made by chopping, or slicing, 2 onions into a spider with a little water and cooking well, then spread on a cloth.

*Remarks.*—This cooking of the onion, accounts to the author, for their not acting as quickly as the turpentine; mash them and lay them on raw, and I think they will act as quickly and as effectually as the others. Her balsam is entirely different from any I have seen, but it will be found very valuable. It is as follows:

III. *Blackberry Balsam and Cordial for Children.*—Take of the small and growing roots of the blackberry, 4 ozs.; bark of the bayberry, 2 ozs.; cranes-bill root (known also as *geranium maculatum* by the profession, and alum root by the people), and cinnamon bark, each 1 oz.; gum myrrh and cloves, each ½ oz.; fennel seed, ¼ oz.; loaf sugar and brandy as given below. DIRECTIONS—The roots should all be cut short, then with the other articles all bruised, and steeped in 2 qts. of water until half is evaporated (4 to 6 hours at least), making up with hot water if too much evaporation; but if steeped slowly, as it should be, or covered, it will be about right; then strain, and for the balsam add loaf sugar, 1 lb., and dissolve by heat.

*For the Cordial.*—Make the same way, but add sugar, ¼ lb., and best French brandy, ½ pt. Each are to be bottled and kept corked for use. DOSE —For children, 1 to 2 tea-spoonfuls, according to age and severity of the disease; repeat every 1, 2 or 3 hours, as needed. For adults—for it is good for them too—1 table-spoonful for a dose, time as above.

*Remarks.*—I can see no reason for making two kinds, balsam and cordial. I should put the full 1 lb. of sugar and the brandy, or good whiskey, as one can get handiest, ½ pt. to the strained mixture, and call it syrup, and be done with it; for the spirit will insure its better keeping and action. Prof. King in speaking of the fruit of this berry family, in which the red raspberry, dew- berry, etc., are all included, says: "The fruit, especially that of the black- berry, is of much service in dysentery, being pleasant to the taste, mitigating (easing) the accompanying *tenesmus* (griping and straining) and suffering of the patient, and ultimately effecting a cure. Blackberry syrup has cured cases of dysentery, even after physicians had despaired of a cure."

**3.** Dr. J. D. Lauers, of Conover, Ohio, adds to the blackberry cordial, made by any good cordial recipe, as follows: "Blackberry cordial, 1½ ozs.; tinct. kino and paregoric, each, 1½ drs., and syrup of ginger sufficent to fill a 3 oz. bottle. DOSE—For an adult, 1 tea-spoonful every hour. For children, ½ tea-spoonful every hour. In severe cases increase the dose."

*Remarks.*—It will need some care about increasing the dose, if given so often, as the kino is quite astringent and might, if the dose is large and given often, have a tendency to produce the opposite condition—constipation. Watch this, and you will be safe, as it is not best to sew one up too tight. As much syrup of rhubarb added, as tinct. of kino, would prevent that condition, and im- prove the syrup for the purpose intended.

**4. Summer Complaint from Teething of Children.**—Sub-car- bonate of bismuth, 36 grs.; Dover's powder, 6 grs. Mix thoroughly, and divide into 12 powders. DOSE—For a child from 1½ to 2 years, 1 powder in a little syrup, every 3 or 4 hours. When the looseness, ordiarrhea, has improved to justify it, give only 2 or 3 daily, when needed, to keep it under control so long as the irritation from the teething causes the continuance of the diarrhea. If properly managed it will control it.

*Remarks.*—I think, in one case, a girl of 1½ years old, I continued its use occasionally for nearly a year. The child being weak and feeble—puny, as the doctors say,—but care and perseverance overcame both difficulties, and at this writing, she is nearly 8 years old and of very good health. Without these powders and the care, I believe she would years ago have been in her grave.

**5. Colic of Infants and Adults, Quick Relief and Cure.**—I. *For Infants.*—Fl. ex. of *dioscorea* (wild yam, also called colic root), ½ dr.; camphor water, 1 dr.; simple syrup, 1 oz. Mix. Dose—For an infant of 2 months or under, ½ tea-spoonful every half hour, or shorter time, if not relieved. "The mixture," says Dr. Harris, of Suwanee, Ga., "gives immediate and permanent relief."

II. *For Adults.*—Prof King, in his *Dispensatory*, speaking of the wild yam, says: "It is a specific in bilious colic, having proved itself invariably successful in doses of ½ pt. of the decoction (tea), repeated every half hour or hour. No other medicine is required, as it gives prompt and permanent relief in the most severe cases." The fl. ex. of this, which is now kept more generally than heretofore, will no doubt prove equally effective, and be easier obtained. Decoctions are made by steeping 1 oz. of the root to 1 pt. of water.

**6. Hernia, or Rupture of Children, To Cure.**—A Mrs. A. A. Benson, of Loveland, Col., communicates the following cure for hernia of children to the *Blade*, which I trust will give as good satisfaction to others as it did to her boy of 11 years. The sooner applied after hernia is known, the more likely it will be to effect a cure. She says:

I. "I wish to give you a cure for 'Hernia,' or rupture, as used on my little boy. He was ruptured when about 3 weeks old on one side, and had to wear a truss. When 2 years old he had a second rupture on the opposite side, and since then has had to wear a double truss. This he could not leave off save when lying down. A woman once told me, when he was a baby, that oil of eggs would cure rupture, but I did not know how to prepare it, and had no faith in it. My boy is now 11 years old, and last summer I was told how to prepare oil of egg, and that it would cure rupture. So I tried it, using it about 3 weeks. For 6 weeks he has not had on a truss. He has pulled beans, helped to cut corn, and done a variety of chores around the farm, and seems perfectly cured. So now to the recipe for making oil of egg. I hope every one so afflicted will try it.

II. *Oil of Eggs to Make, as Used in Hernia of Children.*—"Boil 15 eggs hard, take out the yolks and cut them up in a spider (skillet), put over a slow fire and stir constantly, gradually increasing the heat. It will soon dissolve into a creamy looking substance; then, as the fire grows hotter, it will rapidly turn brown and look almost like coffee grounds. Now stir rapidly all the time; it will smoke and smell terribly, and you will feel sure that it is all burned up, but keep at it patiently, and after a while it will dissolve into a black oil. Now strain it off and bottle it. This quantity will make over an ounce of oil, and I did not quite use up this quantity before my boy was cured, although I should not have been discouraged if I had been compelled to make the second quantity.

Rub this oil on every night after lying down, being sure that the rupture is back in place. Then every morning use the following:

III. *Healing Salve.*—"Melt together a little fresh, unsalted butter with one-quarter as much beeswax, and after melting, add a few drops of oil of spike. This is very healing and prevents its getting very sore on the outside. I continued this treatment a little over three weeks."

*Remarks.*—Let no one, who has a child with hernia or rupture, fail to give it a fair and faithful trial.

**7. Milk-Scab of Children, Cure for.**—Fresh mutton tallow melted and applied very thick, once or twice a day; wash once a week, or oftener, with white castile soap; apply fresh tallow after washing; it will allay the burning and itching; no medicine is needed.

*Remarks.*—These scabs, or crusty eruptions, come out upon the forehead and upper part of the face of nursing children; at first slightly elevated pimples, sometimes becoming pustules, or containing matter, in clusters, the edges more or less red and inflamed. It takes its common name from a supposition that the mother's milk causes it; but I have seen it on children "raised upon the bottle." It is sometimes also called "honey disease," because the scabs look much like a drop of honey dried upon the skin. If it works up into, or upon the head, it would be called "scald-head." Besides washing with pure castile soap, or a weak lye made from wood ashes, and applying the mutton tallow, you can also give a little sulphur and cream of tartar, internally, to gently move the bowels, and after, give less to act on the blood. These should be mixed— half as much sulphur as cream of tartar; then mixed in molasses or syrup. This disease is also known as *tinea capitis* and dow worm; at first it is only an inflammation of the skin, but by neglect, want of cleanliness, and simple means to reduce the inflammation by slippery elm poultices and the cream of tartar and sulphur, it becomes aggravated, mattery, and harder to cure. In such cases use the following:

**8. French Ointment for Scald-Head of Children.**—Rose ointment, 1 oz.; white precipitate, 1 dr.; mix. DIRECTIONS—Wash carefully with mild castile soap and water; dry carefully with a soft dry cloth; then, after a few minutes, rub in a little of the ointment—morning and evening.

*Remarks.*—This originated with Prof. Spielman, at the University of Strasburg, France, and was used by him very successfully.

**9. Scald-Head, Tar Plaster for.** — This plaster has been recommended; but if tar is to be used, let it be only in small proportions, as follows: Boil a qt. of urine, 4 ozs. of lard, and a table-spoonful of tar together for an hour or two; and when only warm, strain and add 1 oz. of sulphur; simmer together and strain again, and it is ready to use, taking all the care of washing, drying, etc., before using, and also not forgetting the aperient of sulphur and cream of tartar, to keep the bowels easy and to act on the skin, which they do.

**10. Bed-Wetting and Urinary Diseases of Children, Certain Remedies.**—The following is from the *Eclectic Medical Journal*, of Cincinnati, O. The article was furnished by Dr. J. Berger, of El Passo, Kansas. He says:

I. "I have been using santonine in difficulties of the urinary organs for a year or more, and it has not failed to have the desired effect in a single case. I have used it in suppression of urine, incontinence of urine, and *dysuria* (see III., below), and also in fevers, When the urine is scant and deposits a 'brick dust' sediment, it is just *the* remedy. In my first case the suppression of the urine was complete, and resisted all treatment as per books, also the reputed *apis mel* (honey bee tea) was tried, and failed. But santonine thoroughly triturated (rubbed) with sugar, in ½ gr. doses every 3 hours, established the secretion in 8 hours, and cured the case in 24 hours. I have used it, in two other cases of suppression, with like results. [Then rub 4 grs. of sugar of milk, if done by a druggist—or, if done at home, in half a tea-spoonful of white sugar—and divide into 8 powders—1 for the dose, as above.]

II. *Enuresis, or Inability to Retain the Urine—Bed-Wetting Proper.*—"The second case was a lad of 8 years. His mother called on me for medicine; said 'Ed.' had worms and would 'wet the bed' 3 or 4 times during the night. I gave santonine triturated, in 2 grain doses, every 4 hours till 6 doses were taken. Followed with tonics of salicine and carbonate of iron in 4 gr. doses, 3 times a day for 4 days. Saw his mother two months after; said 'Ed.' had not 'wet the bed' since taking that medicine.

III. *Dysuria, or Pain and Heat in Passing Urine.*—"The third case was a lady, aged 22 years, troubled with dysuria (pain and heat in passing urine). She was cured with santonine in 2 gr. doses every 3 hours. Continued 12 hours only, triturated as above."

Confirmatory of Dr. Perger's position above upon the use of santonine, Dr. Scudder, in his "Diseases of Children," page 35, makes the following remarks: "We think of santonine as a vermifuge only; yet it has some other desirable properties. One of them is its influence over the bladder in retention of urine. In some diseases there is sometimes a tendency to retention which ordinary remedies will not reach, and which at last proves fatal. Santonine thoroughly triturated with sugar, in doses of from ½ to 1 gr. every 2 hours, affords very certain relief. It is also very effectual in relieving burning, scalding, etc., in passing urine and the tenesmus (pain in passing of urine), and other unpleasant sensations of the urinary passages," adding: "I think santonine is deserving a place among the 'Specific Medicines.'"

IV. *Incontinence of Urine (Bed-Wetting) Remedy for.*—Sulphate of quinine, 7 grs.; tincts. of belladonna and chloride of iron (muriated tinct. of iron), each ½ oz.; water, ¾ oz.; mix and shake when used. DOSE—Give 30 drops, 3 times daily, one being at bedtime.

*Remarks.*—The above dose is for a child of 6 or 7 years; older or younger in proportion. By the time this amount is taken, generally at best, there will be no more "wetting the bed."

**FOR JAUNDICE OF YOUNG CHILDREN.**—See under that head, or "Jaundice in Children, Treatment, etc."

**1. ASTHMA, Quick Relief and Other Remedies for.** — Although a lobelia, or some other emetic, has for a long time been considered the only hope for relief, yet, more recently, the inhalation of chloroform has proved generally a much quicker relaxant, and consequently the more satisfactory remedy. It is not necessary to breathe it to entire unconsciousness, but simply to relieve by putting a bottle of it—an ounce is sufficient to buy at a time—first to one nostril, closing the other with the thumb of the opposite hand, and, the mouth being closed, draw in a long and deep breath to the fullest extent the lungs will allow; then alternate with the other nostril in the same way until you realize the needed relief, or to the number of 2 or 3 times to each nostril. Then if not relieved, wait a few minutes and do the same again. It is better thus than to continue until unconscious. The chloroform is very satisfactorily inhaled from a glass tube inhaler, which see in note following "Acute Phthisic, or Consumption." To be corked up when not in use,

**2. Asthma, Relief in.**—A friend of mine who had had asthma, so that, at one time, he did not go to bed for 5 years, but took his sleep in a rocking chair, has found great relief inhaling the smoke of what he calls the

I. *Nitrated Stramonium for Relief in Asthma.*—He says: "I gather the green leaves of the stramonium, after the plant blossoms, and dry them in the shade. When dry, I soak them a few hours in a strong solution of purified nitre (common saltpeter does not answer), 3 ozs., to soft water, 1 pt. Powder the niter finely, and pouring on the water hot, quickly dissolves it. Soak the previously dried leaves in this solution, re-dry, in the shade, then pulverize the leaves and keep from the air in box or bottle. To USE—Put a rounding teaspoonful of the nitrated powder on a plate, and touch a lighted match to the heap, when, if properly done with the purified nitre, it burns without a blaze, throwing off considerable smoke. Place a small funnel (more generally called a tunnel), over it, and breathe the smoke arising from it by holding the mouth as close to the funnel as possible, to inhale as much as you can of the fumes. It will cause some coughing, at first, but this helps to clear the throat and bronchial tubes of phlegm and soon subsides and gives very great relief.

*Remarks.*—I used this at one time after having taken a severe cold, which settled upon the lungs, and found great relief, as it especially (as the gentleman says above) helped to clear the phlegm from the throat and bronchial tubes, most effectually. If it seems to be going out at any time, raise the edge of the funnel a moment, and it will burn and sputter on again.

II. *Asthma Powder, Improved.*—Some persons think that sage, belladonna and digitalis, the dried leaves of each, with the dry stramonium, all in equal proportions, nitrated, as above (remembering always to use the purified nitre, kept by druggists only), and inhaled in the same manner, is preferable to the stramonium alone. If I were to use them, however, I would not use more than half as much of the belladonna and digitalis as I did of the sage and stramonium.

**3.** Whenever the inhalation of chloroform, or nitrated stramonium, etc., above given, fails, then 20 to 40 drops of laudanum, according to robustness of the patient, or the severity of the case, with 15 to 30 drops of sulphuric ether, put into a glass with a little water, and immediately drank, will almost always give relief at once. This should not be taken often enough to establish the habit of opium eating, which would prove a disease in itself, as bad as asthma and as difficult to cure.

**4. Alterative Relaxing Anodyne, and Curative for Asthma.** —Ethereal tinct. of lobelia and iodide of potash, each, 2 ozs.; tinct. assafœtida (fetta), and laudanum, each, 1 oz.; simple syrup, 4 ozs. Mix. Dose—From a tea to a table-spoonful every hour or two, to relieve a paroxysm, for 3 or 4 doses. As a curative, after the paroxysm has subsided, take the same dose only 3 or 4 times a day.

*Remarks.*—In closing the subject of asthma, I would say in addition only, that according to the condition of the system, any existing difficulty, as costiveness, liver or kidney complaint, must be met and overcome on general principles, that is, to treat them as you would if they existed alone. Do all. as per instructions given under each head referred to, in connection with the above items under this head, and very many cases of asthma will be cured, the general opinion to the contrary, notwithstanding. The condition of the surface, to keep it clean and the blood freely circulating therein, by the salt washings, dry rubbings, etc., (which see), must not, in any case, be neglected in any long standing disease. If neglected, it is at your own peril.

**1. JAUNDICE—Successful Remedies.**— No matter how much the liver may be affected, unless the stools are clay-colored, or, in other words, without color, and the skin and the whites of the eyes yellow, it is not called jaundice. With the yellowness of the skin, there is generally constipation, tongue heavily coated, mouth dry, appetite variable, and sometimes headache, nausea, or vomiting.

*Treatment.*—With eclectics it is claimed that the fl. ex. of chionanthus Virginica (fringe tree), in 10 to 20 drop doses, according to age and robustness of the patient, will cure it.

Dr. Goss, of Marietta, Ga., prefers the tinct. made with 8 ozs. of the bark of the root to alcohol, 1 pt. In answer to some inquirers through the *Brief,* he refers to the fringe tree in the following manner:

"The doctor again asks me about the chionanthus Virginica—fringe tree. I have stated in several journals, and in my "Materia Medica," and also in my "New Medicine," emphatically, that I had never failed to cure simple jaundice with the tinct. of the root (bark of the root is what is used) of the chionanthus, when it was made from the freshly dug root. Several others ask me whether it acts on the liver, or not? I never claimed it as an active stimulant to the biliary secretions in health. It cures jaundice in some specific way, but how, I do not know."

The doctor uses the tincture, made as above, in doses of $\frac{1}{2}$ to 1 tea-spoonful, 3 or 4 times a day. He first cured himself with it, while a student in the University of Georgia. "The faculty," he says, "having failed to cure me, or to ameliorate my symptoms in the slightest degree. In this state of utter despair I finally concluded I must succumb to the malady; but, by accident, I heard of a tailor who had been cured of the jaundice with gin bitters, made of the bark of the chionanthus root, so I procured some, and made me a bitters in gin, by adding 2 ozs. to 1 qt. Of this I took a table-spoonful 3 times a day, and in 10 days I was entirely cured of jaundice; and at the same time I found that it improved my digestion very much, and I continued it for a month or two with much benefit to my digestive organs generally. [In making the bitters in places where it grows plentifully, I should use at least 4 ozs. to 1 qt. of gin, and take the same dose.]

"After that I prescribed it for others, and, I believe, always with success, where there was no complication of diseases. I cured many soldiers in the 'late unpleasantness,' only losing a single case, which was complicated with biliary calculi (gall-stones in the bile-ducts of the liver)." He closed by saying: "Since I published my use of the chionanthus I have seen reports in various medical journals of its success in jaundice and hypertrophy (enlargement of the liver), as well as some reports of its use as a female tonic. I know a case of hypertrophied (enlarged) uterus cured by the use of the chionanthus—used for a considerable time."

**2. Jaundice Cured by the Use of the Chionanthus and Acetate of Potash.**—Dr. Henning, of Redkey, Ind., reports through *The Brief* also (February, 1879): "Twenty years ago I used to give calomel and leptandrin with poor success. But now I give, in all cases, of the fl. ext. of chionanthus (fringe tree) from 10 to 20 drops (of course according to age and robustness of the patient) 4 times per day. This will correct the action of the liver in a short time. But in addition I prescribe the acetate of potassa (potash), 10 grs., 3 times per day, to act upon the kidneys (it is a very valuable diuretic) to pump out and eliminate (throw off) the bilious excrementitious (of the nature of excrement or feces, but here more particularly worn out) matter from the blood. This I follow with the elixir of calisaya (Peruvian) bark with iron and strychnine (kept by druggists) as a tonic, increasing the nutrition and strength. This treatment," he says, "has been very successful in my hands, and I am satisfied it is the true theory of the disease in practice." He thinks it best to "follow up the treatment 3 to 5 weeks to make a permanent cure."

**3. Jaundice in Children, Treatment of.**—J. E. Ball, M. D., of Texas, reports a case which was printed in the April number of *The Brief*, as follows: "I noticed in the February number of *The Brief* 'Treatment for Jaundice,' by John A. Henning, M. D., and as I think my treatment a little more prompt in its action I will give you the full treatment of my last case: Called Feb. 3d to a child 18 months old; skin and eyes as yellow as saffron, urine thick and stained its clothes of that saffron color peculiar to jaundiced urine. Prescribed: Leptandrin, 1 gr.; podophyllin, ½ gr.; pulverized Jamaica ginger, 2 grs.; mix, and divide into 8 powders. Gave 1 powder every 4 hours until the biliary secretions were aroused. Also Tinct. of buchu and sweet spirits of niter, each, 1 dr. Dose—Ten drops every 2 hours.

"Feb. 5th.—First prescriptions acted well. Then prescribed: Fl. ext. of chionanthus (fringe tree) and tinct. of sanguinaria canadensis (blood root), each equal parts. DOSE—Ten drops 4 times per day.

"Feb. 12th.—Little patient entirely relieved; skin and urine as clear as it ever was."

### 4. Jaundice, Allopathic Treatment of—Successful.—I give the

following treatment because it contains calomel and may meet some cases where the chionanthus cannot be obtained, and also because it will lead me to follow it with remarks, showing how a very little calomel will sometimes arouse the action of the liver when, as the saying is, "everything else has failed." This is from Geo. B. Snyder, M. D., of Hays City, Kans. It will explain itself. It was reported in the July number of *The Brief*, 1879. He says:

"In looking over the April number of your valuable journal, I notice an article on the 'Treatment for Jaundice.' As I understand it, the mere presence of jaundice is not a disease, but merely a symptom. The yellow skin indicates the presence or hepatic (liver) trouble, the true character of which I am, in candor, bound to confess is not always easy to determine. The last patient under these circumstances, I was called upon to see, was on August 19, 1878. His symptoms were yellow skin, impaired digestion, excessive restlessness, with eclampsia, etc." [This 'eclampsia,' here, no doubt, refers to an appearance, to the patient, like flashes of light, a symptom of epilepsy.] "My prescription," he continues, "was: Hydrarg chlor. mite (calomel), 4 grs.; podophyllin, 3 grs.; potass chlor. (chlorate of potash, pulverized), 36 grs.; ex. of hyoscyami (hyoscyanius) 3 grs.; mix. Make into 10 powders. DOSE—One powder every 2 hours. On the second day I found my patient so much improved that with a single prescription of bitter tonics with ex. of nux vomica, I dismissed him. His recovery to perfect health was absolute." [A good tonic pill for these cases would be: Quinine, 45 grs.; alcoholic ex. of nux vomica, 2 grs.; mix thoroughly and make into 30 pills. DOSE—One pill only, 4 times a day, for an adult. These pills should not be given to children. But for them 1 gr. powders of quinine might be given as the tonic, without the nux, in cold strong coffee, which hides the bitter taste very much.]

*Remarks.*—Dr. Snyder says, above, "the yellow skin indicates the presence of hepatic, or liver, trouble," but the true character, he "confesses is not always easy to determine." Well, I would ask, why try to determine at all, so long as the *chionanthus*, as given in the foregoing recipe, or even his own combination, will cure it? We know this much, that whenever the skin and eyes are yellow, there is a certain condition of the liver, and it is generally believed, at least, that this condition is always the same, hence, they are always cured, as above indicated, by the same medicines. But there is a certain diseased condition of the liver, attended with considerable uneasiness, sometimes amounting to actual pain, but not having the jaundiced or yellow skin and eyes, when the author has not been able to touch the liver, so as to start the bile, with either the common liver pills, which contain podophyllin, leptandrin, etc., nor with the chionanthus; but very minute doses of calomel, even the 20th of a grain, taken at bed-time, followed with a tea-spoonful of epsom salts, in the morning, has aroused its action, and started the bile freely within the following 24 hours, and was entirely satisfactory and lasting, by repeat-ing the same doses, at an interval of a week, for 2 or 3 times. These were desperate cases, else I should not have ventured upon what I had always considered a desperate remedy—calomel. But, as I have always believed in "giving the devil his due," I have thus set this down to the credit of calomel, notwithstanding I, and my mother before me, as well as eclectics generally, have fought against the use of calomel all our lives. But I would not, even now, use it in large doses, especially when such very small ones have such a decided and beneficial effect. But I always try the ordinary treatment first, and only fall back upon these small doses of calomel when the first plan fails.

But if I fail to "touch" the liver, as the allopaths call it, *i. e.*, fail to arouse its action, by which its usual biliary secretions are produced, with the small doses, I should use them as large as 1 to 3 grs.; or, if need be, blue mass, a 3 gr. pill, followed with the salts, to accomplish the same end. I know several persons who claim, and no doubt believe, that nothing but a 3 grain pill of of blue mass at night, and sometimes for a second night, will act on their liver when out of order. Working off next morning, of course, with salts or some other active cathartic. And I certainly prefer to try this plan rather than to lose the life of my patient, or have him go to a doctor who will use calomel or blue mass from choice; although, by their giving large doses of calomel, they often fail to cure. But I always give this class of patients a 1 to 2 gr. pill of quinine 3 or 4 times daily, after the bilious passages have somewhat subsided; and if much sour eructations arise from the stomach while the bile is being poured out so freely, I give a little bi-carbonate (common baking) soda, in half tea-spoonful doses, in a little water. Certainly, however, there can be no objection raised to Dr. Snyder's doses of calomel, as there would be less than ⅓ a gr. to each powder, while allopaths, in the first time of cholera in the United States, gave it sometimes in ounce doses, and no doubt killed by such treatment more than the cholera itself. But now, as some of them have got down to the 20th of a grain, or even ½ grain doses, I will gracefully cease my warfare upon it, at least, when given in the above, homœopathic, doses. And I am now, more than ever before confirmed in the idea that it was by large doses, and other abuses of its use, that much of the harm it has done was brought about. Where it is used, let it be in small doses only, and its action watched with great care, and I trust the result will be as satisfactory to others, as it has been with myself.

1. **SYPHILIS — Alterative for, Successful in Bad Cases.—** Fl. ex. of stillingia, corydalis, poke root, yellow dock root and burdock root, each 2 ozs.; iodide of potash, ½ to ¾ oz.; simple syrup to make 1 pt. DIRECTIONS—Dissolve the iodide in a little of the mixture, and mix all. DOSE—1 tea-spoonful 4 times daily, one being at bed-time. Large and robust patients may put in the ¾ oz. iodide, weak and feeble ones only the ½ oz.

*Remarks.*—If there is any gonorrhea discharge, every other time it is made, leave out the extract of poke root, and put in the same amount of the fl. ex. of buchu, in its place. In very bad cases of syphilis, when the pint has been all taken, get a pint bottle of Tilden's Elixir of Iodo Bromide of Calcium Compound (kept by druggists), and take it according to the directions upon the bottle, and so alternate, for a year, or longer, unless well satisfied that all the syphilitic poison is eradicated from the system sooner than this. The doctor of whom I obtained this, at Grand Rapids, Mich., told me that in this manner he had cured very bad cases—one where the whole body was covered with scabs and sores, except, fortunately for the patient, his face and hands did not show the eruptions. Upon the scales, or rather around them, he applied an ointment made as follows: Take a pint bottle and put into it nitric acid, 1 oz.; quick-silver, 1 oz., and let stand until the silver is cut; then melt lard, ½ lb., in an earthen bowl, and mix all together and stir with a wooden spatula until cold. This was swabbed on around the scabs (if a little gets on the scab it does not matter; but he thinks it not best to tear off the scabs, but to put it freely around the edges), at first three times a week, then twice, and finally only once a week, till all is smooth as a child's flesh; This case paid him $100, and had previously paid out over $250, without benefit. I have also since cured a very bad case with it, and therefore know its value as an alterative. In the case first given the doctor told me that after the scabs or sores were cured about 6 months, the man wanted to know if he might "marry with safety;" the answer was, "continue the alterative for a year longer, then there will be safety in marrying." He followed it up as directed and then did marry, and never afterwards saw any ill effects from the disease Although the plan of alternating the above alterative with the Tilden prepara tion is especially valuable for syphilis, yet the alterative above will be found very valuable in all the other diseases requiring one.

2. **Gonorrhea—Remedy.**—It consists of an inflammation of the urethra of the male and of the vagina of the female, which causes, generally, a dis charge (which is contagious) of a muco-purulent character, having the appearance of mucous and pus. It is generally caused from impure cohabitation; but it does sometimes arise from the parts coming in contact with this gonorrheal matter, even when partially dry, upon sheets where those having the disease have slept, or from privy seats, and, in fact, husbands sometimes are affected by an inflammation of a similar character taken from the wife who has an acrid leucorrheal discharge, while both are perfectly honest and virtuous towards each other. These points are now well-known by many physicians, but not well understood by the people, which leads me to introduce these recipes as much to point out these facts as to enable people to cure themselves or their friends in like condition. Then, as the disease is well-known, as above remarked, in the manner also described above, let everyone be very careful how they pronounce another guilty of criminal or impure connection, at least until they are positive as to the facts in any particular case. And let me caution every one having this disease, or in treating others who have it, to be very careful not to allow any of the matter to come in contact with any open sore, nor with the eye or nostrils, for all mucous membranes will take on the disease by such contact Keep the hands clean and burn all cloths used for the purpose of cleanliness to ensure safety.

*Other Treatment Necessary.*—In the commencement of the disease, while the inflammation is acute or active, give a full cathartic dose of some cooling purgative—for instance, the compound powder of jalap, with cream of tartar, or a full cathartic dose of any medicine one is in the habit of usiug as a cathartic.

*Compound Powder of Jalap.*—Best Alexandria senna, in powder, 1 oz.; powdered jalap, ½ oz.; powdered cloves, ½ dr.; or powdered ginger, 1 dr.; mix. This forms an excellent cathartic in all cases requiring quick action. It is mild but efficient, stimulating the liver and biliary ducts to a healthy action, and helping materially to reduce all inflammatory diseases. It should not, however, be given in inflammation of the stomach or the bowels, if of a severe character. In pregnancy, painful menstruation, and other like conditions of females, it should be taken only in about half the usual doses; repeat half the dose, if it does not operate in 4 hours in all cases. DOSE—Take one tea-spoonful of the powder in a tea-cup and half fill with boiling water; stir occasionally till cool; stir again and drink all. Sweeten, if desired. In all fevers and in the above cases put into the cup 1 tea-spoonful of cream of tartar, which aids in reducing fevers or inflammations, especially of the character above indicated.

The patient should also take freely of mucilaginous drinks, as gum-arabic water, ½ oz. to 1 oz. to the pint, poured on boiling hot, and the whole drank in the course of the day, or two at most; or, a tea of marsh mallows, 1 oz. to the pint of water daily; or, flaxseed tea made in the same way, as most convenient to obtain. As soon as the action of the cathartic is well over, and one of the mucilaginous drinks have helped to allay the severity of the inflammation, use injections also of an astringent, tonic or antiseptic character, according to the severity of the case, like the following:

**3. Injection for Gonorrhea.**— The following is one of the more common, being principally astringent, for cases where the inflammation and discharge is slight: Sulphate of zinc, 8 grs., to water, 4 ozs. DIRECTIONS—To be injected 2 or 3 times a day at least; but it is well to inject after each urination; but if much purulent or thick matter, use one of the following, first having injected water to cleanse the parts thoroughly, and if this strength causes much smarting or pain, reduce half with water. A glass or rubber syringe is better than the metallic ones for all these purposes.

**4. Injection for Gonorrhea.**—The following combines tonic, astringent, and antiseptic properties, applicable in the severe cases. It was given by Prof. King in his "Chronic Diseases," with the remark, "that he makes it known for the first time": Sulphate of quinine. 20 grs.; elixir of vitriol (which is aromatic sulphuric acid), 1 dr.; mix, and shake to dissolve the quinine; then add camphor water, 1 oz., and distilled water, 3 ozs.; solution of iodide of iron, ½ dr. Inject as the first; and if it causes pain or uneasiness to any extent, reduce a little with water, until the improvement enables it to be borne. I will give one more, which also combines the astringent, tonic, and antiseptic properties necessary to ensure success, and equally valuable as an injection in leucorrhea (which see). It is as follows:

**5. Injection—Valuable in Gonorrhea and Leucorrhea.—**Fl. ext. of golden seal, ½ dr.; sulphate, or acetate, of zinc, 1 dr.; chlorate of potassa, ½ dr.; tannin and sulphate of quinine, each 15 grs., the quinine to be dissolved with 15 or 20 drops of aromatic sulphuric acid before put in; distilled or soft water, 1 pt. Used same as the above.

For leucorrhea it had better be made in double the quantity, and used with a female syringe, cleansing the parts, first, by injecting water as hot as it can be borne, keeping it in the vagina 2 or 3 minutes, by placing the fingers over the external parts to prevent its immediate escape. This is important in all these injections. It is also thought best, by J. W. Burney, M. D., of Des Arc, Ark., for leucorrhea, to give, internally, a tea-spoonful 3 times daily of the fl. ext. of buchu in some flax-seed tea. It will prove valuable as a diuretic in either of these diseased conditions of the system.

**6.** Any of the articles named in these injections have been used alone, in the strength of 2 grs. to the oz. of water, for gonorrhea; and, besides these, strychnia, 1 gr. to the oz. of water, and corrosive sublimate of the same strength, have been used, it is claimed, with success. The acetate, and the iodide of zinc, 1 to 3 grs. of either to the oz. of water, have been used very satisfactorily.

Of late, suppositories have been brought into use, containing a suitable amount of any of the foregoing, or other articles which are desired, to be introduced into the ureter at bed-time, by which, it is claimed, a better action is had, from the fact that the cocoa butter, in which the medicines are held, dissolves slowly, and thus the medicine is held the longer in contact with the diseased parts of the ureter. They are also made of suitable size for the vagina, in leucorrhea and gonorrhea of females.

**7. Gonorrhea Cured Without Injections.—**If the following internal treatment will do what Dr. Given, of Louisville, Ky., claims for it, it is preferable, or, at least, is a less difficult plan to pursue. He states, through the *Brief,* in answer to an inquiry, "How to Cure Gonorrhea Successfully Without the Use of Copaiba, Cubebs or Injections?" as follows:

"The following is my prescription, as published in the *American Practitioner* several years ago. It cures in from 2 to 10 days, if given within the first 24 or 36 hours after the disease has developed. I have never injected a single patient: Spirits of nitric ether, balsam copaiba and camph. tinct. opii (paragoric), of each 1 oz.; tinct. veratrum viride, 1 dr. Mix. Dose—A tea-spoonful 3 or 4 times a day."

*Remarks.*—The author would say in flaxseed tea or some of the other mucilaginous drinks. The more freely the mucilages are taken, the better for the patient. It is generally claimed, however, that those suffering with gonorrhea must be careful about their diet, excluding meats of all kinds, fats, tea, coffee, and absolutely avoid all alcoholic and malt liquors, and tobacco in all its forms, if they hope to get well at all speedily; and also to take a mild cathartic every 3 or 4 days, and that it is also valuable to take a hip-bath 2 or 3 times a day, while the inflammation is considerable, as hot as it can be borne; also to keep as quiet as possible, else support the scrotum with a suspensary bandage to prevent stagnation or accumulation of blood in the parts, to which there is often considerable tendency.

**8. Gonorrhea, the Great French Remedy for.**—In Gunn's "New Family Physician" we find the following, which he says is known as the "Great French Remedy for Gonorrhea" in any stage of the disease, and said to be infallible, without any other medicine:

"Take ¼ oz. each of dragon's blood—to be found at the druggists'—pulverized colocynth and pulverized gamboge; pulverize (better buy the pulverized article if you can) and rub these three articles together in a mortar; then add ½ pint boiling water (rain or soft water preferable) and stir occasionally for an hour with the pestle; then add 2 ozs. each of sweet spirits of nitre and balsam copaiba, and stir again till well mixed; then bottle for use. Dose—Two teaspoonfuls night and morning until it operates thoroughly on the bowels; then 1 tea-spoonful 2 or 3 times a day, or sufficient to keep up a gentle action on the bowels, and continue until a cure is affected."

**9. Gonorrhea in Its Commencement—Cure Without Injection.**—After having written the above, I went to my dinner, and on my return found my *Medical Brief* had been delivered, and, on looking it over, was struck at the simplicity of a recipe for gonorrhea, given in answer to an inquiry for such a cure, by Dr. Hall, of Fairmount, Ga., as follows:

"Spirits nit. dulc. (sweet spirits of nitre), 1 oz.; balsam of copaiba and tinct. of mur. ferri (tinct. of muriate of iron), of each, 1 dr. Mix. Dose— A tea-spoonful in water, milk or wine (I would say in some of the mucilages before mentioned) given every few days, 4 to 6 hours apart. No injections needed in incipient (the beginning of) gonorrhea."

*Remarks.*—He uses the same in ardor urinæ (scalding, or heat in passing urine) with like success; but in this last condition he gives the same dose, repeating in 3 hours, then at longer intervals. From my knowledge of the properties of the article, I recommend a trial, at once, wherever and whenever needed, in either disease. But as some persons will not begin any treatment at once, as they ought to do, letting the disease become chronic, or by mismanagement or carelessness in taking medicine, or by persisting in the use of spirits, fat meats, etc., a gleet, or slight discharge, will continue from the urethra after the inflammatory condition has been subdued. Such a condition will require something of the character given for gleet, after the next item.

**10. Gonorrhea, the Latest and Most Simple Treatment for.**— Some time after all the foregoing had been written, upon this subject, the December number of my *Therapeutic Gazette*, of Detroit, Mich., came to hand, with a treatment for this disease, from Dr. Joseph McChesney, surgeon of the Atchison, Topeka & Santa Fe Railroad Co., at Deming, N. M., which appears so simple and easy of trial, and withal so effectual (he reporting a number of cures in from 6 to 10 days, and some of them of long standing), that I feel constrained to give it, believing it to be as effectual as it is simple. It is as follows: Dissolve corrosive sublimate, 1 gr. only, in water, 6 ozs., injecting a syringe of it every 4 hours.

*Remarks.*—He gave cases of acute, or just commenced, as well as those of long standing, in which it was equally effective. It needs no further comment nor recommendation of mine, only to say I trust too, with him, that in the corrosive sublimate treatment for gonorrhea, I have at last met with the drug that gives such entire satisfaction to the unfortunate, and one that will prove a financial boon to me, and hereby a boon to the unfortunate many, who may never see Dr. McChesney, nor myself.

**11. Gleet, Effectual Treatment for.**—Some of the first above mentioned injections for gonorrhea, may be injected for gleet, or the following, as used by Dr. S. L. Blake, of San Francisco, Cal., who has found it so effectual that he deemed it his duty to place it before the readers of the *Brief*, in 1880, as follows: Sulphate of zinc, 12 grs.; tinct. iodine, 10 drops; distilled water (soft water will do in all such cases), 8 ozs.; mix; inject 4 times a day. Also, fl. ex. uva ursi, 3 ozs.; fl. ex. pareira brava, 1 oz.; fl. ex. cascara sagrada and syrup of orange, each 2 ozs.; water sufficient to make 8 ozs.; mix. [The pareira brava is a native of the West India Islands and the Spanish Main, says King, in his American Dispensatory, "It is a tonic, diuretic and aperient, used in chronic inflammations of the bladder, and various disorders of the urinary organs." The cascara sagrada is valuable in constipation, while the properties of the other articles in these prescriptions are well known to be valuable for what he recommends them.] DOSE—Take a tea-spoonful 3 times a day before meals.

*Remarks.*—This, he says, I consider an invaluable remedy in obstinate cases. Of course the principal readers of the *Brief* are physicians, which shows that Dr. Blake was well satisfied with it or he would not risk the criticism he would receive if it was not reliable.

**12. Gleet, for the Pain and Weakness in the Back.**—For this condition take Venice or white pine turpentine, and work into it as much finely pulverized rhubarb as will make it pill. Make into usual sized pills, and take 2 pills twice daily.

**13. Red Drops, Specific for Gleet, Gonorrhea, Leucorrhea, and Affections of the Kidneys.**—Tinct. of guaiac and compound spirits of lavender, each ½ oz.; oil of cubebs and laudanum, each ¼ oz.; balsam of copaiba, 1 oz.; mix. DOSE—A tea-spoonful 3 or 4 times a day—one always being at bed-time in these cases.

*Remarks.*—Dr. Gunn says of these drops: "A specific (positive cure) for gleet, gonorrhea and leucorrhea, and good for affections of the kidneys." They are all, in a certain degree, of a similar character, *i. e.*, there is an inflammation of the mucus membrane of the parts in each disease; then, what will overcome it in one case, will also do it in any of the others, and yet not be a "cure all," as the mucus membrane is the same everywhere.

**BEE AND WASP STINGS—Sure Cure for.—I.** *Bees.*—Mr. R. L. Aylor, of Waterloo, Ky., in reporting his success in keeping his bees over the winter of 1881-2, sends a recipe to the *Bee Journal*, headed "Bees," claiming it as his own discovery. It is simple, easily obtained, and cheap; and if it proves as quick and successful a cure as he claims, he is the one to have the benefit of "discovery." He gave it in the following words: "Buy from any drug store a small phial of tincture of myrrh; as soon as you are stung apply a little to the puncture, when all pain and swelling ceases instantly. It is also excellent for bites of spiders and poisonous reptiles."

*Remarks.*—Certainly no one would ask it to cure quicker than "instantly." I trust it shall prove as successful as claimed. If it does, nothing else could be desired.

II.  *Wasp Stings, Quick and Certain Cure.* — Cut an onion, scrape and apply the juicy part to the sting. It quickly relieves, and allays the irritation almost as quickly.

*Remarks.*—A correspondent of the *London Times* reports the case of his son, stung in the eyeball by a wasp, and when he reached the house, "looked like death," etc., which made a great commotion, and the sal volatile was gotten, but one of the maids used the onion juice, and the relief was so quick that he got up and went out again to help the men destroy the nest. I have no doubt the onion juice, or scraped onion, is as good for bee stings as for the other; but lose no time in applying it, if a wasp sting, for they are very poisonous.

III.  *Handy Remedy for Bites and Stings of Poisonous Animals and Insects.* —A writer in *Holt's Journal of Health* says: "That for persons about to travel or to go into the country for the summer, an ounce vial of spirits of hartshorn should be considered one of the indispensables, as, in case of being bitten or stung by any poisonous animal or insect, the immediate and free application of this alkali, as a wash to the part bitten, gives instant, perfect and permanent relief, the bite of a mad dog (we believe) not excepted; so will strong ashes-water.

*Remarks..*—I should as soon risk the immediate application of the spirits of hartshorn as any other caustic for a mad dog bite; but it would not do to put it into the eye—as the onion juice referred to.

**SPRAINS, SWELLINGS, CROUP, ETC.—Remedy for.**—Best cider vinegar, 1 pt.; spirits of turpentine, ½ pt.; beat well, 3 eggs, and mix all. DIRECTIONS—Apply to the neck in croup, and to sprains or swellings by saturating (thoroughly wetting) cloths and lay on, or bind on when necessary. "Cures," says Preacher Jones, "on the 'double quick.' It cured a woman's swollen arm in 9 days who had had to give up work and go to begging on account of the swelling."

*Remarks.*—It would be as valuable for animals as for persons. See "Croup, Sovereign Remedy for," for the value of turpentine in this disease. I think the vinegar and beaten eggs will improve it.

**HOP BITTERS—Cheap and Reliable, Without Spirits of Any Kind.**—Hops, 2 ozs.; ginger root, bruised, 1 table-spoonful; water, 2 galls.; brown sugar, 2 lbs.; yeast, ½ cup. DIRECTIONS—Boil the hops and ginger to obtain their strength, strain half an hour; add the sugar and continue the heat, removing all scum that arises; then cool to blood warmth, put in the yeast; let the yeast work over night, or that length of time, then bottle

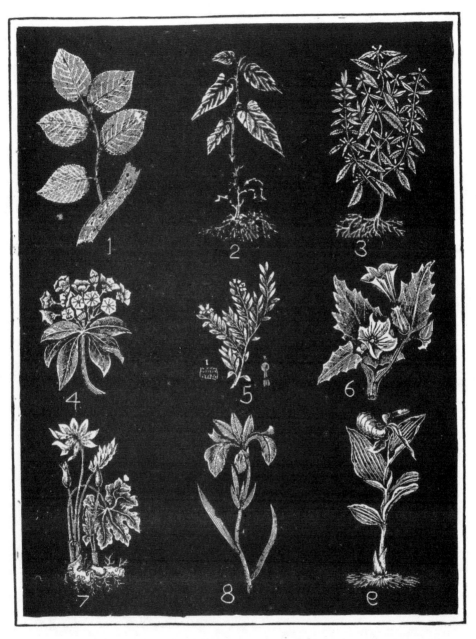

1—Slippery Elm.  2—Virginia Snake Root.  3—Pennyroyal.  4—Mountain Laurel, or Calico Bush.  5—Bear-Berry, or the Upland Cranberry.  6—Jamestown Weed, or Stramonium.  7—Blood-Root, or Red Puccoon.  8—Blue Flag.  9—Ladies' Slipper, or American Valerian.

and keep in a cool place. DOSE—Take 2 or 3 good swallows before each meal, or in amount as found necessary from the following:

*Remarks.*—These bitters are recommended in all cases requiring a tonic action, where there is a tendency to a chronic inflammation, as in catarrhal headache, pain in other parts, kidneys out of order, etc. The gentleman from whom I obtained this, at Grass Lake, Mich., was a kind of "domestic doctor," had a cure for everything. I have used these hop bitters, however, and am well pleased with their action. They improve the appetite and strengthen the diges- tion. One of his cures was for ague, by taking sulphur in molasses every night. He claims to have cured over 100 obstinate cases with that simple rem- edy. He said if the hop bitters did not loosen the bowels after a few days to add a little salts—Epsom—enough of it, for a day or two only, to loosen them.

The following is claimed to be the real Hop Bitters which has made such a stir in the world: Hop leaves, 3 ozs.; buchu leaves, 1 oz.; fl. ext. of dandelion, 1 oz.; fl. ext. of mandrake, 2 drs.; whisky, 1 qt. DIRECTIONS, DOSE, ETC.— Boil or simmer the hops and the buchu leaves in water, ½ gal., for 6 hours, or down to 1 qt., strain, and when cold add the fl. exts. and whisky. DOSE— From 1 to 3 table-spoonfuls 3 times a day, before meals.

*Remarks.*—It will be found a tonic and laxative, and the amount taken must be governed so as not to loosen the bowels but slightly, else its tonic effects would be carried off too readily. I have not used this, but I have the first above, with much satisfaction.

**TOBACCO—Its Use Frequently Injuring Sight and Memory.** —Dr. Mackenzie, in his "Opthalmology," a work on the anatomy and diseases of the eye, expresses his opinion that tobacco is the frequent cause of *amaurosis*, diminution, or complete loss of sight, and says: "One of the best proofs of this being the case, is the great improvement in vision (sometimes complete res- toration), which ensues on the use of that narcotic being abandoned." Tobacco is a powerful narcotic, and often affects the nerves disastrously. This position of Mackenzie, says a French writer, is confirmed by M. Michel, who classes the disease among the two forms of *cerebral*, or brain, *amaurosis* (loss or dimin- ution of sight by the condition of the brain), which are but little known. One of these conditions is seen in heavy drinkers, and is symptomatic of delirium tremens; but the other, he thinks, is brought about by the use of tobacco; and he also believes there are but few persons who have habitually, for a long period, smoked more than 5 drachms, ⅝ of an ounce, daily, without their sight, and often their memory, being more or less enfeebled. Then let those who already realize either of these conditions, or think the prospect good for their occur- rence, abandon the use of tobacco in any form, at once, and forever, and keep their young folks from its use, if possible. Fortunate for the author he could never tolerate its use at all; but one can scarcely see an old man, or even young men, and many boys, even passing along the street, without a cigar in their mouth, or gracefully (?) held in their fingers. If its use continues to increase for the next century as it has for the last decade (10 years passed of this cen- tury) we shall, I greatly fear, be the next thing to a nation of imbeciles; with much larger per cent. of idiots than at this writing. A fearful responsi bility rests upon parents, and governments. Certainly no school-boy should be allowed to use tobacco in any form; but it is law, and vigilant watchfulness of officers appointed for this purpose, with the same care and watchfulness of parents also that will ever prevent it, and that not wholly; for it has a fascination which cannot be accounted for upon any other principle only that of exhilaration, which is, in fact, the reason why it should never be used. It over stimulates the nerves, and thereby destroys, or very much injures them, shortening life, if no more serious catastrophe, as blindness, loss of memory, paralysis, etc., does not set in before.

**EPILEPSY—Remedies Which Have Been Successful.—I.** Chas. VanWye, M. D., of Browning, Mo., reports through the *Brief* the case of a man of 37, who had been troubled from childhood with epilepsy, cured by the use of bromide of potassium, 30 grs., 3 times a day, dissolved in water, half a tumbler or so, until it produced its physiological effects, which are similar to that of iodide of potassium, *i. e.*, it may affect the head like a cold, and if the stomach or alimentary canal are irresistible, it may produce diarrhea, and increase the urine too much, but it may produce *acne* (a pustular affection of the skin), and a person taking large doses very long may have a manifestation of weakening of the mind; then, if any of these occur, stop its use a few days, or a week; or if taking it 3 times daily about meal-time, stop the noon dose, and if this does not relieve that, or either of these conditions, drop to 15 or 20 gr. doses, twice daily, then if not relieved in a few days stop as above indicated. In the case given it was used at intervals, *i. e.*, stopping every fourth week for 15 months, and only one convulsion after beginning its use. But the doctor would not begin unless the man would agree to take it several months at least. He considered it a perfect cure.

*Remarks.*—Dr. King, in his Dispensatory, says: "It has been used suc. cessfully in enlarged spleen and liver, swelling of lymphatic glands (glands of the neck, armpits, front of elbow, back of knee, groins, etc., externally, and along the lymphatic vessels internally), scrofula, epilepsy, nervous depression from masturbation, also nocturnal (night) emissions, irritability of the nervous centers, and in hypertrophy (enlargement) of the ventricles (of the heart). It has proved successful in pertussis (whooping-cough), and also in asthma, in doses of 20 to 30 grs., repeated 2 or 3 times a day," etc. So you see it has been used in as large doses as Dr. Wye prescribes it above; but it has not been used as long, generally, and that is the probable reason that it has not proved more beneficial heretofore. Even in doses of 10 to 15 grs. it has held fits in check, and in such doses may be continued for years safely; watch in all cases, however, for any of the above named bad symptoms and stop or lessen the dose as directed.

II. *Pill for Epileptic Fits in the Early Stages.*—Sulphate of zinc and cayenne pepper, each 60 grs.; rhubarb and ipecac, each 30 grs.; all pulverized and made into 60 pills, with solid ext. of hyoscyamus, enough only to form into pill mass. DOSE—Take 1 pill night and morning one week, then stop a week, and so on every other week.

*Remarks.*—Dr. Gunn, in his "New Family Physician," says of it: "An important remedy, and has cured many cases of epileptic fits, when taken in early stages."

**SALT WASHINGS, DRY RUBBINGS, ETC.—Important in all Chronic Diseases, Especially of an Inflammatory Character.—** In all chronic diseases, and especially diseases of an inflammatory character, as catarrh, throat, bronchial or lung difficulties, inflammation of any or all these parts named, or inflammation of the stomach, liver, kidneys, bladder, urethra, vagina, white swelling, and any or all other swellings or inflammation, and in fact in all conditions and at all times of life, it is of the utmost importance, not only to keep the whole surface clean by bathing or washing, at least twice a week in summer and once a week in winter; but in all chronic or long-standing diseases, it is very important to stimulate the skin by salt-water washings, every other morning (Sunday morning being set for a soap and water washing), followed by brisk rubbing of the whole surface, which equalizes the circulation, helps to break up congestions (an undue amount of blood in any organ or part), putting the whole machinery of the circulatory system (heart, arteries, veins, and the smaller vessels near the surface known as capillaries), into complete working order, without which perfect health cannot be long maintained.

I. *Strength of Salt Water.*—Dissolve ½ a tea-cup of common barrel salt in 3 pints of water (in winter the water should be warm and the bath taken in a warm room; in summer, if the water stands in the room over night, it will do very well without warming); then with a sponge, or what is better, a piece of coarse woolen cloth, wash first the arms, neck and body thoroughly, then the lower limbs and feet, by which time the upper parts will be dry without wiping, when, with another piece of coarse woolen cloth, flesh-brush or hair mitten, rub as hard and long as the friction can be borne, or till the whole surface glows or burns with the heat caused by the free circulation of the blood in the skin. The morning is the best time to do it, as the system is then free from excitement, and, unless you have been too warmly covered, also free from perspiration; therefore, less likely to "take cold." Do not neglect the feet even, but rub all well and thoroughly each time. It is claimed by some physicians that these salt washings and dry rubbings alone will break up and cure many chronic diseases. I know, however, without a good circulation in the skin, health will sooner or later fail. My desire is to impress its importance upon every invalid, for without it not half the speed can be made in curing disease, even with the best of treatment.

II. *Dry Rubbings.*—All other mornings and evenings than those for the salt-water washings, the friction or dry rubbing will materially help to bring about the desired circulation of the blood in the skin, as it draws it away from any inflamed or otherwise diseased organ or part of the system. To be done as you undress for the night, and before dressing in the morning.

III. *Cold Feet.*—In all cases of habitual cold feet, the foregoing plan of washings and rubbings is also of the utmost importance, making the friction, or rubbings, of the lower limbs and feet the most thorough.

**INFLUENZA (A Cold).**—*Symptoms:* A sense of fulness in the mucous membrane of the nose, and a tingling, with dryness, are among the first symptoms of this disease. Sneezing is a common symptom. Shortly, pains are felt in the forehead, and breathing through the nose becomes difficult. The eyes are red and watery, the throat sore, a dry cough, hoarseness, thirst, general languor, chills, and an anxiety to be near the fire. The mucous membrane of the nose, throat, windpipe, and breathing tubes, is inflamed, red, swollen, and occasionally painful.

In a short time water runs from the eyes and nose, and the cough becomes more moist. There is also a slight discharge from the throat and tubes, gradually increasing, and, at length, as the disease becomes less acute, the expectoration is thick and yellow.

An aching of back and limbs, appetite gone, thirst, flashes of heat and chills, whenever the patient is exposed to air cooler than accustomed to, are almost continual attendants upon this complaint.

A slight attack of the above mentioned disease, affecting here and there a person, and lasting but a few days, is called a cold. If it affects a large portion of the community at the same time, lasting days, and even weeks, it is then an epidemic, termed influenza. The latter sometimes sweeps over a whole country, as in 1832, when it extended over a greater part of the universe. In its progress it often shows marked severity, leaving serious results behind.

**Treatment.**—In mild cases treat the disease as you would a severe cold, as only simple treatment is required,—such as remaining in the house for a few days, bathing the feet in warm water, taking a mild sweat, drinking warm infusions of mullein, flax-seed, slippery elm, or warm lemonade, and taking sparingly of vegetable diet. If the bowels are costive, use a gentle physic, likewise a laxative drink will be useful.

When the attack is quite severe, decisive measures must be taken to induce sweating. This may be accomplished by the spirit vapor bath, or by putting bottles of hot water to the patient's feet and sides while in bed, and giving warm drinks, also compound tincture of Virginia snake root. Three drops of the tincture of veratrum viride every three or four hours, will often cause free perspiration, and reduce the inflammation upon the mucous surface.

Emetics are sometimes very useful. Vomiting may be produced by the use of powder of ipecac, ten to twenty grains, or the compound tincture of lobelia.

The inflamed mucous surfaces are soothed very much by inhaling the vapor from half a pint of hot water, with five drops of tincture of veratrum viride, or a like quantity of tincture of aconite root.

If the cough is severe, use the preparations recommended under bronchitis and consumption.

**LA GRIPPE, or Russian Influenza.**—For the last four or five centuries medical observers have noted the occurrence, from time to time, of an epidemic affection characterized by bronchitis (inflammation of the bronchial tubes), it is commonly known by the name of influenza, after a term introduced by the Italian writers in the seventeenth century. The French call it "la grippe." There was a great epidemic of this disease in 1832, and it again made its appearance in the year 1889, being most severe in France, England and the United States. The epidemic is accompanied by more marked and general symptoms than the ordinary influenza.

*Symptoms:* Chills, fever, lassitude, debility, a loss of appetite, and a general prostration. Frontal head-ache is also a prominent feature, but no two persons are affected alike, while some at first are seized with protracted sneezing, others will commence with chills and fever; yet, however, the general run of the disease is the same. It often ends in free perspiration or with diarrhœa. The duration of an attack of "la grippe" is from three to six days, but frequently serious complications arise, such as broncho-pneumonia or capillary bronchitis, and with the old and feeble often proving fatal.

**Dr. S. P. Duffield's Prescription.**—Sulphate quinine, 12 grs.; powdered capsicum, 3 grs. Mix; divide into 12 pills, or put into gelatin capsules. Take one every 3 hours. These pills, if taken at the commencement of the disease, will completely check it. This remedy is well known among the fraternity, and is extensively prescribed.

**1. An Effectual Remedy.**—Sulphate quinine, 20 grs.; sulphate morphine, 1 gr.; powdered capsicum, 3 grs.; tincture aconite root, 6 drops. Mix, and divide in 12 pills or capsules. Take one every 3 hours.

**2. A Good Receipt to Control Fever.**—Liq. Ammon. Acet., 1 oz.; tinct. aconite rad., 12 drops; spirits æther nit., 2 drachms; syr. limonis, enough to make 3 ozs. of the whole; mix. DOSE—1 tea-spoonful with water every hour, until the fever is well under control.

**3. Powders that will Relieve the Headache.**—Acetanilid, ½ drachm. Divide into 6 powders. Take one every 3 or 4 hours, till easy from pain. This is very simple, but the relief that it affords is in some cases astonishing.

**4. A Good Receipt for Children.**—To be taken in doses of one tea-spoonful every 3 hours. This will be found very effective. Sulphate quinine, 24 grs.; wine ipecac, 1 drachm; laudanum, 24 drops; syrup licorice, 3 ozs.

**1. BALM OF GILEAD BUDS, TINCTURE OF—For Cuts, Bruises, etc.**—Take any sized bottle and fill it, loosely, with Balm of Gilead buds, which have been bruised or cut into two or three pieces, then fill with good whiskey or diluted alcohol (half water, half alcohol), cork and shake occasionally for a week or ten days, when it will be ready for use, for wetting bandages applied to cuts, bruises, wounds, sores, etc. (See also "Balm of Gilead Ointment," and remarks following. There is nothing known to be more healing than the Balm of Gilead buds.

**2. For Coughs and Sore Lungs.**—Mix equal parts of honey with the tincture and take 1 or 2 tea-spoonfuls 3 or 4 times a day. It is considered expectorant, diuretic and somewhat stimulant and tonic.

**TUMORS, POISONED WOUNDS, AND WILD VINE POISONINGS—Earth Cure for.**—Take the stratum of clay used for making the best red brick, which lies immediately below the soil, Dry in the sun so it can be put through a sieve; keep in air-tight jars; mix with hot water until of the consistency of putty, and apply warm, with a knife, over the tumor, half an inch thick; cover with light brown paper, then bandage with a good strong bandage, and keep it on 24 to 48 hours. This has caused some wonderful cures, I am told. It is also good for some forms of rheumatism, dropsy and poisoned wounds.—*Housekeeper.*

*Remarks.*—I have no knowledge, only my judgment, as to the value of this for tumors, but knowing the clay cure to be positive in drawing out the poisonous effects, swelling, soreness, etc., when poisoned by ivy, I know it will be valuable in poisoned wounds and, I believe, even good for mad dog bites, if applied quickly after cauterizing; and, therefore, I judge it good for tumors. The clay is very absorbing. I should, however, change it as often as the covering gets dry. (See also Poisoning by Poison Ivy, etc.)

**DIURETICS, VALUABLE.—I.** Buchu and uva ursi, leaves of each, 1 oz.; pareira brava root, 1 oz. Mix and divide into 3 powders or parcels, evenly. DIRECTIONS AND DOSE—Pour upon one of these parts a quart of boiling water, in a covered tin pail or fruit jar. When cool enough to drink, take 1 to 3 moderate swallows every 2 or 3 hours, so as to increase the flow of urine, which will use up the quart in about 2 days. If to be kept longer, 6 ozs of good gin will prevent its souring, if strained from the dregs. Used in catarrh of the bladder, irritation of the kidneys, uretha, etc.

**II.** Take buchu leaves, 2 ozs., and treat as in I.; when cool add 1 tea-spoonful of bi-carbonate of soda, and 30 drops of fl. ex. of hyoscyamus, and drink all in 2 days. Use more than the above in cases where there is mucus of a stringy character passed in the urine. After a day or two, repeat the same until relieved. If much irritation of the uretha, get 1 oz. of sub-nitrate of bismuth and put into 8 ozs. of soft water, and inject ½ oz. into the urethra 3 times daily, shaking before pouring out; else, obtain "Humphrey's Marvel of Healing," and add 3 times as much water as of the "Marvel," and inject in its place. Either is excellent. Retain them 2 or 3 minutes, whichever is used. These are good for any case requiring diuretics.

**HOT WATER CURE—Directions for Using.**—The following instructions as to the manner of using hot water as a means of restoring health to a generally debilitated or exhausted system, I take from the *Medical Brief,* thinking the explanation and directions here given will enable many of our readers to obtain additional helps. over and above what are given under the head of Hot Water in Consumption, Dyspepsia, etc. I have been unable to find where Dr. Salisbury's institute is located, or anything further than given in this quotation, and the different items referred to in this book. as above indicated; but as I have been using it with satisfaction in several cases of dyspepsia I think it will be found generally useful. I will here say that I recommend the water to be heated to 140° F. in summer, and 145° to 150° in winter, in quantity about ½ to ¾ of a pint as a general thing, and taken about ½ to ¾ of an hour before meals. If one should be very thirsty at bed-time, then also, but not unless necessary to allay thirst.

I. *"The Water Must be Hot, Not Cold Nor Lukewarm.*—This is to excite peristalsis (like peristaltic, a successive contraction and relaxing of the muscular coats) of the alimentary canal. Cold water depresses, as it uses animal heat to bring it up to the temperature of the economy (body), and there is also a loss of nerve force in the proceeding. Lukewarm water excites upward peristalsis, or vomiting, as is well-known. By hot water is meant a temperature of 110° to 150° Fahrenheit, such as is commonly liked in the use of tea and coffee. In cases of hemorrhage, the temperature should be at blood heat (98° F.). Ice-water is disallowed in all cases, sick or well.

II. *"Quantity of Hot Water at a Draught.*—Dr. Salisbury first began with one-half pint of hot water, but he found that it was not enough to wash out, nor to bear another test founded on the physiological fact that the urine of a healthy babe suckling a healthy mother—the best standard of health—stands at a specific gravity varying from 1.015 to 1.020. The urine of the patient should be made to conform to this standard, and the daily use of the urinometer (an instrument for telling the specific gravity of the urine, but not generally necessary to have nor obtain except in hot-water cures) tells whether the patient drinks enough or too much hot water.

"For example, if the specific gravity of the urine stands at 1.030°, more hot water should be drank, unless there is loss by sweating. On the other hand, should the specific gravity of the urine fall to 1.010, less hot water should be drank. The quantity of hot water varies usually from ½ pt. to 1½ pts. at one time of drinking.

"The urine to be tested should be the *urina sanguinis*, or·that passed just after rising from bed in the morning, before any meals or drinks are taken.

"The quantity of urine voided in 24 hours should measure from 48 to 64 ozs. (1½ to 2 qts.). The amount will, of course, vary somewhat with the temperature of the atmosphere, exercise, sweating, etc., but the hot water must be given so as to keep the specific gravity of the infant's standard, to wit: 1.015 to 1.020. The urinometer will detect, at once, whether the proper amount of hot water has been drank, no matter whether the patient is present or absent. Another test is that of odor. The urine should be devoid of the rank *urinous* smell, so well known, but indescribable. [The absence of this "rank smell" is a sufficient guide for home tests; take enough to get rid of this rank odor, is all sufficient.]

"The Salisbury Plans aim for this in all cases, and when the patients are true and faithful, the aim is realized. [If a patient will not be true to himself, or herself, you may as well give up trying at once.]

III. *"Times of Taking Hot Water.*—One to two hours before each meal, and half an hour before retiring at night. [I have taken it myself, and so recommended to others, half or three-fourths of an hour, only, before each meal, and have never known vomiting, or even sickness of the stomach to arise.]

"At first, Dr. Salisbury tried the time of one-half hour before meals, but this was apt to be followed by vomiting. [I have not so found it.] One hour to 2 hours allows the hot water time enough to get out of the stomach before the food enters, or sleep comes, and thus avoids vomiting. Four times a day gives an amount of hot water sufficient to bring the urine to the right specific gravity, quantity, color, odor, and freedom from deposit, on cooling. [There is probably something of importance in these points, but I have, as yet, at any rate, only recommended to take it 3 times daily, unless thirsty at bed-time.] If a patient leaves out one dose of hot water during the day, the omission will show in the increased specific gravity (weight, by the urinometer), in the color, etc. Should the patient be thirsty between meals, 8 ozs. (half pint) of hot water can be taken any time between 2 hours after a meal and 1 hour before the next meal. This is to avoid diluting the food in the stomach with water.

IV. *"Mode of Taking Hot Water.*—In drinking the hot water, it should be sipped, and not drank so fast as to distend the stomach and make it feel uncomfortable. From 15 to 20 minutes may be consumed in drinking the hot water. [About 5 minutes time is all the author took in drinking the hot water, and all he recommends; still, if 1 to 1½ pts. are to be taken, a longer time will be needed. But, for ordinary cases of home treatment, I think ½ to ¾ pt. is enough, and especially so if it is taken 4 times daily.]

V. *" The Length of Time to Continue the Use of Hot Water.*—Six months is generally required to wash out the liver and intestines thoroughly. As it promotes health the procedure can be practiced by well people throughout life, and the benefits of cleanliness be enjoyed. The drag and friction on human existence from the effects of fermentation, foulness and indigestible food, when removed by this process, gives life a wonderful elasticity and buoyancy.

VI. *"Additions to Hot Water.*—To make it palatable, in case it is desired, and to medicate it, aromatic spirits of ammonia, clover blossom tea, ginger, lemon juice, sage, salt and sulphate of magnesia (epsom salts), are sometimes added. When there is intense thirst, and dryness, a pinch of chloride of calcium (chloride of lime) or nitrate of potash (niter) may be added, to allay the thirst and leave a moistened film over the parched and dry mucus membrane surfaces. When there is diarrhea, cinnamon, ginger or pepper may be boiled in the water, and the quantity drank, lessened. For constipation, a tea-spoonful of sulphate of magnesia, or ½ tea-spoonful of *taraxacum* (dandelion fl. ex.) may be used in the hot water.

VII. *"Amount of Liquid (Tea, Caffee or Water) to be Drank at a Meal.*—Not more than 8 ozs." [½ pt. or 1 cup of tea or coffee.] "This is in order not to dilute the gastric juice, or wash it out prematurely, and thus interfere with the digestion process.

VIII. *" The Effects of Drinking Hot Water, as indicated, are:*—The improved feelings of the patient. The fæces (passages) become black with bile, washed down its normal (natural, or healthy) channel. This blackness of fæces lasts for more than six months (I have not found this so, but it may be in some cases), or until the intolerable fetid odor of ordinary fæces is abated (this I have found true), and the smell aproximates the smell of healthy infants sucking healthy breasts, and this shows that the ordinary nuisance of fetid (bad smelling) fæces is due to a want of working out and cleansing the alimentary canal from its fermenting contents. The urine is clear as champaign, free from deposit and odor, or coloring, 1.015 to 1.020 specific gravity, like infants urine. The sweat starts freely after drinking, giving a true bath from center to surface. The skin becomes healthy in feeling and looks. The digestion is correspondingly improved, and with this improvement comes a better working of the machine." [Human system as a whole.] "All thirst and dry mucus membranes disappear in a few days, and a moist condition of the mucus membrane, and the skin, takes place. Ice water in hot weather is not craved for and those who have drank ice water freely are cured of the propensity. Inebriety has a strong foe in the use of hot water."

*Remarks.*—The author finds, by personal use of hot water, nearly all the foregoing statements of the *Brief* to be facts, and I especially hope the last statement shall so prove that "inebriety has a strong foe in the use of hot water," and I feel almost sorry I cannot attest to this from a personal knowledge, so anxious am I to do good to my fellow-creatures, knowing, as I do, how much confidence the statement of a fact with which the author has positive knowledge helps one to have faith enough in any certain thing to give it a trial. Let none needing it for that purpose, or any other given here and in other parts of this book, for all purposes indicated here or there, fail to try it. The author, however, can give no greater assurance of his own confidence in the use of hot water than to say that I now arise to go and heat water to take myself, half an hour before my supper, for it does me good, stops all craving for cold drinks and allays all feverishness of stomach, bowels, etc., etc., of this hot day, the thermometer reaching 90° Fahrenheit in my office at 3 P. M:

**MEASLES.**—This is a contagious or "catching" eruption, and would be a disease of less severity were it not sometimes followed by serious results. It is a disease peculiar to childhood, although persons well along in years sometimes have them. As children have them easier than adults, it is advisable to take no special precaution to prevent them. They usually appear in from 7 to 14 days after exposure.

*Symptoms.*—The first symptoms of measles are shivering, succeeded by heat, thirst and languor; then follows running at the nose, sneezing, cough; the eyes water and become intolerant of light; the pulse quickens, and the face swells; there are successive heats and chills, and all the usual signs of catarrhal fever. Sometimes the symptoms are so mild as to be scarcely noticeable, and sometimes greatly aggravated; but in any case, at the end of the third day, or a little later, an eruption of a dusky red color appears, first on the forehead and face, and then gradually all over the whole body. In the early stage of this eruption there is little to characterize it, but after a few hours it assumes the peculiar appearance, which once seen can never be mistaken. The little red spots become grouped, as it were, into crescent-shaped patches, which are slightly elevated above the surface, the surrounding skin retaining its natural color. On the third day of the eruption it begins to fade and disappear, being succeeded by a scurfy disorganization of the cuticle, which is accompanied by an intolerable itching. The febrile symptoms also abate, and very quickly leave the patient altogether, but often in a very weak state and with a troublesome cough. Between exposure to the infection and the breaking out of measles, there is usually an interval of 14 days, which is called the period of incubation; so that it is not uncommon, where there are several children in a family, for the cases to succeed each other at fortnightly intervals.

This disease is often rendered dangerous by complications with others; so that, not in itself of a fatal character, it frequently leads to fatal results. Where there are the seeds of consumption or scrofula in the constitution, they are likely to be called into activity during the debility which follows an attack of measles; dropsy often follows it, as do affections of the air passages, chest and bowels.

**How to Distinguish Measles from Scarlet Fever.**— Measles is a less dangerous disease than scarlet fever, although sometimes mistaken for it in the early stages. In measles the spots are not as deeply colored as in scarlet fever, and are differently shaped and rougher to the touch. In scarlet fever the spots usually appear on the second day after the first symptoms are observed, and in measles on the third or fourth day. The irritation of the nose, sneezing and discharge, that are prominent symptoms in measles, do not occur in scarlet fever.

TREATMENT.—Generally speaking, for simple measles, little medicine is required. Give the patient plenty of diluent drinks; let him have a spare diet, and a moderately warm and well-ventilated room; keep the bowels gently open; if a roasted apple, or a little manna in the drink will not do this, give a dose of castor-oil. Where there is much heat of the skin, sponging with tepid vinegar and water will completely relieve it, and also the itching. When the eruption has subsided, and the desquammation of the skin commenced, a tepid bath will materially assist this process, and get rid of the dead cuticle. On the third or fourth day after the disappearance of the eruption, give a small dose of powder of rhubarb, jalap, or scammony. Care should be taken to protect the patient against change of weather, and to restore the strength by a nourishing diet. Attention should be paid to the cough. Give drinks of flaxseed tea or slippery elm, made slightly acid.

If the attack is severe, attended with high fever, headache, restlessness, etc., the feet should be placed in a hot mustard bath for 10 or 15 minutes, after which place the patient in bed warmly covered, giving every hour until the fever subsides and sweating takes place, Fluid Extract of Aconite, 1 drop to a tea-spoonful of water; and every 2 hours, or until the pulse is reduced in frequency, give 1 drop Fluid Extract of Veratrum Viride similarly diluted.

Cold water may be taken freely with benefit in this as well as all in other eruptive or miasmatic fevers. A very good drink can be prepared by making a bowlful of slippery elm infusion, and adding the juice of a lemon and a table-spoonful of cream of tartar, and using as a drink as the patient desires.

SCARLET FEVER.

MEASLES.

The bowels should be regulated by the Compound Podophyllin Pills, or the Compound powder of Jalap.

The diet should be light, and consist largely of ripe cooked fruits, gruels, broths, and other easily digestible articles.

Sore throat should be relieved by inhalation of hot vinegar, or by a gargle of Carbolic Acid, 2 drops to 1 ounce of water. If the eyes should become irritated and inflamed, they may be relieved by a cool wash of slippery elm, alum curd, rose leaves, or moist tea grounds taken from the pot.

**To Bring them Out.**—In cases where the eruption does not appear, warm whiskey sling or the Compound Tincture of Virginia Snake Root may be given to bring it out.

**2.** Sometimes when warm drinks fail to bring them out, drinking largely of cold water, and keeping warmly covered in bed, will produce the desired effect.

**3.** The following will be found most efficient: Strong balm tea with a little saffron infused, or hot ears of corn, wrapped in a cloth saturated with diluted vinegar, placed about the body.

**Striking in.**—Sometimes the eruption of measles disappears suddenly—then there is cause for alarm, and energetic treatment required; the patient should be directly put into a warm bath, and have warm diluent drinks; if the pulse sinks rapidly, and there is great prostration of strength, administer wine whey, and the following draughts: 10 drops of aromatic spirits of ammonia, or 5 grains of the sesquicarbonate in ½ an ounce of camphor mixture, with a drop of laudanum every four hours; should the prostration be very great, weak brandy and water may be given. The state of the chest, head, and bowels should be closely watched for some time after the patient is convalescent, as disorders of these organs are very likely to occur, in which case it is probable that there may be pneumonia, hydrocephalus, or diarrhea.

**2.** Apply mustard poultices to the feet, ankles, wrists, and over the whole abdomen, letting the poultices remain a few minutes and until they produce considerable redness.

Severe cases of measles are liable to be accompanied with pneumonia, and where there are decided symptoms of this, the Hop Fomentation (see below) should be applied over the whole chest, with warm applications to the feet and legs. The frequent inhalation of the vapor of hot vinegar should be employed.

Chronic sore eyes, diarrhea, a lingering cough, etc., are liable to follow severe cases of measles, and these should be treated according to the indications of each individual case.

**Malignant Measles.**—This is a variety which commences with the above symptoms in an aggravated form; the rash quickly assumes a livid hue, alternately reviving and disappearing, and is mixed up with dark red spots like flea-bites; in this form of the disease we have extreme debility and all the symptoms of putrid fever. like which it should be treated. No time should be lost in procuring medical aid

*Herbal or Eclectic Treatment for Measles.*—A strong tea composed of saffron and snake root always proves beneficial. Decoctions of licorice, marshmallow roots and sarsaparilla are likewise beneficial. Sudden changes should be guarded against, and especially exposure to cold draughts, the room, however, should be kept moderately cool. No animal food should at first be taken. but the patient confined to low, spare diet, such as sage, gruel, etc. A good drink may be made of barley water, acidulated with lemon juice.

**HOT FOMENTATIONS AND POULTICES.**—Hot fomentations are serviceable in treating many forms of disease, and in some they are indispensable. Hops, stramonium or jimson weed, tansy, hoarhound, catnip, lobelia, etc., either in the herb or in tincture, are among the most common agents employed. The herbs should be simmered in water, or vinegar and water, until their strength responds to the liquid, when they should be placed between thin muslin cloths, applied as hot as the patient can bear, and covered with a number of thicknesses of heated cloths. Material should be prepared for two applications, so that as one is removed the other may be applied. The same application may be used over and over, using the liquid in which it was steeped, or adding hot water to keep it moist. They should be changed every 5 to 8 minutes, using care not to expose the part to the cold air during the changes, When using tinctures instead of herbs, prepare a lotion by adding to a sufficient quantity of water, or vinegar and water, or whiskey and water, so much of the tincture as will give it the requisite strength, warm the lotion and place it where it will keep warm, and saturate and wring from it several thicknesses of flannel or muslin, applying hot to the part as in other cases. Vinegar or whiskey should form an ingredient, if practicable, in any fomentation, and hops form a good combination with other ingredients when not used alone.

**Hop Fomentation.**—In bilious colic, inflammation of the lungs, and other cases requiring energetic treatment, the best fomentation is made as follows: Take a quart of vinegar, put in a kettle, and add as much hops as the vinegar will take up; boil them together for 5 or 10 minutes, and stir in as much corn meal as will made the whole into a thick mush. The meal is added simply to give consistence to the mass so as to retain the heat and not wet the bedding. If corn meal is not at hand, shorts, or bran and flour mixed together, will do. Spread this thickly upon an ample piece of muslin cloth (if 2 or 3 inches thick all the better), and apply hot. If too hot to be applied next the skin, lay folds of cloth between. The essential point is to get the heat and the fullest effects of the hops and vinegar as soon as possible, and to hold their effect as long as possible.

**Hot Mustard Foot Bath.**—Prepare a bucket or tub, the same as for an ordinary foot bath, filling it a third to half full of water as hot as the patient can bear with comfort. Put in it about two table-spoonfuls of ground mustard (more or less, according to the degree of strength desired). Provide a reserve of hot water (boiling hot, or nearly so), and after keeping the feet in the bath for a short time, add hot water to keep up the temperature, keeping it as hot as the patient can bear for ten or fifteen minutes. The parts should then be gently dried and warmly wrapped.

**Slippery Elm Poultice.**—Take of slippery elm bark, in powder, half an ounce, and a sufficient amount of hot water to form a poultice of the proper consistence. This poultice is valuable in all cases of burns, scalds, swellings, inflammations, ulcers, painful tumors, abscesses, and wherever a general soothing emollient poultice is required.

**Yeast Poultice.**—Applicable to sores and indolent ulcers. Made by taking 5 ounces of yeast and a pound of flour (or in that proportion), and adding to water at blood heat, so as to form a tolerably stiff dough; set in a warm place (but not so as to scald) until it begins to ferment or to "rise," and apply like any poultice.

**MUMPS.**—This disease, which is a contagious epidemic, consists of inflammation of the salivary or parotid glands, which are situated on each side of the lower jaw.

SYMPTOMS.—It commences with slight febrile symptoms of a general character. Very soon there is a redness and swelling at the angle of the jaw, which gradually extends to the face and neck near to the glands. These sometimes become so large as to hang down a considerable distance, like two bags.

They may come on suddenly, or else be preceded by a few days of general indisposition, which now and then amounts to high fever. A feeling of stiffness about the jaws is soon followed by swelling, often very bulky, and more or less tense. The swelling is apt to extend either at the back of the lower jaw or underneath it. The swelling contains no fluid; dental pain is absent. Generally first one side of the jaw is attacked and then the other; it is rare for both sides to suffer simultaneously. Not uncommonly similar swellings burst out in other localities of the body, the genital organs being most liable to seizure.

TREATMENT.—But little medical treatment is required for this disease when at its height. The patient, from sheer inability to move the jaw, must live chiefly on slops; and it is well for him to be kept low, unless very delicate, in which case a little good broth or beef tea should be given. If there is much pain, the throat should have hot fomentations applied; and, in very severe cases, two or three leeches. Mumps is not a dangerous disorder, unless the inflammation should be turned inwards, in which case it will probably affect the brain or testicles; or, in the female, the breasts. Should the swellings suddenly disappear, and thereby aggravate the symptoms of fever, the following liniment must be applied: Camphorated spirits, 1 oz.; solution of sub-carbonate of ammonia, 2 drams; tincture of cantharides, ½ dram. Mix, and rub in until the swellings re-appear. Take also, internally, nitrate of potass, 1 dram; tartarised antimony 1½ grs. Mix, and divide into six powders, one of which is to be taken every four hours.

**Camphor for Mumps.**—Camphor is said to have been used successfully to reduce the after-swelling in mumps; in the case of males holding the pendant parts in a basin of spirits of camphor, and bathing the adjacent parts freely with it, continuing or renewing the application until relief is had. If it occasion smarting more than the patient can bear, the liquid may be diluted with water.

**CHICKEN POX.**—Chicken-pox is an eruptive disease which affects children and occasionally adults. It is attended only with slight constitutional disturbance, and is therefore neither a distressing nor dangerous affection. The eruption first appears on the body, afterwards on the neck, the scalp, and lastly on the face. It appears on the second or third day after the attack, and is succeeded by vesicles containing a transparent fluid. These begin to dry on the fifth, sixth or seventh day. This disease may be distinguished from variola and varioloid by the shortness of the period of invasion, the mildness of the symptoms and the absence of the deep, funnel-shaped depression of the vesicles, so noticeable in variola. The main distinctions between chicken-pox and small-pox are the absence or extreme mildness of the premonitory fever in the former disease, and the form and contents of the vesicles; those of the latter eruption being filled with dark matter, and having, invariably, a depression in the center.

TREATMENT—Ordinarily very little treatment is required. It is best to use daily an alkaline bath, and as a drink, the tea of pleurisy-root, catnip or other diaphoretics, to which is added from half to a spoonful of extract of smart-weed, or the patient should be put upon spare diet; this, and a dose or two of some cooling aperient, as rhubarb or magnesia, is generally all that is necessary; but should the febrile symptoms run high, give a saline draught, as the following: Carbonate of potash, 1 scruple; citric or tartaric acid, 15 grains; essence of cinnamon, ½ a dram; syrup of orange peel, 1 dram; water, 10 ounces. Shake, and drink while sparkling a wineglassful as a refrigerant. To make it effervescing, add the acid after the draught is poured out. Give plenty of cooling drink, and, if the bowels are at all obstinate, emollient injections. Care must be taken that the skin is not irritated by scratching—as it is, painful and troublesome sores may be produced—and also that the patient does not take a chill. If these precautions are observed, little or no danger is to be apprehended from chicken-pox.

**YELLOW FEVER.**—This disease is peculiar to hot climates and is a species of typhus, which takes its name from one of the symptoms, but which, however, is not an essential one. It is probably caused by a vitiated state of the atmosphere arising from decayed vegetable or animal substances, in hot, sultry weather. It is very contagious and an epidemic.

*Symptoms.*—Costiveness, dull pain in the right side, defect of appetite, flatulence, perverted tastes, heat in the stomach, giddiness or pain in the head; dull, watery, yellow eye; dim or imperfect vision, hoarseness, slight sore throat, and the worst features of typhus.

TREATMENT.—In this disease, good nursing is indispensable. Let the patient have perfect rest and quietness, in a well ventilated room. In the early stages of the disease, the diet must be confined to preparations of sago, arrow-root, barley, etc.; but as the disease advances, give animal broths made of lean

SMALL POX.

CHICKEN POX.

meat, thickened with bread-crumbs, oat-meal, or barley. The strictest attention must be given to cleanliness, and the linen changed frequently. If the stomach be very irritable and the vomiting violent, give the following preparation : Powdered rhubarb, 20 grains; powdered saleratus, 20 grains; powdered peppermint, 1 tea-spoonful; laudanum, 15 drops; brandy, 1 table-spoonful; boiling water, 1 gill. Mix. Sweeten with loaf-sugar, and give a table-spoonful every hour till the symptoms change. The bowels must be kept open as in all fevers. For this purpose use the following: Ginger, 2 ounces; bayberry bark, 4 ounces; cayenne pepper, ½ ounce.

Dose, a tea-spoonful in a little milk, with half a tea-spoonful of powdered rhubarb every hour till it operates freely.

Captain Jonas P. Levy, who has had an extensive experience with yellow fever, states that he never knew a case of yellow fever terminate fatally under the following treatment:

Dissolve a table-spoonful of common salt in a wineglass of water; pour it into a tumbler, and add the juice of a whole lemon and 2 wineglasses of castor-oil. An adult to take the whole at one dose. Then give a hot mustard foot-bath, with a handful of salt in the water. Wrap the patient in blankets until he perspires freely. Remove to the bed, and well wrap the patient's feet in the blanket. Afterward apply mustard plasters to the abdomen, legs, and soles of the feet. If the headache is very severe, they may be applied to the head and temples. After the fever has been broken, taken 40 grains of quinine and 40 drops of elixir of vitriol to a quart of water. Give a wineglass full three times a day. Barley-water, lemonade and ice-water may be used in moderation.

**CHOLERA MORBUS.**—This is a disease prevalent in warm weather. From the great amount of bile secreted it is also called bilious cholera.

*Causes.*—Excessive heat, sudden atmospheric changes, indigestible food, unripe fruits. Dampness, wet feet and violent passions will also cause it.

*Symptoms.*—This disease begins with sickness and distress at the stomach, succeeded by violent gripings, with vomiting of thin, dirty, yellowish, whitish, or greenish fluid, with discharges from the bowels similar to that vomited. The nausea and distress continue between the vomiting and purging, and the pain at times is intense. The pulse is rapid, soon becoming small and feeble, the tongue dry, the urine high-colored, and there is much thirst, though no drink can be retained on the stomach.

TREATMENT.—Apply a large mustard poultice over the stomach and liver. Give large draughts of warm teas, by which means the stomach will be cleansed of all its solid contents. Every half-hour give table-spoonful doses of the compound powder of rhubarb and potassa, until the vomiting is checked. Warm injections must be given frequently, and hot bricks applied to the feet, while the whole body should be swathed in warm flannels. To get up a warmth of the body and the stomach is, in fact, the most important thing in this disease. Hot brandy, in which is a dose of cayenne, is excellent to quiet the vomiting and griping. A few drops of laudanum in the injections may be given, if pain is excessive; but generally it is not needed.

Either of the following have been found useful: Bicarbonate of soda, 12 grs.; common salt, 6 grs.; chlorate of potash, 6 grs. Mix and take in cold water. Or the following: Acetate of lead, 20 grs.; opium, 12 grs. Make into 12 pills and take one every half hour until looseness ceases.

*Eclectic or Herbal Treatment for Cholera Morbus.*—No time must be lost in treating the severe stages of this disease. Give the patient copious drinks of whey, warm barley-water, thin water gruel, or weak chicken broth. Bathe the feet and legs in warm saleratus water, and apply warm fomentations of hops and vinegar to the bowels. In addition to these, apply a poultice of well-stewed garden mint, or a poultice of mustard and strong vinegar will be found of much service. The vomiting and purging may be stopped by the following: Ground black pepper, 1 table-spoonful; table salt, 1 table-spoonful; warm water, ½ tumblerful; cider vinegar, ½ tumblerful. Dose, a table-spoonful every few minutes. Stir and mix each time until the whole is taken.

The evacuations, however, should not be stopped till the patient feels very weak. Nourishing diet should be taken by the patient. A wineglass of cold camomile tea once or twice a day would be very beneficial, as would ten drops of elixir of vitriol three or four times a day, or a tea made of black or Virginia snake-root. Flannel should be worn next to the skin, and the warm bath should be frequently resorted to.

**CHOLERA INFANTUM,** otherwise known as the summer complaint of children, has been by some regarded as belonging exclusively to America. It has been ascertained, however, that this disease prevails in Europe, where it is called by a different name. It usually attacks children under four years of age, and generally between the months of June and October.

*Symptoms.*—There is at first diarrhea and the stools are sometimes of a watery, colorless consistence; at others they have a greenish-yellow appearance; the pulse is quick, the head and abdomen are hot, while the limbs are cold. The child seems to suffer more or less pain, as indicated by its crying, and frequently screams as if suffering acutely. The disease often terminates unfavorably and sometimes within a few hours; again, it continues for several weeks, and the little sufferer becomes very much emaciated, his eyes sunken, countenance pale, and yet a recovery is possible.

*Causes.*—From the fact that it oftener occurs during the summer months than at any other time of the year, it may be inferred that the temperature greatly influences the prevalence of this disease. It more frequently attacks the poorer classes, or those living in unhealthy sections, although the children of the wealthy are likewise subject to it. Teething, change of diet at the time of weaning, and unhealthy, diluted milk, may be the exciting causes of this disease so common to children.

Cholera infantum is more prevalent in our large cities, it being comparatively unknown in rural districts. Often these little sufferers are greatly improved by a trip into the country or to the sea-shore. Pure air and fresh sweet milk, as hygienic and dietetic adjuncts, are necessary for recovery.

TREATMENT.—The first treatment should be *preventive*. The little patient should be placed in a well ventilated room. Next, attend to the diet, and ascertain if the milk be pure and healthy. If the child nurses, then the mother should properly regard her diet. She should not eat unripe or stale fruits or vegetables, but her food should be nutritious and easily digested. She should not overwork, nor heat her blood, neither should she allow herself to become excited and irritable. She should occasionally give the child some milk alkali to obviate undue acidity of the stomach. Scalding the milk, or using a little lime-water in it, is sometimes beneficial. The following can be obtained at almost any drug store: Syrup of rhubarb, 2 ounces; lime-water, 4 drachms (about 4 tea-spoonfuls), and water of peppermint 2 drachms. Give of this mixture, to a child one year old, 1 tea-spoonful every hour until it acts on the bowels as a laxative, which may be known by the changed appearance of the passages. Follow this with small doses of compound extract of smart-weed and cover the bowels with cloths wet with the same. This treatment I have employed with perfect success in my own family and also with the same uniformly happy results in the general practice of medicine.

**SALT RHEUM, or ECZEMA.**—In this disease the minute blood vessels are congested, causing the skin to be more vascular and redder than in the natural state. There is an itching or smarting sensation in the affected parts and the skin is raised in the form of little pimples and a watery substance exudes. This disease usually attacks the hands, and depends very much upon the occupation and habits of the person. Washerwomen, and those whose hands are exposed to the action of flour, soap, wax, resin, etc., are most subject to it.

TREATMENT.—All soaps and alkalies, and lead preparations, should be avoided. Wash the hands only in warm water, to which may be added some oatmeal or cornmeal, or a little oxalic acid or vinegar. The following prescription is an excellent external application: Stramonium ointment, 1 ounce; carbolic acid, 10 grains. Mix thoroughly together. First wash the part affected with warm water and oatmeal and cornmeal, then dry thoroughly, and apply the ointment, bandage, and let remain all night.

2. Make a wash of warm water and oatmeal, cleanse the part with it, and dry with a soft cloth; bathe with tincture of iodine, let it dry, and apply carbolic acid mixed with sweet cream, about 5 drops of the acid to a tea-spoonful of cream.

3. Take of beef marrow, sulphur, black pepper, white turpentine, equal parts; mix, make an ointment, and apply, cleansing as otherwise directed.

**SCALD HEAD.**—This is a disease of the scalp, and at first consists of minute pustules around the roots of the hair. These pustules increase in size and number until the entire scalp becomes covered by one dense and uniform crust. The disease is contagious, and is caused by the presence of parasites.

TREATMENT.—Cut the hair as closely as possible; wash the head with cas-tile soap and water, then apply at night on going to bed a large flaxseed meal poultice and let remain until morning, when the poultice should be removed, and with it all loose incrustations. This poultice should be applied from time to time, if there should any new crusts form. On removing the poultice cleanse the scalp with carbolic acid soap and warm water, then use the following oint-ment: Carbolic acid, 10 grs.; vaseline, 2 ozs. Mix, and apply every morning sufficient to anoint slightly all the diseased parts. Wash the scalp each time with carbolic acid soap before applying the ointment.

To increase the general tone of the system, the muriate tincture of iron in 5 drop doses may be given in 1 table-spoonful of water, 3 times daily.

THRUSH.—This is one of the most common diseases of infancy. It is characterized by a peculiar eruption of minute pustules, and a whitish incrusta-tion of the tongue.

*Symptoms.*—There are generally much thirst, restlessness, languor, acid and flatulent eructations, loose and griping stools, drowsiness, pain, difficulty of sucking, and a copious flow of saliva from the mouth. The stomach and bowels are almost always prominently disordered, and the infant is apt to vomit after taking anything into its stomach. The abdomen is often sore to the touch, and great difficulty of swallowing is experienced. Feeble and sickly children scarcely ever escape this disease; children, also, who are kept in crowded or ill-ventilated apartments are especially liable to it.

TREATMENT.—The first object is to restore the healthy condition of the stomach and bowels, if disordered. Where the ejections from the stomach are sour, and the alvine evacuations of a grass-green color, from 3 to 4 grains of magnesia, with 2 grains of rhubarb, and 1 of powdered valerian should be given every two or three hours until the bowels are freely evacuated. If there is much general irritability and restlessness after this, the tepid bath, followed by a drop or two of laudanum, should be employed. The mucous membrane of the intestines is apt to become highly irritated in severe cases; the alvine evacu-ations in such instances are frequent, watery, and streaked with blood. When these symptoms are present, a large emollient poultice should be applied over the abdomen in conjunction with the internal use of minute portions of Dover's powder, with a solution of gum arabic as drink. Borax is a familiar remedy with nurses and mothers as well as the profession. It may be used either in form of powder or in solution. If the former is employed, 2 or 3 grains of it, mixed with a small portion of pulverized loaf sugar, must be thrown into the mouth every 2 or 3 hours; if the solution be used, a drachm of the borax should be dissolved in 2 ozs. of water, and applied to the mouth with a soft linen rag tied to the extremity of a pliable piece of whalebone, or with a soft feather. The practice of forcibly rubbing off the eruption is extremely reprehensible; for, when rubbed off in this way, the crust is soon renewed in an aggravated form. Where the mouth is very red, livid or ulcerated, we must have recourse to a decoction of bark. A ½ oz. of powdered bark, boiled about 30 minutes in ½ pt. of water, will make a suitable decoction; and of this about the third of a tea-spoonful may be put into the child's mouth every hour or two.

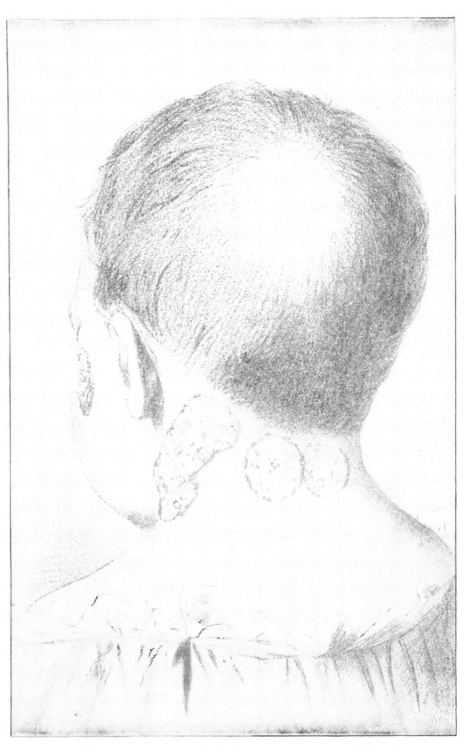

TINEA TRICHOPHYTOSIS CIRCIRNATUS, OR RING-WORM.

1. **WATERBRASH.**—Pyrosis is the medical name for this disease, but it is usually called Waterbrash. It is a peculiar affection of the stomach, in which the patient brings up frequently a considerable quantity of thin watery liquid, sometimes insipid, at others intensely acid. Before the fluid is brought up, often there is more or less pain experienced at the pit of the stomach. This complaint attacks, mostly, persons past the middle age, particularly females, and the fit comes on generally in the morning and afternoon. It usually begins with a severe pain in the pit of the stomach, attended with a feeling of constriction or oppression, and soon after a quantity of thin watery fluid is thrown up, which is sometimes insipid, at other times it has a highly acid or burning taste. The causes of this complaint are various, but whatever disorders the stomach may give rise to it. It appears to be owing to a peculiar state of irritation of the stomach; and is most certainly relieved by the use of the white oxide of bismuth, from 2 to 3 grs. made into pills with extract of gentian, 3 times a day. This medicine will often perfectly cure waterbrash; but attention to the diet, as laid down under dyspepsia, is of much consequence, and will be absolutely necessary in order to render the cure permanent. A diet of plain animal food may be allowed, with which may be united the use of biscuits, home-made bread, and preparations of rice and milk. Daily exercise must also be taken, and frictions, with the flesh-brush, over the region of the stomach and bowels, are of no small service. The bowels must of course be kept open by purgatives, when necessary, even when making use of other curative means.

2. Plump wheat carefully burned to a charcoal, and powdered, a teaspoonful into the nursing bottle before filling it, once a day. The same, taken before each meal, is good for dyspepsia.

1. **RINGWORM.**—A disease of the skin appearing in small circular patches, or rings of vesicles round the circumference of a circle of apparently healthy skin: these vesicles are small, and contain a transparent fluid, which is discharged in three or four days, when little dark scabs form over them. Sometimes there is a succession of the circles on the upper parts of the body, as the face and neck, and the arms and shoulders.

The more formidable and infectious species of ringworm appears in distinct patches of an irregularly circular figure, on the scalp, head, and neck. It commences with clusters of small light yellow pustules, which soon break and form thin scabs over each patch; and these, if neglected, become thick and hard by gathering on one another. If the scabs are removed, however, the surface of the patches is left red and shining, but studded with white elevated points, in some of which, minute globules of pus again appear in a few days. As the patches extend, the hair covering them becomes lighter in its color, and sometimes breaks off short; and as this process is repeated, the roots of the hair are destroyed, and at length, there remains uninjured only a narrow border of hair round the head. It generally occurs in children of three or four years old and upwards, and often continues for several years. It can be considered as about to terminate, only when the redness and exfoliations disappear together, and the hair begins to grow of its natural color and texture.  The disease seems to originate spontaneously in children of feeble and flabby habit, or in a state approaching to marasmus; who are ill fed, uncleanly, and not sufficiently exercised; but it is principally propagated by the actual conveyance of the matter from the diseased to the healthy, by the frequent contact of the heads of children, but more generally by the use of the same towels, combs, caps, and hats.

TREATMENT.—While the patches are in an inflamed and irritable condition, we must be content with regular washing or sponging with warm water, or some emollient fomentation.  Even the operation of shaving, which is necessary to be repeated at intervals of 8 or 10 days, produces a temporary increase of irritation.  At this time, all stimulant lotions and ointments should be avoided.  The disease assumes various forms, and these require a corresponding variety in the treatment; so that no single application can be said to possess any unfailing power against the ringworm.  When the inflammatory state subsides, a dry scabbing and exfoliation ensues, but again the pustular eruption breaks out, and the patches again become red and tender.  In other instances, the surface becomes inert and torpid, while a dry scaly scab constantly appears, and active stimulants are requisite to effect any change in the disorder.  In more irritative states, the milder ointments, with calomel, oxide of zinc, acetate of lead, should be employed, or sedative lotions, or decoctions or infusions of poppy heads or tobacco.  When there is an acrimonious discharge, the ointments of zinc and lead, or the milder mercurial ones, or a lotion of lime-water with calomel, are advantageous.  In a very dry and inert state of the patches, caustic substances are often very successful.  The late Dr. A. T. Thomson strongly recommends the application of a solution of 1 dr. of nitrate of silver in ½ an oz. of diluted nitric acid.  But in the varying forms and degrees of ringworm, the remedies must be varied, and combined, according to the degree of irritation which prevails.  The constitutional treatment is of consequence.  A nutritious diet must be prescribed, containing a due admixture of animal food; the clothing must be warm; regular exercise must be enjoined; and a course of tonic medicines, such as iron or quinine, must be ordered.

2.  Touch it with caustic ammonia,

3.  Apply sulphate of copper, 20 grs., to 1 oz. of water.  The same is good for *Itch*.

PAINTERS' COLIC.—This form of colic is caused by the slow introduction of lead into the system,— generally the carbonate of lead.  It passes under the different English names of painters' colic, Devonshire colic, and dry belly-ache.  The first of these is the name by which it is most commonly known, from its frequent occurrence among painters, who use white lead (carbonate of lead) a great deal in the preparation of their colors.

TREATMENT.— For relieving the pain and opening the bowels, the treatment should be very much the same as that for bilious colic.  There is one article, however, which is thought to have some special influence in curing this disease, after it has become chronic; it is alum.  Fifteen grs. of alum, 2 of aloes, 2 of jalap, and 4 of Dover's powder, may be mixed, and taken for a dose 2 or 3 times a day. If the muscles of the arm be palsied, 1-16 of a gr. of strychnine may be added to the above. The aromatic sulphuric acid, taken as a drink, fifteen drops to the tumblerful of water, is always worthy of trial.

The use of the electro-magnetic machine may be tried for the palsy; or a splint applied to the arm and hand, with vigorous friction applied once or twice a day, will sometimes do much for recovering the use of the muscles.

But the best remedy for the palsied muscles that I know of is the following: Fl. ex. of sarsaparilla, 4 ozs.; fl. ex. of pipsissewa, 1 oz.; water, 1 quart; iodide of potassium, 2 ozs. Mix. DOSE — A table-spoonful 3 times a day. The sulphuret of potassa, 1 oz., dissolved in a quart of water, and taken in tea-spoonful doses, 3 times a day, is also worth a trial. The affected arm should be soaked an hour, once or twice a day, in the same amount of this latter salt, dissolved in a gallon of water. The following is Dr. Gunn's treatment:

TREATMENT.—The treatment in this form of colic should be very similar to the bilious form. The first thing to be done, is to overcome the constipation of the bowels. If there is vomiting, give medicines to allay it. Then make use of strong purgatives, with hot fomentations to the bowels. Narcotics and relaxants are also indicated to relieve the pain, and overcome the spasms. As a narcotic and anodyne use the ex. of hyosciamus; take 20 grs., and form into 6 pills; give 1 every 2 hours. At the same time give the Anti-bilious Physic, and aid the operation with purgative, stimulating and relaxing injections. A portion of the physic, with a little salt, a tea-spoonful of tincture or powder of lobelia and hot water may be used as an injection, to be repeated according to the urgency of the case. Sometimes it will be well to add a little cayenne to it. Apply hot fomentations to the bowels, and if the physic does not operate in 2 or 3 hours, give the croton oil, 2 or 3 drops at a time, in a spoonful of castor oil, or a little milk, and repeat every 2 hours. Also rub a little of the croton oil on the abdomen, over the bowels. In other respects, treat the same as a severe case of bilious colic. It is sometimes well to put the patient into a warm bath, for half an hour, or even longer, in order to relax the muscular system, and overcome the spasm of the intestines. After you have got an operation on the bowels you may give the following pills: Ex. of hyosciamus, 40 grs.; ipecac, 20 grs.; pulverized opium, 10 grs.; podophyllin, 10 grs.; make into 20 pills, and give 1 every 3 or 4 hours. Also Cholagogue as a tonic and alterative.

*Remarks.* — The numerous persons who work in lead, should comb their hair with a fine comb, wash their hands and face, and rinse their mouth several times a day, and also wash the whole person with soap once or twice a week, and with clear water, or saleratus and water, once a day. Their working clothes should be of a kind to admit of being washed once or twice a week, and they should be put off for others when out of the workshop. A paper cap should be worn while at work. The food of the workmen should not be exposed to the vapors or floating particles of lead, and consequently should not be carried into the shop; and when much of the poison is floating in the air of the work room, it is a good plan to wear a mask to prevent its being drawn with the breath into the throat and lungs.

It has been said that those who eat freely of fat meats, butter, and other oily substances are not attacked by the disease, though exposed to the poison. I know not what protection this can give, unless the skin is in this way kept more oily, which prevents the absorption of the poison. This would seem to afford a hint in favor of anointing the whole person once or twice a week with sweet oil.

**STITCH IN THE SIDE.** — This is a spasmodic affection of the muscles of the chest, and is rheumatic in its origin. With this there are not the symptoms of inflammation nor the difficulty of breathing, except that caused by the pain or stich in the side. Exposure to cold or violent exercise will also cause this. Apply warm applications, mustard poultices, or stimulating liniments. The best medicines in this case will be pills of colocynth 3 grs., with ex. of colchicum ¼ of a gr. in each, taken every night; and 3 times a day a seidlitz draught, with 15 grs. of wine of colchicum and 6 of laudanum in each.

**PROUD FLESH.**—The granulations which arise when a sore is in progress of healing, sometimes project beyond the level of the surrounding parts, and form a red excrescence very irritable, easily made to bleed, and sometimes growing fast in spite of all that can be done to prevent it. Caustics of various kinds, as lunar caustic, or the blue vitriol, are to be applied, or red precipitate of mercury, and occasionally pressure, by straps of adhesive plaster or other bandages, is found useful.

**1. BED SORES.**—The constant pressure of certain portions of the body upon the bed or mattress frequently produces in invalids excoriations, which are known by the above name.

TREATMENT.—When the skin becomes red and inflamed, and painful to the touch, immediate steps should be taken to prevent if possible an abrasion of the skin. Mix two tea-spoonfuls of brandy with a wine-glassful of hot water, with 30 drops of tincture of arnica. Dab the part with this, and dry with violet powder. Or, either before or after the skin breaks, dip a camel hair brush into collodion, and brush the inflamed surface over, repeating the operation from time to time until the part is healed.

**2.** Saturate cloths with alcohol and apply; not painful and effects speedy cure.

**3.** Bismuth powder is also good, and is just the thing for *chafing*. Covering the sore with clay dust or ''mineral earth'' is recommended also.

**FITS OR CONVULSIONS IN CHILDREN.**—Most persons have seen a baby in fits; and it is a sad sight,—its little face all distorted and livid; its eyes rolling and squinting frightfully; its hands clenched, and arms bent, and legs drawn up. and body arched backward, and limbs twitching violently,—itself insensible, and unable to see, or swallow, or move. After a time the fit ceases, sometimes by degrees, at other times suddenly,—the child fetching a deep sigh, and then lying quiet and pale, as if it had fainted.

From this state it passes into a sleep, and, on waking some hours later, seems quite well.

Fits may attack a child which is apparently well, and cause death immediately, or it may have fits daily, or even several times a day, and linger on for weeks. A child may have fits from a great variety of causes. Fits, therefore, have a different meaning in different cases. But they always show that the brain has in some way been disturbed.

TREATMENT.—As fits are not a disease in themselves, but only a symptom of some disease, the treatment must have reference to the cause. Sometimes, while the fit lasts, it is wise to do nothing. But, if a fit come on suddenly, in the case of a child previously healthy, it is generally safe to place it in a hot bath, and at the same time to dash cold water on its face, or to pour cold water on its head, or hold on it a large sponge dipped in cold water. The hot bath will draw the blood to the skin, and away from the over-loaded brain. It will quiet the disturbance of the system, and if scarlet fever or measles are about to appear, it will bring them out.

**HYSTERIA—HYSTERICS.**—TREATMENT.—To treat this complaint successfully, it is necessary to search out its cause, and remove that. Like the whites, it is not so much a disease in itself, as a symptom.

The first inquiry to be made should have reference to the real origin of the complaint. Is it dependent upon inflammation of the ovaries or the womb, or to displacement of this latter organ; or does it arise from the low state of the blood, and the weakened condition of the nerves, acted upon by some irritation or heightened sensibility of the sexual organs.

If dependent upon inflammatory disease, that is to be treated according to directions elsewhere; if upon falling of the womb, no remedies will avail until that is put in its proper place. If diluted blood and weakened nerves be the cause, iron and quinine are the remedies. When the complaint arises from deficient menstruation, iron and aloes will be serviceable. The nervous spasm can sometimes be broken up by pouring cold water upon the head, or face, or limbs of the patient.

**The Hygienic and Moral Treatment** are of great consequence. The complaint is very much under the control of the will. Whatever tones the moral nature and strengthens the will, tends to subject this disorder to the control of the patient. Plain wholesome diet, exercise, bathing, and the enforcing, as far as possible, of a rugged, self-reliant habit, generally go far towards breaking its force.

**TONGUE-TIED.**—The tongue is fixed down to the lower part of the mouth by a membranous cord, which prevents too great a degree of motion. Sometimes the cord ties down the tongue of infants so much that they cannot suck. This is supposed by the common people to be the case much oftener than it really happens; and they very often request the surgeon to remove the inconvenience; but so long as the patient sucks there is no occasion for any operation. But it happens sometimes that the tongue is not perceived to be tied till the child begins to articulate, and is prevented from forming certain letters for which a free motion of the tongue is requisite. At whatever time the operation may be necessary it is easily done by a pair of scissors; but the surgeon must be careful not to wound any of the neighboring large vessels.

1. GANGRENE.— TREATMENT.—When the result of cold, the part becomes first white, and a restoration of the suspended circulation should be attempted by rubbing with snow, if it can be procured; if not, with a coarse cloth or flesh-brush. No heat must be applied; even that of the bed-covering will sometimes set up inflammation. Camphorated spirit of wine is, perhaps, the best liniment that can be used. After the rubbing, if it appears to be at all effectual, apply cold poultices. If, in spite of these efforts, a discoloration of the skin shows that gangrene has really commenced, apply to the part a poultice of flaxseed with a little powdered charcoal in it, and also spirit lotions, to keep the disease from spreading. The constitution of the patient must be soothed and supported by some anodyne and stimulant. Cooper recommends from 7 to 10 grs. of carbonate of ammonia, with 20 or 30 drops of tincture of opium, 2 or 3 times a day or more frequently if required. A bolus composed of 5 grs. of carbonate of ammonia, with 10 grs. of musk, may be given every 4 hours, with excellent effect. When the gangrene has proceeded to a sloughing sore, a port wine poultice is a good application, as is spirits of turpentine, to stimulate the parts.

2. Apply yeast poultice mixed with charcoal powder, and renew the poultice often; or keep the part well covered with charcoal powder.

If, however, the gangrene is not stopped in its first stages, it can seldom be after; and the only chance of saving the patient's life is to amputate the limb; and this must be done before the morbific influence has spread far towards a vital part.

BLOODY FLUX.—TREATMENT.—In mild cases, give a table-spoonful of castor oil and 2 tea-spoonfuls of paregoric, mixed, once a day. Sometimes, in place of the above, a dose of Rochelle powder, dissolved in water, with 30 or 40 drops of laudanum, may be taken. A moderate quantity of flaxseed or slippery elm tea, may be taken as a drink, and the bowels be well emptied by an injection of starch.

When there is much pain in the bowels, a mustard poultice laid upon them, will have a good effect. The starch injections should, in such case, have a $\frac{1}{2}$ tea-spoonful of laudanum mixed with it. The compound syrup of rhubarb and potassa will often act favorably, given in table-spoonful doses.

If there is reason to suppose the liver is affected, give podophyllin, or some other liver remedy recommended under the head of "Liver."

The patient should not be allowed to sit up, and must be kept very still, and be allowed only a very scanty diet, as flour porridge, well boiled, rice water etc.

RUPTURE (Hernia).—Children and old people are most liable to this, though sometimes they occur to persons of middle age. If difficult, or impossible to be returned, it is called strangulated rupture, and requires the best assistance.

TREATMENT.—The patient must be laid on the back, the head low, and the buttocks raised; while in this position the gut must be returned by a gentle pressure, if it does not fall back of itself. After it is returned, a piece of sticking-plaster may be applied over the part, and a truss, or bandage, worn for a length of time. If it has been forced down with great violence, or happens from any cause to become inflamed, it is often very difficult to return it, and sometimes impracticable, without an operation, a description of which is foreign to our purpose, but in those cases, until some assistance can be obtained, act as follows: foment with warm fomentations; give clysters; then, when the bowels have emptied, the operator must press and guide the gut back through the aperture, if possible to do so. An adult, after being ruptured, should never neglect wearing the proper truss.

**HAY FEVER.**—This disease is so called on account of its occurring during hay time, or summer, and is thought to be caused by the odor of new-mown hay; but it may be caused by other strong odors. It does not differ very much from the ordinary asthma, except perhaps there is not so much difficulty of breathing, and the attacks last longer in the hay-asthma; the lining membrane of the nose is also much more inflamed and the throat irritated in the latter disease.

The best thing to do is to remain within doors and keep quiet for a few days; take a few doses of Rochelle salts or rhubarb, also a tea-spoonful of paregoric at bed-time for two or three nights, and live on light diet. A dose or two of quinine (1 gr.) may be beneficial, night and morning.

*Remarks.*—Thousands of people go to Northern Michigan annually for this disease, and I have never heard of one that did not get relief—Northern Michigan is the surest cure in the world for Hay Fever.

**VARICOSE VEINS OR ENLARGED VEINS.**—The veins which lie near the surface, especially those of the legs, are apt, by exhausting labor upon the feet, and by strains, to get weakened, so that their valves lose their tone, and their sides stretch and give way in certain places, letting the blood bulge out, and form purple bunches. These bags of blood, lying along upon the surface of the limb, form knotty tumors, looking like blood boils. They occasion a kind of distress, but no sharp pain.

Persons of weak, soft, and relaxed muscles and blood vessels are particularly liable to this complaint. It often attacks women in the family way.

TREATMENT.—Where only a few veins are affected, it may be sufficient, in some cases, to apply firmly over them a few strips of leather, spread with soap plaster. But generally it is better to support the whole limb with a good cotton bandage, or with a laced stocking, which should be applied in the morning before the patient is up. It is generally also well to use friction with some liniment or iodine ointment. Lead water or alum water, or an infusion of white oak bark, may be used with advantage. Burdock and plantain leaves, bound upon the skin, and removed before they are dry, are useful. Showering with cold water strengthens the veins.

**INGROWING TOE NAILS.**—Those who have been afflicted with this affection have often found it to be very troublesome and painful, at least I have found it to be so myself. The edges or sides of the nail are disposed to turn down and grow into the flesh, giving rise to inflammation, ulceration, and often great pain and suffering.

For this difficulty the best remedy I have ever known is to scrape with some sharp-pointed instrument, as the point of a pen-knife, a sort of groove or gutter in the center of the nail, lengthwise from the root to the end. It should be scraped down to near the quick, or as thin as it can be borne. This makes the nail weak, so that it will gradually and ultimately turn up at the sides until the edges come above and over the flesh. Keep up this practice as fast as the nail grows out and grows thicker, and you will eventually succeed in getting the nail in its proper shape and position. It is a good idea to poultice if there is much inflammation, and also apply healing salve. If ulceration, bathe the parts occasionally with tinctures aloes, myrrh, and opium, mixed in equal parts.

**1. FEVER-SORES.**—One lb. fresh lard, ½ lb. red lead, 1 table-spoonful soft water; put in an iron dish and cook until it turns to quite a dark brown; stir most of the time while cooking, and watch to keep it from running over; apply it, spread on a cloth, change twice a day.

**2.** The following has cured some very severe cases of fever sores, and is good for cuts and bruises in man or beast. Take a quantity of the bark of sumac root and boil for two hours; strain and add fresh lard to the liquid, then boil down until the water is all out; anoint the sore three times a day.

*Remarks.*—This salve cured a sore on a son of G. W. Childs, of Petoskey, Mich., from which pieces of bone had been taken. They had tried several things but all but this failed. Uncle Chancy Howard, Chardon, Ohio, cured a fever-sore of long standing, and up to the time of his death, some ten years ago, it had never bothered him. The above is also good for chilblains and ulcers.

**CHOLERA.**—TREATMENT.—There is one important precaution which ought to be observed at all times, but more particularly during the epidemic of cholera: the perfect *purity of the drinking water* should be ascertained, and its freedom from all *decomposing organic matters* made certain.

Care is also to be observed *not to take active purgatives*, especially *salines*, such as Epsom or Rochelle salts, seidlitz powders, etc., which produce watery evacuations; if aperient medicine is required, it ought to be of a warm character, such as magnesia and rhubarb, with some aromatic, (cinnamon or allspice), for whatever produces free action of the bowels apparently increases the susceptibility to attack. For this reason, too, *the slightest tendency to diarrhœa should at once be arrested* by a dose of paregoric or laudanum, or what is preferable, a mixture of prepared chalk, 1 table-spoonful; cinnamon or allspice powdered, 1 table-spoonful; white sugar and flour, 1 table-spoonful each, water, 1 wine-glassful; paregoric, 2 table-spoonfuls; Cayenne pepper, ½ tea-spoonful. Mix, and take a tea-spoonful every half hour, or as may be needed, and the use of milk and farinaceous preparations (corn starch, farina, flour, etc.,) containing gelatine, for food. The speedy adoption of these measures, in places distant from medical assistance, might do much to check the disease. Should the astringents above recommended fail, use the remedies recommended below.

As to the actual treatment of the disease itself, when fully established, many different methods have been proposed and practiced, and few of them, perhaps without apparent advantage in some cases, but as yet no treatment which can be called decidedly successful (a cure), has been discovered.

The treatment which would be safe in the hands of others than medical men would be about the following: When vomiting and purging have set in, with cramps, give the following mixture: Tincture of Cayenne pepper, laudanum, spirits of camphor, of each 1 oz.; spirits of hartshorn, ½ oz.; mix together, and take 1 table-spoonful every hour or half hour according to the symptoms. Or give 1 gr. of opium, 1 of camphor, 1 of Cayenne pepper, (made into a pill with a little flour and water) every hour, or as may be needed.

The patient should be wrapped at once in a blanket, or flannels next the skin. For the cramps use the following as a liniment: Tincture of Cayenne pepper, spirits of hartshorn, chloroform, turpentine, or kerosene oil, 2 ozs. of each. Mix, and rub over the affected parts with a woolen cloth. Be *careful to remove the contents of the chamber from the room immediately and bury it in the ground.* Also mix with the discharges from the stomach and bowels, as soon as voided, some sulphate of iron (common green vitriol), also dissolve some of the green vitriol in hot water, and set the same in vessels around the room and in the different parts of the house; and then throw some down the sinks, privy, cellar, and such places, once every day. Keep the sick chamber well aired, and by all means try to cheer and comfort the patient, so as to keep up his spirits. A mixture of mustard and Cayenne pepper moistened with strong vinegar, applied to the stomach and bowels is good to check the vomiting and purging, or applied to the limbs for cramps.

During the prevalence of this disease the greatest care is necessary in regard to cleanliness, ventilation, etc. It may be mentioned also that warm bricks or warm stones, irons, or hot salt should be applied to the limbs or body where there is coldness or cramps. An injection up the bowels of ½ a tea-spoonful of laudanum, 4 or 5 table-spoonfuls of brandy or whisky, with a little thin starch, is often very beneficial in the active stage of this disease, to be repeated if necessary.

1. **ULCERS.**— A chasm or vacancy formed on the surface of a part, whether external or internal, by the absorbent vessels removing parts back into the system. Ulceration takes place more readily in the cellular and fatty substance, than in muscles, tendons, blood-vessels, and nerves. (For treatment by bandaging, see page 82.)

2. **Simple Purulent Ulcer.**—Some ulcers are covered with matter of a white color, of a thick consistence, and which readily separates from the surface of the sore. There are a number of little eminences called granulations, which are small, florid, and pointed at the top. As soon as they have risen to the level of the surrounding skin, those next the old skin become smooth, and

are covered with a thin film, which afterwards becomes opaque, and forms skin.  The principal thing to be done in the treatment of this kind of ulcer, is to keep the surface clean by putting on a little dry lint, and a pledget over it, covered with very simple ointment.  In some patients ointment irritates and inflames the neighboring skin.  Bandages sometimes irritate the sore, and disturb the healing process; but when they do not, they are useful in giving a moderate support to the parts, and in defending those that are newly formed.

3.  **Ulcers in Weakened Parts.**—Other ulcers are in parts which are too weak to carry on the actions necessary to their recovery.  In them the granulations are larger, more round, and less compact than those formed on ulcers in healthy parts.  When they have come up to the level of the healthy parts, they do not readily form skin, but rising still higher, lose altogether the power of forming it.  When the parts are still weaker, the granulations sometimes fill up the hollow of the ulcer, and then are suddenly absorbed, leaving the sore as deep as ever.  Ulcers are very much under the influence of whatever affects the constitution; so that change of weather, emotions of the mind, diet, and other agents, quickly occasion a change in their condition.  Such ulcers as we have been describing, require general as well as local treatment; bark, wine, porter, and other cordials and tonics are to be given; and the granulations are to be kept from rising too much, by the prudent application of blue vitriol, lunar caustic, and the like, weakened sufficiently by proper admixture of ointment to act as stimulants, and not as caustics.  This will give a proper and healthy action to the granulating surface; whereas the destroying of the rising parts by escharotics seems rather to encourage the growth. Bandages and proper support to the parts are highly useful.  These ulcers, in weak parts, do not seem to be the better of poultices, or other relaxing applications; powders rarely do good, and perhaps the best dressing is the citrine ointment, more or less diluted.

4.  **Irritable Ulcers.**—There are certain ulcers, which may be called *Irritable Ulcers*.  The margin of the surrounding skin is jagged, and terminating in an edge which is sharp and undermined.  There is no distinct appearance of granulations, but a whitish spongy substance, covered with a thin ichorous discharge.  Every thing that touches the surface gives pain, and commonly makes the ulcer bleed.  The pain sometimes comes on in paroxysms, and causes convulsive motions of the limb.  Such ulcers seldom do well without a frequent change of treatment.  Fomentations with poppy heads, chamomile flowers, or hemlock leaves, are sometimes of use in irritable ulcers. When poultices are prescribed, they should never be allowed to rest or bear weight on the sore limb.  Powdered applications are generally too stimulating for irritable ulcers, and bandages also prove hurtful.

5.  **Indolent Ulcers.**—These ulcers are those which have the edges of the surrounding skin thick, prominent, smooth, and rounded.  The surface of the granulations is smooth and glossy; the matter is thin and watery, and the bottom of the ulcer is nearly level.  A great proportion of the ulcers in hospitals are of the most indolent kind.  Indolent ulcers form granulations, but

frequently they are all of a sudden absorbed, and in four and twenty hours the sore becomes as much increased in size as it had been diminished for many weeks. The principal applications required for indolent ulcers are those of a stimulating nature, as the basilicon ointment, and occasional sprinkling with red precipitate. Pressure is to be made by a roller, and by slips of adhesive plaster. Scrofulous, syphilitic, and cancerous ulcers are to be treated according to the methods laid down under these various diseases.

**PALSY.** — A disease in which some part of the body is affected with the loss of the power of motion. It may be of all degrees, from a universal attack of the whole body, or a complete palsy of one of the sides, to the palsy of a single finger, or a few fibres of a muscle. It proceeds from the same causes as apoplexy, and is in reality often a modification or partial attack of that disease. The disease is also brought on by mere loss of nervous power, as when the brain "gives way," in hard-worked literary men. When a patient, by proper remedies, or the powers of nature, recovers a little from an attack of apoplexy, it is very common for him to be seized with palsy.

Palsy sometimes comes on suddenly, at other times there is numbness, coldness, and paleness of the part about to be affected. Sometimes the judgment and memory are impaired; the speech is imperfect from the disease of both body and mind; the mouth and cheeks are distorted, and the countenance is expressive of much anxiety. When the lower extremities are partially affected, the patient drags them after him.

*Causes.*—The same causes that excite apoplexy, occasion palsy when applied in a less degree; therefore tumors, wrong determination of blood, bruises, pressure on nerves, the drying up of usual evacuations, are often found to induce palsy. When one side of the body is palsied, the disease is termed *hemiplegia*, and when the lower part of the body is affected the disease is called *paraplegia*. Certain sedative substances, long applied, produce palsy of some parts of the body, as we see in those who work among lead, and are affected with the Devonshire Colic; one remarkable symptom of which is the palsy of the thumbs and calves of the legs. Palsy is not unfrequently produced gradually by some tumor or other disease pressing on the vertebræ of the back; and this is commonly the cause of the palsy of young people.

*Prognosis.*—It is generally unfavorable. Palsy does not suddenly prove mortal. Its cure is the more difficult the more the senses are injured; and such cases commonly continue till the end of life, often very remote. When palsy follows apoplexy, or happens in old people, it is seldom cured. The palsies of young people are sometimes recovered from. If convulsions occur in the parts opposite to those that are palsied, the danger is great. When palsy occurs from pressure or blows on the spinal marrow, or on any large nerves, it is generally hopeless, and the dragging of the limb is seldom got completely the better of.

TREATMENT.—When palsy comes on suddenly, it is proper to treat it as we do apoplexy sometimes, by bleeding, by purging, by blisters to the head; and when the acute symptoms are in some measure relieved, we apply stimulants to the limbs, or weakened parts, if they are within our reach. When the case is of longer standing, and the constitution is in a state of debility, those evacuating measures would be improper; and instead of them we must be contented with stimulating applications, aided by such exercise as the patient is able to take. It is surprising how much may be done in cases apparently very hopeless. The patient must not be discouraged at the apparent bad success of his first efforts at motion, but must persevere, and his perseverance will probably at last be rewarded. The applications proper for palsied limbs are such as the following: Ammoniated oil, camphorated oil, cajeput oil, when it can be got; turpentine and oil, warm sea-water, warm salt, stinging with nettles, mustard, etc. Great benefit is often derived from strychnia, but this drug is so powerful that it ought to be given only by a medical man. Electricity and galvanism are also frequently had recourse to; also the use of the Bath or other mineral waters pumped upon the palsied limbs. Our choice of internal medicines must be determined by the state of the constitution. If there be any excitement, or inflammatory tendency, or any probability that the palsy may be followed by apoplexy, all internal stimulants must be avoided; and it is only in old cases, unattended by fever, that we are to give such medicines as guaiac, iron, aromatics, or the like. Paralytic limbs should be kept warm, and well covered with flannel. The diet should be light and nutritive. The patient should take what exercise he can; and if he is unable to do it by his own exertions, he must have it by a carriage, or by sailing, or by a swing. In the palsy of the lower limbs from diseases of the spine, issues to the back, or to the neighborhood of the diseased vertebræ, are of great service. (See Apoplexy.)

*Remarks.*—Many astonishing cures have been effected by taking the mineral baths at Mt. Clemens and Ypsilanti, Mich. There may be other places, and I have no doubt there are, where the mineral waters will have the same effect. I only speak of these from my own knowledge.

Palsy in children occurs pretty frequently, and attacks infants and young persons in different degrees. It often attacks one side at first, and gradually comes on the other side. It is generally attended with costiveness and deranged state of the bowels; and, accordingly, a course of purgative medicines of considerable activity, as jalap and calomel, or rhubarb and calomel, in no long time effects a cure. Blistering on the head, or on the palsied limb, may be tried; and leeches to the temples, when the head is much affected. If the palsy is owing to water in the head, it is to be feared the case is hopeless. Tonic medicines and external stimulants are proper, when there is no fever present. Electricity is often a valuable assistant to other remedies.

**SUFFOCATION.**—Is the extinction of life by the function of breathing being violently stopped. This may happen from hanging and drowning; from blood or matter bursting from the lungs into the branches of the wind pipe; from inflammation or croup, producing a false membrane or thickened mucus in the air passages from foreign bodies sticking in the same; from large pieces of meat in the gullet pressing on the back of the wind pipe; and many similar incidents. Where the suffocation is complete nothing can be done; but where it is only threatened the proper means of relief are to be had recoarse to, varying, of course, according to circumstances. Foreign bodies are to be extracted, if possible, from the windpipe, and vomited from the gullet, or pushed down into the stomach; and the means for restoring suspended animation to be employed in the case of hanging and drowning.

**SUFFOCATION FROM HANGING.**—Immediately remove all clothing from the upper part of the body, and follow the directions under Artificial Respiration to restore breathing.

**SUFFOCATION FROM GAS AND OTHER NOXIOUS VAPORS.**—Immediately remove the person into the open air, and throw cold water upon the face, throat and chest, expel the foul gas from the lungs, and restore respiration by means prescribed for Artificial Respiration. As soon as you discover the least breathing, hold strong vinegar to the nostrils. Should the suffocation be from breathing carbolic acid gas, chloride of soda or a solution of chloride of lime, is preferable, sometimes moistening a cloth, with either of the solutions, and holding it to the nose, will produce the desired effect. Oxygen should be forced into the lungs if it can be produced. Excite warmth in the manner prescribed for "Drowned Persons" on pages 80 and 81. Where suffocation is caused by fire-damp in mines, wells, etc., remove the person at once and treat as above.

**SUSPENDED ANIMATION FROM COLD.**—When a person is apparently frozen to death, the body should be handled very carefully, and be very careful not to bend the joints; have the body in a cold place, and rub the same from head to foot with cold water or snow, for fifteen or twenty minutes, until the surface is red, then wipe the body perfectly dry and rub with bare warm hands; it is better if several persons will join in this rubbing, and then wrap the body in a woolen sheet, and follow the directions as in "Artificial Respiration" to restore breathing. This treatment must be continued with energy for several hours if necessary, and until animation and respiration are thoroughly restored. Allow the patient to swallow a little lukewarm water and wine or red pepper, or ginger tea.

**STRICTURE OF THE RECTUM.**—In many cases this is the result of an inflammatory process, simple or syphilitic, from the cicatrization of deep-seated and extensive ulceration; in others, it is due to the contraction of inflammatory material poured out external to the bowel in the sub-mucous tissue; in exceptional instances it may be caused by contraction of the parts external to the bowel, after pelvic cellulitis, and Curling quotes a case where it was the direct result of injury.

The disease, taken as a whole, is twice as common in women as in men, my note book revealing the fact that thirty-two out of forty-eight consecutive cases were in this sex. But syphilitic stricture is more common in the female, and cancerous stricture in the male.

Constipation is the one early symptom, and it is not till some ulceration has commenced, either at the stricture or above it, that others appear, such as diarrhœa, with lumpy stools, containing blood, pus or mucus, straining at stool, and a sensation of burning afterward, with at last a complete stoppage, abdominal distension and dyspeptic symptoms.

An examination with the finger carefully introduced into the rectum will, as a rule, at once reveal the true nature of the case, for about two inches up the rectum the narrowing will be felt, with or without new tissue infiltrating the part or ulceration. In exceptional cases the stricture is beyond the reach of the finger; under these circumstances, however, it may, at times, be brought within reach by pressing with the free hand upon the abdomen above the pelvis.

The examination of a rectum, the subject of disease with a tube, flexible or otherwise, requires the greatest care and gentleness. Fallacies may mislead the surgeon in every way, the end of the instrument striking against the sacrum, or being caught in a fold of mucous membrane, may lead him to suspect obstruction where none exists. But if some warm fluid, as linseed tea, be injected somewhat forcibly through the tube, a place is formed admitting the easy transit of the instrument. In stricture pain is felt when an instrument reaches the point of contraction, and a flexible one is arrested or passed on with more or less difficulty.

TREATMENT.—It is so rare for a surgeon to be consulted about a stricture of the rectum till the ulcerative stage has set in, or nearly complete obstruction has taken place, that he has few opportunities of testing the value of dilatation of the stricture, for, although this practice is clearly useless if not injurious when ulceration exists, it is probably of great value before any breach of the surface has taken place. In cicatricial or inflammatory strictures, indeed, it is the only form of practice upon which reliance is to be placed, but in the cancerous, whether in the ulcerating style or not, it is not wise to make the attempt.

The dilatation is to be effected by mechanical means, and many instruments have been invented for the purpose. The elastic gum bougie, in the hands of the surgeon is, however, the best; forcible dilatation is inadmissible. They are made in many sizes, and the one just large enough to pass through the stricture should be chosen. It should be warmed and well greased, and guided by the finger passed gently through the stricture, and retained for ten or fifteen minutes at a time. When it does not produce any irritation, a second larger, may be passed in two days. But when irritation has set in, the repetition of the operation should be suspended until it has subsided. By these means a simple stricture may be checked in its progress, and even dilated, but rarely cured; this practice may prolong life for years. Mr. Curling has, however, given a case in his book in which he believes he cured an annular stricture in a lady, age 24, by incisions and dilatation.

This dilatation is, however, only a means to an end, and that end is to secure a passage for the intestinal contents. Enemata are valuable aids to effect this purpose, the daily washing out of the bowels with gruel and oil giving great relief, or the daily dose of mist, olei with manna, confection of senna with sulphur, or any other gentle laxative that the patient has found to suit. Cod liver oil in full doses often acts as a laxative as well as a tonic. Care must, however, be observed in the introduction of the tube, for in a cancerous bowel perforation is very apt to occur, and even in a healthy one the same accident has taken place.

How far it is safe to allow a patient to pass a bougie for himself or herself, is another question. I am disposed to think it is an unwise act to allow when the bougie is solid, for I am sure I have seen great irritation and harm follow upon the practice, and in several cases deep seated suppuration. Curling has given a case where the patient caused his own death by perforating the bowel, half an inch in extent, above the stricture. I have, consequently, been in the habit of instructing my patients to use candles as bougies, and have been well pleased with the practice.

There comes a time, however, when this treatment by dilatation ceases to be beneficial; when the stricture has so closed as to render it useless; or ulcerated so as to render it unwise to adopt the practice; or associated with so much distress as to forbid its use; and under these circumstances the practice of *colotomy* is of great value; it gives comfort to a degree that sometimes astonishes, and always gratifies. On convalescence or recovery, it is not found to be practically associated with such inconveniences as surgeons of old have practically surrounded it. It prolongs life and adds materially to its comfort, and little more than this can be said of most operations. But it must not be postponed till the powers of life have become so exhausted as to render the chances of recovery from the operation poor; or till the large intestine has become so distended as to have become damaged or inflamed. It should be undertaken as soon as it is clear that the local disease has passed beyond the power of local treatment with any prospect of good, and the general powers of the patient are beginning to fail; as soon as the local distress finds no relief from palliative measures, and a downward course, with unmixed anguish, is evidently approaching. The difficulties of colotomy are not great, nor are its dangers numerous. When unsuccessful, it is usually made so from the delay in its performance; from want of power in the patient; or death has resulted from the secondary effects of the disease on the abdominal viscera.

When most successful, it gives immediate relief to most of the symptoms, and makes life worth living. When least so, by lessening pain, it renders what remains of life endurable. The operation is now regarded as established, and creditable to surgical art, and according to Curling; but, in the general way, it has been postponed until too late a period to demonstrate its value.

**HYDROPHOBIA.** — TREATMENT. — Cut off the bitten part, or apply dry cupping, or suction, at once. Also the caustic potash. The internal remedies heretofore employed have had little success. Perhaps nothing now known promises more than to keep the patient, for a long time, under the innuence of chloroform or ether. The tincture of scullcap, in 2 or 3 dram doses, will allay the nervous agitation, and is always worth using. It has been proposed to clear the throat of the tough mucus by cauterizing it with a strong solution of nitrate of silver applied with a shower syringe. The remedy is worthy of a trial.

Some of the Western physicians declare the red chickweed, or scarlet pimpernell, to be an absolute remedy for this disease, and cite some quite remarkable cases of its success. Four ozs. of this plant, in the dried state, are directed to be boiled in 2 qts. of strong beer or ale, until the liquid is reduced one half. The liquid is to be pressed out and strained, and 2 drs. of laudanum added to it. The dose for a grown person is a wine-glassful every morning, for 3 mornings. A larger dose is required if the disease has begun to show itself; and if the case be fully developed, the whole may be taken in a day. The wound is to be bathed with the same decoction. The medicine, it is said, produces profuse sweating. It is worth a trial.

Considerable has been said of late of a remedy used in some parts of Europe, and said to be effectual. It is the "golden cenotides" (*cetonia aurata*), or common rose beetle, found in large quantities on all rose trees. A similar insect is said to infest the geranium plant. When collected, they are dried and powdered; and given in this form, relieve excitement (so it is said) of the brain and nerves, and throw the patient into a sound sleep.

**HEARTBURN.** — What is commonly called heartburn is not a disease of the heart, but an uneasy sensation of heat or acrimony about the pit of the stomach, accompanied sometimes by a rising in the throat like water.

*Causes.* — Debility of the stomach; the food, instead of being properly digested and turned into chyle, runs into fermentation, producing acetic acid; sometimes the gastric juice itself turns acid, and causes it; at other times, it arises from bilious humors in the stomach.

TREATMENT.—Take 1 tea-spoonful of the spirit of nitrous ether, in a glass of water or a cup of tea; or a large tea-spoonful of magnesia, in a cup of tea, or a glass of mint-water.

**DISEASES OF THE HEART.** — The heart, from the important part which it plays in the animal economy, is subject to various, serious and often fatal diseases. Like the other viscera, it is removed from the eye, so that but little knowledge of its condition can be obtained by inspection; and hence we must have recourse to other means. The ear is the principal means of obtaining a knowledge of the state of the heart, and by auscultation and percussion we are enabled to detect the existence of various diseases. The heart gives out two sounds, known as the first and second, which are distinguished from each other. The first sound is longer than the second, and the interval between the first and second sounds is shorter than that between the second and first. They have been compared to the two syllables *lupp*, *dupp*. Any manifest alteration in these sounds is indicative of the existence of disease. They may be high or low, clear or dull, muffled, rough, intermittent, etc. Murmurs or regurgitant sounds may arise from disease of the valves. The power of distinguishing between the normal and abnormal sounds of the heart, and of the causes producing the latter, can only be obtained by lengthened experience. Diseases of the heart are usually divided into two classes: first, functional or nervous; and second, structural or organic. Chief among the former are palpitations, syncope or fainting, and angina pectoris. They are chiefly to be met with in persons of a naturally nervous temperament, more especially women suffering from hysteria, or other like complaints, and may be induced by great mental excitement. In such cases great attention should be paid to the general health, and, by means of tonics, sea-bathing, and gentle open-air exercise, the system is to be strengthened. Violent exertion and strong mental excitement are particularly to be avoided. Among the principal organic diseases to which the heart is subject are pericarditis, carditis, endocarditis, atrophy, hypertrophy, dilation and valvular diseases.

TREATMENT.—In all cases of heart disease, the body and mind should be kept as easy and cheerful as possible. The diet should be well regulated,— nourishing but not stimulating. Coffee, tea, liquors, and tobacco must be dispensed with. The feet should be constantly dry and warm, and occasionally rubbed with mustard.

For inflammatory diseases of the heart, the bowels, if costive, may be moved with compound tincture of jalap. To each dose add 10 grs. of cream of tartar. Keep up a perspiration till the pain is relieved, by giving a tea-spoonful of compound tincture of Virginia snake-root; also a warm infusion of pleurisy-root. Mustard-plasters over the chest and spinal column are also to be employed. If the patient is troubled with sleeplessness, give 8 to 10 grs. of compound powder of ipecac and opium.

For palpitation, the tincture of digitalis, 10 or 15 drops 3 or 4 times a day, has been found useful. When the nervous system is affected, give small quantities of wine or spirits, or a few drops of laudanum or ether.

For neuralgia, or breast-pang, give a tea-spoonful of a mixture of equal parts of laudanum, ether, and oil of castor. The powder of Indian hemp-root may also be taken in doses of a small tea-spoonful 2 or 3 times a day. If the stomach is acid, a tea-spoonful of soda in half a tumbler of water will correct it.

1. **INFLAMMATION OF THE LIVER.**—TREATMENT.—When the bowels are confined, usually termed a costive state of the bowels, 1 pt. of warm water, 1 table-spoonful of salt, and 1 tea-spoonful of hog's lard, as a clyster, will give relief; or take one or two of the following liver pills at bed-time:

**Dr. Chase's Cathartic and Liver Pill.**—Take podophyllin, 60 grs.; leptandrin, sanguinarin, ipecac, and pure cayenne, each 30 grs.; make into 60 pills, with a little soft extract of mandrake or dandelion. This is the best pill I have ever used, as a cathartic and liver pill, and to act on the secretions generally. As a purgative the dose is from 2 to 4 pills, for a grown person; and as an alterative and substitute for blue mass, and to act on the liver, 1 pill once a day, or every other day.

*Remarks.*—Should you not wish to go to the trouble of making this pill, inquire at the drug store for it, or send 25 cents to the Chase Medicine Company, Detroit, Mich., for it.

When, from any cause, the languor, sleepiness, furred tongue, etc., give notice of an impending bilious attack, 4 or 5 of the liver pills should be taken at night, and followed in the morning by a dose of infusion of senna and salts, or a dose of castor oil. Extract of dandelion made into pills with 1 gr. of leptandrin to each pill, 1 taken every night, is an excellent remedy. From a long practical experience I have found that the dandelion is a most valuable medicine for this complaint, and there are herbs to cure all diseases provided by our Heavenly Father, if we would but seek them out and test their virtues. But experiments on this subject have been too much neglected to afford us all the information we need. I have found the use of the dandelion in the treatment of this disease to be a most valuable remedy. Indeed I may here observe that in the treatment of liver complaint the same precautionary remarks as those on indigestion, will also apply to this disease—that sick headache, foul tongue, or heaviness in the region of the stomach, will indicate the necessity of giving a mild emetic of ipecacuanha; and should there be great heat, inflammation, or feverishness, the use of warm lemonade or a dose of salts mixed in warm water, and bathing the feet in warm water, so as to produce perspiration or determination to the surface will afford relief. Should the bowels be costive, regulate them with the following valuable pills: Take extract of butternut, 30 grs.; powdered jalap, 20 grs.; soap, 10 grs. Mix. Make 15 pills. Three or 4 is a dose. The extract of butternut has been found one of the best cathartics in fevers, and as a general purgative medicine.

Dr. Wilson, in the *Medico-Chirurgical Review*, says: "The more the dandelion is employed the more certain proofs it will afford of its great virtues," —a fact to which my experience enables me to testify. In my own practice, more than a hundred cases have been cured either by the simple extract of the herb and root, or by taking a tea-cupful of a strong decoction of dandelion twice a day. In almost every instance I have succeeded in relieving and restoring those who have used this most valuable plant of the fields.

**2.** The dandelion is diuretic and aperient, and has a direct action upon the liver and kidneys when languid; and is likewise applicable to all derangements of the digestive organs generally. In chronic inflammation of the liver and spleen, in cases of deficient biliary secretions and in dropsical affections of the abdominal viscera or belly, it will be found very beneficial. The inspissated (thick) extract is the most efficacious and active form of using this plant, and may be purchased at any drug store; the doses of these are from 10 grs. to ½ dr. I have, however, generally used it in a decoction as before mentioned.

**3.** The constant application of hot poultices relieves the pain and hastens cure. This is *good* for inflammation of any of the internal organs.

For disordered liver, good strong thoroughwort (boneset) tea is a mother's cure. For thorough case of biliousness there is nothing better than Dr. Chase's Cholagogue; it combines the antibilious ingredients that act directly upon the liver in a mild and pleasant form, and is very effective in all malarial diseases.

**1. BRAIN—Inflammation or Concussion of.**—The name given to the injury supposed to be received by the brain from great violence inflicted on the head, when there is no organic injury discovered, neither fissure, fracture, nor extravasation, either in the living or dead body. The same symptoms occur when the head has not received any external injury, and when the shock has appeared to have been sustained by the whole frame. A person may fall from a height, light on his feet, and yet be affected with all the symptoms of concussion of the brain. These vary in degree from the slight stunning which follows almost every violence done to the head, to the loss of all sense and motion which is soon followed by death. Dr. Abernethy thinks that the symptoms of concussion may properly be divided in three stages; the first is that state of insensibility and derangement of the bodily powers which immediately succeeds the accident. The breathing is difficult, but in general without stertor or snoring; the pulse intermits, and the extremities are cold. This goes off gradually, and is succeeded by the second stage; in this, the pulse and breathing are better, and though not regular, are sufficient to main-tain life, and to diffuse warmth over the extreme parts of the body. The patient is inattentive to slight external impressions, though he feels when the skin is pinched. As the effects of concussion diminish, he replies to questions put to him in a loud tone of voice, particularly if they refer to his own suffer-ing; otherwise he answers incoherently, and as if his attention was occupied by something else. While the stupor remains there appears little inflammation of the orain, but as the stupor abates, the inflammation increases; and this consti-tutes the third stage. Much caution and prudence are required in the treat-ment of the first stage. A person is knocked down and becomes insensible; many have seen or heard of bleeding being employed when a person has fallen down suddenly, and the bystanders impatiently require that this shall be the first article of the treatment. But the breathing is slow, the pulse intermitting and the extremities cold; and to draw blood in such circumstances as these would be taking the effectual method completely to extinguish life. Again, suppose people were to reason from the resemblance of the state in which the patient is in, to that of a person in a faint, and should as in that case give stimulant liquors by the mouth, or apply pungent substances to the nose, there is danger here, that by such appliances, the subsequent inflammation may be increased. The utmost that should be tried is the endeavoring to restore the heat of the extremities by friction with warm cloths or with stimulating embro-cations; we must wait a little till we see whether the patient recovers from the first stunning effect of the blow, and then be regulated in our future treatment by the symptoms that occur. Those that we are principally to look for are those of an inflammatory tendency; and to prevent the evils arising in the after stages of concussion, we are to employ bleeding and purging, to keep the patient in a dark room, to enjoin perfect quiet, and to put in force the anti-phlogistic (inflaming) regimen.

**2. Brain—Inflammation of.**—Inflammation of the brain and its mem-branes is characterized by very violent feverish symptoms, great flushing of the face, redness of the eyes, intolerance of light and furious delirium; the skin is hot and dry, the pulse hard and frequent, the bowels are costive, and there is a great feeling of tightness across the forehead.

*Causes.*—These symptoms are occasioned by passions of the mind, by drink-ing spirituous liquors; and in warm climates by exposure to the sun forming what is called *sun-stroke.*

TREATMENT.—Quiet both of mind and body with cooling aperient medi-cines, abstinence from all rich and stimulating food and drink is the proper treatment; in those of spare, weakly habit, it is sometimes owing to want of vital energy, and in this case the diet should be rich and stimulating; and the aperients, if required, must be of a cordial nature; but all this should be left to the medical practitioner; the disease too nearly affects the issues of life and death to be tampered with, and a doctor must be called.

**1. THROAT, INFLAMMATION OF.**—Quinsy and sore throat are names of an acute disease, of which the seat is in the mucous membrane of the upper part of the throat, and all the surrounding parts of the muscles which move the jaws. The tonsils or almonds of the ears, are especially affected, and the inflammation extends to the pendulous *velum* of the palate and to the uvula. Commonly, shiverings and other symptoms of approaching fever precede the affection of the throat, which is attended with pain and difficulty of swallowing, the pain sometimes shooting to the ear; there is also troublesome clamminess of the mouth and throat; a frequent but difficult discharge of mucus; and at an early period of the disease the fever is fully formed. The inflammation and swelling are commonly most considerable at first in one tonsil; and afterwards, abating in that, they increase in the other. The disease is not contagious. When the disease is actively treated at an early period, it abates gradually, or is said to end in resolution; but very often it goes on to suppuration, and the pus which is evacuated is of the most fetid and nauseous kind. Very soon after the abscess breaks, great relief is obtained, and the pain and difficulty of swallowing cease.

*Causes.*—The most frequent cause is cold, externally applied, particularly about the neck. It is chiefly the young and sanguine who are affected; and when a person has had sore throat once or more, he is very liable to frequent repetitions of it, so that the slightest exposure to cold, or getting wet feet, will bring on an attack of the disease. It occurs especially in spring and autumn, when vicissitudes of heat and cold are frequent.

*Remarks.*— The principal point in the diagnosis of this disease is to distinguish it from the sore throat which attends scarlet fever; in some varieties of which the rash is inconsiderable, although the disease of the throat goes rapidly on to gangrene, accompanied with a destructive fever of the typhoid kind. The distinction between the two kinds of sore throat is of great importance, as it most materially influences our practice. It is, in general, easily made by proper attention. The smart fever, the difficulty of swallowing, and the bright florid redness of the parts, mark out the inflammatory sore throat with sufficient distinctness; and we are in many cases assisted by observing the person affected to be often subject to the disease, which occurs soon after the application of cold. The dangerous and malignant sore throat is known by the dark and livid color about the fauces, by the appearance of specks on the part, which rapidly spread and form sloughs; and by the circumstance of scarlet fever being the prevailing epidemic. The treatment proper in inflammatory sore throat would be destructive here. And it is probably the knowledge that some sore throats are so dangerous, that makes many people much alarmed when a quinsy seizes themselves or any of their family.

TREATMENT. — When sore throat is threatened, it may in many cases be prevented from coming forward. by using a strong astringent gargle. Of these, there is a great variety. As useful a one as can be made is that with diluted vinegar, a little sweetened with honey or sugar. The infusion of red rose leaves, acidulated with a few drops of sulphuric acid, forms a very elegant gargle. The same purpose may be served by gargling with strong spirits, or with the decoction of oak-bark or diluted spirit of hartshorn not so strong as to hurt the mouth. A blister behind the ear, extending from under the lower jaw to the wind-pipe, will almost certainly prevent the internal disorder of the throat; but it must be put on at the early part of the disease, or it will do no good. If this is not done, Dr. Chase's Liniment should be rubbed on the under jaw, below the chin. An emetic may be given at the commencement of the disease, but a saline purgative is better. Gargles must be used with incessant diligence as long as the disease continues. Jellies of preserved fruits, vegetable acids, or good sharp small beer, may assist the gargles in keeping the mouth clean and allaying the thirst; but the difficulty of swallowing is so great that the patient is very apt to save himself the pain, and let the throat get dry. However, a resolute draught occasionally to quench the thirst, gives little more pain than swallowing the spittle. A little bit of sal ammoniac, or sal prunella, allowed slowly to dissolve in the mouth, is useful. If there is much swelling, and pain in swallowing, 4 or 5 leeches may be applied outside the throat, and afterwards large bran poultices should be assiduously kept on. At the same time marked relief will be got by inhaling the steam of hot water, impregnated with vinegar or any aromatic; and if there is a tendency to suppuration, this is a good way of ripening the abscess, which often forms in the tonsils. As the sore throat and fever are sometimes relieved by perspiration, the patient should keep his bed for a few days. Sometimes the swelling is so great that nothing can be swallowed, and the breathing is impeded. The tonsils have been scarified, or the abscess has been opened, and the operation of opening the wind-pipe may be sometimes required. Happily those very violent cases are of rare occurrence.

2. The yolk of a raw egg is excellent for sore throat of public speakers.

3. Gargle frequently with hot water and vinegar in which black pepper has been boiled.

*Remarks.*—I would add: apply to the throat flannel cloths wrung out of hot water and vinegar, covering them with dry ones. (See receipts for sore throat elsewhere.)

1. **INFLAMMATION OF THE LUNGS.**—This disease requires prompt treatment, and of course, if possible, a physician should be called at the earliest moment. When one is not to be had conveniently, let no time be lost, but pursue the course here marked out, which in a great many cases will be the means of curing the disease, or checking it while medical aid is being procured.

TREATMENT.—Open the bowels by means of an injection, and also giving some mild purgative, such as castor oil, Epsom or Rochelle salts, or rhubarb. Apply leeches, 10 to 20 to the side affected, if they can be procured; if not, scarify (to scratch or cut the skin off) and apply the cups, (cupping is the operation of drawing blood after the skin has been scratched off)after which a warm poultice of bran, Indian meal, or linseed meal or slippery elm, etc., to be sprinkled over with a little laudanum or paregoric; to be applied frequently. Small doses of ipecac, either in powder or the syrup, should be given every 3 hours, just so as to produce slight *nausea but not vomiting.* When this has been continued for about 12 hours, then use the following mixture: Water, 8 ozs. (1 gill); syrup of ipecac, 1 table-spoonful, or 5 grs. of the powder; chlorate of potash, 1 dr., or about 1 tea-spoonful; spirits of nitre, 2 table-spoonfuls. DOSE—A tea-spoonful every 3 hours; if much sickness of the stomach is produced, not so often  Let the patient have plenty of cooling drinks, such as flaxseed tea, gum arabic, or slippery elm water, toast water, etc. The bowels to be moved occasionally by a dose of castor oil.

Dr. Scudder's treatment of this disease is so *short, plain* and *effective,* I will give it in his own words. He says:

" Have the person bathed with an alkaline wash, to prevent undue heat of the skin, and apply a poultice of bran, or corn meal to the chest, changing it twice a day, keeping the patient well covered. Give internally, tinct. of veratrum, 1 dr.; tinct. of aconite, 20 drops; water, 4 ozs.; a tea-spoonful every hour until the fever is *subdued,* and then in smaller doses. On the *third,* or *fourth* day, add a solution of acetate of potash as follows: Acetate of potash, 1 oz.; water, 8 ozs.; simple syrup, 2 ozs.; mix. This will be found an excellent diuretic in fevers and inflammations, headaches, etc., as it helps to carry off the urea, or solid matter that should be carried off by the urine. DOSE— tea-spoonful every 1, 2 or 3 hours as required.

" The patient's bowels should be kept regular, but active physic should be avoided. If the cough is *very severe,* give a sufficient dose of opium to give the necessary sleep. Let the patient's food be light and nutritious. Keep the room *well ventilated,* and everything scrupulously clean."

Thus you have it in a "nut shell." The variations which I make are as follows:

In cases where a good nurse, or plenty of help is not to be had to look after the comfort of the patient, instead of the "bran, or cornmeal poultice to the chest," I use a *bag of hot dry bran,* changing it sufficiently often to *keep it hot,* and *occasionally use a mustard poultice,* having a thin piece of cloth between the poultice and the body, as this means appears, at least, to have as good an effect, and avoids the *wetting* of the bed clothing and the chilly dampness which will arise unless, as above stated, you have *plenty of help and use great care to keep the patient dry and comfortable.*

Also, if the case is taken in hand *at once,* in the commencement of the disease, I take the *sweating* process at first, as you will see below, but if the disease gets some days the *start,* then the "alkaline wash," or spirit sponging, not only "twice a day," but as often as it will add to the comfort of the patient. The temperature of the "wash" must also be governed by the patient's feelings — if he wants it *cool,* have it so, if *warm,* make it to his liking. *The tinctures of veratrum viride, and aconite, in all inflammatory diseases and in fevers, I consider almost an absolute necessity.*

2. **Sweating Process.**—Pleurisy has been cured with but very little other treatment than the *bag of hot dry bran,* being kept upon the side for the greater portion of the day, after the case became severe. As often as one

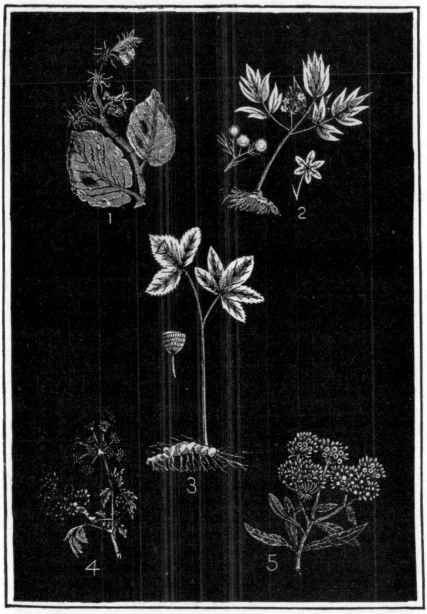

1—Witch Hazel, or Winterbloom.   2—Blue Cohosh, or Papoose Root.   3—Golden Seal, or Yellow Puccoon.   4—Poison Hemlock.   5—Pleurisy Root, or Butterfly Weed.

became at all cool, another was ready to be applied, as hot as it could be borne, by which means a little perspiration was kept up, until the severity of the pain gave way, and the cure was complete—in fact, inflammation nor fever can long exist in the system after a gentle perspiration is fully established, and permanently maintained.

*Remarks.*—There is no alkaline wash equal to that made by leaching ashes in the regular way, as for making soap, then put sufficient of this lye to the water to give it quite a perceptible slippery feeling to the hand. Dr. Beach recommends it very highly in *all fevers* and *inflammations,* when there is any *considerable* fever, to be used as often as the *heat or dry harshness* of the skin calls for it.

3. Sal-soda makes a passable substitute, using of it until the same slip pery feeling is obtained. The putting of sufficient ashes into a pail of water and stirring until a good strength is obtained, then straining off, also answers very well.

4. **Congestion of Lungs.**—Bandage limbs tightly at arm-pit and groin. Keep the blood in the extremities.

5. Apply hot fomentations or poultices to chest; renew frequently and keep covered with dry compress.

1. **ACID IN STOMACH.—Also Inflammation from Gas.—**Chloroform, 10 to 20 drops in a little sweetened water, ten or fifteen minutes after meals.

*Remarks.*—I know from experience that this is an excellent remedy.

2. For pains in the stomach, or old stomach troubles: for an adult, 1 tea-spoonful of fl. ex. of Eucalyptus in milk, before meals, will produce instant relief in most cases.

3. Lying with the head lower than the rest of the body during sleep at night cures headache caused from a deranged stomach.

**INFLAMMATION OF THE STOMACH.**—This is a very much more common disease than the preceding. Though it does not put life in immediate danger, it perverts the feelings of the stomach and causes many of the symptoms of indigestion. Dyspepsia, however, is a different complaint, and not necessarily connected with inflammation.

TREATMENT.—If there be much tenderness, we may apply leeches over the stomach. With less tenderness, counter-irritation will answer,—as blisters, croton oil, mustard poultices, the compound tar plaster, or dry cups.

The skin of the whole surface should receive special attention. The warm or the cold bath should be used often, according to the strength of the patient. When the reaction is good, a cold compress bound upon the stomach every night will do much to bring relief.

The diet cannot be too carefully managed. While there is considerable tenderness, the nourishment must be of the most simple and un-irritating kind, —consisting of little more than the most bland nutritive drinks; and even these should be taken in small quantities at a time. Gum arabic water, rice water, barley water, arrowroot gruel, tea, and toast without butter will be amply sufficient to keep soul and body together, and will, in two or three weeks, generally starve the enemy out of his quarters. After this a more nourishing diet may gradually be resumed.

**INFLAMMATION OF THE BOWELS OR BELLY ACHE.—** Like other chronic inflammations, this may follow the acute form, but it also results from various other causes, as unripe fruit, taking cold, drastic physic, and improper treatment of other diseases.

*Symptoms.*—Red end and borders of the tongue, dull pain in belly, increased by pressure and rough motion, abdomen either swelled or flat, skin dry and husky, feet and hands cold, small frequent pulse, thirst, loss of flesh, low spirits, urine scanty and high-colored, and dirty, slimy discharges from the bowels, from one to four times a day.

TREATMENT.—To begin with blisters of croton oil or mustard poultices if the tenderness is not great, or leeches if it is.

If the bowels are hot and feverish, bind a cold compress upon the belly over night,—covering it well with flannel. The warm bath should be used twice a week.

The diet must be of the most simple, un-irritating kind,—beginning with a solution of gum arabic, rice water, barley water, arrowroot or sago gruel, and gradually rising as the symptoms improve, to beef tea, mutton and chicken broth, tender beef steak, etc.

When the strength will permit gentle exercise must be taken in the open air, but not on horseback or in hard, jolting carriages.

As soon as the inflammation is subdued some mild laxative may be given in connection with an infusion of wild cherry bark, geranium, and Solomon's seal, equal parts.

**1. INFLAMMATION OF THE KIDNEYS. —** TREATMENT. — Avoid everything of a heating or stimulating nature, and let the diet consist chiefly of light, thin broth, mild vegetables, etc.; drink plentifully of balm tea, sweetened with honey, decoction of marshmallow roots, with barley licorice, etc. Nothing so safely and certainly abates the inflammation as copious dilution. Should there be much pain in the back, heat should be applied to the part; and this is done by means of cloths dipped in hot water, re-warmed as they grow cool. Another good plan is to fill bladders with a decoction of madders and camomile flowers, to which is added a little saffron, and mixed with about a third part of new milk. Should there be shivering and signs of fever with considerable tenderness over the kidneys, and no medical advice at hand a few leeches may be applied. After some time the bowels should be freely opened, and the best means of effecting this is with 3 grs. of calomel, and 2 hours afterward ½ an oz. of castor oil; subsequently the following may be given; carbonate of soda, 2 drs.; spirit of nitric ether, tincture of henbane, of each 2 drs.; syrup of tolu, mixture of acacia, of each 1 oz.; camphor mixture 4 to 8 ozs.; mix, and take half a wine-glassful every 4 hours. A very good remedy is the following: Take of tincture of opium, liquor of ammonia, spirit of turpentine, and soap liniment, of each equal portions; mix and rub well into the parts affected. In conjunction with this external application, take of infusion of buchu, 11 drs.; powdered tragacanth, 5 grs.; tincture of buchu, 1 dr.; mix for a draught, and take every morning. If there be much nausea, a clyster should be administered, consisting of a dram of laudanum, with ½ a tea-cupful of thin starch; this to be injected every 2 or 3 hours, or at longer intervals, according to the effect produced. Employ the warm bath, and afterwards warm fomentations to the stomach and loins; drink freely of linseed tea. Take also of sulphate of magnesia 1 oz.; solution of carbonate of magnesia, 1 oz.; tincture of henbane and tincture of ginger, of each 2 drs.; sulphuric ether, ½ a dr.; water, 4 ozs.; mix and give 3 table-spoonfuls every 6 hours. Those who have once suffered from inflammation of the kidneys are very liable to it again; to prevent a recurrence of the attack, they should abstain from wine and stimulants; use moderate exercise; avoid exposure to wet and cold; eat of food light and easy of digestion; not lie too much on the back, and on a mattress in preference to a bed

2. Aconite in minute doses is good for kidney complaint, peritonitis, puerperal fever, etc.

3. Constant application of poultices, as recommended in "2" for the liver, promotes cure and relieves pain.

1. **INFLAMMATION OF THE BLADDER**—Acute.—This disease affects the lining membrane of the bladder,—sometimes its muscular substance. It may attack the upper portion, the middle, or the neck of this organ. It runs a rapid course.

TREATMENT.—If the urine be retained, it is of the utmost importance that it be early drawn off with the catheter, lest a distention of the bladder bring on mortification. Great care is required not to produce irritation by any roughness in introducing the instrument.

Leeches should be applied upon the lower part of the bowels, the perinæum and around the anus. When these are removed, warm poultices should be applied. Cold compresses will often do as well. The bowels must be opened with Epsom salts. Injections of warm water with a few drops of tincture of arnica leaves will act finely as a local bath,—the water being retained as long as possible.

The tincture of veratrum viride will be required in 5 to 10-drop doses, or the compound tincture of Virginia snake root to induce perspiration. Dover's powders may sometimes be used for the same purpose.

Drinks must be taken very sparingly. A small amount of cold infusion of slippery elm bark or marshmallow and peach leaves. This mucilaginous drink must be the beginning and the end of the diet during the active stage of the disease.

2. **Inflammation of the Bladder**—Chronic.—This is much more common than the active form of the disease. It often arises from the same causes which produce acute inflammation of the bladder.

It often passes under the title of "catarrh of the bladder." It is a chronic inflammation of the mucous lining of the bladder, and is a very common and troublesome affection among old people.

TREATMENT.—To reduce the inflammation apply leeches, mustard, croton oil, or a cold compress every night.

As a diuretic give an infusion of buchu, uva ursi, trailing arbutus, queen of the meadow, etc. The compound infusion of trailing arbutus is well recommended. So is the compound balsam of sulphur. An infusion of the pods of beans has been well spoken of, but I have found the following very effective: Pulverized gum arabic, 1 scruple; soft water, 2 ozs., sweet spirits of nitre, ½ oz.; tincture of veratrum viride, 20 drops. Mix. Give ½ a tea-spoonful every half hour.

**3.** An injection into the bladder once a day of a tepid infusion of golden seal root with much care may be of great service; or an infusion of equal parts of golden seal, witch hazel and stramonium. It may be done with a gum elastic catheter and a small syringe.

The bowels must be kept open with the neutralizing mixture or some other mild physic; and the skin bathed with saleratus and water once a day and rubbed well with a coarse towel.

Should there be any scrofulous, gouty, or rheumatic condition of the system, the remedies for those complaints may be used in addition to the above.

**4.** For an adult, 1 pint a day of compound of sarsaparilla is the "boss" cure for gravel, and restores the worn out and wasted system. Try it.

**1. BRONCHITIS.**— TREATMENT.— The patient should, as a matter of course, be confined to bed; warm diluent drinks, such as flaxseed tea, or barley water, with a slice or two of lemon in it; gentle aperients, if required; foot-baths, and hot bran poultices to the chest. The chief dependence, however, is to be placed upon nauseating medicines. Four grs. of ipecacuanha powder, in a little warm water every quarter of an hour until vomiting is produced, and should be kept up at intervals of 2 or 3 hours. Sometimes a state of coma or collapse follows this treatment, and then it is necessary to give stimulants; carbonate of ammonia in 5 gr. doses, or sal volatile, ½ tea-spoonful about every hour. These are preferable to alcoholic stimulants; but should they not succeed, brandy may be tried, with strong beef tea. Should the urgency of the symptoms yield to the emetics, a milder treatment may be followed out. The following is a good mixture: Ipecacuanha wine, 1 dr.; aromatic spirit of ammonia, 2 drs.; carbonate of potash, 1 dr.; water, 8 ozs.; 2 table-spoonfuls to be given every 4 hours. If the cough is troublesome, add 1 gr. of acetate of morphine. The diet should be light and nourishing, and all exposure to cold must be carefully avoided. In children, acute bronchitis does not com-monly produce such marked effects as in adults, although sometimes it is extremely rapid and fatal, allowing little time for the action of remedies, which should be much the same as those above recommended, with proper regard, of course, to difference of age. If the child is unweaned, it must be allowed to suck very sparingly, if at all. The best plan is to give it milk with a spoon, or feeding-bottle, as the quantity can be thus better regulated. Great attention must be paid to the bowels, and also to the temperature of the air breathed by the little sufferer. A blister on the chest, about as big as a large copper cent, may be sometimes applied with advantage if the hot bran does not give the desired relief.

Winter coughs, catarrh, and asthma are very commonly but forms of chronic bronchitis. For the troublesome coughs which almost invariably attend confirmed bronchitis, and especially in the aged, opium is the most effectual remedy. The best form of administration is perhaps the compound tincture of camphor taken with ipecacuanha or antimonial wine—say ½ dr. of the former, with 10 grs. of either of the latter, in a little sugar and water or flaxseed tea, or use Dr. Chase's Cough Syrup. If there are febrile symptoms, add 15 minims of sweet spirits of nitre to each dose.

It is especially during the spring months, and when there is a prevalence of east wind, that bronchitis attacks young and old, often hurrying the former to a premature grave, and making the downward course of the latter more quick and painful. With aged people, in such cases, there is commonly a great accumulation of mucus in the bronchial tubes, which causes continued and violent coughing in the efforts to expel it, which efforts are often unsuccessful. Thus the respiration is impeded; the blood, from want of proper oxygeniza-tion, becomes unfit for the purposes of vitality, and death, often unexpectedly sudden, is the consequence. Such bronchitic patients must be carefully treated —no lowering measures will do for them, but warm and generous diet; opium can not safely be ventured on. Warm flannel next the skin, a genial atmos-phere, inhalation of steam—if medicated with horehound, or some demulcent plants, so much the better—a couple of compound squill pills at night, and during the day a mixture, composed of camphor mixture, 6 ozs.; tincture of squills, wine of ipecacuanha, and aromatic spirits of ammonia, each 2 drs.; with perhaps 2 drs. of tincture of hops. Take a table-spoonful every 3 or 4 hours.

ANOTHER TREATMENT. — To properly introduce the treatment, we will suppose a case, similar to which I have had many a one,—a man (for men have these inflammatory diseases 10 times to women once) comes home at night, with a cough, sore throat, etc., indicating that he has *taken cold*, and that it has set-tled upon the *throat and bronchial tubes*—take no supper, but go right to work, as for common colds, and get up a perspiration, by soaking the feet in water as hot as it can be borne, and pouring in more hot, from time to time, to keep it hot, for 20 to 30 minutes, and if you have one of the *alcohol lamps for sweat-ing purposes*, set it to work at the same time, and take some hot teas to help the work, and if there are no sweating herbs in the house, of course there is some whiskey or other liquor, make about a pint of hot stew, using 1 gill of whiskey, with sugar and hot water; and drink one or two good draughts of this while the feet are in the water, and the rest of it after you get into bed, covering up warm so as to continue the sweating for an hour or two, with hot irons, bricks or stones at the feet, as your conveniences will allow; then, when the family go to bed, take a good dose of physic, so it shall operate well by the next morning, and *ten* chances to *one* you will not need much further treatment. Perhaps some of the *sweating tincture*, and a little of the *cough syrup* and a little *diuretic* may be needed through the following day, or for a few days. But, if this does not work such a decided improvement as to indicate that no serious trouble remains, after the physic has operated, then take an *emetic*, or repeat the previous process, at farthest, on the following evening, when the symptoms, fever, etc., would likely be worse than through the day. But should you deem it best, from the violence of the symptoms, to take an emetic, one of the *diaphoretic* or sweating medicines had better also be taken to keep a tendency to the surface, according to the directions under that head.

But if these cases are neglected, they run on into a *chronic*, or long standing disease, and become very troublesome to cure, and often set up a chronic inflammation of the lungs, and finally consumption is the result.

**2. Bronchitis—Chronic.**—Chronic bronchitis must needs be of a similar character, and treated in a similar manner; but the emetic or sweating need not be repeated oftener than once a week, nor the cathartic, and they need not both be taken the same day; but a cough syrup, or some cough medicine should be taken daily; and a diuretic be taken for a day or two each week, as the case seems to demand, and a little essence of spearmint may be taken, a few drops whenever the soreness or rawness of the throat is troublesome, keeping a vial of it handy to taste, night or day, without water; or a drop or two of cedar oil may be taken on a little sugar, and the throat have some of it rubbed upon the outside as a liniment. The following combination of articles will fulfill all the indications needed, except that of cathartic, which can be used by itself, once in a week or 10 days:

Acetic tincture of bloodroot, tincture of black cohosh, and of the balsam of tolu, and wine of ipecacuanha, of each, ½ oz.; sweet spirits nitre, 1 oz. Mix. Dose—tea-spoonful, in a little water, 3 to 5 times daily according to the amount of irritation present.

**SCARLATINA.—With Severe Fever.**—In other cases of scarlet fever, the febrile symptoms at the commencement are more severe; there is a sensation of stiffness and pain on moving the neck, and it is also painful to swallow; the voice is thick, and the throat feels rough and straitened. The heat of the surface rises in a most remarkable manner; not only to the sensations of the patient or observer does the heat seem greater, but the thermometer shows it to be 108° or 110°, that is more than ten degrees above the natural standard. There is sickness, headache, great restlessness and delirium; the pulse is frequent but feeble, and there is great languor and faintness. The tongue is of a bright red color, especially at the sides and extremity, and the rising points are very conspicuous. The rash does not appear so early as in the milder scarlet fever, as is seen in patches, very frequently about the elbows. Sometimes it vanishes and appears again at uncertain times without any corresponding change in the general disorder. When the rash is slight or goes off early, there is little scaling off of the skin; but in severer cases, large pieces of the skin come off, especially from the hands and feet. The swelling and inflammation of the throat sometimes go off without any ulceration; but at other times slight ulcerations form at the tonsils and at the back of the mouth; and whitish specks are seen intermixed with the redness, from which a tough phlegm is secreted, clogging the throat and very troublesome. This kind of scarlet fever is not unfrequently followed by great debility, or the occurrence of other diseases, as inflammation of the eyes, or dropsy, or an inflammatory state of the whole system or water on the brain.

TREATMENT.—It is in general, proper to begin with giving an emetic, especially if we at all suspect the stomach to be loaded with undigested matter; and we are very soon after to exhibit laxative medicines which are truly one of our most important remedies in this disease. A dangerous and exhausting looseness which takes place towards the fatal termination of an ill-managed scarlet fever, for a long time excited great fears and prejudices against the use of laxative medicines in this disease; but better observation has con-.inced us that so far from being detrimental, laxative medicines, early and prudently begun have the best effect in mitigating the disease and in preventing the collection of that putrid and offending matter in the bowels which is so sure to produce wasting diarrhœa when it is suffered to accumulate. To lessen the burning heat of the skin, nothing is at all comparable in some cases to the free affusion of cold water, which, when employed prudently and at the proper time, cools the surface, and from a state of the most restless irritation, brings the patient to comparative ease and tranquility. The cold affusion, however, is not proper where there is much fullness of blood on one hand or great debility on the other; and in the majority of cases we must trust to the washing or sponging of the whole body with tepid water, or vinegar and water; and till the heat of the body is reduced by these means, it is in vain that we give internal medicines to procure perspiration or to allay restlessness and induce sleep. After washing it is not at all unusual for the formerly harassed patient to fall into a gentle and refreshing sleep, and a mild and breathing sweat comes out over the whole body This supersedes the necessity of sudorific and anodyne medicines; and provided we attend to the bowels, keep away stimulant and nourishing food, give the drink cold or acidulated, and employ proper gargles for the mouth and throat, the drugs we administer may be very few indeed.

The inflammatory state of the system which often follows scarlet fever is not unfrequently accompanied with a swelling resembling dropsical swelling; but we are not to regard this last as a sign of debility, or to be deterred from the use of active remedies. Bleeding from the arm is seldom admissible, but leeches behind the ears may be necessary if head symptoms come on; brisk purgatives are to be freely administered, and the inflammatory and dropsical tendency is to be combated by the use of foxglove and other diuretics. When the inflammatory action has subsided and the dropsy appears to be the principal malady, we are to give tonic medicines and nourishing diet along with such medicines as increase the flow of urine.

**MALIGNANT SCARLET FEVER—With Putrid Sore Throat.**—There is yet another and more fatal form of scarlet fever where the malignant and putrescent symptoms are more rapid and severe, where the general system is much oppressed, and the throat and neighboring parts affected with rapidly spreading ulcerations. It is this which has obtained the name of *putrid sore throat.* This form of scarlet fever begins like the preceding, but in a day or two shows symptoms of peculiar severity. The rash is usually faint, and the whole skin soon assumes a dark or livid red color. The heat is not so great nor so permanent as in the other kinds; the pulse is small, feeble, and irregular, there is delirium and coma, with occasional fretfulness and violence. The eyes are suffused with a dull redness, there is a dark red flush on the cheek, and the mouth is incrusted with a black or brown fur. The ulcers in the throat are covered with dark sloughs and surrounded by a livid base; there is a large quantity of tough phlegm which impedes the breathing, occasioning a rattling noise; and increasing the pain and difficulty of swallowing. A sharp discharge comes from the nostrils, producing soreness, chaps, and even blisters. There is severe diarrhœa, spots on the skin, bleedings from the mouth, bowels, or other parts, all of which portend a fatal termination to the disease. Sometimes the patients die suddenly about the third or fourth day; at other times in the second or third week; gangrene having probably arisen in the throat or some parts of the bowels. Those who recover have often long illnesses from the ulceration spreading from the throat to the neighboring parts, occasioning suppuration of the glands, cough, and difficulty of breathing with hectic fever.

TREATMENT.—The active remedies formerly mentioned are quite inadmissible here. Unnecessary heat is to be avoided, but we are not to think of the cold washing or of purging, lest we oppress the powers of life and bring on a fatal diarrhœa. The system requires support and stimulants from the commencement of the attack. Strong beef tea should be given in as large quantities as possible, and wine and bark should be liberally administered; the throat must be injected with strong cleaning gargles. The infusion of cayenne pepper or the decoction of bark acidulated with sulphuric or muriatic acid, or gargles to which a little tincture of myrrh or of camphor is added, may be usefully employed. Too often, however, all treatment is unavailing, and there is no more fatal contagious disease than malignant scarlet fever.

There is an ulcerated sore throat of peculiar malignity, distinct from scarlet fever, which commonly terminates with the worst symptoms of croup.

**ABORTION, OR MISCARRIAGE—(Abortus.)**—The separation of the child from the womb of the mother at any period before the sixth month of pregnancy; between which period and the full time the same event is called premature labor.

*Symptoms.*—Abortion may be described as consisting of three stages, each of which should be carefully studied; because in the two first much may be done by the patient herself or by the judicious management of friends about her.

In the first stage the woman merely " threatens to miscarry;" there is pain in the lower part of the belly, or about the back and loins, with unusual depression of spirits and faintness without any apparent cause. If these symptoms do not pass off, they are succeeded by a discharge of blood from the external parts, sometimes light, at other times profuse and alarming; accompanied or succeeded by sharp pains in the back, the loins, and the lower part of the belly, not constant, but intermitting, like those of regular labor. Often there is vomiting, sickness, or pains of the bowels, and headache; and from the quantity of blood lost, fainting fits frequently occur, and there is commonly a sense of weakness, much greater than can be accounted for by the copiousness of the discharge. This is the second stage; and in it the child has become partially separated from the womb. If by the efforts of nature or the assistance of art these symptoms abate or cease, the embryo may be retained, and many continue to grow. But in other cases the discharge of blood continues and the signs of approaching expulsion of the contents of the womb become more evident. Regular pains ensue, there is a feeling of bearing down, with a desire to make water; and at last the fœtus comes away, either surrounded with its membranes, if the whole ovum be small, or the membranes break, the waters are discharged, and the fœtus comes away, leaving the after-birth behind. This constitutes the third stage, in which the child is altogether separated and must be expelled.

*Causes.*—1. Abortion may be caused by external violence, as kicks or blows, a fall, or violent action, as dancing, riding, jumping, or much walking. Women in the state of pregnancy should avoid many of the domestic operations so proper at other times for good housewives to engage in. As our aim is to be practically useful, we venture at the risk of exciting a smile, to mention some exertions that ought to be avoided, viz., hanging up curtains, bedmaking, washing, pushing in a drawer with the foot, careless walking up or down a stair. 2. Straining of the body, as from coughing. 3. Costiveness. 4. Irritation of the neighboring parts, as from severe purging, falling down of the gut, or piles. 5. Any sudden or strong emotion of the mind, as fear, joy, surprise. 6. The pulling of a tooth has been known to produce a miscarriage; and though toothache is occasionally very troublesome to women in the pregnant state, the operation of drawing teeth should, if possible, be avoided at that time. 7. Women marrying when rather advanced in life are apt to miscarry. It would be hazardous to name any particular age at which it is too late to marry, but the general observation is worth attending to. 8. Constitutional debility from large evacuations, as bleeding or purging; or from disease, as dropsy, fever, small-pox. 9. A state the very opposite of this is sometimes the cause of abortion, viz., a robust and vigorous habit, with great fullness of blood and activity of the vascular system. 10. The death of the child.

TREATMENT.—Miscarriage is always an undesirable occurrence, and is to be prevented by all proper means, as a single miscarriage may irretrievably injure the constitution, or give rise to continual repetitions of the accident.

Unless we have reason to believe that the child is dead, it is desirable that miscarriage should be prevented, and that the woman should go on to the full time, if possible; but if the motion of the child should cease, if the breasts of the mother should become soft, after disease or great fatigue, and signs of miscarriage come on, it would be improper to endeavor to prevent the embryo coming away; and we must direct our efforts to relieve any urgent symptoms, and do what we can to conduct the patient safely through the process.

In the first stage of abortion, when it is merely impending or threatening, and even in the second stage, when the child has become partially separated, it is proper to attempt to check the discharge and prevent the consequent expulsion. The patient must cease from all exertion in walking, or even sitting upright, and must lie on a bed or sofa; all heating food or liquors must be avoided; whatever is taken should be rather cool, and cold applications must be made to the back, the loins, and neighboring parts. A lotion useful for this purpose is 1 part of vinegar to 2 or 3 parts of cold water; cloths or towels dipped in this are to be applied as directed above. The fainting which so often occurs requires to be relieved by a very moderate use of cordials, as a little wine and water, or even brandy and water; but in this much caution is required, lest feverishness or inflammatory symptoms be brought on, which in a weakened frame are apt to occur, from causes too slight to have the same effect in a healthy one.

As abortion sometimes takes place from too great fullness of blood, and from that state of the constitution well known by the name of high health, it is right in such cases to enjoin abstinence, to order a cooling diet, as light puddings, preparations of milk, or boiled vegetables; and to give gentle laxatives, as castor oil, senna, small doses of purging salts, magnesia, and rhubarb. If, under such treatment, the discharge from the womb stops, if the pains cease, and the sickness, headache, and constitutional symptoms are relieved, we may hope that the woman will not part with her offspring, but bring it to the full time. She must make up her mind to be in the reclining posture for some time, and must consider herself as liable to be again affected by the same symptoms and the same danger, if she uses the smallest liberty with herself.

If the discharge, however, still continues, and if there is little likelihood of the pregnancy going on, everything must be done to assist the woman in the safe completion of the process. We must introduce a soft cloth dipped in oil into the birth, so as to fill the lower part of it. By this means the blood has time to form into clots, and the contraction of the womb throws down the embryo along with them. We should not hastily use any force by the hand to bring it away; but the time when this may be done is to be left to the judgment of the medical person in attendance. As the after-birth in the early months bears a larger proportion to the contents of the womb than it does in the later months, it is often retained long after the child is expelled; but it must be remembered, that the womb will not contract till every thing is out of it, and therefore the bleeding will continue till the after-birth is off. It may happen to lie partly out of the womb, and if so, the practitioner is to attempt gently to remove it by the hand; but if it be wholly in the cavity of the womb, its expulsion is to be promoted by clysters of gruel, with the addition of salts, or with senna, or even a little of the tincture of aloes; or by a cautious use of the ergot of rye.

Patients should be careful not to throw away any thing discharged, on the supposition that they know what it is, but should uniformly show every clot to the practitioner, that he may be enabled to distinguish with certainty whether the child and after-birth are thrown off. When the womb is emptied, the belly is to be tied up with a binder, as after delivery at the full time; the same rest and quiet is to be ordered; the diet must be light and nourishing; heating food, all spirituous and malt liquors, are to be avoided, till the practitioner judges it proper to allow sulphuric acid, bark, and wine, or porter, to assist in recruiting the strength, which in the event of abortion is generally so greatly exhausted.

A very strong reason for enjoining rest and quietness after a miscarriage is this, that when twins or three children have been conceived, the embryo of one of them may be thrown off, and the other may be carried to the full time. Any premature exertion might, therefore, endanger the life of more than one child. When the woman is in some degree recruited, her recovery is to be completed by moderate exercise, by proper diet, by the use of the cold bath or sea-bathing, and by taking stomachic medicines, as the bark and wine, preparations of iron, or the elixir of vitriol. Few incidents have so pernicious an effect as a miscarriage, on certain constitutions; sometimes the health is irreparably injured, or a habit is begun which prevents the woman from ever carrying a child to the full time. In every future pregnancy particular caution is requisite; especially at the period when the miscarriage formerly happened, which is very generally between the eighth and twelfth week. For a considerable time before and after this, the woman should lie in a reclining posture, should attend to keeping the bowels easy by such mild laxatives as have been already mentioned; and if too full, should lose a little blood.

Sometimes, for wicked purposes, it is attempted to procure abortion, either by strong and acrid medicines, by violent exercises, or by direct application to the parts concerned; but it should be generally known that there is no medicine which directly and certainly acts on the womb itself; and that to procure abortion by any drug or mechanical violence, is to run the risk of speedy death, or inducing madness, or causing irreparable injury to the constitution, besides being punishable by law as a crime.

**DISEASES OF WOMEN.**—Women, in all civilized nations, have the management of domestic affairs; and it is very proper they should, as Nature has made them less fit for the more active and laborious employments. This indulgence, however, is generally carried too far; and women instead of being benefited by it, are greatly injured, from the want of exercise and free air. To be satisfied of this, one need only compare the fresh and ruddy looks of a milk-maid with the pale complexion of those females whose whole business lies within doors. Though Nature has made an evident distinction between the male and female with regard to bodily strength and vigor, yet she certainly never meant, either that the one should be always without, or the other always within doors.

The confinement of women, besides hurting their figure and complexion, relaxes their solids, weakens their minds, and disorders all the functions of the body. Hence proceed obstructions, indigestion, flatulence, abortions, and the whole train of nervous disorders. These not only unfit women for being mothers and nurses, but often render them whimsical and ridiculous. A sound mind depends so much upon a healthy body, that where the latter is wanting, the former is rarely to be found.

I have always observed that women who were chiefly employed without doors, in the different branches of husbandry, gardening, and the like, were almost as hardy as their husbands, and that their children were likewise strong and healthy.—But as the bad effects of confinement and inactivity upon both sexes have been already shown, we shall proceed to point out these circumstances in the structure and design of woman, which subject them to peculiar diseases; the chief of which are their *Monthly Evacuations, Pregnancy,* and *Child-bearing.* These indeed cannot properly be called diseases, but from the delicacy of the sex, and their being often improperly managed in such situations, they become the source of numerous calamities.

**MONTHLY TURNS OR MENSES.—First Signs of the Menstrual Discharge.—**Women generally begin to menstruate about the age of *fifteen,* and leave it off about *fifty,* which renders these two periods the most critical of their lives. About the first appearance of this discharge, the constitution undergoes a very considerable change, generally indeed for the better, though sometimes for the worse. The greatest care is now necessary, as the future health and happiness of the woman depends, in a great measure, upon her conduct at this period. It is the duty of mothers and those who are entrusted with the education of girls, to instruct them early in the conduct and management of themselves at this critical period in their lives. False modesty, inattention, and ignorance of what is beneficial or hurtful at this time, are the source of many diseases and misfortunes in life, which a few sensible lessons from an experienced matron might have prevented. Nor is care less necessary in the subsequent returns of this discharge. Taking improper food, severe nervous strain or catching cold at this period is often sufficient to ruin the health, or to render the woman ever after incapable of procreation.

If a girl about this time of life be confined to the house, kept constantly sitting, and neither allowed to romp about, nor employed in any active business, which gives exercise to the whole body, she becomes weak, relaxed, and puny: her blood not being duly prepared, she looks pale and wan; her health, spirits, and vigor decline, and she sinks into a valetudinary for life. Such is the fate of numbers of those unhappy women, who, either from too much indulgence, or their own narrow circumstances, are at this critical period, denied the benefit of exercise and free air.

A lazy, indolent disposition proves likewise very hurtful to girls at this period. One seldom meets with complaints from obstructions amongst the more active and industrious part of the sex, whereas the indolent and lazy are seldom free from them. These are, in a manner, eaten up by the *chlorosis*, or green-sickness, and other diseases of this nature. We would therefore recommend it to all who wish to escape these calamities, to avoid indolence and inactivity, as their greatest enemies, and to be as much in the open air as possible.

Another thing which proves very hurtful to girls about this period of life is unwholesome food. Fond of all manner of trash, they often indulge in it, till their whole humors are quite vitiated. Hence ensues indigestions, want of appetite, and a numerous train of evils. If the fluids be not duly prepared, it is utterly impossible that the secretions should go properly on. Accordingly we find that such girls as lead an indolent life and eat indiscriminately are not only subject to obstructions of the *menses*, but likewise to glandular obstructions, as the scrofula, or King's evil, &c.

A dull disposition is also very hurtful to girls at this period. It is a rare thing to see a sprightly girl who does not enjoy good health, while the grave, moping, melancholy creature proves the very prey of vapors and hysterics. Youth is the season for mirth and cheerfulness. Let it therefore be indulged. It is an absolute duty. To lay in a stock of health in time of youth, is as necessary a piece of prudence as to make provision against the decays of old age. While therefore wise Nature prompts the happy youth to join in sprightly amusements, let not the severe dictates of hoary age forbid the useful impulse, nor damp with serious gloom the season destined to mirth and innocent festivity.

Another thing very hurtful to women about this period of life, is tight clothes. They are fond of a fine shape, and foolishly imagine that this can be acquired by lacing themselves tight. Hence by squeezing the stomach and bowels, they hurt the digestion, and occasion many incurable maladies. This error is not indeed so common as it has been; but, as fashions change, it may come about again; we therefore think it not improper to mention it. I know many women, who to this day, feel the direful effects of that wretched custom of squeezing every girl into as small a size in the middle as possible. Human invention could not possibly have devised a practice more destructive to health.

**RETENTION OF THE MENSES.**—After a woman has arrived at that period of life when the *menses* usually begin to flow, and they do not appear, but, on the contrary, her health and spirits begin to decline, we would advise instead of shutting the poor girl up in the house, and dosing her with steel, asafœtida, and other nauseous drugs, to place her in a situation where she can enjoy the benefits of free air and agreeable company. There let her eat wholesome food, take sufficient exercise, and amuse herself in the most agreeable manner, and we have little reason to fear but Nature thus assisted, will do her proper work. Indeed she seldom fails, unless where the fault is on our side.

This discharge in the beginning is seldom so instantaneous as to surprise women unawares. It is generally preceded by symptoms which foretell its approach; as a sense of heat, weight, and dull pain in the loins; distention and hardness of the breasts; headache; loss of appetite; lassitude; paleness of the countenance; and sometimes a slight degree of fever. When these symptoms appear about the age at which the menstrual flow usually begins, everything should be carefully avoided which may obstruct that necessary and salutary evacuation; and all means used to promote it, as sitting frequently over the steams of warm water, drinking warm diluting liquors, taking hip baths, &c.

**SUPPRESSION OF THE MENSES.**—Cold is extremely hurtful at this particular period. More of the sex date their disorders from colds, caught while they were out of order, than from all other causes. This ought surely to put them on their guard, and to make them very circumspect in their conduct at such times. A degree of cold that would not in the least hurt them at another time, will at this period be sufficient to entirely ruin their health and constitution.

After the *menses* have once begun to flow, the greatest care should be taken to avoid everything that may tend to obstruct them. Women ought to be exceedingly cautious in what they eat or drink at the time they are out of order. Everything that is cold, or apt to sour on the stomach ought to be avoided; as fruit, butter-milk, and such like. Fish, and all kinds of food that are hard of digestion, are also to be avoided. As it is impossible to mention every thing that may disagree with individuals at this time, we would recommend it to each one to be very attentive to what disagrees with herself, and carefully to avoid it.

The greatest attention ought likewise to be paid to the mind, which should be kept as easy and cheerful as possible. Every part of the animal economy is influenced by the passions, but none more so than this. Anger, fear, grief, and other affections of the mind, often occasion obstructions of the menstrual flow, which proves absolutely incurable.

From whatever cause the flow is obstructed, except in the state of pregnancy, proper means should be used to restore it. For this purpose we would recommend sufficient exercise, in a dry, open, and rather clear air; wholesome diet, and, if the body be weak and languid, a good tonic, (see Mrs. Chase's Magic Tonic;) also cheerful company and all manner of amusements. If these fail, recourse must be had to the physician.

When obstructions proceed from a weak relaxed state of the solids, such medicines as tend to promote digestion, and assist the body in preparing good blood, ought to be used. The principal of these are iron and Peruvian bark, with other bitter and astringent medicines. The bark and other bitters may either be taken in substance or infusions, as is the most agreeable to the patient.

When obstructions proceed from a viscid state of the blood; for women of a gross or full habit, evacuations, and such medicines as attenuate the humors are necessary. The patient in this case ought to bathe her feet frequently in warm water, to take now and then a cooling purge, and to live upon a spare thin diet.

When obstructions proceed from affections of the mind, as grief, fear, anger, &c., every method should be taken to amuse and divert the patient. And that she may the more readily forget the cause of her affliction, she ought, if possible, to be removed from the place where it happened. A change of place, by presenting the mind with a variety of new objects, has often a very happy influence in relieving it from the deepest distress. A soothing, kind, and affable behavior to women in this situation, is also of importance.

An obstruction of the *menses* is often the effect of other maladies. When this is the case, instead of giving medicines to force that discharge, which might be dangerous, we ought, by all means, to endeavor to restore the patient's health and strength. When that is effected the other will return of course.

1. For *Suppressed menstruation,* as soon as possible use the tepid foot-bath. At the same time sit over a vessel of warm water, in which has been boiled some bitter herbs, till a profuse perspiration is produced. Then retire to a warm bed and take every hour or two a tea-cupful of warm tea made from the root of bervine. If this is not successful, give a little pulverized mandrake root, with a little cream of tartar, on an empty stomach; after which penny-royal or motherwort tea may be drank freely.

2. Aromatic spirits of ammonia taken in doses of 20 to 30 drops in sweetened water several times a day is almost sure to relieve suppression and is good for painful menstruation.

3. Mrs. H. Y. Johnson, of Iowa, once told my wife that oil of cotton seed, one dram daily, was unfailing. I have used it in my practice with success and have also used it to spur up *labor* when it dragged, with good success.

4. Crushed ice placed to the back in oil cloth or rubber bag—place low down—is also good for suppressed menses. It is also valuable sometimes in restoring *falling womb* and cures leucorrhea.

**MENSES, TO RESTORE.**—Fl. ex. of ergot, and fl. ex. of gossypium (cotton root), each ½ oz.; fl. ex. of black cohosh, 1 oz.; simple syrup, 2 ozs. Mix. DOSE—Take 1 tea-spoonful 4 times daily, for a few days; then if the menses are not restored, stop its use till 4 or 5 days before the regular period for their return, and take it up again, with the help of warm hip baths daily, and daily sitting over the steam of bitter herbs, etc., as the grandmothers knew so well how to do. In the meantime, doing anything needed to tone up the system, by taking tonics; overcoming constipation by laxatives, and in a similar manner endeavoring to overcome any other irregularity, if any exist; and it is thus—or by such means—you will succeed in restoring the general health.

**PROFUSE MENSTRUATION.**—The menstrual flow may be too great as well as too small. When this happens, the patient becomes weak, the color pale, the appetite and digestion are bad, and swelling of the feet, dropsies, and consumption often ensue. This frequently happens to women about the age of forty-five or fifty, and is very difficult to cure. It may proceed from a sedentary life; a full diet, consisting chiefly of salted, high-seasoned, or acrid food; the use of spirituous liquors; excessive fatigue; relaxation; a dissolved state of the blood; violent passions of the mind, &c.

The treatment of this disease must be varied according to its cause. When it is occasioned by any error in the patient's regimen, an opposite course to that which induced the disorder must be pursued, and such medicines taken as have a tendency to restrain the flow and counteract the morbid affections of the system from whence it proceeds.

To restrain the flow, the patient should be kept quiet and easy both in body and mind. If it be very violent, she ought to lie in bed with her head low; to live upon a cool and slender diet, as veal or chicken broths with bread; and to drink decoctions of nettle-roots, or the greater comfrey. If these be not sufficient to stop the flow, stronger astringents may be used, as Japan earth, alum, elixir of vitriol, the Peruvian bark, &c.

Two drams of alum and 1 of Japan earth may be pounded together, and divided into 8 or 9 doses, one of which may be taken 3 times a day.

Persons whose stomachs cannot bear alum, may take 2 table-spoonfuls of the tincture of roses 3 or 4 times a day, to each dose of which 10 drops of laudanum may be added.

If these should fail, half a dram of the Peruvian bark, in powder, with 10 drops of the elixir of vitriol, may be taken in a glass of red wine, 4 times a day.

**2.** Oil of erigeron 1 to 5 drops every ½ hour or hour, dissolved in a little alcohol, arrests flooding, or hemorrhage of the womb, promptly. A very severe case of "flooding to death" was saved by putting hot sand bags under the back of the head and heart—hotter than the hand could bear, frequently renewed.

**LEUCORRHEA, FLUOR ALBUS, OR WHITES.**—The *uterine flow* may offend in quality as well as in quantity. What is usually called the *fluor albus*, or "whites," is a very common disease, and proves extremely hurtful to delicate women. This discharge, however, is not always white, but pale, yellow, green, or of a blackish color; sometimes it is sharp and corrosive, sometimes foul and fetid, &c. It is attended with a pale complexion, pain in the back, loss of appetite, swelling of the feet, and other signs of debility. It generally proceeds from a relaxed state of the body, arising from indolence, the excessive use of tea, coffee, or other weak and watery diet.

To remove this disease, the patient must take as much exercise as she can bear, without fatigue. Her food should be solid and nourishing, but of easy digestion; and her drink pretty generous, as red port or claret, mixed with lime-water. Tea and coffee are to be avoided. I have often known strong broths to have an exceeding good effect; and sometimes a milk diet alone will perform a cure. The patient ought not to lie too long a-bed. When medicine is necessary, we know none preferable to the Peruvian bark, which in this case ought always to be taken in substance. In warm weather, the cold bath will be of considerable service.

**1.** Moisten a sponge with glycerine, roll it in fine powder of boracic acid and push up in the mouth of womb daily—a tape or ribbon may be tied to the sponge to remove it.

**2.** Obstinate cases of "whites," or leucorrhea may be cured by insufflation of powdered vegetable charcoal.

**3.** Pond's ex. of witch hazel, 1 table-spoonful in a tea-cupful of warm water, injected well up into the vagina, 3 times a day—cures the worst cases in a few weeks.

**4. Leucorrhea, Injection for.**—Pulverized golden seal, 1 oz.; boracic acid, ½ oz.; pulverized alum, ½ oz.; sulphate of zinc, 20 grs. DIRECTIONS —Mix thoroughly together, and keep in a well stopped bottle, or suitable covered box. At tea time put 1 tea-spoonful of the powder into a cup of hot tea—green tea is preferable. Stir 2 or 3 times during the evening, and at bedtime strain it and inject, with a female syringe, every night, if bad, or every second night in ordinary cases. First cleansing the parts by injecting 1 pt. to 1 qt. of water, as hot as it can be borne. (See also "Injection, Valuable in Gonorrhea, or Leucorrhea." See also "Red Drops for Gonorrhea, Leucorrhea, etc.")

*Remarks.*—Dr. Mason says this has proved a splendid remedy in every case where he has used it. I have also used it with success. But as quinine and tannin have latterly been used considerably in these cases of leucorrhea, with almost entire success, I will give one containing them, which I have also tried with great satisfaction as follows:

**5. Leucorrhea, Valuable Injection for.**—Fl. ex. of golden seal and chlorate of potash, pulverized, each 1 dr.; sulphate of zinc, 2 drs.; tannin and sulphate of quinine, each ½ dr.; distilled or pure soft water, 1 qt. Inject morning and night; first cleansing the parts by injecting, once or twice, water as hot as can be borne. DIRECTIONS—In mixing these ingredients, dissolve the sulphate of zinc in ½ pint of water, then put the quinine in a mortar, with a little aromatic sulphuric acid to dissolve it, then add to the zinc water. Put the tannin into another ½ pint of the water, and stir until dissolved, then mix the two and add the other articles, and the balance of the water, to make 1 qt.; shake when used; and use only enough to fill the vagina once, holding it in place 2 or 3 minutes, by placing the fingers of one hand over the vulva, or external part, having first used the hot water, as directed in the last recipe above; keeping it in place also 2 or 3 minutes, each time, in the same manner as here directed, is of the utmost importance, as this plan distends and cleanses the whole vagina, while in the old way, the injections flowed out alongside of the tube, cleansing but very little indeed. Use enough of the hot water to distend it twice at least, before using the tea or other injection, and the cure will be quick and satisfactory.

*Remarks.*—With this, Dr. J. W. Burney, of Des Arc, Ark., says he has had more success than with any other; but with this he also gives 1 tea-spoonful 3 times daily of the fl. ex. of buchu internally, in a little flaxseed tea. The plan and remedies are excellent, as I have tested them.

**CESSATION OF MENSES, OR TURN OF LIFE.**—That period of life at which the *menses* cease to flow is likewise very critical to the sex. The stoppage of any customary evacuation, however small, is sufficient to disorder the whole frame, and often to destroy life itself. Hence it comes to pass, that so many women either fall into chronic disorders, or die about this time; such of them, however, as survive it, without contracting any chronic disease, often become more healthy and hardy than they were before, and enjoy strength and vigor to a very great age.

If the *menses* suddenly cease, in women of a full habit, they ought to abate somewhat of their usual quantity of food, especially of the more nourishing kind, as flesh, eggs, &c. They ought likewise to take sufficient exercise, and to keep the bowels open. This may be done by taking, once or twice a week, a little rhubarb, or an infusion of hiera picra in wine or brandy, or purgatives recommended elsewhere, and if complicated with other diseases, call a doctor.

**DEFICIENT AND PAINFUL MENSTRUATION.**--The amount of suffering among women from this disease is alarming, and far greater than in our "grandmothers' days." It seldom appears until they have menstruated some time with considerable regularity, and little or no pain; afterward, they begin to suffer more or less pain, which increases until it becomes grinding and more severe than those of labor.

It soon affects the general health, destroys the complexion, and ruins the disposition. The pain generally begins in the back, extends to the loins and hips, and is followed by pressing down pain, resembling in severity, those of labor. At first a slight discharge takes place, but suddenly ceases, after some time is renewed and becomes more plentiful, which, together with the pain gradually ceases. The discharge differs from that of a healthy menstruation in appearance, being mixed with lumps, and clots of flaky matter, having the appearance of membrane or skin. The breasts frequently swell and become painful. Women seldom have children who have this disease in a severe form.

Strictly avoid the use of all spirituous liquors, and keep the bowels well open a few days before the expected attack. The patient should be kept in bed, drink freely of tea made either of pennyroyal, catmint, sage, or the leaves of spruce pine, until the discharge be fully established; after which the pain seldom returns for that period. Sometimes 1 or 2 grains of powdered ipecac, or ½ tea-spoonful of the syrup taken every 2 hours, will bring on the flow freely, when other means fail. Keep up the warm baths for some time.

1. In painful menstruation, great benefit is received from the use of the warm bath; and apply hot water in bottles to the whole surface of the abdomen, with hot bricks to the feet; or apply a hot poultice or fomentation of hops, tansy, or boneset and take the following:—Pulverized camphor, 25 grs.; macrotin, 25 grs.; ipecac, 25 grs.; cayenne, 12 grs.; opium, 12 grs. Mix, and make into 24 pills, with ex. of hyoscyamus, and take 1 pill every 2, 3, or 4 hours, according to the urgency of the case.

2. Take warm hip baths ½ hour at a time. Hot fomentation low down on the back will arrest *overflow of menses*.

3. Take ¼ gr. codeia night and morning. You won't need anything else.

4. **Painful Menstruation and Other Pains, Remedy for.**— Dr. King, of Toledo, thinks very much of the following remedy, not only in painful menstruation, but also for pain in the stomach or bowels, colic, cholera-morbus, diarrhea, etc. The author has used it in the latter cases with so much satisfaction that he has faith in its virtues in the first named: Oil of cloves, cinnamon, anise and peppermint, each 40 drops (⅔ drs.); put these into 3 ozs of alcohol, and add sulphuric ether and laudanum, each 1 oz. DOSE—In bad

cases, 1 tea-spoonful in cold, sweetened water; repeat in 10 to 20 minutes, if needed, and at longer intervals as long as needed. For children, in stomach or bowel difficulties, according to age and severity, from 10 drops to ½ tea-spoonful, as required to meet all cases.

**5. Painful Menstruation and Nervous Debility, Stimulating Tonic for.**—Quinine, 60 grs.; morphine and arsenious acid, each 1 gr.; strychnine, 1 gr.; alcoholic ex. of aconite (or if this is not on hand, the same amount of the ex. of hyoscyamus may take its place), 3 grs. of the one used. Mix very thoroughly, and make into 30 pills. Dose—Take 1 pill only, every 6 hours, until relieved. Women troubled with painful menstruation, should keep them on hand for use, as soon as the least pain is manifested; but do not take them any oftener than 1 once in 6 hours.

*Remarks.*—This pill I obtained from an old physician, whom I have known over 40 years, and I know him to be in every way reliable. Some will say: "They contain poisonous articles." So they do, and so do very many of our best medicines. It depends wholly upon the amount taken as to their injurious effects; here we have 2 grs. of quinine, ½ gr. of the ex. of aconite, $\frac{1}{30}$th. of a gr. of morphine and arsenious acid, and $\frac{1}{30}$th. of a gr. of strychnine, only, in each pill. If they are taken as directed, as to dose and time—1 pill, 6 hours apart—there is not the least danger in their use, as these articles are all sometimes, given in doses twice as large as here given. It is indeed, a happy combination of our most reliable remedies, for cases requiring the properties named—something to allay pain and strengthen the system. After the 30 pills have been taken, if not cured before, wait a week, at least, before having any more made. By that time some of the chinoidine, or cinchonidia pills, found among the Ague Remedies or the tonic pills for Debility following Leucorrhea, may be taken, with good results.

**DISEASES OF THE WOMB, UTERUS**—The organ in which the embryo lives and grows until the time of birth. It is shaped something like a pear, with the broad end uppermost. Its broadest part is called its *fundus;* it has also a body and a neck; its mouth opens into the vagina. In the unimpregnated state, it would hardly contain a kidney-bean, but at the full time, it expands sufficiently to contain one or more children, with their waters, membranes, and after-births. At the upper part of the womb, two broad membranous expansions arise, and are the means of its attachment to the sides of the pelvis; in the doublings of these expansions are situated the ovaria, the receptacle of certain vesicles, which are afterwards animated; and also the tubes, through which one or more vesicles pass down into the uterus, there being an opening at each side of the fundus. Sometimes the embryo grows in one of these tubes, instead of getting into the uterus. Such extra-uterine conceptions are generally fatal to the mother and child. From the womb proceeds the Monthly Discharge.

The sympathies of the womb with the other parts are of the most general and extensive kind. Not even the stomach itself has more influence on the rest of the system. When the state and contents of the womb are altered by pregnancy, the stomach, the bowels, and digestive functions are in very frequent instances exceedingly deranged. The brain and nervous system, the function of respiration, and the state of the breasts, are all very much influenced by the condition of the womb.

The womb is subject to a variety of disorders, the most common and important of which are as follows:

1. **Bearing Down or Falling Down** signifies that the womb is lower than it ought to be. The first symptom is an uneasy feeling in the lower part of the back, while the patient is standing or walking; with a sense of pressure or bearing down. As the complaint increases, a swelling appears to come in the way of the discharge of urine, which the patient cannot pass without lying down, and pushing aside the tumor which prevents it. In more advanced and severe cases, the womb is forced altogether out of the parts, as a hard and bulky substance hanging between the thighs. In many cases the protruded parts are ulcerated, and give great uneasiness by their being fretted. Many complaints arise in other parts of the system from this local disease. There is sickness and other disorders of the stomach and bowels, with hysterics and nervous affections; while the inability to take exercise is itself a great evil, and tends to impair still more the general health.

*Causes.*—Every woman should know these, and avoid them as far as possible. Whatever tends to weaken the general system or the passage to the womb, may give occasion to its falling down. In the unmarried state, all violent or long continued exercise when the person is unwell, has a tendency to bring on the complaint; hence, young women at these times should avoid dancing, riding, and long walking or standing. Married women have it brought on by frequent miscarriage, improper treatment during labor, and taking much exercise too soon after delivery.

TREATMENT. When the disease has occurred recently, and is not very bad, the system is to be strengthened by nourishing diet, by the cold bath, by moderate exercise; and a mild astringent fluid is to be thrown into the passage. This may be made of 20 grs of white vitriol to 1 pint of rose-water. But when the complaint is of longer standing and more severity, the patient must be confined to the horizontal posture; bark and wine, and chalybeate medicines must be employed, and a stronger astringent, as a decoction of oak-bark, with some acid added to it, must be thrown up. Sometimes these means are all ineffectual, and an instrument of wood or ivory, called a pessary, must be worn, to fill the outer passage and prevent the womb from falling down. This instrument should be removed every two or three days, and cleaned. Sometimes this soon effects a cure; but, in general, it requires to be worn for years. If a person liable to this disease becomes pregnant, it disappears about the third or fourth month; and if proper measures be taken after delivery, the return of the complaint may be prevented in many instances.

2. **Tumors or Polypi in the Womb and Vagina.**—These are of various sizes and consistency; they are sometimes broad and flat at their base, sometimes they have a narrow neck. They occasion a discharge of blood at

times; but when small, they are not productive of much inconvenience. But if they become large, they give rise to symptoms both troublesome and dangerous. There is violent bearing down pain, discharges of blood, or of fetid dark-colored matter from the vagina, pain or difficulty of making water, irritation of the rectum, and a frequent desire to go to stool. When very large, the polypus hangs out from the passage. If the disease be not relieved, the pains become more violent, the constitution is affected, and the continual discharge greatly weakens the patient.

TREATMENT.—As the patients themselves cannot distinguish tumors from other diseases producing similar symptoms, their existence must be ascertained by the examination of a physician; and their removal effected by a surgical operation, either by the knife or by ligature, performed by a surgeon well acquainted with the structure and connections of the parts. No internal remedies will do any good till the tumor is removed. When this is accomplished, the general health is to be improved by proper diet and tonic medicines.

3. **Cancer of the Womb.**—This, when in a state of ulceration, constitutes one of the most deplorable diseases which can afflict humanity. Cancer of the womb most generally attacks at the decline of life, though not exclusively so. At first the patient has an uneasy feeling of weight at the lower part of the belly, with heat or itching. Afterwards shooting pains occur; then a pain, giving a gnawing burning sensation, seems fixed in the region of the womb. This pain is attended by the discharge of ill-colored, sharp matter, which irritates and corrodes the neighboring parts. As the disease continues, almost every function of the body becomes disordered. Sickness and vomiting comes on, the bowels are torpid and irregular, hectic fever, and great emaciation ensue, and the spirits are dejected and desponding. Swellings of various glands, and watery swellings of the limbs, not unfrequently occur. Symptoms resembling those of the early stages of cancer, may arise from other complaints in the womb, as from polypus growths; the nature of the disease should therefore be, if possible, ascertained at an early period, that the one may be removed, and the other kept from rapid advancement and ulceration, so far as we are able. Cancer in the womb appears to begin with a thickening and hardness of that organ; which we suspect when there are pains in the thighs and back, a bearing down when the patient is using exercise, and occasional discharge of clotted blood.

TREATMENT.—Of the nature of cancer of the womb, we are as ignorant as of cancer in any other part of the body; and when the disease is established, we are as destitute of any remedy. In the periods of deplorable suffering which terminate the life of the patient, we can do little more than palliate symptoms; and the whole tribe of narcotic medicines have been brought into requisition on such occasions. Opium, belladonna, hemlock, and various others have been tried, and failed. Mercury, in every shape, is absolutely pernicious in cancer.

The melancholy distress to which patients are reduced by cancer of the womb, disposes the minds both of themselves and their friends to listen with eagerness to the promises of relief, which ignorant and interested empirics so liberally make to them.   But all such promises must be met with the most obstinate incredulity.   The learned, the experienced, and the candid members of the medical profession declare, that, as yet, no drug has been found capable of curing cancer by acting on the constitution; and whoever suffers herself to be deluded by the boasts of those whose only aim is to vend their nostrums, loses the time that might be better employed, and neglects those suggestions which might palliate, though they cannot cure, her complaints.

**4.   Inflammation of the Womb.**—This seldom happens, except in the puerperal state.   It may occur at any time of life, especially during the years of menstruation.   Like other inflammations, it is ushered in by shivering, followed by great heat, thirst, quick hard pulse.   Pain is felt in the womb from the beginning, with a sensation of fulness and weight; also a burning heat and throbbing.   The exact spot where the pain is felt varies according to the part of the womb that is inflamed; it may be towards the navel, or over the share-bones, or shooting backwards, or down the thighs; or it may affect the bladder with pain and suppression of urine, or difficulty of passing it.

It is distinguished from after-pains by the constancy of the pain, by the heat and throbbing of the part, and by the pain being much increased on pressure at the region of the womb.

*Causes.*—Inflammation of the womb is induced by cold, direct injury external or internal, from medicinal or instrumental means to produce abortion, by difficult or tedious labor, by officious interference during labor, or by forcing the expulsion of the child and after-birth; by too much strong food or heating drinks; by exposure to cold during perspiration, or by using cold drinks.

TREATMENT.—It requires very prompt and active interference, as its progress is very rapid, and its event uncertain and dangerous.   If assistance is procured in time, it may be stopped by blood-letting, both general and local, by leeches, low diet, diluent drinks slightly acidulated; with laxative medicines or clysters, and fomentations to the belly.   A copious sweat, and a flow of the lochia, with relief from pain, mark the success of this plan of treatment.   But we are not always so successful; for the pain sometimes becomes more acute, with throbbing, and an increase of fever, sickness, delirium, and restlessness.   In these cases there is risk of mortification; and this is shown to have come on by a languid pulse, low deliriun, and cold clammy sweat.   Such termination happens chiefly in bad constitutions, or in those who are much debilitated.   The discharge does not escape and there is absorption.   A physician should be called at once as there is great danger.   When the discharge commences, the strength of the patient is to be supported by nourishing diet, the bowels are to be kept open, and bark and wine to be given.   Much attention must be paid to cleanliness.

# MISCELLANEOUS RECEIPTS FOR FEMALE COMPLAINTS IN GENERAL.

**1. Female Debility, Tonic Pill and Infusion for.**—In cases of female debility from uterine difficulties, often also connected with ague or chills and fever; but whether chills and fever or not, the following pill and infusion will be found valuable:

I. *Pill.*—Sulphate of quinine, 1 dr.; citrate of iron, 2 drs.; solid, or alcoholic ex. of nux vomica, 16 grs. Mix thoroughly, and make into 64 pills. Dose—Take 1 pill only, half an hour before each meal and at bed-time.

II. *Tonic and Alterative, or Infusion.*—In connection with the above pill much additional benefit will be derived in these cases by the use of the compound infusion of gentian, made as follows:

Gentian root, ½ oz.; orange peel and coriander seed, each, 1 dr.; dilute alcohol (half alcohol and half water), 4 ozs.; cold water, 12 ozs., to which in these cases add nitro-muriatic acid, 1 dr. Directions.—All the articles to be dry and coarsely ground or bruised; then put on the diluted alcohol and let stand 3 or 4 hours; then put on the water and let stand 12 hours, and strain; then add the acid and shake well. "An excellent way," says Dr. Warren, " for using gentian." This plant comes from Germany, growing in the Alps, Apennines and Pyrenees mountains. It excites the appetite and invigorates the digestive powers, and is used in all cases of debility. It is much used in dyspepsia and during recovery from all exhaustive diseases. Dose—Take 1 table-spoonful half an hour after each meal.

*Remarks.*—If in any case there are ulcerations at the neck of the womb or vagina, let there be taken ½ tea-spoonful doses, 3 times daily, of the syrup of iodide of iron, an hour or two after the infusion is taken; and in these cases of ulceration it is best to submit the case to a physician and have him make such caustic applications as will kill the ulcers. The Monsel salts is a good thing to be applied to them. The fact of ulceration may be known by a sensation of heat, and perhaps pain, at the point of ulceration, the discharge of matter, etc. This combination of treatment is well known to be exceedingly valuable. The nitrate of silver (lunar caustic in stick) is often used, and I have applied it—just touching the surface of the ulcer once in 4 or 5 days, has soon cured them, but more recently I have introduced the Monsel salts upon them, and also along the vagina as the speculum was withdrawn, with very satisfactory results, except that this salt contains iron, and consequently stains the clothing; hence, again, I have applied the sub-nitrate of bismuth, which does not stain, and I cannot see but it does equally well if put on pretty freely twice a week, night and morning, using the injections as given in leucorrhea (which see).

**2. Mrs. Chase's Magic Tonic Bitters for Weak and Debilitated Females.**—Best red Peruvian bark, prickly ash bark, and poplar-root bark, each, 4 ozs.; cinnamon bark, 1 oz.; cloves, ½ oz.; whiskey and clear worked cider, each, 2 qts. Directions, Dose, etc.—Grind all coarsely, or bruise with a hammer, and put into the jug or bottle with the spirits and cider, (or water, if no good cider can be had, but the cider is much the best), and shake daily for 10 days; take out the dregs, either filter, or strain and press out, as you choose, and take a wine-glass of it immediately after each meal. The dregs steeped in 1 qt. of water will yield considerable more strength, which may be added to the tonic bitters when strained off.

*Remarks.*—I have made this for my wife several times, and I did not fail to help her dispose of it occasionally myself. Her remark has often been: "Oh! what an appetite it gives me," etc. It is a very valuable tonic, and, from the spices, very pleasant to take.

**3. Sore Nipples, Remedy.**—A mixture of honey, borax, alum and strong sage tea.—Mrs. Mary Blake, of Parsons, Kan., in *Blade.* Knowing a similar mixture to be valuable as a gargle for sore throat, I believe it will be equally valuable for sore nipples. About ½ tea-spoonful each of powdered borax and alum, and 1 tea-spoonful of strained honey to 1 cup of strong sage tea.

*For a Gargle.*—A heaping tea-spoonful, each, of the powder, and 2 tea-spoonfuls of honey to ½ pt. of the strong sage tea, will be sufficient, and be found excellent; and for the gargle it would be all the better, if 1 to 2 cayenne peppers (such as pepper sauce is made of), or small red pepper, was steeped with the sage in making the tea. Children, however, cannot tolerate the pepper; then, for children, leave them out. Gargle at least 6 times a day, and for the nipples, wash off the saliva, and apply afte. each time of nursing. (See also the following, and "Sore Nipples, Breasts, etc., to Avoid and to Cure," below.)

**4. Sore Nipples, Efficient Remedy.**—A medical writer informs us that nitrate of lead, 10 grs., in 1 oz. of glycerine, or brandy, applied after each nursing, and washed off before each nursing, is an efficient (certain) remedy.

*Remarks.*—As he leaves it optional to use one or the other, the author would say use ½ oz. each of brandy and glycerine, to the 10 grs. of nitrate of lead.

**5. Milk, Suppression of, While Nursing—Treatment to Restore.**—I. As this difficulty quite frequently occurs with nursing mothers, and is also sometimes slow in its first secretions after child-birth, I will give an item from the *L'Union Médicale*, a French publication, which will prove valuable when needed. It says:

"When the milk secretion is slow in appearing, in a lying-in-woman (woman in confinement, or child-bearing), or when it ceases from mental or moral causes (not from inflammation of the breasts or other actual disease), it may be made to return by cataplasms (poultices), or fomentation of castor leaves applied to the breast, or by suction of the nipple, or by means of electricity. The mammary gland (the breast), is to be slightly compressed between two sponge electrodes (also known as the poles of a battery), and a feeble current passed through the gland for 10 or 15 minutes twice a day, after the first few electrizations, the breasts become full, the large veins appear on the gland, and the milk secretion is set up.

*Remarks.*—I have only had an opportunity to test this in one case, which began to improve by the third day. The poultice should be warm, and if the castor-bean leaf can be got (many people raise them as an ornamental plant in the garden), they, too, should be put on as hot as can well be borne. The poultice or the leaves used in connection with the electricity make it more likely to succeed.

II. It is well, also, in suppression of the milk which occurs most generally, if at all, when the child is only a few weeks old, to give acetate of potash, 1 oz., in water, 8 ozs.; adding a little tinct. ess. or fl. ex. of sassafras to flavor. Give in doses of 1 to 2 tea-spoonfuls, in a little more water, 3 times daily, to act on the kidneys, which are generally at fault, governing the dose by this action, not to make too free a flow of urine. As this also helps to relax the secretory functions of the breasts as well as the kidneys, weak coffee with plenty of milk and loaf sugar, and the old-fashioned chocolate, with milk and sugar plenty, drank alternately with the coffee, through the day, is also excellent, says an old doctor who has had large experience; and also rub upon the breasts freely, Trask's ointment, or what he thinks better, the bitter-sweet ointment, given below, all that will be absorbed.

**6. Sore Nipples, Breasts, etc.—To Avoid and Cure.**—Sore nipples are sometimes caused by wearing the dress or corsets too tight, but most generally by neglecting to wash them with cool water, and properly drying with a soft towel, after every nursing. When there is the least tendency to soreness of the nipples, dust on a little powdered magnesia or starch, kept generally as a baby powder, to prevent soreness in the groins or other folds of the skin. A very little mutton tallow, or, better still, lamb tallow, which is much softer, will prevent chafing when applied to any part liable to chafe. But if they become sore and irritable, make the following:

I. *Bittersweet Ointment.*—Bark of the root, with the outside scraped off a little, ¼ lb.; mutton tallow or lamb tallow, ½ lb.; stewed carefully together; then strain while hot, and box or bottle for use. Apply a little after washing and drying the nipples as above at each nursing.

II. *Smartweed Ointment.*—In places where the bittersweet can not be obtained, take smartweed and tallow, the same amount, and make the same way, and use in the same manner as the Bittersweet Ointment.

[The bittersweet makes a most valuable ointment for all healing purposes, and I know of only one thing at all comparable with it for similar purposes, and that is an ointment made with Balm of Gilead buds, same amount, and made the same as the bittersweet. (See also Tinct. of Balm of Gilead Buds for Cuts, Bruises, Wounds, etc.) But the smartweed ointment is considered much the best to prevent breasts from inflaming and going on to suppuration.] So if there is danger of this, use the smartweed, if obtainable, or the following:

**7. Sore Breasts, to Prevent Breaking, etc.**—As soon as there is inflammation and swelling of the breast, indicating any danger that suppuration will take place, send to the druggist and obtain fl. ex. (remember, fl. stands for fluid and ex. for extract,) of poke root, 4 ozs., and apply to the breast by wetting cloths with the extract and keeping upon the breast. Also take internally of the same, in doses of 5 to 10 drops, in a little water, every 3 hours, until you see improvement has commenced; then every 4 or 5 hours, lessen the dose to 3 to 8 drops. (A large, fleshy and robust woman will take the 10 drops; small and feeble ones, the 5 only.) Re-wet the cloths, at least, as often as taken internally.

*Remarks.*—This is from Dr. Duncan (referred to in II., for Milk, To Dry Up), who says of it: "If administered early, it will in 12 hours begin to give relief, and in 36 hours all traces of inflammation will have subsided and disappeared." He has used it in numbers of cases, and always with success, when begun as soon as inflammation set in, and before suppuration began. He thinks it, in such cases, specific (positive cure).

But if it is seen that the inflammation of the breast will go on, in any case, to suppuration, poultice with slippery elm, or bread and milk, as warm as can be borne, till they break without lancing, if possible; but when it comes to lancing, this calls for a physician. So I will leave the further treatment of that condition to him, simply remarking that a weak tinct. of myrrh and aloes, or a weakened tinct. of the muriate of iron, make good injections into the orifices; if they do not heal kindly, with some of the healing ointments, as Bittersweet, Balm of Gilead, etc., which are good to heal any sore on persons or domestic animals.

**8. Itching of the External Genital Organs.**—The delicate internal lining of the external organs of generation sometimes becomes the seat of a most distressing itching, to relieve which the parts may be so irritated by friction as to become violently inflamed. Leeches have been used sometimes with benefit: so has the application of cold, such as ice-water, or even lumps of ice introduced into the vagina. When there is an eruption like that in the sore mouth of children, injections of a strong solution of borax have been very useful; thick starch water, with a solution of sugar of lead, injected into the vagina and retained for an hour or two, have been also of great utility in a few cases under our care. This irritation sometimes arises from disease of the womb, pregnancy, the presence of a stone in the bladder, or worms in the bowels. The original affection must first be attended to in these cases.

**9. Milk, To Dry Up—Camphor and Soap Liniment for.**—Take a pint bottle and put into it alcohol, 12 ozs.; gum camphor, 1 oz.; and when dissolved, fill the bottle with good soft soap; but if no soft soap can be obtained, put in castile soap(shaved finely), 2 ozs., and fill the pint bottle with alcohol. Either has to be shaken when used; apply by wetting cloths and laying on 3 or 4 times a day, after having rubbed the breast thoroughly each time. Before rubbing, however, apply a little of the Bittersweet Ointment, or a little mutton or lamb tallow, to enable the hand to glide over the breast easily. Careful rubbing is good alone—with the hand, or a soft, dry towel, properly gathered in the hand, so it shall not slip. The friction must always be gentle, but continued some time. If you want to avoid a broken breast, see "Sore Nipples, Breasts, etc., to Avoid."

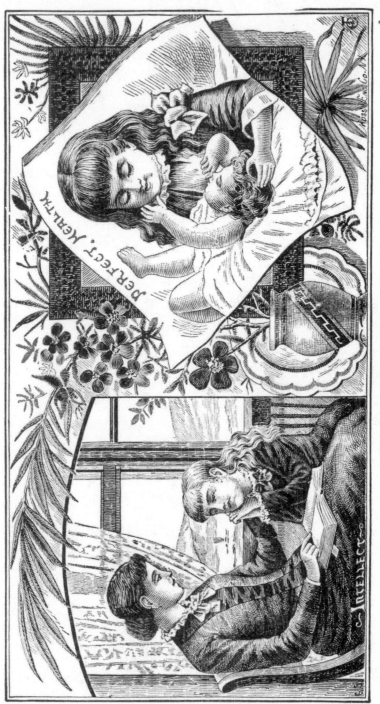

HEALTH AND INTELLIGENCE.

D. P. Duncan, M. D., of Waynesboro, Ga., says that mint leaves, steeped and applied to the breast, will at once stop the secretion of milk, even of one breast alone, leaving the other with its usual flow of milk, if desired. The poultice should be applied hot, and changed when getting cold.

**10. Sore Nipples.**—Nothing better than pulverized gum acacia applied every night, or as often as convenient.

**11. Prevent Flooding.**—Put your bandage on early and secure it firmly with good, strong safety-pins; as time and labor advances tighten the bandage.

**12. Hemorrhage Pill.**—Sulphate of berberine made into 5 gr. pills; take every 2 hours if necessary. Women suffering from *excessive flow* may rely on these pills, and should always keep them on hand. The same cures itching of the vulva.

**13. Offensive Urine**—10 to 20 grs. of boric acid will remedy it every time.

**14. Vomiting during Pregnancy**—1 drop of chloroform in hot sweetened water stops it.

**15. Leuchorrhea or Whites.**—Back ready to break. Take pulverized egg shell (burn the shell so as to pulverize it) 10 grs. with sweetened milk.

**1. BABY'S RECEIPTS.—Sore Mouth.**—Wash with cold water, with a drop of alcohol in it.

**2. Colic.**—Aromatic spirits of ammonia, 2 to 4 drops in milk is as good a thing as I ever discovered.

**3. Nursing Baby's Colic.**—Let the mother take 1 gr. pill of asafoetida every morning for a week; baby will take more comfort. Anise tea taken by the mother increases the flow of milk and prevents colic. Fennel seed tea has the same effect.

**4. Baby's Sore Mouth.**—Borax mixed in honey and applied to the sore.

**5. Baby's Food.**—Boil sugar of milk, 1 oz. in ½ pint water 15 minutes, then add ½ pint fresh cows' milk and boil again. Always give from bottle lukewarm. If bowels are loose add a tea-spoonful of ground barley, and if bowels do not move freely, use oatmeal instead, boil 15 minutes. Do you want to " make the baby fat," bring fresh milk just to a boil, add 1 table-spoonful each of corn starch and white sugar, and continue to boil until it thickens.

**6. Baby's Diarrhea.**—In the course of 24 hours give the white of an egg well beaten and stirred into 5 or 6 ozs. of water that has been boiled, add 3 to 5 drs. condensed milk. Increase the quantity if necessary.

**7. Spasms of Children.**—Apply a rag wet with ice water, or ice itself to the back of the neck, just below the base of the brain. Never apply it to the head.

**8. Fretful Baby.**—Give it onion tea. The same is also good for colic, also colds.

# MIDWIFERY—NURSING.

**THE EARLY SIGNS OF PREGNANCY:** Cessation of Menses —Morning Sickness — Changes in the Breasts—Enlargement of the Abdomen— Calculation of the Probable Date of Confinement.

**First Signs of Pregnancy.**—The first circumstance to make a woman suspect that she is pregnant is generally the non-appearance of her usual monthly discharge. This is called the cessation of the *menses*, or monthlies, and is one of the most constant signs of pregnancy. Cases, do, indeed, now and then occur, in which, notwithstanding pregnancy, the customary flow takes place for the first few months just as usual, and in certain still rarer instances it has been known to appear regularly throughout the pregnancy.

On the other hand its absence is by no means a sure indication of pregnancy, as it may be due to many other causes; such, for example, as an attack of severe illness, a condition of general weakness, or even strong emotional excitement.

**Another Symptom.**—The next symptom to attract attention is usually a feeling of sickness, often most distressing in the early morning, and sometimes accompanied with vomiting. This commences about the fourth or fifth week, and continues to the middle of pregnancy, when it generally ceases. Occasionally it lasts to the end of the pregnancy, while, on the other hand, in some women it is entirely absent throughout.

Shortly after pregnancy has commenced, a sensation of weight and fullness is felt in the breasts. A little later these organs enlarge, and the nipples become more prominent; the skin, too, just around the nipples becomes darker in color, an alteration most marked in women of fair skin and light complexion. Of course these changes are most noticeable in women who are pregnant for the first time; for when they have once occurred, the breasts never quite resume their original appearance, so that subsequent changes are less observable. The breasts *may* increase in size, and *may* even contain milk, without pregnancy; as, for example, in the case of certain diseases of the womb.

**Enlargement of the Abdomen.**—About the end of the third month the abdomen begins to enlarge, and continues to do so from that time forwards; by the end of the seventh month the hollow of the navel has generally disappeared It need scarcely be said, however, that the abdomen may enlarge from many other causes, so that not one of the four signs above described affords, when taken alone, positive proof of pregnancy; although, when two or more of them are found to be present, there is good ground for a strong suspicion. Whenever it is important that the question of pregnancy should be established beyond a doubt, a doctor should be consulted.

278

**Probable Date of Confinement.**—The usual method of reckoning the probable date of confinement is to learn on what day the last monthly flow ceased, then to count three months backwards (or nine months forwards) and add seven days. This is, in practice, the best plan that has been suggested, and will generally give a date within a very few days of actual confinement, frequently the very day. The following example will show how the calculation is made:—A woman, we will say, wa‹ last unwell on March 10; counting three months back from March 10 gives December 10; add seven days and it will give December 17, which is the probable date of her confinement. If it is not the actual day, labor will in all probability take place within three or four days before or after it.

**Movements of the Fœtus.**—The movements of the fœtus are not perceived by the mother until between the fourth and fifth months—that is, until pregnancy has advanced about half-way. Not very uncommonly the occurrence of the first definite movement of which the mother is conscious is accompanied by a sensation of nausea and faintness. It is this fact which gave rise to the opinion long held, and still prevalent amongst the ignorant, that the fœtus then for the first time becomes living, an opinion that finds expression in the word "quickening," the use of which, like that of many other words, has outlived the theory in which it had its origin. As a matter of fact, the fœtus is living from the very commencement of pregnancy, and the reason why movements are not felt during the earlier half of pregnancy is to be found in the fact that the womb itself is not sensitive, and that it is not until the middle of pregnancy that that organ has enlarged sufficiently to bring it in direct contact with a part fully endowed with sensibility—namely, the inner surface of the abdominal wall. From the moment when they are first perceived, the movements of the child become more and more distinct as pregnancy advances, and constitute one of the most important of the later signs of that condition. When from any cause it is impossible for the probable date of confinement to be calculated according to the rule laid down in the preceding paragraph (as, for example, when the date of the last menstruation is uncertain, or when one pregnancy succeeds another so quickly that menstruation has not been re-established in the interval), it may be approximately arrived at by reckoning it as four and one-half months after the date of "quickening."

**MANAGEMENT OF PREGNANCY: General Rules—Constipation—Piles—Hardening the Nipples—Swollen Breasts—Varicose Veins—Falling Forward of the Womb—Obstinate Vomiting—Difficulty in Passing Urine, &c.**

**Proper Treatment of Pregnancy.**—The proper treatment of pregnancy consists for the most part in paying increased attention to the laws of health. A pregnant woman requires a full allowance of rest, and should therefore be careful to avoid late hours. She should take plenty of outdoor exercise whenever the state of the weather permits; and, while avoiding all unnecessary strain, such as the lifting of heavy weights, or reaching things from a height, she may engage in the lighter duties of her house, not only without risk, but with actual gain of health and strength. Her food should be taken with the utmost regularity, and should be plain and simple in its nature. Good new milk should form a considerable part of her every day diet. Stimulants are entirely unnecessary, except when taken under special medical direction.

As the abdomen enlarges it is of the utmost importance that the clothing should not be tight. A foolish regard for appearances has led many a woman into most lamentable mistakes on this point.

During pregnancy the mind should be attended to as well as the body. All unnatural excitement is to be carefully guarded against, and *distressing sights are to be especially shunned.*

**Action of the Bowels.**—Great care must be exercised to ensure a daily action of the bowels. An excellent plan is to set apart a certain hour of the day for attending to this function, whether the desire for relief be urgent or not. Perhaps the most convenient time for most people is immediately after breakfast. By following this simple rule, a habit is established which will go far to obviate the necessity for aperient medicine. When such medicine is required, it should be of the simplest possible kind; for example, a compound rhubarb pill, or a little castor-oil. When constipation is associated with piles, the aperient chosen should be a tea-spoonful of sulphur in a little milk every morning, or a similar quantity of the compound liquorice powder made into a paste by mixing a little water with it; and the patient should be instructed to make her daily visit to the water-closet immediately before retiring to bed for the night. By these means the aching pain which, under such circumstances, is apt to follow every action of the bowels, may be considerably diminished. Injecting half a pint of cold water into the bowel, immediatly before the bowels are moved, often proves highly serviceable. Should the piles become inflamed or unusually painful, the patient must keep her bed for a day or two, and bathe the parts with warm water from time to time. Where these measures are required, however, the medical attendant should be consulted.

The nipples, especially in first pregnancies, should be hardened by bathing them daily during the last month or two with a mixture of equal parts of eau-de-Cologne and water, in order to render them less liable to crack and become sore and painful on the application of the child. Inflammation and abscess of the breast often originate in cracked nipples.

**Sore Breasts.**—When the breasts become swollen and painful, they should be frequently fomented with flannels wrung out of hot water, and, in the meantime, should be supported, as in a sling, by a broad handkerchief passing under the arm of the affected side and over the opposite shoulder.

Sometimes the veins of the legs, thighs, and lower part of the body become swollen and uncomfortable. Under these circumstances, the patient should lie down as much as possible every day, and at once discontinue the use of tight garters.

In women who have borne many children, the abdominal walls are apt to become relaxed, and the pregnant womb, being insufficiently supported, is then in danger of falling forward, so as not only to produce deformity, but to prove a hindrance during labor. A flannel binder, or one of the abdominal belts sold for the purpose, should in these cases be constantly worn during the daytime.

Now and then the sickness, already alluded to as a common accompaniment of the early months of pregnancy, becomes so troublesome and incessant as to cause serious loss of strength. Under such circumstances consult a physician.

**The Urine.**—Towards the end of pregnancy it is not at all unusual for there to be some difficulty in passing urine, and for the desire to pass it to become very frequent. Should these symptoms, however, occur during the earlier months, and especially during the third and fourth, a medical man should be consulted; as they may be due to a displacement of the womb, which requires immediate attention.

Troublesome heartburn, diarrhœa, palpitation, persistent neuralgia, salivation, itching or swelling of the external parts, swelling of the face or ankles, all require prompt attention, and if severe, the personal care of the medical attendant.

**UTERINE HEMORRHAGE DURING PREGNANCY: Its Usual Significance and Temporary Treatment—Placenta Prævia—Precautions after Previous Abortions—Treatment after Miscarriage.**

**Uterine Hemorrhage,** or a discharge of blood from the womb, during pregnancy, is usually a sign that miscarriage is threatening, and hence requires prompt medical attention. In summoning a doctor under these circumstances it is always desirable to send a note, rather than a verbal message, and to state clearly the nature and urgency of the case. Meantime an endeavor should be made to restrain the hemorrhage by causing the patient to lie down, with the head low and a pillow under the hips, by admitting plenty of cool, fresh air into the room, and by ensuring perfect quietness.

If possible, the services of a trained nurse should be obtained at once, and she, with perhaps one other person, should alone remain in the room. Cloths, dipped in cold water or in vinegar and water, must be applied to the external genitals for a few minutes at a time, the application being frequently repeated. If wet cloths are kept on for a longer period, they are sure to become warm, and so, by acting as a poultice, defeat the object in view, and indeed tend rather to increase than to check the flow of blood. When the hemorrhage continues, or becomes very profuse, the nurse must not hesitate to send for the nearest doctor as well as for the ordinary medical attendant. In such cases it will be desirable for her to take a dry napkin or two, and, having folded them in the form of a pad, to press them forcibly against the external genitals and hold them there. All the discharges, whether solid or fluid, should be carefully retained for the inspection of the medical attendant.

These alarming hemorrhages are often brought about by accidents, such as blows or falls, or by the lifting of heavy weights. But when flooding first makes its appearance, at the seventh month or later, and there has been no such accident to account for it, the probability is that the case is one of *placenta prævia*, in which the after-birth is in an unusual position — namely, over the mouth of the womb, constituting a very dangerous complication. The temporary treatment of flooding due to this condition in no way differs, however, from that already described.

When previous pregnancies have been cut short by miscarriage, it is very necessary that the greatest precautions should be observed to avoid the repetition of such an accident. Now, we know from experience, that miscarriages are most apt to take place at those times which, in the absence of pregnancy, would have been the ordinary menstrual periods. It is on these occasions, therefore, that preventive measures are most needed and most likely to be useful. Every month, then, during the time that the patient would, under other circumstances, have been unwell, she should maintain the recumbent posture, if not in bed, at any rate on a couch. If this simple rule were attended to, many a miscarriage would be averted. A woman known to be liable to abortion should, moreover, be specially careful to avoid all its most common causes; she should abstain from exciting entertainments, violent exercise, fatiguing or rough journeys, strong purgative medicines, and exposure to cold. And, lastly, as it is very doubtful whether any of the causes I have named are sufficient in themselves to bring on abortion, without a predisposition thereto from some local or general weakness or disease, it is very desirable that patients who have formed the so-called "habit" of aborting, should consult their medical attendant at the commencement of pregnancy with a view to being placed under a regular course of treatment.

The after-treatment of patients who have miscarried is a most important matter, and one which receives far too little attention. It is no uncommon thing among patients of the laboring and middle classes for women to go about their ordinary duties as early as the second or third day, and some do not even rest for more than a few hours. Now, although this neglect of proper precaution may not result in any immediate ill-effects, it frequently lays the foundation of chronic disease with much attendant misery and suffering. Whenever nurses have an opportunity they should tell their patients what there is in store for them if they resume their ordinary duties too soon after such an occurrence. No absolute rule can be laid down as to the length of time during which rest is necessary; it depends so entirely on circumstances that vary in different cases. Thus, in a case of abortion during the early months, for instance, where the loss has been small and the health has not suffered, four to six days' absolute rest in bed, followed, during the next ten to fourteen days, by the greatest care and prudence, will, in the absence of special directions from the medical attendant, be generally found sufficient. When the health is unaffected it becomes very irksome to lie in bed for the time here indicated; nevertheless, this rule cannot be neglected without running grave risk.

Should the pregnancy be further advanced, or the circumstances less favorable, a longer period of rest will be required. Where there has been severe or long-continued flooding, a patient is frequently reduced to a condition of weakness quite equal to that following an ordinary confinement. In such cases it is only reasonable to expect the same care to be exercised as after a labor at full term.

On no account should a patient leave her bed, after a miscarriage, so long as any discharge of blood continues, as, while that persists, it is uncertain whether there is not some portion of the after-birth or membranes still remaining in the womb, and rendering the patient liable to further attacks of flooding.

**PROCESS OF NATURAL LABOR:** Signs of Approaching Labor—Its Division into Stages—Labor-Pains,—The "Bag of Waters"—Description of First Stage—Of Second Stage—Of Third Stage.

**Approach of Labor Pains.**—Towards the latter part of the ninth month, certain changes take place which give warning that labor is not far off. One of the earliest of these is sinking of the abdominal swelling; the upper end of the womb, which at the beginning of the ninth month, reaches as high as the pit of the stomach, now falls a little below that point. Great relief to the breathing follows this alteration, as the pressure upon the organs within the chest is thereby greatly lessened. On the other hand, owing to this change in the position of the womb, certain new inconveniences arise from the pressure of its lower portion on the various important parts contained in the pelvis. Thus, walking becomes more difficult, the bladder requires relieving more frequently, and piles are apt to form.

A sign that makes it probable that labor is actually about to commence is the appearance of a slight discharge of mucus, streaked with a little blood. This is spoken of, in the lying-in room, as the "show."

**Labor is Divided, for the Sake of Description, into Three Stages.**—*The first* of these is called the stage of dilatation of the mouth of the womb; *the second* lasts from the moment when that dilatation is completed up to the birth of the child; while *the third*, or last stage, includes the time from the birth of the child to the coming away of the after-birth, or placenta.

The so-called pains of labor are, in reality, contractions of the muscular wall of the womb. At the early part of labor they are slight, occur at long intervals, and are felt mostly in the lower part of the front of the abdomen; as labor advances, they become longer and more energetic, follow one another more quickly, though always with a certain regularity, and are generally felt chiefly in the back and loins. Each pain is comparatively feeble at its commencement, increases in intensity until it reaches its height, and then gradually passes off. This character, together with the regularity of their recurrence, serves to distinguish pains really due to uterine contraction from colicky and other pains, for which they are sometimes mistaken.

The bag of waters consists of the membranous coverings of the fœtus, enclosing within them what the doctors call, the *liquor amnii*, in which the child floats. During pregnancy this fluid serves to preserve the child from injury; during labor it forms a pouch at the mouth of the womb, which it acts upon like a wedge, and so assists in dilating. Experience tells us that, when the waters escape early, labor is rendered more tedious. The explanation of this is to be found in the fact that the bag of waters, being round and even, and pressing on the mouth of the womb (*os uteri*) equally all around, the mouth of the womb is opened out more rapidly and easily by this even pressure than by the uneven surface of the presenting part of the child.

As the *os uteri* opens, and the end of the first stage draws near, the pouch formed by the protruding membranes is pushed further into the front passage, or vagina, and, the pains becoming more violent, the membranes at last give way during a pain more severe than the rest, and so the waters escape. In natural labors this usually happens as soon as the mouth of the womb is fully opened and thus the *first stage of labor is ended.*

The head of the child now begins to pass through the *os uteri*. After a certain time, usually much shorter than that occupied by the first stage, it reaches the vaginal opening, through which it gradually escapes, and thus the child is born, and the *second stage is completed.*

The pains of the first stage are called "grinding pains," and are different in character from those of the second stage, which are known as "forcing" or "bearing pains." The cry which is called forth by the pains during the first stage is also different from the groan which escapes from the patient when the pains of the second stage commence. An experienced nurse knows from this circumstance alone that the first stage is over, and as the sending for the doctor ought on no consideration whatever to be delayed beyond this period, it is a point of great practical importance.

The pains now become stronger and more frequent; the patient, holding her breath and bearing down at each return of the pain, becomes hot and flushed, and breaks out into a profuse perspiration. At the end of each pain the head of the child goes back a little, which prevents the strain from being so continuous as to be hurtful and exhausting. Nevertheless, almost every pain marks an advance upon the one preceding. This slight withdrawal of the head is frequently perceived by the patient herself, and unless explained to be natural and necessary, is apt to make her think she is not making any progress. There eventually comes a point, however, when the head is so far expelled that it no longer recedes between the pains. The intervals become shorter, and the pains more severe, until at last the head slips out altogether, and then the most painful part of the labor is over. The uterus usually now rests for a moment. Then the face of the child makes a little turn towards one of the patient's thighs, generally the right, in order that the shoulders may be brought into such a position that they may pass with the least difficulty. With another strong pain the shoulders are expelled. The rest of the body gives little trouble, for no part of it is as broad as those which have already passed.

The contractions of the womb now cease for a short time, varying from five to ten or twenty minutes, when a little pain is again felt, and the after-birth and membranes are discharged, along with a small quantity of blood, with which a few clots are generally mixed.

Such is a brief account of the order of events in a perfectly natural labor.

**DUTIES OF A NURSE DURING LABOR**—Articles Needed in the Lying-in Room—Preparation of the Bed—Personal Clothing of Patient—Number of Persons in the Room—Caution in Conversation—Attention to the State of the Bladder—Food—Vomiting—Cramp—Fomenting the Perineum in First Labors.

If the nurse is not already in the house, the appearance of the first discharge or "show" is a sufficient warning that she should be summoned. No time should be lost in obeying the call, for many women, especially if they have borne children previously, pass through all the stages of labor very quickly. On arriving at the house the nurse should make the necessary changes in her dress, and appear before the patient ready for duty. An opportunity will soon occur of forming a judgment as to whether the patient is really in labor, and, if so, how far it has advanced. If labor has actually commenced, the patient will, before long, cease speaking, suddenly grasp the nurse's arm, or the back of a chair, or whatever happens to be at hand, and exhibit other signs of suffering. The nurse will know, by the characters enumerated on a previous page, whether this is a genuine labor-pain or not, and will observe how long it lasts and the degree of its severity. When it is over, she should inquire when the pains began, how often they return, whether the waters have been discharged, and other similar questions, in order that she may know what kind of message she is to send to the medical attendant, who ought at once to be informed that his patient is in labor.

Let me now suppose that the nurse has made sure that her patient is in labor, and that she has acquainted the medical attendant.

If the bowels have not been freely opened within the last six hours, it will be desirable to give a simple enema of soap and water. The emptying of the lower bowel will facilitate the labor, and will save both the patient and attendant the annoyance caused by the passing of fæces during a later stage. This having been attended to, the patient may be allowed to sit up in a chair or walk about the room, according to her inclination, provided it is clear that the labor has not yet reached its second stage. If it is night-time, however, it is better for her to remain in bed, in order that she may, if possible, get a few moments' sleep between the pains. During the early stage of labor it is of no use for patients to "hold their breath and bear down" during each pain, as they are often urged to do by untrained and inexperienced nurses. It must always be left to the medical attendant to decide when bearing-down efforts have become desirable and ought to be encouraged.

It is often a great relief to a patient for the nurse to support her back with her flat hand during a pain. In the meantime she should see that all things are in readiness for the actual confinement. The following are always wanted:—

Basins.
Binder.
Napkins.
Needles and Thread.
Nursery, or safety, pins
Olive-oil.
Pieces of old linen.
Receiver.
Roller-towel.
Scissors.

Sponges.
Thread, or strong worsted, for tying cord.
Towels.
Vaseline, cold cream, or lard.
Water, hot and cold.
Waterproof sheeting.
Puff-box, and complete set of clothes for the baby.

In addition to the above it is advisable to have in the room some good brandy, a fan, a syringe, a foot-bath, and a nursing-apron.

**The Binder** usually consists of two pieces of stout twilled cotton, each two yards long and of good width, the edges of which are stitched together so as to make the binder of double thickness. On an emergency, a small table-cloth or cotton sheet, suitably folded, answers the purpose very well.

**The Receiver** should be of flannel made of double thickness, and large enough to wrap the child thoroughly. The flimsy receivers sometimes used are only fit to protect a doll. A good thick flannel petticoat, or a cot-blanket, is as good as anything.

**The Thread or Worsted for Tying the Cord** must be made ready in the following way: Twelve equal lengths, measuring about a foot, are to be laid side by side and arranged evenly. Six of these lengths, are then to be knotted together at a distance of about two inches from each end, and the remaining six in the same way. Having been thus prepared, the threads must be laid on the dressing-table, and a pair of good scissors by the side of them, ready for handing to the medical attendant at the proper moment.

**The Preparation of the Bed** is a matter of considerable importance, and ought to be attended to during the early part of labor. Women are usually delivered lying on the left side, with the knees drawn up towards the abdomen. The right side of the bed, therefore, is the one which requires preparing, and that part of it near the foot is preferable because the upper part of the bed is thus kept clean and comfortable for the patient when the labor is over, and because of the help derived from being able to plant the feet firmly against the bed-post during the pains.

The mattress being uncovered, a large piece of rubber cloth is to be spread over it, and upon this a sheet folded several times. Next to this should come the clean under-sheet, on which the patient is to lie, and upon that another piece of waterproof sheeting, large enough to reach above the hips. Over this upper rubber, and ready to be removed with it after the labor is over, are to be then placed a folded blanket, and, lastly, a folded cotton sheet, both of which should reach well above the hips, so as to absorb the discharges.

Two pillows are then to be put in the centre of the bed, so that the patient may lie with the upper part of the body directly across the bed, the hips being as near the edge as possible. The upper bed-clothing during labor should consist of a sheet, one blanket, and a thin counterpane, which should completely hide from exposure every part of the patient's person, except the head and neck. A long roller-towel should be fastened to the bed-post at the patient's feet. Nurses often make the mistake of fixing this to the post at the opposite corner, or even to one of the posts at the bed's head. A very little consideration, how-ever, will make the inconvenience of this arrangement apparent. By grasping the end of a towel, attached in the way I have recommended, the patient pulls herself still closer to the edge and foot of the bed; whereas, by pulling at a towel fastened to one of the posts on the further side of the bed, she drags herself away from the very position which it is desirable she should preserve. The same objection, of course, applies to supplying the place of the towel by means of the hands of an attendant standing on the left side of the bed. This should never be encouraged, as it always has a tendency to displace the patient, and to render it difficult for the medical attendant to give needful assistance.

As labor advances, and it becomes necessary for the patient to be placed in bed, she should put on a clean chemise and night-dress, which should be rolled up under the armpits out of reach of the discharges, while the soiled chemise and night-dress should be slipped down from the arms and shoulders, and loosely fastened round the waist. (Amongst the working classes it is still too much the custom for women to be confined in their every-day dress. It is a practice that ought always to be discountenanced.) The hair should be dressed in such a way that the continuous lying in bed after the confinement will not drag upon or entangle it more than is inevitable.

It is very undesirable for a woman in labor to be surrounded by a number of friends and neighbors. In most cases the nurse herself is the only attendant that is really needed, although the presence of one other person (the husband) should not be objected to, if the patient wishes it.

No nurse should ever allow herself to be teased into prophesying that the labor will be over by a certain hour. If such prophesies turn out incorrect, as they are most likely to do, the patient loses courage and confidence. All gossip is to be avoided, and nurses should be particularly careful to make no reference to their past experiences, especially such as have been unfavorable. A good, kind nurse will not be at a loss for a few helpful and encouraging words as labor goes on, and will not need to have recourse either to foolish promises or dismal anecdotes.

Every now and then the patient should be reminded to pass water, lest the bladder should become so full as to hinder labor. This point is often neglected, partly because the attention is so preoccupied that the desire to empty the blad-der is scarcely perceived, and partly because when the waters have broken, the escape of a little gush of amniotic fluid during each pain often misleads the patient, making her think she has passed urine when really she has not.

**Food for the Patient.**—In the early part of labor when pains are slight and the intervals long, there is no reason for interfering either with the character or regularity of the patient's ordinary meals, provided there exist the desire for solid food. During the later stages, however, it is wise to confine her to fluids, such as beef-tea, gruel, milk, and tea, and to administer them in small quantities at a time, so as not to overload the stomach and excite sickness. Patients often ask for a little cold water, and many nurses, influenced by old traditions, fear to gratify the wish. A sip of pure water can never do harm, only it must be a "sip" and not a tumblerful, the patient being assured that small draughts, frequently repeated, assuage thirst far better than larger quantities. On no account must stimulants be given, except when expressly ordered by the medical attendant.

Vomiting is a troublesome symptom and distresses the patient, but its influence on the progress of the labor is in no way unfavorable. Should it, however, be excessive, it is well to give a little iced effervescing water from time to time.

**Cramps During Labor.**—Many patients suffer very severely from cramp during labor. Relief can frequently be obtained by stretching the limb straight out, and at the same time bending the ankle so as to put the muscles of the calf well on the stretch. Gentle rubbing of the affected part with the hand also affords great comfort.

In the case of patients who have not borne children previously, it is an excellent plan to diligently foment the perineum from the very outset of labor, so as to render the skin softer and more yielding, and lessen the risk of tearing.

**DUTIES OF A NURSE DURING SECOND STAGE OF LABOR: —What to do in the absence of the Medical Attendant— Supporting the Perineum—Assisting at the Birth—Tying the Cord—Breech Cases—The Third Stage—Application of The Binder, &c.—Convulsions—Fainting—Falling Forward of the Womb.**

When the pains alter in character, compelling the patient to make efforts to bear down, and the face begins to get flushed and the skin to become moist with perspiration, the nurse may feel pretty well assured that the first stage is over; and if the medical attendant has not arrived, she should request him to be summoned without delay. In the meantime, the patient must be put to bed, and encouraged to bear down and assist the pains. The binder, napkins, and receiver must be spread near the fire in readiness.

Should the child's head press upon the perineum before the arrival of the medical attendant, a warm folded napkin may be placed in the palm of the nurse's left hand and held against the bulging perineum, the fingers being directed backwards, so that the front edge of the perineum may receive the chief support. The object of this is to prevent the child's head passing too quickly and suddenly forwards to the vaginal outlet and to preserve the perineum from being torn. The great point at this stage is to avoid doing too much. Nothing but harm is likely to result from attempts to enlarge the opening by stretching the lips apart with the fingers, or to push back the edge of the perineum in the hope of facilitating the escape of the head. Contrary to the popular belief, the attendant's duty is rather to keep back the head by gentle pressure, than to hasten its expulsion. Above all things there should be no pulling; Nature is to be allowed to do her own work.

If the medical attendant be still absent when the head is born, the nurse must spread the flannel receiver close up to the vaginal orifice, and receive the head of the child upon her right hand, still keeping up the gentle pressure upon the stretched perineum until the shoulders have passed out. Even then the body and legs must be left to follow of themselves, the nurse meanwhile holding up the parts which are already born. The upper bed-clothes should be now turned back sufficiently to allow the child to breathe, without causing any exposure of the patient herself. If the navel-string is found coiled around the child's neck, it must be slipped over its head as quickly as possible, lest the life of the child should be sacrificed owing to a stoppage in the circulation of the blood through the cord. Very occasionally it happens that the child is born with the membranes unbroken; they will in such cases be found drawn tightly over the little face, and will cause death from suffocation, unless quickly torn open and the mouth freed. Amongst some people this occurrence is known as being born with a *veil* or *caul*.

The cry which a child usually utters as soon as it is born, helps to fill the lungs with air, and is on that account rather to be encouraged than checked. If the child does not cry, the nurse must examine the mouth to ascertain whether there is anything either over it or within it, preventing the breathing. Sometimes there is some frothy mucus in the mouth which can be cleared away with the finger. It is often useful, also, when breathing is delayed to turn the child on its face, and give it a few gentle slaps on the back with the flat hand.

The navel-string must not be tied until the breathing is established, unless it is quite evident that the child is still-born. The first ligature must be tied an inch and a half from the navel, and the knot must be pulled tightly two or three times so as to squeeze out of the way the jelly-like material which surrounds the blood-vessels of the cord; otherwise the vessels may not be closed by the ligature, and bleeding from the stump may occur to a fatal extent while the nurse is attending to the mother. The second ligature is placed an inch further from the child than the first one, and the cord is then divided with scissors mid-way between the two. All this must be done outside of the bed-clothes, lest some other part than the cord be cut in mistake.

Now and then it happens that a nurse has to take the temporary charge of cases where not the head, but the breech, passes out first. Delivery with the child in this position is full of danger to the life of the child. The nurse must not hasten matters by pulling, even when the legs are already born; but, when the whole of the child's body has passed except the head and arms, and when these parts appear to be arrested, she may endeavor to assist Nature by bringing down the arms from the sides of the child's head in the following manner: — Passing her forefinger up the child's back, and over its shoulder, she draws the arm gently down across the front of the chest by hooking her finger into the bend of the elbow. The same manœuvre is repeated with the other arm. The head will then be the only part remaining unborn. It is possible that, now that the arms have been brought down, the efforts of Nature may be equal to the task of expelling the head. Should the pains, however, prove ineffectual, the nurse may render further assistance by pressing with the fingers of one hand against the back of the child's head and so tilting the head forwards, while with the two first fingers of the other hand, placed 'one on each side of the nose, she endeavors to draw down the face. This plan is generally preferable to the one, not unfrequently adopted, in which traction is made by placing the fingers in the child's mouth. In all breech-cases a warm bath should be in readiness, in the event of the child requiring to be resuscitated.

The child, having been now separated, is to be wrapped in the receiver, with the face alone exposed, and placed out of harm's way on the other side of the bed. The patient must be warned to lie perfectly still, and to wait patiently for the one or two insignificant pains which accompany the expulsion of the after-birth. These generally occur from five to twenty minutes after the birth of the child. Meanwhile the nurse must provide the medical attendant with a basin or other vessel, previously warmed before the fire, to receive the after-birth, and one or two warm napkins.

Should the medical attendant, however, be still absent, the nurse must place her hand upon the abdomen of the mother and ascertain whether there is another child. If she should find such to be the case, she must convey the news to the mother very cautiously, assuring her that the second child will be born with much less pain than the first. If there is no second child to be felt, the nurse will do well to keep her hand laid upon the mother's abdomen until a slight pain occurs, when she must spread out her hand like a fan and gently press the uterus so long as the pain continues. Meantime, she is to hold a suitable vessel in her left hand ready to receive the placenta when it is expelled, taking care on no account to pull the cord. Sometimes the placenta and membranes are expelled during the first pain; more frequently two or three pains occur before this takes place.

If the uterus can be felt, under the hand, hard, firm, and as small as a good-sized cricket-ball, the placenta, if it has not already made its appearance, will in all probability be found lying in the vagina. In order to make sure about this, the hand may be withdrawn from the front of the abdomen, and the fore-finger passed gently up by the side of the cord. If the insertion of the cord into the after-birth can be easily and distinctly made out, it is pretty certain that the placenta has escaped from the uterus into the vagina, and it may, therefore be carefully hooked down with the finger. As the placenta passes out, it is a good precaution to twist it round once or twice, so as to make a wisp of the membrane and bring them all away at the same time. A slight discharge of clotted and fluid blood usually accompanies the termination of the third stage.

When the placenta and membranes have come away, the hand should again be placed over the uterus, in order to make sure that it is firm and well contracted. If, instead of this being the case, it is felt to be large, soft, and uncontracted, firm pressure should be continued, so as to excite contraction and prevent flooding, which, in such circumstances, is greatly to be feared.

Should a gush of blood make its appearance in spite of the pressure, the hand must still be kept over the uterus and the pressure increased, cold wet cloths being in the meantime repeatedly applied with suddenness to the external genitals. Of course, if the medical attendant has left the house, he must be again summoned at once.

The uterus being firmly contracted, and the flow of blood having ceased, the thighs and surrounding parts are to be gently sponged with warm water and dried by means of a soft warm napkin.

If there has been no flooding, the soiled chemise and night-dress may now be drawn down, and, along with the folded sheet, blanket, and upper rubber, removed from beneath the patient, who must not be permitted to make the slightest effort while this is being done. Then she may be slowly rolled over on to her back, to allow of the application of the binder. The binder, well aired, must be rolled up to half its length, and the roll passed underneath the lower part of the patient's back. Being caught on the other side, it is then unrolled, and having been smoothed out free from wrinkles, it is so applied as to encircle the hips tightly, and the overlapping end is then secured by means of three or four good safety-pins. All this is to be done with as little exposure of the patient as possible. The pillows having been duly replaced, the patient may now be carefully lifted into her usual position in bed; a fresh warm napkin being applied against the vulva, and the clean chemise drawn down into its place.

If, however, there has been any flooding, the patient, must still remain undisturbed for some time after the discharge has ceased, the nurse from time to time examining the napkins to make sure that there is no return of the bleeding.

When the medical attendant is present, he will probably prefer to undertake many of these duties himself; at any rate he, being the responsible person, will give instructions according to the requirements of each individual case, which instructions it will be the nurse's simple duty to obey.

During the passage of the child's head, it facilitates matters if the patient's knees are separated. This is sometimes effected by placing a pillow between them, but the pillow is apt to be in the way, and a better plan is for the nurse to pass her hand beneath the right knee, and keep it well raised during each pain.

Sometimes the medical attendant desires the nurse to make pressure upon the womb during the third stage of labor, to assist it in expelling the after-birth. To do this she should stand behind the patient at the doctor's left hand, and passing the hand under the bedclothes, she should place it on the abdomen, where she will feel the round, firm body of the uterus above the pubes. Spreading out her hand over this organ, she should keep up a steady pressure downwards and backwards as long as the attendant desires it.

**Convulsions,** coming on during labor, are always alarming, and place the patient's life in great danger. Should they occur before the arrival of the medical attendant, no time should be lost in sending for him. In the meantime all that the nurse can do is to keep her patient lying flat down; to see that there is no tight clothing about her head and chest; to prevent biting the tongue by pushing it, if possible, behind the teeth, and placing a cork or piece of India-rubber between them; to admit plenty of fresh air into the room; and, lastly, to restrain the meddlesome interference of bystanders. It is altogether worse than useless to attempt to force water or stimulants down the throat while the patient is struggling and unconscious; and although sprinkling the face with water, rubbing the hands, and applying smelling salts to the nose, can do no harm, it is more than doubtful whether they ever produce any benefit. When the fit is over, should the medical attendant not have arrived, the nurse may administer a soap-and-water enema with advantage.

**Fainting** during labor should always lead to a suspicion that there is some loss of blood going on, and the medical attendant ought to be immediately summoned, even if there is no blood to be seen externally, for internal bleeding may be going on, notwithstanding. The important point to remember about fainting is, that the patient is on no account to be raised up, however much she may desire it. The level posture, plenty of cool, fresh air, sprinkling a little water on the face, and firm, steady pressure with the hand over the uterus, comprise all that it is desirable for a nurse to do in the way of treatment. If there is external hemorrhage, an endeavor must be made to control it in the manner described later on.

Some women, who have previously borne children, suffer from a falling forward of the womb, causing an unusual prominence of the lower part of the abdomen. Such persons require to be put to bed at a very early stage of labor, and should either be allowed to lie flat on the back, or be supported in the half-sitting posture. The late Dr. Radford, of England, to whom I am indebted for the recommendations contained in this paragraph, has recorded two fatal cases in which this condition was present, and in each of which rupture of the uterus took place at the very moment of the patient rising to her feet during labor.

He suggests that, in order that the uterus may be safely guided into, and maintained in such a position as will facilitate labor, the nurse should, in all such cases, put on a broad bandage at a very early period of the labor, and tighten it as labor advances. After the membranes have ruptured and the waters have been discharged, this bandage should be applied as follows:—The end lying upon the bed is to be fastened to the side of the bed, so as to constitute a fixed point, while the other end is held obliquely by the nurse, and gradually tightened as the child descends into the pelvis. The direction of the pressure will thus be slightly upwards as well as backwards.

This mode of support, by what he terms a "regulating bandage," effectually assists the entrance of the child's head into the pelvis.

## MANAGEMENT OF THE NEWLY-BORN CHILD: Washing and Dressing — Feeding and Feeding-bottles — Aperients — Sleep — Warmth and Fresh Air — Separation of Navel-string — Swelling of the Breasts in the Newly-born — The "Thrush."

After making the mother comfortable, the next duty of the nurse is to attend to the washing of the child. This should be done, if possible, before the medical attendant leaves the house, in order that he may have an opportunity of examining the child thoroughly. For the washing, a foot-bath is required, or a basin at least one foot broad, one foot deep, and two feet long, so that the whole body, with the exception of the head, may be placed in the water for a minute or two. The nurse must also be provided with a piece of soft flannel, some olive-oil, a piece of good, unirritating soap, and, for the dressing, in addition to the clothes, a needle and thread, some safety-pins, and a piece of linen rag six inches square, with a hole cut in its centre large enough to admit the navel-string. Sitting at a convenient distance from the fire, she then proceeds to unfold the flannel wrapper and anoint the child's skin with warm olive-oil wherever it is covered with the white greasy material usually present. This having been done, the child is to be put into the water, the temperature of which should be about 90°, and the head supported on the left hand out of the water. After having rested there for about two minutes, it is to be taken on the lap and washed with soap and flannel, the eyes being carefully cleaned first, then the head, and afterwards the remainder of the body, great pains being take to cleanse the little wrinkles at the various joints. After gently drying the skin with a soft warm towel, it must be well powdered, and especially those parts near the joints where chafing is most likely to occur; viz., under the knees and armpits, in the groins, and between the thighs. The piece of flannel used for the first washing should be burnt.

The skin having now been well washed, dried, and powdered, the square of old linen is to be held near the fire for a minute and slipped over the remains of the navel-string, which is to be folded in it and turned upwards upon the child's abdomen, where it is to be retained by means of the flannel binder until its separation, which usually takes place about the fourth or fifth day.

Up to the time of this separation, the child must be washed from head to foot on the nurse's lap, night and morning. Afterwards, when there is no longer any fear of injuring the navel, the child should be placed in the water for two minutes during the morning washing, the evening washing being done on the nurse's lap as before. Whenever a napkin is removed, the parts protected by it must be well cleansed by sponging with a little soap and water, and then thoroughly powdered, so as to prevent the skin becoming sore. This rule holds good even if the napkin has only been soiled with urine, though it is of course still more necessary when there has been also an action of the bowels.

It is part of a nurse's duty to wash and dress the child during the time she stays in the house, and she should, for this purpose, be provided with a large soft flannel apron, which must be carefully dried each time it is used.

The child's clothing should be warm without being heavy, and should fit loosely so as to allow the organs free play, and the blood to flow unhindered. The body-binder should be of flannel, as it is impossible to prevent its being soiled with the urine, and flannel, when wetted, does not chill the skin so much as other materials. None but patent safety-pins should be used about a baby, and even for them it is better to substitute two or three stitches wherever it is possible.

The medical attendant must always be informed, when he makes his first after-visit, whether the infant has passed urine and whether the bowels have acted; also as to any marks or other peculiarities that may have been noticed. The state of the eyes, too, should be narrowly watched, and any unhealthy appearance or the least sign of discharge at once reported.

It is most undesirable to give a newly-born child butter and sugar, or other similar compound. For the first twelve hours at least, and indeed for a much longer time, the child will take no harm if left unfed. The proper course, however, is to apply it to the breast a few hours after birth—that is, as soon as the mother has recovered a little from the fatigue of labor. The breasts will probably not fill with milk for twenty-four or thirty-six hours, or even a little longer; but there is generally a little thick secretion of creamy fluid, called *colostrum*, much earlier than this, of which it is good for the mother to be relieved, and which acts as a gentle laxative upon the child. The early application of the child to the breast also helps to form the nipples, and renders the flow of milk easy from the first; it teaches the child how to suck, a lesson learnt less readily if it has previously been fed with a spoon; and, lastly, it provides it, in the majority of cases, with all the food it requires during the first day or two, and obviates the necessity of artificial feeding.

The child should be put to the breast with clock-like regularity. Until the flow is fairly established, the interval should be four hours; afterwards, for the first month, an hour and a half or two hours in the daytime and four hours in the night. In the daytime the child may be awakened at the feeding-hour; in the night he should on no account be disturbed out of his sleep. Many infants will sleep continuously for six hours in the night, and suffer no harm from the long fast.

If it is important that a child should be fed as often as is here stated, it is no less important that he should not be fed oftener. Young infants very soon learn habits of regularity, and, besides, their stomachs need rest between their meals, just as in our own case, except that, of course, the intervals required are shorter. Many women put the child to the breast whenever it cries, forgetting that this is the only way in which it can express its sense of discomfort, from whatever cause arising, and that it is quite as likely to be crying because it is in pain, or because its napkin wants changing, as from hunger.

It is important from the first to apply the child to each breast in turn.

When the secretion of milk is long delayed, and it becomes consequently necessary to feed the infant, the proper food is good cow's milk, boiled, so as to prevent its being a carrier of infection, then mixed with about an equal quantity of water, and sweetened. Bread and oatmeal gruel are not fit food for newly-born infants. They irritate the stomach and bowels and cause griping and flatulence. In short, during the first month of life no other food than the mother's milk or diluted cow's milk should be given, except under medical advice.

When the mother has not enough milk to satisfy the child, nursing may be combined with hand-feeding, which is generally preferable to hand-feeding alone. The additional food should consist of good milk, boiled, diluted with an equal quantity of water and sweetened. After the first month the quantity of added water requires to be gradually lessened.

In case the mother cannot nurse her child, the next best way of feeding it is to obtain a good, healthy wet-nurse, whose child is not much older than the one she is to nurse. The medical attendant should always be consulted in regard to the health and suitability of a wet-nurse, before she is engaged.

It may be that a wet-nurse cannot be obtained, and then hand-feeding becomes necessary. For this purpose good milk (from one cow if possible), boiled, diluted, and sweetened, as already directed, is for the first few months all the food that is required. Arrowroot, cornstarch, and bread are all unsuitable at this tender age, and afford far less nourishment than milk.

Now and then a child is found with whom fresh milk does not agree, the curdy character of the stools showing that it is only partially digested. Should a change of dairy not suffice to set matters right, it will be desirable to try the concentrated Swiss milk, which, though greatly inferior to fresh milk, is the best of all artificial substances. Failing success with this, a malted preparation, known as Mellin's Food for Infants, may be tried, at any rate until the digestive powers become sufficiently improved to return to milk.

The custom of using feeding-bottles with India-rubber tubes has become exceedingly prevalent. These tubes are difficult to keep clean, and a mere drop or two of milk left adhering to the bottle or tube will often be sufficient to turn the next supply sour. Hence have arisen flatulence and indigestion, and much sickness and suffering. Another objection to the use of tubes is, that nurses are tempted to place children in the cot with the bottle of milk by their side and the tube in their mouth, a practice which is highly objectionable on several grounds. It does away with all regularity in feeding, and is very liable to cause the milk to be turned sour owing to the heat given off from the child's body. Feeding-bottles without tubes, and fitted with teats only, have the advantage of requiring to be held in the nurse's hand, and are on every account to be preferred. There should always be two, for alternate use, one being kept under water while the other is in actual use. Immediately after the child has had a meal, the bottle must be thoroughly washed in warm water.

It is an unnecessary and injurious practice to administer castor-oil to the newly-born. The first milk (or *colostrum*) from the mother's breast generally relaxes the bowels sufficiently, and if not, no aperient should be administered except under the advice of the medical attendant.

Children should not sleep in the same bed with an adult, but should, from the first, be placed in their own separate cot. Attention to this rule would annually save many lives which are now sacrificed. The number returned every year as having been found dead in bed is astounding. Sometimes both mother and child fall asleep, while the child is at the breast, whereupon the child's face gets pressed so closely against the mother's body that both nose and mouth are covered, breathing becomes impossible, and the child is smothered; sometimes fatal asphyxia is produced by the child nestling down in the bed and going to sleep with its head completely covered by the bedclothes; and sometimes, though of course very rarely, the cause of death in these cases is over-lying. These dangers are best avoided by letting the child sleep by itself.

During the first month or two a healthy child sleeps the greater part of both day and night.

Children should not be allowed to form the habit of being put to sleep on the nurse's lap, but should be placed in their cot awake, and soothed to sleep there. This is a lesson learnt without difficulty, if taught from the earliest days.

On no account should any kind of soothing medicine be given, except under medical advice.

Young babies require to be kept very warm, and yet need abundance of fresh air. Nursery windows should be opened very frequently, and the room kept pure and wholesome. After the first two or three weeks children should be carried in the arms out of doors every day in fine weather. In winter they should be well wrapped up, and in summer the head should be carefully protected from the rays of the sun.

When the navel-string is an unusually long time in separating, no force is to be used; all will go on properly if left to Nature. Separation having taken place, a small round piece of linen should be covered with a little vaseline or simple ointment, and applied to the navel. If the process be accompanied or followed by bleeding, the medical attendant should be informed without delay, as children occasionally die from this cause. He should also be told if, after the separation, the navel is found to project more than usual.

It is by no means an unfrequent occurrence for the breasts of newly-born children to become swollen and inflamed, and sometimes they are even found to contain a few drops of milk-like fluid. In either case the nurse must carefully avoid rubbing or squeezing them. The swelling will gradually disappear, and the fluid become absorbed under soothing treatment—as, for example, the ordinary water dressing; whereas rough manipulations, such as have just been mentioned, increase the inflammation, and are apt to result in the formation of abscess.

The appearance of a number of little white spots on the tongue, inside the lips and cheeks, and on the roof of the mouth, known in the nursery as "the thrush," is an almost certain sign that the child's food is in some way unsuit.able, and ought, therefore, invariably to be reported to the medical attendant. In the meantime the affected places should be painted several times a day with glycerine of borax, by means of a camel-hair brush.

## MANAGEMENT OF THE MOTHER AFTER LABOR: Treatment During the First Few Hours—The Lochia—Necessity of the Level Posture—Care when First Sitting-up—Change of Room—Going out of Doors—Changing the Linen—The Binder—Washing, &c.—Avoidance of Excitement—Occupation—Diet—The Bowels—Flooding—Rigors—Suckling—Sore Nipples—Abscess of Breast—Dispersion of Milk in the Event of Not Suckling.

After the patient has been made comfortable in the manner already described, it is above all things desirable that she should have several hours of undisturbed rest, and, if possible, sleep. There used to be a curious notion prevalent amongst nurses that a woman ought not to be allowed to fall asleep directly after delivery. This is altogether a mistake; sleep is to be encouraged by every possible means. To this end the room should be kept exceedingly quiet, and the blinds drawn down so as to subdue the light. In this way the patient will be best enabled to recover from the exhausting effects of labor. In the meantime the nurse should keep an eye on the patient's face, and if she observe that it is becoming unusually pale, she must at once ascertain whether there is any flooding.

For the first few days the patient will suffer more or less from after-pains, which only require to be brought under the notice of the medical attendant in case they are very severe or interfere with sleep. As a rule, no after-pains occur after a first confinement.

**The Proper Food** to be given directly after labor is a cup of tea, gruel, or warm milk; but if the patient prefers to wait a little before taking anything at all, there is no harm in allowing her to follow her inclination. When the patient has had a few hours' rest, and has recovered from her exhaustion, the child should be applied to the breast. The nipples can be drawn out much better before the breasts become filled with milk than afterwards.

Not more than six hours should elapse after labor before the patient is reminded to pass water. She should not be allowed to wait until she feels a desire to do this for, under these circumstances, the bladder may be quite full without the patient having any inclination to empty it. At the end of six hours, then, if it has not been already asked for, the slipper-pan should be passed, a little hot water having previously been poured into it and the vessel itself warmed before the fire. If she finds herself unable to use the slipper-pan, she may be allowed to turn herself gently on to her hands and knees, in which position she will almost always succeed, an ordinary chamber utensil being in in that case substituted for the slipper-pan. Should she, even after changing her position, still be unable to pass urine, she must not make forcing efforts, but lie down again, rest a little, and then make a further attempt. The patient herself frequently imagines that she has passed urine, when she has not; hence the nurse, knowing this, must not be satisfied without seeing for herself the contents of the vessel after its removal.

Should no urine be passed during the first twelve hours, something to aid the patient to do so must be given, as recommended elsewhere; and probably it will be necessary to call a doctor to draw it off by means of the catheter.

For the first few hours after delivery the vagina and external genital organs are very sore and painful, and the discharge consists of pure blood. Ten or twelve napkins are required during the twenty-four hours succeeding labor. On the second day the discharge becomes less, and each day the quantity diminishes, the discharge itself gradually changing from pure blood to a thick dark fluid, and lastly to a thin serum, like soiled water. The discharge always possesses a peculiar and distinctive odor, but if the odor become offensive the medical attendant should be informed. Similarly he should be told if, after having once ceased to consist of pure blood, the discharge should again assume that character.

The discharges after labor are termed the *lochia;* they sometimes last only a few days, and at other times continue for three or four weeks. They vary, too, in quantity in different women, even when they are quite natural and healthy. When they have passed through the changes I have named, they ought presently to cease, and if, instead of doing so, they continue, and if, especially, they become purulent in character—that is, if they contain matter like that of an abscess—an examination is necessary and the medical attendant must be informed.

On the other hand, it is not very unusual for the lochia to cease rather early and suddenly, and although this often causes alarm both to patient and nurse, it need not do so provided there is no other sign of ill-health, such as shivering, thirst, and feverishness.

For the first three days after confinement a patient should on no account be raised to a sitting posture lest an attack of flooding should come on, or fainting and even sudden death occur. There is not the same danger in allowing her to turn on to the hands and knees; indeed, I have already said that this posture may be resorted to in the event of any difficulty in using the slipper-pan in the ordinary way.

After the first three days, provided all is going on favorably, this rule as to the level position may be relaxed a little, by allowing the patient to be propped up by means of pillows or a bed-rest while she is taking food. At all other times, however, she must continue to lie down until the ninth day, when she may be assisted or carried to a couch and allowed to remain upon it for an hour or an hour and a half. At first very little dressing ought to be attempted on these occasions, the patient being protected from cold by wearing a warm dressing-grown, or by having a good blanket thrown over her. The length of time she is allowed to be out of bed may be increased day by day; and on the twelfth or thirteenth day she may be fully dressed. The temperature of the room must be regulated most carefully when the patient first leaves her bed, it being much more important for the room to be well warmed then, than during the time she remained in bed.

Should there be a suitable sitting-room on the same floor, the patient may take advantage of it as early as the fourteenth day; the lying-in chamber being meanwhile thoroughly freshened by opening the windows, spreading out the bedclothing, and leaving the mattress or bedding uncovered for some hours. If, on the other hand, the only available room is downstairs, it will be prudent to postpone the change for a few days longer.

If it happens to be mild, bright summer weather, and the patient's recovery has been rapid and satisfactory, the medical attendant may, in an exceptional case, consent to her taking a short walk or drive, at the end of three weeks.

After confinement a patient's linen requires to be frequently changed, both for health's sake and her own comfort. The patient must on no account be allowed to sit up or make any exertion while the clothes are being changed; the nurse must take off the soiled clothing by drawing down the sleeves from one arm, gathering up the clothes on that side into a handful, passing them gently over the head, and then drawing off the sleeves from the opposite arm. The clean linen, well aired, must then be put on as the patient lies.

The first binder should always be placed next to the patient's skin; after the first twenty-four hours this is a matter of less consequence. Each morning during the first week a clean binder should be applied with moderate tightness, the nurse re-adjusting it from time to time during the day in case it should become wrinkled or loose.

The patient's hands and face should be washed, and her hair straightened, as far as is possible without raising her, every morning. The hands and face having been attended to, the external genitals should be thoroughly cleansed over a bed-bath by means of a sponge and some water. In the absence of a bed-bath, a large slipper bed-pan may be made to answer the purpose, and if neither is obtainable, the patient must be made to turn on to the left side, with the thighs close to the edge of the bed, and the knees drawn up, when, the bed being duly protected by means of a rubber and warm folded sheet, the nurse can proceed with the sponging in the manner ordinarily adopted immediately after labor. For the first few days, while the lochia are somewhat abundant, it is well to repeat this process again in the evening.

Should the nurse while bathing the patient, discover a wound or raw surface, or any unusual swelling, she must quietly mention it to the doctor at his next visit; and so, too, if she finds any piles protruding. In the event of the patient complaining of severe pain from piles, the nurse must frequently foment the part, or apply a bread-poultice, until she receives instructions from the medical attendant.

Vaginal injections and douches are only to be used under medical direction.

The mind requires rest equally with the body. No painful news, or other exciting or disturbing influences, should be allowed to reach her. The visits of friends to the lying-in room must be entirely forbidden, except in the case of those who have obtained special permission.

It should never be forgotten that a peculiar and distressing form of mental derangement is liable to attack lying-in patients. Hence, if a nurse finds her patient irritable in temper and difficult to manage, she must avoid anything like contention or direct contradiction. By a firm, quiet, decided manner, a good nurse will be able to carry her point without exciting her patient.

As the patient grows a little stronger, there can be no objection to her occupying herself while in bed, if she is wishful to do so, with a little plain sewing or fancy work, and now and then with a little reading, so as to make the time pass more agreeably.

With regard to diet, many medical practitioners have rules of their own, which the nurse must always be prepared loyally to carry out. It is not now generally thought necessary for patients to be restricted to tea and gruel for a whole week. When a nurse is left to her own discretion she will find her patients recover their strength most rapidly by being allowed some variety in their food from the beginning. Boiled milk should always enter largely into the dietary of a woman who intends to suckle her child. An occasional cup of good black tea is generally very grateful, with or without a little biscuit, toast, or bread-and-butter. From the first, beef-tea, chicken, mutton, or veal broth, rice-caudle, milk or oatmeal gruel, and other simple fluids, are perfectly allowable. If all is going on well, and the bowels have acted, there is no harm —in case the patient expresses a desire for more solid food—in giving, even on the second or third day, a slice of chicken, or tender roast beef, or a mutton chop. The diet, indeed, at this time needs to be nutritious and plentiful, while its kind may safely be regulated very much according to the patient's inclination. No stimulants of any sort, however, must be given, except under medical direction.

A nurse should not give opening medicine on her own responsibility. The medical attendant will order what is necessary and state when it is to be given. Very often, instead of medicines, he will prescribe a simple enema of soap and water.

**Flooding after Delivery.**—Whenever an attack of flooding comes on during the period of lying-in, the nurse must at once send for the medical attendant, stating clearly her reasons for sending, in order that he may know what will be required. In the meantime she must unfasten the binder, and make firm pressure with her outspread hand on the womb, which she will have no difficulty in finding, as it will not yet have returned to its natural size and position. She must also apply cloths dipped in cold water, or in vinegar and water, to the external genitals, keeping them applied not longer than a minute or two at a time. Where the flow is great it will be right for the nurse to try to check it by taking a dry napkin and pressing it firmly with her hand against the external parts, while the other hand is still engaged in compressing the womb from above. The patient must, of couse be kept all this time strictly lying down, with the head and shoulders low, and cool, fresh air must be admitted through the open window.

The occurrence of a shivering fit, especially if it is a severe one, or is followed by others, ought always to be regarded seriously. No time should be lost in acquainting the doctor, and the nurse must meanwhile do all in her power to produce a feeling of returning warmth in her patient. With this object, a warm bottle should be put to her feet, an additional blanket thrown over her, and a cup of warm tea administered. This event is often the sign of approaching illness that, when it has shown itself, the patient should be watched with the utmost anxiety.

The secretion of milk is not usually established until the second or third day; now and then, however, it makes its appearance earlier. This event is sometimes accompanied with a little constitutional disturbance, which soon subsides. When the breasts are becoming so full and hard as to be painful, great relief will be afforded by fomenting them every few hours, and supporting them, in the meantime, as in a sling, by a handkerchief tied over the opposite shoulder. (See page 193.) This condition will generally soon subside if the child be applied at regular intervals. Nurses must beware of meddling too much with the breasts, and especially avoid rubbing them, except under special direction from the doctor. The nipples and surrounding parts should be carefully washed each time the child leaves the breast, and should be excluded from the air by covering them with a small piece of linen rag on which a little vaseline or simple ointment has been spread.

As soon as it becomes clear that the supply of breast-milk is insufficient, it is unwise to keep putting the child to the breast, as this only produces irritation and is very liable to set up inflammation and abscess. Similarly, if the nipples are extremely sore, so that, even when they are protected by a nipple-shield, the application of the child is attended each time with intense pain, or if they are so depressed that neither the efforts of the child nor the cautious use of the breast-pump will draw them out, it is running a great risk of exciting breast-abscess to persevere beyond twenty-four hours in an attempt to suckle.

If the nurse notices a patch of redness on a patient's breast, and finds that the skin at that spot is painful and tender to the touch, she should take means to acquaint the medical attendant as soon as possible, for an abscess has actually formed; it should be opened with as little delay as possible, lest it spread and become much more formidable.

**Still-Born.**—When the child is still-born, or when, from any other cause, it is not going to be suckled, there is often great anxiety expressed about the dispersion of the milk. It is astonishing, however, how quickly it becomes absorbed if left to Nature. If the patient will only submit to the discomfort arising from the fullness of the breasts for a few hours, without insisting on their being partially emptied from time to time by the use of the breast-pump, or other similar means, whereby the breasts are stimulated to fresh secretion and the evil is aggravated, she will soon have the satisfaction of finding them softer and less painful, and will be amply rewarded for her patience. Should the feeling of tension be excessive, it will be best relieved by hot fomentations applied every few hours; if not excessive, the application for a few days of belladonna plasters with a hole in the centre for the nipple, is often all that is necessary. In ordering these plasters the nurse should furnish the druggist with paper patterns showing the size required.

# FOOD FOR THE SICK.

**THE SICK-ROOM.**—Its Location—A Good Nurse—Fresh Air—Light—Warmth—Cleanliness—Quiet—Food, Drink and Delicacies, and the Faithful Administration of Medicines, are of the utmost importance, and will each receive consideration. But, in accordance with the design of this work, the *essentials* only will be pointed out, the *minor details*, or little things, must be left to the judgment and "common sense" of the nurse or head of the household, to be met as best they can by the conveniences at hand or the means of obtaining them.

**I. Location of the Sick-room.**—In summer, if it be possible, let the sick-room be on the north side of the house; in winter, upon the south—to avoid the mid-day heat of summer and the cold blasts of winter. And also, if there is a room in the house having a fire-place, give it the preference, as it is considered the best means of aiding ventilation and providing artificial warmth when needed. And, if the windows do not admit of *lowering* the upper sash as well as to *raise* the lower ones, prepare them at once to allow this movement. Further on, you will see, under the heads of "How to Produce the Temperature of Sick-rooms," and "Ventilation of Sick-rooms," where the necessity of this is fully explained.

**II. A Good Nurse.**—We have so often heard the expression: "If Mr. Blank had not had the best of nursing, he would never have got well." Knowing that very much depends upon it, I say, get the best nurse that your means can obtain; then see and know for yourselves that they carry out your, or the physician's directions faithfully; for a physician's prescriptions, nor your own desires or directions, are of any account unless they are faithfully followed: But, of course, much of the details must be left to the nurse, hence the necessity of getting one of sound judgment and considerable experience, if possible.

**III. Fresh Air.**—Although fresh air is essential in a sick-room, yet a draft must not be allowed to strike upon the patient; hence the necessity, in small rooms especially, of having the means of raising and lowering the sash, either for ventilation or to reduce the temperature. The temperature of the sick-room, in all ordinary cases of diseases, had better be kept as near 60° to 65° Fah. as possible, by opening or closing windows, or by raising the fire or lessening it—either, or both,—as the necessity of the case requires. And, let me say, the day has gone past when the great "bug-a-boo" against "night-air" has any weight—pure night-air, properly managed in the season of the year requiring it, is far better than the stifled or suffocating air of

302

a close sick-room; ventilate and reduce the temperature always as needed, and, of course, with proper care. Keep the air pure by carrying out of the room any and all vessels *de chambre* as soon as used, no matter how small the discharge may be. Never bring a slop-bucket into the sick-room, as the pouring out, rinsing, etc., is not only very contaminating to the air, but annoying to the patient.

**IV. Light.**—If a room for the sick has been chosen which will allow proper ventilation and fresh air, as needed, through the windows, the light can easily be governed by the curtains; and it is only necessary to say: allow all the light that is agreeable to the patient; and, except in nervous or eye diseases, but little exclusion of light will be necessary, unless the room is on the south or western side of the house, which is not desirable, generally.

**V. Warmth.**—Under this head it will be necessary to include the temperature of the patient's surface as well as that of the room. The warmth or temperature of the room being about 60° to 65° Fah. if the limbs are cold, rub them with the dry naked hand, or wrap in hot, dry woolen cloths, or place hot bricks, or bottles or jugs, filled with hot water, or, what is still better, small bags of dry, hot sand, made for this purpose, whichever is most convenient or necessary to keep them comfortable. Comfort is to be sought, no matter how much labor and trouble it causes; for, unless a genial warmth can be maintained, health will seldom be regained. On the other hand, in fevers and inflammatory diseases, the surface must be cooled by means of sponging with cool or cold water with a little whiskey, or what is better, whiskey with bay-rum in it—sponging sufficiently often to keep down extreme heat. Especially overcome all extremes of heat or cold.

**VI. Cleanliness.**—It is claimed that "cleanliness is next to Godliness." Whether this be a fact or not, it is absolutely necessary, if it is desired to restore the patient to health in the least possible time, that not only the sick-room be kept clean, but the bed, bed-clothing and wearing apparel be kept neat and clean; and the patient, also, must have such frequent washings or spongings as will keep the pores of the skin open, that the general exhalations, perspiration sensible or insensible, as when sick an odor, also, may not only pass readily through the pores, but to provide, in disease, for the escape not only of a larger amount than usual but that of a more offensive and injurious character, if left to be re-absorbed from the surface or clothing.

**VII. Quiet.** If the patient is very sick, absolute quiet is very essential. If a person is once admitted to the sick-room who is found to annoy the patient by long talking, or, in fact in any manner, they must not only be asked to retire but never be admitted again. What is necessary to say, speak in a mild but perfectly distinct voice, and never allow whispering in a sick room for any purpose whatever. If there are any secrets to be kept from the patient, no hint of them, or whispering about them, should ever occur in his hearing; yet if it is believed the patient can not live very long, I would most certainly inform them of this belief—'tis cruel and unjust to withhold it. Any continuous noise, although slight in itself, soon becomes annoying to any nervous person, and there are but few sick persons, indeed, who do not soon become more or less nervous. Be firm, but kind, in all your relations with the sick. Give them to understand you know best, and what you know to be best to do you are going to do; and what you know they ought not to do, you are not going to allow them to do, but in all the kindness possible, and their acquiescence may soon be expected. Rustling silks, squeaking shoes and the rattling of dishes must not be allowed in a sick-room.

**VIII. Food, Drink and Delicacies.** While the patient's condition will allow them to use plain and substantial food, and the usual drink, as tea and coffee, not too strong, it is best they should have them; but with the weak and debilitated the delicacies must take their place; and I desire to call especial attention to, and to give my sanction and advice, that if any special thing is craved, be it food or drink, I would most positively allow it, in moderation. We have all heard of the cravings, in olden times, of fever patients for cold water, and the cures brought about from its having been obtained stealthily against the commands of the physician; but there has recently come to my knowledge a case wherein the life of a typhoid fever patient was saved by drinking two quarts of hard cider, which he had craved and repeatedly called for, and when he got hold of the pitcher he would not let it go until it was empty. I do not call this, however, "in moderation," but the patient was stouter in his desperation than the nurse and the physician who had allowed it to be brought, so no one could have been blamed even if it had killed rather than cured the patient. Do not understand this, however, even in desperate cases, to be a pattern drink—A small glass, and often, as long as the craving continues, would be the safer plan with any drink. But both food and drink should be given regularly in reasonable quantities. And to aid the nurse or family in this, the following recipes, or receipts, may be resorted to with confidence and general satisfaction. To purify sick-rooms, see " Disinfectants."

## BEEF TEA, ESSENCES OF BEEF, ARTICLES OF DIET, DRINKS, ETC., FOR THE SICK.

**1. Beef Tea.**—Take lean beef, $\frac{1}{2}$ lb.; cold water, $\frac{1}{2}$ cup; a little salt, pepper, mace, or nutmeg. DIRECTIONS—Cut the beef into small bits—$\frac{1}{4}$ or $\frac{1}{2}$ inch squares—and see that no particle of fat adheres to it; put into a bottle with the water and cork, placing the bottle in a pan of cold water upon a stove, and as soon as it reaches the boiling-point, move it back, but keep it near the boiling-point for 2 hours; then strain, pressing out the juices, and season with a little salt and a sprinkle of pepper, mace or nutmeg, as preferred by the patient.

**2. Beef Tea—Improved Flavor, by Broiling.**—Take a nice steak and remove all the fat. Have a gridiron, perfectly clean—all particles of burned steak may easily be removed from the bars by placing it in hot water a few minutes when first taken from the fire; then scrape, or what is better, use a stiff brush, kept for this purpose. Have a very nice fire of coals, and place the steak upon the gridiron and broil, as usual, till it is ready to turn; then take off, having at least a qt. bowl with 1 pt. of boiling-hot water in it, and keep it standing by the fire, or on the back part of the stove, to keep it hot. Place the steak, when the first side is nicely broiled, in this bowl of hot water, and press it with the knife and fork—a stiff spoon is the best—to extract the juices of the meat. Repeat this broiling and pressing several times, turning the steak each time, till all the juices and strength of the steak are extracted; and if, at the last, the steak is cut into squares of an inch or a little more, and each piece pressed in a lemon-squeezer, its virtue, or strength, will all be obtained. It looks much like wine of itself; but still, if a teaspoon or so of wine is added to what may be taken at any one time, it will not injure the most delicate stomach, but will be borne, even by a delicate stomach, better than bread-water, while it, of course, is much more nourishing; and, if properly seasoned, as suggested in No. 1, it will be relished by the patient—much more so from the broiling.

3. **Essence of Beef.**—The real essence, or nourishing properties of beef, is obtained the same as directed in No. 1, except that no water is to be put into the bottle, and the boiling may need to be continued an hour or two longer; then the juice or essence pressed out, and a little wine added when desired or needed; also a touch of salt and pepper; or, if mace or nutmeg is preferred, there is no reasonable objection that can be offered against their use.

*Remarks.* The foregoing are the plans which have been heretofore followed in extracting the strength or essence from beef for the sick. But as the science of medicine, especially the chemical department thereof, advances, it has been prolific in improvements, among which that of not boiling, but steeping, either in cold water, or using heat only of a moderate degree, or not above 100° to 135°, so as not to cook the albuminous (like white of egg) portions of the meat in making beef tea, or extracting its juice.

4. **Beef Tea for the Sick—New Process.**—Beef tea, if rightly made, may be received with benefit by a stomach which would reject any nourishment; but skill in preparing it, is not universal among nurses. The two following receipts may be relied on as among the best that can be devised:

**Beef Tea** (with moderate warming up after cold steeping).—Take 1 lb. of the best beef; cut in thin slices and scrape the meat fine; put with a salt-spoon of salt into 1 pt. of cold water contained in an earthen bowl, and let the mixture stand 2 or 3 hours, stirring it frequently; then place it in the same vessel covered, on the back part of the range or stove, and let it come very gradually to a blood-heat and no more. It has been found that 135° of heat does not set or cook the albumen—blood-heat is only 98°. Any higher temperature would injure the nutriment, or nourishing properties; then strain it through a fine sieve or muslin bag, and it is ready for use. The making of beef tea is not a cooking process, but a steeping process. Some chemists think it better to be made without heat, with the addition of the muriatic acid, which is a component part of healthy gastric juice, as follows:

5 **Beef and Other Meat Teas Without Heat.**—Take ⅓ lb. of fresh beef, mutton, poultry or game (the lean part only), minced very fine;

place it in 14 ozs. of soft cold water (2 or 3 tablespoons less than 1 pt.) to which has been added a pinch or about 18 grs. of table salt, and three or four drops of muriatic acid; stir all with a wooden spoon, (on account of the acid, which rusts iron) and set it aside for 1 hour, stirring it occasionally; then strain it through gauze, or a sieve, and wash the residue left on the sieve by means of 5 additional ozs. of cold soft water, pressing it so that all the soluble matter will be removed from the residue; mix the two strainings and the Extract is ready for use. It should be drunk freely every two or three hours.

*Remarks.*—The properties taken from these last two receipts are largely borne out by a well known article made at Richmond, Va., by Mann. S. Valentine, called "Valentine's Preparation of Meat Juice," which, in using, is not to be heated above 130° F., and that only upon a water-bath to avoid the possibility of over-heating—the preferable way being to use it cold, even with ice when this is desirable. Stale bread is recommended by him to be crumbled into the Meat Juice as a savory diet for the sick, as one becomes able to digest more solid food. This, of course will hold good with any of the above or other juicy foods, or soups, or essences, etc., prepared from any meats whatever. The greatest objection that can be raised against Valentine's Meat Juice is its cost. He claims to have concentrated the strength, or virtues, of 4 lbs. of beef into a 2 oz. bottle which, usually, retails at $1.25, which would certainly prevent its use by the sick poor — the sick rich, of course, can indulge it. But from its array of testimonials from the most popular physicians in America and Europe, and by those connected with insane asylums, hospitals, etc., it must have proven an exceedingly valuable preparation; and I will close my remarks upon this subject by saying I have not referred to it for the benefit of the manufacturer (for he knows not of this reference at all), nor am I paid for it, only as it may do good to the people in observing the value of the cold process, as it may be called, of the last two receipts, and being "posted," as the saying is, upon the best ways or plans of preparing food for the sick. This Meat Juice was on exhibition and received awards at the International Exhibition in '76 at Philadelphia, and in '78 at Paris, and although he does not give its mode of preparation in his circulars, yet this must have been given to the commissioners at these exhibitions, for the awards were:

"For excellence of the method of its preparation, whereby it more nearly represents fresh meat than any other extract of meat, its freedom from disagreeable taste, its fitness for immediate absorption and the perfection in which it retains its good qualities in warm climates."

The method is undoubtedly by maceration (softening by steeping), and then by pressure, having used but little water, and leaving a heavy pressure to accomplish the separation of the juices of the meat, to avoid the necessity of heat to condense by evaporation. There is no doubt of the value of this article as a food for the sick, and as only from ½ to 2 teaspoonfuls of it are required as a dose. or meal, those who can afford to use it will prefer to do it rather than prepare any of the others above given, unless they have a skillful nurse; and, in that case, I shall have done the good I intended by calling attention to it. See also Beef Water, Broths, etc., below.

**6. Oyster Essence.**—Take ½ doz. (or any number, according to the necessity, or ability of the patient to take the essence) of large, nice oysters, with their share of juice; put in a stew-pan, and place on the stove, or over the fire, and let them simmer slowly, until they smell, or become plump or full—3 to 5 minutes according to the heat; then take off, strain and press out the juices without breaking the oysters, and serve hot. Light, stale, bread crumbs, very light, dry biscuit, or crackers, as preferred or convenient, will give additional relish and strength when the patient is able to have them.

*Remarks.*—Most people say, "put in salt," when they give directions to prepare oysters; but I know it is best not to put in the salt, or other seasoning, until just as you are about to remove them from the fire.

**7. Chicken Broth.**—Cut up half of a young chicken, removing the fat and skin; sprinkle a little salt upon it and put it into 2 qts. of cold water and set it over a quick fire; when it comes to a boil, set it back on the stove or range, where it will only simmer. When entirely tender, take out the white parts, letting the rest remain until it is boiled from the bones. Mince the white part and pound it fine in a mortar or suitable dish; add this to the broth, adding boiling water, if necessary, to make it thin enough to drink readily. Put again in the sauce-pan and boil a few minutes. Some persons will desire a slight addition of salt and a little pepper: but use just as little pepper as will satisfy them, a light sprinkle, however, will hurt no one. It is very nutritious, and hence should be taken only in small quantities. A little rice may be boiled in some of this broth, either for its taste or greater nourishment; and a little stale bread, or a cracker or two, may be broken into some of it at another time, for the same reason, and for changing the flavor also. A little parsley may be added to flavor any of these broths, waters, or drinks, if desired, or any other pot-herbs.

**8. Mutton Broth.**—Take 1½ lbs. of chops, from the neck of a lamb or young sheep (old and strong mutton is never to be used for the sick); cut into small bits, removing all the fat possible; put bones, as well as the lean meat, into a stew-pan, with 3 pts. of cold water and a little salt; put where it will stew gently till all scum is removed as it rises. In 30 to 40 minutes some may be poured off for the patient, if he is impatient for it. Continue to stew it slowly an hour or two, seasoning to taste while hot; when cool strain, and when cold, remove all the tallow or fat from the surface. After this it may be given cold or hot, as suits the patient. A slice of bread, as in the chicken panada, may be toasted nicely and broken into a plate; then pouring on some of this broth, as in that case it is more strengthening, and gives another variety of broth to meet the varying tastes of the sick; or stale bread, without toasting, is generally preferable.

**10. Veal Broth.**—Veal broth is generally made by some chops of veal, as in the mutton broth above, or a joint of veal, with suitable amount of meat upon the joint, in about 3 qts. of water, 2 oz. of rice, a little salt, and a piece or two of mace; stew till the water is about half evaporated.

**10. Beef Broth or Water.**—Take a piece of perfectly lean steak (from the rump or shoulder is preferable) the size of your hand; cut it into small bits, and put into a stew-pan with 1 pt. of cold water; bring it to a boil and skim; then set it back and simmer 20 to 30 minutes, occasionally pressing each piece with a spoon to obtain the full juice, or strength of the beef. In hot weather any of these broths or drinks will be relished well if ice-cold. by setting upon ice what was not taken hot when first made; otherwise it is better to re-heat them when called for.

**11. Vegetable Broth.**—Let all the articles named be of medium size only: potatoes, 2; carrot, turnip and onion, 1 each; slice (of course after washing and paring); boil 1 hour in 1 qt. of water, adding more boiling water from time to time to keep the original quantity good. Add a little salt and pepper, and any pot-herbs, as parsley or other herb, as preferred, to flavor; strain, or allow to settle. This is a good substitute for the animal broths, when they can not be borne, or at distances from where fresh meats can be obtained; or as an additional variety when sickness is long continued.

**12. Milk Porridge, with Raisins.**—Stir 2 tablespoons of flour with sufficient cold milk to make smooth; then stir this into 1 qt. of boiling milk; break or cut into halves 20 or 30 nice large raisins, and boil 20 minutes. Strain and add a little salt.

**13. Oatmeal Porridge, or Gruel.**—Mix 2 tablespoons of the finely ground oatmeal with a little cold water, then stir it into 1 pt. of boiling water and let it boil 15 to 20 minutes. Add a little salt and sugar, to taste; if desired a small quantity of wine and nutmeg may also be added.

**14. Cornmeal Gruel, or Porridge.**—One of the most common gruels is made with cornmeal and a little flour. Half a cup of cornmeal and ½ a tablespoon of flour wet to a smooth paste, then stirred into 1 qt. of boiling water, and the boiling continued slowly for 30 minutes. Seasoned with salt and a little sugar, makes it the most palatable to most people; and some add a little butter; but if any is used it should be a very little, and that of the choicest kind. This is not only nourishing for the sick, but is mildly laxative, and aids the action of cartharic medicine; but if it is intended to aid a cathartic do not use any flour in its make. A bit of cinnamon or nutmeg, as preferred, may be added to any of these gruels or waters. But if any astringent is desired, or a gruel to aid astringent remedies, use one of the two following:

**15. Browned Cornmeal Gruel, or Cakes, for Weak Stomachs, and for Summer Complaints of Children.**—Brown corn the same as you roast coffee; grind it fine in a coffee-mill, and make a gruel as with common cornmeal. Make some into a mush, or batter, and bake, in thin cakes, to a light brown. Very feeble stomachs will retain the gruel; or the cakes, as preferred. See also "Corn Coffee for the Sick."

**16. For Diarrhea of Children, or Others.**—Parch the corn nicely; grind it into meal, and boil it in skim milk. This is claimed to be a sure cure for summer complaints.

**17. Milk and Rice Gruel.**—Rice flour, or very finely pulverized rice, 3 table-spoonfuls, wet smoothly with cold milk, and stir into 1 qt. of boiling milk, and stir all the time it is boiling—10 to 15 minutes, or till it tastes *done.* Nutmeg is a very nice flavor for this gruel, and a little sugar, if desired. It is very acceptable for children.

**18. Tamarind Whey—Cooling and Laxative.**—Dr. John King, of Cincinnati, says:

"A convenient and cooling laxative is Tamarind Whey, made by boiling 1 oz. of the pulp of the Tamarind in 1 pt. of milk, and straining the product."

*Remarks*—Tamarinds grow on quite large trees, principally in the East and West Indies. They are put up in kegs with syrup for importation; and on being received in the United States are often put up, by wholesale druggists, in bottles for their better preservation as, like other fruits, they keep better in air-tight bottles. I trust their value as a cooling and thirst-allaying fruit may, hereafter, be more fully appreciated, especially in fevers, inflammation and dyspepsia.

**19. Tamarind Water, for Fever Patients—To Allay Great Thirst in Hot Weather, and for Dyspeptics.**—Take nice Tamarinds (kept by druggists in large cities, and sometimes, also, by grocers), 1 qt. —3 lbs will about equal 1 qt.—place them in an earthen jar and pour upon them 3 qts. of boiling, soft water; cover, and let stand three or four hours; then, with the hand squeeze the pulp out of the bird-nest clusters, in which the seeds and pulp are held; then strain through stout muslin; bottle and cork tightly; and put into a cool cellar. In three or four weeks it will be ripe and fit for use.

*Remarks.*—In hot weather, especially with dyspeptics, there is often experienced very great thirst. With such, I am not aware of any other article or drink equal to this to relieve them of the excessive craving for drink. Then take a wine-glass of this in as much ice-cold water, sweetened to taste, and you will have a healthy and most agreeable nectar, and one of the most powerful extinguishers of thirst ever discovered. The author has tested it and knows whereof he speaks. It settles by standing and becomes as clear and pure as champagne. I have taken a glass of it when very thirsty, ice-cold, as above mentioned, and the relief would be so perfect I would not think about drinking again for 2 or 3 hours. The properties of the tamarind are very peculiar, as it contains not only small quantities of sugar, but pectic, citric, tartaric and malic acids, and also the bi-tartrate of potassa; is nourishing, refrigerant (cooling), calmative and laxative; hence its great value in fevers. But, of course, to prepare it for a drink in fevers, you cannot wait for it to purify itself by standing, yet it should be bottled all the same, and a bottle of it placed at once upon ice; or if no 'ice is at hand, stand a bottle of it in a bucket of cold water, so as to have it as cool as possible; then add as much cold water to what you use of the tamarind water at each time, and sweeten to taste. Let the patient partake of it as freely as desired, so long as it agrees with the stomach, and does not prove too laxative.

**20. Wine Whey.**—Put 1 pt. of sweet milk in a suitable basin upon the stove, and when it comes to a boil, pour into it a gill (about 5 or 6 table-spoonruls) of wine, and when it has again boiled about 15 minutes, remove from the fire; let it stand a few minutes, but do not stir it; then strain or remove the curd, and sweeten to taste; flavor with cinnamon, or nutmeg, or any other spice or fruit, as orange or lemon peel, etc. It is used for very weak and feeble patients.

**21.  Sour Milk Whey.**—Where wine is not to be had, and a whey is needed, bring a cup of sweet milk to a boil, and add the same amount of sour milk, and the result is a very nice whey.  Season or flavor, as desired.

**22.**  If no sour milk, a table-spoonful of good vinegar will do the same thing if not curdled, by standing a few minutes, stir in a little more vinegar, strain and season to taste.

**23.  Chicken Water.**—Take half of a young chicken, divest it of the skin, remove the feet, and break all the bones.  Put into 2 qts. of water and boil for half an hour; strain through muslin, and season with a little salt and pepper, if desired.  It quenches the thirst and is quite nourishing for use when the strong teas or essences cannot be borne by the stomach.  Straining through muslin removes or absorbs any oil or fat upon the surface, which cannot be dipped off.

**24.  Barley Water.**—Pearl barley, 1 oz.; wash in cold water, and pour off; then boil it a few minutes, and pour off again, which removes a certain rank taste; now pour on boiling water, 1 qt.; and boil, in an open dish, until half evaporated; strain and season to the taste of the patient.  It is nourishing and pleasant, hot or cold, as desired.

**25.  Chicken Panada.**—Toast a slice of stale bread (bread not less than two days old) to a very nice brown (be careful never to burn bread in toasting for the sick, for scraping off does not remove the burned taste,) and break into a soup plate, pouring over it some chicken broth, boiling hot; cover the plate and let it stand till cold enough to eat, or drink, according to the condition of the patient

**26.  Plain Panada.**—Split 5 or 6 Boston, or other very light crackers, put into a bowl with a very little salt, nutmeg and sugar to taste; pour boiling water over them and cover till cool; it makes a nourishing drink—and still more nourishing if the patients digestion will allow them to eat the crackers, or a portion of them.

**27.  Plain Panada, With Bread.**—Put into a bowl, in small pieces, 1 slice of stale bread (not less than 2 days old), leaving out the crust; put in a small piece of nice butter, and pour upon it ½ pt. of boiling water.  Sweeten, if desired, and flavor also if preferred, with nutmeg and a little wine also, if desired.

**28.  Corn Coffee, for the Sick, or for a Nauseous Stomach.**—Take nice, sweet, dry corn (I do not mean sweet corn, but nicely dried field corn); be careful in browning it, not to burn it, as it injures its flavor, as much as it does to over-brown coffee for general use—makes it bitter rather than pleasant.  To 1 coffee cup of this ground, as coffee, stir in 1 beaten egg; put into the coffee pot, and pour on boiling water, 1 pt. or a little more; steep and season also as coffee, with cream and sugar. It is nourishing and sufficiently stimulating to allay a nauseous stomach before vomiting has taken place. See also browned corn meal gruel for weak stomachs.

**29. Corn Tea.**—Make the same as the corn coffee above, except not to use the egg. It is pleasant, hot or cold, but not quite as nourishing, lacking the egg; hence adapted to very weak patients (see also the herb teas), but as there will be found patients in every condition of strength, or want of strength, it becomes important that a variety of receipts should be given, and hence the following:

**30. Rice Coffee, Especially Nice for Children or Weakly Patients.**—Brown the rice carefully, as you would the coffee bean, or corn, above; then grind, or mash in a mortar, and to 1 cup of this pour on 1 qt. of boiling water, let it stand 15 minutes; strain if it does not pour off clear. Sweeten all these coffees with loaf or granulated sugar, and use boiled milk with them, as freely as relished. It may be drank as freely as the stomach will bear. Children are very fond of it; and it is better for them, or for weakly persons, than common coffee. The same holds good, also, of the corn preparations above.

**31. Common Teas.**—A rather weak tea (never a strong one) may be made of any of the ordinary green or black teas, when craved by the sick sweetening and using milk as desired; for we believe it better to allow a mild beverage of this kind to any sick person rather than to allow their minds to worry over a refusal, for all excitement is to be avoided if reasonably possible, for amendment seldom begins, nor does it continue long, after any dissatisfaction arises, no matter what the subject, nor how slight the dissatisfaction may be; hence indulge all opinions, or even whims, that have not in themselves an absolute wrong.

**32. Eggnog for the Sick.**—Beat the yolk of 1 egg with 1 table spoonful of pulverized sugar to the consistency of cream; grate in a little nutmeg; add 1 large table-spoonful of brandy and 2 of Madeira wine. Beat the white of the egg to a stiff froth, and mix in with 1 cup of nice sweet milk.

*Remarks.*—This is palatable, and for weak and feeble patients will be found very invigorating and strengthening, the true "Madeira" being rich in its tonic and invigorating qualities. The original formula ran thus: "The yolks of 16 eggs, and 16 table spoonfuls of pulverized loaf-sugar (the day of this "loaf-sugar" is over, except in small cubes or squares) beaten to a cream; 1 grated nutmeg; ½ pt. of good brandy or rum, and 2 glasses of Madeira wine. The whites beaten to a stiff froth and put in, finishing with 6 pts. of milk made cold." This would indicate that it was being made for general or hospital use, or the patient must have been expected to live on it for a week at least, or otherwise to have many visitors. But this was a universal practice in an early day, and finally whiskey took the place of the brandy and the wine. No party or evening gathering was considered to be well provided for unless a large supply of milk punch or eggnog was prepared and set before the guests, when every one was expected to help themselves, from time to time, to all they desired; but it is one of the most dangerous forms in which liquor can be placed before young men, and especially so if there are to be frequent evening parties. I speak from the experience of my early life, where this beverage was freely supplied by a man of social disposition, having plenty of means, to induce about a dozen of us young men to spend our evenings in his society at least two or three evenings in the week. But, for one, I soon discovered that the days were too long, and that I desired the parties would suit me better every night .ather than only two or three in the week, and on the days upon which a party was to gather in the evening, I wanted night to come even before supper-time, which opened my eyes to the danger of these nightly meetings while I yet had moral courage and strength of mind to say: "Excuse me, I shall meet with you no more,"—and I did not, notwithstanding the jibes and jeers of my associates in labor through the day. To this decision, made very soon after my marriage, I owe a life of great industry and labor, in which, I humbly believe, I have done at least some good to my fellow creatures; for which I feel very grateful to Him to whom we all have to render an account. Then allow me to say to everyone, but especially so to every young man: "Touch not any liquor as a beverage, as you hope to spend a life of usefulness here, and of happiness in the better land beyond the river."

33. **Negus for the Sick.**—Barley-water, 1 pt.; wine, ½ pt.; lemon-juice, 1 table-spoonful; nutmeg and sugar to suit. DIRECTIONS—Make the barley-water, as before given; then mix.

*Remarks.*—Nourishing and stimulating. Used by weak patients like Col. Negus, from whom it takes its name.

34. **Raw Egg and Milk for Convalescents.**—A fresh egg; milk, 1 cup; a little port or other wine, and a little sugar. DIRECTIONS—Use only the yolk, beating thoroughly; then add the milk, and beat till foamy; then sugar and wine.

*Remarks.*—Have this ready to be taken by convalescents when they feel the least fatigue on returning from exercise.

35. **Milk Punch for the Sick.**—Nice sweet milk, ½ pt.; white sugar, 2 table-spoonfuls, best brandy, 2 table-spoonfuls; ice. DIRECTIONS—Dissolve the sugar in the milk, and add the brandy, stirring well.

*Remarks.*—This punch has maintained the life of very sick persons when nothing else could be taken for several days, or until the natural forces returned to the rescue. Make cold with ice, or keep it on ice.

36. **Milk Punch, with Eggs, for Weak Patients.**—If the patient is very weak, it is more strengthening to beat a fresh egg (in fact, none but freshly laid eggs should be used with the sick) thoroughly, and stir into the above punch before the spirit is added.

*Remarks.*—The white of a fresh egg beaten with 1 table-spoonful of white sugar, then a table-spoonful of best brandy added and again beaten, was fed to me by a Methodist clergyman—a special friend—in tea-spoonful doses, which sustained me 2 or 3 days, and, no doubt, saved my life, when even the consulting physician declared it would send the disease to the brain and soon destroy me. The occasion for its use arose from typhoid pneumonia of the right lung—the exhausting discharges from the bowels and the change of position necessary producing such sinking spells that life must have soon given out. The attend·ing physician had determined to administer the brandy; but the consulting one (a much older man, and hence more set in the "old fogy" idea that brandy would excite inflammation of the brain) was contending with him in the parlor, as I was afterwards informed, that it would not do; when the clergyman came in, as he was in the habit of doing in my sickness, and heard their argument, he came in to see my condition; as soon as he saw my exhaustion—he having been raised from the same condition by a physician in another city, went back to the doctors and said: "I will take the responsibility of this case to-day," thus agreeing with the advance in science, as shown by the younger physician; he did as above indicated, personally attending to me all that day and night till 5 o'clock in the morning; pronouncing the danger past, he called my dear wife (since passed to the "better land"), whom he had compelled, as it were, to lie down for a few hours, which she had not before done for several days and nights (getting all her rest and sleep in a chair, notwithstanding there was plenty of help, through her anxiety for me—such is a true woman's love). The brandy was truly the hinge on which the case turned back to life, when scarcely a hope was entertained that such could be the result. Why should not this, then, or some other of these punches, eggnogs, etc., save others when in such extremely weak conditions? If I did not so believe, I would certainly not take such pains and so much space to explain and recommend them. But do not understand me as recommending these stimulating drinks, only in these exhausting diseases, where the diffusive as well as the stimulating power of the spirit is demanded to aid the strength and stimulate the recuperative powers of nature to rally to the rescue. My reasons for opposing stimulation generally, is more fully shown in the remarks following "Eggnog."

**37. Claret Punch.**—Claret, 1 bottle; ice-water, ¼ as much as wine; sliced lemons, 2; powdered sugar, ½ cup. Put the sugar upon the sliced lemons for a few minutes; add the ice-water and stir well for a minute or two, then pour in the wine. Put plenty of ice into each glass as served  For the sick come as near to the proportions as practicable, for why should not the sick have their share of the good things, as well as those who only use them for the enjoyment? These fixtures are only additions to improve flavor, and make more palatable; hence let the sick have the advantage of them by all means.

**38. Currant Shrub for the Sick.**—A lady writer says: "Make the same as jelly, but boil only ten minutes; then bottle, and cork tightly. Put 2 table-spoonfuls of the shrub (jelly) to ½ glass of ice-cold water, and have some bits of ice in it."

*Remarks.*—This would be pleasant and grateful to the taste, but it is not shrub—that always contains spirits of some kind, to prevent souring; or, for its stimulating effects; see the following:

**39. English Shrub, for the Sick.**—"One sour" (lemon juice) "two sweet" (sugar), "three strong" (rum, or other spirit), "four weak" (water).

*Remarks.*—The measure might be a tea cup, or a pint measure, as desired, but each article was to be measured in the same dish. For those patients needing any stimulants, I would add ¼ as much good whiskey, or Bordeaux, preferably, as is used for the jelly. Any common acid jelly, properly diluted with ice-cold water, makes a pleasant drink for fever patients, or those sick from other diseases. Or, any of the following may be used, as needed.

**40. Acid Drinks From Raspberry Vinegar Jelly, is Nourishing and Pleasant for Invalids.**—Take 4 qts. of red raspberries and cover them with good cider vinegar, and let them stand 24 hours; then scald, strain and add sugar, 1 lb., to each pint of the juice; boil 20 minutes, or until it jells; bottle and cork, or can, air tight, and it will keep well, or is ready for present use. A table-spoonful of this to a glass of ice-cold water, taken a little at a time, makes the patient, if a reasonable one, feel very grateful, when sick, or convalescing. So also does:

**41. Toast Water.**—Make by nicely browning (not burning in the least) stale bread; then pouring boiling water upon it, and letting it stand upon ice, if you have it, then squeezing in a little lemon juice.

**42. Raw Egg Drink for Invalids—Strengthening, Restorative and Pleasant.**—A fresh, raw egg, being both strengthening and restorative, may be made into a pleasant drink, for the feeble, by breaking a freshly laid egg into a bowl, and beating it well, with 1 or 2 table-spoonfuls of sugar, then adding a little ice-cold water, and a tea to a table-spoonful of spirits, or wine, as prepared, or at hand.

**43. Drink for Great Thirst of Fever Patients.**—Cream of tartar, ½ oz.; white sugar, 4 ozs.; confection of orange peel, 3 ozs.; boiling hot water 3 pts.

[*Confection of Orange Peel.*—Take the external rind of nice fresh oranges, separated by rasping (grating), 1 lb.; white pulverized sugar, 3 lbs. (or in these proportions). Directions.—Beat the rind in a stone. or wedge-wood mortar, then add the pulverized sugar, and continue the beating till perfectly incorporated together. Keep in cans.]

Directions.—Pour the hot water upon the other ingredients; when all are dissolved, set aside to cool. When cold drink as freely as the thirst of the patient demands. (See fevers, preventative and cure.—Dr. Buchanan.)

*Remarks.*—This confection is tonic, and stomachic, and is principally used as a vehicle for the exhibition of tonic powders, drinks, etc.—*Cooley's Cyclopedia.*

**44. Pectoral Drink.**—Common barley and stoned raisins of each 2 ozs.; licorice root, bruised, ½ oz.; water, 2 qts. Directions.—First boil the barley, then add the raisins and continue the boiling until the water is one-half evaporated, and add the licorice. When, cool strain.

*Remarks.*—Dr. Buchanan, an old English physician, made it the usual drink in all pectoral (chest) difficulties, to be drank freely.

**45. Herb Teas, for the Sick Room.**—Dried sage leaves, or any of the mints, or balm leaves, ¼ oz.; boiling water, ½ pt.; steep and strain, or pour off, when cool enough to drink. A little sugar may be used with any of them when desired.

**46. Sage Tea,** Made as above, with ½ tea spoonful of pulverized alum dissolved in it and sweetened with honey, is especially valuable as a gargle for sore throat.

**47. Mint Teas,** From the dried or green leaves crushed, with a little sugar, are agreeable to the taste, and soothing to a nauseous stomach, and to an irritated condition of the bowels of children.

**48. Catnip Tea,** However, is considered, by old nurses, as the greatest panacea for infant ills, known among them.

**49. Pennyroyal Tea,** Is equally well known as the best 'thing to break up colds, and to restore a checked perspiration from exposures, damp feet, etc.

**50. Gentian Root** and chamomile flower teas are both valuable tonics, and may be taken hot or cold, as preferred, and with or without sugar, but as both are quite bitter, sugar will make them more palatable.

**51. Strawberry Leaf Tea,** From the green leaves, is considered valuable in canker of the mouth of infants, and with the alum, as in the sage, for adults, as a wash or gargle.

**52. Blackberry Tea,** Made from the roots are considered valuable in bowel difficulties; and that from the raspberry are believed to be equally valuable; and a syrup from these fruits are valuable in bowel complaints, and also make agreeable drinks in fevers and inflammatory diseases.

**53. Mint Tea, Juleped.**—It would be hardly right to close the subject of herb teas without giving an idea that something besides teas can be made from the mints. Take, then, a few sprigs of green mint (if any urinary difficulty, or in case of fever let it be spearmint, as that is more diuretic and febrifuge than peppermint, while the peppermint is the most carminative and antispasmodic), and bruise them in a glass with a spoon—mashing considerably—adding sugar freely, and cold water to half fill the glass, with a table-spoonful or two of wine, or brandy, and pounded ice to fill, shaking, or stirring well, and if quaffed quickly you will think there has been a hail storm in the neighborhood, of an agreeable character—a little of which is not bad to take by sick or well people.

## PUDDINGS, TOAST, PAP, JELLIES, STEAKS, CHOPS, ETC., FOR THE SICK.

**54. Rice Pudding—Baked.**—Rice ½ lb.; water, 1 pt.; milk, 1 qt.; sugar 1 cup; 3 eggs; salt, 1 tea-spoonful; lemons, nutmegs or vanilla to flavor. DIRECTIONS—Wash the rice and boil in the water 30 minutes; then add the milk and boil 30 minutes longer; beat the eggs, sugar and salt together, and stir into the rice. Bake in a nicely buttered dish for half an hour. To be eaten with a very little nice butter, or sauce, if preferred.

*Remarks.*—Although a little of this is very appropriate for the sick, yet, I think, most families will be willing to help them dispose of the surplus, if it comes from the oven just at dinner-time

**55. Tapioca, Cream Pudding.**—Tapioca, 3 table-spoonfuls; water and milk, 1 qt.; 3 eggs; a little salt; lemon or vanilla to flavor. DIRECTIONS— Cover the tapioca with water and let soak 4 hours; pour off what water is left. Put the milk over the fire, and as soon as it boils stir in the beaten yolks of the eggs and the salt, then the tapioca, and stir till it begins to thicken. Make a frosting of the whites and brown a moment only, having added the flavoring. This is very palatable and very nourishing.

**56. Graham Pudding—Steamed.**—Boiling water, 1 pt.; graham flour, salt; hot milk, 1 pt.; 1 egg. DIRECTIONS—Stir into the boiling water sufficient graham flour to make a stiff paste; adding the egg, beaten, and a little salt; then stir into the hot milk and steam ¾ of an hour—the steam being up when the dish is set in the steamer. Serve with maple syrup, or nice cream and sugar, or any other sauce preferred.

**57. Egg Toast.**—A fresh egg, nice bread, not less than one day old, salt and hot water. DIRECTIONS—Toast the bread only to a light brown; break the egg into hot water on the stove, and cook only to "set" the white; put a little salt into sufficient hot water, dip the toasted bread, quickly, into it, and place it on a hot plate, and put on the egg, adding a sprinkle of salt only.

*Remarks.*—It is presumed that if this is done nicely, according to directions, and the patient is able to digest this kind of food, it will be found enjoyable. At another time a soft toast, with water or sometimes with milk, of course, hot, in either case will give the needed varieties, to meet different tastes and circumstances.

**58. Pap, of Boiled Flour—For Diarrhea of Children.**— Tie 1 cup of flour closely in a cloth, and boil 5 hours; when cool grate off a table-spoonful of it, and mix smoothly in a little cold milk; then stir this mixture into 1 pt. of boiling milk, and boil a few minutes, and sweeten with loaf sugar, and add a little nutmeg, if desired. Very valuable in diarrhea of children or adults.

**59. Wine Jelly.**—In places where none of the common fruit jellies are obtainable, the following will make an excellent substitute: Boil white sugar, ½ lb. in 1 gill of water. Have dissolved isinglass, 1 oz., in a little water, and strain into the syrup; and when nearly cold add ½ pt. of wine; mix well in a bowl or suitable dish; cover. For convalescents or those getting up from exhausting diseases, this will be found as nutritious as it is palatable. If too thick at any time, add a little milk or water, as preferred, or convenient.

**60. Arrowroot.**—Mix 2 table-spoonfuls of arrowroot to a smooth paste with a little cold water; then add to it 1 pt. of boiling water, a little lemon peel, and stir while boiling. Let it cook till quite clear. Sweeten with sugar, and flavor with wine or nutmeg, if desired. Milk may be used instead of the water, if preferred.

**61. Beefsteak—Broiled.**—Have a small piece of rather thick surloin-steak; a perfectly clear, coal fire should be ready, to avoid the possibility of the taste of smoke, and the gridiron must be perfectly clean; 3 or 4 minutes to each side, if the patient likes it at all rare, will be sufficient, being very careful to avoid burning. Season with a little salt and very little pepper. Place on a hot plate and serve immediately.

**62. Mutton or Lamb Chops.**—These must be trimmed free of fat, and broiled the same as beefsteak, except that they must be a little better done, and hence should be cut a little thinner to allow cooking through. Season and serve the same. But if any patient, at any time, desires any modification in cooking or seasoning, let it be done to suit him, unless known to be injurious.

**63. How to Reduce the Temperature of Sick-rooms and to Keep them Cool.**—In very warm weather it is often desirable, for the comfort of the patient to have the room considerable cooler than the natural atmosphere. In such cases raise the lower sashes entirely upon the side of the room from which the breeze comes; then have a piece of muslin soaking wet, squeeze slightly, and tack it on so as to make all the air come in through the wet muslin, which will reduce the temperature of the room 5 or 6 degrees in a few minutes. This is done by the absorption of a part of the heat in the atmosphere by the passing of the water in the muslin from its liquid to a gaseous state (a principle well known in philosophy), and the air of the room becomes more moist also, which makes it more endurable.

*Remarks.*—It only needs trying to satisfy the most incredulous, and it will benefit the very feeble patient more than enough to pay everyone for the trouble taken. As the cloths become dry, replace them with others; or keep them well wet with a sponge.

**64. Ventilation of Sick-rooms and Sleeping-rooms—Avoiding the Draft over the Patient.**—Have a piece of board made just as long as the width of the window; then raise the lower sash, and place the board under it. The width of the board may be 3 or 4 inches only, as this will allow a current of air to pass up between the glass and sash, breaking the draft that otherwise enters directly into the room when the sash is raised. In this way air may be admitted even at the head or back side of a sick-bed, for the curtain may be lowered to break the current from passing directly upon the patient. This plan is equally important in small and ill-ventilated sleeping-rooms. This much fresh air, at least, should be admitted into every sleeping-room, excepting the extremely cold and windy days of winter.

# PART II.

---

# GENERAL DEPARTMENT.

For anything in this department, or outside of the Medical Department, see GENERAL INDEX, page 844. For anything in the Medical Department, see MEDICAL INDEX, page 833.

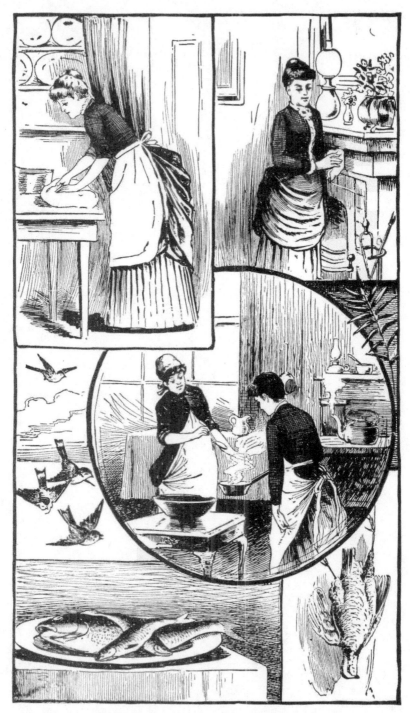

THE KEY TO A HAPPY HOME.

# CULINARY RECIPES.

## BREAD, PUDDINGS, PIES, CAKES, SOUPS, MEATS, AND VARIOUS DISHES.

## BREAD.

*Remarks.* — If the simple word "bread" only, is spoken, it is always understood to mean white, or bread made from wheat flour. Other kinds always have a descriptive attachment, as Graham, Indian, brown, Boston brown, corn, etc. Two things are especially essential in good bread—lightness and sweetness. If bread is heavy—not light and porous—or if it is sour, it is only fit for the pigs. And it is important to know that good bread cannot be made out of poor flour. In the following these points are nicely explained, together with full and complete instructions in the three necessary processes of making good bread—making sponge, kneading, and baking.

**How to Make Good Bread.**—A loaf of perfect bread, white, light, sweet, tender, and elastic, with a golden brown crust, is a proof of high civilization, and is so indispensable a basis of all good eating that the name "lady," or "loaf-giver," applied to the Saxon (English, as now understood, for England was overrun and conquered by the people of Saxony, in northern Germany, in an early day, so that now, to say a "Saxon," or of the Saxon race, refers to the English, descended from them, more often than to the people of Saxony itself —and especially Anglo-Saxon always means English) matron, may well be held in honor by wife or maiden. But do all the gracious ladies who preside in our country homes see such loaves set forth as daily bread?

Inexperienced housekeepers and amateur cooks will find it a good general rule to attempt at the beginning only a few things, and learn to do those perfectly. And these should be, not the elaborate dishes of special occasions, but the plain every-day things. Where can one better begin than with bread? The eager patronage of the over-crowded, carlessly served, high-priced Vienna bakery at the Centennial gave evidence that Americans appreciate good bread and good cofiee, and had, perhaps, some effect in stimulating an effort for a better home supply. To make and to be able to teach others to make bread of this high character is an accomplishment worth at least as much practice as a *sonata* (a piece of music); and the work is excellent as a gymnastic exercise. With good digestion, honest personal pride, and the grateful admiration of the family circle as rewards, surely no girl or woman who aspires to responsibilities and joys of home, will shrink from the labor of learning to make bread.

The whole art and science of bread-making is no mean study. The *why,* as well as the *how*, should be aimed at, although exact knowledge or science, even in bread-making, is not so simple a matter as some might fancy. Varying conditions, even the temperature of the kitchen, work confusion in the phenomena of a batch of bread as surely as in the delicate experiments of a Tyndall or a Huxley. Fortunately, an exhaustive knowledge is not essential to practical success. Skillful manipulation will come with experience, and I have taught the actual art to a succession of uneducated cooks so that, with a little supervision, they satisfactorily supplied an exacting family. But the mistress, the house-mother, who must give intelligent direction, will not be satisfied without going to the root of the matter. Let her not rest upon her laurels without making sure that her table is constantly supplied with such delicious loaves of "the staff of life" as, with the fragrant, highly-flavored butter of May or June, shall make a fit repast even for the good women whose hand have prepared them.

**Good Flour Essential.**—The first requisite to good bread is good flour (and *sifted*, to enliven it and make it mix more readily). If the very best seems too expensive, make up the difference in cost by eating less cake. With really delicious bread you will do this naturally, and almost unconsciously.

**The Yeast, to Make.**—In the country, where fresh yeast from breweries is out of the question, the first process must be making yeast; and it is well to begin there, and know every step of your way. The commercial yeast cakes must form a basis; from them it is easy to make the potato yeast, which is perhaps the simplest and best of several good forms of soft yeast. Dry yeast cake used directly will not make bread of the first quality. For the yeast, soak *three yeast cakes* in a cup of tepid water, while *six* or *eight* fair-sized potatoes are boiling. When they are perfectly soft, put the potatoes, with a quart of water in which they were boiled, through a colander, and add a teaspoonful of salt and two of sugar. When tepid, add the yeast cakes, rubbed with a spoon to a smooth paste, and place the whole in a stone jar, and keep the contents at blood heat for twelve hours, when a lively effervescence should have taken place. The yeast will be in perfect condition the next day, and will remain good for ten days or more if kept in a cool celler in a closely covered jar.

**Setting the Sponge.**—Many New England housekeepers make a great mistake in setting their sponge over night. One secret of good bread is that every stage of the process must be complete and rapid. Every moment of waiting means deterioration. At the precise moment *when the sponge is fully light* the bread should be kneaded, and the process of rising ought not to require more than *three hours* at most. Set your sponge, then, as early in the morning as you like, by taking in the bowl or basin kept for the purpose (and you will soon learn just how high in it the sponge should rise) two quarts of *sifted* flour. Make a hole in the middle with the stirring spoon; pour in half a pint of the soft yeast, first thoroughly stirring it from the bottom, then mixing with the flour; add tepid water, stirring constantly, until a smooth, stiff batter is formed, which stir and beat vigorously with the spoon for at least five minutes after it is perfectly mixed. Cover lightly, and set in a warm place until thoroughly light, almost foaming; but be sure not to delay kneading until it begins to sub-side.

**Kneading.**—Sift the flour, say 6 qts., in a pan, make a hole in the mid-dle, pour in the sponge; add a pinch of salt, and, dexterously mingling the flour with the soft sponge by the hand, gradually add a quart of warm milk or warm water, quickly incorporating the whole into a smooth, even mass. Cover the kneading-board with flour, place upon it the dough, which must not be soft enough to stick or stiff enough to make much resistance to pressure, and knead vigorously and long. Half an hour's energetic kneading is not too much for a family baking. By that time the bread should be elastic, free from stickiness, and disposed to rise in blisters. Cover with a soft bread-cloth folded to four thicknesses, and set it where a temperature of about blood-heat will be main-tained.

In two hours it should have risen to fully twice its volume. Place it again upon the board; divide with the hands (which may be floured, or, better, but-tered) a portion of the size which you wish for your loaves, remembering that it will rise again half as much more; lightly mold it into a smooth, shapely loaf, with as little handling as possible, and place in a well-greased pan. Set the loaves back in their warm corner for half an hour, when they should be very light and show signs of cracking. Bake at once in a hot oven, with a steady heat, from 45 minutes to 1 hour, according to the size of the loaves. Take immediately from the pans and wrap in soft, fresh linen until cold.

**Biscuit From Some of the Dough.**—A portion of the dough will make a pan of delicious biscuits by adding a piece of butter as large as an egg to sufficient dough for a small loaf, mixing it lightly but thoroughly, and molding into small round balls, set a little distance apart in the pan. They will soon close up the space, and should rise to twice their first height. The swift, sure touch which makes the work easy, rapid, and confident, will come with practice; but the necessary practice may come only with patience and determi-nation.

**To Make Bread Crust Soft and Delicate.**—Take a cup of cream off the pan, and put it into your bread when you are about molding it, and it will cause the crust to be very soft and delicate.

*Remarks.*—Knowing this to contain good sound sense, from the fact that I know the Vienna bread has a softer and more delicate crust than common bread, I mention it, believing that one reason, at least, for this is that the Vienna bread is made richer with milk than the common, as you will notice, by com-parison. Bread should not be made too thin and soft, in kneading, nor too stiff and hard; but of such a consistence that when you press the doubled hand upon the mass of dough the depression will quickly rise up again to nearly its former shape. Let beginners be a little careful in all the foregoing points of instruction, and the author has no fears in guaranteeing a bread that they, even, shall not be ashamed of. If bread, or rather the sponge, becomes sour from being set over night (although it is conceded not to be best to set it over night), or from neglect to knead it at the right time (when just fully light), dissolve a teaspoonful of soda (baking soda is always meant) in a little warm milk or water and work it in, which will correct it. If there is danger at any time, in baking, of burning, or over baking, cover the bread with thick brown paper, or a folded newapaper, until the loaf is done through; and if too hot at the bottom to endanger burning, put the oven grate, or a few nails or bits of iron, under the pan, which will prevent it from burning by the admission of air under it. By observing these points you are always safe.

**Bread, Cakes and Pies, to Stand in the Cook Room, After Baking, Till Cool.**—Bread and cakes, as soon as baked, should be taken out of the pans, wrapped in suitable cloth and stand till cool in the cook room; pies the same, or simply covered, if too juicy to take out of the pans; for, if put too soon into a cold closet, they are liable to fall, by chilling. After they are cool, put in jars or boxes and keep from the air as much as possible.

**Vienna Bread, or Yeast.**—Since the Centennial there has been much said about the Vienna, or yeast bread—called yeast bread from the fact that it is made with the compressed brewers yeast, known by various names, such as "German Pressed Yeast," "Patent Yeast," etc , in place of ordinary yeast, differing from common bread principally in use of a larger proportion of yeast, to the flour used, and also in its being made in smaller loaves. Below you will find, under the head of "The Best Yeast Known," the way the Vienna, or pressed, yeast is made. The following is the process, or way the bread is made at Vienna, and by the bakers who make it in this country, since the Centennial at Philadelphia, where, so far as I know, it was first introduced in the United States. And as I find a very plain description of how to make it given, at the time, in *Peterson's Ladies National Magazine*, I will give it in their words. It says:

"Sift in a tin pan 4 lbs. of flour; bank it up against the sides, pour in 1 qt. of milk and water (half-and-half), and mix into it enough of the flour to form a thin batter; then quickly and lightly add 1 pt. of milk, in which is dissolved 1 oz. of salt, and $1\frac{3}{4}$ ozs. of compressed yeast. Leave the remainder of the flour against the sides of the pan; cover the pan with a cloth, and set it in a place free from draught, for three-quarters of an hour; then mix in the rest of the flour, until the dough will leave the bottom and sides of the pan, and let it stand two hours and a-half. Finally, divide the mass into 1 lb. pieces, to be cut in turn into 12 parts each. (This, you will see, is for biscuit; for bread this last division is not to be made, and more recently, it is made into rather long, narrow loaves.) This gives square pieces about $3\frac{1}{2}$ inches, each corner of which is taken up and folded over to the centre, and then the cakes are turned over on a dough-board to rise for half an hour, when they are put into a hot oven, that bakes them in 10 minutes, or till done."

**For a Breakfast Loaf.**—"Take 1 lb. of the above dough, 2 ozs. of butter, 2 ozs. powdered sugar, 2 eggs; beat all well together, in a basin, in the same manner as eggs are beaten, only using the hand instead of the whisk; set in a plain mould to rise for three-quarters of an hour, then bake in a quick oven. When cut, it should have the appearance of honeycomb. This is a very nice breakfast-cake, and will make delicious toast when stale."

*Remarks.*—I see that some of the ladies who have been trying the Vienna bread recommend putting a tablespoonful, or two, of sugar into the sponge, when they begin to knead it. The author does not think it amiss in any kind of bread.

**Vienna Yeast, or the Best Yeast Known.**—A writer. in describing how the compressed, or Vienna, yeast is made, first says: "Vienna bread is the best in the world. It owes its superiority to the yeast used, which is prepared in the following manner: Indian corn, barley and rye (all sprouting) are powdered and mixed, and then macerated in water at a temperature of from 149 to 167° Fah. Saccharification (production of sugar) takes place in a few hours, when the liquor is racked off and allowed to clear, the fermentation is set up by the help of a minute quantity of any ordinary yeast. Carbonic acid is disengaged during the process with so much rapidity that the globules of yeast are thrown up by the gas and remain floating on the surface, where they form a thick scum. The latter is carefully removed and constitutes the best and purest yeast, which, when drained and compressed, can be kept from 8 to 15 days, according to the season."

*Remarks.*—Although but very few people may engage in the manufacture of compressed yeast, yet it is a satisfaction to almost every one to know how it is done.

**Potato Bread.**—Boil 6 or 8 good sized potatoes, mash fine while hot, then add 1 qt. sweet milk, ½ cup of white sugar, a good pinch of salt, ⅓ of a cup of good yeast; have ready a pan of sifted flour, make a hole in the middle, stir in the ingredients; do this about 6 o'clock, and if it gets light before you retire at night, stir it down, sprinkle flour over the top and let it stand until morning, then mix it down again, and when light the third time, knead into loaves. Try this, and if your yeast is good you will never have poor bread.—*Mrs. S. T. Dolph, McBride, Mich.*

*Remarks.*—It will not be amiss to say here, that new potatoes are of no value in bread making. Only those that are fully ripe can be used.

**About Setting Sponge Over Night.**—It will be observed that the above recipe for potato bread, as well as most of the following ones, contrary to the instructions of the first recipe, directs to set the sponge over night; but those who may use them, must act upon their own judgment as to doing so, or in beginning in the morning, depending upon its being cold winter weather, warmth of the room, etc.; and also depending upon whether they can give it their watchful care during the day, or until the sponge is risen and the whole process completed and the bread baked, thus avoiding all possibility of souring, as it often does if set over night; for, although to a certain extent, by the use of soda, this condition is corrected, yet, after once souring, the bread will never be as good as if kneaded and baked at just the right time, *i. e.*, as soon as light in each process, not having stood to overwork in either case.

**Hop Yeast Potato Bread.**—Another lady writer says: "I would like some of the ladies to try my way of making hop yeast bread. Set a sponge at night and be sure to put in a dozen good-sized potatoes. In the morning put half a tea-spoonful of grated alum in half a tea-cupful of water and add to the sponge. Mix quite hard in the pan and let stand till light; then mix down in the pan once more before putting in the tins. It makes the puffiest bread you ever saw."

*Remarks.*—Much has been said against the use of alum in making bread but in the quantity here given for a batch of 3 or 4 loaves, the author would have no fears of using. It gives an additional lightness to bread, and that is the only object of its use. Potatoes also help in this respect, while they also, as well as milk, make bread more rich and nourishing, and which also keeps moist longer than without them. It is well to use both if you have them.

**Rice Bread.**—Rice prepared as follows, makes another variety of bread, which will please many tastes at the seaport table: Take 1 pt. of well-cooked rice, ½ pt. of flour, the yolks of 4 eggs, 2 spoonfuls of butter, melted; 1 pt. of milk, ½ teaspoonful of salt. DIRECTIONS—Beat these altogether; then having beaten the whites of the eggs to a stiff froth, beat them in also. Bake in shallow pans, or gem tins.

**Naples Bread or Biscuit.**—Flour, 1 lb. (3½ cups); nice fresh butter, 1 oz. (1 rounding table-spoonful), worked into the flour, with 1 egg, a little salt, good yeast, 2 table-spoonfuls, and 1 pt. of milk. Mix all well and let it rise one hour; then do not work it down, but cut it in suitable sized pieces and form into biscuit and bake in a quick oven. If baked in a loaf, you have Naples bread.

**Currant Sweet Loaf.**—Mix 2 heaping tea-spoonfuls of cream of tartar with 1 pound of flour; then rub into it 4 ozs. of butter, as for pastry; add 8 ozs. of currants, 6 ozs. of sugar, and 1 pt. of milk, in which 1 heaping tea-spoonful of soda has been dissolved; add a little salt; spice to taste, and bake. The addition of 2 beaten eggs and 4 ozs. of citron makes a rich loaf.

*Remarks.*—This baked in biscuits, or rolled out and cut in strips 1 or 1½ x 4 inches, makes a nice tea or breakfast cake.

**Graham Bread, Western Rural's.**—When the author can find arguments in favor of any point, whether it be the making or use of Graham bread, or upon any other subject of value to the public, and perhaps written better than he could do it, he considers that by quoting them, giving the proper credit, which he always does, if the originator is known, the public, as well as himself, are materially benefitted; and in this case, especially, the well-known popularity of the *Western Rural* will undoubtedly influence many persons to use more Graham bread than they otherwise might do, whereby their health will be greatly improved, and certainly no one harmed; and it is by this course that the author in his two former books, as well as in this the third and last which he will ever write, has done and still is enabled to do a greater good than he otherwise could. I fully agree with the principles and suggestions, and the way of making, and hope that every family into whose hands this book shall come, will adopt them and keep their tables supplied with this delicious and health-giving bread. The editor says:

" We are seldom without Graham bread on the table, and have noticed that our friends and visitors almost invariably prefer the brown bread to the white. We have often wondered why more people do not use it, especially when we take into consideration the fact that it is less trouble to make, being much more wholesome, and yielding a greater amount of nourishment. Some people who are habitually constipated, only need unbolted wheat in some form once a day, with plenty of fruit, to entirely obviate this difficulty. You want good, finely ground Graham flour, and good yeast to begin with. Take your mixing bowl, put into it two table-spoonfuls of any kind of molasses or brown sugar, a table-spoonful of salt, a little over a pint of warm water, and yeast in the same proportion that you would for white bread. We use the compressed yeast, and use a little less than 2 cents' worth to make 2 pie-pan loaves. Stir in Graham flour to make a sponge and beat it a few minutes hard, then add a pint of white flour, adding Graham to make it stiff enough to mould, taking care not to get it too stiff. Better have to add a little flour in molding. Let it stand only long enough to get quite light. Mold and put into pans, and when it is light, bake in a moderate oven. Graham requires a few moments longer to bake than white. All bread should be kept at a rather low but even temperature while rising, away from drafts, as a higher temperature produces what is known among chemists as false yeast, which is an advanced stage of fermentation or decomposition, and is unwholesome."

*Remarks.*—This last point, as to the temperature being too high, causes the bread, or sponge, to become sour by over working, and would call for soda to correct it whenever this occurs. I will give another wherein the sponge is set with white flour, and also a small amount more added in the morning, which some prefer to an all Graham. There is a caution, too, near its close, against a too hot oven at the beginning, by which the crust is set so soon, the center of of the loaf must necessarily be soggy, as it had not time to rise—because tight—before it was bound down by the setting of the crust from the over-heat. But if you ever find that your oven is too hot, see plan of covering the bread with paper, as directed with the white bread at first given. I am unable to give the proper credit for the origination of the following, but I know it will make a nice bread if carefully done.

**Graham Bread.**—For 4 loaves of bread take 1½ cups of good fresh yeast. Sift white flour and mix to rather a stiff sponge with moderately warm water, beat well; add the yeast and beat again; set in a warm place over night. In the morning, when light, add salt, a heaping pint of sifted white flour, and then stiffen with graham, this being the first graham which is put into the bread, Allow it to rise again, and when light, mold into loaves, working as little as possible. When these have raised sufficiently, bake well in a moderately heated oven, If the stove be too hot when the bread is first put in, the crust forms too quickly and the inside of the loaf is apt to be moist and soggy,

**Graham Bread, One Loaf.**—Wheat flour, 1 cup; Graham flour, 2 cups; warm water, 1 cup; soda, 1½ tea-spoonfuls, dissolved in water; yeast, ½ cup; molasses, ⅓ cup; salt, 1 tea-spoonful. Stir with a spoon, let it rise once, and bake very slowly about 1 hour, or a little longer, as needed.

**Graham Bread with Soda, Started after Breakfast for Dinner, Baked or Steamed.**—Graham bread that can be started after breakfast and baked before dinner, is made of 1½ pts. of sour milk; 2 scant tea-spoonfuls of soda, dissolved in a little hot water; ½ cup of New Orleans molasses; 1 tea-spoonful of salt; and as much Graham flour as can be stirred in with a spoon. Grease a large bread tin very evenly, as the molasses in the bread renders it liable to stick, put into the oven and bake 2 hours. Have the oven hot when the bread is put in, and toward the last half of the last hour let it cool gradually. Or, this bread may be steamed 1¾ hours, and be dried off in the oven 20 minutes. When it is taken from the oven, wrap a towel around the loaf, the tin and all, and in 10 minutes remove from the tin, and keep the loaf wrapped in the cloth until it is sent to the table.

*Remarks.*—I am sorry I can not give credit for the originator of this plan, but it is too good to lose on that account, especially as it will help some person who may find in the morning that they have not bread enough for dinner.

**Rye Bread.**—Set in the evening, with good hops or other good yeast, and mold it in the morning, just the same as wheat bread, only a little stiffer. Let it rise and mold it down again. This makes it spongy. After this it will come up very quick. Shape it into loaves, and, when light enough, bake it in a moderate oven a little longer than ordinary wheat bread.

**Rye and Indian Bread.**—Take Indian meal, 2 cups, make in a thick batter with scalding water; when cool add a small cup of white bread sponge, a little sugar and salt, and a tea-spoonful of soda, dissolved. In this stir as much rye flour as is possible with a spoon; let it rise until it is very light; then work in with your hand as much more rye as you can, but do not knead it, as that will make it hard; put it in buttered bread tins, and let it rise for about 15 minutes; then bake it for 1½ hours, cooling the oven gradually for the last 20 minutes.

**Wheat and Indian Bread, Steamed.**—Molasses, 1 cup; sour milk, 2 cups; soda, 2 tea-spoonfuls; flour and Indian meal, of each 1 pt. DIRECTIONS —Beat well together, put into a buttered pan and steam 2 hours.—*Mrs. Carrie Case.*

*Remarks.*—Perfectly reliable, for I have eaten it of her own make, and I shall never forget the "jolly time" we had while eating it the first time.

**Brown, or Rye and Indian Bread, Steamed.**—Indian meal, 1 qt.; rye flour, 1 pt.; stir these together and add sweet milk, 1 qt.; molasses, 1 cup; soda, 2 tea-spoonfuls; a little salt, and steam 4 hours.

**Brown, or Wheat and Indian, Baked.**—Indian meal, 2 cups; stir into it ½ cup of cold water; stir well, and add 1 qt. of boiling water, allowing it to cool; then add 1 cup of molasses and a small soaked yeast cake; then stir in sifted flour to make it as thick as possible with the spoon and let rise over night; knead lightly in the morning, and bake slowly.

**Brown Bread, Rye and Indian, New England Style; or Steamed and Baked.**—Rye flour, 4 cups; Indian meal (the yellow is generally used in making any of the brown breads), 3 cups; molasses, 1 small cup; cream tartar, ½ tea-spoonful; a little salt; mix very soft with sour milk or buttermilk; steam four hours, and then bake two.

**Boston Brown, Baked.**—Take 4 cupfuls of Indian meal and 4 cupfuls of rye meal (not flour); sift through a coarse wire sieve; add 2 tea-spoonfuls of soda, a little salt, 1 cupful of molasses; 1 cupful of sour milk, and water sufficient to make a soft dough. Bake 4 hours in a moderately heated oven, or what would be better, 2 hours in a brick oven.

**Brown, or Minnesota Corn Bread, Steamed and Baked.**—Corn meal and flour, each 2 cupfuls; sweet and sour milk, each 1 cupful; molasses, ½ cupful; salt and saleratus, or soda, each 1 tea-spoonful. Put into round tin cans, and steam 1 hour and bake ½ an hour.

**Brown, or Indian Bread, Baked for Tea.**—Sour milk, 1 pt.; sweet milk, ½ pt.; molasses, 1 cupful; butter, ½ cupful; eggs, 3; saleratus, 2 tea-spoonfuls, or its equivalent in soda; salt, 1 large tea-spoonful; Indian-meal, 1 qt.; flour, 1 pt. Mix all according to general rules, and bake in a deep basin, with oven same heat as for cake, for 1½ hours, or thereabouts.

**Indian Bread, Baked.**—Take 2 qts. Indian meal, add 1 large spoonful of butter, 1 of sugar, a little salt; mix together; pour upon the whole 1 qt. of boiling water; then cool with cold water sufficiently to add ½ cupful of good yeast. Let it rise for 2 hours, then add wheat flour (if the dough is not thick enough) so as to give it the consistency of "pound cake." Put it into deep dishes, let it rise for 1 hour. Bake in a stove oven. You will find it delicious. —*Mrs. L. B. Arnold, Ithaca, N. Y.*

**Indian Bread, Extra, Steamed.**—Buttermilk, sweet milk and Indian meal, each 3 cups; flour, 2 cups; soda, 2 tea-spoonfuls; salt, 1 tea-spoonful. Mix, put into a greased or buttered pan (as all should be), and steam 3 hours.

**Old-Fashioned Indian, or Corn Bread.**—This is from Mrs. S. N. Ross, Sparta, O., in Toledo *Blade:* "The recipe which I have is the nearest to the old Dutch-oven corn bread of anything that can now be baked: Two pt. cups of Indian meal, 1 pt. cup of flour, 2 pt. cups of sweet milk, 1 pt. cup of sour milk, ½ pt. cup of sugar, 1 tea-spoonful of salt, 1 tea-spoonful of soda. Mix, and bake slowly 1½ hours."

**Corn Bread, Southern, Far-Famed.** — The following recipes, obtained through the *Blade*, give you the different plans of making the celebrated "Southern Corn Breads" and "Southern Corn Dodgers," and will be found very satisfactory, as well as a very healthful form of bread. The first is from the "Old Lady" who always knows how to do things in the "Household" line, while the second claims to be an improvement upon that, and the third, the latest style of corn dodger, *i. e.*, baked on tins or in a pan, while the old style or plan was to wrap them in corn husks, or paper, wet, and then bake them in the embers or upon the hot hearth. The "Old Lady" says:

"Take 2 eggs, beat them well; add 1 pt. of water, and stir well; put in 1 tea-spoonful of salt, same of yeast powders, and add meal enough to make a batter that will pour out of the pan. Put a table-spoonful of lard into the baking pan, set it in the oven and let it get hot; pour the batter in it and bake a nice brown. I assure you you will never make any other kind after eating this."—*Old Lady, Mobile, Ala.*

**Corn Bread, Southern, Improved.**—This writer says: "In the *Blade* I saw a recipe for the 'far-famed Southern Corn Bread.' I was raised in the South, and have a few times eaten bread made in that way; but it is not the way we make our bread—and as I think there is an 'excellence' about *ours*, I send you the recipe. Take 1 egg, a tea-spoonful of salt and 1 of soda (if the milk is very sour it will take more soda), and 1½ pts. butter-milk; then put in white corn meal enough to make a nice tolerably thick batter. It is very nice baked in a bread pan, but we like it best baked in gem irons, or muffin irons, as some people call them. Whatever it is baked in must be well greased and smoking hot when the batter is put in. Serve while hot. Corn bread never was intended to be eaten cold."—*Hawthorne, La Place, Ill.*

*Remarks.*—It will be noticed that "Hawthorne" calls for white corn meal. The Southern people raise the white corn only, or, at least, almost wholly so; and some people, even in the North, think it makes the best bread. It would be well, then, to give it a thorough trial in the North, and if it proves more valuable than the yellow, let it be raised especially for cooking purposes. I would say in regard to the idea that "corn bread was never intended to be eaten cold," I think it to be an error. I like it best warm, still I have eaten it many hundred times cold, and enjoyed it very much, although I believe it to be healthful while warm, and I know it is rather more palatable and pleasant warm; still, if there is any left over, I should by no means throw it away, but warm it up by steaming, else eat it cold, as preferred, or most convenient.

**White Corn Dodgers.**—Take 1 pt. of Southern corn meal (white corn meal), and turn over it 1 pt. of boiling water, add a little salt and 1 egg well beaten up and stirred into the batter when nearly cold. Butter some sheets of tin and drop your cakes by the table-spoonful all over the pan. Bake for 25 minutes in a hot oven.

*Remarks.*—Do not think for a moment, that because you may not have white corn meal, therefore, you can not make corn bread or corn dodgers, for you can; although the yellow meal may not be quite as nice, yet it does make excellent bread, as well as griddle cakes, too, by using a very little white or graham flour with it.

**Salt-Rising Bread, How to Make.**—Knowing my propensities for gathering valuable recipes, a gentleman friend said to me one day: "Doctor, the finest bread I ever ate in my life was at Mrs. J. A. Marks' in Detroit. I wish I had asked her for the recipe, especially for you." As my friend seemed so enthusiastic over the elegant bread eaten at the table of Mrs. Marks I took her name and address and wrote her, asking for the recipe. Here it is in her own words: "Early in the evening I scald 2 table-spoonfuls of corn-meal, a pinch of salt and 1 of sugar, with milk enough to make a mush; then set in a warm place till morning; then scald a tea-spoonful of sugar, 1 of salt and ⅓ as much soda with a pint of boiling water; then add cold water till lukewarm, and thicken to a thick batter with flour, then add the mush made the night before and stir briskly for a minute or two. Put in a close vessel in a kettle of warm water, not too hot. When light, mix stiff, add a little shortening, and mold into loaves  It will soon rise and will not require as long to bake as yeast bread—25 to 30 minutes in a good oven.  Great care is required to keep the sponge of a uniform heat (the water should be about as warm as the hand will bear)  The finest patent process flour is not as good as a little coarser grade— I prefer Knickerbocker—for this kind of bread.  All dishes used in making should be perfectly clean and sweet, scalding them out with saleratus or lime-water."

*Remarks.*—My wife has made many loaves after this recipe, and, like my friend, I must say " it is the finest bread I ever ate."

**Salt-Rising Bread No. 2.**—A Mrs. Bruce, although she does not give her whereabouts, tells " Aunt Nancy," who inquired through the *Blade,* how to make salt-rising bread as follows, which will speak for itself, and as many people prefer this kind, I give it a place: " Set your rising in a pitcher, a sugar bowl, or a new tin dipper.  Either must be sweet.  Have ready a crock or pot with warm water enough to come even with the rising and just hot enough not to burn the finger.  Put a plate in the bottom of the crock, so the rising does not scald.  Set on the back of the stove or anywhere to keep an even heat.  I set my rising about 5 o'clock in the morning, and about 10 o'clock I add 1 table-spoonful of flour and stir.  If successful, your rising will be ready to make into loaves about 2 o'clock in the afternoon.  To set rising, take 1 table-spoonful of sifted corn meal, scald it by pouring over it 1 pt. of boiling water and stir quickly.  To this add cold water until just hot enough not to scald.  Then add a large tea-spoonful of coarse salt, a pinch of soda, a pinch of sugar, and flour enough to make a stiff batter.  When risen, sift 4 or 5 qts. flour into the bread bowl.  Make a hole in the center and put in a table-spoonful of sweet lard or butter.  Pour over this 3 pts. of warm water.  Then add your rising.  Mix and work in loaves; grease on top.  This makes 3 large loaves.  When risen to top of pan, bake.  Bake in long, deep tin pans, and from a ½ to ¾ of an hour. When done, let remain in the oven about 10 minutes to soak.  Do not wrap it up, but lay on the table until cool.  Then put away in a large stone jar.  Cover closely, and you will have nice moist, sweet bread.  I use coarse flour to set rising and fine to make it up when I can get both.  I have had 18 years' experience, and my bread is No. 1."

**Apple Bread, Pumpkin Bread, etc.**—A very light, pleasant bread is made in France by a mixture of apples and flour (meaning wheat flour, of course), in the proportion of one of apples to two of flour (say cups or pints, as you please).  The usual quantity of yeast employed as in making common bread, and the yeast is beaten with the flour and warm pulp of the apples (dried) after they are boiled and mashed, and the dough is then considered " set;" it is then allowed to rise from 8 to 12 hours, then baked in long loaves. Very little water is needed.

*Remarks.*—This will make nice and very pleasant flavored as well as healthful bread, but I must caution against giving it too long a time to rise. " Keep an eye on it," and when properly risen make into loaves and bake, lest some one should go by the " 8 to 12 hours."  Use judgment in all cases, and there will be but few failures.   I have known my mother and my wife to use pumpkins in a similar manner, even with corn meal as well as flour, which gave a pleasant relish to the bread.   And if I was a woman I should try peaches which had been peeled before drying, believing that I should get a still finer flavored bread.   Not the sourest, but a medium tart apple or peach only should be used.   I think the proportion of apple above given is greater than is generally used of pumpkin.   About 1 cup to each loaf of bread would, in my opinion, be enough, instead of 1 of apple to 2 of flour or meal or rye and Indian, etc.   It is used with either or all kinds of bread, when desired, except the Vienna.

# PUDDINGS.

**PUDDINGS.**—*General Remarks and Directions.*—Puddings are much like cake, and require about the same manipulation (skillful hand-working), and much the same ingredients. Eggs should be well beaten, and usually the whites and yolks are beaten separately although not quite so essential; but if so beaten the yolks should be beaten into the sugar before creaming in the butter, then the whites, having been well beaten; saving the whites of a sufficient number, when desired, to frost the top of a pudding—latterly called a *méringue,* made by whipping the whites of three or four eggs to a froth, with a tablespoon of powdered sugar to each egg used, with a little lemon juice, or such other fruit juice, as orange, etc., or some of the flavoring extracts, as rose, cinnamon-waters, etc., as you have or prefer; the pudding, when just done, to be carefully drawn to the mouth of the oven and covered with the frosting, or *méringue,* and a few minutes more given to nicely brown it; then taken hot to the table—nothing, it seems to the author, is so out of place as to pretend to have a pudding, just baked, come to the table only luke-warm (half cold); for me, I tell them: "Save this for me till tea-time, as I love cold pudding very much." But, of course, I would not add: "I dislike a half-cold one," but I do dislike them "all samee." Bread puddings, or those made with corn-starch, rice, or fruits, require only a moderate oven to bake them; while butter or custard puddings require not only a quick oven, but should go into it as soon as all the ingredients are mixed in with a final thorough beating, or stirring, and placed in the oven at once. The pudding-dish should always be well buttered, and, if to be a boiled pudding, the cloth must be first dipped into boiling hot water, then well floured on the outside. If boiled in a basin or mold, it must be buttered, and if a cloth is to be tied over it, it is to be treated the same as for boiling in a cloth; then when done, either way, dip into cold water, which will allow it to be emptied at once, without sticking, into a suitable dish to place upon the table; but always keep covered with the cloth or a napkin until placed upon the table, but there ought to be no delay in serving after it is emptied out of the cloth. It is usual to direct that "puddings be tied loosely," but you will see in the first receipt, that this plan is wrong, as it gives too much chance for water to get in and make them "soggy." Steam puddings often swell up and crack open—a sure sign of tightness. In boiling a pudding, remember this, the water must be boiling before the pudding is put in, and not allowed to slacken lest it becomes clammy or "soggy," as the sailor calls it in the first receipt. Keep the pudding also well covered all the time by pouring in boiling hot water, if needed, from time to time. To prevent the pudding from adhering or sticking to the kettle, cloth or dish, while boiling move it occasionally or else put a tin cover of some other dish into the bottom of the kettle, to make at least half an

331

inch space from the kettle—the rim around the cover does this.   To show the
real value of the old English plum pudding, I take my first one from the New
York *Times,* as related by a sailor—the second mate on a ship from New York
to Liverpool—in which case, of course, even the half of the Christmas plum
pudding saved (?) the ship and quickly brought all safely to their desired
haven.   Note well the instructions given in the receipt part of the item, as they
will all be found correct and worthy to be followed, on land as well as on the
sea.   I take the item from the Detroit *Free Press,* but it originated with the
*Times,* as credited above.   It is as follows:

**English Plum Pudding.**—It was about the stormiest voyage I ever
see.   We left the Hook on November 5, 1839, in a regular blow, and struck
worse weather off the Banks (New Foundland), and it grew dirtier every mile
we made.   The old man was kind of gruff and anxious like, and wasn't
easy to manage.   This ain't no Christmas story, and ain't got no moral to it.   I
was second mate and knowed the captain pretty well, but he wasn't sociable,
and the nearer we got to land according to our dead reckoning (for we hadn't
been able to take an observation) the more cross-grained he got.   I was eating
my supper on the 24th, when the steward he comes in, and says he, "Captain,
plum pudding to-morrow, as usual, sir?"   It wouldn't be polite in me to give
what that captain replied, but the steward he didn't mind.   All that night and
next day, the 25th of December, it was a howling storm, and the captain he
kept the deck.   About 3 o'clock Christmas day dinner was ready, and a
precious hard time it was to get that dinner from the galley to the cabin on
account of the green seas that swept over the ship.   The old man, after a bit,
came down, and says he, "Where's the puddin'?"   The steward he come in
just then as pale as a ghost, and says he showing an empty dish: "Washed
overboard, sir."   It ain't necessary to repeat what that there captain said.
Kind of how it looked as if the old man had wanted to give himself some
heart with that pudding, and now there wasn't none.   I disremember whether
it wasn't a passenger as said "that, providing we only reached port safe, in
such a gale puddings was of no consequence."   I guess the old man most bit
his head off for interfering with the ship's regulations.   Just then the cook
he came into the cabin with a dish in his hand, saying: "There is another
pudding.   I halved 'em," and he sot a good-sized pudding down on the table.
Then the old man kind of unbent and went for that pudding and cut it in big
hunks, helping the passenger last, with a kind of triumphant look.   He hadn't
swallowed more than a single bit than the first mate he comes running down,
and says he: "Lizard Light on the starboard bow, and weather brightening
up."   "How does she head?"   "East by north." "Then give her full three
points more northerly, sir, and the Lord be praised."   And the captain, he
swallowed his pudding in three gulps, and was on deck, just saying, "I
knowed the pudding would fetch it," and he left us.   We was in Liverpool
three days after that, though a ship that started the day before us from New
York was never heard of.   This here is the receipt for that there pudding:

Take six ounces of suet, mind you skin it and cut it up fine.   Just you use
the same quantity of raisins, taking out the stones, and the same of currants;
always wash your currants and dry them in a cloth.   Have a stale loaf of
bread, and crumble, say three ounces of it.   You will want about the same of
sifted flour.   Break three eggs, yolks and all, but don't beat them much.   Have
a teaspoonful of ground cinnamon and grate half a nutmeg.   Don't forget a
teaspoonful of salt.   You will require with all this a half pint of milk—we
kept a cow on board of ship in those days—say to that four ounces of white
sugar.   In old days angelica root candied was used; it's gone out of fashion
now.   [Angelica grows all over the United States, as well as Europe, has

a peculiar flavor, and was, at least, once believed to be a very valuable medicine, but used more, of late, merely for the agreeable flavor it imparts to other medicines. The root is of purplish color, and is to be sliced up and cooked in sugar, if "candied," as referred to above, the same as citron or lemon, etc., are done. King sets it down as "aromatic, stimulant, carminative, diaphoretic, expectorant (this often used in cough or lung medicines), diuretic and emenagogue." Used in flatulent colic and in heartburn. It is said to promote the menstrual discharges. In diseases of the Urinary organs, as calculi and passive dropsy, it is used as a diuretic, in decoction with *uviursa* and *eupatorianum purpuseum* (queen of the meadow). Dose—of the powder 30 to 60 grs.; of the decoction (tea), 2 to 4 ozs, 3 or 4 times a day. There are several species, or kinds, of it, any of which may be used medicinally as a substitute for other kinds.] Put that in—if you have it—not a big piece, and slice it thin. You can't do well without half an ounce of candied citron. Now mix all this up together, adding the milk last in which you put half a glass of brandy. Take a piece of linen, big enough to double over, put it in boiling water, squeeze out all the water, and flour it; turn out your mixture in that cloth, and tie it up tight; good cooks sew up their pudding bags. It can't be squeezed too much, for a loosely tied pudding is a soggy thing, because it won't cook dry. Put in 5 qts. of boiling water, and let it boil 6 hours steady, covering it up. Watch it, and if the water gives out, add more boiling water. This is a real English plum pudding, with no nonsense about it.

*Remarks.*—It has always appeared to the author that an occasional incident like the above sea voyage, in connection with a recipe, or receipt, (recipe is the proper spelling, but receipt is much the more common manner of speaking), not only gives relief to the mind from the sameness of the receipts, or descriptions, but also helps one to remember the *modus operandi* (manner of operation) of the whole instructions and directions of the receipt.

An incident like this one here given will also give a subject for conversation, and also call for the relation of other incidents known, or passed through, by some of those who may be gathered around the Christmas board, when the old English plum pudding, "with no nonsense about it," will be reproduced, if at no other time in the whole year. So I trust to be excused for the space the story part of the receipt occupies. I think, generally, there is no instruction to remove the dry membrane, or skin, as the sailor calls it, from suet; but it ought to be done, as it is not only indigestible, but hard to chop, becoming more or less stringy and troublesome while chopping. I will give a few more plum puddings, for variety's sake. It is to be understood that when plum pudding is mentioned, it always means a pudding to be boiled.

**Plum Pudding No. 2, and Sweet Sauce for Same.**—Bread crumbs, 1 lb (3½ cups); sweet milk, 1 qt.; eggs, 6; sugar, 1 cup; suet, chopped; English currants, and raisins, each, 1 lb.; sliced and chopped citron, ½ lb.; cinnamon, cloves, nutmeg and allspice, each, ½ teaspoonful; sifted flour to make a thick batter; pour into the flannel cloth (see general directions), tie, leaving very little room for swelling, and plunge into a large kettle of boiling water, and boil for 7 hours, in a well covered kettle, pouring in boiling water, if needed, to keep the pudding covered all the time. This pudding, says a lady writer, in the *Free Press,* will keep for several weeks, and is nearly as good steamed, as when first boiled.

**Sauce for Same.**—Sugar, 4 tablespoonful, rubbed to a cream with butter, 2 spoonfuls, and 2 of flour; then add boiling water, 1 pt., or still better, some of the boiling water in which the pudding was boiled, same amount flavored with lemon or vanilla. "A tin fire-pan, or small tin cover, bottom upwards in the bottom of the kettle," she says, "will prevent the pudding from burning."

*Remarks.*—This, to the author, only seems to lack a teaspoonful of soda, and 2 of cream tartar, but if light enough without them, all right. Of course any other extracts as orange, rose-water, or cinnamon-water, can be used, if preferred, with any sauce. But the author would like to see the family in which the above or the following pudding, (made to Englishmen's taste, in rhyme,) "will keep for several weeks," unless put "under lock and key."

### Plum Pudding to Englishmen's Taste, No. 3, In Rhyme.—

To make plum-pudding to Englishmen's taste,
So all may be eaten and nothing to waste,
Take of raisins, and currants, and bread-crumbs, all round;
Also suet from oxen, and flour a pound,
Of citron well candied, or lemon as good,
With molasses and sugar, eight ounces, I would,
Into this first compound, next must be hasted
A nutmeg well grated, ground ginger well tasted,
With salt to preserve it, of such a teaspoonful;
Then of milk half a pint, and of fresh eggs take six;
Be sure after this that you properly mix.
Next tie up in a bag, just as round as you can,
Put into a capacious and suitable pan,
Then boil for eight hours just as hard as you can.

**Plum Pudding, No. 4.**—Sifted flour, 3 cups; eggs, 3; a wine-glass of molasses to color it; milk, ½ pt.; finely chopped suet, 1 large cup; English currants and raisins, each 1 cup; mace, cloves, and cinnamon, ½ teaspoonful each, or to taste; soda, 1 teaspoonful; cream of tartar, 2 teaspoonfuls; boil for at least 2½ hours 3 is still better. The 2½ are sufficient to cook, but the other half-hour's boiling gives a certain lightness to the pudding, which is greatly to be desired. Eat with any good sauce. The following either with the vinegar or brandy is good:

**Pudding-Sauce—Fast or Spirituous.**—Sugar, 2 cups, dissolved in boiling water, ½ pt.; flour, or corn starch, 2 tablespoonfuls, worked smooth, in cold water, 1 cup, and stirred into the boiling sugar, with nice butter, the size of an egg, (hen's egg); then add two or three tablespoonfuls of good vinegar (more or less as a sharp or mild taste is preferred); or brandy, or good wine, in like quantities to suit the taste of self or guests, with cinnamon, nutmeg, or other flavor, as you like.

**Plum-Pudding, No. 5.**—Suet, chopped fine, English currants and raisins, each 1 lb.; flour, 1½ lbs. (about 5 cups); cloves, cinnamon, and nutmegs, each ½ teaspoonful; salt, 1 tablespoonful. Mix all well together and add molasses, 1 cup; sugar, 2 cups; eggs, 7; sweet milk, ½ pt. Make over night, in the morning tie in a cloth and boil 4 hours. To be eaten with sweet sauce. Any of the above sauces are known as "sweet sauce."

*Remarks.*—Salt, the author considers, as important in puddings as in bread or cakes, although it is not always mentioned. [See, also, "Suet Puddings, Steamed."]

**Christmas Plum-Pudding, No. 6, Old Style.**—Stone 1½ lbs. of raisins, wash, pick and dry ½ lb. of currants, mince fine ¾ lb. of suet, cut into thin slices ½ lb. of mixed peel (orange and lemon), and grate fine ¾ lb. of bread-crumbs. When all these dry ingredients are prepared; mix them well together, then moisten the mixture with 8 eggs, well beaten, and one wine-glass of brandy; stir well, that everything may be thoroughly blended, and press the pudding into a buttered mould; tie it down tightly with a floured cloth, and boil 6 hours. On Christmas day a sprig of holly is usually placed in the middle of the pudding, and about a wine-glass of brandy poured round it, which, at the moment of serving, is lighted, and the pudding thus brought to the table encircled in flames.

*Remarks.*—With half-a-dozen plum-puddings none need go without a Christmas day, certainly. The only point that seems to me unreasonable is the long boiling, 8, or even 6 hours, which appears to be more than is needed. A circle of three ladies, to whom I referred the matter, gave it as their judgment that 3 hours would be sufficient. Let English people stick to the old custom, but Americans will find that from 3 to 4 hours will cook them perfectly. [See the Paradise Pudding below, which is only to be boiled 2 hours.] A wine-glass, at least, of brandy is almost universally put into the sauce upon Christmas occasions.

**Paradise Pudding.**—Pare, core and mince 3 good-sized tart apples into small pieces, and mix them with ¼ lb. of bread-crumbs, 3 eggs, 3 ozs. of currants, the rind of one-half lemon, ½ wine-glass of brandy, salt, and grated nutmeg to taste. Put the pudding into a buttered mould, tie it down with a cloth, boil for 2 hours, and serve with sweet sauce.

*Remarks.*—These fancy names, no doubt, are calculated to convey the idea that the article is to be very nice. The author would prefer to see more common names used, but he takes them as he finds them, so long as the article itself, like this pudding, is really nice. "Angels' Food" has been recently advertised; so these dear creatures will not have to "live on air" much longer.

**Cottage Pudding, or Pudding Baked as Cake, No. 1, and Sauce.**—Eggs, 3, well beaten; sugar, 2 cups; butter, ½ cup; sweet milk, 1½ cups; baking powder, 1 tea-spoonful; flour to make as cake batter, to dip with spoon into a cake pan to bake. To serve, cut into suitable pieces, for a saucer or side-dishes, with the following sauce:

*Lemon Sauce for the Pudding.*—Boiling water, 3 cups; sugar, ½ cup; butter, half the size of an egg. Mix. Boil a lemon and cut it into small pieces and add to the sauce, putting at least one piece to each dish of pudding in serving.

*Remarks.*—I first ate of this pudding at the City Hotel, Winfield, Kans., kept at that time by S. S. Major, and was so well pleased with it that I got him to take me to the cook, who kindly gave me the recipe, as above, which has proved itself many times since, and it will please all who try it carefully

**Cottage Pudding, No. 2, With Sauce for Same.**—Sifted flour (flour should always be sifted), 1 pt.; white of 3 eggs, beaten to a stiff froth; butter, 3 table-spoonfuls; sugar, 1 cup; sweet milk, 1 cup; baking powder, 3 teaspoonfuls. Mix, and sprinkle granulated sugar over the top.

*Sauce for the Same.*—Sweet milk, 1 pt.; sugar, ½ cup; yolks of 2 eggs, beating and stirring well while being boiled together; flavor with lemon. Of course, any other flavor can be used.

**Cottage Pudding, Quickly Made, No. 3, With Sauce for Same.**—Sugar, raisins and sour cream, each 1 cup; flour, 2 cups; soda, 1 tea-spoonful; 2 eggs; ½ grated nutmeg; bake in long cake tin.

*Sauce for Same.*—Sugar, 1 cup; butter, ½ cup; flour, 4 heaping table-spoonfuls; rub all well together, and grate in the other half of the nutmeg and pour on boiling water, 3 pints; let it boil up once, and it is ready for use. Use freely, as there is plenty of it; and light cottage puddings take up sauce as freely as a toper does whiskey—all he can get. I can take the sauce freely, but beg to be excused on the whiskey, although I do not object to a little spirits in pudding sauce. Sugar makes it palatable, if but little is used.

**Cottage Pudding, No. 4, Steamed.**—Sugar and sweet milk, each 1 cup; melted butter, 3 table-spoonfuls; 1 egg; flour, 1 pt.; soda, 1 tea-spoonful; cream tartar, 2 tea-spoonfuls. Steam in suitable dish 1½ hours. Serve with any sauce desired.

**Custard Pudding.**—Sweet milk, 1 pt.; peel of 1 fresh lemon; lump sugar, ¼ lb.; eggs, 4. DIRECTIONS—Shred (cut in long thin strips) the lemon peel very fine, and put it into the milk, bringing to a boil; then take out the peel and add the sugar and pour the scalding milk upon the eggs, which have been well beaten. Put into a basin or tart dish, and set in a sauce pan with boiling water to reach only half way up. Do not boil the water, but keep it at bubbling heat for 20 minutes, or until the custard sets.

*Remarks.*—Very nice, hot or cold. Orange or other flavoring may take the place of lemon, if preferred.

**Pudding with Chopped Eggs, a la Creme.**—Boil 6 eggs hard, chop fine; have grated bread sufficient. Put into a buttered dish, alternate layers of the chopped egg and grated bread to fill the dish, or nearly so; put butter in small bits, 1 table-spoonful over the top; a little salt and pepper; then pour on boiling sweet milk, 1 pt. Bake to a light brown. To be served warm with very nice butter.

**Cream, or Custard Pudding, No. 1.**—Sweet cream, 1 pt., into which stir smoothly fine sifted flour, 1 cup; put over the fire and stir until quite thick, take off, and when cool, stir in 4 well beaten eggs; white sugar, 2 cups, and chopped citron, 1 cup. Bake till set only. If a custard is baked too long it becomes watery, which is considered to spoil them. To be eaten cold, with or without sauce as preferred.

**Custard Pudding, "Dandy," No. 2.**—Sweet milk, 1 qt.; flour, 2 table-spoonfuls; white sugar, 5 table-spoonfuls; a pinch of salt and a little mace. DIRECTIONS—Mix the flour, salt, mace and 4 spoonfuls of the sugar with the milk; beat the yolks of the eggs and stir in also, and place in the oven to bake, stirring with a spoon 2 or 3 times after putting it into the oven, which prevents the flour from settling; beat the white of the eggs with the other spoonful of sugar and spread on the top, just before done; replace in the oven to cook the eggs and to give the top a nice brown. Serve with a little granulated or pow-dered sugar.

*Remarks.*—The word "dandy" here simply means "tip top," or very nice.

**Snow Pudding, With Gelatine, Very Nice—No. 1.**—Pour boil-ing water, 1 pt., over ½ box of Cox's gelatine; add sugar, 2 cups, to the juice of 2 lemons; put peel and all in, and mash all together. Let simmer till the gelatine is dissolved; when only lukewarm, strain through a thin cloth into the dish in which you are to send it to the table. When cold and formed, or hard-ened, beat the whites of 3 eggs to a stiff froth, with 1 table-spoonful of pow-dered sugar, and place on top. And if, on especial occasions, you would give variety, make a soft-boiled custard with the yolks of the eggs and spread a layer over the white; then put bits of any jell, or bits of different-colored jells, thickly—*i. e.,* ½ to 1 inch apart—over the top of all, so that each guest will have several bits in the dish.—*Miss Tillie Bratshaw, Detroit.*

The following sauce is from the same person:

**Snow, or White Pudding Sauce.**—Beat powdered sugar, 1 cup, with butter, ¾ cup, till white and foamy. Just before sending to the table, add 2 tea-spoonfuls of boiling water, no more, no less. If rightly made, it will drop from the spoon, white and light as snow.

*Remarks.*—The lady who gave me these recipes was the daughter of a special friend of mine, with whom I have frequently dined, and therefore know her ability and taste in getting up very nice dishes.

**Pudding Sauce, Strawberry Color and Flavor.**—Rub butter, ½ cup; sugar, 1 cup, to a cream, adding the beaten white of 1 egg and 1 cup of nice ripe strawberries, thoroughly mashed. This, in the season of strawberries or other berries, gives a nice color, as well as flavor, to the sauce.

**Snow Pudding, with Corn Starch, No. 2.** — Dissolve, or rub up smoothly, 3 table-spoonfuls of corn starch with cold water; then pour on 1 pt. of boiling water; beat well the whites of 3 eggs and stir in, it all being done in a suitable earthen dish, to steam it in 10 or 15 minutes.

*Sauce for Same.*—Beat the yolks of the eggs into 1 cup of sugar, then the same amount of sweet milk, and 1 table-spoonful of butter; boil till quite thick. If enough is made to leave over, it is nice cold at tea-time; many prefer it cold.

**Sauce for Puddings—The Author's Favorite.**—The best sauce to suit me is made by using rich cream with plenty of pulverized sugar, so the spoon will fetch it up from the bottom of the "boat," or bowls, at every dip—and I like to dip deep every time; milk does very well, but it is well-known that it is not so rich as cream; but half-and-half does excellently. Use any flavor-ing you please; grated nutmeg is the most common with cream sauce.

**Tapioca Pudding, No. 1.**—Sweet milk, 1 qt.; tapioca, 1 cup; eggs, 2; sugar, 4 tablespoonfuls; butter, half the size of an egg; a little salt, nutmeg to taste. DIRECTIONS—Put a part of the milk upon the tapioca for 1 hour; beat the eggs and sugar together; mix all and bake.

**Tapioca Pudding No. 2.**—Tapioca, 2 cups; sweet milk, 4 cups; eggs, 4; butter, 1 heaping table-spoonful; sugar, 1 cup, or to taste; a grated lemon peel improves it. DIRECTIONS—Soak the tapioca in the milk 1 hour; then put into a rice kettle, or tin pail, set in an iron pot, or kettle, of hot water, and cook till soft. When soft, or done, put into the baking dish, with the butter, eggs well beaten, sugar, lemon peel, etc., and bake about ½ hour. Orange peel may be used in the same manner, or it may be flavored with any fruit extract desired. [A rice kettle is a double dish, or double kettle, on the same principle as a glue-pot (generally made of tin), smaller at the top than bottom, to allow another one made smaller at the bottom than at the top, to set inside of it. The inner dish has a cover, and the outer one a lip, or nose, to allow pouring in water, as may be necessary, while cooking the rice or other articles which burn easily, if not surrounded with water. Tinners know them as rice kettles. They are exceedingly handy for cooking, not only rice, but tapioca, sago, oat meal, etc.]

**Tapioca Pudding, with Apples, No. 3, Without Milk or Eggs.**—Tapioca, 1 cup; water, 1½ pts.; apples, 6 good sized tart ones; sugar, lemon or nutmeg. DIRECTIONS — Soak the tapioca in water over night. Pare and punch the cores from the apples, with a tin apple corer—a piece of tin rolled into cylinder shape, about ⅝ of an inch in diameter, and soldered together—(at the proper time to have the pudding ready for dinner), and place them in a pudding dish, fill the holes with sugar and sprinkle some over them, grate on nutmeg, or put on powdered cinnamon, or other flavor, as preferred, pour over a cup of water and bake till quite soft; then pour over the tapioca in the milk, and bake ½ to 1 hour. (See also " Danish or Tapioca Pudding.")

*Sauce for Same, Hard.*—Butter, 1 cup; powdered sugar, 2 cups; wine, ½ cup, or brandy, 2 table-spoonfuls; the juice of 1 lemon or orange, and nutmeg, 1, grated. First beat the sugar and butter to a cream, then add the wine or brandy, and the lemon or orange juice, and the nutmeg, stir all well together and set on ice to cool, if you have it. The wine, or brandy, and the fruit juice may be left out, and still you have a nice sauce, good enough for anybody; but as some persons will use them we have to give them.

**Sago Pudding.**—Sago, 3 table-spoonfuls; milk, 1 qt.; peel of 1 lemon; nutmeg, ½ of 1; eggs, 4; a little salt. DIRECTIONS—Boil the sago in the milk, in the rice kettle (double kettle) till done; remove from fire, and when cool stir in the beaten eggs, salt and seasoning, and bake about 1 hour.

*Sauce for Same.*—Eat with sugar and cream, if you have it, if not rub 1 butter to 2 sugars, with a little nutmeg, if the pudding is not highly flavored. Almost any pudding is nice to be eaten with plenty of sugar and rich cream. Even milk does pretty well, if rich with sugar and nutmeg (most people like the flavor of nutmeg), at least I have yet to find the first one who does not.

**Orange Pudding.**—Peel and slice 4 large oranges, lay them in your pudding dish and sprinkle over them 1 cup of sugar. Beat the yolks of 3 eggs, ½ cup of sugar, 2 table-spoonfuls of corn starch, and pour into a quart of boiling milk; let this boil and thicken; then let it cool a little, before pouring it over the oranges. Beat the whites of the eggs and pour over the top. Set it in the oven to brown slightly.—*Mrs. R. McK. of Jackson, Mich., in Farm and Fireside.*

**Pop-Corn Pudding.**—Sweet milk and pop-corn, each 3 pts. (each kernel must be popped white, and not a bit scorched); eggs, 2; salt, ½ teaspoonful. Bake ½ hour.

*Sauce for Same.*—Sweetened cream or milk.

**Chestnut Pudding.**—Peel off the shells, cover the kernels with water, and boil till their skins readily peel off. Then pound them in a mortar, and to every cup of chestnuts add 3 cups of chopped apple, 1 of chopped raisins, ½ cup of sugar, and 1 qt. of water. Mix thoroughly, and bake until the apple is tender—about ½ hour. Serve cold with sweet sauce.

*Remarks.*—Whoever loves chestnuts (and who does not) will like the flavor of this pudding. Take out a chestnut from the boiling water, and drop it into cold water a moment, and if the dark skin will rub off with the thumb and finger (which is called blanching), they have boiled enough.

**Salt Pork Pudding.**—Chop very fine 1 large cup of salt pork, which has been sliced and soaked in milk over night. Add to it 1 cup of molasses, with 1 tea-spoonful of saleratus or soda stirred into it. Three-fourths cup of sweet milk; 1 cup of stoned raisins or currants; 1 tea-spoonful each of ground cinnamon, cloves and nutmeg. Add flour enough to make as stiff as a berry pudding. Steam in a cloth or boil for 4 hours.

*Sauce for Same.*—For a sauce take 1 cup of white sugar and pour over it the same quantity of boiling water; when melted stir in two well beaten eggs. Flavor with vanilla or lemon.

*Remarks.*—If made nicely it will equal rock cake, and keep well, if made in large quantities.

**Fig Pudding, Boiled.**—"Cooking for Invalids" directs fig puddings to be made as follows: Chop ½ lb. of figs very finely; mix with them coarse sugar, ¼ lb.; molasses, 1 table-spoonful; milk, 4 table-spoonfuls; flour, ½ lb. (1¾ cups); suet, chopped, ½ lb.; 1 egg and a pinch of grated nutmeg; put the pudding into a buttered mould, and boil 5 hours.

*Remarks.*—Nothing said about a sauce; but any of the "sweet sauces" would be nice for it; or the "sweetened cream," as the prune pudding below.

**Prune Pudding.**—Prunes, ½ lb., boiled soft and thick; remove the pits, chop fine, and stir in coarse sugar, a scant cup; the whites of 6 eggs, beaten stiff. Bake a light brown. Serve with sweetened cream or milk, with nutmeg to suit.

**Apple Pudding, No. 1, Dutch.**—Flour, 1 pt. (1¾ cups); salt, ½ tea-spoonful; baking powder, 2 tea-spoonfuls, or 1 of cream of tartar; soda, ¼ tea-spoonful. Rub 1 tablespoonful of butter into the flour. Beat 1 egg and add to it, and ¾ of a cup of milk. Mix the flour into a dough thick enough to spread ½ an inch thick in a baking tin. Peel and cut in eighths 4 apples and place them in rows in the dough, narrowest edge down. Sprinkle over it 2 table spoonfuls of sugar and bake in a quick oven 20 minutes. Serve with the following:

*Lemon Sauce for Same.*—One cupful of sugar and 2 cupfuls of water put on to boil; 3 tea-spoonfuls of corn starch into a little cold water and stir into the boiling syrup; cook about 8 minutes, adding a little more water when thick; juice and grated rind of ½ a lemon, 1 tablespoonful of butter; stir until the butter is melted and serve at once. ITEMS—It is well to have the pan buttered and everything ready before wetting up the dough. If the dough is too soft it will rise and fall; just thick enough to drop and to spread.—*Blade Household.*

**Apple, Peach, or Other Fruit Pudding-Pie, or Pie-Pudding, No. 2, Yankee Style.**—Sweet milk, 1 cup; 1 egg; butter, 1 table-spoonful, heaping; baking powder, 1 tea-spoonful; flour, 1 cup, or sufficient to make rather a thick batter ("batter" means like cake—better to handle with a spoon, or to pour out); a little salt; tart, juicy apples to half fill an earthen pudding-dish, DIRECTIONS—Stir the baking powder into the sifted flour; melt the butter, beat the egg and stir all well together; having pared and sliced the apples or peaches, buttered the dish and laid in the fruit to only half fill it, dip the batter over the fruit to wholly cover it, as with a crust; the dish should not be quite full, lest as it rises it runs over in baking. Bake in a moderate oven to a nice brown, to be done just "at the nick of time" for dinner. Turn it bottom up upon a pie-plate, and grate over nutmeg or sprinkle on some powdered cinnamon or other spices, as preferred; then sprinkle freely of nice white sugar over all and serve with sweetened cream or rich milk, well sweetened. Peaches, pears, strawberries, raspberries, blackberries, etc., in their season, work equally as well as apples.—*Mrs. Sarah A. Earley, Mt. Pleasant, Iowa.*

*Remarks.*—This plan avoids the soggy and indigestible bottom crust of pie; and it matters not whether you call it pie or pudding, it eats equally well, even cold, with plenty of sugar and milk, having the cream stirred in.

**Apple Short-Cake Pudding, No. 3, With Sour Cream and Buttermilk.**—Fill a square, deep bread-tin ½ or ¾ full of pared and sliced tart apples; make a thick batter of ½ cup each of sour cream and buttermilk, 1 tea-spoonful of saleratus, a little salt, and flour, sifted, to make quite stiff, a little stiffer than for cake; turn this over the apples; bake 40 minutes, and serve with sauce, or cream and sugar with nutmeg.

*Remarks.*—Other fruit, as peaches, etc., will do nicely with this as well as the No. 2, above; nor would an egg in the batter hurt it a bit.

**Sweet Apple Pudding, No. 4.**—Sweet milk, 1 qt.; eggs, 4; sweet apples, pared and chopped, 3 rounding cups; a lemon, nutmeg and cinnamon; soda, ½ tea-spoonful; vinegar enough to dissolve the soda; flour to make as cake batter. DIRECTIONS—Grate off ½ the rind of the lemon, using all the juice; beat the yolks very light; add the milk, seasoning and stir in flour to make rather a thick batter, and stir hard 5 minutes; then stir in the chopped apples, then the beaten whites, and finally the soda, dissolved in a little vinegar, mixing all well. Bake in 2 shallow dishes, to ensure cooking the sweet apples, which require more cooking than tart ones—about 1 hour—covering the top with paper the last half hour. To be eaten hot with cream, or milk and sugar.

**Apple Charlotte, or Bread Pudding With Tart Apples, No. 5.** —Butter your pudding-dish, line it with bread buttered on both sides; put a thick layer of apples, cut in thin slices, or chopped, sugar, a little cinnamon and butter on top, then another layer of bread, apples, sugar, cinnamon and butter last. Bake slowly 1½ hours, keeping the basin, or dish, covered till a little before serving, to let the apples brown on top.—*Blade Household.*

*Remarks.*—No matter whether there is any *Blade* about it or not, it will be found nice and healthful.

**Apple Custard Pudding, No. 6.**—Good-sized tart apples, pared, and the cores punched out with a tin cutter [see "Tapioca Pudding, No. 3," for description], sufficient only to cover the bottom of a large earthen pudding-dish, buttered; set the apples on end, so as to fill the holes with sugar; grate over them a little nutmeg, and cinnamon powder, if liked; then make a rich custard, say with 4 or 5 well-beaten eggs to 1 qt. sweet milk and 1 to 2 cups of sugar, according to the sourness of the apples, and pour over the apples Bake till the apples are tender; serve with sweetened cream or milk. One apple to be placed in each dish in serving. Very delicious and healthful.

**Bird's-Nest Pudding—Several Styles.**—Tart apples, pared and the cores punched out, sufficient to cover the bottom of an earthen pudding-dish; fill the holes with sugar and grate on some nutmeg; having mashed, say 4 heaping table-spoonfuls of sago, mix with cold water to properly fill the dish; pour it upon the apples and bake in a moderate oven about 1 hour.

*Remarks.*—Ripe peaches, pears, cherries, prunes, etc., with the proper amount of sugar, may take the place of apples, and tapioca may take the place of sago; time for baking the same. Serve either with cream and sugar, or milk with the cream stirred in. Palatable, healthy and not expensive, as good brown sugar may be used with any colored fruits.

**Dried Peach Pudding.**—Dried peaches, 1 pt.; wash, sweeten with sugar, 1 cup, and stew till nicely done, using water sufficient to have plenty of the juices; then, having made a batter with buttermilk, 1 small cup, and ½ tea-spoonful of soda and a little salt, thicken with flour very stiff; drop in spoonfuls among the peaches while boiling. Continue the boiling about 20 minutes. An egg and ½ a cup of sugar would improve this puffy paste. Serve with cream and sugar, or sweet sauce, as you choose. Be careful not to burn the peaches in stewing.

**Yorkshire Pudding, English.**—Sweet milk, 1½ pts.; flour, 7 table-spoonfuls (as you lift them up out of sifted flour); a little salt. DIRECTIONS— Put the flour into a basin with the salt and sufficient of the milk to make a stiff, smooth batter (that is, to be no lumps); then stir in two well-beaten eggs and the remainder of the milk; beat all well together, and pour into a shallow tin which has been previously rubbed with butter. Bake for 1 hour; then place it under the meat for ½ an hour to catch a little of the gravy as it flows from the roasting beef. (This is the English way, where they "spit" the beef in roasting. See remarks below for the American way, and also about serving on a napkin.) Cut the pudding into square pieces and serve on a hot folded napkin with hot roast beef.—*Warne's Model Cookery, London, Eng.*

*Remarks.*—The plan of putting the pudding under the roasting beef, where they roast it upon spits (a pointed bar of iron, or several of them, to roast before a fire), as our grandmothers used to roast a goose, turkey or spare-rib, was a very convenient way of moistening the top of the pudding with the rich juices of the beef; but in place of that we, here in America, have the pudding 10 or 15 minutes longer in the oven, but baste it frequently during this time, with the meat drippings; make this pudding only when you are roasting beef; and we serve it upon the plates with the beef, and not upon napkins, which makes too much washing for our wives and daughters. In England, with plenty of "servants," they care not for this extra work. "A hot oven, a well beaten batter, and serving quickly, are the secrets of a Yorkshire pudding," to which the author will add, also a rich meat gravy.

**Hunters' Pudding, Boiled—Will Keep for Months.**—Flour, suet finely chopped, raisins chopped, and English currants, each, 1 lb.; sugar, ¼ lb.; the outer rind of a lemon, grated; 6 berries of pimento (all-spice) finely powdered; salt, ¼ tea-spoonful; when well mixed add 4 well beaten eggs, a ½ pt. of brandy, and 1 or 2 table-spoonfuls of milk to reduce it to a thick batter, boil in a cloth 9 hours, and serve with brandy sauce. This pudding may be kept for 6 months after boiling, if closely tied up; it will be required to be boiled 1 hour when it is to be used.—*Farm and Fireside.*

*Remarks.*—This, for hunters going out upon a long expedition, would be a very desirable relish to take along. There is not a doubt as to its keeping qualities, as it contains no fermentive principles; and the fruit and brandy are both anti-ferments, while the long boiling is also done to kill any possible tendency to fermentation. I should, however, boil it in a tin can, having a suitable tight-fitting cover, if intended for long keeping, on the principle of air-tight canning, as well as to be safe from insects, and convenience in carrying. Do not think, however, but what it would be very nice for present use with only 4 or 5 hours' boiling, using the sauce freely, as it is made so dry for the purpose of long keeping.

**Danish, or Tapioca Pudding.**—Tapioca, 1 cup; water 3 pts.; salt, ½ tea-spoonful; sugar ½ cup; any high-colored jelly, 1 tumblerful. DIRECTIONS —Wash the tapioca in the evening, and soak over night in the water; in the the morning put into a double boiler (see Tapioca Puddings No. 2—Note—for the Rice, or double kettle, a rice-boiler is what is wanted), and cook 1 hour, stirring occasionally; then add salt, sugar, and jelly, and mix thoroughly; then turn into a mold or serving-cups which have been dipped into cold water, and put in a cool place to "set" for dinner or tea, with cream and sugar. (See also Tapioca Puddings.)

**Naples, or Duke of Cambridge Pudding, with Candied Peel.**
Candied lemon, orange and citron, each, 1 oz,; butter and pulverized sugar, each, 6 ozs.; yolks of 4 eggs; rich puff-paste, or well-buttered bread, to line the dish. DIRECTIONS—Chop the candied peel finely, put the rich crust or paste into the dish, else line it with bread well buttered on both sides; then put in the chopped mixture; warm the butter and sugar together, adding the well-beaten yolks, stirring over the fire until it boils; then pour this over the other and bake in a slow oven 1 hour; or, in place of the butter, beat the whites of the eggs also with the yolk, and make a custard with milk, 1 qt.; sugar the same, and pour over, and bake ¾ hour. This makes you two puddings for variety's sake—make one way at one time, and the other way next time.

**Chester, or Almond Flavored Pudding, English.**—Lemon, 1; sweet almonds, 20; bitter almonds, 6 only; butter, 1 heaping table-spoonful; sugar, 1 cup; eggs, 4; puff paste. DIRECTIONS—Blanch the almonds and chop them, or what is better, cut into long strips, or shreds, with a sharp knife. Put the butter into a sauce pan over a slow fire, and as soon as the butter melts put all in, except the whites of the eggs, and beat together thoroughly, having the pudding dish already lined with the light paste, pour in the mixture, and bake in a quick oven. To be sent to the table on a folded napkin, with the whites of the eggs beaten to a froth with a spoon of powdered sugar, and laid upon the top. [To blanch almonds, pour boiling water on the meats, and let stand till the skin will rub off easily, between the thumb and finger, throwing them into cold water as the skin is removed, to whiten; then drain off the water and chop, or slice up into shreds, with a sharp pen-knife, or pound in a mortar, as directed in the recipe. Never let them dry, as that brings out their oiliness.]

*Remarks.*—Being an American, I would say put the whites beaten on top, and brown a few moments before serving, and serve in saucers, or suitable side dishes. (See remarks following the "Yorkshire Pudding," about serving on napkins, etc.)

**Sponge Cake Pudding.**—Butter a mould, and having cut in halves, large raisins, ¼ lb.; fill the mould ¾ full, loosely, with sponge cake which has been cut in long strips—square form—crossing each tier, strips a little distance apart, cob house fashion, to allow space for the custard; then pour in a custard made with 3 eggs to rich milk, 1 pt. (rich milk means milk with the cream stirred in), or 5 eggs to 1 qt., with ½ to 1½ cups, as to whether liked very sweet or not; flavored with nutmeg or any extract desired. Set the mould in a kettle of water to come up ⅔ or ¾ only; up the sides, and boil 1 hour; or set in a steamer, if you have one (and they are very convenient in every family), and steam 1 hour, properly covered, to prevent the condensing steam from dripping from the cover into the pudding.

*Sauce for Same.*—Sugar, 1 cup; butter, ½ cup, whipped to a cream; then pour in boiling water, 1 cup, setting the same dish on the stove, to continue to scald, but not to boil, while 2 or 3 tea-spoonfuls of corn starch are rubbed up with a little cold water and stirred in; then a well beaten egg, and lastly a wine-glass of wine; or still better, a wine-glass of brandy. Serve while both are hot. I wonder if the English would not say, "On a folded napkin."

*Remarks.*—A napkin will be needed to wipe the lips, after smacking them; for there are but few persons who will not smack their lips for more of it.

**St. James' Stale Bread Pudding.**—Grate a stale loaf of bread (*i. e.*, 2 or 3 days old) into crumbs; pour over them 1 pt. of boiling milk; let stand 1 hour; then beat to a pulp; then beat, sugar, 1½ cups, to a cream with 4 eggs, and butter, 2 table-spoonfuls; grate in the yellow of a lemon, and a bit of nutmeg, and a pinch of cinnamon, if liked; beat all well together, and pour into a pudding dish lined with nice puff paste, and bake about 1 hour. The juice of the lemon to be used in making whatever sauce you prefer, as there are many already given.

*Remarks.*—The author feels very sure you will ask St. James to call again. Bread, buttered well on each side, may be substituted for the puff paste to line the dish.

**Baron Brisse's Rice Pudding.**—Wash 1 cup of rice and boil it in as little milk and water, half-and-half, in a rice kettle (which see) as will swell it soft. When thus cooked, add 6 well-beaten eggs, leaving out the whites of 4; butter, 3 heaping table-spoonfuls, and a little salt. Butter a tin baking-mould well and sprinkle over it finely-powdered bread-crumbs, or cracker-crumbs, thickly at bottom and all that will adhere on the sides. Whip the whites to a stiff froth and stir in last; then pour into the mould and bake ½ an hour. Turn out upon a dish and serve as if it was a loaf of cake.

*Remarks.*—I do not know who Baron Brisse is, or was, but I do know this pudding is nice. It matters not what a pudding is called, but it does matter whether it is good or not when you are "called" to eat it. I will vouch for the Baron's; still I think he might have allowed 1 cup of sugar to the mixture, as the author has a "sweet tooth." Yet it does very well without, if served with a sauce of 1 butter to 2 sugars, whipped nicely together, and flavored with grated nutmeg or other flavor, as preferred.

**Queen Mab's Pudding, With Gelatine.**—Soak a sixpence packet (about 1 oz.) of gelatine, in warm water enough to cover it, for 2 hours; then boil a fresh sliced lemon-peel (better a candied one, nicely chopped) in 1 pt. of milk and add to the gelatine, continuing the heat till the gelatine is dissolved; then sweeten to taste, pouring in gently the beaten yolks of 4 eggs; place the saucepan again upon the stove and simmer as a custard (which it is) over a slow fire, not allowing it to boil; when thick enough, remove from the fire and stir in preserved cherries (preserved blackberries, or black-caps), and stir occasionally till nearly cold, and pour into a mould or cups for serving. Set on ice, if you have it, till served.

**The Queen of Puddings, With Bread-Crumbs.**—Bread-crumbs, 1 pt.; sweet milk, 1 qt.; the yolks of 4 eggs, well beaten; butter, the size of an egg; sugar, 1 cup; the grated rind of 1 lemon. Mix and bake till done, but not watery; then, having beaten the whites with a cup of white sugar (powdered always for this) to a froth, replace for a few moments to brown. If needed for a dinner-party, it improves the appearance by spreading on the top of the pudding, when taken from the oven, a layer of preserves or jelly and then the sugar and whites of the eggs over the jelly; set it back in the oven and bake slightly, to be served when cold; cut in slices it is very beautiful.

*Remarks.*—Butter and sugar creamed, and the juice of the lemon creamed in, is not amiss when served, especially for the dinner-party. But sifted sugar over it does nicely.

**Cracked-Wheat Pudding.**—Unskimmed sweet milk, 1 qt.; sugar and cracked-wheat, each 1 cup; a bit of cinnamon; stir together and place in an oven of medium heat. When about half done stir in the crust already formed, and leave it to form another, which will be sufficiently brown. Try when it is done by tasting a grain of wheat, which must be very soft. This, served hot or cold with sweetened cream or rich milk, is not only delicious but a very healthful pudding. So is the following, with the same sauce:

**Poor Man's Pudding, Boiled.**—Molasses, water, chopped suet and raisins, each 1 cup; saleratus or soda, 1 tea-spoonful; salt, 1 teaspoonful, and sifted flour to make a stiff batter. Tie in a prepared cloth [see general directions] and boil 2 hours. Of course, it must be put into boiling water and kept boiling all the time. [See last remarks for a sauce.]

**Floating Island Pudding, No. 1 — Very Nice.**—Eggs, 8; sweet milk, 1¼ qts.; sugar, 5 heaping table-spoonsful; vanilla and lemon extracts, or any other two kinds of extracts. DIRECTIONS—Separate the whites, and make a custard of the yolks with 4 spoonfuls of the sugar and the milk, flavored pretty freely with one of the extracts; and when properly made, put into a suitable glass dish and set in a cool place, to be ready for the "floats," to be made with the whites of the eggs and the other spoonful of sugar, and slightly flavored with the other extract, as follows: Beat the whites, with the spoonful of sugar and slight flavor, to a stiff froth; have a shallow pan of water—or milk is best, if you have it—boiling hot when the froth is hot; then, with a wet spoon, take up this white froth and poach (boil the same as poaching eggs, which see) them in the water or milk, turning once to ensure cooking both sides, and when all is poached, carefully place these, the large end outwards (if properly done, they will keep their oblong shape), on top of the yellow custard. Each piece of the "floats" may have a bit of colored jell upon them, if you choose, for ornamentation.

*Remarks.*—You may say, this is too much trouble Of course, it is considerable labor; but you can't have nice things without a certain amount of labor, and as this would only be expected upon occasions of the presence of especial friends, it might be a pleasure to make it; otherwise, take the following, No. 2—the more common plan. If not so large a supply is needed, take half the quantities.

**Floating Island Pudding, No. 2.**—Ingredients and quantities the same as No. 1, lining the dish, however, with strips of cake, pour in the yellow custard, when properly cooked, and place the beaten white froth upon the top, as a whole, and put on a few bits of colored jell, if you like; but if it is in a dish which you can set in the oven 3 or 4 minutes, to slightly brown the frosting, do so before putting on the bits of jell.

**Blanc-Mange, or Substitute for Pudding.**—Sweet milk, 1 qt.; corn-starch, 1 cup; sugar, ½ cup; salt, 1 tea-spoonful. DIRECTIONS—Heat the milk to a boil, and stir in the salt and corn-starch, and boil 10 minutes (in a farina, or rice-kettle), and stir it all the time, so it shall not burn. Remove from the fire, and stir in the sugar and flavoring extract to taste. Pour into cups, and set in a cool place. Eaten cold, with sugar and milk, or powdered sugar, as you prefer, or have.

*Remarks.*—If you want it richer, beat 3 eggs, yolks and whites separately, and stir in the yolks 3 minutes before removing from the fire; and the whites, after removing and stirring in the sugar. It does nicely without the eggs. I have so eaten it many times, with a tea-spoonful or two of sugar dipped on, then pouring over a little milk. Irish moss, gelatine, tapioca, etc., can be used in place of the corn-starch, to make blanc-mange; but this is nice, and the easiest made.

**Quick Pudding, Baked.**— Eggs, 1; sugar, 1 cup; melted butter, 1 table-spoonful; sweet milk, 1 cup; soda, ½ tea-spoonful; flour, 3 cups; bake in a quick oven, about ½ hour, or a little more. Eat with any sauce preferred; or the quickest is, butter, 1, and sugar, 2 spoonfuls, creamed together.

**Strawberry Float No. 3—A Substitute for Pudding.**—Cap and sugar to taste 1 pt. of nice fully ripe strawberries, and set aside one hour; then mash them through a colander; beat the whites of 6 eggs to a stiff froth, and stir into the mashed berries; whip all till the spoon will stand erect in them. Serve with rich cream.—*Good Cheer.*

**Float No. 4, With Corn Starch or Flour.**—"M," of Mason, Mich., in answer to "Kitties'" inquiry in the *Blade* for a float, sends the following, which she says is simple and easy to make and good—very desirable points: "Take 2 pts. sweet milk and put in a large spider or saucepan on the stove. When it boils have the whites of 2 eggs beaten to drop in the milk. While they are scalding, beat up the 2 yolks with ½ cupful sugar and 1 table-spoonful corn starch or flour wet with a little cold milk. Take out the whites with a skimmer to drain, and stir in the above mixture. Set away in the cellar until tea-time."

*Remarks.*—Of course, when cold or cool, the whites of the eggs are placed on top of the float. If put into cups or glasses to be ready to serve when cold, the white is cut up and a part placed on each cup. Or, the white may be cut into dice and scattered on top when partially cool; or ripe berries of any kind, or pieces of cake, or lady-finger cakes (which see) may be laid upon the edge of the dish, when it is cooled in a large one, for variety's sake.

**Batter Pudding No. 1, Boiled or Steamed, with Sweet Milk.** —Flour, 1 cup; sweet milk, 1 qt.; eggs, 6; salt, 1 tea-spoonful. DIRECTIONS— Rub the flour smooth with a little of the milk, adding the balance, salt and well-beaten eggs. Turn this into the pudding-cloth and tie tight, leaving room for it to swell one-third. Boil 2 hours; serve with liquid sauce. Great care must be taken in boiling puddings to have the water boiling when you put the pudding in and to keep it boiling all the time. Steaming is the safer way.

Always keep a kettle of boiling water to fill up as it boils away from the pudding. For a pudding-cloth get ¾ of a yard of white drilling. Keep an old saucer in the bottom of the kettle to save the pudding from burning.—*Christian Union.*

*Remarks.*—Steaming is not only the safer way, but it is, of late, much the more common way, and no doubt, much the most healthful way, Any of the sweet sauces, heretofore given, will be nice for this or any of the following batter puddings, unless otherwise directed.

**Batter Pudding No. 2, with Sour Cream, Baked.**—Sour cream, flour, and sweet milk, each, 1 cup; eggs,3; a little salt, and soda, ⅔ tea-spoonful. DIRECTIONS—First rub the flour smooth with the cream, then add the milk and the well-beaten eggs, salt and soda, and bake in a quick oven. To be eaten with highly sweetened cream or milk to make up for the absence of sugar in the pudding.

**Batter Pudding, No. 3, with Sweet Cream, Baked.**—Sweet cream, ½ cup; sweet milk, 1 cup; eggs, 2; flour, 4 table-spoonfuls; butter, 1 table-spoonful; sugar, 1 cup; 1 lemon. DIRECTIONS—Work the same as the last above, grating in the yellow rind of half the lemon, and putting in half the juice, saving the other half for flavoring the butter and sugar, to be creamed to serve it with; bake in a moderate oven.

**Fruit Batter Pudding, No. 4, with Sour Milk, Baked or Boiled.**—Sour milk and sugar, each 1 cup; flour, 1 pt. (1¾ cups); cream tartar, 1 tea-spoonful; soda, ½ tea-spoonful; home-made dried fruit, English currants or raisins, as most convenient, or preferred, 1½ cups; eggs, 2, well beaten; a little salt and the flavoring extract preferred, 1 table-spoonful. Bake in a moderate oven ¾ to 1 hour, or boil in a mould, cloth, or tin pail, covered, 3 hours. To be eaten with cream and sugar, maple syrup, or any other sauce preferred.

**Batter Pudding, No. 5, Without Milk or Sugar, Except in the Sauce, Baked.**—Flour, 1 cup; eggs, 3; a little salt, and soda, 1 tea-spoonful; mix on general principles. Bake in a reasonably hot oven, and serve with the following:

*Sauce for Same, or Any Other Pudding.*—A table-spoonful of flour rubbed smooth in a little cold milk; pour it into 1 cup of boiling milk, having sugar, 1 cup, rubbed well with butter, ½ cup, and as soon as the milk comes to a boil again put in the creamed sugar and butter, and continue to boil 2 or 3 minutes only, and serve, both pudding and sauce, hot.

**Batter Pudding, No. 6, Rich with Sweet Milk and Eggs.**—Sweet rich milk, 1 qt.; eggs, 8, beaten separately, very light; flour, sifted, 12 table spoonfuls; a little salt. Beat the batter perfectly smooth, and bake in a quick oven, and serve immediately, with butter and sugar creamed, and flavored to suit each maker's taste, or preference.

**Batter Pudding, Extra, No. 7, with Pork and Raisins, Steamed.**—Sifted flour, 3 cups; sweet milk, 2 cups; chopped raisins, 1 cup;

molasses, ½ cup; chopped, fat, salt pork, ⅔ of a cup; soda, 2 tea-spoonfuls. Steam 3 hours.   Serve with any sweet sauce, dipped on freely.—*Fostoria Review.*

*Remarks.*—I have found their "domestic recipes" reliable every time, which is more than can be said for many newspapers; but I know the value, or worth- lessness of a recipe, for the last 15 years, as quickly as I read it; hence blame the author if the recipes he gives fail in any case.

**Suet Pudding, No. 1, with Sour Milk, Splendid, Steamed.** —Julia M. M. writes to the *Western Rural,* as follows, upon the suet pudding question; and as ladies make all their explanations before they give the recipe, I will let her speak for herself, simply saying she headed it, "Splendid Suet Pudding," and then proceeded by saying: "Our suet pudding for dinner was so very nice, and gave such general satisfaction, that I send the recipe for the benefit of my *Rural* sisters, as it may be new to some of them.   It is particu- larly nice and convenient for house-keepers, as it will keep nicely a month or two in a cool, dry cellar in earthen jars or a tin box, and a part of it may be sliced off and steamed from time to time, as needed—when, with suitable sauce, it will be found as good as when newly made.   Take suet, chopped fine; rais- ins, chopped; syrup and sour milk, each 1 cup; English currants (of course washed and picked over, to free them from dirt and little gravel stones), ½ cup; soda, 2 even tea-spoonfuls.   Mix the suet, raisins and currants well into the syrup; then add the sour milk, next the soda, pulverized and well mixed in a handful of dry flour.   Stir until it begins to foam; then add flour enough to form a stiff batter.   Steam 1½ hours.   For a large family double the quan- tity, and steam 2 hours.   Serve hot, with the following:

*Sauce, Lemon, for Same.*—Butter and sugar, ½ cup, each; beat these together with flour, 1 heaping table-spoonful.   Pour into it, a little at a time, stirring all the while, boiling water, 1 pt., and let it simmer on the stove a few minutes.   Add lemon extract, 1 tea-spoonful, and the juice of 1 lemon.   Or the following:

*Lemon Sauce for Any Pudding.*—One large cup of sugar; nearly ½ cup of butter; 1 egg; 1 lemon, all the juice and half the grated peel; 1 tea-spoonful nutmeg; 3 table-spoonfuls boiling water.   DIRECTIONS—Cream the butter and sugar, and beat in the egg whipped light; the lemon and nutmeg.   Beat hard 10 minutes, and add a spoonful at a time the boiling water.   Put in a tin pail, and set within, or upon, the uncovered top of the kettle, which you must keep boiling, until the steam heats the sauce very hot, but not to boiling.   Stir con- stantly.

*Remarks.*—I see this is modified, slightly, from one of Mrs. Harland's, in "Common Sense in the Household," still it will be found a very nice sauce, for any pudding,

The principles given by "Julia" are all correct, but most people use twice as much sugar as butter in making sauces.   Cooks can suit themselves. See "Hunter's Pudding" for corroboration as to the keeping properties of this or any pudding which has plenty of these dry fruits in them and are made with a "stiff" batter, when well covered and kept in a dry, cool cellar, or other cool place,

### Suet Pudding, No. 2, With Sweet Milk and Crackers, Baked.

—Suet, chopped fine and freed from strings (to skin the membrane of the suet is to "free it from strings;" see the first, or "English Plum Pudding," and the remarks following it, as to "skinning" suet to save time), ½ cup; fine cracker-crumbs, 1 cup; sugar, 3 table-spoonfuls; eggs, 3; sweet milk, 3 cups; salt, 1 tea-spoonful. DIRECTIONS—Beat the yolks with the sugar: add to them the cracker and milk; then the suet; whip the whites and add lastly, leaving out the white of one to whip for the frosting; bake about 1 hour; make the frosting by beating, and adding 1 table-spoonful of powdered sugar; spread your frosting on when the pudding is baked; set it back in the oven to give it a brown, watching closely; and, before sending it to the table, ornament with dots of currant jelly.—*Letters of Experience.*

*Remarks.*—"Experience" is necessary to do things well. The author, when he began his work of making "receipt books," had great difficulties to overcome; but twenty years of experience enables him to tell at a glance now what formerly would take a long time, and often several tests to accomplish. Stick to your life-work as I have to mine, and 99 in every 100 will succeed as I have done. See, also, "Plum Puddings," which are generally made with suet, in place of other shortenings.

### Stale Bread Pudding, With or Without Fruit.

—Stale bread (dry bread or hard crusts), grated, 2 qts.; eggs, 5; sugar, raisins and English currants, each 1 cup; butter, ½ cup; spices to suit. DIRECTIONS—Soak the bread in water sufficient to cover it (milk is much better); whip the eggs, then the sugar into them; pick over the raisins, mash and look over the currants, melt the butter, and mix all nicely together, having mashed the bread-crumbs into a pulp; and if not sufficiently moist, add a little more water or milk, whichever you are using, to make a suitable batter. Having lined the pudding-dish with a nice crust, pour in the mixture and put a thin crust over of the same; bake in a moderate oven about 1 hour; serve with any of the "sweet sauces" preferred.

*Remarks.*—Home-made dried fruit may take the place of the foreign kinds, remembering that home-dried currants require double the amount of sugar. If no fruit is used, you will still have a nice pudding. And if you cut prunes in bits from the "pit," you also have a nice pudding.

### Bread Pudding, Aunt Rachel's.

—"Aunt Rachel," in the *Rural New Yorker*, says: "A pudding may be made of small pieces of bread, if the family taste does not rebel. [I never see the family taste rebel against so good a pudding.] The bread should be broken fine, covered with milk, and set on the stove where it is not too hot, until it becomes soft. Remove and stir in a table-spoonful of sugar, 1 of butter, a small tea-spoonful of salt, also a pinch of cinnamon, or allspice, and, if liked, ½ cup of chopped or cut raisins, or dried raspberries. When cool enough, stir in an egg, well beaten, and bake 1 hour in a moderate oven. To be eaten with cream and sugar, or pudding-sauce, as preferred"

*Remarks.*—This is like what my wife used to make, except she used to put the raisins in whole, to which I should never object; nor did I, as above remarked, "ever see the family taste rebel against it."

"Aunt Rachel" adds: "I knew a lady who kept all the broken pieces of bread in a bag, that was hung where they would dry and not mold, and she had the material for a pudding always at hand. The price of flour and cost of living would determine whether such economies would pay." It would pay, unless it may be for farmers, who raise their own wheat and have fowls to feed the broken pieces of bread to.

**Quick Pudding.**—When hurried, butter a pudding-dish well, and put in a layer of stoned raisins, cut into halves; then fill up with small bread-crumbs, or rolled crackers; beat an egg, and add a little milk, a pinch of salt and a spoonful of sugar; stir well and pour over the crumbs and bake in a moderate oven. Turn out upon a plate just at time of serving.

**Honey Pudding.**—Best honey, ½ lb., with 6 ozs. butter, to a cream, and stir in a cup of bread-crumbs; beat the yolks of 8 eggs, then beat all together for 10 minutes; pour in suitable dish to set in water and boil, or steam, 1½ hours. Make a sauce with arrowroot or corn starch, and flavor with extract of orange.

**Blackberry Pudding, Baked or Boiled, and a Jelly, or Jam, as Sauce for Same, and a Cordial for the Children.**—A writer in the *Western Rural* gives the following very nice ways of using this delicious fruit in its season. For the pudding: Take nicely ripe blackberries and sweet milk, each 3 pts.; eggs, well beaten, 5; sugar, 1 cup; a little salt: yeast powder (the author would say baking powder, as it acts quicker), 2 tea-spoonfuls, and flour to make a suitable batter to handle with a spoon, if to be baked; and as stiff as can be worked if to be boiled. To be eaten with any sauce, or the following jelly or jam:

*For the Jelly.*—Place perfectly ripe blackberries in a porcelain kettle with just water enough to keep from burning, stirring often, over a slow fire, until thoroughly scalded; then strain or drain through a jelly-bag, the berries having been well mashed by the stirring in scalding—twice through, if necessary to make it clear;—measure, and put the juice on the stove and boil briskly 10 minutes; then add equal measures of nice white sugar, and continue to boil until a bit of it dropped into a glass of very cold water sinks at once to the bottom, instead of dissolving much in the water, when it is done, and makes a splendid sauce for the pudding.

*For the Jam.*—To each pound of the berries put, for present use, half as much light brown sugar, and boil to thoroughly cook the fruit, and use as sauce for the pudding; but for longer keeping, for winter use, use berries and sugar equal weights, and cook carefully 1 hour, stirring constantly to avoid burning. It is a cheap and excellent preserve, of which the children are very fond; and it is valuable for the younger ones having the least tendency to bowel complaints, and may be given half-and-half with the cordial, flavored highly with cinnamon, of which most children are very fond.

*For the Cordial.*—Take the very ripest blackberries, mash them in a suitable tub or pail, pressing out the juice through a stout piece of muslin: and to each quart put 1 lb. of best loaf or lump sugar, also in a porcelain kettle, pouring on the juice, and as soon as softened place on the stove and boil to a thin jelly only; and when cold add brandy, ½ pt. to each pound of sugar used. If this is to be given to very young children, the jelly may be used in place of the jam, in equal parts, thus avoiding the seeds. For a child of 2 to 5 years, put 2 or 3 table-spoonfuls of each into a glass with a tea-spoonful of essence or extract of cinnamon, mixing thoroughly, and giving a tea to a table-spoonful of it as often as they like, or every half hour until relieved.

*Remarks..*—This shows the great value and variety of ways in which the blackberry may be used. (See also the Blackberry Cordial in the Medical Department.)

**Whortle (Huckle) Berry Pudding, Boiled.**—Eggs, 4, well beaten; sweet milk, 1 pt.; salt, 1 tea-spoonful; nicely assorted and fully ripe whortle-berries, 3 pts; stir all well together, then stir in sifted flour to make a stiff batter, tie tightly in a properly prepared pudding-cloth, mold or dish, and boil or steam 2 hours. To be served with any sweet sauce, or sugar and butter creamed.

**Beefsteak Pudding, Boiled.** — Cut into small pieces tender, round beefsteak, 2 lbs.; season with a little salt and pepper; celery, or celery salt (an article now in the market), and summer savory, each, 1 tea-spoonful; a few sprigs of parsley, if you have it, chopped, and if you use fresh celery, chop it, too; and 1 small onion, chopped very fine (if you tolerate them at all); mix the seasoning well together; having lined the pudding dish with a crust or paste, as directed below, put on a layer of the steak, and sprinkle on some of the seasoning, and so fill in all with alternate layers of steak and seasoning; then dip over with a spoon sufficient hot water, and cover in with a top crust, and lay upon this a buttered paper, covered with a suitable plate; stand it in a basin of boiling water and let it continue to boil 2 hours; then remove the plate and paper, and set in a hot oven a few minutes to brown. Sufficient for 5 or 6 persons.

*For the Paste.*—Flour, 1½ cups; salt, ½ tea-spoonful; eggs, 1; butter, or what is better for this paste for meat, beef, or other drippings, 2 table-spoonfuls; water, about ¼ cup, to properly wet up the flour.

**Meat and Rusk, or Bread Crumb Pudding, Baked.**—Chop any kind of cold meat, with an equal amount of cold salt pork, or better still, season it well with butter, pepper and salt, and add 2 or 3 beaten eggs. Then put into the buttered dish a layer of rusk, or bread crumbs; wet with milk; or in place of these, cold boiled rice, or hominy, and so fill in, in alternate layers; crumbs, or rice, or hominy being first and last; cover with a plate, and bake ¾ of an hour; remove the plate to brown the top, and serve hot, in place of other meat. (See also Potato Pudding, No. 2, below.)

**Potato Pudding, No. 1, Baked.**—Large mealy potatoes, 6; eggs, 6; sugar, 2 cups; butter, 1 cup; flour, ½ cup; milk, or if you have it, cream, 1 pt.; 1 lemon, and a little salt. DIRECTIONS—Boil, or steam, the potatoes and mash nicely, stirring in the yolks of the eggs; beat the whites to a froth and stir in the sugar, flour, milk, or cream, the grated rind of the lemon, and salt; squeeze out the juice, and stir all together, and bake about 1½ hours. Sugar and cream, or sugar and butter sauce. **Very nice.**

**Potato Pudding, No. 2, with Meat or Fish, Baked.**—Steam and mash mealy potatoes, and season with butter, cream, salt and pepper, or for eating, butter; butter the dish and place a layer of the potatoes on the bottom; then, having finely chopped meat, or finely picked fish, put a layer of the one used, and so on alternating, finishing with a layer of bread or cracker crumbs, with a few bits of butter and a little water, or milk to moisten, at last; cover, till nearly done, with a paper, and bake about 1 hour. If fish is used stir into it a beaten egg. " Very nice " does not express the full parts.

**Sweet Potato Pudding.**—A writer in the *Blade Household* gives us the following ingredients: Buy sweet potatoes, 2 lbs. (they are sold by the pound now almost wholly); brown sugar, ½ lb.; butter, ¼ lb.; cream, 1 gill (¼ pt.); 1 grated nutmeg; a small piece of lemon peel; eggs, 4; flour, 1 table-spoonful. DIRECTIONS—Boil the potatoes well and mash thoroughly, passing it through a colander; and while it is yet warm mix in sugar and butter; beat the eggs and mix in when cool, with the flour, grated lemon peel, nutmeg, etc., very thoroughly; butter the pan and bake 25 minutes in a moderately hot oven. May be eaten with wine sauce. I would say yes, or any other sauce, and still be good, very good.

**Indian Pudding, No. 1, Baked.**—This pudding was made at the Cataract House, Niagara Falls, by Mrs. Polk, for thirty-six successive seasons: One quart of milk put on to boil; 1 cup of meal, stirred up with about a cup of cold milk; a piece of butter, about the size of an egg, stirred into the hot milk, and let boil; beat 6 eggs, or less, with 1 cup of powdered sugar, and add a tea-spoonful of ginger and nutmeg; then stir the whole together, and have it thick enough to pour into the dish, buttered. Bake in a quick oven.

*Sauce for Same.*—One cup powdered sugar; ½ cup butter, beaten to a cream. Flavor with nutmeg and a little wine or brandy, to taste.

*Remarks.*—Myself and family spent several days at the above hotel, in 1874, where we were so well pleased with this pudding—as has always been my custom, in my travels, if I found some particularly nice dish upon the table—I made an effort (through the waiter) to obtain the recipe, and, by " oiling the machinery," at both ends of the route—paying waiter and cook—I succeeded. I have given it word for word as dictated by Mrs. Polk (colored), who was highly gratified because we were so much pleased with her pudding, assuring us she " had made it in the same house for thirty-six seasons, without missing one." The family having made it many times since, I can, therefore, assure every one " it is genuine," and very nice indeed. Coarse meal is considered better than fine for baked puddings; and if the milk is rich by stirring in the cream so much the better. They are made without eggs, molasses taking the place of sugar, as No. 2.

**Indian Pudding, No. 2, Without Eggs, Baked.**—Indian meal, 1 cup; butter, or lard, 2 table-spoonfuls; molasses, 1 cup; salt, ½ tea-spoonful; cinnamon, or ginger, as preferred, 1 tea-spoonful; mix all these nicely, and pour in boiling milk, 1 qt., mixing thoroughly, and put into a buttered dish; and when ready to set in the oven stir in cold water, 1 cup; bake ¾ to 1 hour.

*Remarks.*—The water, it is claimed, gives the same lightness as the eggs—certainly it can not give the same richness.

**Indian Pudding No. 3, Old-Fashioned, Baked.** — Scald milk, 1 pt., and pour it upon Indian meal, 1 cup; add a beaten egg; molasses, ⅔ cup; salt and cinnamon, to taste; add cold milk, 1 pt., and bake about 2 hours, stirring 2 or 3 times while baking to make it wheyey.

*Remarks.*—This, it will be seen, has more meal in proportion to the milk, and consequently is not quite so much of a custard, but more of a pudding—the more eggs and milk, the more they are like custards.

**Indian Pudding No. 4, Steamed.**—Sour milk, 2 cups; Indian meal, 1½ cups; wheat flour, 2 cups; soda, 1 tea-spoonful, dissolved in a little of the milk; a little salt, and chopped raisins, ½ cup. Mix all, and steam 2 hours. To be eaten with any sauce preferred.

**Indian Pudding No. 5, With Sweet Apples, Baked.**—Sweet milk, 2 qts.; scald 1 qt., and stir in Indian meal, 10 rounding table-spoonfuls; molasses, ½ cup; salt, 1 tea-spoonful; then stir in chopped sweet apples, 1 cup, and bake 3 hours in a moderate oven.

**Corn Starch Pudding.**—Sweet milk, 1 qt.; corn starch 4 table-spoonfuls, nicely rounding; eggs, 5; sugar, 1½ cups; ½ grated nutmeg, or other flavor to suit. DIRECTIONS—Put the milk in a suitable dish to set in water to boil (it is always safer to boil milk in this way); when it boils stir in the beaten yolks, corn starch, 1 cup of the sugar, and flavor, and continue the heat to cook the starch; then put into the baking dish and set in the oven 15 or 20 minutes, having the whites beaten with the ½ cup of sugar, and a little flavor if desired; put on top and brown nicely.

**Cream Pudding.**—Stir together 1 pt. of cream, 3 ozs. of sugar, the yolks of 3 eggs, a little grated nutmeg, add the well-beaten whites, stir lightly, and pour into a buttered pie-plate, on which has been sprinkled the crumbs of stale bread to the thickness of an ordinary crust; and over the top also sprinkle a layer of the grated crumbs, and bake. Very nice. (See also cream pies.)

*Remarks.*—And now, it appears to the author, that with about sixty recipes for puddings—a different one for each Sunday in the year, Fourth of July, and Christmas, too,—some very rich, and others plain, there need be no family which can not select one to suit special occasions, as the visits of friends, holidays, etc., and also such as shall meet the demands, with plain puddings in places where the richer materials are not to be had, or when, although everything might be obtained, yet, the pocket-book does not allow it, or the health, or rather, the want of health, will not allow rich food. Every condition as well as desire can be met satisfactorily. So we will next see what we can do in the line of pies.

# PIES.

**PIES. —The Pie of Our Fathers—Minced Pie.**—*General Remarks.*
—Any pie, to be good, ought to have a light and flaky crust, or "pastry," as more recently called, and the filling should be put in sufficiently thick to remove all suspicion of stinginess on the part of the maker, both of which points are most eloquently brought out in the following communication of Jennie June's, to the *Baltimore American,* written more particularly as a defence of the minced pie, or "the pie of our fathers," as she calls it, against which so much has not only been said, but written. It is so rich in thought, eloquent in argument, and correct in its principles of instruction, it is worthy of a perusal, at least on Christmas occasions, by all lovers of minced pie, who have not "abused their stomachs," as she puts it, "until they have become dyspeptics." Such persons may feel grieved that they cannot allow themselves to indulge in this luxury any more, but they should have been reasonable in an earlier day, then they would not feel a necessity for complaint. Some writers claim that minced pies are bad, only, when eaten just before retiring. Such a plan with any food, to be made a habit of, is bad. The stomach needs, and must have rest, as well as the body, or it will sooner or later make a complaint, never to be forgotten. She says:

"I feel moved to say a word in defense of not only the pie in general, but the pie in particular—the symbolic *mince pie,* which the people who have abused their stomachs until they have become dyspeptics unite in abusing. The mince pie is a very ancient institution, and the only pie that has religious significance. The hollow crust represents the manger in which the Savior was laid; its rich interior, the good things brought by the wise men as offerings and laid at His feet. A good mince pie is not only better for digestion than a poor one but it has a representative character of its own—it symbolizes our love and devotion to the divine principle to which the Christmas festival is consecrated. Mince pies should be prepared with a due sense of their character and importance. They should not be eaten often; but they should be well-made of fine and abundant materials, and, when served, received with due regard and given the place of honor. Thin layers of impoverished mince, inclosed in flat, ceramic (hard, like earthenware) crust, are *not* mince pies; they are the small-souled housekeepers substitute for the genuine article. The true mince pie is made in a brown or yellow earthen platter, is filled an *inch thick* with a juicy, aromatic compound, whose fragrance rises like incense the moment heat is applied to it, and it comes out the golden brown of a russet which has been kissed by the sun. No common or nerveless hand should be allowed to prepare or mix the ingredients for this sum of all pastry. Every separate article should be cut, cleansed, chopped, sifted, with strong but reverent touch, and the blending should be effected with the sweetest piece of the apples, reduced by boiling with the sirup of the maple and sacramental wine. Thus the spices of the East, the woods of the North, the sweetness of the South, and the fruit of the West is laid under tribute, and the result, if properly compounded, is a pie that deserves the esteem in which it was held in ancient times, and does credit to the skill of our foremothers, who brought it to its present state of perfection and to the good judgment of our forefathers, who appreciated and ate it. Let us defend and sustain one of our time-honored institutions against the attack of a weak and effete generation, which, having demoralized itself by indulgence in many more obnoxious pleasures of the table, makes the "pie" the scapegoat, and especially the "mince pie," which, when deserving of its name, is a revelation of culinary art—a kitchen symphony—deserving the respect and consideration of all who understand and appreciate a combination and growth which has achieved the highest possible result."

**Pastry, or Crust, No. 1, for Minced and all other Pies.**—As it is of the utmost importance to have a light and flaky crust for minced pies, as well as all others, I will give two or three plans of making. The first is the celebrated Soyer's Receipt given by "Shirly Dare," in the *Blade Household;* and, although it is some labor to make it, it will pay to follow it whenever a very nice, flaky crust is desirable. It is as follows:

"To every quart of sifted flour allow the yolk of 1 egg, the juice of 1 lemon, 1 saltspoonful of salt, and 1 lb. of fresh butter. Make a hole in the flour, in which put the beaten egg, the lemon and salt, and mix the whole with *ice water* (*very cold* water will do) into a soft paste. Roll it out, put the butter, which should have all the buttermilk thoroughly worked out of it, on the paste, and fold the edges over so as to cover it. Roll it out to the thickness of a quarter of an inch; fold over one-third and roll, fold over the other third and roll, always rolling one way. Place it with the ends toward you, repeat the turns and rolls as before twice. Flour a baking sheet, put the paste in it on ice or in some very cool place half an hour, roll twice more as before; chill again for a quarter of an hour; give it two more rolls and it is ready for use.

"This is very rich paste, and may be made with *half* the quantity of butter only, chopped fine in the flour, rolled and chilled, forming a very light puff paste that will rise an inch, and be flaky throughout."

*Remarks.*—The object of chilling the pastry, by putting it upon ice or into a cold place, is to keep the butter cold, so it shall not be absorbed into the crust, but keep its buttery form, which makes it flaky, by keeping the dough in layers, while the many foldings and rolling out makes them thin, like flakes of snow. But it is only in *hot* weather that this chilling becomes necessary, and not then, unless you desire it to be flaky. In making pie by the last paragraph above, using only ½ lb. of butter to 1 qt. of flour, for common use, the lemon juice, and egg too, may be left out, using the salt however. Still the yolk of an egg gives some richness, but more especially a richness of *color*. And even *half* lard, or "drippings" may be used, as indicated at the close of the 1st receipt below, and be good enough for all common purposes, using the egg, or not, as you choose.

It has always seemed to me, however, that pie-crust ought to have soda or baking-bowder in it to make it light; and to be certain about it, I have just called on one of our best bakers in the city and asked him about it. He tells me that some bakers keep flour, sifted with baking-powder or soda, ready for use; and, in making crust, they take one-fourth of the amount of flour to be used from that having the baking-powder or soda in it, to make the crust rise a little, and help to prevent any soggyness from using a juicy pie-mixture;

but he says it depends more upon the heat on the bottom, or rather from the want of a proper heat at the bottom of many stoves. With the uniform heat of the bottom of a baker's brick-oven they have no trouble, generally, in baking the bottom crust so it is done, and hence not soggy. To do this in a stove-oven, move the pie occasionally to another part of the oven, where the heat has not been absorbed or used up in heating the plate or tin—in other words, see that the bottom of the oven is kept as hot as it ought to be, and you have no soggy or under-done crusts. Pies, not to be eaten the day they are baked, should be baked harder than those for immediate use, to prevent the absorption of the juice of the pie or dampness from the air.

This baker also gave me the following as the best glaze to prevent the escape of the juices of very moist pies, as apple, peach, pie-plant, etc., of any thing that can be used.

**Pie-Crust Glaze—To Prevent Escape of Juices.**—Dust flour all around the outer edge of the crust, after the mixture is put in; then wet this completely, with a brush or otherwise, before laying on the top crust, and pinch together, and no juice can possibly escape; but if any place is not wet, there the juice will escape. He thinks it far preferable to the white of an egg or anything he knows. Bakers keep a small soft-haired brush for this purpose. But I guess the women will find a way to do it, even if they tie a bit of cloth on a stick, and keep it for that purpose. However, I will guarantee that to wet up a little flour into a rather thick, smooth paste, and apply a little of it with the swab, finger, or brush, will do the same thing, in less time and with greater certainty of touching every part, than by using the dry flour and depending on wetting every part of it—this much for the Doctor's inventive genius. I believe, also, this glaze will be just as nice, or nicer even, than the egg, to have a light coat of it put over the crust of minced or other juicy pies, as named above, and allow it to dry a minute or two in the oven or to stand a few minutes upon the table, before putting in the pie-mixture, to prevent the under-crust from becoming soggy by absorbing the juices before the baking is completed. We use the word pastry as synonymous, or meaning the same as pie-crust, probably from the fact that these mixtures, in an early day, were baked in a crust, or paste, without a dish or tin, and were called "pasties," or "pasty"—like paste—on the same principle that we now make turn-over pies, frying in hot fat; as Shakespeare says: "If you pinch me like a pasty," etc. So "pinching" is the thing to do, to prevent the escape of any of the mixture or juice from the swelling or puffiness, caused by the necessary heat to bake the pie properly.

**Cream Pastry or Pie-Crust, No. 2.**—This is the most healthy pie-crust that is made. Take cream, sour or sweet; add salt, and stir in flour to make it stiff; if the cream is sour add saleratus in proportion of one teaspoonful to a pint; if sweet, use very little saleratus.

*Remarks.*—Soda will do very well in place of the saleratus, when that is not to be obtained.

**Pea Pie-Crust, No. 3.**—Stew the split peas as for dinner. Strain through a colander or coarse sieve. Then add equal parts good wheat meal (sifted Graham will do nicely) and fine corn meal sufficient to make a soft dough. Knead well for fifteen minutes, adding mixed meal enough to make a moderately stiff dough, then roll out and use as any other pie-crust. As it cooks very quickly, it is not best to put in for a filling, any fruit that requires long cooking.

*Remarks.*—This is undoubtedly of German origin, as they make great use of the split pea soup, etc. But you may be assured of its healthfulness, for the Germans, with their plain cookery and hard labor manage to be healthy and long-lived people.

**Baking the Pastry Before Putting in the Pie Material.** —It has always seemed to the author that to bake the under crust before putting in any juicy pie, as mince, custard, lemon, etc., as it will be seen in the cream pie, No. 1., below, would ensure a light and more healthy crust, by preventing the absorption of the juices, and consequently, a soggy and indigestible crust, which I never eat. I think there is nothing that will pay better in pie making than this, and especially so with any not to be eaten the day they are made. It will take but a few minutes to do it, pricking the crust the same as you would crackers, to prevent their blistering, or puffing up, in some part of them.

**Minced Pies, No. 1.**—Boil a fresh beef's tongue (or very nice tender beef in equal amount, about 3 lbs), remove the skin and roots (any remains of the wind-pipe, blood vessels, etc.) and chop it very fine, when cold; add 1 lb of chopped suet; 2 lbs of stoned raisins; 2 lbs of English currants; 2 lbs of citron, cut in fine pieces; 6 cloves, powdered (½ teaspoonful powdered cloves); 2 teaspoonsful of cinnamon; ½ teaspoonful of powdered mace; 1 pt. of brandy; 1 pt. of wine, or cider; 2 lbs of sugar; mix well and put into a stone jar and cover well. This will keep some time. When making the pies, chop some tart apples very fine, and to 1 lb of the prepared meat put 2 bowls of the apple; add more sugar if taste requires it, and sweet cider to make the pies juicy, but not thin; mix and warm the ingredients before putting into pie plates. Always bake with an upper and under crust, made as follows:

**Crust.**—Lard, butter and water, each 1 cup; flour, 4 cups.

*Remarks.*—To which I would add, the yolk of an egg and a little salt. As a general thing, I do not think so much brandy and wine are used, and although I do not object to eating, occasionally, of such a pie, yet, as many persons do, they can leave them out, substituting boiled cider—3 to 1—in the place of the brandy or wine; or pure alcohol, ½ pt., would be as strong in spirit, and cost less than half as much, while the difference in taste would not be observed. Each person can now suit themselves and be alone responsible. I will guarantee this much, however, no one will be led into habits of drink from the amount of spirit they will get in a piece of pie thus made—possibly one-fourth of a teaspoonful. Nearly all receipts for minced pies contain wine or brandy; they can be used or left out, as any one shall choose, by using the cider more freely.

**Minced Pie, No. 2, for Ready Use.**—One beef's tongue, suet, and currants, each 1 lb.; raisins (stoned), and citron, each ½ lb.; large tart apples, 8;

juice of 1 lemon; wine, 1 qt.; and spices to taste—cinnamon and cloves are generally used; but it always seemed to the author that black pepper should have a place in them. Sweet cider may take the place of the wine; but boiled cider is better, because there is more spirit in it. Of course, all to be properly chopped, mixed, etc, and put in, at least, half to three-fourths of an inch thick.

**Mock Minced Pies, No. 1, with Bread Crumbs.**—Bread crumbs, sugar, molasses, vinegar, boiling water, raisins, and currants, each 1 cup; butter, ½ cup; spices to taste.

**Mock Minced Pies, No. 2, with Cracker Crumbs.**—Cracker crumbs, sugar, molasses, boiling water, and raisins, each 1 cup; vinegar and butter, each ½ cup; 2 beaten eggs; nutmeg and cinnamon, each 1 tea-spoonful; cloves, ½ tea-spoonful. Either of them will make 3 pies.

*Remarks.*—English currants can be added to this, if desired, or dropped from No. 1, as one may choose. To imitate minced pies, of course, they must have upper as well as under crust. (See Pastry, for making the crust.)

**Mock Minced Pies, No. 3, with Apples.**—Crackers, double handful; tart apples, medium size, 8; raisins, 1 cup; butter and molasses, each ½ cup; ground cinnamon, cloves, and allspice, each 1 tea-spoonful; salt, 1 salt-spoonful; sugar and cider. DIRECTIONS—Roll the crackers; pare, core and chop the apples, melt the butter, and mix all, using cider to make sufficiently moist, and if the cider is not quite tart, add 1 or 2 table-spoonfuls of vinegar, with sugar enough to give the requisite sweetness, which each must judge for himself, as tastes vary so much.

*Remarks.*—The apples give these pies a much greater resemblance to the real, than as formerly made without apples. If they are made with a light biscuit crust, which is made with at least 1 tea-spoonful of baking powder; then wetting the bottom crust with the beaten white of an egg before the mixture is put in, even the dyspeptic may eat them, if he can eat ordinary food. They are healthful, as well as very palatable. Give the author the one with the apples when he calls upon you.

**Lemon Pie, Quickly Made.**—One lemon; melted butter, 1 table-spoonful; water, 6 table-spoonfuls; corn starch, 1 table-spoonful (flour will do, but not quite so good); eggs, 2; sugar, 6 table-spoonfuls. DIRECTIONS—Grate off the yellow, or zest of the lemon, as it is called—peel off the white part and throw it away—then grate up the pulp, if you have a coarse grater, or chop it fine having picked out the seeds. Put starch or flour in the water, and stir as for gravies; then stir in the melted butter and 3 spoonfuls of the sugar, and the beaten yolks of the eggs with the grated yellow and pulp of the lemon. Make with one crust only, and when baked properly, having beaten the whites of the eggs with the balance of the sugar for frosting, put it on and give it a nice brown. Powdered sugar is the best for frosting.

*Remarks.*—The advantage of this pie is it can be made in a hurry, as it is all made cold, except the butter. Lemon pies are quite often made with flour in place of the corn starch.

**Lemon Custard Pie, Extra.**—Sweet milk, 1 pt.; 3 eggs; 1 lemon; ⅔ cup of sugar. DIRECTIONS--Mix the beaten eggs, sugar and milk together, as for a custard; remove spots, stem, and flower end from the lemon, and chop perfectly fine, and stir into the custard, and bake at once.—*Mrs. Eastman, Toledo, O.*

*Remarks.*—Having eaten of this pie several times while boarding there, and considering it a very nice custard pie, except in its lemon flavor, I enquired as to using lemons to flavor them without spoiling the custard, and received the above instructions from the lady herself, and can recommend it as an " extra " indeed worthy of all confidence. One lemon gives a nice flavor to 3 pies.

**Lemon and Raisin Pies No. 1.**—Two small lemons, prepared as above; sugar, 1 coffee-cupful; 1 egg; butter, 1 rounding table-spoonful; flour, 3 table-spoonfuls; boiling water, 2½ coffee-cupfuls; raisins, 1 coffee-cupful; a little salt. DIRECTIONS—Stir the flour smooth in a little cold water, and mix all, putting in the beaten egg last, not to scald it. This mades 2 or 3 pies, according to your liberality in filling or size of your plate. Bake with 2 crusts.

**Lemon and Raisin Pies, No. 2.**—Raisins, 1 lb.; 1 lemon, prepared as in the " Extra " above; sugar, 1 cup; flour, 2 table-spoonfuls. DIRECTIONS —Stew the raisins 1 hour, leaving just water enough to cover them; then, having rubbed the flour smooth in a little cold water, mix all and make 3 pies.

*Remarks.*—Either of these may be baked with or without upper crust, as you choose, generally without. We have so many lemon pies we must next have an

**Orange Pie.**—One good-sized orange, grate the rind, and chop or slice the inside, removing the seed; 3 eggs, ½ cup of sugar, 1 cup of milk, 1 heaping table-spoonful of corn starch; no upper crust.—*"Keystone," Bradford, Pa.*

*Remarks.*—The author cannot see why any person who can make as nice a pie as this recipe does should blush by dropping her name and taking an artificial one. So it is with some people. I can tell if the recipes are good as soon as I read them, even if they have no name at all attached to them. Hence I take the best I can find anywhere and everywhere, giving the proper credit, for the good of the many people who have so far patronized "Dr. Chase's Book," not because they were Dr. Chase's, but because they were good. And I will here remark that I have often wondered that I did not see more orange pies, even to the lessening of the lemon. For, if you get nice juicy oranges, the flavor is delicious, and less sugar is required than for lemons. They may be frosted the same as lemon, if desired. What is more delicious than a nice juicy blood orange—certainly there is but one thing which can equal it—a luscious peach.

**Cream Pie, No. 1, Crust Baked First.**—For each pie to be baked take 2 small eggs; sugar, ½ cup; corn starch, 3 table-spoonfuls, or half flour; milk, 1 pt. DIRECTIONS—Make your crust and have it ready baked (pricking with a fork to prevent blistering); put the milk on to boil; beat the yolks of the eggs, stir the corn starch in a little cold water, smoothly; then add sugar, and stir all into the boiling milk, and continue the heat until the custard is set, or thick; then put into the baked crust and bake 15 or 20 minutes, having beaten the whites with 1 tea-spoonful of cream or butter and 2 table-spoonfuls of sugar; spread on top and brown nicely in the oven.—*Henry Crane.*

*Remarks.*—Having eaten of this pie many times, I know it is very nice. The pumpkin pie below is from the same gentleman, and is equally nice of its kind. See, also, "Cream Pudding," which is mixed like a pie:

**Cream Pie, No. 2.**—Sweet cream, 1 cup; sugar, 3 table-spoonfuls; flour, 1 table-spoonful; butter, the size of an egg; a little grated nutmeg, all creamed together; bake like a custard, or put strips of crust across the top.—*Eliza Watts, Croton, Iowa, in Toledo Blade.*

**Boiled Custard Pie.**—"Mrs. B. H. H.," in *Farm and Fireside*, gives the following directions for making: Morning's milk, a qt. Let it simmer—not boil; stir into it sugar, 1 cup; the yolks of 3 eggs; flour, 3 table-spoonfuls, and a little nutmeg. When it becomes thick, pour it into the crusts—which should be previously baked—and when just done spread with frosting made of the whites of the eggs with sugar, 3 table-spoonfuls, with a little nutmeg, and brown slightly. This makes 3 pies.

**Pumpkin Pie.**—Stewed pumpkin, 1 heaping pint; 6 eggs; flour, 6 table-spoonfuls; butter, size of an egg; sugar, 1½ cups; cinnamon, 2 level tea-spoonfuls; ginger, ½ tea-spoonful; ½ a grated nutmeg. DIRECTIONS—Rub the pumpkin through a colander, adding the butter, sugar and spices, and make hot, then the beaten eggs and flour; mix smoothly together, and while hot put into the dish, having a thick crust to receive it, and bake in a moderate oven. —*Henry Crane, Frost House, Eaton Rapids, Mich.*

*Remarks.*—This makes a thick, salvy pie, very nice. If fearful of a soggy crust, bake it before putting in the pie mixture. If a pint of milk was added, it would be more like the old-fashioned pumpkin-custard pie, softer and not quite so rich, unless an additional egg or two, with an extra cup of sugar is put in. If milk is plenty, and pumpkin scarce, take this latter plan.

**Pumpkin and Squash, Best for Pies, Prepared by Baking.** —Ruth H. Armstrong, in the *Housekeeper*, says: If all housekeepers who make pumpkin pies knew how much better and easier it is to bake the pumpkin first, they would no longer worry over cutting up and peeling it, but just cut it in halves, take out the seeds, lay it in the oven and bake until soft, when it can be scraped out and used as usual, and is so much better for not having water in it. Winter squash makes a much richer pie when treated in the same way.

**Squash Pie, Very Rich.**—Stew a medium sized crook-necked (or other equally rich) squash, and rub the soft part through a colander, as for the pumpkin pie, above; butter, ½ lb.; cream and milk, each 1 pt., or milk with the cream stirred in, 1 qt.; sugar, 2 cups; 1 dozen eggs well beaten; salt, mace, nutmeg and cinnamon, 1 tea-spoonful each, or to taste.

*Remarks.*—Of course the mixing and baking, the same as for the pumpkin pie above; and if less is needed for the family keep the same proportions as in that also. I think good squash makes a richer pie than pumpkin, while some persons claim the reverse, and call for an egg or two extra. If a poor quality is used, this would be so; but crook-necked, or Hubbard, are much nicer than pumpkin, both in quality and flavor, and I like this pie much the best, but can get along very nicely even with a good rich pumpkin pie.

**Potato Custard Pie.**—Nicely mashed potatoes, 1½ cups; sugar, 2 cups; milk, 1 qt.; eggs, 5; a little salt, and any flavoring desired. DIRECTIONS —Beat the eggs well, mix all, and dip into the pans made ready with the usual paste, or crust, and bake the same as custard pie.

**Sweet Potato Pie.**—Sweet potatoes make an equally nice pie, for all who, like myself, are fond of them, treated the same as their Irish brethren above.

*Remarks.*—Sweet potatoes make a richer pie than the common potato, as much so as good squash makes a pie richer, in quality and flavor, than common pumpkin; but as the Irish potato keeps the best, a pie can be made of them, after the sweet ones are out of season.

**Apple-Custard Pie.**—Moderately tart apples, stewed, and treated the same as the potatoes, above, make a custard pie, of very excellent flavor; using sugar according to the sourness of the apples, with cinnamon, nutmeg, or other spices as you like, baked with one crust only, in all kinds of custard mixtures. Bars, or strips, as mentioned in cream pie No. 2, above, may be put upon any of them, if one choses to do so. But I think they muss, or mar the pie, in cutting them for the table, hence I think them nicer without bars.

**Apple, Peach, and Other Fruit Pies.**—Pare and slice, ripe, tart apples from the core, or peaches from the pit, for as many pies as you wish to make at one time; line your plates, or tins, with a crust, having a little baking powder or soda in the flour (one-fourth as much only as for biscuit; see remarks following Pastry, No. 1), wetting, or not, as you choose, with the flour paste, to prevent the juices from soaking into the crust; put on a layer of the sliced fruit, and sprinkle over light brown sugar according to the sourness of fruit; then another layer of fruit and sugar, for at least 3 layers, using cinnamon, nutmeg, or any other spices preferred, freely on the last layer, and 2 or 3 spoonfuls of water, unless the fruit is very juicy; cover with a crust secured from the escape of the juices, with the flour wet, and a few ornamental cuts through the top crust; bake in a moderate oven, and you will have a pie "fit for a king," especially so, if you sprinkle freely of powdered sugar over the top before serving. Blackberries, raspberries, strawberries, cranberries, whortleberries, and stoned cherries, in their season, make an equally nice pie, with the same treatment, remembering this, the sourer the fruit the more sugar. But it is important to remember this also, that pies, not to be eaten the day they are baked, ought to be baked a little longer, or harder, than those to be eaten at once, which prevents their absorption of dampness from the air, as well as from the moisture of the pie-mixture. By canning or drying, and stewing when needed, pies from any of the above named fruits may be had at any time of the year.

**Grandmother's Apple Pie.**—Line a deep pie-plate with plain paste. Pare sour apples—greenings are best—and cut in very thin slices. Allow 1 cup of sugar and a quarter of a grated nutmeg mixed with it. Fill the pie-dish heaping full of the sliced apple, sprinkling the sugar between the layers. It will require not less than six good-sized apples. Wet the edges of the pie with cold water, lay on the cover and press down securely that no juice may escape.

Bake three-quarters of an hour, or even less if the apples become tender. It is important that the apples should be well done, but not over-done. No pie in which the apples are stewed beforehand can be compared with this in flavor.

**Chicken and Other Meat Pies.**— According to the number in the family, 1, 2, or more, young and tender chickens, cut up, washed and put into a stew-kettle, with water enough to nicely cover, and a very little salt, and stew till perfectly done, and if pork or small pieces of any cold meats are to be used, stew also with the chicken; when entirely tender, rub a spoon or two of flour smooth, in cold milk or water, and stir in as for gravy; add salt and pepper to taste. Set back on the stove to keep hot while you make the pastry or crust.

**Pastry or Crust.**—If for 1 chicken in a 2 quart basin, or pie dish, use 1 pt. of flour with 1 tea-spoonful of baking powder, and 1 table-spoonful of lard, and a little salt. For a 4 quart or 6 quart dish double the amount of all the articles, and if half butter is used, it will be nicer and require a little less salt. It is designed to have a light, but thick crust when baked. Put the chicken, with its gravy, enough to nicely cover it, into the dish, without a bottom crust; but roll out the pastry of such a thickness as to just cover the dish nicely, cut a few fancy slits through the top, to allow the steam to escape, and place in the oven at once, and bake about 30 minutes, or long enough to cook the crust nicely. Serve hot, with mashed potatoes, made rich with milk and butter, or cream, if you have it. Some put potatoes in the pie, but it is out of fashion, and, thank the Lord, there is one fashion, at least, which is conducive to health, as water-soaked potatoes are not.

Beefsteak, cold roast beef, veal, lamb, prairie hens, and other wild game, may be treated in the same way, with like success; but prairie hens should have the skin removed before cooking. Any meats not tender must be stewed tender, or done, before putting into the pie dish, as you cannot depend on the baking to cook the meats, it would spoil the crust.—*Mrs. Catherine Baldwin, Toledo, Ohio.*

*Remarks.*—Having had my office in this lady's house for about two years, and boarded in the family most of the time, I am able to say, if you follow these instructions, you will have no reason to complain. A closing, word, only, milk, for wetting up pastry, as bread, makes them richer than water, hence use is when you have it plenty, but do not make pastry too soft, but rather stiff.

**Chicken and Ham Pie.**—Season sufficient slices of boiled ham, with pepper and salt, if needed, and put a layer upon the paste, which should be ½ inch thick; then a layer of chicken, which has been jointed and cooked till tender, upon the ham, and also the yolks of some hard-boiled eggs, sliced; a couple layers of each should properly fill the dish; putting in some gravy made with water in which the chicken was boiled, adding, if liked, ½ cup of tomatoes to the gravy; cover with another crust, and bake only to bake the crust; or it may be baked without the gravy, and I think this the better way, the gravy being made to dip upon the pie, and mashed potatoes, with which it is to be served. If no eggs and tomatoes, make it without, and still it will be very nice, if the meats have been cooked tender before putting into the pie.

**Rabbit Pie, Fricasseed and Roast.**—Cut up the rabbit, remove the breast bone and bone the legs. Put the rabbit, a few slices of ham, a few force-meat balls, and 3 hard-boiled eggs, by turns, in layers, and season each with pepper, salt, 2 blades of pounded mace, and ½ tea-spoonful of grated nutmeg. Pour in ½ pt. water, cover with crust, and bake in a well-heated oven for 1½ hours. When done, pour in at the top, through the middle of the crust, a little good gravy, which may be made of the breast and leg bones, flavored with onion, herbs and spices.

*Fricasseed.*—Rabbits, which are in the best condition in midwinter, may be fricasseed like chicken in white or brown sauce.

*To Roast.*—Stuff with a dressing made of bread-crumbs, chopped salt pork, thyme, onion, and pepper and salt, sew up, rub over with a little butter, or pin on it a few slices of salt pork, and a little water in the pan, and baste often. Serve with mashed potatoes and currant jelly.

**Oyster Pie.**—Small oysters, 1½ qts.; cracker crumbs, 1 cup; salt and pepper to suit. DIRECTIONS—Drain the oysters in a colander, and throw away the juice, unless you wish to cook it, seasoning properly and eating it as "soup," with some crackers; there will be juice enough from the oysters. Line the sides of a deep buttered pie-dish with a crust made as for the chicken and other meat pies above; put a layer of the oysters, salt and pepper to suit; then a light sprinkling of the cracker-crumbs, and so fill the dish; put over the top some bits of butter to season nicely, and cover with a crust; bake in a quick oven. As soon as the pastry is done the oysters will be cooked also.

*Remarks.*—By using the juice the pie is made too mushy, or soggy.

**Escaloped Oysters, or Oyster Pie With Crackers.**—Oysters, 1½ qts.; crackers, sufficient; pepper, salt and a little mace. DIRECTIONS—Drain the oysters as above; butter the dish and put a layer of the oysters over the bottom; then, the crackers being thin, butter one side lightly, and place a row of them around the dish in place of a crust; season the oysters, each layer as you go along, then sprinkle on some cracker-crumbs, else split crackers, buttered, does nicely in place of crumbs, and so fill the dish, or until the oysters are all in, putting another tier of crackers up the side, if needed, as you fill up to the top of the first tier, and cover the top with a layer of buttered crackers, putting on the butter pretty freely on the top crackers; which melts down into the dish and makes a crispy cover or crust, without the trouble of making pastry.

*Remarks.*—If this new plan is done carefully you will be pleased with the result. If not, you can take the old crusty, mushy way again; but I know you will not.

**Minced Turn-Over Pies, Fried or Baked.**—For the pastry, or crust, sugar, 1 cup; 2 eggs; butter, ½ the size of an egg; sour milk, 1½ cups; soda and salt, each, 1 teaspoonful; flour. DIRECTIONS—Beat the eggs, butter and sugar together; put the soda into a bowl with a tea-spoonful of water, mash it and dissolve, then pour the milk upon it, and mix all together, stirring in what flour you can with a spoon, then mix with the hands; work in only enough to make a soft dough, as for fried cakes. Cut off a piece as large as a good sized egg, rolling out in round form; then put 2 table-spoonfuls, or a little more, of minced pie meat (which see), which is not very moist. Spread it over one-half only, of the crust, leaving an edge margin of ½ inch; then turn over the other half, and with plenty of flour on the fingers pinch or crimp the edge firmly together, to keep in the juices. Fry in hot lard, turning carefully when one side is done. Take up carefully also, using a knife to assist, lest they fall from the fork, placing them on plates, separately, until cold; but if done just before dinner, at our house, several of them never get cold. If the juice works out while frying the hot lard will sputter and fly around lively; hence, be sure to pinch the edges well together. Bake when you prefer to do so.

*Remarks.*—If the pastry is made as soft as it can be rolled by dusting freely it will be very light, and the turnovers very nice. They are very nice, too, to bake them.

**Apple Turn-Overs, Fried or Baked.**—Dried apples, 1 pt.; raisins, 1 cup; cinnamon and allspice, or nutmeg, each, 1 tea-spoonful. DIRECTIONS— Stew the apples and raisins together, leaving as little water as possible. Mash the apples to a pulp (but I prefer to find the raisins whole), and put in the seasoning. Make the paste and otherwise treat the same as the mince turn-overs. Of course, the apples may be used without the raisins, but they suit me better with them. These, also, may be baked as well as fried, when you choose. Other fruit, as peaches, berries, etc., may be used in the same way.

**Apple Turn-Over Pudding, Baked**—Apples, sugar, butter, nutmeg, a little salt, and pie-paste. DIRECTIONS—Sufficient nice tart apples to fill such a pudding-dish as the family demands; peel, slice and put into the dish, which has been buttered; cover with good pie-paste, and bake in a quick oven. When done, "turn-over" upon a suitable plate, and spread upon the apples 3 or 4 table-spoonfuls of sugar, and butter half the size of an egg, and a pinch of salt, mixing with a spoon a little on the top; then grate on some nutmeg. Serve hot. The sugar, butter, and nutmeg on it form the sauce, but milk or cream passed with it will suit some better. Of course, this may be "turned over" with peaches as well as with apples.

*Remarks.*—Although this is a dish to be "turned-over-upon-a-plate," yet I have placed it here among the "turn-overs" proper, as it makes but little difference where we find or place a good dish. It is nice. I speak from knowledge.

# CAKES.

**CAKE-MAKING, BAKING, ETC.**—*General Remarks and Explanations.*—To make good cake every article used must be good, of its kind—flour, sugar, or molasses, butter or lard, eggs, spices, or flavoring extracts, fruit, cream of tartar and soda, or saleratus, or baking-powder, milk, etc.

But to save repeating the explanation with every cake receipt given (many of which must be very similar, if not absolutely the same), I will make such an explanation in connection with each of the articles mentioned as entering into cake-mixtures that persons can soon familiarize themselves with, all that is necessary, to a full and complete understanding of the whole subject, without the repetition referred to.

**Flour.**—It being understood, then, that all the articles, or material used in making cake shall be good, I need only say: The flour will be the better if put into the oven and thoroughly dried—stirring a few times while drying—then sifted; and if cream of tartar with soda, or baking-powder are to be used, they—or the one to be used—should be stirred into the flour before sifting.

**Sugar and Butter.**—Use your own judgment at to whether white or light brown sugar may be used. For common purposes the light brown will do very well; but if a delicate cake, for any particular occasion, is to be made, use pure white sugar and very nice butter. If sugar is at all lumpy, crush by rolling, then the sugar and butter should always be creamed together, *i. e.*, beaten together until they are completely blended into a mass, much the appearance of cream, hence the word "creamed" has been appropriately applied. And this creaming of the butter and sugar is a very important part of cake-making; for, by this process, the oiliness and consequent indigestibility of the butter is overcome, the cake rises brighter, and is much more healthy and digestible than by rubbing the butter into the flour, which has heretofore been the more usual custom.

In cold weather it may be necessary to place the butter in a warm place a short time to soften—not to melt—to enable the creaming to be properly done.

**Lard and Drippings.**—Neither lard nor drippings are as good as butter, but, for family use, half the amount may be very satisfactorily put in the place of half of the butter named.

**Molasses.**—When molasses is used the cake will scorch quickly if the oven is too hot; hence for these, and for cakes having fruit in them, bake in a moderate oven, especially such as fruit loaf-cakes, they being generally thick, require a longer time for baking. Then, if there is danger of burning the top, in any case, cover with brown paper, until nearly done.

**Eggs.**—Eggs must be fresh and well-beaten; and it is claimed that all cakes are better if the yolks and whites are beaten separately. This may be true, to a certain extent, but my wife who has made cake for me (or seen that it was done as she desired) for over forty years, claims, and I have no doubt of the fact, that the difference, for general use, is not sufficient to pay for the extra trouble; while, for nice cake, for special occasions, it may be best to beat separately.

**Spices** are always to be ground, or very finely pulverized, where the old fashioned mortar is still in use.

**Flavoring Extracts,** kept by dealers may be used, or those made by receipts given in this work, which will be found under proper headings, using only sufficient to obtain a fair flavor of the fruit represented.

**Fruit** requires care in selection, or purchase, and also in its preparation for use.

**Raisins** need to be looked over to free them from any remaining stems, and from small gravel-stones, which are often found among them, then washed drained, dried and floured, and used whole, or they may be seeded and chopped after washing and draining, then rubbed—"dredged"—with flour, which largely prevents them from settling to the bottom of a cake or pudding.

**English Currants** require picking carefully to free them from gravel, dirt, etc., and several careful washings, for the want of proper care in curing. They also require drying and flouring, the same as raisins, for the same reason.

**Home-dried Fruit.**—Currants, raspberries, blackberries, whortle ("huckle") berries, etc., may be substituted for foreign fruit very satisfactorily when desired, or when they are plenty.

**Citron,** when used, is to be "shred," *i. e.*, cut into long narrow strips, or chopped, as preferred. If chopped, however, leave it the size of peas, so that one eating the cake can tell what it is without too close scrutiny.

**Almonds** are to be blanched, *i. e.*, boiling water is to be poured upon them and allowed to stand until the thin skin will rub off easily, then chopped as citron, or pounded finely in rose water—preferably chopped.

**Cream of Tartar and Soda** are always to be stirred into the flour before it is sifted, the same as baking powder. The proportions in using should always be two of the first to one of the latter. They are usually kept in separate boxes and mixed when used, by taking out 2 teaspoons of the cream of tartar to 1 of the bi-carbonate of soda (baking soda), but they may be purchased in quantities of ½ lb. of the cream of tartar to ¼ lb. of the soda (or in these proportions) and all mixed at once, if dry, and kept in an air-tight box in a dry place, and thus you have always ready for use a better baking powder than you can buy.

**Saleratus,** when used, is to be dissolved in a little hot water, or in a little of the milk, by rolling finely on the table or moulding-board before putting 'nto the cup to dissolve. After the same is dissolved, add it to the cake mixture.

**Soda,** when used alone, is to be treated the same as saleratus.

**Baking Powder** should always be mixed into the flour, the same as cream of tartar and soda, before the flour is sifted.

**Milk** is always to be sweet when baking powder, or cream of tatar with soda are to be used. Sour milk or buttermilk when soda, or saleratus only are to be used.

**Making Up or Putting Cake Together.**—The eggs being properly beaten, the flour sifted, the sugar and butter creamed, everything to be used being placed within reach, little by little add the milk to the creamed sugar and butter, stirring constantly, then the yolks of the eggs (when beaten separately), after which the sifted flour, having the proper amount of baking powder, or cream of tartar and soda in it, and then the fruit (if fruit is to be used), spices or flavoring extracts; but, now, if saleratus is being used, it is to be dissolved and stirred in, and lastly the beaten whites of the eggs, stirring but little after these are added; but the more thorough the stirring together, previous to putting in the whites, the better.

**Baking—Heat of the Oven, etc.**—To bake cake nicely, the heat of the oven should be uniform throughout the whole time of baking; and for light, thin cakes (and that covers nearly all, except those having fruit in them) a quick oven is required, so that by the time the cake is properly raised the baking shall commence; for if the heat is not uniform throughout the baking there will be a soggy streak shown in the cake, because if the cooking slackens much the cake begins to "fall," and although the heat may be again raised, yet what has settled together will not rise again; while if you get too great a heat simply cover the cake with brown paper to prevent burning the top, and partly close the damper to prevent too much heat from passing under the bottom; but the oven door must not be left open in cake baking, or else the cake will "fall," the same as if the heat had fallen off for want of fuel. Avoid, as much as possible, also, the moving of cake after it is placed in the oven and has began to rise, as the motion may cause the escape of gas, leaving the cake heavy, and especially is this important with cake containing grated or dessicated cocoanut.

**Pans.**—Pans should always be well buttered, except for thick, or loaf cake, which requires the bottom of the pan to be covered with a buttered piece of white paper, buttering the sides, unless deemed safest to paper the sides also, especially if the cake is a thick fruit cake, and in this case the top must be covered with brown paper until nearly done.

**To Know When a Cake is Done,** pierce it with a clean broom splint. If it comes out free of the cake mixture it is done; but a few minutes more had better be given it than to have it at all under done.

**Hints and Suggestions.**—If attention is given to the above explanations and a moderate degree of experience is brought to bear upon the following recipes, I have no fears of a failure; and those who have not been instructed as they should have been by their mothers,, or those having the care of them in their minority, and now find it necessary to make cake for themselves and their husbands, must begin with the cookies, and other smaller and plainer cakes, lest a failure should too greatly discourage them; and should they fail a few times, take the mottoes, "don't give up the ship," but "try, try again," and ultimate success must follow.

**Special Explanations.**—If any special explanations are needed, they will be given in connection with the recipe.

**Lastly—Keeping Cakes.**—Keep cakes in the cook-room until cool; then wrap and place them in boxes with covers to exclude the air. Jelly cakes, however, had best not be removed from the plates upon which they have been built up, but need to be wrapped and placed in boxes, the same as others, which insures their moisture much longer than if not put away in boxes. Fried cakes, cookies, etc., after becoming cool, may be put into stone jars, and a cloth of several thicknesses be put upon them, pressing it down around the edge, then another cloth over the top of the jar, with a plate upon it will keep them sufficiently moist. It is not best to make large amounts of them at a time. Bread needs the same care to keep it nicely moist.

**Table of Explanations and Comparative Weights and Measures.**—When white sugar is called for, "A," or first-class coffee sugar is intended.

The cup intended to be used is the common sized tea-cup, but if larger amounts are needed for large families, double the number, or use the larger coffee-cup.

1 lb. white sugar equals about 2½ cups; 1 lb. butter, 2 cups; 1 lb. lard, 2 cups; 1 lb. wheat flour, 3½ cups; 1 lb. graham, 3½ cups; 1 lb. Indian meal, 3½ cups.

**Icing, Boiled, for Cakes.**—Powdered sugar, (and this is the right kind to use for all Icings), 2 cups: boiling water, 1 gill; whites of 2 eggs; flavoring to suit. DIRECTIONS—Pour the boiling water upon the sugar in a suitable dish, upon the stove, and boil until it readily creams, then pour this hot upon the beaten whites, and beat till cool, when it is ready to use, the cake being cold, or, at least, cool; add vanilla, lemon, or orange extract, rose or cinnamon water, or essence, a teaspoonful to a tablespoonful, to suit, and dip upon the cake; smoothing, if necessary, with a knife wet in cold water,

**Icing, Boiled, that will not Break.**—White sugar, 1 cup; white of 1 egg; put water enough into the sugar to dissolve it; put it on the fire and let it boil till it will "hair." Beat the white of the egg to a stiff froth; pour the heated sugar on to the froth and stir briskly until cool enough to stay on the cake. The icing should not be applied until the cake is nearly or quite cold. This quantity will frost the tops of two common sized cakess.—*Godey's Lady's Book.*

**Boiled Icing—Quick to Harden.**—To 1 cupful sugar, take 1 egg. Put sugar in pan and a little water over it, and let boil 20 minutes. Beat white of egg stiff and gradually beat boiling sugar into egg. Flavor. Apply to cake quickly, as it soon becomes hard.

**Icing, Old and Confectioner's Plan, or Without Boiling.—** Icing or frosting for cakes was formerly done by beating the whites of eggs to a stiff froth, then beating in white sugar till stiff, or as hard as desired; but if it is not desired to boil it, as above, a better plan is to take the white of 1 egg for each medium-sized cake, and at the rate of ¼ lb. of powdered sugar for each egg to be used; and first, throw in some of the sugar, then begin to beat, and, from time to time, throw in more of the sugar, continuing the beating until the sugar is all in, and the icing of a smooth and firm consistence—nearly or about half an hour will be required: The piece of a lemon or an orange, or any of the extracts, may be used to flavor, allowing sugar extra to absorb it.

*Remarks.*—If beaten together as above, it hardens on a cake quicker than if the eggs were beaten, as of old, before the sugar was added; and if made as thick and as hard as it ought to be with the sugar, one coat will suffice; while in the old way it almost always required two. If in a hurry to have the cake ready, this may be set two or three minutes in a moderate oven to harden,

**Icing to Color Different Shades.—**Any icing may be colored, if desired, a yellow with lemon or orange, and pink with strawberries or cranberries. Grate the yellow of a lemon or orange, squeeze some of the juice upon the gratings, put into a stout muslin and press out the coloring into the icing. Strawberries and cranberries are to be pressed in the same way, or their syrups used. If considerable is used, add powdered sugar to make them thick before stirring in.

**Icing Chocolate for Cakes.** Flavored chocolate, 4 ozs.; whites of 3 eggs; powdered sugar, 20 tea-spoonfuls; corn starch, 4 tea-spoonfuls; extract of vanilla, 2 tea-spoonfuls. DIRECTIONS—Beat the eggs and add the sugar and corn starch, stirring together; then, having grated the chocolate before you began the other work, add it and beat to a smooth paste; then spread it upon the cake, the top layer as smoothly as possible, and place the cake in the oven a moment, turning it around, and the icing will become nice and glossy.

**Icing, Almond.—**Blanched almonds, ½ lb. (for two ordinary cakes), rosewater, sufficient. DIRECTIONS—Rub the almonds to a smooth paste (in a mortar) by adding a little rosewater from time to time to moisten sufficient only to form the paste; and then mix with any of the icings having no other flavor.

**Icing With Gelatine.—**More recently some cooks have been using gelatine in making icings. Where no eggs are to be had it will make a good substitute. For each cake, soak gelatine, 1 tea-spoonful, in cold water, 1 table-spoonful, till soft, or about ½ hour; then pour upon it hot water, 2 table-spoonsful, stir to perfectly dissolve it; then stir in, while warm, pulverized sugar, 1 cup, continuing to stir until perfectly smooth, and spread upon the cake.

**CAKES—Martha's Cake.—***Remarks.*—As my wife's name is Martha, I trust I shall be excused for beginning the cake list of my " Third and Last Receipt Book " with her favorite, especially as it is plain and not expensive, and by little changes, and flavoring, such a variety may be made out of it, as loaf cake, jelly cake, etc. Sugar, 2 cups; butter, 1 cup; 6 eggs; flour, 2 cups; sweet milk, ½ cup; cream of tartar, 2 tea-spoonfuls; soda, 1 tea-spoonful. DIRECTIONS—Familiarize yourself with the general remarks and explanations, at the head of this subject, then you will be able to make any ordinary cake— the articles, and proportions, only being mentioned. I only mention here the different ways this may be flavored, baked, etc.

This may be baked in a loaf, or in jelly cake tins (shallow pans) and, when cold, laid up with fruit jelly spread between the layers, and you may ice the top, or not, as you choose—sometimes with—sometimes without. Sometimes flavor with the juice and grated yellow of a lemon, again with an orange, or the extracts of one or the other, and again without either, being plain. And thus you can have a cake differing from the leopard's skin in this—its spots may be changed, and that as often as you like, giving a great variety of cake without change of composition, except in flavoring, icing, etc., or in not flavoring, or not icing, baking in loaf, or for jell cake, or by baking in patty pans. as you choose, or as occasion may call for. Mrs. Chase occasionally ices them when baked in the little pans, especially so if the icing is being made for large cakes, at the same baking.

**Ribbon Cake.**—I. Sweet milk, ½ cup; butter, ½ cup; 3 eggs, flour, 2 cups; cream of tartar, 1 tea-spoonful; soda, ½ tea-spoonful. DIRECTIONS— Dissolve the soda in the milk: mix the cream of tartar in the flour; beat the eggs, sugar and butter well together; then the milk and flour.

II. Take of the above mixture, 1 cup; molasses, 1 tea-spoonful; cinnamon, cloves, allspice and nutmeg, each ½ tea-spoonful: citron, almonds or walnut meats, each ¼ lb.; raisins and English currants, each ½ cup. DIRECTIONS —Chop the citron, and almond or walnut meats (whichever you prefer to use), dredge the raisins and currants with flour, and mix with the molasses and spices into the cup of batter taken from the first. Use shallow tins for baking, putting in a strip of the white batter lengthwise of the tin; then a strip of the dark beside it, and so cover the tins; thus you have a "marbled cake," which has ribbon-like strips.

*Remarks.*—By leaving out the citron and fruit, and putting into pans, as the marble cake next following, you have another variety of composition for marble cake.

**Marble Cake.**—*Light Part:* White sugar, 3 cups; whites of 6 eggs; butter, ½ cup; flour, 2 cups; sweet milk, ½ cup; baking powder, 2 tea-spoonfuls. *Dark Part:* Yolks of 6 eggs; butter, 1 cup; brown sugar, 3 cups; sweet milk, 1 cup; cinnamon, cloves, allspice and nutmeg, each 1 table-spoonful; flour, 3 cups; baking powder, 3 tea-spoonfuls. DIRECTIONS—Beat the butter, sugar, milk, eggs, and spices together in each part (they will work best if put in in the order named); then mix the baking powder in the flour for each part, stirring in the flour with the baking powder in it last, and one quickly after the other, for when baking powder is used, the cake must be placed into a hot oven as soon as can be done, to insure lightness. Cover the bottom of the pan with the light part, and dip the dark over it, in spots; then level up with the light, and so on till the pan is properly filled, allowing room to raise.

**Marble Cake—Chocolate.**—Make any plain cake and pour out half of it; then, having shaved up 2 table-spoonfuls, or a sufficient amount of chocolate, and dissolved it in as little water as practicable, boil it a minute or two; then mix it with one of the parts, and put into the pan the same as the receipt above.

**Watermelon Cake.**—I. White sugar, 2 cups; butter and sweet milk, each ⅔ cup; whites of 5 eggs; flour, 3 cups; baking powder, 1 tea-spoonful. DIRECTIONS—Beat the eggs, sugar, butter and milk together; put the baking powder into the flour before sifting it in, and mix.

II. Red sugar (kept by confectioners), 1 cup; butter and sweet milk, each ½ cup; flour, 2 cups; baking powder, 1 tea-spoonful; whites of five eggs: raisins (nice large ones), ½ lb. DIRECTIONS—Beat together in the same order as the first, cut the raisins into halves, the longest way, and mix in last; then put some of the first into the pan, hollowing it in the center to receive all of the second or red part, if it is sufficiently stiff to allow it, piling it up in the round form as neatly as possible, to represent the red core of the melon; then cover with the balance of the white, so you have a white outside and a red core, like a watermelon, if neatly done.

**Watermelon Cake, No. 2.**—*White Part:* White sugar, 2 cups; butter, 1 cup; sweet milk, 1 cup; flour, 3½ cups; whites of 8 eggs; cream of tartar, 2 tea-spoonfuls; soda, 1 tea-spoonful; dissolve the soda in a little warm water; sift cream of tartar in flour; mix.

*Red Part:*—Red sugar, 1 cup; butter, ½ cup; sweet milk, ⅓ cup; flour, 2 cups; whites of 4 eggs; cream of tartar, 1 tea-spoonful; soda, ½ tea-spoonful; raisins, 1 cup; mix. Be careful to keep the red part around the tube of the cake-dish; the white part outside; best to have two persons fill in, one the red and the other the white, going around the tube till full.—*Mrs. S. O. Johnson, in Inter Ocean.*

**Lemon Cake With Milk.**—Butter, 1 cup; sugar, 3 cups; 5 eggs; flour, 4 cups; sour milk, 1 cup; soda, 1 tea-spoonful; the juice and grated yellow (the white has a bitter taste,) of one lemon. DIRECTIONS—Study well the General Remarks and Explanations, and also the Making-Up, or Putting Together, and you will then be prepared to proceed with the work of cake-making.

*Remarks*—In making cake, double the amount, or only half may be used, to suit the size of the family. But in taking half, if 5 eggs are called for, always use 3 in the reduction, as eggs are absolutely necessary to maintain the lightness of the cake.

**Lemon Jelly Cake, Without Milk.**—Sugar, 3 cups; flour, 2 cups; cold water, ½ cup; 5 eggs; cream of tartar, 1 tea-spoonful; soda, ½ tea-spoonful; 1 lemon or orange. DIRECTIONS—Beat all the yolks and the whites of 2 of the eggs for the cake, and cream with 2 cups of the sugar, butter, etc. Bake in 4 jelly cake tins. Grate off the yellow of the lemon or orange, peel off the white and throw away (this part of these fruits is bitter); then squeeze out the juice and chop up the pulp; having beaten the whites of the other 2 eggs, mix and stir in the other cup of sugar, or sufficient to make of proper thickness to put between the layers in place of jelly.

*Remarks.*—When lemons or oranges are used in making the cakes or the jelly, avoid the seeds.

**Lemon Jelly Cake.**—Butter, ½ cup; sugar, 1½ cups; milk, ½ cup; 3 eggs; flour, 2 cups; baking powder, 1½ tea-spoonfuls; 1 lemon; water, ½ cup. DIRECTIONS—Cream the butter with 1 cup of the sugar, stirring in the beaten whites of the eggs, and the milk; then sifting in the flour in which the baking powder was mixed, and bake in jelly cake tins. To the beaten yolks of the eggs add the other ½ cup of sugar, and the water, and juice of the lemon, and boil till thick enough to spread between the layers.

*Remarks.*—You will observe this receipt calls for baking powder, the one above for soda and lemon juice in place of cream of tartar. This enables you to choose between them, either from taste, or from having the soda and not the baking powder, or *vice versâ.*

**Orange Jelly Cake.**—Sugar, 4½ cups; butter, 1 cup; milk, 1 cup; 5 eggs; baking powder, 1½ tea-spoonfuls; flour, 2 cups; 2 oranges. DIRECTIONS —Cream 2½ cups of the sugar with the butter, beat the yolks of the eggs and stir in, then the milk, and sift in the flour, having the baking powder in it. Bake in jelly cake tins.

*For the Jelly.*—Beat the whites of the eggs and whip in the other 2 cups of of sugar, adding the juice of the 2 oranges. Put between the layers.

**Orange Jelly Cake.**—Sugar, 1 cup; 3 eggs; milk, ½ cup; flour, 1½ cups; baking powder, 1½ tea-spoonfuls; salt, 1 salt-spoonful; 1 orange. DIRECTIONS—Make up the cake as above, and bake in 3 layers. Grate the yellow of the orange, peel off the white and throw it away, beat the white of an extra egg and beat in 3 table-spoonfuls of the extra sugar, then the grated yellow and chopped pulp of the orange. Lay up with this and strew sugar upon the top thickly.

**Orange and Lemon Jelly Cake.**—Mix 2 cups of sugar with the yolks of 2 eggs; then the whites beaten to a froth, then a large table-spoonful of butter, then 1 cup of milk, and flour enough to make a batter that may be lifted upon a spoon (like cup cake). Bake in jelly cake tins.

*Jelly for Same.*—Grate the yellow from 1 lemon and 2 oranges, add the juice of the same, and add 1 cup of water, 1 of sugar, 1 table-spoonful of corn starch, and boil till smooth. When cool put between the cakes.

*Remarks.*—The boiling makes a harder jelly, not so likely to soak into the cake, the same as in boiling the icings.

**Delicious Filling or Jelly for Any Layer or Jelly Cake.**— Take 1 cup of white sugar, put it into a tin basin with enough water to dissolve it; let it boil until it will harden in cold water; have 1 cup of stoned and chopped raisins ready; then beat the white of an egg to a stiff froth, and mix with the raisins into the boiling sugar; stir briskly, and while warm put between the layers of cake, having taken them from the tins and laid on a cloth, selecting the brownest done for the bottom and the smoothest one for the top.—*Michigan Farmer.*

**Orange—Sponge—Jelly Cake.**—Sugar, 2 cups; 5 eggs, cold water, ½ cup (sweet milk is better); flour, 2½ cups; baking powder, 2 tea-spoonfuls; salt, 1 pinch; 1 orange. DIRECTIONS—Beat the yolks and whites of 2 of the eggs for the cake, and make up as others and bake in jelly cake tins.

*Jelly.*—Beat the whites of the other 3 eggs with 7 large table-spoonfuls of additional sugar, and all the grated yellow and the juice of the orange; spread this between the layers.—*Mertie Odell, Spartansburgh, Va.*

**Orange Jelly Cake—Rich.**—Sugar, 1 cup; butter, 1½ cups; cold water or milk, ½ cup; flour, 2 cups; baking powder, 2 tea-spoonfuls; 3 eggs, 1 orange. DIRECTIONS—Make the cake as usual and bake in jelly cake tins; reserving the whites of 2 of the eggs for frosting, using ⅔ cup of powdered sugar: grate off the yellow of the orange, to be sprinkled between the layers; but use the juice and chopped pulp of the orange in the cake mixture.

**Chocolate Jelly Cake—French.**—Butter, 1 table-spoonful; sugar, 1¼ cups; 2 eggs; milk, 1 cup; flour, 2¾ cups; soda, 1 small tea-spoonful; cream of tartar, 2 tea-spoonfuls; vanilla, 1 tea-spoonful.

*Jelly.*—Milk, 1 cup; corn starch, 2 table-spoonfuls; cold water, ½ cup; Baker's flavored chocolate, 2 ozs.; yolk of 1 egg; powdered sugar, 1 cup; extract of vanilla, 3 tea-spoonfuls. DIRECTIONS—Warm the butter a little, if necessary, to cream with the sugar and the beaten eggs; then sift in the flour with the cream of tartar therein, and the milk with the soda therein; then the vanilla; bake on 4 jelly cake tins in a quick oven. For a jelly or paste to go between the layers: Bring the milk to a boil, and while boiling add the corn starch which has been stirred smoothly in the water; then add the chocolate, grated, and the beaten yolk of the egg, stir all these over the fire and remove, and when a little cool stir in the powdered sugar and vanilla and put between the layers.

**Chocolate Jelly Cake.**—Butter, ½ cup; sugar, 2 cups; flour, 3 cups; milk, 1 cup; 4 eggs; baking powder, 1 tea-spoonful.

*Jelly.*—Milk, 1 pt.; grated chocolate and sugar, each 1 cup; corn starch, 1 table-spoonful. DIRECTIONS—Cream the butter and sugar, eggs and milk, as usual (in the order here named); then sift in the flour and baking powder and bake in jelly cake tins. For the jelly: Bring the milk to a boil and stir in the grated chocolate and sugar, and, having rubbed the corn starch smooth in a little cold water, stir it in and boil until it forms a smooth jelly, or paste, as some call it; when a little cool put between the layers.

*Remarks.*—In boiling milk it is safest to set the tin containing it into a larger pan containing a little water, which removes the danger of burning—otherwise, it requires constant watching and stirring. Allow me to say that this is my favorite chocolate cake, as it has no other flavoring, while it seems that many of the recipes call for vanilla or lemon or orange, etc.; but for me, give me a single flavor only in any cake. But it may be vanilla to-day and the next day lemon, then orange, and then chocolate; but a mixture of flavors only leaves one to wonder what the cook had been trying to imitate; but persons can suit themselves. A recipe is no sign that that flavor must be used. If you have not.got what is called for, but have some other; or if you prefer some other flavor, the cake will be just as nice if you accommodate yourself to the circumstances or to your preferences. There is another point, also, which calls for an explanation: If you have fruit jellies on hand, they may sometimes be used in laying up any of these "jelly cakes," instead of those which are called for in the recipe. This also extends the varieties which may be made.

**Chocolate Jelly Cake.**—Butter, 2 table-spoonfuls; sugar, 1 cup; 1 egg; milk, ½ cup; flour, 2 cups; cream of tartar, 1 tea-spoonful; soda, ½ tea-spoonful. Jelly: grated chocolate, 1 cup; milk enough to mix in. Lemon or vanilla to flavor. DIRECTIONS—Cream the butter, sugar and egg; then sift in the flour with the cream of tartar therein; dissolve the soda in the milk and stir in also, and bake in 3 jelly cake tins. For the jelly, moisten the chocolate and sugar with the milk, and bring to a boil, stirring until smooth; remove from the stove and when cool put in the flavor, and lay up the cake with it, before it gets cold.

*Remarks.*—To boil milk, see remarks in next recipe, above.

**Chocolate Jelly Cake.**—The following recipe is from Bertha Stanley, Decatur City, Iowa. I give it in her own words: Two cups sugar, 1 cup butter, the yolks of five eggs and the whites of two; 1 cup of milk, 3½ cups of flour, 1 tea-spoonful of cream of tartar, ½ tea-spoonful of soda. Spread on 8 tins and bake in a quick oven. Use the following mixture for filling: Whites of 3 eggs, 1½ cups of sugar, 3 table-spoonfuls of grated chocolate, 1 tea-spoonful extract of vanilla. Beat well together and spread between the layers and on top of the cake.

*Remarks.*—If it is preferred, at any time, any cake, although directed to be baked in layers, may be baked in a loaf, or loaves, by putting the chocolate, grated or dessicated (dried), cocoanut, orange, lemon, etc., into the cake mixture, instead of putting them into the jelly, as directed when the cake is to be baked in layers. With a little practice, in both ways, you can make a great variety of cakes with but few recipes.

**Chocolate Cake.**—Sugar, 2 cups; butter, 1 cup; 3 eggs; sweet milk, ¾ of a cup; flour, 3 cups; cream of tartar, 2 tea-spoonfuls; soda, 1 tea-spoonful. Bake in jelly pans. For the icing or jelly: Chocolate, ¼ cake; sugar, 1½ cups; sweet milk, ¾ of a cup; lemon extract, 2 tea-spoonfuls. Let boil until it thickens, so as to spread between the layers.—*Farm and Fireside.*

**Cocoanut Cake—Jelly and Loaf.**—Sugar, 1 cup; butter, ½ cup; 3 eggs; milk, ¾ of a cup (if a fresh cocoanut is used let it be a good sized one, then the milk of the cocoanut may take the place of the milk); flour, 2½ cups; baking powder, 2 tea-spoonfuls. Jelly: Whites of 2 eggs; pulverized sugar, ½ lb.; cocoanut, 1 good sized one, grated, or dessicated (dried) cocoanut ¼ lb. DIRECTIONS.—Cream sugar and butter; then having beaten all the yolks of the eggs and the white of 1, stir them in and the milk (or the milk of the cocoanut in its place), and sift in the flour with the baking powder therein, bake in jelly cake tins. For the jelly: Beat the whites of 2 eggs, saved for this purpose, to a froth, and stir in the pulverized sugar, and beat properly. Put this between the layers; having grated the cocoanut, strew this over the jelly in laying up the cake; or, if dessicated is used, strew it in place of the fresh. In this way the full flavor of the cocoanut is obtained. If baked in loaf all the eggs are to be used in the body of the cake, and the cocoanut also stirred into the cake just before putting it into the oven, being careful not to jar it after putting it into the oven, as it is more likely than other cakes to fall, if jarred.

**Cocoanut Jelly Cake.**—Sweet milk, butter, corn starch, each 1 cup; white sugar and flour, each 2 cups; whites of 5 eggs; cream of tartar, 2 tea-spoonfuls; soda, 1 tea-spoonful. Bake in 3 layers. For the jelly: White sugar, 1 lb., and boil until candied; when cold stir in the beaten whites of 2 eggs, and 1½ cups, rounded, of grated, or 1 cup dessicated, cocoanut, saving some for the top.

**Cocoa Cones.**—Whites of 5 eggs; powdered sugar, 1 lb.; ½ or ⅔ a grated cocoanut, having pared off the dark coating which adheres from the shell, before grating. DIRECTIONS—Whip well the whites, then, from time to time, sprinkle in a little of the sugar, till all is whipped in; then beat the grated cocoanut, and mold with the hands into cones, and set them on buttered paper, not to touch each other. Place in a pan and bake in a very moderate oven—if too hot they will melt down.—*Farm and Fireside.*

**Cocoanut Drops.**—One cocoanut; the white of 1 egg; powdered sugar. DIRECTIONS—Grate the cocoanut, weigh it, and take ½ its weight of the sugar; beat the white of the egg to a stiff froth; stir all together; then with a dessert, or small spoon, drop upon buttered white paper, or tin sheets, and sift sugar over them. Bake in a slow oven 12 to 15 minutes.

**Roll Jelly Cake—Fancy Way of Making.**—Take the whites of 6 eggs, 1 cup of white sugar, same of flour, 1 tea-spoonful of butter, 2 table-spoonfuls of sweet milk, 2 tea-spoonfuls cream tartar and 1 of soda. Bake in a large oblong dripping pan, so the cake will be very thin; meanwhile stir another batch, making just the same, with the exception of using the yolks instead of the whites; when both are done, spread when warm with jelly, or preserves of any kind; put together, bring the largest side of the cake towards you, and roll immediately; or cut in four or eight parts, put together alternately, putting jelly between each layer, and frost lightly over the top. Another method is to make three pans, making the third layer of ⅓ red sand sugar, proceeding the same as for the other layers; in putting together let the first layer be the yellow, made of the yolks, then the red, and lastly the whites. Nicely frost the top, and you have a beautiful as well as delicious party cake. They are very pretty made into rolls.

**Jelly Rolls.**—Sugar, ½ cup; 3 eggs; flour, 1 cup; cream of tartar, 1 tea-spoonful; soda, ½ tea-spoonful (or in place of the tartar and soda, use baking powder, 1½ tea-spoonfuls). DIRECTIONS—Bake in thin cakes, spread with jelly and roll up (jelly side in); cut across the roll.

**Roll Jelly Cake.**—Sugar, 1 cup; 4 eggs; flour, 1 cup; cream of tartar, 1 tea-spoonful; soda, ½ tea-spoonful; salt, 1 pinch. DIRECTIONS—Mix the powders and salt with the flour, beat the eggs, light; add the sugar and flour, and beat up light again. Bake in a square pan, turn upon a towel, spread on the jelly, and roll immediately.

**Jelly Cake.**—Sugar, 1 cup; butter, ½ cup; sour milk, ½ cup; 2 eggs; flour, 2 cups; soda, ½ tea-spoonful; jelly. DIRECTIONS—Bake in 4 cakes. When cold spread the jelly and lay up.

*Remarks.*—Grated cocoanut and sugar are very nice in this, or any other jelly cake, in place of the jelly, which is generally used. Remember this, also, when shortening (butter) is used in a jelly cake, it cannot be rolled.

**Corn Starch Cake.**—Sugar, 1½ cups; flour, 1½ cups; butter, ½ cup; corn starch, ½ cup; milk, ½ cup; whites of 6 eggs; baking powder, 1 tea-spoonful; extract of lemon, orange or vanilla, 2 tea-spoonfuls, or to taste; or if your taste says none, use none. DIRECTIONS—Cream the sugar and butter, then the beaten whites of the eggs; wet up the corn starch with the milk and stir in; then sift in the flour wherein the baking powder has been mixed. Bake in a moderate oven.

*Remarks.*—See general remarks upon cake making, baking, etc., to test when done; but another test is a cake generally loosens from the edge and sides of the pan when it is done.

**Lady Cake.**—Whites of 8 eggs, beaten to a froth; white sugar 2 cups; butter, 1 cup, creamed with the sugar; flour, 3 cups; cream of tartar, 1 tea-spoonful in the flour; sweet milk, ½ cup, with soda, 1 tea-spoonful in it; then heat all together and bake in a mold or small pans, as you please. Season, if desired, any flavor preferred.

**Lady Cake, No. 2.**—Sweet milk, ½ cup; powdered sugar and flour, each 2 cups; 4 eggs, whites only; baking powder, ½ tea-spoonful.

**Lady-Fingers.**—One-half lb. pulverized sugar and 6 yolks of eggs, well stirred; add ¼ lb. flour, whites of 6 eggs, well beaten. Bake in lady-finger tins, or squeeze through a bag of paper in strips two or three inches long.

**Lady Fingers, as Made in India.**—Sugar, 1 lb.; 8 eggs; flour, 1 lb. DIRECTIONS—Sift sugar and flour; beat the yolks separately, then beat with the sugar for 20 minutes; then beat in also the beaten whites, then, slowly, the flour, and drop upon white paper, long, to resemble the finger; dust sugar over them and bake in a hot oven.—*Indian Domestic Economy and Cooking.*

*Remarks.*—These will be found equal in delicacy to a true "lady's finger," even with an engagement-ring upon it. I should say moderate oven, lest they melt, if too hot, in baking.

**Love Knots for Tea.**—Little cakes folded over in the form of love knots are nice for tea. Flour, 5 cups; sugar, 2 cups; butter, 1 cup; a piece of lard the size of an egg; 2 eggs; sweet milk, 3 table-spoonfuls; soda, ½ tea-spoonful; a grated nutmeg, if liked, or as much cinnamon. DIRECTIONS—Sift the soda in the flour, then rub in the butter, lard and sugar, and then the beaten eggs, milk and spices, if any are used; roll thin and cut in strips an inch wide and 5 or 6 long, and lap across in a true love knot. Bake in a quick oven. *Ann Arbor Register.*

**Charlotte Polonaise—Iced Cake.**—Powdered sugar, 2 cups; butter, ½ cup; 4 eggs, beaten separately; cream, 1 cup, or rich milk with a little cream; prepared flour (an article now in the market), 3 cups.

*The Custard.*—Powdered sugar, 1 small cup; 6 eggs; flour, 2 table-spoonfuls; cream, 3 cups; chocolate, 1 small cup; almonds, ½ lb.; citron, ¼ lb.; macaroons, ½ lb.; apricots, ¼ lb.; candied peaches, or other candied fruit in their place, ¼ lb.; cold milk. DIRECTIONS—Beat the yolks very light; mix the flour with the cold milk, then stir in the cream, then the yolks, slowly; boil for 5 minutes, stirring constantly. Now pour out the custard into 3 equal parts.

First part—The chocolate being grated and the macaroons crumbled, stir them, with 1 table-spoonful of sugar with the first and boil for 5 minutes, stirring all the while; then pour out and whip 5 minutes with the egg-beater (if you have none, beat with a spoon), flavor with vanilla and set away to cool.

Second part—The almonds having been blanched (the skin removed by soaking in water until it will slip off with the thumb and fingers), chop them, then pound them in a Wedgewood mortar (same as druggists use, the name coming from the man who first made them from a mixture made for this purpose), putting in a few only at a time, adding a little rosewater from time to time. Chop the citron and mix with the pounded almonds, adding sugar, 3 table-spoonfuls, and stir into the second part, heating to a boil; flavor with extract of bitter almonds, then set aside as the first.

Third part—Chop the peaches, or other candied fruit, fine, and stir into the last custard, which will not need flavoring. The cake being baked in 4 layers, you have a custard, or jelly, of different color or flavor to go between each, the top to be iced with lemon ice or frosting.

*Remarks.*—This makes 2 loaves, and although it is not presumed that this cake will be made for every-day use, yet, for an evening party or other especial occasions, the nicety of the cake will pay for the extra trouble. The name, Polonaise, means simply, in three parts, like music having three crotchets in a bar.

**National Cake.**—White part—Cream together 1 cup white sugar and ½ cup of butter, then add ½ cup of sweet milk, the beaten whites of 4 eggs, ½ cup of corn starch, 1 cup of flour into which has been mixed 1 tea-spoonful of cream tartar and ½ tea-spoonful of soda. Flavor with lemon extract.

Blue part—Cream together 1 cup of blue sugar sand an ½ cup of butter, then add ½ cup of sweet milk, the beaten whites of 4 eggs and 2 cups of flour, in which mix 1 tea-spoonful of cream of tartar and ½ tea-spoonful of soda. No flavor.

Red part—Cream together 1 cup of red sugar and ½ cup of butter, then add ½ cup of sweet milk, the beaten whites of 4 eggs and 2 cups of flour, in which mix ½ tea-spoonful of cream of tartar and ½ tea-spoonful of soda. No flavor. Place in a bake pan, first the red, then the white, and last the blue. Bake in a moderate oven.

**Kansas Puffs.**—One cup of sugar, ½ cup of butter, ½ cup of molasses, 1 cup of sour milk, 1 tea-spoonful of soda, 1 cup of chopped raisins, and 1 cup of currants. Flavor with cloves and cinnamon. Make a little stiffer than you would cake and bake in little gem pans.—*Ella J. Shirley, Larned, Ks.*

*Remarks.*—Following our National colors, or red, white and blue, it is proper to give one of black and white, or the Union Jack (perhaps red and white would have been better, but we take them as we find them), for the Prince of Wales, by Miss E. R. Bruckman, of Tioga, Ill., in *Blade:*

**Prince of Wales Cake.**—Black part—One cup of brown sugar, ½ cup each of butter and sour milk, 2 cups of flour, 1 cup of chopped raisins, 1 tea-spoonful of soda dissolved in warm water, 1 table-spoonful of molasses, the yolks of 3 eggs, 1 tea-spoonful each of cloves and nutmeg.

White part—One cup of flour, ½ cup each of corn starch, sweet milk and butter, 1 cup of granulated sugar, 2 tea-spoonfuls of baking powder, the whites of 3 eggs. Bake all in 4 layers. Put together with icing, a black, then a white, alternating.

**Corn Starch Cake.**—Sugar, 1 cup; flour, 1 cup; corn starch, ½ cup; milk, ½ cup; butter, ½ cup; whites of 3 eggs; cream of tartar, 2 tea-spoonfuls; soda, ½ tea-spoonful. DIRECTIONS—Make same as the first, above, except the cream of tartar goes into the flour, and the soda to be dissolved in the milk.

**Corn Starch Cake.**—May Millbank, of Barnhart's Mills, Pa., vouches for the following: One-half cup of butter, 1 cup pulverized sugar, ½ cup of milk, ½ cup of corn starch, 1 cup of flour, ½ tea-spoonful of soda, whites of 2 eggs. DIRECTIONS—Make the same as the first.

**Ginger Snaps.**—Brown sugar, 1 lb. (see table of number of cups to the pound); butter, 1 lb.; New Orleans molasses, 1 qt.; Babbitt's saleratus, 1 oz.; cloves, 2 ozs.; ginger, 1 oz.; cinnamon, 2 ozs. DIRECTIONS—Cream sugar, butter and molasses; dissolve the saleratus in a very little hot water, and stir in, then the spices, of course, all ground; then sift in winter wheat flour, to make a stiff, very stiff, batter; no water, excepting the least possible to dissolve the saleratus.

*Remarks.*—Having to stay over night at Howard Station, Ill, I found so nice a ginger snap on the breakfast table, I inquired how they were made, and found that they were made by a baker within a short distance of the hotel, who, upon my introducing myself, very kindly gave me the recipe, as above. But in my hurry, lest being left by the cars, I missed taking his name, so I cannot give him the proper credit, which I ought to do, as bakers will very seldom part with their plans, or recipes, for doing their work. He charged particularly that spring wheat flour, such as was generally used in his neighborhood, would not do. Whether it is chargeable to their mills, or whether it is applicable to all spring wheat flour, I am not aware; a test in the north-western states will have to settle this point, as I have never had any of the flour to test it with.

**Ginger Snaps, Evangeline's.**—This lady says: Somebody wanted a ginger snap recipe that would stay hard, and not get soft. One cup of butter,

1 cup of lard, 1 cup of brown sugar, 1 pt. of molasses, 1 table-spoonful of ginger, 1 cup of sour milk, 2 tea-spoonfuls of soda, 1 pt. of flour—use more, if needed. Melt lard and butter together, stir in the ginger, sugar and molasses; dissolve the soda in the milk; stir all together, put in the flour, roll out thin, cut and bake in a quick oven.

*Remarks.*—If made sufficiently stiff, properly baked, allowed to get cold, then kept from the air, they will keep hard a very long time.

**Ginger Snaps.**—Here is the way they make them in the Old Bay State (Massachusetts), and they consider them very excellent: Molasses, 1 cup; butter, 2 table-spoonfuls; ginger, 1 table-spoonful; saleratus, 1 tea-spoonful; flour. DIRECTIONS—Boil the molasses and stir in the butter, ginger and saleratus, rolled fine; and stir the flour in while hot; roll out thin, cut and bake.

**Ginger Snaps.**—Sugar, 2 cups; 2 eggs; fried meat gravy, 1 cup; cider vinegar, 1 table-spoonful; ginger, 1 table-spoonful; soda, 1 large tea-spoonful; flour enough to roll; bake in a quick oven. Mrs. R. S. Armstrong is responsible for this.

**Ginger Snaps.**—I will give you another from the "Indiana Dutch Girl," of Tillmore, Ind.; Lard or butter, 1 cup; New Orleans molasses, 1 cup; ginger, 1 table-spoonful; soda, 1 heaping tea-spoonful; flour enough to make a stiff dough; roll quite thin, cut with cake cutter and bake quick.

**Ginger Drop Cake.**—Shortening, ½ cup; sour milk, 1 cup; brown sugar, 1 cup; molasses, ½ cup; 2 eggs; ginger, 1 tea-spoonful; soda, 1 rounding tea-spoonful; flour enough to make a thick batter, to drop from a spoon, in drops as large as an egg, in a bread pan, far enough apart not to touch. To be eaten warm.

*Remarks.*—In this, and the foregoing "snap" recipes, you have a sufficient variety for the hard or drier kind of ginger cakes; hence I now take up the softer gingerbread, for which I have several excellent recipes.

**Gingerbread for Training.**—This recipe was sent to the Detroit *Tribune* by a "Mrs. D.," of Atchison, Kan., in answer to "Uncle Ben's" inquiry for a recipe for making "training" gingerbread; and although she was not positive that it was ever used to "train" by, yet she thinks it good enough: "Molasses, 1 cup; butter, ½ cup; boiling water, ½ cup; ginger, 1 tea-spoonful; soda, 1 tea-spoonful; flour. DIRECTIONS—Pour the water on to the butter and when cool add the rest and flour enough to roll. When baked wet the top with molasses, diluted considerably with water, and sprinkle with sugar. It will be found toothsome."

**Gingerbread, Alice's.**—This was furnished to the "Household Department" of the *Blade* by Elizabeth Kent, of Burlington, Vt., but for a plain, small cake or loaf, with quite a ginger flavor, it can be depended upon: "Molasses, 1 cup; boiling water, 1 cup; butter, 1 table-spoonful; ginger, 1 table-spoonful; soda, 1 tea-spoonful; thicken to pour."

*Remarks.*—Pouring the hot water upon the butter, and then putting in the molasses to help cool it, as in the next recipe above, and when cool, the other articles, and baking in a moderately hot oven, is the order of proceeding.

**Gingerbread, Mrs. Rice's.**—This recipe is from Mrs. Rosella Rice, quite an extensive writer for the *Blade* "Household." It was given in answer to an inquiry for her gingerbread recipe, which, she says, "I give with pleasure." I take pleasure, also, in giving it a place, for I know it is good. She says: "Take 1 cup of sugar, 1 of butter, 1 of West India molasses, 1 of sour milk or butter milk, 2 eggs, 1 table-spoonful of ginger, 1 tea-spoonful of cinnamon, and one of soda, dissolved in hot water. Take flour enough to make a good batter, say 4 or 5 cupfuls, but don't make it too thick; stir the spices, sugar butter and molasses together, keeping the mixture slightly warmed; then add the milk, then the eggs, beaten their lightest, then the soda, and then the flour, last. Beat it long and well, and bake in a large buttered pan; or, if for cakes, in patty pans. If you want to add raisins, dredge them with flour, and put them in the last thing."

*Remarks.*—Here you may have a loaf cake with or without raisins, or may bake in small cakes if you choose.

**Gingerbread, Soft.**—Molasses, 3 cups; butter or lard, 1 cup; sour milk, 1 cup; 4 eggs; ginger, 2 table-spoonfuls; soda, 1 table-spoonful; flour, 7 cups. DIRECTIONS—Stir butter, sugar, molasses, and ginger together; then the milk and eggs well beaten; then the soda dissolved in a little hot water; then the flour.

*Remarks.*—This writer to the *Blade* "Household" only gives the name "Jessie," but assures her friends that "I know this to be good, for I have used it over twelve years," but the reading of it satisfied me it was good, hence I give it a place. Having given my whole life to the observation and test of practical items of a general character, I know as quick as I read a recipe whether it is reliable or not. At least, for several years past, I have tested but very few recipes which proved a failure; while, in my earlier experience, the failures were frequent. Such I now throw aside on their first reading.

**Gingerbread, Poor Man's.**—Molasses, 1 cup; sugar, ½ cup; 1 egg; buttermilk, ⅔ cup; lard or butter, 1 table-spoonful; ginger, 1 table-spoonful; cinnamon, 1 tea-spoonful; soda, 1 tea-spoonful; flour, 2 cups. "A. Y. E.," of O'Brien, Iowa, says of it: "Good and very cheap. [See, also, "Poor Man's Cake."]

**Ginger Cakes, or Bread.**—"Mrs. S. E. H.," of Circleville, O., gives the *Blade* "Household" the following, which I give in her own words: "I give a good ginger cake recipe—one that has taken the premium at our county fair for the last five years: One pt. best Orleans molasses, 1 pt. of sour buttermilk, 1 large table-spoonful of ginger, 1 of lard, 1 of soda; dissolve the soda in the buttermilk; flour enough to make soft as you can handle, the softer the better. Turn on the bread-board, roll, cut into cakes, and bake in a quick oven. Try this. If you prefer it baked in pans, add 2 eggs, well beaten, and mix as other cake. A small lump of alum, dissolved, improves the cake."

*Remarks.*—Most people object to the use of alum in baking powders; then why not objectionable to use it here? I think it is not at all necessary; but if it is used, "a small lump" is too indefinite. I would say not more than half to a tea-spoonful, at most. If pulverized, it dissolves quicker, using a little hot water.

**Ginger Cookies.**—Sugar, ½ cup; molasses, ½ cup; shortening, ½ cup; boiling water, ⅓ cup; soda, ½ tea-spoonful; ginger, 1 large tea-spoonful; salt; flour. DIRECTIONS—Have the shortening very hot and the water boiling; dissolve the soda in the water and put into the creamed sugar, shortening and molasses; use only flour enough to make as soft a dough as you can roll, dusting freely.

*Remarks.*—This recipe is from Sarah Green, of Portageville, N. Y., who indicates it to be nice, if properly made. The two following are also hers:

**Sugar Cookies.**—Sugar, ⅔ cup; butter, ⅔ cup; 1 egg; cream of tartar, 2 tea-spoonfuls; soda, 1 tea-spoonful; hot water, ½ cup, to dissolve the soda; flour, sufficient

*Remarks.*—Make from general directions, at the head of this subject, also the following:

**Sugar Cookies.**—Sugar, 1 cup; butter, 1 cup; sour milk, 1 cup; soda, 1 tea-spoonful. Mix soft as possible. Caraway seed, she says, is the best seasoning for sugar cookies.

**Sugar Cookies, No. 2.**—Sugar, 1 cup; butter, 1 cup; 1 egg; essence of lemon; flour to roll and cut out.—*Mrs. C. W. Phillips.*

**Excellent Cookies.**—Meat fryings, 1 cup, or butter, ½ cup, and lard, ½ cup; sugar, 1 cup; cold water, 1 cup; soda, scant tea-spoonful; nutmeg to taste. Mix quickly, roll very thin, and cut with teacup or goblet. The cookies will not curl; bake in a quick oven.

**Cookies, With Carbonate of Ammonia.**—Carbonate of ammonia, 1 oz.; sugar, 1 pt , sweet milk, ½ pt.; sweet cream, ½ pt.; flour, enough to roll them out nicely. Bake quick. They are better to let them stand 2 or 3 days. So says "Fannie C.," of Medina, Wis.

**Cookies, With Ammonia.**—Lard, 1 lb.; sugar, 5 cups; milk, 1 qt.; carbonate of ammonia, 1½ ozs.; caraway seed, a little salt, and flour to make stiff enough to roll. DIRECTIONS — Dissolve the ammonia in the milk and add to the lard and sugar, previously rubbed together. For small families, one-half or one-fourth the amount may be used. Hope Humason, of Brookside, Conn., says: "It has been tried and approved."

*Remarks.*—It will be observed that where more than one recipe is given for making any cake, or other article, they are always different; so that persons who have not the articles called for in one may have those called for in another, thus enabling everybody to be accommodated. And I may properly say here that I give none which my own judgment, from my long experience in studying and testing practical recipes, does not at once consent to the appropriateness of the ingredients to produce, if properly combined, the cake, or whatever other article the recipe calls for.

**Custard Jelly Cake.**—Sugar, 1 cup; 3 eggs; flour, 1½ cups; cream of tartar, 1 tea-spoonful; soda, 1 tea-spoonful; cold water, 2 table-spoonfuls; make 4 layers.

*Custard for the Cake.*—Sweet milk, 1 pt.; 2 eggs; sugar, 1 cup (light brown is best); corn starch, 2 table-spoonfuls, beaten with a little milk; butter, ½ cup. DIRECTIONS—Put the milk in a tin pan on the stove and let it come to a boil; then stir in the sugar, then the butter, then the eggs, then the corn starch; it must be stirred rapidly all the time, so as not to burn. Let it boil until it is about as thick as jelly. When cold flavor with lemon extract. Do not make the cake until you make the custard, as the custard must be put on the cakes as soon as they are taken from the oven.—*White Lily, Wilseyville, O.*

**Cream Cake.**—Sugar, 1 cup; butter, ½ cup; whites of 4 eggs; sweet milk, ½ cup; soda, 1 tea-spoonful; cream of tartar, 2 tea-spoonfuls; flour 2 cups. Bake in round tins.

*For the Cream.*—The yolks of 3 eggs; sweet milk, ½ pt.; butter the size of an egg; corn starch, 4 teaspoonfuls; sugar to suit the taste, as for custard. DIRECTIONS—Boil the same as custard, and when a little cool, flavor with lemon, orange, or vanilla, and spread between the layers.

**French Cream Cake.**—I will give it in their words: Beat 3 eggs and 1 cup of sugar together thoroughly; stir 1 tea-spoonful of baking powder into 1½ cups of flour (sift the flour in), stirring all the while in one direction. Bake in 2 thin cakes. Split the cakes while hot, and fill in the cream prepared in the following manner: To 1 pt. of new milk add 2 table-spoonfuls of corn starch, 1 beaten egg, and ½ cup of sugar; stir while cooking, and when hot, put in butter, size of an egg; flavor the cream with lemon, vanilla, or pineapple. The milk for cream must be put in a pail and then heated in a pot of hot water—same as one does blanc mange.

**Boston Cream Cakes.**—Water, 2½ cups; flour, 2 cups; butter, 1 cup; and 5 eggs. Boil the butter and water together; stir in the flour while boiling; after it is cool add the eggs well beaten. Put a large spoonful in muffin rings, and bake 20 minutes in a hot oven.

The cream for them is made this way: Put over the fire 1 cup of milk, add not quite a cup of sugar; 1 egg, mixed with 3 tea-spoonfuls of corn starch and 1 table-spoonful of butter. When cool add vanilla to the taste; boil a few moments only. Open the cakes and fill them with the cream. They are easily made, and are delicious.

**Snow or Tea Cake.**—Mrs. R. H. De La, Brough, Iowa, makes these remarks in introducing this cake recipe. She says:

"I often make a cake which I think is the nicest tea cake, or for dyspeptic persons (as it is not a rich cake), that I ever saw. One and a half cups of nice white sugar and 1 cup of flour, rubbed well together; add 1 tea-spoonful of cream tartar, and stir until thoroughly incorporated; whites of 10 eggs (or 7 make it very nice when eggs are scarce), beaten to a stiff froth, stirred with the other mixture, just enough to mix evenly; bake in a moderate oven."

**Saratoga Tea Cakes.**—To each pound of flour allow a dessert-spoonful of yeast powder, 1 egg, ½ pt. of milk, 2 spoonfuls of melted butter, 2 spoonfuls of sugar. Rub the dry ingredients together, then quickly mix in the milk with the butter, then the beaten egg; cut out into biscuit form, and bake quickly in buttered pans.

**White Cake.**—Contributed by Laughing Ora, Morris, Ill. Two cups of sugar, ½ cup of butter; beat the butter and sugar till like cream; stir in 1 cup of sweet milk; add 3 cups of flour and 2 tea-spoonfuls of baking powder; beat the whites of 5 eggs and stir in with the flour. Do not bake too fast.

**White Mountain Cake.**—Sugar, 2 cups; butter, 1 cup; flour, 3 cups; sweet milk, ½ cup; whites of 10 eggs, beaten very stiff (or the whole of 5 eggs, if the shade from the yolks is no objection); cream of tartar, 2 tea-spoonfuls; soda, 1 tea-spoonful. DIRECTIONS—Bake in 3 deep jelly tins, or 6 thin layers. If iced, take the whites of 4 eggs; white powdered sugar, 16 table-spoonfuls; flavor to taste, if desired.

**White Mountain Cake, Iced.**—Granulated sugar, 3 cups; butter, 1 cup; 5 eggs; sweet milk, 1 cup; flour, 3 cups; cream of tartar, 2 tea-spoonfuls; soda, 1 tea-spoonful; salt, 1 pinch. DIRECTIONS—Beat the butter, sugar, and yolks of the eggs to a cream; mix soda in the milk and the cream of tartar in the flour; add the whites just before the flour. Bake in jelly cake tins, browning a little.

*In Place of Jelly.*—Take the whites of 2 eggs, a little water, and the proper amount of powdered sugar, beat together and with a knife spread over the top of each cake. Grate a fresh cocoanut and mix it with more sugar, and sprinkle it over the cakes; then lay-up, finishing the top the same.

*Remarks.*—Especially applicable for use upon occasions when ice cream is to be served.

**Loaf Cake.**—Butter, 1 cup; sugar, 2 cups; 4 eggs; sweet milk, 1 cup; cream of tartar, 2 tea-spoonfuls; soda, 1 tea-spoonful.

**White Cake, With Sweet Milk.**—Sugar, 2 cups; butter, 1 cup; sweet milk, 1 cup; whites of 5 eggs; baking powder, 2 tea-spoonfuls.

**White Cake, With Butter Milk.**—Fine white sugar, 3 cups; butter, 1 cup; butter milk, 1 cup; whites of 10 eggs: baking powder, 3 tea-spoonfuls; lemon, to taste; flour, 4 cups. DIRECTIONS—Let some one beat the whites of the eggs to a stiff froth while you cream the sugar and butter, etc., mixing in the whites last.

**Tea Cake Instead of Biscuit—Without Sugar.**—Butter (or half lard), 1 cup; sweet milk, 1 cup; 4 eggs; salt, 1 pinch; flour, 1½ pts.; baking powder, 2 tea-spoonfuls.

*Remarks.*—It will be found excellent.

**Tea Cake.**—Sugar, 1 cup; butter, 1 table-spoonful; 1 egg; buttermilk, 1 cup; soda, ½ tea-spoonful; flour to make a tolerably stiff batter.

*Remarks.*—"Aunt Margaret" always makes this when she finds a visitor to tea, and only half an hour to make and bake the cake in; also, because it is good cold.

**Tea Cakes.**—Sugar, 2 cups; butter, 1 cup; sour milk, or buttermilk, 1 cup; soda, ½ tea-spoonful; flour, nutmeg or caraway. DIRECTIONS—Beat the sugar and butter together and add the milk. Dissolve the soda in a little water and add, with as much flour as will make a stiff dough, grating in a little nutmeg, or sprinkle in some caraway seed, as you choose. Roll and cut in small cakes, baking a light brown.

**French Loaf Cake.**—Sugar, 2½ cups; butter, 1½ cups; flour, 1½ cups; 8 eggs; sour milk, 2 table-spoonfuls; soda, ¼ tea-spoonful; 1 lemon. DIREC-TIONS—Cream the butter and sugar together, then stir in the yolks (the French always beat the yolks and whites separately), then the whites; and, having grated off the yellow of the lemon (peeled off the white and thrown away), and also grated up the inside upon a coarse grater and picked out the seeds, stir this in, then the flour, and having dissolved the soda in the sour milk stir it in and bake in a moderate oven. An orange or two may be used instead of a lemon, for variety's sake, if desired or preferred.

*Remarks.*—It may not be amiss to say that the French not only beat the yolks and whites of eggs separately, and for a long time, but they also make their cakes very rich. If it is desired to have cake like theirs we must follow their directions.

**French Loaf Cake—Plain.**—Sugar, 2 cups; butter, ½ cup; sweet milk, 1 cup; flour, 3 cups; 3 eggs; baking powder, 3 tea-spoonfuls. DIREC-TIONS—Cream the sugar and butter together with the hand; beat the eggs well and stir in; then add the milk; stir the baking powder into the sifted flour and mix in thoroughly, and bake in a moderate oven two fair-sized cakes.

*Remarks.*—Flavoring of any kind may be used; but the first time I ate of it was at my own table, made by one of my married daughters, without flavoring. If flavoring is used, of course it is not plain, and it certainly is very nice with any flavoring.

**Delicious Cake.**—White sugar, 2 cups; butter, 1 cup; sweet milk, 1 cup; 3 eggs; soda, ½ tea-spoonful; scant tea-spoonful of cream of tartar; flour, 3 cups. DIRECTIONS—Beat eggs separately and bake in rather a hot oven.

**Delicate Cake.**—Flour, 3 cups; sugar, 2 cups; butter, ½ cup; sweet milk, ¾ cups, and 1 tea-spoonful of cream of tartar (or ¾ cup of sour cream), ½ tea-spoonful of soda. Beat well, then add the whites of 6 eggs beaten to a stiff froth, flour to taste.

*Remarks.*—This is in the words of the "Belle" of Libertyville, Iowa, and will be found delicate as belles in general.

**Delicate Cake, Cheap and Easy to Make.**—Butter, ¾ cup; sugar, scant 2 cups, stirred to a cream; flour, 3 cups; baking powder, 2 tea-spoonfuls, run through a sieve twice; sweet milk, ½ cup; whites of 6 eggs; flavor with lemon.

*Remarks.*—This makes a delicate jelly cake baked in layers.

**Jumbles.**—Mrs. Phœbe Jane Rankin, of Illinois, gives the following recipe for a very nice jumble: Sugar, 2 cups; lard, 1 cup; beat to a cream, then add 2 eggs; sweet milk, 1 cup; soda, 1 tea-spoonful; cream of tartar, ½ tea-spoonful; then stir in flour till about as stiff as pound cake; put plenty of flour on the board; dip out the dough with a spoon; flour your rolling pin well; roll to about ¼ inch thick; sprinkle sugar over the top; cut out and bake in a quick oven; when done set on edge to cool; the softer they are rolled out the better they will be. Add a little lemon extract if you like.

**Jumbles, or Sand Tarts.**—Sugar, 2 cups; eggs, 4; sweet milk, ½ cup; baking powder, 2 tea-spoonful; flour. DIRECTIONS—Use flour enough, only, to make as cookies; then sprinkle on sugar, cinnamon and nutmeg, and bake in a quick oven.

*Remarks.*—Sprinkling the sugar and spices upon the surface gives them a sandy appearance, and hence some cooks call them sand tarts.

**Soft Jumbles.**—Butter, 1 cup; sugar, 2 cups; 2 eggs; sour or sweet milk, 1 cup; flour, 4 to 4½ cups; soda, 1 tea-spoonful, scant; cream of tartar, 2 tea-spoonfuls; vanilla ex., 1 tea-spoonful. DIRECTIONS—Cream the sugar and butter, and add one-half the milk, in which the vanilla has been put; then one-half the flour, then the beaten eggs; then the other half of the flour into which the cream of tartar has been mixed by sifting together; lastly the other half of the milk in which the soda has been dissolved. Make in small cakes and bake quickly

*Remarks.*—Jumbles are always to be sprinkled with sugar, or rolled in sugar. For me the more sugar the better is the jumble.

**Rich Jumble.**—Sugar and butter, 1 lb. each; cream together, with 4 eggs; then mix in 1½ lbs. of flour. DIRECTIONS—Roll in powdered sugar, lay on buttered tins and bake in a quick oven.

*Remarks.*—Coffee sugar, 2½ cups, equal 1 pound. Butter, 2 cups, equal 1 pound; and flour, 3 cups, make 1 pound. Common sized tea-cups are intended. But, for large families, the largest coffee cup may be taken, as the proportions would be the same, except that the soda and cream of tartar (when used) should be increased accordingly.

**Muffins for Tea.**—Flour, 3 cups; baking powder, 2 tea-spoonfuls; 3 eggs; melted butter, 2 table-spoonfuls; sweet milk, 1 pt.; a little salt. DIRECTIONS—Sift flour and baking powder together, stir in the egg and butter, then the milk. Bake in rings, in a quick oven.

**Muffins.**—Milk, 1 pt.; yeast, ½ cup; salt, a very little; flour, sufficient to make a batter. DIRECTIONS—When light, cook in rings upon the stove.

**Mush Muffins.**—Take cold mush, made in the ordinary way, thin with milk, 1 qt.; 7 eggs, and butter the size of an egg; a little salt; then bring to the proper consistency with wheat flour. Bake in rings.

*Remarks.*—Very nice and healthful to thicken with graham flour. If these are not as light as some may choose, put a little baking powder in the flour.

**Hermits.**—Brown sugar, 1½ cups; 3 eggs; butter, 1 cup; raisins, chopped, 1 cup; sour milk, 2 table-spoonfuls; soda, 1 tea-spoonful; cinnamon, nutmeg, cloves, and allspice, of each ½ tea-spoonful; flour enough to roll out; cut as in cookies.

**Apple Fruit Cake.**—Dried apples, 1 cup; molasses, 1 cup; 1 egg; sugar, ½ cup; milk, ½ cup; flour, 2½ cups; baking powder, 1 tea-spoonful. DIRECTIONS—Soak the apples over night, then steam until soft; then simmer them slowly in the molasses, until well cooked; when cool, add the other ingre dients and bake.

**Apple Fritters.**—Prepare the batter as for fritters, having washed, and sliced the apples, crosswise, and if you have a corer the core should have been taken out. Have the lard boiling hot. Drop the slices into the batter and see that every part is well covered; fry until brown, then turn and fry until done.

*Remarks.*—These instructions are from Miss Arabell, of Knox City, Mo. I say Miss because, as she gives no "sir" name, I take it for granted she had not found the "sir." I will guarantee the fritters, however, to be found nice.

**Coffee Cake.**—Brown sugar, 2 cups; 4 eggs; butter, 1 cup; molasses, 1 cup; cold coffee, 1 cup; raisins, 2 cups; cloves, 2 tea-spoonfuls; ½ a nutmeg; soda, 1 tea-spoonful; flour, 4 cups.

**Coffee Cake.**—Brown sugar, butter, cold, strong coffee and molasses, each 1 cup; 3 eggs; raisins, 2 cups; baking powder, 2 tea-spoonfuls; flour, 2 cups.

**Raisin Cake.**—Sugar, 1½ cups; butter, ⅔ of a cup; milk, ⅔ of a cup; flour, 3 cups; chopped raisins, 1 cup; 3 eggs; baking powder, 1½ tea-spoon-fuls. Bake as a whole or in sheets.

**Raisin Cake, Without Sugar.**—Flour, 1 cup; cream, 2 cups; butter, 1 cup; 4 eggs; raisins, 1 lb., not chopped; candied lemon, 1, chopped; soda, 1 tea-spoonful; a little cloves and cinnamon may be added. Stir well.

**Fig Pound Cake.**—Brown sugar, chopped figs, raisins and flour, each 1 lb.; butter, ¾ lb.; cream or milk (sour), ½ pt.; 7 eggs; soda, ½ tea-spoon-ful; 1 nutmeg.

*Remarks.*—One tea-spoonful of alum, pulverized, is added, by some, but I would prefer cream of tartar.

**Currant Cake.**—Butter, 1 cup; sugar, 2 cups; 4 eggs; flour, 3½ cups; sour milk, 1 cup; English currants, 2 cups; saleratus or soda, 1 tea-spoonful; flavor with lemon or other extracts, as you choose.

**Fruit Cake, Plain.**—Sweet milk, 1 cup; molasses, ½ cup; brown sugar, 1 cup; butter, ½ cup; 2 eggs; raisins and currants, each, ¼ lb.; salt, 1 tea-spoonful; cloves and cinnamon, each, 1 table-spoonful; nutmeg; baking powder, 2 tea-spoonfuls; flour, 3 cups. See directions in next cake.

**Premium Fruit Cake.**—Sugar, 3 cups; butter, 1½ cups. 6 eggs; sour cream, 1½ cups; saleratus or soda, 2 tea-spoonfuls; currants ½ lb.; raisins, ¾ lb.; citron, ¼ lb.; 1 nutmeg; flour. DIRECTIONS—Beat the eggs thoroughly; then add sugar and butter, and beat till smooth. Dissolve the saleratus in a little warm water and put it in the cream, and make the cake quite thick with flour to prevent the fruit from settling to the bottom. Do not chop the raisins, but cut them in halves and remove the seeds, else use "seedless" raisins; then scald a few moments to soften, drain and flour (dredge) them before putting into the cake. Cut the citron in thin slices, and as you fill in a layer of cake put the citron over evenly, then more of the cake mixture and another layer of the citron; and so on, until the citron is evenly divided through the whole.

*Remarks.*—Mrs. John Rice, of Seneca county, Ohio, who originated this recipe, says: "If any one will follow this recipe she may do as I did—get the first premium at the coming fair

**Fruit Cake that will Keep for Months.**—Butter, sugar, molasses, and sweet milk, of each, 1 cup; currants, 4 cups; 8 eggs; baking powder, 2 tea-spoonfuls; citron, chopped, ½ lb.; 2 grated nutmegs, and cinnamon to taste. Bake 2 hours.

**Fruit Cake, Very Nice.**—Butter, brown sugar, sifted flour, and citron, of each, 1 lb.; 12 eggs; raisins, stoned, and English currants, of each, 3 lbs.; molasses, ½ cup; cinnamon, mace, cloves, and allspice, of each, 1 table-spoonful; 1 nutmeg; grated rind of 1 lemon; baking powder, 4 tea-spoonfuls. DIRECTIONS—Beat the yolks, butter and sugar together till very light; then stir in the molasses, spices and the grated rind of the lemon, also the stiff-beaten whites of the eggs; then the flour, into which the baking powder has been mixed by sifting; when, after thoroughly mixing, the raisins and currants are to be added and evenly mixed in. The citron having been shaved and chopped finely, and a suitable pan well buttered, and a buttered paper also having been put into the pan, dip in a layer of the batter; then sprinkle on a thin layer of the citron, until all is put in, the top layer, of course, having no citron upon it. Bake in a moderate oven, covering with paper if necessary to avoid burning the top. It will require about 4 hours to bake it

*Remarks.*—This will be found a very nice cake to have been given to the *Blade* by the "Sunflower," of Farragut, Ia. It will keep well, and will be all the better if not cut for some weeks. And now, although either of the above fruit cakes will make nice wedding cakes, yet I must give one which is so called, and a very good one, too, the baking, manner of preparation, etc., being about the same as in the foregoing:

**Wedding Cake, Very Rich.**—The finest and nicest flour, 5 lbs; very nice butter, 3 lbs.; English currants, nicely washed, dried and dredged, 5 lbs.; sifted loaf sugar, 2 lbs.; nice sweet almonds, blanched, 1 lb.; nutmegs, 2; mace, ¼ oz.; cloves, ⅛ oz.; lemon and orange peel, each ½ lb.; wine and brandy, each ¼ pt.; very nice fresh eggs, 16. DIRECTIONS—See the directions in the recipes above and the general directions. I will say, however, if made in one, or even into two cakes, it will take 4 hours to bake them, as the oven must not be over hot, and care, by covering with paper, etc., not to burn them.

**Coffee Cake.**—Strong cold coffee, butter and raisins, of each 1 cup; sugar, 1½ cups; flour, 3½ cups; cinnamon, cloves, nutmeg and soda, of each 1 tea-spoonful; eggs, 2 DIRECTIONS—Make it upon general principles. Other fruit may be used in place of the raisins, and it will be nice even without any fruit at all.

**Molasses Cake.**—Molasses, 1 pt.; brown sugar, 3 cups; sour milk, 1 pt.; 4 eggs; soda, 2 tea-spoonfuls, flour, 7 cups; cinnamon, or any other spice, or ginger, to taste.

**Soft Molasses Cake.**—Molasses, ⅔ cup; brown sugar, 1 table-spoonful;

butter or lard, the size of an egg; sour milk, ½ cup; soda, 1 tea-spoonful; flour, 2 cups.

**Mrs. Chase's Sponge Cake.**—Sugar, 1 cup; 4 eggs; sweet milk, 3 table-spoonfuls; flour, 2 cups; baking powder, 2 tea-spoonfuls; salt, 1 pinch; orange or lemon extract (home-made), 2 tea-spoonfuls. DIRECTIONS—Beat the eggs, then beat in the sugar, add the milk, salt and flavor; and, having mixed the baking powder into the flour, sift it in, beat all together and bake in a quick oven.

*Remarks.*—This will make 2 cakes if baked in the round tin, or 1 in the square. I have eaten of this many times with great satisfaction, and expect the same in eating of the one which, I am just informed, is ready for tea  Yet I give several others to meet all circumstances and desires. Sponge cake is credited with being the most healthful of any form of cake, for the reason that, as a general thing, no butter or other shortening is used, although of late, as will be seen below, some people are beginning to introduce them; but, for myself, I am very fond of one of the above, coming warm from the oven at tea-time, having some very nice butter to eat with it.  Those who are dyspeptic had better forego this luxury. My next is from " Fern Leaves," of Oswego county, N. Y., who told the *Blade* "Household " that it would make " roll jelly cake," " cup cake," or "plain cake." It is as follows:

**Sponge Cake.**—Sugar, 1 cup; flour, 1 cup; 3 eggs; water, 2 table-spoonfuls; baking powder, 2 tea-spoonfuls; salt and spice to taste.

The following is from somebody's lady friend, as the result of long experience: "Flour, 1 cup; sugar, 1 cup; baking powder, 1 heaping tea-spoonful; cold water, 3 table-spoonfuls; flavor with lemon or vanilla. DIRECTIONS—Beat the whites and yolks separately, and add the water the last thing before baking.

**Improved Berwick Sponge, or Custard Cake.**—Sugar, 2 cups; 4 eggs; flour, 3 cups; cream of tartar, 2 tea-spoonfuls; soda, 1 tea-spoonful; salt, a pinch; cold water, 1 cup; the juice of 1 lemon. DIRECTIONS—Beat the eggs well, then beat in the sugar and half of the flour, in which the cream of tartar has been mixed; the soda and salt being dissolved in the water, add in with the lemon juice, and lastly the balance of the flour, stirring well together, and bake in cakes to be fully 2 inches thick.

*For the Custard.*—Milk, a scant ½ pt. (take out a little to wet up 3 tea spoonfuls of flour); sugar, 1 scant cup; butter half the size of an egg; 1 egg, well beaten; flavor with the grated peel of the lemon.  Mix all, and cook for 15 minutes in the rice-boiler (a tin dish made to fit inside of another, in which the water is placed, on the same principle as a glue kettle, which saves the labor of constant watching and stirring to prevent burning) then set aside to cool.  This should be done so as to be cold by the time the cake is done.  Split the cake with a sharp knife, and spread the cold custard between.

**Molasses Sponge Cake.**—Molasses, 1 cup; melted butter, 1 table-spoonful; 2 eggs, well beaten; sweet milk, ½ cup; cream of tartar, 1 tea-spoonful; soda, ½ tea-spoonful; flour, 1½ cups; ginger, to taste.  Makes a good loaf, or it may be baked in layers and laid up with jelly for variety

**Butter Sponge Cake.**—Butter, 1 cup; sugar, 2 cups; flour, 1½ cups; 6 eggs; cream of tartar, 1 tea-spoonful; soda, ½ tea-spoonful. DIRECTIONS— No special directions given, except to dissolve the soda in a table-spoonful of the milk, and mix the cream of tartar evenly with the flour, which is in accordance with my general directions.

*Remarks.*—But as this recipe shows how a farmer's wife of White Church, Kansas, makes sponge cake, I thought I would give her directions in full. It will be noticed that this cake is rich in eggs and butter; but if the Kansas farmers can not afford it I do not know who can.

**Lemon Sponge Cake, with Butter.**—Sugar and flour, each, 1 cup; 3 eggs; sweet milk, 3 table-spoonfuls; melted butter, 2 table-spoonfuls; baking powder, 2 heaping teaspoonfuls; extract lemon, ½ tea-spoonful.

**Cream Sponge Cake.**—Gertie, of Kewanee, Wis., prefers cream in hers, as follows: Beat 2 eggs in a tea-cup, fill up the cup with thick sweet cream, 1 cup of sugar, 1 cup of flour, 1 tea-spoonful each of cream of tartar and soda.

**Sponge Cake.**—Sugar, 1 cup; 1 egg; sweet milk, 1 cup; butter the size of an egg; baking powder, 2 tea-spoonfuls; flour, 2 cups; season to taste.

*Remarks.*—The more frequent use of sponge cake, as compared with other kinds of cake, is the reason of my giving so large a number of them, that everybody may be suited.

**Pound Cake.**—Sugar, 1 lb. (2½ cups); butter, 1 lb. (2 cups); flour, 1 lb. (3 cups); 10 eggs; soda, 1 tea-spoonful. DIRECTIONS—Beat the yolks and whites separately; and if you wish a fruit cake, use raisins, or currants, 1 lb.

*Remarks*—It keeps moist a long time, if properly covered. For varieties sake, flavoring extracts may be sometimes used, or take the Imperial next below, for the variety.

**Imperial Cake.**—Sugar, flour, butter, eggs (10), raisins, currants, figs, almond meats, peel (½ citron, ¼ lemon, ¼ orange), of each 1 lb., except as explained about the peel, baking powder, 3 tea-spoonfuls. DIRECTIONS—No flavoring, nor spices, are to be used. The butter and sugar rubbed together, then the beaten eggs (10 eggs average a pound); add baking powder to the flour and put it in after the eggs; add only one kind of the fruit at a time—no flour on the fruit—but the peel and figs are to be chopped fine, the almonds blanched and split. Stir well when all is in, and bake in square tins.

*Remarks.*—I should think it would be rich enough for any imperial family of Europe, or for the wedding of an American, but, in this case, the company to be large, the amounts may be doubled, or trebled.

**Dark Cake.**—Brown sugar, 2 cups; molasses, 1 cup; butter, 1 cup; raisins, chopped, 2 cups; sour milk, 1 cup; saleratus, 2 tea-spoonfuls; 3 eggs; flour, 5 cups; cloves and cinnamon, of each, 1 table-spoonful; allspice, 1 tea-spoonful; 1 small nutmeg, all well beaten.

*Remarks.*—Mrs. C. B. Greely, of Alpena, Mich., says: This makes two good sized loaves. Is splendid! Don't get too much butter in, take large cups of flour, etc.   The compiler needs not to add a word, he knows it will be found plendid.

**Charity Cake.**—Sugar, 1 cup; butter the size of an egg; 1 egg; stir to a cream; add sweet milk, 1 cup; flour, 2 cups; cream of tartar, 2 tea-spoonfuls; soda, 1 tea-spoonful.—*Emily A. Hammond.*

*Remarks,*—No other place so appropriate for a poor man's cake, as to let it follow charity cake, for who needs charity any more than a poor man is likely to.

**Poor Man's Cake.**—One cup of sugar, 1 cup of milk, 1 table-spoonful of butter, 1 tea-spoonful cream of tartar, ½ tea-spoonful of soda dissolved in the milk, 1 egg, a little cinnamon, and flour to make it as stiff as pound cake.

**Potato Cake.**—"S. A. M." (Sam), of Mogadore, O., claims this to be a new kind of cake.   She says:   Mashed potatoes, 1 cup; sugar, 1 cup; risings, 1 cup; ⅔ cup of shortening, and 3 eggs.   DIRECTIONS—Stir well together about 5 o'clock P. M., and at bedtime stir all the flour in the mixture you can with a big spoon; keep in a warm place, and in the morning put it in gem dishes and let rise again.   Bake in a slow oven, and you will have a cake that children and invalids can eat without harm.

**Potato Cake, Without Eggs and Quick Process.**—Mashed potatoes, 3 cups; flour, 1 cup; melted butter and sugar, of each ½ cup; a little salt; milk to make a paste of proper consistence to roll; roll rather thin, and bake in a quick oven.   If not light enough first time, add a little soda to the flour next time.

**Potato Puffs.**—Take mashed potatoes and make them into a paste, with 1 or 2 eggs, roll it out with a dust of flour and cut round with a saucer; have ready some cold roast meat (any kind) free from gristle and chopped fine, seasoned with salt, pepper, thyme, or pickles cut up fine; place them on the potato and fold in over like a puff, pinch or pick it neatly around and bake for a few minutes.—*Detroit Free Press.*

*Remarks.*—The author would say, "no pickles in his," but cold ham would be very nice.

**Spanish Fritter Puffs.**—Powdered sugar, 1 table-spoonful; butter, 2 ozs. (2 table-spoonfuls); salt, 1 tea-spoonful; water, 1 cup; yolks of 4 eggs; flour.   DIRECTIONS—Put the water into a saucepan, add the sugar, salt and butter, and, while it is boiling, stir in flour enough to have it leave the pan; then stir in the one-by-one, the yolks of the eggs; now drop a tea-spoonful at a time into boiling lard and fry to a light brown.   If nicely done they will be very puffy.

**Philadelphia Cream Puffs.**—Butter, 2 cups; 10 eggs; flour, 3 cups; water, 1 pt.; soda, 1 tea-spoonful.   DIRECTIONS—Boil the water, melt the butter in it, stir in the flour dry while the water is boiling; when cool, add the soda and the well-beaten eggs; drop the mixture with a spoon on buttered tins and bake 20 minutes.   CAUTION—Do not open the oven door more than twice while they are baking.

**Cake Without Eggs.**—Sugar 1 cup; butter, ½ cup; sweet milk, 1 cup; cream of tartar, 2 tea-spoonfuls, soda, 1 tea-spoonful. Flavor to taste.

**Cider Cake, Requires Neither Eggs Nor Milk.**—Sugar, 1½ cups; butter, ¾ cup; sweet cider, 1⅓ cups; flour, 4½ cups; soda, 1 tea-spoonful; cinnamon and cloves, of each 1 tea-spoonful.

*Remarks.*—Although this from the "Young Lady." of Tontogany, O.. it will make a nice cake, better than some old ladies make.

**Scotch Cake.**—Brown sugar, 1 lb.; flour. 1 lb : butter, ½ lb.; 2 eggs; cinnamon. 1 tea-spoonful; roll very thin and bake. [See, also, "Scotch Oat-cake."]

**Buffalo Cake.**—Sugar, 1 cup; butter, melted, 1 table-spoonful; 1 egg, beaten to a froth; soda, 1 tea-spoonful, dissolved in sweet milk, ⅔ cup; cream of tartar, 2 tea-spoonfuls; flour to make so it will pour on tins. Bake like jelly cake, and put custard or jelly between.

*Remarks.*—Mrs. J. A. Heister, of Denver, Col , says. ' It is cheap and good enough for any one." And I cannot account for the name, unless it is because the Denver people take it with them when they go out to hunt buffalo.

**Buckeye Cake.**—Sugar, ¾ lb ; butter, ½ lb.; 6 eggs, well beaten; sweet milk, ½ pt.; 1 lb. of "prepared" flour: flavor with vanilla. Good for Ohio people, where they use this kind of flour.

**Boston Cake.**—Sugar, 1 cup; milk, 1 cup; butter. 1 table-spoonful; 1 egg, flour, 2½ cups; cream of tartar, 2 tea-spoonfuls; soda, 1 tea-spoonful; flavor with lemon or nutmeg. Nutmeg is their favorite: so much so, some of them have been accused of making wooden ones.

**Vanilla Cake.**—Sugar, ½ cup; 4 eggs; sour cream, 4 table-spoonfuls; salt, 1 tea-spoonful; cream of tartar, 1 tea-spoonful; soda, ⅛ tea-spoonful, flour, 1½ cups; flavor with vanilla—is the way "Jenny" makes hers at Irving, Mich.

**Nutmeg Cake.**—Sugar, 2 cups; butter, 1 cup; 3 eggs; 1 nutmeg; flour, 4 cups; milk, 1 cup; cream of tartar, 2 tea-spoonfuls; soda, 1 tea-spoonful; rind of 1 lemon. DIRECTIONS—Beat sugar and butter together, then add half of the flour and half of the milk, then the beaten eggs, grated nutmeg and grated rink of the lemon, then the balance of the flour, having the cream of tartar mixed into it, and lastly, the balance of the milk with the soda dissolved in it. Beat all thoroughly and bake in bread pans, buttered and prepared.

**Choice Cake.**—Sugar, 1 lb.; flour, 1 lb ; butter, ½ lb.; 7 eggs; cream, 1 cup; saleratus, 1 tea-spoonful; nutmeg, to taste. DIRECTIONS—Beat sugar and butter to a cream, add the eggs, then the cream, with the saleratus dissolved in it; then flour and nutmeg. It requires much beating. Bake in a quick oven. —*Godey's Lady's Book.*

**Rock Cakes, To Make.**—Break 6 eggs into a dish, and beat till very light; then add powdered sugar, 1 lb. (2½ cups), and mix well; then dredge in gradually flour, ½ lb. (1¾ cups), and English currants, ¼ to ½ lb., which have been nicely washed and dried. Mix all well together; then put on to a baking tin (size to suit) with a fork, to make them look as rough as you can.  Bake in a moderate oven, about half an hour.  When cool store them in a box and keep them in a dry place, and they will last as long as you keep them in the box, but if placed on the table at meal times they will not keep a great while

**Cold Water Cake.**—Flour and white sugar, each, 1 cup; 2 eggs; butter, 1 heaping table-spoonful; cold water, 3 table-spoonfuls; baking powder, 1 heaping tea-spoonful.  Not expensive but nice.  Make on general principles.

**German Crisps.**—Sugar, 2 cups; butter, 1 cup; 3 eggs, and the rind and juice of 1 lemon; flour  DIRECTIONS—Mix thoroughly with hand or spooon, adding sufficient flour to roll out.  Roll out very thin  Cut in small cakes. Place in the pan and rub the tops with egg and sprinkle on white sugar.  Two eggs are enough for the tops.  They will bake in a few minutes. — *Harper's Bazar*.

**Common Cake.**—Sugar, 1 cup; butter, ½ cup; sour cream, 1 cup; 2 eggs; soda, 1 tea-spoonful; ½ a nutmeg, and as much flour as needed  DIRECTIONS—Beat the sugar and eggs together, then add the cream and butter, then the nutmeg and soda, and lastly the flour, are the instructions given by Mrs. A. M. McCrary, of Kirwin, Kan.

**Raised Cake**—Light dough, 2 cups; butter, 1 cup; sugar, 2 cups; 3 eggs, beaten light,  Mix all well together, add fruit and spices, as you wish.  It is good without either, but better with plenty of both.  DIRECTIONS—Put in a pan and let stand till light before baking.

**Spiced Cake.**—Butter and cold water, of each, 1 cup; flour, 3 cups; sugar, 2 cups, 3 eggs; soda, 1 tea-spoonful; cinnamon or other spices, as preferred, 2 tea-spoonfuls; chopped raisins, 1 cup; currants, 1 cup.  DIRECTIONS Sarah F. Purdy, of Belmont, Iowa, says: "Beat butter and sugar, adding the beaten eggs, then the cold water  sift the soda into the flour  and add the spice and fruit."

**Aunt Lucy's Spice Cake.**—Sugar, 2 cups; butter, ⅔ cup; 2 eggs; butter milk, 1 cup; soda, 1 tea-spoonful; cloves, 1 tea-spoonful; cinnamon, 1 table-spoonful; ½ of a nutmeg; "rising flour," 1 cup, or to make thick.

*Remarks*—Who ever knew a cake-making aunt that did not make a good cake?  This will make a nice cake, however, even if common flour is used, as the soda will make it light.

**Spiced Cake, Very Fine.**—Sour milk, molasses, and brown sugar, of each, 1 cup; butter, ⅔ cup; 3 eggs; soda, nutmeg, and cloves, of each, 1 tea-spoonful; cinnamon, 1½ tea-spoonfuls (or if any other flavor is preferred to be the most prominent, use the 1½ tea-spoonfuls of that, and of the cinnamon only 1), flour, about 3 cups, or to make the batter pretty thick, as spice cake is disposed, if too thin  to run or spread before the baking begins to set it.  Make as the others.

**Sally Lunn Cake.**—Sugar, 1 egg cup; sweet milk, 1 pt.; butter, 1 table-spoonful; 4 eggs; flour, 4 coffee cups; yeast powder, 3 tea-spoonfuls. DIRECTIONS—Warm the milk and melt the butter in it; beat the whites of the eggs to a stiff froth; the yolks and sugar together, and stir into the warm milk; the yeast powder having been mixed in the flour, sift it in; then the whites of the eggs; pour into a buttered cake mold, and bake in a quick oven 30 minutes.

**"Sallie-Long," or Tea Cake.**—Flour, 1 qt.; baking powder 3 tea spoonfuls; sweet milk, 1 pt.; eggs, 3; butter and lard, of each 1 table-spoonful pulverized sugar, ½ cup. Mix the baking powder into the dry flour; beat the eggs, and stir them and the milk, butter, lard and sugar together, then the flour, mixing all thoroughly; baking in a moderate oven.

*Remarks.*—This cake I suppose to be an own cousin of Sally Lunn, but why it should have been called Long, when, in fact, it is so nice and short, I cannot tell. I give it as I received it, and will make no complaint about its "Long" name, so long as it fills the bill as well as it has done, with my family, for a long time. It is, no doubt, a first cousin of Sally Lunn, above.

**Apees, or Cake Without Eggs or Yeast.**—Fresh butter, 1 lb. (2 cups); sifted flour, 2 lbs. (7 cups;) powdered sugar, 1 lb. (2½ cups); mixed spices (nutmeg, mace and cinnamon), 1 tea-spoonful; caraway seeds, 4 tea-spoonfuls; wine (white is best), 1 large glass; cold water to make a stiff dough. DIRECTIONS—Cut the butter into the flour and rub fine, or smooth, mixing in the sugar and spices, then put in the wine, and water to work stiff, with a broad knife, or knead with a wooden potato masher. Roll thin (less than ⅛ inch), and cut into small cakes. Place in long tins, slightly buttered, not to touch each other. Bake in a quick oven till they are a pale brown.

*Remarks.*—They are quickly made, requiring no eggs nor yeast, and are very nice, resembling, somewhat, the German crisps.

**Cream Cake.**—Sweet milk, 1 pt.; butter, 1 table-spoonful; salt, a pinch; flour, 3 cups. DIRECTIONS—Melt the butter in milk, put in the salt and then mix in the flour, only enough to make a stiff dough. Roll out rapidly, several times, on the board, cut into squares and bake on a griddle, or in a hot oven.

**Cookies, Plain.**—Sugar, 1 cup; butter, ½ cup; soda, ½ tea-spoonful; warm water, ½ cup; flour enough to roll. DIRECTIONS—Dissolve the soda in the warm water; mix, roll very thin, cut and bake in a quick oven.

**Plain Cookies, with Ammonia.**—Sugar, 2 cups; butter, 1 cup; milk, 1 cup; 2 eggs; carbonate of ammonia, ½ oz.; flour, 1 qt. (3½ cups.) DIRECTIONS—Pulverize the ammonia and mix it with the flour, and mix the butter in well, then the other ingredients; use only flour enough to allow you to handle (not stiff); roll thin, cut and bake in a suitable oven—in fact all cookies require quick handling and a quick oven.

**Cookies—Rose Flavor.**—Sugar, 3 cups; butter, 1 cup; 3 eggs; milk, ½ cup; rosewater, 2 table-spoonfuls [see "Tincture of Rose"]; flour, enough to roll out well. DIRECTIONS—Beat the eggs very light, rub the butter, sugar and rosewater together, then the eggs, soda in the milk, flour, etc.; roll thin, bake quickly.

**Carraway Cookies.**—Sugar, 2 cups; butter, 1 cup; 2 eggs; milk, ½ cup; soda, ½ tea-spoonful; caraway seed, 1 table-spoonful, or to taste. I like them to be put in freely.

**Nice Plain Cookies, Without Eggs.**—Sugar, 2 cups; butter, 1 cup, or salt pork drippings; sweet milk (all milk is to be sweet unless sour is called for), 1 cup; cream of tartar, 2 tea-spoonfuls; soda, 1 tea-spoonful; flour to make a dough. DIRECTIONS—Roll thin, bake in a quick oven, but not to scorch. If you have no milk, cold water will do quite well.

**Ginger Cookies, With Molasses.**—Molasses, 2 cups; butter, 1 cup (lard or salt pork drippings do well); hot water, 4 table-spoonfuls; ginger, 1 table-spoonful; salt (unless salt pork drippings are used), 1 tea-spoonful; flour enough to roll out; soda, 1 tea-spoonful.

*Remarks.*—As the ladies say: " It is just splendid."

**Spiced Cookies.**—Orleans molasses, 1 cup; sugar, 1 cup; warm water, ½ cup; soda, 1 large or rounding tea-spoonful; butter, ⅔ cup; cloves, cinnamon and ginger, of each 1 tea-spoonful. DIRECTIONS—Mrs. S. M. Ferguson, of West Holbach, Ill., is the originator of this, and says: " Dissolve the soda in the water, mix soft, roll thin, bake quick, etc. If made nicely and not over baked they will please old people and young children."

**Spiced Cakes.**—Yolks of 4 eggs, well beaten; baking powder, 2½ tea-spoonfuls, in flour, 2½ cups; brown sugar, 1 cup; syrup, milk and butter, of each ½ cup; powdered cloves, 2½ tea-spoonfuls; allspice and cinnamon, powdered, of each 1 tea spoonful. DIRECTIONS—Rub the baking powder and spices well into the flour, add the syrup after the sugar and butter are creamed together, then the beaten eggs, then the milk, and lastly the flour, and prepare at once for a moderate oven. Given me by a sister-in-law after making them many times.

**Macaroons, or Drop Cake.**—Sugar, 1 lb.; blanched and pounded almonds, ¼ lb.; whites of 3 eggs. DIRECTIONS—Mix, sprinkle sugar on paper, then drop the mixture thereon and bake quickly. Very nice.

**Farmers' Gems.**—White sugar, 1 cup; sour cream, 1 cup; soda, 1 tea-spoonful; flour, as for cookies. DIRECTIONS—Roll thin, cut and bake quickly. Sue Perrin makes them in this way. If you expect them to last long, however, you will have to double the quantity of material.

**Drop Cake.**—Powdered sugar, 1 cup; butter, 1 cup; flour, 2 cups; 3 eggs; juice and rind of 1 lemon. DIRECTIONS—Mix butter and sugar to a cream, add the well-beaten eggs, then the flour, and lastly the lemon. Drop on buttered paper and bake in a quick oven.

*Remarks.*—Nice making and nice baking make nice cake, whether plain or delicate cake are being made.

**Drop Cakes.**—Put 6 well-beaten eggs into a pint of thick cream; add a little salt, and make it into a thick batter with flour. Bake it in rings or in small cups 15 or 20 minutes. The same may be made with graham flour

**Rye Drop Cup Cake.**—Wheat flour, 1 cup; 3 eggs, well beaten; new milk, 1 pt.; salt, 1 tea-spoonful; sugar, 1 teaspoonful; rye flour, enough to make a stiff batter; half fill earthen cups, put them in a pan and bake 1 **hour** in a moderate oven.

*Remarks.*—Equal to rye and Indian bread. If you wish them lighter, use baking powder or sour milk and soda. Have them come out just at tea-time, and have some freshly-made butter if you wish to appreciate a good thing.

**Pork Cake.**—Fat salt pork, 1 lb.; strong coffee, 1 pt.; brown sugar, 4 cups; stoned raisins, 1 lb.; citron or English currants, ½ lb.; flour, 9 cups; soda, 1 table-spoonful; 1 nutmeg and 1 table-spoonful of cinnamon. DIREC-TIONS—The pork is to be weighed free of rind and chopped very fine; then pour the coffee, boiling hot, upon it and set on the stove a few minutes before adding any of the other ingredients. The spices are all to be ground, and if citron is used, it is to be finely chopped. The raisins and other fruit are to be dredged with flour to prevent settling. Fit a piece of white paper to the bottom of the pan or pans and cover the top with paper also, to prevent burning. Bake in a moderate oven until a splinter can be thrust into it and pulled out without the cake sticking to it.—*Mrs. Carrie Case, Toledo, O.*

*Remarks.*—This will be very palatable, and will keep as long as you will allow. It is excellent.

**Buns.**—Flour, 6½ cups; sugar, 1 cup; butter, ⅔ cup; milk, 1 cup; currants, 2 cups; yeast, 1 table-spoonful. DIRECTIONS—Dry and sift the flour, melt the butter in the milk; the currants to be washed and dried beforehand. Mix all, and stand in a warm place till it rises, before baking.—*Peterson's Magazine.*

**Buns, Better Than Bakers'.**—Warm milk, 3 cups; sugar, 1 cup; yeast, ½ cup. Stand over night. In the morning add another cup of sugar, 1 cup of butter, knead stiff and let rise again; then cut into 60 pieces, roll in the hand and put into pans just to touch each other, let rise again, then rub with whites of eggs, and bake to a light brown. Currants or raisins improve them. These are much better than bakers' buns.

*Remarks.*—They will be excellent if not allowed to stand so long as to sour before baking—if so, soda will correct it.

**Easter Buns, or "Hot Cross Buns" of the London Criers.**—Sweet milk, 3 cups; yeast, 1 cup; flour, to make a thick batter. Set over night, and in the morning add sugar, ½ cup; ½ a nutmeg; 1 salt-spoonful of salt, and flour enough to roll out like biscuit dough. Knead well and set to rise 5 hours. Roll ½ inch thick, cut and set in a well-buttered pan; when they have stood a ½ hour make a cross with a knife upon each, and instantly put in the oven; bake to a light brown, and brush over with the whites of eggs beaten with white sugar.

*Remarks.*—"Mrs. A. M. S.," of Junction City, Kansas, says: "These are the 'Hot Cross Buns' of the London criers." I know they are nice enough to be that same.

**Breakfast Buns.**—Sugar, sour milk or butter milk, of each, 2 cups; 2 eggs; melted butter, ⅔ cup; soda, 1 tea-spoonful; flour and salt. DIREC-TIONS—Break the eggs into a suitable dish to make the cake in, and beat them well; then put in the sugar, butter and a little salt, and beat all well together; having dissolved the soda in the milk, add it; then sift in sufficient flour to allow handling it upon the molding-board or table, leaving it as soft, however, as you can roll it.  Roll out to half an inch in thickness, and cut with a goblet or a large cutter, as it is intended to have a large and thick bun when done.  If made sufficiently soft they will rise up in the center to fully an inch in thick-ness, and be very nice with coffee as a breakfast dessert.  Put in a stone jar and cover over to prevent their becoming dry.

*Remarks.*—Bakers make a bun, also, having English currants in them. One cup, washed and drained, will be enough for this amount, if evenly mixed in.  Mrs. Chase makes them, sometimes with and then without the fruit, per-haps because the baking has to be done more often when the fruit is in.

**Rusk.**—On putting your light bread in pans save 2 or 3 lbs of dough, and take 5 or 6 eggs, lard or butter, ½ lb.; brown sugar, ½ lb.; mix, and add flour to make dough as stiff as for bread; keep warm, and rise again.  When light, make into rusk the size of a hen's egg, stick a hole in the center of each, place in a pan and when they have risen ½ an inch prime the top with the yolk of an egg beaten with sugar, and bake.

*Remarks.*—This is the plan adopted by " Mrs. J. A. W.,' of Polona, Ill., and this is the only woman, of which I have heard, who could '' jaw' without scolding—j-a-w spells *jaw*; but, to set joking aside, the rusk are nice.  The children like them better. however, if a large raisin is stuck into the center of the top, in place of the hole.

**Rusk With Few Eggs.**—Mrs. Lettie Larsen, of Fair Haven, Minn. makes excellent rusk in the following manner: " New milk, 1 pt.; hop yeast, 1 cup, and flour to make a batter, setting over night; in the morning adding ½ pt. more of new milk, 1 cup of sugar, 1 cup of butter and 1 egg, seasoning with nutmeg, and flour to make quite stiff.  Let it rise, then rolling it out, cutting it it into small cakes, rising again, and baking.  Have ready 1 tea-spoonful of sugar, with an egg well beaten, and just before done, brush over the top with this, replacing till lightly browned, to keep the crust moist."  If she wants extra nice, she adds 1 cup of raisins.

**Rusk Without Eggs.**—When making light bread take 1 pt. of the sponge, 1 cup of sugar, 1 cup of butter, and mix with flour enough to make as for biscuit; spice to taste.  Let set till it rises like bread, then mold into small biscuit and stand till light before baking.

*Remarks.*—Mrs. Etta Wilson says this meets the wants of her people, at Lawn Ridge, Marshall county, Cal.  With nice butter, I haven't a doubt of it.

**Rolls.**—Sweet milk, 1 cup; whites of 2 eggs. butter, ⅔ of a cup; ½ cup of yeast; sugar, 2 table-spoonfuls; flour to make a thick batter.  DIRECTIONS —Raise over night, not putting in the butter nor eggs until morning, working in sufficient more flour to make a soft, or limber dough; form into rolls, place in the pans, and bake as soon as they rise again.

*Remarks.*—For variety's sake, sometimes use water in place of milk, again, and especially if to be eaten with meat, leave out the sugar; and if eggs are scarce make without; but if for "tea," it is better with them all in.  I make such remarks, occasionally, to set cooks to thinking for themselves, for it is by thought and experiment that hundreds of varieties may be made from the few pages of recipes here given—the same will hold good throughout the book, provided the principles of chemistry are not interfered with, *i. e.*, if sour milk or buttermilk is used, the soda must never be left out, it neutralizes the acid and thereby produces a gas (carbonic acid gas), which gives lightness to the rolls, or cakes.

**Parker House Breakfast Rolls.**—Sifted flour, 2 qts.; sugar, butter and yeast, of each ½ cup. DIRECTIONS—Mix with new milk until the consistence of a nice light bread dough. If for tea, stand in a warm place 4 hours; if for breakfast, let stand in a cooler place over night. When light, in either case, take enough off for a roll, and roll it out to any desired size. Spread on one-half of the piece ½ tea-spoonful of melted butter, and lap over the other half, place in a pan to rise again, and as soon as light bake in a quick oven.

*Remarks.*—If as nicely done as at the Parker House, Boston, they will be very nice indeed. I have tried them there and at home.

**Heating the Oven for Cake Baking.**—So much depends, in baking cake, upon the heat of the oven, it is probably best to repeat here some of the instructions given in the general directions, and, perhaps, an additional thought or two upon the subject. In baking cake the oven should always be hot, unless the directions give something especially to the contrary; yet, if the oven is too hot, a few nails may be placed under the pans, and the paper doubled over the top, and a cover may be removed from the top of the stove; but the oven door must not be left open any longer than is absolutely necessary, to follow the above hints. The drafts may be entirely closed (should always be partially closed when baking cake) for a short time, or until the temperature is right. To tell when the cake is done, pierce it with a broom splint, and if the splint comes out free of the cake mixture, it may be considered done, but it is better to leave it in a few minutes over, rather than to remove it a minute too quick, the same holds good also with short cake, bread, pies, etc.

**Short Cake, Sweet, with Soda.**—Flour, 3 cups; butter, 3 table-spoonfuls; sour cream, or rich clabber (milk becoming thick), 1½ cups; 1 egg; sugar, 1 table-spoonful; soda, 1 tea-spoonful; salt, 1 tea-spoonful. DIRECTIONS—Dissolve the soda in a little warm water and add it and the beaten egg to the milk; having put the salt in the flour, cut the butter in small pieces, and work it in smoothly also; mix all, handling as little as possible. Roll quickly and bake in a hot oven. The soda and sour cream will take care of the rising.

**Shortcake, Plain, from Light Dough.**—Prepare the dough as for biscuit, doubling the amount of butter; roll out to make a cake of good thickness; let rise and bake in a quick oven.

**Strawberry Shortcake, in Layers.**—Make the cake as for the sweet above, but roll in 2 sheets, ½ an inch thick for the upper, the lower less; spread a very little butter upon the thin one, placing it in the pan, put the other upon it, and bake. When a little cool, lift off the top one and place a good layer of strawberries upon the other, and replace the top, spreading as many berries upon the top as will lie; serve with sweetened cream or milk—of course the first is the best.

*Remarks.*—My family find that raspberries, blackberries, etc., are also very nice used in the place of strawberries.

**Strawberry Shortcake, Old Way.**—Mix as for biscuit, roll about 1 inch thick, and bake, When done, have the strawberries mixed with sugared cream; split the cake with a sharp knife spread lightly with butter the lower half, then put in a thick layer of the fruit, replacing the top, and covering the top also. Some persons then replace in the oven for a few minutes; but this, I think, make it more like pie than fresh berry shortcake. Other berries or pie-plant may be used, but pieplant must be stewed and no cream used.

**Mother's Strawberry Shortcake.**—I believe the Household and the editor will agree with me in thinking Puck never ate any strawberry shortcake. We are 50 years old, but don't we remember, as well as if it was but yesterday, the dear, delightful ones made by mother in our childhood, and don't we know just how they were made, too; we heard her tell so many times, as every one wanted her recipe. She made them as follows: Sour cream, 1 cup; cream of tartar, 1 tea-spoonful; soda, ⅔ tea-spoonful, with flour to make a suitable dough to roll ½ an inch thick, baked nicely; split open and spread each piece with the sweetest, freshest butter; then pour on to one of the halves, not 6 or 7 gritty, mussy berries, but 2 whole cups of those large, luscious ones from the south side of the garden; put on the other half for a cover, and pour over sweetened cream when eaten.—*Aunt Lulu, Red Willow, Neb.*

*Remarks.*—The author loves all these aunts, because they know how it is done; but he would love them better if they were not ashamed of their real names. This is about as my own mother used to make them, so I know it will prove good and worthy to be followed by all who have the nice " sour cream." But good rich milk with soda—no cream of tartar—will do very nicely. Of course, any berries, fresh or canned, at all suitable for a short cake, ripe, nice peaches, or even a nice, thick custard, may take the place of strawberries when they are not plenty, or for the sake of variety. See the remarks also following "Pumpkin Shortcake," below.

**Pumpkin Shortcake, With Graham Flour.**—"Stewed and strained pumpkin or squash, ' C' oatmeal porridge and water, each 1 cup. Beat these up together, and then stir in 3 cups of Graham flour. Mix thoroughly, spread ½ an inch thick on a baking-tin, and bake half an hour in a good oven. Cover for 10 minutes, and serve warm or cold."

*Remarks*—Our readers will see by the quotation marks (" ") that this is not my own, nor do I known who to credit it to But I have given it for the sake of a few explanations, or remarks, which, I think, will be for the general good; and first, you will see that a porridge is called for made from " C " oat-meal; what does the " C " mean here? It means the grade of fineness of the meal, as known to dealers, the same as "A" coffee sugar means the best—"C" coffee sugar is not quite so good While with the oatmeal it means not quite so coarse a meal as "A" would be For Scotch cake the finest kind is used, and, I should think, would be the best to make into a porridge. Second, some persons never use oatmeal porridge; then, unless people will use a little of good common sense, they, or persons living where they cannot get oatmeal, could never have those nice short cakes; but by using, or calling up this common sense, and reasoning a little, they may say, "now I have not got the oatmeal, nor can I get it; but I will take milk in its place; and even, if no milk, I will take water, and by adding a little butter, lard or drippings, I will have just as good a cake"—and so they would. Now, please judge, in the same manner, in all cases, where such difficulties may of necessity arise, then these remarks will have their intended effect. I will add this word, only, additional, those who don't know anything more than simply to always confine themselves to, or follow a recipe, or receipt, as generally called, (never changing it at 'all) will never amount to much, to themselves, or to the world. The above recipe says "pumpkin, or squash"—everybody ought to know that squash will make the richer cake.

**Apple Shortcake.**—Season well stewed apple sauce with sugar and nutmeg, or mace, make any of the nice shortcakes, above given, open, or split, as the case may be, butter nicely and spread on a thick layer of the prepared sauce, and replace the top; serve with well sweetened cream.

*Remarks.*—You will need to have quite a quantity, if you satisfy the taste and desires of the family, and the guests. The following from dried apples, will enable families to have apple shortcake all the year round, says a writer in the New York *Post.*

**Apple Shortcake From Dried Apples.**—I will tell you of something that makes an agreeable filling for a shortcake. You will not believe it until you try it, but for those unfortunate ones to whom the acid of the strawberry is as poison, it can not be too highly recommended. Take some nice dried apples, wash and soak, and cook them until they are tender; then rub them through a sieve or a fine colander, add sugar and the grated rind and juice of a lemon; then make a shortcake in the ordinary manner and use this in place of the berries.

**Scotch Oat-Cakes.**—Put 3 ounces of drippings with a small tea-cup of water into a pan, and let it boil. Pour it over 1 lb. of oatmeal. Stir it; roll it out at once, very thin; cut with a small round cutter; bake in the oven till done.

*Remarks.*—As suggested in the remarks following pumpkin shortcake, the Scotch cake is nicest made with oatmeal that is ground the finest, which is, as I think, that which is bolted, or sifted out from the coarse, in fact, a flour, rather than meal. I like them done quite crisp.

**Biscuit, Plain and Light.**—Take enough light bread dough to make what you desire; for each square bread pan full, work, or knead in, 1 tablespoonful of butter, lard, or pork drippings, mold into biscuit, place in the pan, or pans, and, when risen again, place in a moderately hot oven—the heat increasing—as for bread. If biscuit or bread are put into a hot oven, the crust is soon set and the rising is, thereby, greatly prevented.

**Light Biscuit, Sweet.**—If a sweet biscuit is desired, prepare the dough as for rusk, and follow the same directions.

*Remarks.*—Mrs. Chase furnishes us with nice, light biscuit by following the directions she has here given me. I have given them a place here because they seem to belong to the rusk and shortcake family, rather than among the breads.

**Biscuit with Baking Powder, Quickly Made.**—Flour, 3½ cups; baking powder, 3 tea-spoonfuls; butter, or nice lard, 1 table-spoonful (rounding); sweet milk. DIRECTIONS—Stir the baking powder into the flour and sift; work in the butter smoothly; then use milk enough to have a soft dough; mold into biscuit by using flour, dusting freely; bake in a hot oven at once.

*Remarks.*—Do not knead biscuit made with baking powder, nor make them stiff, in this lies the secret of making nice light biscuit with baking powder, so says "my good woman," and she knows from an experience of 40 years of married life. In cold weather the butter will work in easier, if warmed. Water may take the place of milk by doubling the amount of butter or lard, to make then equally rich.

**Biscuit With Soda, Cream of Tartar, and Sweet Milk.**— Flour, 1 qt. (3½ cups); cream of tartar, 2 tea-spoonfuls; soda and salt, of each, 1 tea-spoonful; butter, lard, or "drippings," 1 table-spoonful, and sweet milk to wet it up properly. DIRECTIONS—Roll the cream of tartar and soda finely and sift together with the flour; mix in the shortening, and wet up with the milk to a proper consistence, mixing with the hand quickly, till it can be rolled out, cut, and place in tins, and into a hot oven at once, if you wish them to be "light" and "puffy," which they will be if this is all properly and quickly done. For as soon as the soda and cream of tartar are mixed into the flour and wet they begin to produce the gas which gives the biscuit or cake its lightness. The oven may be tempered down a little, if thought best, after the baking is fairly begun, to avoid burning. *Mrs. Catharine Baldwin.*

*Remarks.*—The author has seen nothing in the biscuit line so light, nice, sweet, and good, for his eating—when cold. Most people, however, prefer them hot. Half milk and half water does very well. When no milk is to be had, a very little more shortening will fill the bill.

**Breakfast Biscuit.**—To 3 cups of buttermilk add 1 of butter, 1 tea-spoonful of cream of tartar, ½ a tea-spoonful of soda, sufficient salt, and flour enough to make the dough just stiff enough to roll out into biscuit. These will be wonderfully light and delicate.

**Biscuit or Bread, Quick.**—Flour, 1 qt, (3 or 3½ cups); salt, scant tea-spoonful; baking powder, 2 tea-spoonfuls; sift together. Sweet milk makes soft dough. Work quickly as soft as can be handled, and bake immediately.

The next five recipes I take from the New York *Tribune*, headed "Some Southern Recipes," which will prove valuable to some people, no doubt, in the North as well as in the South. and as they are all in the nature of biscuit or cakes, except the last one—"Velvet Cream,"—I will keep them together as found in the *Tribune*.

**1. Southern Biscuit.**—Two cups of self-rising flour, 1 spoonful of lard; mix with warm milk; knead into soft dough, and roll; cut with a biscuit cutter and prick each with a straw. Cook in a hot oven 10 minutes.

**2. Palmetto Flannel Cakes.**—One pt. of buttermilk, 2 well-beaten eggs, flour enough to make a stiff batter—the flour to be mixed, half wheat and half corn flour. Put a tea-spoonful of sea foam into the flour and cook on a griddle.

**3. Breakfast Muffins.**—For a small family, use 1 pt. of milk, 3 gills of wheat flour, 3 eggs, and a pinch of salt. Beat the eggs very light, add the milk, and lastly stir in the flour. Bake in rings or small pans and in a quick oven. They are very light.

**4. Breakfast Waffles.**—After breakfast stir into the hominy that is left 1 tea-spoonful of butter and a little salt. Set it aside. The next morning thin it with milk and add 2 eggs, beaten well. Stir in flour enough to make the right consistency, and bake in waffle-irons.

**5. Velvet Cream.**—Two table-spoonfuls of gelatine, dissolved in ½ a tumbler of water; 1 pt. of rich cream, 4 table-spoonfuls of sugar; flavor with sherry, vanilla extract, or rose water. This is a delicious dessert, and can be made in a few minutes. It may be served with or without cream.

*Remarks.*—See the remarks above "Southern Biscuit."

**Rusks.**—Rusks require a longer time for rising than ordinary rolls or biscuits. If you wish them for tea one evening, you must make all your preparations and begin them the day before; In cold weather, to make up 2½ qts. of flour, prepare early in the afternoon a sponge in this manner: Mix into a paste with 1 pt. of boiling water 2 table-spoonfuls of sugar, 3 of flour, and 2 large potatoes, boiled and mashed smooth. At 7 in the evening make up your dough with this sponge, adding 3 well-beaten eggs, ¾ of a lb. of sugar, and ½ a pt. of sweet milk. Set it away in a covered vessel, leaving plenty of room for it to swell. Next morning after breakfast work into the risen dough, which should not be stiff, a ¼ of a lb. of butter and lard mixed. Make into rolls or biscuits, and let the dough rise for the second time. Flavor with 2 grated nutmegs, or ½ oz. of pounded stick cinnamon When very light, bake in a quick, steady oven till of a pretty brown color; glaze over the top with the yolk of an egg, and sprinkle lightly with powdered white sugar.

**Rusk.**—Boil and mash 2 good-sized potatoes, 1 qt. rich milk, 1 compressed yeast cake, dissolved, and flour to make a stiff batter; mix at noon; in the evening, when quite light, rub together ½ lb. of sugar, ¼ lb. of butter, and beat very light 2 eggs; stir these into the batter with ½ a grated nutmeg; mold up soft, put in a warm place, and when quite light break off pieces about the size of an egg, form them into small cakes laying them closely together in the pan; when very puffy wash over the top with a little sweetened milk and a little sugar if desired. Sugar is generally used on the top of rusk, but not on biscuit. Bake in a moderately quick oven.

**Indian Rusk.**—Two light cups Indian meal, 1 cup flour, 1 tea-spoonful saleratus, enough sour or buttermilk to dissolve, 1 cup sweet milk; stir in ¾ cup molasses. Bake at once.

**Muffins, No. 1, Very Light and Nice.**—Flour, sifted, 1 qt.; sugar, 1 cup: eggs, 1; sweet milk, 2 cups; lard, 1 heaping table-spoonful; salt, 1 tea-spoonful; baking powder, 2 tea-spoonfuls. Mix on general principles; put into muffin rings, set in a pan, or, what is better, cast-iron muffin rings made in sets, and hot when dipped in, and placed at once into a quick oven.—*Mrs. Catharine Baldwin, Toledo, O.*

*Remarks.*—This amount will make about 1½ dozen, so you 'can judge by the size of the family to use more or less material, as needed. Eaten in place of bread, with the meat course, then with butter and syrup, they are splendid. I think the nicest I ever ate. Very nice also cold. Although they are so light and dry, I do not object to eating them hot:

**Muffins, No. 2. With Eggs.**—Sugar, ⅓ cup; butter or lard, 1 large table-spoonful; salt, 1 tea-spoonful; sweet milk, 1 qt. (if water is used, double the shortening); yeast, ¾ cup; 3 eggs; flour to make a batter. DIRECTIONS—Make over night; in the morning beat the eggs nicely and stir into the batter, and bake in muffin rings in a quick oven. If the oven is sufficiently hot they will bake in 20 minutes.

**Muffins, No. 3, Without Eggs.**—Sweet milk, 1 cup; flour, 2 cups; baking powder, 1 heaping tea-spoonful; bake in cup tins, in a hot oven.

**Muffins, No. 4, With Cream.**—Nice sweet cream, 2½ cups; flour, 2½ cups; 3 eggs; butter, 2 table-spoonfuls; salt, 1 tea-spoonful. DIRECTIONS—Beat the eggs very light, adding the cream, salt and butter; then stir in the flour, stirring only sufficient to mix evenly. Only half fill the rings and bake in a hot oven, serving as soon as done.

*Remarks.*—Muffin rings should always be well buttered. '

**Graham Muffins, No. 5.**—Graham flour, 2 cups, or 1 of graham and 1 of white, as you prefer, only even full; sweet milk, 2 cups, a little scant; eggs, 2, well beaten. Bake in a hot oven; about 15 minutes will be required.

**Corn Meal Muffins, No. 6.**—Corn meal and flour, each 2 cups; baking powder, 1½ tea-spoonfuls; eggs, 3, beaten with sugar and butter, each ½ cup; sweet milk, 1 pt.; salt, a little. DIRECTIONS—Mix the baking powder into the mixed meal and flour, beat eggs, sugar and butter together, then the milk; stir in the meal, having the muffin rings set in a pan, fill properly and place at once in a hot oven.

**Graham Gems.**—Sour milk, 2 cups; sugar, ½ cup; soda, ½ tea-spoonful; graham flour, to stir thick; bake in cups, or iron gem pans, in a hot oven.
*Remarks.*—Both light and healthful.

**Graham Gems, With Sour Milk and Eggs.**—Sour milk, 1 pt., 1 or 2 eggs, well beaten, with one or 2 table-spoonfuls of sugar; soda, 1 tea-spoonful, and nice fresh graham flour to make a stiff batter; if 1 egg only 1 spoon of sugar. Put into heated iron gem pans and bake in a hot oven, and they will be light and nice.

**Graham Gems, With Sweet Milk and Cream.**—Sweet cream, 1 cup; sweet milk, 2 cups; salt, 1 salt-spoonful; graham flour, to make a batter, only a little stiffer than for griddle cakes. Beat thoroughly and drop into hot gem pans, while standing on the stove. Bake quickly, but be careful not to burn. If no cream, use milk in its place, with a very little butter to get the same richness.—*American Farm Journal.*

*Remarks.*—If any one fails to get light gems, next time add a little soda.

**Graham Gems.**—I have been watching your papers to see if they gave any recipe for graham gems as good as mine. I have seen none. Take 1½ good pt. of graham flour, 1 pt. of sweet milk, mix them well together, beat the whites of 2 large eggs to a stiff foam, add yolks, beat well, heat gem pans hot, grease, have oven pretty hot, mix eggs in the last thing, carefully and quickly, as soon as they are beaten. Bake from 7 to 10 minutes.—*Mrs. M. P. Bush, Saline, Mich.,, in Detroit Post and Tribune.*

**Graham Gems with Sour Milk or Buttermilk.**—Graham flour, 1 qt.; 1 egg, well beaten; butter, 1 table-spoonful, melted; soda, 1 tea-spoonful; a little salt, sour milk or buttermilk, as below. Put the flour, beaten egg, butter and salt into a pan, dissolve the soda in a cup of the milk, and stir it with more sour milk, sufficient to make a stiff batter. The gem pans being warm, or hot, and buttered, dip in the batter to half fill them, for, if properly prepared, they will raise to fill the pans. This will be about sufficient to fill two sets of pans. Bake in a quick oven. These and graham griddle cakes are the only warm bread which the doctor allows dyspeptics to eat. Other bread should always be one day old before eaten by dyspeptics. Except warm corn bread, or breakfast corn cakes may also be eaten in moderation by dyspeptics, if it does not disagree with the stomach, as shown by rising after eating.

**Graham and Wheat Pop Overs.**—For the graham, use fine graham flour and milk, each 4 cups; eggs, 4; well beaten together; and the gem irons being hot, dip in, and bake in a ready hot oven.

For the wheat use the milk and eggs, and white flour enough to make a soft batter. Bake the same. Nice butter, and any nice fruit sauce, as berries, peaches, etc., make either kind very enjoyable.

**Corn Cake with Soda.**—Indian meal and wheat flour, of each 1 cup; butter the size of an egg; 2 eggs; sugar, ¾ of a cup; milk, 1 cup; cream of tartar, 1 tea-spoonful; soda or saleratus, ½ tea-spoonful. Bake in a moderately hot oven.

**Corn Cake, Set Over Night.**—Put 1 pt. of meal in a dish with 1 tea-spoonful each of butter, sugar and salt; then pour over them 1 cup of boiling milk; when cool enough to bear the finger well, add yeast, ½ cup, the same of flour and 2 beaten eggs; now, thin with water until a proper consistence for baking nicely. If kept quite warm it will rise in 2 or 3 hours. Bake in a moderate oven. Corn cakes require nearly double the time to bake, and less heat than flour; still they require good steady heat.

**Vermont Johnny Cake.**—Sour milk, 1 cup; soda, 1 tea-spoonful;

butter or lard, 1 table-spoonful; Indian meal to make a thin batter.    Bake in a hot oven.—*Elizabeth Kent, Burlington, Vt.*

**Plain Corn Cake, to Bake at Once.**—Three cups sour milk, or buttermilk; 3 cups of Indian meal; 3 table-spoonfuls of molasses; 1 egg; a pinch of salt; 1 tea-spoonful of soda, and a heaping table-spoonful of flour. Bake in a quick oven.

**Kentucky Corn Dodgers.**—Place your griddle where it will heat, for this is much better than a bread pan, there being less danger of scorching at the bottom.    Take an even pint of sifted meal, a heaping table-spoonful of lard, a pinch of salt and a scant half pint of cold water; mix well and let it stand while you grease your griddle and sprinkle some meal over it.    Make the dough into rolls the size and shape of goose eggs, and drop them on the griddle, taking care to flatten as little as possible, for the less bottom crust the better.    Place in the oven and bake until brown on the bottom.    Then change the grate and brown on top, taking from 20 to 30 minutes for the whole process.    To be eaten while hot, with plenty of good butter.

**Corn Bread or Breakfast Corn Cake.**—Some years ago business called me to pass through Toledo several times, and I staid over night, each time, at the Island House, where I found so much better corn bread at the breakfast table than I had ever eaten—according to my custom when traveling and finding some dish extra nice—I obtained the recipe, through influence of the waiter girl, as "mail carrier," (paying a price equal to the price of this book,) who wrote it out for me in my diary while I ate my breakfast; here it is: One quart of corn meal, 1 cup of flour, or a little less; 1 table-spoonful of baking powder; milk, to wet; beating in 1 or 2 eggs, a little sugar and salt; put into a dripping pan, and put, at once, into a hot oven, but do not dry it up by over-baking.    (See Corn Dodgers among the breads.)

*Remarks.*—I think I have eaten of it more than 100 times since, but I have never seen corn cake to excel it.    It should be 1 to 1½ inches thick when baked.

**Oatmeal, or Scotch, Cake.**—Into 1 qt. of cold water stir the finest oatmeal enough to make it about as thick as hasty pudding.    Be sure that the meal is sprinkled in so slowly, and that the stirring is so active, that the mush will have no lumps in it,    Now, put it on the buttered pan, where it can be spread out to half the thickness of a common cracker, and smooth it down with a wet case knife.    Run a sharp knife across it, so as to mark it into the sized pieces you wish, and then place it in a warm oven and bake slowly, being careful not to brown it.    Salt.

**Waffles, With Yeast.**—Sweet milk 2 cups; flour, 2 cups; yeast, 3 table-spnonfuls; 2 eggs; melted butter, 1 table-spoonful; salt, 1 salt-spoonful. DIRECTIONS—Set the sponge over night; in the morning beat and stir in the eggs and butter; bake in waffle-irons.

**Rice Waffles.**—Cold boiled rice, 1 cup; sweet milk, 2½ cups; 2 eggs; butter, 2 table-spoonfuls; cream of tartar, 1 tea-spoonful; soda, ½ tea-spoon-ful; use flour to make the batter.    Bake in waffle-irons.

**Fried Cakes, Nut Cakes, Doughnuts, Crullers, or Twist Cakes, etc.**—It does not matter which you call them, but Mrs. J. M. Venoy, of Wayne, Mich., informs the Detroit *Tribune* that for 10 years she has made fried cakes in the following manner without a failure: Sugar, 2 cups; cream and buttermilk, of each 1 cup; 2 eggs; soda and salt, of each 1 tea-spoonful.

**Raised Doughnuts, or Fried Cake.**—Bread sponge, equal to 1 qt.; warm water, 1 pt.; 2 eggs; sugar, 1 cup; salt, a pinch; lard or fryings. 3 tea-spoonfuls; cinnamon, 1 tea-spoonful. DIRECTIONS—Mix same as bread; when light roll out and cut in any desired shape, and fry in hot lard. Mrs. J. F. Bayles, of Salina, Kans., furnishes this recipe to the *Blade*, and says: "If made without sugar, they are nice with coffee. I never object to the sugar, even with coffee."

**Doughnuts, as Made by "Peggy Shortcake."**—Sugar, 1 cup; 1 egg; sour milk, 1 cup; soda, ½ tea-spoonful; flour to mix as for biscuit. DIRECTIONS—"Peggy" says: "Roll pretty thin; have your lard boiling hot, and fry a nice brown. No dyspepsia about these; try 'em, if you want such as grow 'way down East.'"

**Doughnuts.**—Sugar, 1 cup; butter, ½ cup; 4 eggs; flour, 3½ cups; milk, 1 cup; cream of tartar, 2 tea-spoonfuls; soda, 1 tea-spoonful; salt, 1 tea spoonful; nutmeg, to taste. DIRECTIONS—Beat sugar and eggs together, with the cream of tartar and butter in the flour; dissolve the soda in the milk, then add it to the eggs and sugar, then the flour; roll out thin, cut and fry in hot lard.

**Crullers, With or Without Eggs.**—Buttermilk or sour milk, cream and sugar, of each ½ cup; saleratus or soda, 1 tea-spoonful; spice and salt, to taste; a little yeast, and flour enough to mold, and let rise before frying; or, if an egg is at hand, beat and put in; the yeast may be left out, and the cakes molded, cut and twisted to suit and fried at once. But care must always be given in the frying, heat of the lard, etc.; for if not done they are spoiled, as much so as if scorched or over-done. Done nicely, any of these will be nice of their kind.

**Fried Cakes.**—Sugar and sweet milk, of each 1 cup; 2 eggs; baking powder, 1½ tea-spoonfuls; melted lard, 6 table-spoonfuls; salt, 1 salt-spoonful, or to taste; flour to make as soft as can be rolled. Cut it into any shape desired and fry carefully. The author prefers his the next day after made, and so on as long as they keep without becoming too dry and hard; but if any of these cakes become dry and hard—the same with biscuit or slices of bread—steaming softens them very nicely.

**Norwegian Breakfast Cake, Fried—Very Nice.**—Put into a pan 4 eggs and 4 table-spoonfuls of sugar, and beat very light. Then add 1½ cups of sweet cream, and 1 tea-spoonful of salt, flour enough to roll very thin. Cut in diamonds, and have ready a frying-pan of hot lard. The lard should be about half an inch deep in the pan. Lay the cakes in and turn quickly. They should fry fast. If you want them very nice, roll them in pulverized sugar as you take from the lard. In making them be careful not to roll the cakes up as you put them into the frying-pan, but keep them nice and flat.—*Fannie T. Bradley, Fossum, Minn., in Blade.*

**Rye and Indian Fried Cakes, or Drop Cakes.**—Indian meal, 1 pt.; rye meal, ½ pt.; molasses, 2 table-spoonfuls, and a little salt; cold milk to make a smooth batter, and drop from a spoon into hot lard. If not as light as desired, use a little soda next time. To be eaten with syrup.

**Fritters, Plain—Quick.**—Sweet milk, 1 pt.; 4 eggs; salt, 1 tea spoon-ful; baking powder, 1 table-spoonful; flour. DIRECTIONS—Beat the eggs well, stir in salt and milk; then put the baking powder into 2 or 3 cups of flour and stir in, using as much more flour as will stir in well; drop into hot lard. To be eaten with maple syrup, or syrup made by dissolving granulated sugar.

*Remarks.*—"Ivy," of West Jefferson, Ohio, calls these Johnny Jumpup Cakes, because they jump up from the bottom of the hot lard so quickly and lightly.

**Fritters, Sweet, Quick.**—Make as above, with the addition of 1 table-spoonful each of sugar and butter.

**Fritters, Light.**—Warm water, 1 pt.; yeast, 2 table-spoonfuls; salt, ½ tea-spoonful; stir in flour to make a thick batter. When light, drop into hot lard and fry brown. Eat with syrup or honey, while warm.

**Cream Fritters.**—Milk and cream, of each, 1 pt.; 6 eggs; ½ of a nut-meg; salt, 1 tea-spoonful; flour, 1½ pts.; baking powder, 2 tea-spoonfuls. DIRECTIONS—Mix in the usual manner, stirring in the sweet cream last; let the lard be pretty hot when dropped in.

**Orange Fritters.**—Take 3, or as many large smooth oranges, as needed, take off the peel and the white skin also, then slice them, crosswise, ¼ inch thick, pick the seeds out, and dip the slices in a thick batter made according to any of the foregoing recipes; fry nicely, placing them in layers, on a plate, as fried, sifting sugar over each layer. Serve hot.

**Cheese and Apples, or Sandwich Fritters.**—Wash and slice as many tart apples as needed, and cut half as many slices of cheese; beat 2 or 3 eggs, or according to the amount needed, and season rather highly with salt, mustard and pepper. Soak the cheese, a few minutes, in the egg mixture, then place a slice of the cheese between two slices of the apple, and dip them into the mixture also; then fry in hot butter, turning carefully, the same as oysters are fried. Serve hot, for breakfast, or Sunday tea, as there is too much labor for more than once a week.

**Corn Fritters.**—One qt. corn meal; 1 table-spoonful of lard; 2 eggs; 1 table-spoonful of salt; scald the meal with the lard in it with boiling water, cool with a little milk, add the eggs (beaten light); beat very hard for 10 min-utes; make them thin enough with cold milk to drop off the spoon and retain their shape in boiling lard; have the lard boiling hot when you drop them in. Serve hot.

**Buckwheat Griddle Cakes, Aunt Essy's.**—Warm water, 3 pts.; salt, 1 dessert-spoonful; ⅓ cup of good jug yeast; buckwheat flour to make a batter. DIRECTIONS—Set in a warm place over night, and bake on a hot griddle. Serve warm, with good butter and syrup, made of sugar—maple is best—and she says you will need but little else for breakfast.. The author would have at least some potatoes, and nice steak, and plenty of butter gravy with his breakfast; does not even re fuse nice ham with plenty of ham gravy with his buckwheat cakes.

**Buckwheat Griddle Cakes, "Arf and Arf."**—Buckwheat and wheat flour, of each 1 pt.; molasses, 2 table-spoonfuls; a little salt; mix with water, and just before baking stir in a heaping table-spoonful of yeast powder.

*Remarks.*—"Sunshine," of Bridgeton, N. J., says they are nice made with wheat flour alone. I have no doubt of it; there might be some shortening added, but if to be eaten with meat, having plenty of gravy, it is not needed.

**Buckwheat Griddle Cakes, in Rhyme.**—For ordinary buckwheat cakes, we will give one in rhyme, from one of the muses of the Detroit *Free Press,* which may be relied upon as safe to follow:

> If you fine buckwheat cakes would make
> One quart of buckwheat flour take;
> Four table-spoonfuls then of yeast;
> Of salt one tea-spoonful at least;
> One handful Indian meal and two
> Good table-spoonfuls of real New
> Orleans molasses, then enough
> Warm water to make of the stuff
> A batter thin. Beat very well;
> Set it to rise where warmth do dwell.
> If in the morning, it should be
> The least bit sour, stir in free
> A very little soda that
> Is first dissolved in water hot,
> Mix in an earthen crock, and leave
> Each morn a cupful in to give
> A sponge for the next night, so you
> Need not get fresh yeast to renew.
>
> In weather cold this plan may be
> Pursued ten days successfully,
> Providing you add every night
> Flour, salt, molasses, meal in right
> Proportions, beating as before,
> And setting it to rise once more.
> When baking make of generous size
> Your cakes; and if they'd take the prize
> They must be light and nicely browned,
> Then by your husband you'll be crowned
> Queen of the kitchen; but you'll bake,
> And he will, man-like, "take the cake."

*Remarks.*—When buckwheat cakes are made without molasses, as is often done, if a small spoonful of molasses is added, each morning, to the cake batter, they will take a much nicer brown, being careful, however, not to burn them.

**Mock Buckwheat Cakes.**—To make mock buckwheat cakes, warm 1 qt. skimmed milk to the temperature of new milk; add 1 tea-spoonful of salt and 3 table-spoonfuls of good lively yeast; thicken to the consistency of real buckwheat cakes with graham meal, in which 3 small handfuls of fine corn meal have been mixed. Very coarse middlings, such as one gets from country mills, answers quite as well, and none but an expert would know the difference between the imitation and the real.—*Indiana State Sentinel.*

*Remarks.*—Why not have mock buckwheat cakes as well as mock minced pies? Certainly these will be found very nice and healthful. And any person can eat these, while with some persons real buckwheat cakes eaten as steadily as many do in the winter, causes an irritable condition of the skin, these will not, with anyone.

**Buckwheat Batter, To Keep Sweet.**—Keeping buckwheat batter sweet is sometimes very troublesome, especially in mild weather. It is said the only way to keep it perfectly sweet is to pour cold water on that left from one morning to another. Fill the vessel entirely full of water and put it in a cool place. When ready to use pour off the water, which absorbs the acidity.— *Lansing Republican.*

**Buckwheat and Graham Griddle Cakes, Also Oatmeal Griddle Cakes.**—Buckwheat cakes are improved for some people by mixing the buckwheat with graham flour. Put about one-third of graham with it. Start the cakes at night with yeast—a small tea-cupful of yeast to 1 qt. of flour; mix with cool, not cold, water, and set in a warm corner. Griddle cakes can be made of oatmeal by putting one-third of wheat flour with it. They require more time for cooking than buckwheat cakes do, and should be browned thoroughly.

**Bread Griddle Cakes.**—Take your pieces of dry bread, and pour over them boiling water; stir and beat to a smooth paste; put in flour enough to make them the consistency of buckwheat cakes; add a little salt, 1 tea-spoonful of soda, and 3 eggs, well beaten. They are delicious for breakfast or tea. If the weather is cold, it will be better to soak the bread over night Milk is better than water to soak the bread in.

**Bread Griddle Cakes, Richer.**—Soak a loaf of bread, or its bulk in stale bread, in milk over night; in the morning stir in 1 cup of flour, 2 eggs, beaten till light, a table-spoonful of butter or lard; soda, 1 tea-spoonful, and a little salt Mix smooth and drop 2 spoonfuls upon the hot griddle for each cake.

**Pancakes or Griddle Cakes With Dry Bread.**—Crumble the bread and soak in cold milk until soft, then add soda or saleratus, and salt, according to amount, and flour to make a batter.

**With Rice.**—Cold, boiled rice, 1 cup; flour, 3 cups; 2 eggs, beaten; salt, 1 tea-spoonful; milk to make a thick batter; baking powder, 1 tea-spoonful; beat well together—hot griddle.

**Rice Griddle Cakes.**—Left over rice may be used; but if it is to be boiled purposely, take rice, 2 cups, well washed, and boil in about 1 qt. of water till nicely done and the water about all evaporated; then add milk, 1 qt. wheat flour, 1 cup, and 1 beaten egg.

**Indian Griddle Cakes.**—White Indian meal, 2 cups; flour, 1 cup; yeast, ½ cup; salt, 1 tea-spoonful; milk to make a stiff batter; put in a warm place over night, as sponge for bread; stir in the morning, and make of a suitable consistence by adding milk or meal with a little flour, which ever may be needed.

**Graham Griddle Cakes.**—For a family of 4 or 5 persons, take sour buttermilk, 2 cups, with a small tea-spoonful of soda; 2 eggs, well beaten, and added with a pinch of salt; then stir in graham flour to make a batter a little thicker than usual for cake batter. Fry upon a hot griddle, and keep in a tureen or other covered dish.

*Remarks* —By some people griddle cakes are always called "pancakes." It matters not which you call these; but they take the place of bread during the meat course for breakfast, after which with a little nice butter and a home-made syrup, by dissolving granulated sugar by putting in a little water and bringing to a boiling heat—I like the syrup to be pretty thick; and I greatly prefer these for general use to those made from buckwheat, both in flavor and for healthfulness, as they never cause an eruption upon the skin as buckwheat often does. With those having rich cream and maple sugar, they will prove a rare dish, not soon abandoned if tried. If graham bread, graham biscuit, or gems, are left over until they become dry, let them be broken into sour milk or buttermilk over night, then mashed with a spoon or a clean hand in the morning, and thickened with a little graham flour, and the cakes will be very light and nice by using a little soda, as first mentioned. These, like warm graham biscuit or gems, may be eaten in moderation even by dyspeptics, by which you may know, as the author has proved, they are healthful.

**Crackers.**—To 1 qt. of light bread dough—about enough for 1 loaf of bread—work in shortening, 1 cup, and soda, ½ tea-spoonful; then knead in flour to make a stiff dough; roll and pound with the rolling-pin for 15 or 20 minutes, then knead and roll thin and cut with a small cutter, put in a dripping pan, pick with a fork and bake. Graham crackers may be made in the same way.—*Farm and Fireside.*

# MEATS.

CURING, SMOKING, KEEPING, ETC.—Curing Hams, Smoking, Etc., as Done in Pennsylvania.—Good for All Places and Kinds of Meat.—The following is the plan pursued in Pennsylvania, where it is well known that they have the very nicest hams:

After the hams are nicely trimmed, lay them upon slanting boards, to carry off the dripping brine, and rub well with pure fine salt, working it into every part; then let them lay 48 hours. Then brush off the salt with a dry cloth or brush-broom, and have ready a mixture of powdered saltpeter, 1 teaspoon; brown sugar, 1 dessertspoon, or a small tablespoon, of red pepper; use 1 teaspoonful of the mixture for each ham or shoulder, and rub well into the fleshy parts; then pack in a tub or barrel, skin-side down always; put also a good sprinkling of nice, pure salt on the bottom, and between each layer, as packed. Let them stand thus 5 days; then cover with pickle made as follows:

To each pail of water required put 4 lbs. of pure, coarse salt; saltpeter, ¾ to 1½ ozs., and brown sugar, ¾ to 1½ lbs. The pickle should be made beforehand, so as to remove all skum arising, and to be cold when poured on. According to the size of the hams, let them lay 5, 6 or 7 weeks.

**For Beef,** 10 to 15 days only, according to size of pieces, in the same strength of pickle, and same treatment. Hang up a few days to dry nicely before smoking.

*Remarks.*—It will be noticed that there is a margin given in the amount of saltpeter and the sugar; it is because some persons prefer more than others. The least amounts given would be enough for me. I will remark here, for all, that the smoking and putting away for summer use should always be done while the weather is yet too cold to allow a fly to be seen, so there need be no annoyance from them, nor from bugs, if packed according to direction.

The following for hams or beef is from a lady, a name-sake of mine, Jennie Chase, of Elsie, Mich., differing a little from the above in that she uses a little saleratus, which is said to prevent meat from becoming dry and hard. I will give it, as some of the ladies know more about such matters than their brothers or husbands. I do not know, however, that this one has either, for I have never seen her, but would be glad to, and thank her for not being ashamed to give her name with her information. She says:

**Hams or Beef—Pickle for.**—"For 200 lbs. of meat, use 14 lbs. of salt, 1½ lbs sugar, 6 oz. saltpeter, 2 oz. saleratus; dissolve by boiling in three pails of soft water; skim, and when cold, pour over your meat. Sprinkle a very little salt on when you put down your meat. As soon as the weather is warm, scald the brine, and add a little fresh salt."

*Remarks.*—The plan of scalding on the approach of hot weather, and **add**

410

hig a little more salt, is certainly desirable for keeping meat over summer in the pickle.

**Curing Ham, or other Meat for Smoking, without Pickle—Warranted to Keep all Summer.**—This plan is from Mrs. S. Weaver of Columbiana, O., who says it has been in use in their family eight years, while, if not good, one year would have been sufficient. I will give it in her own language. She says:

"Take 1 lb. of saltpeter, 1 lb. of pepper, 3 lbs. of brown sugar and 10 qts. of salt to 1000 weight of pork  Dissolve the saltpeter in a very little hot water: mix all the ingredients well, and then rub it on and into the meat—hams, etc.—with the hand, until it is everywhere covered.  Insert your finger under the center bone in hams and shoulders, and then fill that opening with the mixture.  Then lay in a cool place for about two weeks, not allowing it to freeze, when it will be ready to smoke.  This recipe has been tried and tested by a number of people, and is a preventive in keeping off all troublesome insects, and the meat will be sweet and tender, and warranted to keep all summer."

*Remarks.*—The plan of pushing the finger in alongside the bone, and filling with the salt mixture, is valuable.  A butcher-knife pushed in along-side of the bone, would be the easier way for many to do.  If used on beef, one week would be long enough to lay instead of two for pork, as it takes salt or other seasoning quicker than pork.

**Pork and Beef for Farmers, or Others, to Have Fresh in Hot Weather, Without Cooking to Keep it, as Heretofore—Tested for Several Years.**—It has been known for some time past that if fresh meat was pretty well cooked, seasoned as for present eating, and packed in jars in its own fat, it would keep a whole season as well as canned fruit, it being upon the air-tight principle; but a writer in the New York *Times*, after a fair test, gives us the following plan, without the cooking, which most persons will, no doubt, prefer, then do the cooking when it is wanted for the table. He says:

"There is no good reason why farmers and their families should eat so much salt pork, leaving all the fresh to the inhabitants of cities and villages, when the following method will keep meat fresh for weeks even in the warmest weather.  I have tried it for several years.  As soon as the animal heat is out of the meat, slice it up ready for cooking.  Prepare a large jar by scalding it well with hot salt and water (strong brine).  Mix salt and pulverized saltpeter. Cover the bottom of the jar with a sprinkle of salt and pepper.  Put down a layer of meat, sprinkle with the salt, saltpeter and pepper the same as if it was just going to the table, and continue in this manner until the jar is full.  Fold a cloth or towel and wet it in strong salt and water in which a little of the saltpeter is dissolved.  Press the cloth closely over the meat and set it in a cool place.  Be sure and press the cloth in tightly, as each layer is removed, and your meat will keep for months.  It is a good plan to let the meat remain over night, after it is sliced, before packing.  Then drain off all the blood that oozes from it.  It will be necessary to change the cloth occasionally, or take it off and wash it first in cold water, then scald in salt and water as at first.  In this way farmers can have fresh meat all the year round,  I have kept beef that was killed the 12th of February till the 21st of June  Then I packed a large jar of veal in the same way during the dog days, and it kept six weeks.  This recipe alone is worth the price of any newspaper in the land."

N. B.—If you have not a cool dry place to keep the jar, run about two inches of lard over the top of the meat and then put on the cloth.

*Remarks.*—This writer is certainly correct in the idea "that there is no good reason why farmers and their families should eat so much salt pork," for it is destructive to good health, besides it is not so palatable and pleasant as to have it fresh, at least once daily, and as much oftener as they will take this little additional labor of putting up. The pieces should be cut of a uniform thickness, and also cut to fit the jar as nearly as possible, small pieces being cut to fill each layer nicely, to keep it level; and no more salt and pepper put on than would be required for present eating. A heaping teaspoonful of powdered saltpeter will be enough for 1 pt. of salt. This writer does not give his proportions. Of course, a brine is formed by the juices of the meat, salt, saltpeter, pepper, etc.

To show you that this writer is not alone in this plan of keeping meat, I will give an item from another, who says:

**Beefsteaks — To Keep Fresh a Long Time.** — "Have the steaks cut about the usual thickness. Mix together some salt, sugar and some finely-powdered saltpeter. In an earthen jar lay a steak, and sprinkle it with the mixture; put on another, and sprinkle the same as before, and over all turn a plate with a heavy weight on it. This will form a brine of its own, and the meat will keep sweet in this way a long time. You can take it out and broil in the usual way. This is a very good receipt for people who live away from cities. Do not let it freeze."

*Remarks.*—He says: "Do not let it freeze." Of course, anybody ought to know that this would keep steaks fresh in cold, freezing weather; but it will do it, too, in warm weather. He does not give the proportions; put on only as much seasoning as if just going to cook it for the table; say, for each pound of steak 1 teaspoonful each of salt and sugar, with 1 teaspoonful of saltpeter and black pepper to each 4 or 5 lbs. of steak, on the principle of one of the plans of seasoning sausage below; for me, if 1 teaspoonful of summer-savory was also put in for each 4 lbs. of steak, so much the better.

**To Keep Hams After Being Smoked.**—After Hams are smoked, and ready to be put away, a writer in the Toledo *Blade* says:

"First fill a large kettle or boiler full of water and let it come to a boil, then dip your hams in and let them remain three minutes, then remove to a board or table and cover them with a thick paste made of flour, water and cayenne pepper. Have the paste red with the pepper. Let them lay in the sun until dry. Then put in paper sacks and tie closely, and hang in a dark place. This will keep them nice the year round if they are put up before fly time. This is a tried recipe and can be relied on."

*Remarks.*—There is no doubt of the reliability of this plan; for the simple wrapping of hams in brown paper, then tieing up in flour-sacks, will secure them against flies, bugs, etc.; still, the above additional labor will certainly give a positiveness that no fly nor bug can pierce this peppery paste. I would put that on, even if I did not dip them in the boiling water. But the dipping makes, as it were, an oily case, or cover, of the outer surface, which, with the paste, is really an air-tight protector, as much as if put into an air-tight can.

Even by packing hams in open barrels, secured on every side with wheat or oat straw, a writer in the Iowa *State Register* claims to have kept hams perfectly sweet and free from flies and bugs. I should greatly prefer the stout paper sacks, either with the paste above or wrapping in several thicknesses of brown paper, secured with twine, before putting into the sack.

**Curing Hams, as Done by Packing Houses.**—A Mr. Backus, who used to carry on the packing business in Adrian, Mich., with whom I afterwards became well acquainted in Toledo, both of us doing business in the same block, gave me his plan, with which he was very successful, as follows: Use pure salt, enough to make the brine to float a medium sized potato half an inch out of the water; and for 280 to 300 lbs of ham to be packed with salt in a 40 gallon cask: good rich molasses, 1 qt., and 3½ ozs. of rock niter (saltpeter), which has not been adulterated with salt. He thinks it better to not put in over 280 pounds to such a cask, head up, then bore a hole and put in the brine and let settle and fill up again, leaving some on top of the head to insure the cask to be full when driving the plug. Bore with 1-inch augur after the head is put in. Six weeks will cure, but no harm if they stand for months before smoking.

*Remarks.*—I have given this in his own form of expression, and am well satisfied of the nature of his instructions. After smoking properly, packing house men always wrap well in paper, then cover with canvas, to secure against insects. This same strength of brine, with the molasses and pure saltpeter, will be equally valuable for side meat to be kept " all the year round."

**Beef Pickle, and an Excellent Plan of Keeping Sweet and Juicy.**—For 200 lbs., or a barrel of beef, the best, pure salt, 15 lbs.; saltpeter, 4 ozs.; molasses, 1 qt., and brown sugar, 3 lbs.; soft water to fill the barrel, 6 to 8 gals., if well packed. DIRECTIONS—The beef, having been properly cooled and cut into sizable pieces, of 5 to 8 lbs., rub a little salt on the cut edges, that has 1 table-spoonful of powdered saltpeter to 1 qt. of salt, and lay them, singly, upon a table or bench over night to draw out the blood. In the morning put the water and saltpeter, as above, into a large kettle and bring to a boil. And now, having a suitable wire hook or two, dip each piece of beef into the boiling water and hold while you count 20 naturally, *i. e.*, not hurrying, nor being slower than usual in counting, which closes the pores against the escape of the juices of the meat into the pickle when barreled; on the same principle that meat should be put into boiling water when to be cooked for the table, and into cold water for soups, so the juices will flow out into the soup. When this is all done, put in the other ingredients, as above, to the water and dissolve, and as it begins to simmer begin to skim before it boils, pouring in a little cold water, if needed, to allow all the skum to be taken off before it boils; then let stand till cold; the beef having, in the meantime, been packed with a little salt in bottom of the barrel, and between the layers, strain the cold pickle upon it through muslin. If the blood was properly drawn off, as first directed, it will seldom be necessary to scald the pickle before May 1st to 15th, then adding 2 or 3 lbs. more of salt, skimming well, re-packing with a little more salt, putting on the pickle cold.

*Remarks.*—This needs no further comment nor explanation. If done as directed, I will guarantee its safe keeping and juiciness. It takes a little more labor to ensure success with beef than it does with pork, but it pays· for what is nicer than a piece of corned beef with the "biled dinner" occasionally? Nothing. Some persons like soda in their beef. believing it helps to keep the pickle sweet and the beef more tender. The following contains it:

**Dr. Warner's Recipe for Curing 100 Pounds of Beef.**—Six qts. salt, 6 lbs. sugar, 6 ozs. soda, 4 ozs. saltpeter. Mix all together, and rub well into the meat, having previously removed the bones. This makes its own brine.

*Remarks.*—I should prefer to draw out the blood, over night, as in the next recipe above; then rub this mixture into the 100 lbs. of beef and keep weighted down, and be sure of success.

**Pressed Beef.**—Take any amount you choose of the cheaper pieces of beef, as the neck, say 8 or 10 lbs., and of the flank, or "skirt" pieces, that has some fat, to make it show a marbled appearance when pressed. Let it lay in a weak brine over night; rinse and boil until it will fall to pieces when you attempt to lift it, or from the bones, if any in it, keeping closely covered to retain as much of the flavor as possible; using only water enough to avoid burning, adding boiling water, at any time, if needed. Take up the beef, and when cool chop it finely, skim off all the grease from the liquor; and it is all the better to add to this liquor, a table-spoonful of good gelatine for each 4 or 5 lbs. of beef, the liquor being boiled down properly, and when the gelatine is dissolved and the liquor quite jelly like, mix it with a little salt and suitable spices (the mixed spices as now kept by most grocers are very good), into the chopped beef and pack in jars, and put a plate upon the top, and at least 15 pounds weight on the plate. When cold it is ready for slicing, for breakfast or tea, and if properly seasoned, is easily digested, is very nourishing as well as economical, and very convenient when in a hurry. It will keep several days, in spring and fall, and a month or so in winter. Garnished with a lemon sliced thin, so a slice can be taken by each guest, gives a zest to ones lagging appetite, although, with this, but few appetites need coaxing. To avoid any possibility of moulding, a cloth, two or three thicknesses, wet in salt water, may be pressed upon the top of the jar, after the plate is removed, and against the side when sliced off.

**1. SAUSAGE—Amount of Seasoning to Suit Most Tastes.** —Pork, 20 lbs., ¾ lean, ¼ fat; salt, 6 ozs.; pepper, 1 oz.; sage, 1½ ozs. DIRECTIONS—Chop the meat fine, or grind, if you have a grinder, mash the salt, if lumpy, pepper and sage ground nicely, and all mixed in evenly, and put in cases, or in clean muslin sacks, as you prefer. Muslin works very nicely cut in strips about 10 inches wide and sewed up gives a sack about 3 inches in diameter—cut off about 15 inches long, one end tied, then, they being perfectly clean, and wet, pack in the sausage meat, and press in with the potato masher, or one made for the purpose, as they need pressing closely to keep well. Tie the other end, pack closely in a jar, or firkin, and cover with a weak brine, for present use—a stronger brine if to keep long, or the sacks may be well rubbed with lard, or butter, and hung up. To use, open one end, turn the sack back, and slice off about ¾ of an inch thick, for frying, is a very nice way. To keep into the summer as much as ½ lb. of salt may be needed: and some persons may like more, and some less, sage. Those who like but little sage use only 1 oz. to the 10 lbs , and those who like it quite strong of sage use 2 ozs. But the 1½ ozs. will suit most tastes. With these variations all tastes can be be met with very little trouble. It saves all this trying, tasting and guess work  Having tested these in this way, and submitted them to the taste of many others, I know whereof I speak. Those who like beef in their sausage can put in 1 lb. of the lean to each 10, which will be found plenty. It makes the sausage dryer and firmer.

*Remarks* —For small amounts of sausage Mrs. M. E. Kellogg, of Brighton, Mich., says. " For each pound of meat put 1 tea-spoonful of salt, 1 of pepper and 1 of sage. These proportions are just right and easily got at." Heaping, of course.

**2. Sausage, to Can, or Put in Jars for Long Keeping.**—A writer, in one of the "Household Departments," gives the following instructions for doing this. She says: If partly fried, packed in jars, and covered with its own dripping, it remains delicately fresh for a long time. We like the method of packing sausage in muslin bags about 3 inches in diameter—just the thinnest old, clean muslin will answer—and the slices are so round and dainty. Rub the surface with lard before hanging away, as an aid to preservation.

**3. Sausage to Keep Through the Summer and Ham the Year Round.**—The above is confirmed by O. S. Cohoon, of Belvidere, Ill., with the additional thought of preserving ham, through the Detroit *Tribune*, in answer to a lady who inquired for a recipe to keep sausage through the summer, which, if properly done, can't fail. The writer says: After the sausage has been made from 24 to 48 hours, slice and cook about two-thirds done and pack in good stone jars, allowing the jars to stand on the stove hearth, or in some warm place while cooking and packing  Have plenty of hot lard in the pan while cooking  When done, place a light weight on the meat and cover with hot lard  The meat must be kept covered with the lard. This is also the best way to preserve ham—the year round.

*Remarks* —To have nice fresh sausage or ham, at all times, handy, is worth a little extra labor  Keep covered with lard, as taken out, to avoid mould.

**1. BOLOGNA SAUSAGE—Fine, as Made in Germany.**—The London, England, *Farmer* claims to have obtained this from the classic land of sausages. I think it will be nice enough for the people of our country, as well as England and Germany. It is as follows: Lean beef, freed from gristle, is to be chopped up very fine and mixed with ⅓ or ½ its weight of lean pork similarly treated. To this mixture is added an equal bulk of fat bacon, cut in strips as thin as the back of a knife, and then chopped into pieces about the size of a pea. For every 12 lbs. of this mass are required ½ lb. of salt, 1 dr. of saltpeter, ½ lb of powdered sugar, and 1 table-spoonful of whole white pepper. The block on which the meat is to be chopped should be previously rubbed over with garlic, but none of this must be mixed with the sausage mass. In filling the sausages the meat must be well crammed home with suitable appliances, as pressure with the hand alone is quite insufficient to keep out the air, which is sure to spoil the result. After hanging for 2 or 3 weeks to dry, the red color of the meat and the white bits of fat will be visible through the skin of the sausages, and then it is time to smoke them. By careful attention to these directions, sausages thus prepared will keep well for at least a year and a half, and the delicacy of their flavor increases as they get older. The great secret of their keeping qualities is to put in plenty of bacon.

*Remarks.*—Where the word "bacon" is used here, and above "fat bacon," they mean simply fat pork, fresh, of course, the same as the beef must be, not "bacon," as we understand the word in the United States to mean cured and smoked sides—not at all—this is not it, but fresh, fat pork.

2. **Bologna Sausage Americanized.**—Somebody has Americanized the above, as follows, but I don't know who; still, it will be nice for those who like cayenne (and, by the way, if we would all use more cayenne or red pepper, and less of the black, it would be the better for us); but I should try only 1 spoonful at first, and if more would be tolerated by the children (who, as a general thing dislike it very much), and only a small onion, increasing or lessening either, as found most agreeable:

"Lean pork, 6 lbs.; lean beef, 3 lbs; beef suet, 2 lbs.; salt, 4 ozs. (I should say 6 ozs.); 6 table-spoonfuls of black pepper, 2 table-spoonfuls of cayenne pepper, 2 tea-spoonfuls of cloves, 1 of allspice, and 1 minced onion. Chop or grind the meat, and mix well the powdered spices through it. Pack in beef skins as you do those of pork, tie both ends tightly and lay them in strong brine. Let them remain one week, then change them into a new brine. Let them remain another week, frequently turning them. Then take them out, wipe them, and send them to be smoked; when smoked rub the surface well with sweet oil or butter and hang them in a dark, cool place."

*Remarks.*—It strikes me that 1 table-spoonful of cayenne will be found enough for most persons, especially children, who are very fond of "Bologna."

After all this mincing for sausage, "Bologna," etc., it may not be amiss to close with a mixture for Christmas pie, aside from those in the department of "Dishes for the Table," etc., to have always ready for use through the winter, as follows:

**Minced Meat for Pies.**—Chopped beef (the neck does very well if boiled very tender—any part should be thus boiled), 5 cups; suet (uncooked), chopped, after freeing it from the membrane and stringy portions, 2 cups; stoned raisins, unchopped, 3 cups; English or dried currants, and cherries, if you have them, each, 1 cup; brown sugar, 5 cups; nice cider, 6 cups; or, if no cider is to be had, water, 3½ cups, and good vinegar, 2½ cups; but these are not equal to the cider; citron, chopped, 2 cups; cloves, cinnamon, nutmeg, mace, allspice (all in powder), and salt, each, 1 table-spoonful (more of all, or any one of these spices, or salt, if desired, on tasting); the grated yellow and juice of 2 lemons; nice, tart, chopped apples. DIRECTIONS—As this amount will make more than many families will wish to make into pies at one time, for each 2 cups of this mixture that you wish to bake take 3 cups of apple, as above, and mix nicely, and if not as juicy as desired (and mince pie to be good needs to be quite juicy), put in cider to suit, or its substitute as above, and bake with light, porous crusts, the "filling" meat being not less than a plump half to three-fourths of an inch in thickness, so it may be said of the cook, as it often is when she cuts her bread pretty thick, "You would make a good step-mother," which will be as great praise as can be bestowed upon her, and if she does it all nicely, she will deserve it.

*Remarks.*—Some people will have brandy or wine in their mince pies, let such put in 1 cup of brandy, or 2 cups of wine, into the above amount. It is each one's privilege to suit themselves, or the demand of the majority, or the head of the house, as the case may be. What is not baked up when made, pack nicely in jars and cover well with cloths and a plate with a light weight upon it, or other cover, not adding the apples only as used, as the meat keeps better without.

# SOUPS, BOILING MEATS, ETC.

*Remarks and General Directions.*—The most nourishing soups are made of fresh meats; but whatever meat you use should be put in cold water, well covered, and kept at a low temperature and never allowed to boil, for at least one hour, after which a bubbling boil may be allowed. Remembering that the first hard boil hardens the surface and locks up the juices of the meat, which is important to draw out in soup-making. For economy's sake, a knuckle-joint or a shin-bone is preferable; but there should be sufficient meat attached to give the required nourishment and flavor of the meat used. However, after the first hour slow stewing has passed, any cold meats or bits of fowl which have been left over, may be added, having been cut in small slices. It is well, also, with fresh meats to cut small, and bones to be well cracked, or sawed across to allow the marrow and juices to escape. Vegetables should be cut fine or sliced thin, or grated upon a coarse greater, as preferred. Salt helps to harden and lock up the juices, and hence should not be put into soups until the vegetables are added, about an hour before serving. But soup meats should be put over the fire as soon after breakfast as possible, so as to give 4 or 5 hours to its preparation.

**In Cold Weather** soup-plates should be well heated before serving the soup in them from the covered tureen; and in fact, all plates in cold weather, from which meats or gravies are to be eaten, should be well warmed before bringing to the table. Soup properly " warmed up," *i. e.*, put on just before dinner-time, so as not to be to long upon the stove, is equal if not better than the fresh made; and this is especially so when beans enter into its make.

**Straining and Filtering not at all Necessary.**—The fancy "Cook-Books" talk about straining soups, and some even of filtering through a hair sieve after straining. The straining will remove fully one-half of the nourishing properties used, but if "style is preferable" to the strength which would otherwise be obtained from the thicker parts of the soup, by all means both strain and filter them. One point more, and I am done with the general ideas of soup-making—it is this: for healthy people it is not essential to trim off the fat from soup meats, nor the oily particles from the top of soups; but for invalids both these must be done, either by making the day before and removing the fat when cold from the top, or by dipping off as much as possible while hot. As soups always come on the table before the other dishes, we will let them also go before " Various Dishes" in making up the book.

**Boiled Dinner—How to Get It Up.**—To get up a " boiled dinner" it is of the same importance to keep the juices in the meats that it is to draw them out in making soups, therefore as putting into cold water and heating slowly draws them out, so putting into boiling water, properly salted (when fresh meat is used), and continuing to boil briskly shuts up the pores and keeps the juices and nourishing properties in the meats, which is the whole secret of success. And nothing more can be said except what would repeat, in some manner, this only important difference. So the author will now trust to the common sense of the people for who he writes, and has for over twenty-five years written, only adding: never let the boiling stop when getting a boiled dinner, nor never allow hard boiling when making a soup.

**Bean Soup.**—As I look upon bean soup as the *best* of old soups, I will give a receipt taken from " A Book of the Sea," which, having had it made several times, I can say it can be depended upon. And when I say it was given by a sailor, the phraseology needs no further explanation. He says:

" The fact is, that bean soup at sea is such a stand-by that the sailor-man on shore sometimes gets quite mad when it's offered him, and still, bean soup is a mighty good thing, and all according to the way you make it. Now, you get a lot of swells on board, and make 'em soup, and call it *haricot* (in England, this name is still used for beans) and not beans, which is vulgar, and if you know how to turn it out, they will take three platefuls.

" First, you get a *pint and a half* of good sound beans — I don't think there is much difference in beans, whether they are *big* or *little* — and pick 'em over and stand them for an hour in a bowl of cold water. Take three pounds of meat or a shin-bone, and put the beef in 4 quarts of cold water, and let it boil. Fry an onion and put that in, with say 6 whole cloves and a dozen peppers (the small cayenne peppers, the same that are used in making pepper sauce), and some parsley, with a tablespoon of salt. Let it boil for two hours, and you keep skimming. As fast as the water boils away, you keep adding a little hot water. When the concern is cooked, take a colander and strain your soup through it, mashing up the beans and keeping out the meat and the bean skin. If you want to be superfine, you can hard boil an egg, and slice white and yellow through, and put them in the tureen; likewise some slices of lemon. Bits of toast don't go bad with it. If you happen to be cruising south, just you use, instead of the New England bean, the Georgia or South California cow-pea."

*Remarks.*—The author never had any soup he liked better than this, although the following is very nice.

**Bean Soup with Cream or Milk.**—Take 1 pt. of beans, parboil and drain off the water, adding fresh. Never put cold water upon beans which have been once heated, as it hardens them—boil until perfectly tender, season with pepper and salt, and a piece of butter the size of a walnut, or more if preferred; when done skim out half the beans, leaving the broth with the remaining half in the kettle, now add a teacup of sweet cream or good milk, a dozen or more of crackers broken up, let it come to a boil, and you have a dish good enough to offer a king.

**Corn and Bean Soup.**—Take 2 lbs. of fresh beef, 1 lb. of fresh pork, and 1 pint of black or navy beans (I think white ones will do just as well), soak over night, one large onion, a small carrot, a head of celery   Put the above ingredients into the soup pot with a gallon of cold water, and let simmer gently for five or six hours. Take off and let get cold; remove the grease, and place on the stove to boil again. About an hour before dinner add a quart of canned corn. Strain the soup, season with cayenne pepper and salt, and serve it with or without the addition of boiling cream.

*Remarks.*—Excuse me from the straining, but give me the cream, if you have it, by all means. And I have not a doubt but what salt meats, properly freshened, would make a soup hard to tell from that made with fresh; and sweet corn, iu its season, cut from the cob, 1 qt., will do as well as canned. I know this from the nature of things upon general principles. So let others judge, in all things from their own common sense—Think. I have made these remarks to set people to thinking upon common things in the way here indicated, for themselves, which is the true way to all improvements. Instead of straining, sometimes, you may rub the beans and the corn, when perfectly tender, through a colander, as indicated in the sailor's plan above, and thus get rid of the skins of the beans, and the hulls of the corn. This last is from more of the same kind of thinking. Put the *puree,* (any soft, mushy mass) back into the soup, and make hot when served.

**SOUP, TOMATO—Very Nice.**—To canned tomatoes, 1 pt., or 4 large, ripe raw ones, scalded, peeled and sliced, add boiling water 1 qt., and boil till thoroughly soft, then add cooking soda, 1 teaspoonful, and stir well; when done foaming, immediately add sweet milk 1 pt,; with salt and pepper to taste, and 1 tablespoonful of butter; and when it boils again have 8 or 10 common crackers rolled fine which add, and serve hot. Some 'think this equal, or better, even, than oyster soup. As the girls often say of a new bonnet: "It is just splendid." Try it, by all means.

**2. Tomato Soup with Milk.**—Take nice ripe tomatoes, scald, remove the skins, and slice up 1 qt., and stew ½ hour in 1 pt. of water; then add a level teaspoonful of baking soda, stir till done foaming, and put in 1 qt. of hot sweet milk; and as soon as it boils again add salt and pepper to taste; with a bit of butter and a few broken crackers if you want it richer. A small slice or two of salt pork makes a nice substitute for the butter. And if you desire a meat flavor, put in some steak from the soup-jar. It should be made so that the milk addition is put in just as you are ready to serve it. This is often called economical or mock-oyster soup.

**Potato Soup.**—Thinly slice enough potatoes to make 1 pt., with 1 to 4 small onions (to obtain a little or more flavor, as you prefer) and boil in 1 qt. of water until perfectly tender; add 1 pt. of rich milk, and season with salt and pepper to taste. Serve hot. The potatoes and onions may be skimmed and rubbed smooth through a colander, if you like.

**Milk Soup.**—Same as the last without the onions, using 1 pt. of water to boil the potatoes in, then add 1 qt. of milk instead of 1 pt.; simply using half as much water and twice as much milk. Use with either crackers or not, as you choose.

**Chicken Soup, Delicious.**—Take 1 chicken, 4 qts. of water, 1 table-spoonful of rice, an onion, potato and turnip, 1 of each, ½ cup of tomatoes, 2 stalks of celery, pepper and salt. DIRECTIONS—Joint the chicken and boil very tender; pour through a colander and return the soup to the kettle, adding the rice, which has been soaking; chop the potato, onion and turnip and add ½ an hour after. Cut the celery in dice and add 20 minutes before serving; the tomato and seasoning last. If well done it will be very delicious; with milk or cream more so, if ½ pt. of either are put in just in time to get hot when ready to season.

2. **Chicken, Cream Soup.**—The best way to get the virtue out of an old, tough chicken is to properly dress and joint it, then boil it with 1 onion in 4 qts. of water till only 2 remain. Take it out and cut off the breast, chopping it fine with the yolks of 2 hard-boiled eggs, returning to the soup and simmering a few minutes more, then adding 1 cup of heated cream, or ½ pt. of rich milk, boiling hot, seasoning to taste and serving hot from a covered tureen.

3. **Soup, Chicken Currie, as Made in India.**—A pair of nicely dressed chickens, butter, currie powder, flour, salt and cayenne pepper and some rice, to be nicely boiled by itself. DIRECTIONS—Boil the chickens carefully, keeping always covered with water, till perfectly tender, removing scum and oily fat as it rises; then bone them and have a skillet ready for frying the meat in enough hot butter, first dredging the meat with flour before laying in the hot butter; brown nicely, keeping hot. Take 1 pt. of the chicken broth, which is to be kept hot, and stir in 1 table-spoonful of flour, 2 of butter, 1 teaspoonful of salt, and a little cayenne pepper and 2 table-spoonfuls of currie powder, and, when all is well mixed in, add this to the balance of the hot soup in the kettle and simmer a few minutes, then add the hot browned meat and serve hot, and with the hot boiled rice.

*Remarks.*—This is a very nice soup for those loving currie. Is very healthful from the warming nature of the currie. It would still be more warming to the stomach if a spoonful of currie is put into the meat when frying, and some prefer to put into the soup only half of the fried meat, serving the rest as a fry with the rice, I like it either way, because I like the currie.

**Soup, Celery, Rich and Creamy.**—A shank of beef, 1 large bunch of celery or two small ones, and rich cream, 1 cup; a little flour. DIRECTIONS —Make a rich broth of the shank, always putting into cold water, skimming off all the fat as it rises; when ready take up the meat and thicken the broth with a spoon or two of flour, first rubbed in a little cold water; have the celery cut fine and boil it in the soup till tender; then add the cream, salt and pepper to taste, and serve at once.

**Green Corn Soup.**—Cut the corn from a dozen good-sized ears (real "sweet" corn is the best in all cases), lay the cobs closely in the kettle and cover with water—not less than 3 pts. or 2 qts. if needed—and boil half an hour; then take out the cobs and cook the corn in the same water till tender. Now add 1 pint of rich sweet milk, if you have it, and boil a few minutes longer; season with salt and pepper, and if no milk beat 2 eggs and stir in, and con tinue to stir 2 or 3 minutes just as ready to serve. It will be found delicious, if nicely done.

**Barley Soup.**—Take a 2 or 3 lb. shin of beef, well broken, pearl barley, ¼ lb.; 2 small onions, sliced; 2 small carrots, chopped; salt and pepper. DIRECTIONS—Put all into a soup kettle, cover nicely with cold water and heat up slowly for an hour, then continue 3 or 4 hours of more brisk boiling; and if you have celery, a stalk or two, cut and put in 15 or 20 minutes before serving improves the flavor very much. The old plan of simply putting in a little barley requires a fife and drum to call the very much scattered nourishing properties together.

**Macaroni (Italian) Soup.**—To 2 qts. of boiling beef-broth, or soup (made as for the carrot beef soup, above, without the vegetables), add 6 or 7 sticks of macaroni and allow it to cook ½ or ¾ of an hour; then, just when ready to serve, grate in ¼ lb. of nice cheese. (The macaroni should be broken up and soaked in water a couple of hours before cooking with the broth.)

**Beef Soup.**—A knuckle-joint or shin-bone, having sufficient meat attached for a family of 5 or 6 persons; six medium-sized potatoes, 3 or 4 small onions, ½ of a small head of cabbage, salt and pepper. DIRECTIONS—If a joint it should be cut through by the butcher; and if a shin, it should be sawed 1 or 2 times across to allow the escape of the marrow and juices. Put this into sufficient cold water and place upon the stove as early as practicable to allow it to be pretty thoroughly done an hour before dinner, at which time the cabbage, having been finely chopped, should be put in. The potatoes and onions, having been properly prepared, should now be chopped finely together and added to the soup, with the salt and pepper to taste. Some persons are fond of adding a few bits of red pepper to their soups; but if much is put in children usually dislike it. If used, it should be put in with the vegetables.

*Remarks.*—A well-made soup is very healthful, and they ought to be made much oftener than they are in most families.

**Rice Soup.**—The fore leg and brisket of a lamb or very young sheep; rice, ½ to 1 cup, according to size of family; water, sufficient. DIRECTIONS—Wash the rice early in the morning, and put to soak in warm water to wholly cover it. The bones being broken, stew the meat until tender, then put in the rice with the water in which it has softened, and continue the boiling until the rice has become perfectly soft, having set back the kettle where there is no danger of burning.

**Seasoning for Soups.**—A rice soup is usually seasoned with salt and pepper only; but a little celery, summer savory, thyme, parsley or marjoram may be added, when desired, to any soup. All these herbs ought to be raised by all who have gardens, for they add much to the taste of many other dishes as well as soups.

*Remarks.*—There is probably no soup equal to rice generally for the sick. The seasoning may be made to suit their taste, but usually the plainer the seasoning the better it suits them. Certainly nothing but a little salt and pepper should be put in without consulting the patient. There may be some satisfaction in knowing that what is considered best for invalids is good enough for general use. Beef soup is also excellent made with rice occasionally in place of other vegetables.

**Scotch Broth (Soup).**—Take 2 lbs. of the scraggy part of the neck of mutton. Cut the meat from the bone, removing all the fat; cut the meat into small pieces, and put into a soup pot with a large slice of a turnip, 2 small carrots, 1 onion, 1 stalk of celery, all sliced, and ½ cup of pearled barley, water, 3 pts. to 2 qts., and boil gently 2 hours. On the bones put 1 qt. water and boil gently the same length of time; then drain this into the soup. Cook 1 spoonful each of flour and butter together until perfectly smooth, then stir this into the soup with a spoonful of chopped parsley, season with salt and pepper and serve at once.—*Free Press Household.*

*Remarks.*—While we are with the Scotch, we will give a "Scotch Girl's" Porridge, from Tilden, Ill., as it is near enough like soup to go with them. She says:

**Scotch Porridge.**—"If the family consists of 6 persons, take 3 qts. of water, and bring to a boil, take your *spurtle* (the Scotch for pot-stick or mush-stick), keep the pot on the fire, take the oatmeal in your left hand (of course, only right-handed girls can make this), and let it drop gently through your fingers into the boiling water, stir briskly for 10 minutes, and you will have a most delicious dish; salt to taste."

*Remarks.*—It strikes the author that this would not only be more "delicious" if made pretty thick with the oatmeal and then thinned with 1 qt. of rich milk, all made hot together, but more nourishing also. I always like to get the greatest possible good out of a dish, in fact, out of every thing, while it is on hand or being made.

**Soup, Scotch or Mutton, Excellent.**—A leg of mutton, 4 lbs.; water, 1 gal.; pearl barley, 1 cup; small carrots, 5 or 6; small turnips and onions, each, 2; a small head of cabbage, a handful of parsley, if to be had, pepper and salt. DIRECTIONS—Put the mutton and barley into a suitable kettle with the water, cold; slice the onions, turnips, and 2 of the carrots; grate the other carrots, chop the cabbage fine, and when the water comes to a good bubbling simmer, add all the vegetables, keep covered and simmering for 3 or 4 hours, or until all is perfectly tender; add salt and pepper, and serve hot, when all lovers of soup will say "excellent."

**Noodle Soup, and Noodles, To Make.**—By putting noodles into any soup it thereby becomes noodle soup. See carrot and beef soup for the "stock" or manner of making the soup for the noodles. They will cook in 15 or 20 minutes, hence should not be put in only this length of time before serving.

*To Make the Noodles.*—Put 1 cup of flour upon the molding board, making a hole in the center into which put a well-beaten egg with a little salt. Knead and roll as thin as possible, dredging with a little flour, roll up snugly and slice from the end; then shake out the strips and place on plates until perfectly dry. This may be done in the oven, when not too hot, with both doors left open. They may be added to any rich soup, or one made purposely for them as indicated above.

*Remarks.*—How this name ever got applied to this article for soups, I can not imagine, as noodle signifies a simpleton. I know it is a favorite dish with the Germans, although I would by no means consider them simpletons from that fact. Still, I do think that flour dough in this form, or in the form of dumplings boiled in water or soup, is a very indigestible mass, and in no way fit for an invalid. Still, I know, also, that our German population are much more healthy than Americans, and, therefore, they are better able to digest noodles and dumplings than we are. It is from their more simple and plainer style of cookery, no doubt.

**Mock-Turtle or Make-Believe Terrapin Soup, From Bob, the Sea Cook.**—He says: "Of course, its a sham, for there ain't nothing in this world that can take the shine out of a real terrapin (turtle); still, if you ain't got none of these nice creeturs, you can manage to make shift with a calf's head. You don't want the whole head of a calf, but boil it just the same, but don't sluice it with all the water in the reservoir, only enough to cover it, and in that water put a couple of onions and salt and pepper. When boiled tender, take, say, half the meat, half the tongue and a table-spoonful of the brains. Cut it up, but not too fine. Put into a frying-pan a ¼ lb. of the best butter, and bring it up to a light brown, mixing in a very little sifted flour when it is off the fire, and a little cayenne pepper, and just a touch of sweet marjoram. If you put herbs into hot, boiling butter it makes a bitter taste. Then stir the sauce with a little of the water the calf's head was boiled in. Then put in your chopped-up calf's head. Place it on the fire again—not to cook, but to get hot only—and last of all pour in 2 wine-glassfuls of Madeira, but if you have not that let it be sherry- Though it ain't terrapin, it's good all the same."

*Remarks.*—Turtle soup being a favorite with saloon men, of course, wine is always used but home-made will "fill the bill" in any case where wine is always called for. Excuse me from using the brains. If one has not enough of his own, it is no use to try and make it up by using those of a calf. For oyster soup, see Oyster Stew, etc., as made at Delmonico's. For marjoram and other seasoning herbs for soups, see Seasoning for Soups, in connection with the Rice Soup.

The following Prussian, Green Pea, and Asparagus Soups and the Broths, or "Stocks," Veal and Lamb, are from the "Indian Domestic Economy and Cookery," quoted from in some other places, an explanation of which will be found in connection with the Chicken Currie. The recipes are plain, and will be found a valuable addition to those of our own country. See also Mock Oyster, and some other soups in the Miscellaneous Department.

**Prussian Soup, as Made in India.**—Celery, 4 heads; carrots, turnip, onions, and lettuce, 2 of each. DIRECTIONS—Cut them all into small pieces, and fry in a little *ghee* (butter or drippings). Take a *geer* (2 lbs.) of mutton, cut it into slices, put it all together in a large saucepan and keep it sweating for an hour without any water; then pour on water, 2 qts., and shut the lid close and simmer gently for 2 hours longer, and serve. (See explanation of this and the following in the last remarks above.)

**1. Green Pea Soup of India.**—Nice, freshly picked and shelled peas, of a green color, 3 pts.; nice butter, ¼ lb.; parsley and green onions, a handful of each. DIRECTIONS—Boil, as they call it, all these in the butter over a slow fire till thoroughly stewed (fried, as we say); then pound in a mortar (rub through a colander), and put in *consommé* (" stock ") to suit the number for dinner, and leave it on the corner of the fire, for if it boils the peas will lose their green color. (In India the cooking is generally done over a fire-place.) We would say set it back on the stove, merely to simmer. At the moment of sending to the table put in sippets of bread (bread cut into dice-shaped pieces and nicely fried in *ghee* (butter), and serve.

*Remarks.*—It strikes me if ⅓ or ¼ of the peas were saved, and boiled in water with a little salt to fairly cook them, then put into the pea soup when about to serve, it would be a little nicer flavor and show more plainly what it was made of, especially so if the bread "sippets" were thought too much trouble to prepare.

**2. Green Pea Soup, American.**—Take lean, fresh beef, 2 lbs.; green, shelled peas, 2 qts.; water, 2 qts. DIRECTIONS—Boil the pods in the water ½ an hour, then skim them out and put in the meat and simmer slowly till half an hour before serving, adding boiling water to make up for evaporation; then add the shelled peas, and when tender, thicken with a little flour or corn starch, and season with chopped parsley, if you can get it; salt and pepper just before serving

**Asparagus Soup of India.**—This is made only with the green part of the tops. Prepare a veal or lamb broth, which see below, for each 2 qts. needed take 1½ pts. of the green tops and cut about 2 inches long and boil in water with a little salt; then rub two-thirds of them through a sieve or colander and put into the broth; the other one-third, chop as nearly the size of peas as may be (about ¼ inch long), and put into the soup just before serving, which leaves them quite firm.

**Turkey Soup, From the Bones and Left Over Meat.**—I do not know who to credit for thinking out the plan of obtaining the flavor of turkey in a soup, by breaking the bones (instead of throwing them away, as usually done), and putting, with the left over pieces, into a kettle with 2 qts. of cold water, and a table-spoonful of rice, covering closely, and setting on the back of the stove to simmer for an hour; then let boil slowly till the rice is done; and pour into an earthen jar, and set in a cold place till next day. When wanted for dinner remove the layer of fat (and this is a good plan with any soup); then heat, and serve hot, with crackers and pickles.

*Remarks*—So you may do with the remains of 2 or 3 chickens, leg of lamb, veal, rabbits, ets., not forgetting to break all bones containing marrow, or, for using rabbits, see next recipe.

**Game Soup.**—Two rabbits, ½ lb. of lean lamb, 2 medium sized onions, 1 lb. of lean beef; fried bread; butter for frying; pepper, salt, and 2 stalks of white celery cut into inch lengths; 3 qts. of water. DIRECTIONS—Joint the game neatly; cut the lamb and onion into small pieces, and fry all in butter to a light brown. Put into a soup pot with the beef; cut into strips and add a little pepper. Pour on the water; heat slowly and stew gently 2 hours. Take out the pieces and cover in a bowl; cook the soup 1 hour longer; strain, cool, drop in the celery and simmer 10 minutes. Pour upon fried bread in the tureen.

**Carrot Soup, from Stock.**—The day before this soup is required boil 3 lbs. of good soup beef in 1 gallon of water until reduced one-half; when cold skim off all fat. The next day add salt and replace on the fire. Scrape your carrots and cut them into small dice (except one, to be grated, as below): put these in the soup with cayenne pepper, 1 table-spoonful each of burned sugar, sharp vinegar and grated carrot. Boil till the carrots are tender and serve.

*Remarks.*—Much is said about "stock" by nearly all who give directions for making soup. The plan here given is the true way to have a soup rich and nourishing. A jar can be kept for this purpose, if soup is to be made every day, otherwise, the above plan is the better way. When a jar is kept for this purpose all marrow bones, bits of meat, fowl, etc., shall be put in and heat up every day, by placing the jar upon the stove for that purpose, and to draw out the juices of the tit-bits, broken bones, etc., which are added from time to time; observing, however, if a jar is kept for this purpose, it must be scalded out once or twice a week—according to whether the weather is hot or cold—to keep it perfectly sweet.

**Split Pea Soup.**—Make a broth of some water that corned beef or salt pork has been boiled in, and some beef bones. Do not let it be too salt; in that case use half water. Put 1 qt. of the split peas in enough of the water to cover them; when they have stewed soft, mash them through a colander, and then mix with them 2 qts. of the broth, in which the bones have been boiling; add 1 onion, and 1 turnip, chopped up, and 1 carrot, grated. Just before serving put small pieces of toast in the soup.—*Peterson's Ladies' Magazine.*

**Green Pea Soup.**—Boil 1 pt. of green peas in salted water with a slice of onion, a sprig of parsley and a few leaves of mint. When done draw off the water and pass the peas through a sieve. Dilute this purée to a proper consistency with some good stock. Just before serving make it very hot, put in a piece of fresh butter, and if you have it half a cup of cream. If the color is not a sufficiently bright green add a few drops of spinach greening. Serve with small pieces of fried bread.

*Remarks.*—If a broth, or soup, is used, as made for the carrot soup, above, in place of the salted water, as here directed, the soup will be that much richer and better. It is "stock" itself.

**Broths, as Made in India—Veal or Lamb.**—Take a joint of veal, or the fore leg of a lamb, crack the bones nicely, make clean and put into a stewpan and cover with cold water; watch and stir well, and the moment it begins to simmer skim carefully; then add a little more cold water to make all the skum rise; skim again, and when the scum is done rising, and the surface of the broth is quite clean, have properly prepared the following: A medium-sized carrot, 1 head of celery, 2 turnips and 2 onions. Put these into the broth, cover closely and simmer very gently, not to evaporate the broth, for 4 or 5 hours, according to the amount of the meat, strain, and, if not to be used the same day, set in a cool place.

*Remarks*—This may be used for all soups, brown or white, made of beef, lamb or veal, as a knuckle of beef can be used in preparing the broth or stock, if you choose, in place of the veal or lamb.

"**Stock,**" **Explanation of and How to Make.**—The meaning of this, now common, word is the unthickened broth from any meats to form the basis, or strength, of all soups; also often added to gravies to enrich them or to increase the quantity. Made as follows:

*Brown Stock.*—To make the common stock for brown soups, gravies, etc., get a "hock" or "shin-bone" and about 4 lbs of extra soup meat; cut the meat into small pieces, saw the bone off inside the joints and split, to obtain the marrow; slice an onion and fry it, with the cut beef, in the marrow to a nice brown; now put the fried meat and onion with the hock into cold water, 2 gallons, and let it simmer 6 to 8 hours, and pour through a sieve and strain through a cloth into a perfectly clean and sweet earthen crock, and in the morning skim off all the grease. This is used for any brown soups or brown gravies. For white, or uncolored soups or gravies, omit the frying. If kept in a cool place in ordinary weather this stock will keep a week; when the crock or jar in which it is kept must be thoroughly scalded out and aired in the sun or before a hot fire or stove. See, also, remarks at the beginning of soups upon "Stock."

**Onion Soup—The Best Saved to the Last.**—An onion soup nicely made is one of the most healthful, consequently the best soups made. Take 6 medium-sized onions, sliced, and brown slightly in a suitable dish, with a table-spoonful of butter, adding 3 medium-sized potatoes, also sliced, and a little pepper and salt, and let all then cook an hour or two, putting into cold water, and simmer slowly. Add stock, 1 pt., season to taste, and serve hot, as all soups should be.

*Remarks.*—Onions, if peeled under water, saves the tears for other occasions, and does not leave an odor upon the hands.

**Oatmeal Gruel, for Invalids and Children.**—Take oatmeal, 2 table-spoonfuls, and pour upon it boiling water, 1 pt., or a little more; let it boil until quite like jelly; then strain, or pour through a small fine sieve, kept for such purposes. To a coffee cup of this add sugar, 1 tea-spoonful, and 2 tea-spoonfuls of cream, when it will be fit for a king. For very young children or very weak invalids of a dyspeptic tendency make thinner with water while boiling, or with cold fresh milk after done boiling.

*Remarks.*—Although a little out of place, 'tis valuable anywhere and good for anybody, even in health. For those who are sensible enough to take a light tea or supper, this, with some bread or crackers, will "fill the bill" nicely, even with straining.

# VARIOUS DISHES.

**MEATS, POULTRY AND FISH — With Suitable Gravies, Sauces, Etc.**—*Remarks.*—Most beginners in house-keeping will not only find it well to have a few receipts for cooking meats, poultry, fish, etc., in their more common ways, but particularly valuable to know how to be economical in saving what may be left over from a meal, or several meals; with which a dish may be prepared not only as savory and palatable as the original, but often more so. We trust both these points will be found true in the following receipts. And, as we so often hear the question asked by the housewife: "What shall I get for dinner?" or whatever the next meal may be, I will start out in the "dish" line, with a "bill of fare" for a week, so everyone may know what will be proper, remembering, however, they can make any change they choose for the day or for a single meal, as suits their pleasure or desire, according to what they may have on hand.

**A Week's Bill of Fare.**—This list was taken from a note-book, kept by a city lady for her own convenience. It will be found to be as well adapted to a village or country housewife as for a lady of the city. The amounts to be cooked or purchased for cooking to depend upon the number of persons to be at the table; always remembering that it is better to have something over rather than to be short, especially if you have company. Besides the articles named in the daily lists for breakfast there may be oatmeal or cracked wheat, milk or water toast, corn, graham, or buckwheat cakes, tea, coffee or cocoa — as you choose; for dinner, as many of the vegetables of the season as you like, with tea or coffee also; and for supper, such side dishes as you choose, made up from any of the meats, together with canned or fresh fruits, according to the season:

SUNDAY. — Breakfast, beefsteak; dinner, turkey, chicken or other fowl, plenty to leave over, with vegetables, pie or pudding, or both.

MONDAY.—Breakfast, the left-over turkey, or fowl, broiled; and for dinner, what is still left over, fricaseed, warmed up or fried, with the gravy.

TUESDAY.—Breakfast, chops of lamb, mutton, veal or pork, as preferred, dinner, beef-soup, vegetables, and pudding.

WEDNESDAY.—Breakfast, ham and eggs; dinner, boiled corned beef, or pork and beans, and pie.

THURSDAY.—Breakfast, hash or any of the made-up dishes from left-over corned beef, etc.; dinner, soup, with its surplus meat, vegetable etc.

FRIDAY.—To suit catholic " help," be sure to have fish for breakfast and dinner, and any other meats desired by any others of the family.

SATURDAY.—Breakfast, veal cutlets or chops of other meat, as preferred, and buckwheat or other griddle cakes; dinner, beefsteak, mashed or fried potatoes, and pie or pudding.

428

**HINTS IN COOKING MEATS AND FISH.—Boiled Meats.—**
For cooking they should always be put into boiling water. which sets or closes the pores and keeps in the juices: after which slow boiling until tender. And if corned boiled beef. to be eaten cold, is left to stand in its water over night, it will be sweeter and more juicy.

**For Soups** always put into cold water, which leaves the pores open and allows the juices to escape into the soup which is desired. After it begins to boil keep it boiling slowly—not merely to simmer, but to boil.

**The Same for Fish,** using only water sufficient to cover it.

**For Roasting Meats and Poultry,** a hot oven, the door to stand a little open, covering the meat well with drippings or butter before putting into the oven, which keeps the surface moist and also helps to retain the juice of the meat.

**For Frying Fish** always have fat or butter hot, and plenty of it; and the fish should always be well drained after soaking, or the moisture absorbed with a napkin before putting into the pan to fry.

*Remarks.* As sometimes in warm weather meat and fish are liable to get " tainted," I will next give a receipt for correcting this difficulty. This receipt also relieves the pain of burns, etc., and is a great disinfectant.

**Putid, or Ill-Smelling Meats, Poultry Fish, Butter, etc. to Correct:** Permanganate of potash, 1 oz.; water that has been boiled and become cold. 1 qt. DIRECTIONS: Put into a bottle, cork, and shake well, to dissolve the permanganate, and it is ready for use. Put from a teaspoon to a tablespoonful of this (according to the size of the piece of meat), into sufficient cold water to cover the meat in a suitable sized jar or crock; stir with a stick (as it stains the hand or clothing): then put in the meat, chicken, duck, or fish, as the case may be, washing every part thoroughly and letting it remain ten minutes in the water; then rinse thoroughly which will remove all " taint " or ill-smell.

**For Butter.—**Slice it off thin, wash carefully in the same strength, rinse nicely in pure water, then mold again, wrap in muslin, and cover with nice brine.

**For Burns.—**Take 1 teaspoonful of the mixture to ½ pt. of water; wetting cloths in it, laying on and keeping them wet is said to relieve the pain immediately; it is also good for bruises, to relieve pain. See the remarks below as to how to treat extensive scalds and burns and for a general disinfectant.

*Remarks.* Observe the heading is putid, not putrid. The first comes from the Latin word, *putere*, to have an ill-smell; the second from *putrere*, to be rotten. It will not restore rotten meat, but it will correct ill-smelling meat. Actual decomposition (rottenness) cannot be restored. This mixture is claimed to be the same as

**Condy's Fluid,** which is claimed to be the best disenfectant known; and Dunglison, the great Medical Dictionary man says: "Condy's Disinfect ing fluid, is supposed to be a concentrated solution of permanganate of potassa," etc., which is the same as " potash," above. Mr. Condy, in a pamphlet published by himself in 1862 says "half a tumbler of his fluid in a good sized bath (this is supposing a person to be scalded all over, or at least much of his surface), will give instant relief in these frightful scalds and burns,

**Driving away Flies with It.**—The writer of "Hints and Helps," published in the *Blade* in 1879, from which the author gathered and condensed these items, claims that a little of this mixture, in a soup-plate of water, will drive away flies, even those big buzzing ones which are so troublesome when fresh meat is around. This is easily tried, but knowing the permanganate to be a powerful disinfectant, I have no hesitation in recommending the mixture for all the purposes for which it is claimed to be valuable.

**BEEFSTEAK.—How to Cook It.**—As beefsteak is, probably, more often cooked than any other dish, I will begin with it; and as I have, in rhyme, by a Layman contributor to the "Home Department" of the Toledo *Commercial*, the way it was cooked by an English *"beefsteak fluke"* in 1734, and which has continued to be the plan, until very recently, and still is the plan pursued by most people. I will give it, and afterwards make such explanations, in the remarks, as shall give the true, and better way, of cooking beefsteaks. The rhyme referred to is as follows.

> " *Pound well your meat till the fibres break,*
> Be sure that next you have, to broil the steak,
> Good coal in plenty; nor a moment leave,
> But turn it over this way, and then that;
> The lean should be quite rare—not so the fat.
> The platter now and then the juice receive,
> Put on your butter, place it on your meat,
> Salt, pepper, turn it over, serve, and eat."

*Remarks.*—This "contributor" asked: "Can any correspondent of the "Home Department" furnish a better rule?" to which I answer, yes. Simply leave off the first, or italicised line, and you have the better rule, except the steak be very tough, that is the only reason why pounding should be resorted to, as it lets out the sweet juices of the meat, and removes, if broiled, (broiling is the true way to cook a steak) much of the nourishing properties, and spoils its delicacy of flavor. Some people broil, or rather cook, their steak on top of the stove. This is not delicate, nor so advisable as to cook in the hot skillet, or spider, without butter, as mentioned below; but I will give you the plan which my family pursued for a number of years before my companion was taken away by death.

**BEEFSTEAK.—Broiler, to Make.**—I went to a tinner and told him I wanted a kind of "Griddle Ring Broiler," made of suitable sized wire—cross-barred, of a size to drop into the stove, by taking off a cover. The holes being 9 inches, he made a ring of No. 9 wire, 8½ inches in diameter; and cross-barred it with No. 15 wire, to lay the steak upon. Then, for a handle, he took a piece of the No. 9, or possibly No. 8, which is still larger, about 4 or 4½ feet long.

and *b*ent it, in the centre, parallel, about 2 inches apart, looping, or bending **the** two free ends of this wire for the handle, around one side of the ring, **or** frame, part of the circular griddle, on the under side, fastening these two wires, forming the handle, to the opposite side of the ring, with smaller wire, to keep the handle in place, then bending these two wires up, at right angles, with the griddle ring, and bending 6 inches, or thereabouts, of the top of this handle off again at right angles, to take hold of with the hand when broiling; the handle to be long enough to carry the upper bend at least 1 foot above the top of the stove, supposing it, the griddle, to be down in the stove hole 6 inches or **m**ore, with the steak upon it, which will prevent burning the hand while broiling with it. In this way, properly seasoning, and turning two or three times, a steak is very quickly cooked, retaining all the juices, if you did not pound it, to let them out. With this kind of a griddle broiler you can get down close to the coals and save much trouble. We have used this over a coal fire with about the same satisfaction as over a wood fire, if the fire is pretty well burned down. I think almost any tinner can get up such a broiler from the above description, if so, they will be found very convenient for all who love a nicely broiled steak. It is equally as nice for broiling veal, lamb, chicken, etc. Of course seasoning properly, having a hot plate to put it upon, with a moderate amount of butter upon the steak to form the gravy. Cover with another hot plate, if not to be served immediately.

*Remarks.*—Either of the above plans make a nice dish, or, if after the water is poured off the beef, a little milk, or if no milk, a little more hot water is put on, and after cooking a few minutes, thickening a little with flour, rubbed smooth in a little cold water, makes an agreeable change, a very nice dish in-deed. Or the sliced dried beef may be minced fine or sprinkled into a salad, or mixed with potatoes and eggs for a breakfast dish: or heated with steam, or eaten with fresh or canned peas, or with stewed onions and potatoes. Thus it may be used in many ways, to suit the taste; or be utilized with such things as may be on hand or obtainable.

**BEEF BALLS.—With Uncooked Meat, Fried.**—Chop very fine raw beef, 2 lbs, or as much as needed, with ¼ lb of suet, skinned or chopped; season to taste with salt, pepper and a little cloves; mix in a handful of flour, and mould into balls and fry in hot drippings, or lard, (drippings is best for this) to a nice brown, turning to brown both sides. Serve hot; but they are good cold. For the author a tablespoonful of powdered sage helps the flavor much.

**BEEF OR OTHER MEAT BALLS.—From Left Over Meats.**—Chop cold, or left over meats of any kind, with the same bulk of potatoes, add a little onion to flavor slightly. Then take dry bread, pour hot water on it, to moisten sufficiently, having bread enough to make the mass adhere, so it can be fried in cakes or balls (a nice brown), in a skillet, with a little butter or drippings, as you would fry meat. Nettie Hines-Wood, of Janesburg, Mo. in *Blade.*

*Remarks.*—She called them "noodles," but, although I can see a nice dish in them, I do not see "the chuckling grin of noodles." 'Tis too nice to have been made by a "simpleton."

**Cold Meats Economically Used.**—Chop any cold meats, as for hash, and warm up in milk, the more cream in it the better. When about ready for the table, season and break in an egg, if you like; some like it better without. To be eaten with nicely baked potatoes, or potatoes warmed up in a little milk and a bit of butter.

**Cold Beef—Another Way.**—Mince it fine with pepper, salt and onions and some rich gravy, and put it into tins three parts full; fill them up with mashed potatoes and brown in the oven.

**Cream Croquettes—Delmonico's Substitute for "Hash."**— Mr. Delmonico describes croquettes as the attractive French substitute for American hash, and tells how to make them. "Veal, mutton, lamb, sweet- breads, almost any of the lighter meats, besides cold chicken and turkey can be most deliciously turned into croquettes. Chop the meat very fine. Chop up an onion, fry it in an ounce of butter, add a table-spoonful of flour; stir it up well; then add the chopped meat and a little broth, salt, pepper, little nutmeg; stir for two or three minutes, then add the yolks of 2 eggs, and turn the whole into a dish to cool. When cold mix well together again, divide into parts for the croquettes; roll into the desired shape in bread-crumbs, dip in beaten egg, then in bread.crumbs again, and fry crisp to a bright golden color. The cro- quettes may be served plain, or with tomato sauce or garniture of vegetables." —*New York paper.*

*Remarks.*—Thus it will be seen that any kind of cold meats may be eco- nomically "turned," as the women say of re-making a dress, into a new dish, which may even have a nicer relish than in its first form or "dress" The fol- lowing is the manner in which "Winifred," of Toledo, saves her

**Cold Beef and Dry Bread, or Biscuit Balls.**—Chop your beef very fine (pork will not do), then soak your bread in cold water till it is soft, then take it in the hands and squeeze as much of the water out as you can, having two-thirds as much bread as meat; then mix the bread and meat thoroughly together, beat 3 eggs well and mix in; add salt to taste, and grate in enough nutmeg to season nicely; make out in balls about the size of a small biscuit, and fry slowly in butter or cooking fat, till brown on both sides.

**Beefsteak, Broiling in a Spider or Skillet.**—A writer who knows about how to cook a steak says: When steak is bought see that it is not cut more than 3/4 of an inch thick, and that it is of the same thickness all through. Have the skillet on the stove until it gets hot, lay the steak on it, without pounding (she certainly learned the secret of not pounding); turn it immediately, and keep turning for two minutes, or longer, if you do not wish it very rare. Be sure and have the skillet hot enough before you begin; perhaps you may be afraid it will stick or burn, but it will not, if you manage right. Meantime have a plate in the oven heating, and when the meat is done lay it on the plate, with a little butter over it, season with pepper and salt to taste, place in the oven for one minute and it is done.

*Remarks.*—I can see no use of putting in the oven for one minute, unless it is to melt the butter, but if the plate and steak are both hot that will soon melt without putting in the oven, unless you have to wait for something else, which ought not to be, as a hot steak is the way to have it; let it be the last touch to finish getting the meal. It is very proper, however, to cover with another hot plate to send to the table. If the steak sticks to the skillet, at first, loosen it with a knife. Trim off any membrane around the steak that would cause it to curl, or turn up at the edge. This gives you a crisp and brown surface, with all the juices retained. Pepper and salt to taste, in all cases.

**Beefsteak Smothered With Onions.**—Broil the steak, as above, having 2, 3 or 4 onions, according to size of family, nicely chopped, and put into a skillet, or frying pan, with drippings, or butter, stirring to avoid burning until done. Put them upon the steak, in a hot plate, and turn another hot plate over them, for a few minutes, to allow the steak to absorb their flavor; serve hot. Those who do not like the onions can have their steak served without them.

*Remarks.*—Some people boil their onions, first, until tender, then mash, or chop, frying the steak in butter, or drippings, taking up the steak and then frying the onions in the gravy and pouring over the steak. This makes them softer and a little more mushy, and the steak not quite so digestible.

**Beefsteak and Salt Pork Smothered With Onions.**—Fry a few slices of salt pork brown; take out the pork then put in the steak and fry also —any tender steak will do; when done take up and put in the onions, sliced thin, cover and cook slowly, stirring occasionally. Put pork, then steak, then onions upon the dish. Make a gravy by adding a little water, flour, butter and salt, if needed, and pour over the whole.

**Beefsteak Fried in Cracker Crumbs.**—A writer in one of the papers asks, and directs as follows: Do any of you have to get up early in the morning, and get breakfast in such a terrible hurry that you can't wait for nice coals to broil the steak? If so, just have a little very hot butter in the pan, and after pounding or hacking the steak lightly, salt and pepper it, roll in finely crushed cracker crumbs, and brown quickly in the butter. You will find it a decided improvement on the leathery substance called fried steak, and a very palatable substitute for broiled.

*Remarks.*—To have the steak cooked in this way, done, without burning the cracker crumbs, it would seem to me necessary to have the steak cut very thin, say split ordinary steak, with a sharp knife, which will enable it to cook through much quicker than if thick. Steak, as well as pork, is improved by the dipping into cracker crumbs, or batter, and frying quickly, when to be fried at all. I like even broiled pork better than fried, unless the fat, or butter is very hot—sozzling (long soaking) any meat in half hot fat, spoils it for digestion, whether dipped in crumbs or not.

**Dried Beef With Eggs.**—Slice, or buy it of the grocer, cut into thin chips, dried beef ½ lb. Put into a frying pan, well covered with hot water, upon the stove; and when it comes to a boil pour off the water, which freshens

It, now put in butter, a good table-spoonful (lard or drippings will do), add a dash or two of pepper, and let it cook a few minutes, over a quick fire; then break and add 3 or 4 nice eggs, and stir until the eggs are done. Serve hot; or, dredge the beef with flour just as it is done frying, and fry the eggs by themselves, and serve as with ham.

*Remarks.*—Another lady writer uses up her cold meats in the following way:

**Nice Meat Balls.**—Take a quantity of cold meat sufficient for a meal, bone and chop fine, season with salt and pepper, nutmeg and allspice; soak about one-third as much of white bread in cold milk, press out, and mix with the meat; add beaten egg—one egg is enough for three persons—and lump of butter the size of a walnut, mix thoroughly and roll into balls; fry in hot lard. Pile in a pyramid on a flat dish and serve.

**A Dish of Scraps.**—Take some cold potatoes, a few pieces of dry bread, some scraps of cold boiled or fried meat; chop it all quite fine in the chopping-bowl; season with salt, pepper and sage; put in a piece of butter and cook it the same as hash. It is much better than potatoes alone warmed over.—*Mrs. A. M. Fellows, Prairieville, Mich.*

**Beef or Veal Head Cheese from Bony Pieces, or With Chicken.**—Take the bony or cheap pieces of beef or veal and boil them until perfectly tender; remove the bones and chop it fine, as for hash; season with butter, pepper and salt, a few crackers rolled fine, a little sage or sweet herbs of any kind to suit the taste, add a little of the broth in which it is cooked, stir it well together and press it into a tin basin or deep dish, cover with a plate (with weights upon it), let it stand until cold, then slice it as you would head-cheese. It is very nice for supper and lunch, or for your hungry boys and girls who carry their dinners to school. Chicken or turkey prepared in the same way, omitting the herbs, is very nice.—*Melissa W.*

*Remarks.*—This will be just as good a dish as though "Melissa W." had given her full name. Still the author would prefer to give full credit, but it is impossible in all cases. I know it will make a nice dish prepared from any of the articles named.

**Venison Steaks, Broiled.**—Cut them thin and broil nicely by turning frequently, having seasoned to suit the taste; put into a hot dish or plate, with a bit of nice butter upon each steak; keep hot. 'Tis customary to serve venison with cranberry sauce or jelly. No meat equals venison for the author's taste. But rabbits treated as next given are also very nice:

**Rabbit Cutlets.**—Cut the different limbs into the size of cutlets; such as the shoulders cut in half; also the legs, with the ends of the bones chopped off, and pieces of the back, even to the half of the head. Have ready some bread-crumbs and the yolk of an egg beat up. Drop each cutlet into the egg, and then into the bread-crumbs, as for veal cutlets. Fry them a nice brown, and when you dish them pour round them some rich brown gravy, which may be flavored with tomato sauce, if approved, and put round them pieces of fried bacon, if liked.

**Liver Hash.**—"Hash" made of beef is such a common dish we have thought to get up something new, and very nice for those who are fond of liver. Boil the liver until thoroughly tender—there must not be even a suspicion of hardness about it. Then mince it finely with a chopping-knife. Heat the mince very hot in a sauce of butter and browned flour. The seasoning is pepper, salt, a dash of lemon, or a little piquant sauce, such as mushroom or other catsup.

**Chicken Hash.**—This is the proper way to serve for breakfast whatever roast or boiled chicken may be left over from dinner. Mince the cold chicken, but not very fine, and to a cup of meat add two table-spoonfuls of good butter, a half cup of milk, enough minced onion to give a slight flavor, and salt, mace and pepper to taste. Stew it, taking care to stir it, and serve with a garnish of parsley, it you like it. Every particle of bone must be extracted.

*Remarks.*—If prepared cold, press it instead of stewing and serving hot.

**Beef Liver, to Fry.**—Cut the liver in thin slices, dip each slice in wheat flour or rolled crackers, and fry in hot lard, beef dripping or butter; season with pepper and salt. It must be thoroughly cooked and a fine brown; served hot.

**Calf's Liver Head-Cheese, or for Eating Cold.**—Take a calf's liver and put into a saucepan with just water enough to cover it and cook till tender; then bruise it with a spoon, or mash it with a potato masher; add a cup of cream and season with salt, pepper, a little cloves and sweet majoram, if you have it; if not, a little sage, if you like it. Mix nicely and put in a wet dish, or mold, and weight it tightly till cold, when it is ready for tea or lunch at any time, and a very nice dish it makes.

*Remarks.*—It is more delicate and palatable than beef's liver fried in butter as steak, *i. e.*, without the trouble of making into head-cheese; but the head-cheese, too, is nice fried.

**Beef to Roast or Bake.**—A "Farmer's Wife" informs us—and they know how to do it—"to lay the meat on some sticks in a dripping-pan, the sticks to be thick enough to allow ½ an inch of water in the pan without touching the meat. Season with salt and pepper, and put in the oven 3 or 4 hours before it is wanted for the table. Baste it often with the water in the bottom of the pan, renewing it as often as it gets low. This makes sweet, juicy baked beef. The great secret of it is, not to have the meat touch the water in the bottom of the pan, and to baste it often. Tough, unpromising pieces of beef are best cooked by steaming them an hour and a half, or so, and then putting them in the oven and baking as much longer."

*Remarks.*—If the sticks nor the water are used, to prevent burning beef place a dish of water in the oven, the steam from which removes the danger of burning the meat. But the basting with the water and juices as they drip from the meats is a very nice way indeed. The following will also be found a very nice way of roasting a kind of half roast and half stew:

**Beef, a Pot Roast or Stew.**—Slice thin salt pork, ½ lb., and lay it on the bottom of a dinner-pot; peel and slice a medium-sized onion and lay it over the pork; then put into the pot a rather square, solid piece of the round of beef, weighing about 6 lbs.; season it with a table-spoonful of salt and a table-spoon-ful of pepper; add sufficient hot water to reach one-fourth up the side of the meat; cover the pot and set it where the meat will cook slowly; about ½ hour to each pound of meat is generally the time required for cooking. Turn the meat occasionally and cook it very slowly until it is brown and tender; take care to keep only sufficient water in the pot to prevent burning. When the meat is done keep it hot in the oven, while a table-spoonful of flour is boiled for two minutes in the gravy; then serve the gravy and pork on the dish with the pot roast.

**Salad Dressing for Any Kind of Meat, Chicken, etc.**—A scant pint of cold boiled or roast meat cut in small dice. Veal, lamb or chicken can be used, or even two kinds of meat if you have not enough of one. Twice as much cabbage as meat. Only that part of the cabbage which is white and brit-tle should be used, and it should be chopped fine.

*The Dressing, or Salad.*—Take good vinegar, ½ pt.; 1 heaping table-spoon-ful of sugar; 1 tea-spoonful of dry mustard; 2 eggs, a little salt and pepper and butter the size of an egg. DIRECTIONS—Heat the ingredients, the butter excepted, over boiling water, or by setting the basin into a pan of boiling water; stirring all the time to prevent curdling the eggs; as soon as it thickens remove from the hot water, then add the butter, stir it in, and pour, while hot, over the meat, stir and let stand till cold; then stir in the chopped cabbage.

*Remarks.*—This makes a dish for tea rarely excelled.

**Corned Beef, To Boil with Cabbage.**—A 6 to 8 lb. piece will require 3 to 4 hours slow boiling. Put it into cold water, and remove all scum that rises. If allowed to boil quick, at first especially, it will never become as tender as to cook slowly. The slower it boils, the better or more tender it will be, and the better, also, the flavor. If cabbage is to be cooked with it, split a young head into halves and pour boiling water upon it; then, after a few min-utes, pour off the water, which carries with it much of its rank odor and taste. An hour will cook the cabbage nicely. It is said that a bit of red pepper, the size of your finger ends, dropped into boiling meat or vegetables, will kill all unpleasant odors. It is worth a trial, and for me, I like the red pepper flavor, if a small-sized one is put in, whether it carries off the odor, or not.

If is to be used cold, let it stand in the water in which it is boiled over night, or until cold, which makes it more juicy and sweeter to the taste.

**Mock Beef Tongue, or Savory Beef, Baked.**— Lean, raw beef, 3½ lbs.; square soda crackers, or their equivalent, 6; butter, size of an egg; sweet cream, ½ cup; eggs, 3; salt, 4 tea-spoonfuls; pepper, 2½ tea-spoonfuls; powdered sweet marjoram (if you have it and like it, if not, summer savory will fill its place, wherever this is called for, or sage, if liked), 1 table-spoonful. DIRECTIONS—Chop the beef fine and also pound it, removing strings or gristle; roll the crackers fine, warm the butter a little so it will mix nicely, break the eggs over the pounded meat and mix all together with the hands; now make into 2 loaves or rolls like beef tongues, press closely together, put into a pan, and bake 1½ hours, basting with water and butter, nicely browning both sides. What is left, sliced thin for tea, gives a delicious relish.

**Cold Roast Beef Broiled.**—Cut thin slices from the under-done parts of the roast, season with salt and pepper, place upon the gridiron over nice coals, turn them 2 or 3 times quickly, as it broils quicker than if entirely raw, and serve as soon as done, while very hot, with a bit of butter on each slice.

*Remarks.*—Our wire beef-steak broiler, which see, will be very nice for this, as you can drop it into the stove hole, close down to the coals, as it requires quick heat.

**Flank of Beef Rolled and Corned for Eating Cold.**—A lady writing in the *Blade* to a Dr. Utter, who had given a plan of how the Cincinnati butchers prepared their beef for corning, gives what she calls "a better way," as follows:

"For rolled corned beef we take the flank, bone it, sprinkle salt, pepper, and a little saltpeter on one side; salt it, beginning with the thickest end; when rolled, tie firmly and securely with a strong cord around and lengthwise; lay in strong brine 10 to 14 days, remove and boil in fresh water several hours, or till done. On taking from the fire it must be pressed immediately, by laying a board on top, put a heavy stone on the board for a weight, keep the weight on till the next day; when pressed well it cuts up in slices like ham. Hope the doctor will try it and tell me how he likes it."

*Remarks.*—I did not see the "Utter" Doctor's report of how he liked it; but, as the author likes it, and knows that others will, who like a nice slice of cold boiled beef for supper or a lunch, that is enough. It will be found very nice. Summer savory, marjoram, etc., can be added in the seasoning, which will improve its flavor to those who like them, or sage.

**Fresh Beef, To Cook for Use When Cold.**—Take flank, or parts where there is no bone, but streaks of lean and fat; salt and pepper to taste, and roll like jelly cake; then wrap twine around it, tie tightly, and boil till done; when cold, slice as you would cake.—*Mrs. Emma Weatherwax, Cedar Rapids, Iowa.*

*Remarks.*—It will be seen by this that it is not necessary to wait to corn it, but that fresh does equally well, only for those who prefer the corned. Each can suit himself.

**Beef's Heart, to Bake With Dressing.**—Remove the "deaf ears," and all the superfluous strings, fat, etc., washing inside and out, to remove all blood in the heart. Put into the pot and cover with boiling water—boiling until tender. Take up and cut out the inside partitions, to make room for the dressing, or stuffing, made the same as for chicken or turkey, adding a little extra butter, to make up for the leanness of the heart. Bake about 1½ hours.—*Mrs. A. W. Smith, Sheridan, Montana, in Blade.*

*Remarks.*—If this is nicely done a baked heart makes a dish of which the author is very fond. Would be glad to help eat one once each week. If any is left, slice it, and warm up, next morning, in the gravy with what stuffing there may be left; if none, some bits of bread do nicely, warmed in the gravy.

**Beef's Tongue, Potted.**—Boil a tongue which has been salted, but not smoked, with nice veal, 1 lb. Remove the skin from the tongue and chop it finely with the veal; then pound it nicely with the steak pounder, adding 3 or 4 table-spoonfuls of nice butter, a little cayenne, mace, nutmeg and cloves finely ground. Mix all thoroughly, and press into small jars, or bowls, and pour a little melted butter over the top, which helps its keeping. It does nicely without the veal, but is preferable with. May be eaten cold, or fried brown, in hot butter.—*Our Fireside Friend.*

**Scotch Potted Meat.**—Boil an ox cheek and 2 calves-feet, slowly, till the meat comes off the bones freely; chop fine, season with pepper and salt; mix moist with some of the gravy, or broth, in which it was cooked; put into molds. If well cooked and carefully seasoned it will keep a week. Or if covered as the tongue, above, with butter, much longer. The Scotch eat this with a fresh lemon and mustard. If the family is large, both cheeks and 4 feet may be used. The cheek is tender; meat from other parts may be used, by longer boiling to make equally tender.

**Scotch Collops, With Veal.**—Cut the remains of some cold roast veal into about the thickness of cutlets, rather larger than a silver dollar, flour the meat well, and fry a light brown color in butter; dredge again with flour, and add ½ pt. of water, pouring it in by degrees; set it on the fire, and, when it boils, add an onion and a blade of powdered mace, and let it simmer very gently for ¾ of an hour; flavor the gravy with a table-spoonful of mushroom, or other catsup or Worcestershire sauce. Give one boil and serve hot.

**Shoulder of Veal or Lamb, Stuffed—"Dutch Turkey."**—Take a shoulder of nice veal (and it you are buying it of the butcher have him) carefully remove the bones, cutting only at the ends, to leave the opening for the stuffing to be introduced, wash and wipe dry with a cloth by pressing it upon the meat. Grate 1 to 1½ pts. of bread crumbs, season with salt and pepper, a tea-spoonful of sweet marjoram, sage, sweet basil, or parsley, as you have or prefer, made fine; after having been dried; and if onion is liked chop a medium sized one, and put it in a saucepan with as much butter, and stew 5 to 8 minutes, then pour over the crumbs, and mix thoroughly. Press this stuffing all through the length of the leg, from which the bone was removed, and secure the ends with skewers, or by sewing with stout, uncolored, linen thread. Season the outside with salt and pepper, dust with flour and bake about 2 hours, or till done, in a rather hot oven, basting from time to time with the water, and a little butter, put in the pan for the purpose; and if 2 or 3 sticks are put in the pan to keep the meat out of the water, so much the better. If likely to brown too much, put a piece of paper, or a flat pan over it. Keep up the supply of water—about ½ pt.—in the pan, to make a gravy with by thickening with browned or unbrowned flour, as you prefer. A leg of young mutton, or even the hind leg, may be done in the same way; or they may be thus roasted, without the boneing and stuffing, when you have not time for that. Cranberry sauce, or any tart jelly, may be served with either of these; but for lamb the following sauce is generally served.

**Mint Sauce for Roast Lamb.**—Finely chopped green mint, 3 table-spoonfuls; the same amount of granulated sugar, and good vinegar, 6 table-spoonfuls; make and serve hot.

*Remarks.*—I used to have a German butcher prepare the veal shoulder for me in this way in Ann Arbor, Mich., and he always called it "Dutch Turkey," so I am not to be charged with a slight or any disrespect to the Germans as a class, as it originated with one of their own people.

**Meat Loaf, from Beef, Veal, Mutton, or Ham, Left Over.**—Chop fine all such meats as you have left over from previous meals, fat and lean together, with a chopped onion, if allowable; a few slices of dry bread which have been soaked in milk, pressing out the superfluous milk; an egg for each person, and mix all together with pepper and salt as needed. Make into a loaf and bake nicely for breakfast or tea. Mashed potatoes, or fried, sliced from raw ones, are very nice with this relish.

**Minced Meat Fritters.**—Regular minced meat, 2 cups (or you may mince cold beef and veal, and if a little cold ham in it, so much the better, chopping in a good-sized tart apple with these meats, to imitate "minced;" and and fine bread crumbs, 1 cup; 2 eggs, well beaten, and the juice of half a lemon. Mix well, using a little spice if you get it up from left-over meats. Fry in hot lard; drain, if need be, in a colander, and serve hot. If made thin they cook quicker.

**PORK.**—We now come to the question of pork; and I will say that, although many, perhaps most, physicians object to the use of this article of diet, yet the author has always eaten more or less of it. People must judge largely for themselves, and from their conditions of health—eat no food that rises on the stomach, but whatever digests well will give strength. Probably the largest amount of pork is cooked by frying. I will, therefore, first direct how this should be done to be the most palatable as well as the most digestible. Of course, these remarks refer to salt, or "pickled" pork:

**Salt Pork, How to Fry.**—A lady who is competent to instruct in the manner of cooking this article, after saying that " None of my family like salt pork, they say, yet we manage to make a barrel of it disappear yearly. Here is one of my ways of cooking it in the spring, when I want it extra nice. I soak it for a few hours in sweet milk; ordinarily I take skim milk or fresh buttermilk; then drain it, and fry brown."

*Remarks.*—If it is dipped in flour first, it will be crispy and nice. Rolled cracker crumbs make it nice, too. If cut into dice and fried with eggs, as the Omelet with Ham, below, it is also remarkably nice.

**Ham, to Bake, and an Omelet From the "Odds and Ends."**—Take a medium sized ham—8 to 12 lbs.—and soak it 12 to 24 hours in cold water, changing once. Then put it into a suitable kettle that will allow its being covered with boiling water, adding good vinegar, 1 pt., with a little summer savory, sage, thyme, or parsley—parsley seed does well—using any two of these if you have them, and boil slowly for 2 or 3 hours, until very tender. When cool enough to handle remove it from the water, take off the rind and all fat exceeding ½ inch in thickness, and the dark outside from the part not covered by the rind; put into the dripping pan, sprinkle on a little powdered sugar, grate over it a little bread crust, and place in a rather hot oven, about ½ an hour, or until nicely browned. If you can bring it out just at dinner time, it is splendid hot; and it is also " just splendid " cold.    The sugar improves its taste and preserves and increases its juices.

For the omelet take the " odds and ends," chop them fine, and for each pint of the chopped ham, break in 3 eggs and fry a nice brown, makes a delicious dish for breakfast.

*Remarks.*—This is the proper plan to prepare a ham to chop finely, for sandwiches; but for this purpose most, or all of the fat part may be left on, and all chopped together, putting on, or mixing in, as you choose, a suitable amount of mustard, and sufficient of the water in which it was boiled, to make sufficient moist for the sandwich mince.    I prefer it to those made with beef or veal.    If these dishes are nicely made, I should like to see the doctor, or any other person, who would refuse to eat of them, in moderation, although, of course, they are "only pork."

**Omelet With Ham, Raw or Cooked.**—Cut raw ham into small dice (chopped coarsely).    Put a suitable amount of nice butter into a frying pan, on the stove; beat the eggs (1 or 2 for each person to be served, as you wish), putting in a little salt.    Then put the chopped raw ham into the butter, and when nearly fried turn the beaten eggs over the ham, the fire being brisk, will soon cook the omelet.    Cut into suitable pieces to take up and serve.    To make the omelet with boiled ham put the beaten eggs upon the ham as soon as the ham is put into the hot butter, as the ham will be nicely hot as soon as the omelet is cooked, by dipping some of the hot butter upon it, until done.

**Ham Balls.**—Chop fine cold cooked ham; add an egg for each person and a little flour; beat together and make into balls; fry brown in hot butter.

**Ham and Eggs, Extra Nice.**—A cook sends the following to the *Country Gentleman:* Cut the ham not quite ½ inch thick, boil in plenty of water till barely cooked through; put in a pan and brown the fat part slightly; remove from the fire, take out the meat and pour off the fat into a cup; wipe the pan till it shines like a mirror.    Then put in a spoonful of the clear part of the fat, break in the eggs, and set the pan in a place scarcely hotter than boiling water, cover and let the eggs cook slowly, for four or five minutes, taking them out as soon as they can be lifted.    Place them around the dish of ham, but do not put the fat on the dish.    Eat with mashed potatoes.

**Fried Ham With Poached Eggs.**—Fry the ham as usual.    Poach the eggs by putting into a frying pan with boiling water, over a gentle fire; put in the eggs, which should be broken into a dish separately to avoid bad ones, cover the pan 4 to 5 minutes.    Take up with a skimmer, on to the ham, or a separate plate, as you choose, sprinkling over a little pepper and salt, and a bit of butter.    Serve hot.

**Broiled Ham.**—If the ham is very salty freshen it a little in hot water, as salt pork is freshened, except to remove from the stove as soon as it boils, and let it soak about 20 minutes.    Drain nicely, and broil as beefsteak, which see.    Turning 2 or 3 times; season with pepper and a little butter upon it. To be served at once, while hot.

**Ham and Tongue Toast.**—Cut the slices of bread rather thick.    Toast carefully, and butter well on both sides. Chop the ham or tongue pretty finely; put into a pan with a little butter and pepper (the author likes a sprinkle or two of cayenne in it), and a beaten egg for each piece of bread; and as soon as the egg is done spread upon the toast and serve at once.

**Ham Cakes, Baked, for Breakfast or Tea.**—Take the remnants of a boiled ham, fat and lean together. Chop fine, and pound with a steak-pounder, or, if you have one, run it through a sausage machine. Soak a large piece of bread for each person to be served in milk; a beaten egg, also, for each person, a little pepper, and all mixed together, put into a suitable pudding-dish and bake a nice brown. Call this ham pudding if you prefer. It will pass for either. Some may prefer the next one with its mixture of veal.

**Ham and Veal Odds and Ends Economically Used.**—Take equal quantities of cold boiled ham and veal; chop fine, separately; have some hard-boiled eggs, ½ dozen, or more, according to the amount of meats, also chopped fine; then, in a buttered pudding-dish, put a layer of veal, with pepper and salt to suit, and moistened with a little water and a few splashes of Worcestershire sauce, or any of the catsups; then treat a layer of ham in the same way; and then of the eggs, with pepper and salt; and so keep on until all is in; when, if the ham had fat upon it, no butter will be needed, otherwise, lay a few bits of nice butter on the top, and bake slowly about 2 hours; then it may be served hot for any meal, or put away till cold, with a plate and weights upon it, so it will slice nicely.

**"Scrapple" in Place of Head-Cheese.**—"Lorinda," of Anoka, Minn., gives the *Blade* the plan of using up hogs' heads with some cornmeal, which she learned of a Dutch woman in Illinois, which she testifies to the value of from 25 years' experience. It needs only a trial to satisfy any one of its palatableness and economy in using up hogs' heads. She says:

"Soak the head, or heads, in water over night. In the morning clean thoroughly, cutting out the eyes and ears deeply; then boil until tender; take out and let stand till cold; remove all the bone and chop fine. Drain off all the water it was boiled in, to get out all the bits of bone; rinse out the kettle, and put back the water drained off, and put on the fire to get hot; in the meantime, season the chopped meat and put in with additional water, to about half fill the kettle, or to be quite thin, and when it begins to boil thicken with cornmeal to the consistence of mush; take out into pans while hot, make it level on the top, and when cold, pour melted lard over it to prevent the top getting dry and hard; it will also help it to keep longer. When wanted for use, cut out in slices about half an inch thick and fry in a little hot lard or butter until a nice brown; then turn, brown again, eat hot. If any one thinks this is too fat, or greasy, they can put in the heart and tongue."

**Pork Chops Fried with Apples, Very Fine.**—Put the fresh chops in the frying-pan, salt, pepper, and sage, if you like it, or any other sweet herb, to be scattered over, and fried; if not fat enough to make plenty of gravy, add butter or drippings. When the chops are nicely done, having sliced the apples, fry in the same dish, and when nicely browned put them over the chops or in a dish by themselves, as some may not like them, although the author, and probably most others, will be very fond of them. Use nice tart apples only. Chops of fresh pork, fried and seasoned the same way, are splendid, if nicely browned, even without the apples.

*Remarks.*—We will close the pork question with directions for properly cooking and serving pigs' feet, ears, etc., as suggested by the great showman, P. T. Barnum. He is admitted to be "the greatest showman on earth," and why should he not have learned something about good victuals? I should think he had, judging from his size and well rounded face. Being taken from the Bridgeport *Standard* (Barnum's home) it is no doubt reliable. I know "from the nature of things" he is correct.

**"Broiled Pigs' Feet, a la Barnum,"** is one of the dishes printed on the Sturtevant House bill of fare in New York. Barnum says: "Pigs' feet, properly cooked, were given to me to eat long before I was permitted to partake of any other animal food. When old and young feet are boiled together for 2½ hours, as usual, the old ones are tough and worthless. If they were boiled 3½ hours, the young feet would burst and the gelatine swim away. Now, the secret is to wrap each foot in a cotton bandage wound 2 or 3 times around it and well corded with twine. Then boil them 4 hours. Let them remain in the bandage until needed to broil, fry or pickle. The skin will hold them together while being cooked; and when you eat them you will find them all tender and delicate as possible."

*Remarks.*—The *Standard* said there was a hotel in their State (Connecticut) where pigs' feet were a special feature of the bill of fare; cooked as described above by Mr. Barnum. I know very well that pigs' feet as generally cooked, are a nuisance, so far as tenderness and ability to eat them are concerned. This wrapping and long cooking will make a new feature in serving them. I say, "Hurrah for Barnum!" as he has now done the public some real good, that will last, too, as long as pigs' feet grow. The 2½ hours are long enough to cook the ears, which the author has always preferred to the feet, because they were more tender and delicate, from the fact that they did not require so long boiling as the feet, and hence would be tender while the feet remained tough and gristly, for the want of the very knowledge how to cook them.

**Stews of Mutton, Chicken, etc.**—Take the neck, or any part of the forequarter of mutton, not so old as to be strong, cut into rather small pieces, and place in a pot having a well fitting lid, and cover the meat with cold water. boil slowly, removing scum as it rises, till perfectly tender; then set away, keeping covered. Next morning remove the fat, or tallow, from the top; then, at the proper time to get it ready for dinner, place again on the fire, adding salt and pepper to taste, and any herbs, if desired, and pour in hot water to well cover the mutton; and when boiling nicely put in dumplings made of light bread dough or biscuit dough, and fail not to keep up the boiling until the dumplings are done. Serve in a covered tureen that will hold the gravy, or juices, as well as the meat, dumplings, etc. If properly managed, when the meat and dumplings are taken up, there will be only juices enough left to thicken with a trifle of flour, rubbed smooth in a little cold water, or milk for the gravy.

*Very Tough Mutton, and Chickens* which have worn themselves out by laying eggs and raising many broods, by longer stewing the first day can be made very tender and palatable in the same manner.

**Mutton and Pork Stew.**—Neck, or other cheap parts of mutton, 3 lbs.; salt pork, ½ lb.; 1 onion; salt and pepper; and parsley, thyme or summer savory, if on hand and liked. DIRECTIONS—Cut the mutton into small pieces, ¾ or 1 inch square; the pork into small thin slices; break or slice the onion, dividing the rings if sliced. Put the mutton into a covered stew pan with cold water to cover it. Heat it gradually and stew 1 hour; then add the slices of pork, and bits of onion, the salt and pepper to taste, and continue the stewing until the meats are perfectly done, at which time, if desired, have ready some pastry, as for meat pie crust; (for 1 qt. of flour 3 table-spoonfuls of lard; 2½ cups of milk; salt and soda, 1 tea-spoonful each; cream of tartar, 2 tea-spoonfuls, work quickly and don't get too stiff, or in these proportions;) roll out ½ an inch thick, and cut into squares, or diamonds, and put in just long enough before taking up to cook the pastry, 10 to 15 minutes will be enough; and just before taking up add the sweet herbs, if they are to be used—if put in at first their flavor will be too much evaporated. When done thicken a cup of milk with a table-spoonful or two of flour and stir in just before taking into the tureen. In place of the pastry, or dumplings, ½ a can of sweet corn; or, in sweet corn time, the corn cut from ½ a dozen ears, previously cooked, may be stirred in, as an equivalent. Either plan is excellent.

*Remarks.*—Lamb, veal, beef, or young pork ribs, or other lean parts, make a healthful, cheap, easily digested, and a very satisfactory dinner at any season of the year.

**Value of Sweet Herbs for Stews, etc.**—If the people generally knew how much nicer stews are with these herbs, parsley and thyme especially, for flavoring soups and stews, it seems to the author they would raise them for this purpose, as much as sage and summer savory are for sausages and roasts; and as pennyroyal should be, as an herb drink to promote perspiration, break up colds, etc. (See Seasoning Food, etc., after dishes.)

**Irish Stew.**—Mutton cutlets, or chops, 2 lbs.; potatoes, 4 lbs., or enough for the family; 1 onion; pepper and salt. DIRECTIONS—Cut the chops into small pieces, cracking the bones, if any; peel and slice the potatoes; shred, or chop the onion finely; butter the bottom of a stew pan, and place a layer of the sliced potatoes over the bottom, with a proper proportion of the onion upon them, and season each layer with salt, and a very little pepper; then a layer of the chops, etc., until all are in; then put on 1 pt. of cold water, cover the pan and simmer 2 hours, or until done. Serve hot, and keep hot as long as dinner lasts, by keeping the tureen covered.

*Remarks.*—Notwithstanding this is called an Irish stew, if it is done nicely it is quite good enough for an American. It is a very popular dish at hotels and boarding houses, and any kind of cold meats, not too fat, may be utilized in this way, remembering that if made of cooked meats, only about half the time will be required, enough only to cook the potatoes.

**Irish Stew from Left-Over Steak and Potatoes.**—Cut the left-over steak and potatoes into squares of half an inch. Stew the steak in a covered stew-pan until very tender; cut an onion, and add the potatoes with a little of the left-over gravy from the steak; season with pepper, and a little salt if needed, thyme and summer savory.

*Remarks.*—Be certain to have just enough juices of the stew left, as a gravy, *i. e.*, do not cook it too dry, and it will be fit for a king. At least, the author first found a dish of it good enough for him, seasoned as above, at Florence, Kan. Try it if you like a good thing, and can get the thyme and savory. The only fault I ever found, or heard about it, was "I want a little more of that stew."

**Potato Stew.**—For a potato stew, lay 3 slices of salt pork—fat and lean—in the bottom of your stew kettle. Let it fry. If there is too much fat pour off a part. Slice an onion and fry with the pork. When it browns put in the potatoes sliced, not too thin, and hot water, not quite enough to cover. When nearly done, set on top of the stove to simmer. Add pepper, butter, and a cupful of sweet cream. Milk thickened with flour can be used in place of cream.

**Parsnip Stew.**—Salt pork, ½ lb., cut in slices; beef or veal, 1 lb., in small pieces; stew in a saucepan with suitable amount of water. Scrape the parsnips, wash and cut into slices; also ½ dozen medium-sized potatoes, in halves. Put all into the pan or pot together, cover closely for half an hour, or till all are tender; then add a small bit of butter, and pepper pretty freely, dredge in a little flour, and a few minutes more is needed to cook the flour into a gravy, and serve hot. (See also Parsnips Stewed in Milk, among the Vegetable Dishes.)

**Escaloped Parsnips.**—Mash 1 pt. of boiled parsnips. Add 2 table-spoonfuls of butter, 1 tea-spoonful of salt, a little pepper, 2 table-spoonfuls of cream or milk. Mix the ingredients. Stir on the fire until the mixture bubbles. Turn into a buttered dish, cover with crumbs, dot with butter, and brown in the oven.

*Remarks.*—This gives us a new way of cooking parsnips, as well as a very nice dish.

**Venetian Stew.**—Take 1 table-spoonful each of chopped onion, parsley, flour, and Parmesian cheese (cheese made in Parma, Italy, but the author thinks any good old American cheese will do just as well, at least good enough for Americans); a little salt, pepper, and ground mace; spread between some thin slices of veal; leave for some hours; then stew in rich broth with a goodly amount of butter.

*Remarks.*—If the veal had been boiled the day before in a small amount of water, it will be nice for the broth. We should not be complete in the line of stews, if we did not introduce an oyster stew, and as we have Delmonico's, together with his manner of frying and baking, we will put them all in this con. nection as follows:

### Oyster Stew, Fried and Escaloped, According to Delmonico.

—Oysters sufficient, and their liquor; rolled crackers, salt, pepper, and milk. DIRECTIONS—Put the liquor in a stew-pan (a tea-cupful for 3), and add half as much water, salt, a good bit of pepper, and a tea-spoonful of rolledcrackers to each person. Put on the stove and bring to a boil. Have your oysters in a bowl, and the moment the liquor boils pour in all your oysters, say 10 to each person, or six will do. Watch carefully, and as it boils, take out your watch, or count 30, and take your oysters from the stove. Have a big dish ready with 1½ table-spoonfuls of milk for each person. Pour the stew upon this milk and serve immediately. Never boil oysters in milk if you wish them good.

### Oysters, To Fry.

—Oysters sufficient, nice light crackers, eggs, salt, pepper, and cornmeal. DIRECTIONS—Roll the crackers, and mix a little salt and pepper into them; beat the eggs; then first dip the drained oysters into the cracker crumbs, then into the egg, and then into the cornmeal, having sufficient butter pretty hot in a frying pan, put them in as quickly as you can; then, as soon as the first side is nicely browned, turn them carefully, and serve hot. If any of the cracker and egg is left, mix them together, fry, and serve with the oysters. Parsley is a nice relish with them.

### Oysters, Escaloped.

— Oysters, nice crackers, salt and pepper (and, if you desire, a little pulverized mace and cloves), butter, milk with the cream stirred in, else a beaten egg or two may supply the place of the cream. DIREC-TIONS—Roll or pound the crackers finely; apply butter freely to the bottom of the pan in which they are to be baked; then cover it well with oysters and sprinkle them with salt and whatever seasoning you use; then a good layer of crackers, over which put pretty freely small pieces of butter, and wet slightly with the juice of the oysters, which has been mixed with the milk and cream, or egg. So fill the dish, the last layer being cracker, and double the thickness of the others, upon which put more butter and sufficient of the wetting mixture to well moisten. If the dish is deep it will require about 40 minutes to bake sufficiently; and if the dish is covered while baking remove it a few minutes before done to allow the top to be nicely browned.—*"S. E. N."* in *Country Gentleman*.

*Remarks.*—To good judges, it is not necessary to say that this will be very nice, even if a glass of wine is not added to the wetting mixture, as in the original. Some prefer it with, and many, I think, without; each can suit him selves. It is well known that Delmonico led the "ton" in the city of New York for a great many years; and there are so many points—20 different—in the plans of cooking these dishes, as prepared at his restaurant, it will pay for all who like nice digest to heed well these instructions, as I have not a doubt of their origination with him, or, rather, his French cook. To follow them is to ensure success, as the author has tested the stew many times, and the others enough to know their superiority over the old way. The four following recipes for cooking oysters, and the corn oysters, are from the Toledo *Post*, and will be found very nice.

**Chicken Oyster Pie.**—Cut the chicken in suitable pieces for fricassee, and prepare it as for that dish. Line a deep pie dish with a rich crust, and put in a layer of chicken with its gravy, and a layer of raw oysters; sprinkle the latter with salt, pepper and bits of butter. Proceed thus till the dish is full, and cover with a crust of pastry. Bake from $\frac{1}{3}$ to $\frac{3}{4}$ of an hour. Serve with gravy, made with equal parts of chicken gravy and the oyster juice, thickened with flour and seasoned with salt and pepper.

**Oyster Flitters.**—Drain the liquor from the oysters, and to 1 tea-cupful add the same quantity of milk, 3 eggs, pinch of salt, and flour enough for a thin batter. Chop the oysters and stir them in the butter, and fry in half butter and lard rather hot, and send quickly to the table.

**Oyster Omelet.**—Twelve large oysters, 6 eggs, 1 cup of milk, 1 tea-spoonful of butter, salt and pepper, and parsley, if agreeable; chop the oysters. Beat the whites and yolks of the eggs separately, as for cake. Heat 3 table-spoonfuls of butter, pour the milk, yolks of eggs, oysters and seasoning in a dish and mix, and add the whites of eggs and 1 spoonful of melted butter, with as little stirring as possible, then cook to an appetizing brown, turning the omelet carefully.

**Broiled Oysters.**—Drain and wipe the oysters and dip them in melted butter; then broil them on an oiled griddle over a moderate fire. Season to taste.

**Corn Oysters.**—Take young sweet corn; cut from the cobs into a dish. To 1 pt. of corn add 1 well-beaten egg, small tea-cupful of flour, $\frac{1}{2}$ gill sweet cream, $\frac{1}{2}$ tea-spoonful of salt; mix it well. Fry like oysters by dropping into hot drippings or butter by spoonfuls about the size of an oyster.

**DUCKS—To Bake Wild or Tame, to Avoid their Naturally Strong Flavor.**—DIRECTIONS—After having prepared them for stuffing, first parboil them for 1 hour, having an onion cut into 2 or 3 pieces, according to its size; put a piece inside of each duck while parboiling, which removes their strong flavor; then stuff with bread-crumb dressing, in which half of a common-sized onion, chopped fine, has been added for each duck. Bake in a hot oven, leaving the oven door $\frac{1}{2}$ inch ajar to carry off the strong flavor which may be left. Baste often with water and butter kept on the stove for that purpose, as the water first put in is to be poured off, to get rid of the duck-oil, which at first comes out very freely and contains much of the rancid or strong flavor of the duck, which it is our design hereby to avoid. After this the water and butter may be put into the pan for basting and for the gravy. The object is to get rid of all the oil possible.

*Another Plan*—and some people like them better with wholly an onion dressing—is as follows: Peel and wash 4 medium-sized onions for each duck, slice them, and have some water in a saucepan, boiling as hard as may be, throw in the sliced onions (onions can be peeled and sliced under water without affecting the eyes), with a little salt, and boil for 1 minute only after they begin to boil, which removes the acrid oil, or strong taste of the onions; remove from the fire, pouring off the water and draining nicely (this should always be done in cooking onions, even as an onion stew in milk); chop the onions finely, and season with salt and pepper to taste and 1 tea-spoonful of powdered sage for each duck; stuff, and bake as above.

*Remarks.*—This instruction was obtained of a boarding-house keeper, who had many years experience besides. I have had them tried several times myself and will say that for me I prefer at least half the dressing to be bread-crumbs, although the onion dressing alone, prepared as above, is very fine. If bread is used, of course butter is also to be added in all cases. Remember this, also, that in baking ducks, or any other wild game or poultry, they should be basted every 5 to 10 minutes while baking, if you desire them to be tender and sweet. Have plenty of water in the pan, with quite a bit of butter, for the purpose, and for the gravy after the oil has been poured or dipped off.

**Ducks to Roast and Stuff With Potato Stuffing.**—The roasting to be the same as above; but for the stuffing, boil potatoes and mash them finely. Prepare 1 onion at least for each duck, as also above directed (by boiling 1 minute with a little salt and pouring off the water), then chopping fine and mixing with the potato sufficient for the number of ducks to be stuffed, seasoning with salt and pepper and a very little ($\frac{1}{2}$ tea-spoonful to a duck) of thyme, and when filled with this potato and onion mixture, roast as before directed; and as soon as the oil is got rid of, rub over with butter, dredge on a little flour, put in more hot water, and baste often. Put the giblets into the same pan, and when done chop fine, and put into the gravy.

**Duck and Oyster Croquettes, or Balls, to Fry.**—Stuff a young and tender duck with oyster dressing (4 to 6, chopped, for a duck), roast, basting well to keep moist and from burning. When cold remove the bones and chop finely, and mix with the dressing, season with cayenne (if tolerated, else black pepper) and salt. Moisten with catsup and a well beaten egg, and stiffen properly with more bread or cracker crumbs, if needed. Make into croquettes, or balls, and brown nicely in hot butter or drippings. Put a sprig or two of parsley, if you have it, with each one, in serving.

**Mock Duck, With Veal or Beefsteak.**—Take veal steak, or cutlets, from the round; or the round from a young tender beef, and remove the rings of bone. Make a dressing with bread crumbs or rolled cracker, seasoning with a little onion (to imitate duck dressing, proper), which is always used with duck, to help overcome their peculiar tastes, moistening with an egg; adding salt and pepper of course, and a little thyme if you have it. Spread this stuffing, good thickness, over each steak; then roll them as much into the shape of a duck as possible, tying with twine, to keep in place. Baste well, and frequently, while roasting, to prevent their drying up too much. If done nicely you have a nice dish. Of course, making a gravy as for duck. Beef is not generally quite as tender as veal, but is more tender than the general run of ducks.

**Codfish, to Boil.**—Codfish, as generally cooked for dinner, is left so salty that too much water is craved after eating it to be healthful. To avoid this, put to soak in plenty of water the first thing in the morning. It is said, "skin side up," but I think this makes but little, if any, difference. · When breakfast work is done, scale and clean well. Put to soak again in a warm place. About 20 minutes before dinner time, put the whole fish in a deep spider or shallow kettle with water enough to cover and boil gently for about 15 minutes, or until tender. Drain off dry and slip on a deep plate, spread thickly with butter, adding plenty of pepper, and pour over all a cupful of sweet cream, or not, as you choose. If to be prepared for breakfast, soak an hour, after supper, then scrape and clean, and soak over night. Otherwise the same. Remnants can be picked to pieces, and make a gravy with milk, or cream, for dinner, or supper; or be made into balls, as below. If codfish, or other salt fish are properly freshened, they are very healthful food.

*Remarks.*—The author is very fond of codfish when properly freshened, being laid on top of potatoes that are being boiled with their "jackets" on, then a gravy made of the water in which it was cooked, by adding butter and pepper only. This gives you the pure flavor of the fish.

**Codfish or Other Fish Balls.**—Codfish left over from dinner is just as nice for this purpose as to freshen it purposely. Remove all the bones and skin; picking it into fine pieces, or shreds (long fiber-like pieces.) Have twice as much bulk of nicely mashed potatoes as fish; making the potatoes rich with butter and milk, if you have it, as for the table, and a beaten egg or two, according to the amount being prepared; season with pepper (the author likes a sprinkle or two of cayenne in them); flour your hands and make into balls, or rather flat, more like biscuit, and fry in hot butter, or drippings, as you choose, turning carefully when the first side is nicely browned. Drain off any superfluous fat before sending to the table.

*Remarks.*—They may be made perfectly plain, simply fish and potatoes, and still be good; but the hotels pursue the above plan, some of them also adding some boiled or chopped onion to the mixture. Any large fresh fish, even, left over, may be made into balls for the next breakfast, in the same manner, using a little salt in the seasoning. They may be put into pork, which is about half fried, and so give a nicer flavor to the pork, and eaten together; especially nice in this way if you use potatoes a little more freely than used in making the fish balls.

**Codfish and Eggs.**—We have ham and eggs, why not codfish and eggs, as well? Properly soak and pick the fish to pieces, and to each cup of fish put in 2 eggs and beat well together, and drop from a spoon into hot butter, or half-and-half butter and lard, or drippings, and fry a nice brown on both sides.

*Remarks.*—If tried once, they will be again, and again, which is the best praise that can be given any dish.

**Baked Whitefish and Shad with Dressing.** — Clean, rinse and wipe dry with a napkin, a whitefish or any other good-sized fish, weighing 3 lbs. or more. Sprinkle salt and pepper inside and out; then fill with dressing, as for chicken or turkey, only having it pretty dry; sew up and lay on some sticks in the dripping-pan; put in water and butter, dredging the fish with flour before putting in; and, if you have it and like it, put a few thin slices of fat pork on the fish—if no pork, then rub well with butter. Bake 1½ hours, basting frequently to avoid burning. Shad will be done the same, garnishing with a few pieces of lemon, sprigs of celery, or with the lemon sauce below.

**Shad or Other Fish, To Fry.**—Dress nicely, cut in pieces, rinse and absorb the water with a napkin, or drain a few minutes; rub in salt and a little pepper, roll in flour or cornmeal, having fat from salt pork quite hot in the pan, lay in the fish, first the inside down; when browned nicely, turn, cooking rather slowly to avoid burning. Some persons are very fond of grated horseradish with fish. If not serve with potatoes plain, or the sauce given below.

**Broiled Mackerel.**—Put mackerel to soak immediately after dinner the day before they are wanted for breakfast. Always put the skin side up in the tub of water. Change the water at 3 or 4 o'clock, and at tea-time pour off and rinse; then just cover with milk, if you have it, till bed-time; then take out and hang up to dry till morning, when they will be dry enough to broil nicely, the same as beefsteak, which see. They may be fried, but are not so nice, if broiled without burning.

**Stuffed and Baked Fish.**—Take out the backbone of the fish, leaving the head and tail on. Chop fine 2 small onions, and fry them in a table-spoonful of butter then add sufficient soaked bread to fill the fish, the yolk of an egg, and season with salt, nutmeg and parsley chopped fine. Stuff the fish with the mixture; pour over the whole some melted butter, and bake. If the oven is very hot, lay over it a greased paper, taking it off to allow the ·fish to become a nice brown.

**Sauce for Baked Fish.**—If there is not gravy enough from the water and butter with which the basting has been done, add a little more hot water and butter, and the juice of a lemon, with a spoonful of browned flour rubbed smooth in cold water, bring to a boil and serve hot. If you have parsley, a little chopped, or a little chopped spearmint, will add relish.

**Sauce for Meats, Delmonico's.**—The following is Delmonico's favorite sauce: "Take an ounce of ham or bacon, cut it up in small pieces and fry in hot fat. Add an onion and carrot, cut up; thicken with flour, then add a pint or quart of broth, according to quantity desired. Season with pepper and salt, and any spice or herb that is relished (better though without the spice), and let it simmer for an hour, skim carefully and strain. A wine-glassful of any wine may be added if liked."

*Remarks.*—Cold roast or broiled beef or mutton may be cut into small squares, fried brown in butter, and then gently stewed in the sauce above described, and served as a stew.

**The Famous Rhode Island or St. James' Chowder for Six.**—The Providence *Journal* says that some of its readers will recall the late James Brown, whose social sayings have come down to the present, and shall not be gainsaid. The following is his recipe for a chowder very famous in his day, and not altogether forgotten in ours:

"Take 6 slices of good pickled pork (pig preferred), and fry them in the bottom of a good-sized dinner-pot, turning the slices until they are brown on both sides. Take out the slices of pork, leaving the drippings in the pot. Take 7 lbs. of tautaug (a favorite fish along the New England coast) dressed (leaving the heads on) or 10 lbs. of scup (tautaug to be preferred), and cut each in 3 pieces, unless small, when cut them in two. Place in the pot, on the drippings, as many pieces of fish as will fairly cover the bottom of the pot. Throw into the pot, on the fish, 3 handfuls of onions, peeled and sliced in thin slices. Do not be afraid of the onions! Put in over this salt and pepper to taste, as in other soups. Then lay on the six slices of pork, on the top of the pork the rest of the fish; cover this with 3 handfuls more of onions peeled and sliced. (9 or 10 onions in both layers will suffice, though more will not injure it.) More pepper and salt, to taste. Then pour into the pot water enough just to come fairly even with the whole, or partly cover the same. Put the cover on the pot, place it on the fire. Let it boil gently and slowly for 30 minutes. It is to boil 30 minutes, not merely to be on the fire 30 minutes, and at all events let it boil until the onion is done soft. Pour in at this point about a quart (a common bottle) of best cider or champagne, and a tumbler full of port wine, and at the same time add about 2 lbs. of sea biscuits.

"*Note.*—If, when the onion is done, you find there is not liquor enough in the pot, soak the sea-biscuit in water for a few moments before putting them in, I would recommend the practice generally.

"After the cider, wine and crackers are put in, there is no harm in stirring the whole with a long spoon, though it is not necessary. Then let the whole boil again (not merely be over the fire) for about 5 minutes, and the chowder is ready for the table. Before dishing up let the cook taste it and see whether it lacks pepper and salt, when, if it does, it is a good time to add either.

"*Note.*—Also, never boil a potato in chowder. If you want potatoes boil them in a separate pot, and serve in a separate dish."

**Chowder, the More Common, With Fish or Clams.** — Slice some fat salt pork quite thin; put a layer in a suitable pudding dish, and strew over it sliced, or chopped, onions, with plenty of pepper; then cut a haddock (a species of codfish, but smaller), fresh codfish, or any other firm fish, into steaks, or slices, and put on a layer; then a layer of slightly soaked crackers; then pork, fish and crackers, until the dish is properly filled; pour over a suitable amount (a pint or more) of water, and bake in an oven, or where you have heat at bottom and top (used to bake chowder in a pit of well heated stones, all around, under and over). Clam chowder is done the same, substituting clams for the fish.

**Egg Muffins.**—Heat a dripping pan with as many muffin rings on it as you desire. Butter them, and break an egg into each, put on a little salt, pepper, and a bit of butter to each, and put into the oven and brown nicely. Serve hot and you will find them nice, although not original with the author, nor does he know with whom they originated, although he knows them good—a new dish.

**Frogs, How to Cook.**—Somebody writes to the *Blade* how to cook frogs, and does it so nicely I will use his own words for it. He says: As pot-pies, stews and chowder they are a failure. The only legitimate way to cook a frog is to fry him brown in sweet table butter. As a preliminary he must be dipped in a batter of cracker dust, which should adhere closely when cooked, forming a dainty cracknel of a golden brown color, with a crisp tang to it when submitted to the teeth. The tender juices thus retained lose none of their delicate flavor, and the dainty morsel needs no condiments to give it an additional zest. Next to the pleasure of sitting on the borders of a frog-pond at eventide and listening to their sweet, melancholy ch-r-r-r-k is that of reviewing a plate heaped high with the mementoes of a finished feast—the bones of the "Frog that would a wooing go," and a goodly portion of his kindred.

*Remarks.*—Having eaten them done thusly, I can say try them every chance you can get. They are splendid.

**Roast Turkey, a Nice Way to Avoid Burning.**—Having dressed him carefully, rub the inside well with salt, and hang up to drain an hour; then wipe dry with a napkin the crop and inside just as your dressing is ready to be put in; fill the place of the crop with the dressing and sew up, then the body and sew also. The dressing may be simply fine bread crumbs, seasoned with salt and pepper and a little butter, moistened with water or milk and a beaten egg, and you may add sage, onions, oysters, raisins, etc., any or all of them; or sage, thyme or marjoram or summer savory, as you like, have on hand or can get; tie the legs to the body, so that they shall not sprawl by the heat. When ready for the oven, melt a little lard and spread it over a clean white cloth and lay over the turkey; then grease a paper the same way and lay over the cloth, and a piece of thick dry brown paper over all; put a cup of water in the pan, and roast the turkey without basting, as the greased cloth and papers will keep it moist and from burning. If the top paper scorches, replace it with another until the turkey is nearly done; then remove all covering for a few minutes to allow it to brown. Having stewed the giblets (heart, liver, gizzard, etc.) in a little water while the turkey was baking, chop them fine, and with water or broth in which they were stewed added to the gravy in the pan, thicken a little with browned or unbrowned flour, as you prefer, rubbed smooth in a little cold water, seasoning to taste; serve in a "boat" or bowl, as you have.

*Remarks.*—If a turkey, or other fowl or meats, are not covered in this way they must be basted often to prevent burning, and you must also be more careful for the first half hour or so not to have the oven as hot as you may if covered. One-and-a-half and two hours, according to the size of the turkey and the heat of the oven, would be required to bake them nicely. Some people stew and chop the giblets before hand and mix them into the dressing. Each can suit herself in this free country; and a good many also, as well as the author, like quite a sprinkling of cayenne pepper in the dressing, as it seems to remove a peculiar fresh smell coming from the inside of the turkey.

**Turkey, to Boil and to Fry, as in England.**— *To Boil.*—In England turkeys are as often, if not more often, boiled than roasted, and eaten with a sauce called "Golden Rain." Truss (tie the legs and wings firmly) as, for roasting, to prevent their sprawling out by the heat, Have a kettle or boiler large enough to hold water to fully cover the turkey, in which there has been put a carrot, an onion, and a bunch of sweet herbs (if you are to do as the English do), the water being boiling. Put in the turkey, breast down. After it has boiled a minute or two, briskly, move back the boiler to simmer gently from 1 to 2 hours, according to size of the turkey.

*The Sauce, or Golden Rain.*—Boil 3 eggs 10 minutes, and when cold throw the whites and two of the yolks into cold water to keep their color. Melt butter, 1 table-spoonful, in a saucepan; then remove from the fire and stir in a spoonful of flour (about 1 oz.); stir, or beat with a wooden spoon, till smooth; put over the fire again and add ½ pt. of milk and stir till it thickens, adding now a gill of cream, cutting the whites and the yolks of the eggs in the water into dice; stir in, but do not break up the dice by too hard stirring, which would spoil the golden as well as the white rain; bring to a boil after putting in the egg-dice. Take up the turkey in time to drain nicely; then rub the yolk of the other egg over the breast and in spots over the rest of the turkey, or rub it through a sieve, thus in spots, to make it more golden. Pour the same upon it, or serve it in a "boat" or bowl, as preferred.

**Turkey, To Fry.**—Not every one, however, knows how to fry turkey Cut in neat pieces the remains of the turkey, make a batter of beaten eggs and fine bread crumbs, seasoned with pepper, salt, and pounded mace or nutmeg, add a few sprigs of parsley; dip the pieces into this and fry them a light brown. Take a good gravy, thickened with flour and butter, and flavored with mushroom or other catsup, and pour over them. Serve with sippets and sliced lemon. Few breakfast dishes are more delicious.—*Confectioner.*

**Turkey and Other Poultry Hash or Breakfast Dish.**— Cold fowl of any kind may be turned into a hot breakfast dish as follows: Chop the the meat very fine; put ½ a pt. gravy into a stew-pan with a little piece of butter rolled in flour, a tea-spoonful of catsup, some pepper and salt, the juice and peel of half a lemon shred very fine, if you like it; put in the turkey or chicken, and shake it over a clear fire until it is thoroughly hot. The above proportions are calculated for one cold turkey. It may be served with two or more poached eggs. If there are not enough eggs to allow one for each guest, they should be broken with the spoon and mixed with the hash just before serving. It should be served piping hot.

**Italian Cheese, or to Prepare Veal, Chicken, Turkey, etc., for Picnics.**—Take a 4 or 5 lb. piece of veal, boil it perfectly tender, then remove all the bones, and chop the meat fine; add a grated nutmeg, as much cloves, allspice, pepper and salt to suit; strain the liquor in which it was boiled, and mix all together, put over the fire and simmer till the liquor, on cooling a little of it, will jelly; then put in molds or bowls till the next day, when it may be sliced for sandwiches for the picnic or for company tea. Chicken or turkey may be done in the same way. If you like, you can line the molds, or bowls, with hard-boiled eggs, sliced, which adds to its appearance as well as its richness.

**Chicken Fricasseed, Upon Toast and Without.**—Cut up a chicken and put on to boil in a small quantity of water. Add a seasoning of salt and pepper, and onion if you like. Stew slowly (covered) until tender; then add rich milk, ½ pt. (cream is all the better), with a little butter; and if you have parsley, add a little of it chopped, just as ready to serve. Have the bread, which has been cut thin, nicely toasted and lightly buttered, arranged on a platter; then pour over the fricassee, and serve at once. Without the toast, it is the common fricassee.

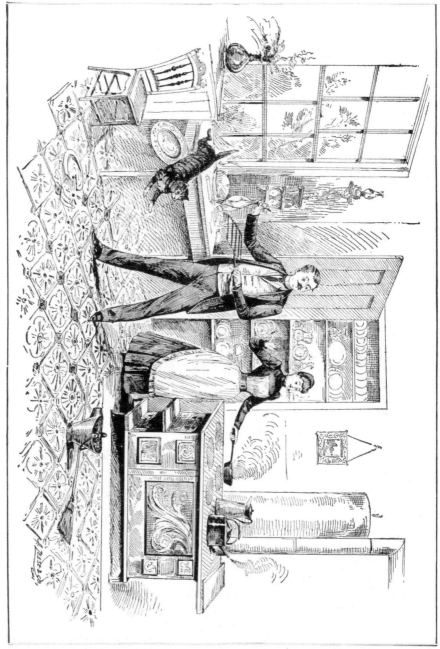

PATIENT HUSBAND.

"Well, our daughter must be taught how to cook if you were not."

*Remarks.*—A young turkey, or a nicely dressed rabbit, treated in every way the same as the chicken, will also make a nice fricassee. But our chicken dishes would hardly be complete without a chicken currie, and perhaps, also, chicken with green peas, both of which I have obtained from a book entitled "Indian Domestic Economy and Cookery," which I borrowed from a Mrs. Bronson, whose husband, Dr. Bronson, had spent over 40 years in India, as a missionary, but whose age and debility required him to return home, and he was then (1881) living at Eaton Rapids, Mich. Dr. Bronson was very anxious, if his health would allow, to return to his work; but being about 70 years old, I told him I thought he had done all that duty required of him in that far off country, and I doubted much if his health would ever allow his return. This lady was his third wife, a faithful and true helpmate in his work. I received several items of information from her in relation to the Indian customs, in cooking, etc., which helped me to understand the work above mentioned, much better than I otherwise would, their ways are so different from ours. These items I shall mention in the different places where needed, in the recipes I shall give from this work. They were married in India, where she had lived several years before their marriage. The book was printed in Madras, in 1853, at the "Christian Knowledge Society Press," and the copy she brought with her showed signs of having been much used. My acquaintance with her was, as some say, purely accidental, others, providential. I was standing in the door of the Frost House, Eaton Rapids, where I was stopping for the benefit of the mineral springs and rest, when Mrs. Bronson, in passing with a baby carriage, having twin babies in it, stopped to talk a few moments with the landlady, who, with some other ladies, were also standing about, when one of them knowing that Mrs. B. had recently come from India, asked her where the children were born, to which the answer was: "In Assam," when I at once became interested (as I had a cousin in that province of India), to know if they had met; when, on learning his name (Mason) they had been neighbors and co-workers for some years; hence my acquaintance with Mrs. B. and her husband, and I thus obtained access to the book from which I take the next recipe, and a few others which are credited as above indicated.

My cousin had then been in Assam about seven years, in the mission work. His health, and that of his wife, having already begun to fail considerably, so that during the following year (1882) he had to come home, more especially, however, on his wife's account, whose health continued to fail very fast, and although she seemed to recruit a little on her first arrival, or soon after, yet her health had been so undermined by her stay in India, she died within a few months after reaching her friends in America. But, notwithstanding the lives of American women who go out as missionaries, are short in India, yet they generally are so devoted to their work, or to their husbands, they seldom make any complaint—they give themselves, and their lives, cheerfully, for the Master's cause. Let none fail, therefore, to do their duty, although it should call them to India.

**Chicken Currie, With Rice, as Made in India.**—Cut the chicken into as many joints as possible. Take 1 onion and slice it finely and fry in a table-spoonful or more of *ghee* (the word used in India for butter, but drippings, or even lard, my informant, Mrs. Bronson, says is often used), sprinkling over the onion, 1 tea-spoonful of currie powder (which see). When the onion is nicely browned put in the jointed chicken, and salt sufficient, and put on a tea-spoonful more of the currie powder, and fry until nicely browned; then pour on sufficient hot water (see in remarks that milk, or the milk of cocoanuts may be used) to cover the chicken, and stew (covered) until perfectly tender. [Some of the native cooks boil the chicken tender before frying in the currie, but my informant says this is not the best way.] Serve with plain boiled rice, either in separate dishes, or, preferably, put the boiled rice on the platter, pushing it out around the edge, then pour the currie into the middle, the whiteness of the rice making fine contrast with the browned currie.—*Indian Domestic Economy and Cookery.*

*Remarks.*—Young mutton, lamb, veal, and fish, when cut into suitable pieces, Mrs. Bronson informs me, treated every way the same as chicken, makes an equally nice currie, and are more frequently used as such in India than chicken; but we Americans think there is nothing equal to chicken. This lady gives me the plan of cooking the rice in India, and the use of the water in which it is cooked, as follows:

**To Boil the Rice India Fashion.**—Wash it through 3 or 4 waters. Have plenty of boiling water in a large kettle, put in the rice and boil very briskly until tender; then pour in a cup of cold water, and pour into a colander; when well drained, return to the kettle to steam a short time to dry out the surplus water; then serve on the platter, or separate dish, as above.

The rice water poured off is, says this lady, the best kind of starch, and is used for that purpose by the washermen—men in India doing the washing wholly. What a blessed thing it would be for some of the over-worked women of our country if their husbands had to do the washing, instead of spending their time, and often the money their wives have earned by washing, for whiskey! How long shall it continue?

**The Milk of Cocoanuts** is often used in India, says our informant, and I think it would be very nice here, as well as there, instead of the water or milk in which, or with which, to cook the currie, whether it be chicken, veal, lamb, or fish; and they also scrape out the meat of the nut, having a tool for that purpose much like a scraper to remove letters from a box or barrel by shippers, except that the edge is rounding to fit the inside of the nut, and has sharp teeth like a saw, which makes the pulp fine and fit to mix into the gravy of the currie. Such a tool could be very easily made by an American blacksmith, taking him a cocoanut that he might get the shape for the toothed edge and knowing what it was to be used for.

At a subsequent time, while in Eaton Rapids, I was invited to take tea with Dr. Bronson, that I might partake of a currie prepared as above, by his wife and an Indian gentleman, who had been several years in the University at Ann Arbor, qualifying himself as a physician to go back to his country for the good of his countrymen. He understood Indian cookery, and between them they made a most excellent currie; and although it was pretty warm—I might say hot—with the currie powder, yet I liked it very much, and should be glad to have a chance to eat of one every day in the week if not at every meal. It warmed up my stomach nicely, and it is said to be a cure of dyspepsia. If found too hot on the first trial to suit any one, use less currie powder next time, and you can soon work to suit the taste of any family. I believe it to be healthful, and they suit my taste exactly.

**Chicken in Peas, as Cooked in India.**—Cut the chicken into joints, as for a fricassee or currie, and put into a sauce-pan with about a quart of young shelled peas, a spoonful or two of *ghee* (butter), a small sliced onion, and a nice sprig or two of parsley, and moisten more with drippings if thought best; put on the fire, dusting with a little flour, and stew (covered) until done; and add a little salt, and a little sugar, if relished, just before serving.—*Indian Domestic Economy and Cookery.*

*Remarks.*—Their plan of making a fricassee is so much like ours above, I need not give it.

**Young Chickens, Nice Way to Cook.**—Dress and joint them as usual; place in a dripping-pan and just cover with sweet cream, season with a little salt, pepper, and a little butter; and now set in the oven to cook, and by the time the cream is almost cooked away the chicken will be done. They are splendid done in this way.—*Mrs. Wetsel, Harverville, Kan.*

*Remarks.*—That is just what the author says: "They are splendid done in this way." I should like to pick such a leg, or two, every day. Have just cream enough left to put over the mashed potatoes as a gravy.

**Chicken Relish, for Journeys, Picnics, or for Company.**—Dress as many as the occasion will require, joint and boil tender in as little water as possible, salting nicely just before they are done; take up and remove the skin. Remove all the meat from the bones; break the bones and boil them and the skin a little while longer in the water; then strain it to have ready to moisten with. Place a layer of dark meat, then a layer of white in a bowl, seasoning with pepper and a little additional salt to each layer as put in, and moisten with the juices or water in which they were cooked, and put on weights till cold, when, with a very sharp butcher-knife, it may be cut in slices for the picnic, journey, or the tea-table when company is present—too much labor for common, as they are good enough for general use without so much labor. Chicken meat is so tender and soft it is very difficult to chop it, hence we do not advise it, unless the chopping-knife is sharper than they are usually found.

**Roast Pigeons and Bread Sauce for Same.**—Dress, wash and wipe dry, *i, e*, absorb all the water you can with a napkin or towel, unless you have plenty of time to drain them dry. Truss them, secure the wings and legs to the body by skewers or twine; mix salt and pepper together and rub them well on the inside, and also put a piece of butter into each, the size of a large shell-bark hickory nut. Lay upon sticks in the dripping-pan, put in hot water and butter to baste with, and put into a quick oven, covering with brown paper, if needed, to prevent burning. If the oven is hot enough, 30 to 45 minutes will do them nicely, if basted often enough.

*Bread Sauce for Same, and for all Poultry, Meats, etc.*—Milk, ½ pt. to 1 pt., according to the amount needed; fine bread crumbs, 1 cup; an onion, small or large, whether you use ½ or 1 pt. of milk; butter, 1 to 2 table-spoonfuls, as you take it out of the lump not melted; salt, pepper, mace, and parsley, if you have them and like them. DIRECTIONS—First boil the sliced onion 1 minute in water, then pour that off and put in the milk and cook it well; then put in your bread crumbs; or, if you wish to be very nice, strain out the onion; put in seasoning with the butter, and let the bread crumbs have time to soften; stir well, and bring to a boil, adding boiling milk or boiling water if too thick.

*Remarks.*—The drippings from the pigeons or other poultry may be put in in place of the milk or water. The onion, of course may be left out, if not relished, and any other flavor substituted, as summer savory, thyme, marjoram, lemon peel and juice, etc., or nothing, so as to suit everybody.

But now I have an animal to introduce, the name of which I am so unfamiliar with I hardly know where to place him, whether among the meat-producing beasts, or the family of fowls; still, I know so many will like to try a few of his "rare-bits," I will give him a place among the choicest recipes I have in the nature of dishes. But as he is taken partly from the beast and partly from the fowls, we will call him the

**1. GOLDEN BUCK, OR WELSH RAREBIT—English Style.** —A golden buck is, in other words, simply a Welsh rarebit, with a poached egg on his back. I will first give the true one, as directed by Warne's (English) Model Cookery: Time, 10 minutes; ½ lb. of cheese; 3 table-spoonfuls of ale; a thin slice of toast. Grate the cheese fine, put to it the ale, and work in a small saucepan over a slow fire, until it is melted. Spread it on the toast, and send it up boiling hot. Now for the "buck" part of it:

**2.** Take fresh, but rather rich cheese and cut into small even-sized pieces, the amount to be regulated by the number of rarebits needed, and melt upon a rather slow fire. If the cheese be dry, add a small quantity of butter. A little—say a wine-glass full to each rarebit—sour ale; or, in its absence, fresh ale, should be added as the cheese melts. After the cheese is thoroughly melted and the above ingredients stirred in, add a small quantity of celery salt, and immediately pour upon a piece of toast previously placed upon a hot plate. By placing a poached egg upon this it immediately becomes a golden buck. The further addition of a slice of broiled bacon renders it a Yorkshire buck.— *New York Review.*

*Remarks.*—For those with good digestion either of the "bucks" will be found nice. For me, I should prefer not to have the ale sour, but fresh, and nice, so I think, would most others. I will give a few more recipes for a plainer, or more Americanized way of making the Welsh rarebit (generally called rabbit), which will be less troublesome to make, and also more easily digested. A young, but experienced housekeeper, of Brinton, Pa., gives the following:

**Welsh Rarebit.**—Chop fine, with a knife, pieces of dry cheese (sharp cheese is best), and to 1 pt. of this allow 1 pt. of milk. Have the milk boiling hot and stir into it the cheese, stirring all the time until it becomes pretty well dissolved, then add a beaten egg, a little salt, and when it has all come to a boil your rarebit is done. Some persons prefer browning in the oven before sending to the table, but it is best eaten as soon as cooked, as the cheese is apt to separate from the milk if allowed to stand long after it is ready.

**Welsh Rarebit, Plain.**—Rich, crumbly cheese, ½ lb.; butter, 1 table-spoonful; rich milk, 1 gill; toast. DIRECTIONS—Put the milk and butter into a frying pan, and crumble in the cheese upon the stove, constantly stirring until all is dissolved together; then pour upon thick toast that has been dipped, quickly, in and out, of boiling milk; served hot it is a rare dish for a healthy stomach. And for a healthy man a poached egg may be put upon each piece of toast, as served, which will make it a second cousin, at least, to the golden buck, given above.

**Welsh Rarebit, Excellent.**—Fresh cheese, the size of a tea-cup; a large cup of sweet milk; a table-spoonful of butter; a pinch of dry mustard; a little red (cayenne) pepper; 2 soda crackers; 1 egg. DIRECTIONS—Roll the crackers; beat the egg; cut the cheese in thin, small slices; place them in the frying pan with the milk; add beaten egg, butter, mustard and pepper; stir in the rolled cracker gradually. As soon as all is thoroughly mixed turn the mixture out, and send to the table in a covered dish. To be eaten with dry toast.

**Welsh Rarebit, Delicious.**—The New York *Post* says that Welsh rarebit is delicious when made after this rule: Half a pound of cheese, 3 eggs, 1 small cup of bread crumbs, 2 table-spoonfuls of melted butter, mustard and salt to taste. After beating the cheese in an earthen dish add the other ingredients, then spread on the top of slices of bread, toasted or not, as you choose, and set in the oven to melt.

*Remarks.*—I will close with one which is more particular in its quantities, and also has a caution or two in the use of seasoning, avoiding skim milk cheese, etc.; and although it recommends the Parmesan cheese, yet, I will say, our good, rich, new milk cheese, having some age, will be found nice enough for all common purposes. If a very nice dish is desired, get the Parmesan, as mentioned below. It is as follows:

**Welsh Rarebit With Parmesan Cheese.**—Boil ½ pt. of milk; have the cheese rich enough to melt; chop ½ tea-cupful of it to every ½ pt. of milk; the yolk of 1 egg is lightly beaten with a fork, and have it ready when the cheese is melted; turn the cheese into the boiling milk and stir until the former dissolves. Welsh rarebit cannot be made from skim milk cheese. Parmesan cheese makes delightful dishes, but is expensive. Stir in the yolk of the egg, adding salt and pepper, and serve on toast or alone. Cheese dishes require little seasoning, and the salt and pepper should be used sparingly.

*Remarks.*—This Parmesan cheese is made in Parma, Italy, but I think our best American cheese is all that need be required, but each must please herself—you certainly have the opportunity of choosing, from the variety given; but, as it is the man who furnishes the largest number of the best recipes, for any given department, who makes the best receipt book, the author, in keeping with his "First and Second Receipt Books,' has endeavored, and he thinks, succeeded, in making his "Third and Last," the best even of his own writing; and far better than any with which he is acquainted, by any other author.

**Minced Veal, With Poached Eggs.**—Mince cold roast, boiled or broiled veal quite finely; fry a chopped shallot (a small bulbous plant much like a garlic, but if as strong as a garlic the author would prefer a small onion in its place) in plenty of butter; when it is a light straw-color, add a large pinch of flour and a little stock; then the mince meat, with chopped parsley, pepper, salt and nutmeg to taste; mix well; add more stock, if necessary, and let the mince gradually get hot by the side of the fire. When quite hot, stir into it, off the fire, the yolk of an egg and the juice of a lemon, to be strained and beaten up together. Serve with sippets of bread, fried in butter, round it, and 3 or 4 poached eggs on top.

*Remarks.*—The sippets of bread are first dipped into milk, or a beaten egg, before frying; and bread is a very nice thing thus fried for a breakfast dish, with fried meats of any kind, whether eggs are used or not.

**Escaloped Veal.**—Chop cold cooked veal fine, put a layer in a baking-dish, alternating with a layer of powdered crackers, salt, pepper and butter, until you fill the dish. Beat up 2 eggs, add a pint of milk, pour it over the veal and crackers. Cover with a plate and place in the oven until nicely heated through, then remove the plate to brown it nicely before serving.

Oysters may be treated the same way, baking longer to cook them through; the same of chicken or any other cold meats that are very tender; all make a nice dish if properly done. So, also, veal in the following manner:

**Jellied Veal.**—Wash a knuckle of veal and cut it into pieces. Boil it slowly until the meat will slip easily from the bones. Take it out of the liquor, remove the bones, and chop the meat fine. Season with salt and pepper, spices, and sweet herbs. Put back into the liquor and boil until almost dry. Turn into a mold and let it remain until next day. The juice of a lemon stirred in just before taken from the fire improves it. Garnish with parsley and thin slices of lemon, if you have them and like them.—*Buffalo (N. Y.) Express.*

**Curried Veal or Chicken.**—Nice veal cutlets, 2 lbs., or a good plump but tender chicken will require about 2 cups of milk, 1½ cups of pounded crackers, 1 egg, butter the size of an egg, salt, dry toast, and 1 tea-spoonful, more or less, as you like it hot or not, of the cayenne and other spices in the currie powder. DIRECTIONS—Chop veal or chicken (cold from previous boiling) finely, put the milk on the fire, with the cracker-crumbs, salt and curried powder, and as soon as it boils up add the meat, and when the meat is hot the egg and butter. Serve hot on the dry buttered toast.

*Remarks.*—This will be found remarkably fine for lovers of currie; and it will be fine also simply to cut the veal or chicken in pieces suitable for frying, then season the same, using the milk or not; if used, seasoning it as before and stewing in it for a time, then finishing by frying in the butter and using the milk as a gravy for potatoes, etc. I am very fond of the curried chicken; the veal I have not tried, but know I should like it for the curries' sake.

*Gravy or Sauce for Veal or Chicken.*—Put a table-spoonful of butter into a hot frying-pan. When it begins to brown dust a table-spoonful of flour into it, stirring constantly with a spoon; add salt and pepper; then stir in 1 pint of milk—cream, if you have it—let it boil 5 minutes, and it will be ready to pour over these fried meats, or to serve with roasts. Some people think that a little stewed tomatoes in the gravy for roast or fried meats is an improvement. The author prefers them without it.

EGGS—How to Boil for Health.—The objection to the common way of boiling eggs is this: The white under three minutes rapid cooking becomes tough and indigestible, while the yolk is left soft. When properly cooked eggs are done evenly through like any food. This result may be attained by putting the eggs into a dish with a cover, and then pouring upon them boiling water, 2 quarts or more to a dozen eggs, in a covered tin pail, and set them away from the stove for 15 minutes. The heat of the water cooks the eggs slowly and evenly and sufficiently, and to a jelly-like consistency, leaving the center or yolk harder than the white, and the egg tastes as much richer and nicer as a fresh egg is nicer than a stale egg, and no person will want to eat them boiled after trying this method.

*Remarks.*—I have tried this writer's instructions, although I do not know who he was, and find him correct for my taste, and I think it the true way to boil eggs, and mostly of general adoption. I will also add an item from a writer in a medical journal upon the healthfulness of hard-boiled eggs in dyspepsia, hoping and believing that it is a true account of what they have done, although the writer's name is not given, nor the place the journal was published. The writer says:

Healthfulness of Hard-Boiled Eggs in Dyspepsia.—"We have seen dyspeptics who have suffered untold torments with almost every kind of food. No liquid could be taken without suffering. Bread became a burning acid. Meat and milk were solid and liquid fires. We have seen those same sufferers trying to avoid food and drink, and even going to the enema syringe for sustenance. And we have seen their torments pass away, and their hunger relieved by living upon the white of eggs which had been boiled in bubbling water for 30 minutes. At the end of a week we have given the hard yolk of the egg with the white, and upon this diet alone without fluid of any kind we have seen them begin to gain flesh and strength and refreshing sleep. After weeks of this treatment they have been able with care to begin upon other food. And all this," the writer adds, "without taking medicine." He says that hard-boiled eggs are not so bad as half-boiled ones, and ten times as easy to digest as raw eggs, even in egg-nog.

*Remarks.*—See the remarks just above, and let none who are suffering in a similar manner fail to give this a faithful trial. See, also, "Voltaire's Food for Dyspeptics" in this work.

Remarkable Use of Long Boiled Eggs, for Typhoid Fever Patients.—After having written the two above items, I was speaking of them to a homeopathic physician of our city—Toledo, O.—June 19th, 1883, when he said : "I have given three eggs which had been boiled an hour, at one time, to a patient just recovering from typhoid fever, without the least distress or suffering, digesting well and improving the patient's strength, while those only boiled 15 minutes did give distress," etc. This to me was remarkable indeed ; but, nevertheless, I have not a doubt of its correctness. He claimed that, like cooking meats, 15 minutes only, "sets," or toughened the albumen (the white of an egg is pure albumen, much like that part of veal which will form jelly, by long boiling), and, hence, that no stomach could digest it ; while an hour's boiling cooked it done, as we say of boiling veal, or other, naturally young and tender meat, chickens, etc. The reasoning is good, and may be tried with safety, 1 egg, only at a time, at first, with weak typhoid, or other patients.

**Egg Gruel, Mulled Jelly, etc., for the Sick.**—Beat the yolk of 1 egg with a table-spoon of sugar till very light ; on this pour ⅔ of a cup of boiling water ; on the top put the white of the egg beaten to a stiff froth, with a tea spoon of powdered sugar ; flavor with something as unlike other flavors the invalid has had as you can give him. Mulled (to mull is to soften by heat, adding hot water, spices, etc. As Gay says : "Drink new cider, mulled with ginger warm" (it is not hard to take, even if not sick); jelly is another drink which may be taken with pleasure, *i. e.*, beat a table-spoon of red or black currant jelly with the white of an egg and a little sugar ; pour over this a small cup of boiling water ; break a cracker in it, or a thin slice of toasted bread.

*Remarks.*—This would properly belong with drinks for the sick, which see; but it had been placed with the other egg receipts, so I give it a place here.

**Eggs, Some of the More Common Ways of Cooking.— Poached.**—It is now well understood that to poach an egg is to break it into boiling water and to dip some of the water, with a spoon, upon it, or them, as the case may be, until cooked to suit; then lift with a skimmer, upon a plate, or upon slices of buttered toast, or into egg cups, in which a bit of butter has just been put, and let each, otherwise, season to suit themselves.

**Eggs, Scrambled.**—Put a tin basin upon the stove, in which you have put a table-spoon of butter, for ½ doz. eggs; when the butter is melted, the eggs having been broken into a dish (to see each is good) put them in, and as soon as cooked upon the bottom a little, begin to stir, or lift them with a spoon from the bottom, till all has had its turn upon the bottom, and consequently done, or thickened to suit. Serve hot, generally, for Sunday's tea, with bread and butter.

**Egg Omelet.**—A French writer says the "secret of an omelet is the know how !"—I wonder if that is not the secret of doing anything well? He then gives us the Bordeaux, or French fashion, which is good. He says: "Tilt the pan, to allow the eggs to run to the lower side, and scrape down from the upper half perfectly clean, pushing all the egg to the lower half. Pepper and salt. When set, turn over back on to the clean half of the pan, brown and serve. But if you do not put a table-spoonful of cold water to each egg in making an omelet, it will be leathery (tough). If you put milk or flour it is not an omelet, but a pancake. To take up, take hold of the pan with the palm uppermost, place your plate over the pan and turn it quickly."

*Remarks.*—Most people have been in the habit of using milk, or flour, or both, while the Frenchman's plan leaves them tender and digestible.

**Egg Omelet with Green Corn or Bread Crumbs.**—Boil 1 dozen ears of nice corn 25 minutes, split the rows lengthwise with a sharp knife, then with a dull knife press out and scrape easily, to leave the hull as much on the cob as possible; add to this pulp 5 well-beaten eggs, season to taste, and fry to a nice brown in a little butter, turning over as a whole, or as the Frenchman above, on a clean half of the pan. In the absence of green corn, 1½ cups of bread crumbs will make a good omelet.

*Remarks.*—Omelets should be served at once when done, as they fall if they stand after being dished up.

**Egg Omelet with Oysters.**—An egg omelet with oysters may be a new dish to some cooks, but I can assure them that it will be a favorite, if the family like oysters. Stew a dozen oysters in their own liquor, if possible, if not, use a very little water; roll 2 or 3 lumps of butter the size of butternuts in flour, and put in and let it come to a boil; salt it well, and add black or cayenne pepper to suit your taste. Take out the oysters and chop them, and, if necessary to make them thick, add a little flour; then put the oysters in again and set the saucepan in which they are back on the stove while the eggs are being fried. Beat 6 to 10 eggs until very light, and add to them 2 table-spoonfuls of cream or rich milk; fry in a well-buttered frying-pan. When done remove to a hot platter or deep plate and pour the oyster sauce over it. Serve while hot.—*New York Evening Post.*

**Eggs-in-the-Nest—A Nice Dish for Breakfast or Tea.**—Beat to a froth the whites of 6 eggs; a little pepper and salt; pour into a buttered baking tin, dip upon it 6 table-spoonfuls of nice cream, 1 only in a place; upon each spoonful of cream drop 1 of the yolks whole (being careful not to break them); place in a moderately hot oven to cook, and serve hot, as omelet should be.

*Remarks.*—I am very sorry I can not give credit to the originator of this dish, as her name ought to have gone with it, as it will be found especially nice, if neatly done. Where I first saw it there was no name given.

I will now close the meat and egg dishes with directions how to take care of pigs' heads, sausage, etc.; then take up the vegetable question.

**Head-Cheese, Souse, etc.**—For the head-cheese, take the pigs' heads, feet, ears, etc., and after soaking and cleaning nicely, cut off the lower jaw (some cut this off first, as it is very nice cooked with cabbage); boil until the bones can be easily removed; then chop fine with onions, 1 or 2 for each head, add salt and pepper, and place in molds till cold. It is usual, however, when these are cooked, to make a meal off them, and chop up the balance for the head cheese, and some persons prefer to eat it all as sauce cold, rather than take the labor of chopping, seasoning, etc. Every one can please themselves. They should all be soaked over night in salt water before cleaning them.

*Remarks.*—My own choice is for an ear, or some other part having plenty of skin, but not much fat. I am a great lover, also, of sage or summer savory in seasoning any kind of fresh meats, in preference to any other of the "sweet herbs," as they are called.

**VEGETABLE DISHES—How to Cook.**—I will first take up the sweetest (?) vegetable we have—truly, however, one of the most healthful, if not the most healthful, of all our vegetables. It is very much used, but ought to be used more extensively than it is in every family in the land. I refer to the well-known

**Onion, How to Cook It with Milk or Cream, Avoiding the Strong Flavor.**—Peel, wash, and slice (under water to prevent affecting the eyes), 3 to 6, according to the size of the family, put into boiling water and boil 1 to 2 minutes, and drain off the water (which removes the acrid oil in which their peculiar sweet flavor resides); then pour over them a cup of scalding milk (cream is better still), in which a pinch of soda has been dissolved; put in a table-spoonful of butter, and cook till tender; pepper and salt, and stir ½ a tea-spoonful of corn starch or flour in a little cold milk and stir in, continuing to simmer a minute or two longer; then, if you have parsley, chop a little of it—½ dozen sprigs—and put in the last moment before dishing up, and if you don't say it is a sweeter and more palatable vegetable than you supposed, the author will be very much disappointed.

**RICE—Its Value and How to Cook It.**—Rice is being used much more, of late years, than formerly. It is very often substituted for potatoes, even at dinner, as it is much more nourishing, and more easily digested; and although it may cost a little more than potatoes generally, yet it is relatively cheaper than oatmeal, and other grain grits, and certainly more palatable. It should always be cooked in a rice kettle, (which see, described in a note following Tapioca Puddings; some people call them farina kettles, because equally valuable to cook farina, oatmeal, or any article liable to burn in an ordinary kettle. The rice, or farina, is put into an inside dish having a cover, and itself forming the cover of the outside one, which contains the water), which prevents any possibility of burning, on the same principle as a glue kettle. Only water enough is put upon the rice to moisten it nicely, which really steams it rather than boiling proper, in the usual, or large amount of water. If boiled in a common kettle, as formerly, 2 cups of water are required to every 1 cup of rice, with a little salt, in either case. When done, remove the cover, to allow the steam and water to escape—to dry it off, for a few minutes only, and the rice comes out a mass of snow white kernels, separate and distinct from each other; and as much superior to the soggy mass, of the old way, as a nice, dry and mealy potato is better than a water-soaked one. With the rice kettle to boil it in, 1 cup of water is enough for 1 cup of rice; and after it begins to boil, 20 minutes is the usual time. It should be taken out, poured into a deep dish or tureen (so it may be covered when steamed dry) and let it stand, uncovered, before the fire, in only a moderately warm oven, with the door open, a few minutes, to dry off the surplus water, sending to the table hot. To be eaten with butter and sugar, or these to be creamed together, half as much butter as sugar, if prefered. The Chinese, or East India cooks, you will see by referring to the remarks following Chicken Currie, boil their rice in a large amount of water, drain it off to use as starch, then put the rice back into the kettle and put over the fire again, to dry off the steam, or surplus water. See next recipe for the old way of cooking rice in the south, which is much the same as the India plan, above referred to. Using so much water to boil it in, then pouring it off, would seem to me, at least, to take away much of its nourishment; but still as they use this water in place of starch, like the India washerman, they may have the best of us after all, as the southern ladies are very much in favor of stiff dress skirts, judging by the rustle of those who staid this summer in the north. This is, probably, as cheap a way as they can get their starch, as they raise the rice in the south.

**Rice, Southern Mode of Cooking.**—Pick over the rice and wash it in cold water; to 1 pt. of rice put 3 qts. of boiling water and ½ tea-spoonful of salt; boil it just 17 minutes from the time it begins to boil; turn off all the water; set it over a moderate fire with the cover off, to steam 15 minutes. Take care and be accurate   The rice water first poured off is good to stiffen muslins.

**Rice Merange, Baked.**—Rice, 1 cup; milk, 1 qt.; 4 eggs; 2 lemons; powdered sugar, as below. DIRECTIONS—Boil the rice 10 or 15 minutes, in the milk in a rice kettle, or tin pail, as mentioned before, and pour into a buttered pudding dish; grate in the yellow of the lemons; add the yolks of the eggs, beaten slightly, with 5 table-spoonfuls of the sugar, and place in the oven to bake, ½ to ¾ of an hour. To make the merange, or meringue, beat the whites with 7 table-spoonfuls of sugar, and the juice of 1 lemon. Place this upon the top to brown nicely, just before serving. May be served with butter, 1 spoonful, to 2 of sugar, rubbed together; or cream sauce, as preferred. The juice of the other lemon will make a nice lemonade.

**Rice Muffins.**—To 1 qt. of sour milk 3 well beaten eggs, a little salt, 1 tea-spoonful of soda and enough of rice flour (or cold mashed rice) to thicken to a stiff batter. Bake in rings.

**Rice Snow.**—Five table-spoonfuls of rice flour; 1 qt. milk; 4 eggs—the whites only—whipped light; 1 table-spoonful of butter; 1 cup powdered sugar; a pinch of cinnamon and same of nutmeg, vanilla or other extracts for flavoring; a little salt. DIRECTIONS—Wet up the flour with cold water and add to the milk when the latter is scalding hot; boil until it begins to thicken; put in the sugar and add spice; simmer 5 minutes, stirring constantly, and turn into a a bowl before beating in the butter; let it get cold before flavoring it; then whip a spoonful at a time, into the beaten eggs; set to form in a wet mold; put sweet cream around it. This is delicate and wholesome fare for invalids; if you wish to have it especially nice, add ½ pt. of cream, whipped light and beaten in at the last.

**Rice Custard.**—Into 1 qt. of boiling water stir 2 table-spoonfuls of rice flour, dissolved in a little cold milk; add 2 well beaten eggs to boiling mixture; sweeten and flavor to taste.

**Rice Blanc Mange.**—Sweet milk (¼ cream if you have it), 1 qt.; rice flour, ⅔ of a cup; vanilla or lemon extract, or rose water, to taste; cream and and sugar, or raspberry or other jelly to serve with. DIRECTIONS—Heat the milk to the boiling point before stirring in the rice flour; and continue to stir constantly for ½ an hour, or until cooked so thick that you know it will harden in the cups, or molds, to avoid burning, unless it is cooked in a rice kettle. Flavor the last thing, when a little cool.

**Red Rice, a Danish Dish.**—Take ripe, red currants, 1½ pts.; very ripe raspberries, 1 pt.; water, 1 qt.; rice flour, 1 cup; sugar to taste, according to the acidity of the currants. DIRECTIONS—Stew the currants until the juice flows freely, add the raspberries just before the currants are ready to strain; then return to the sauce pan, add the sugar; then the rice flour, stirring smoothly, and pour into molds; and when cold turn out upon a glass dish. Thicken with cream and sugar if desired. It may be made with red currant jelly, and raspberry jelly, in place of the fruits, out of their season.

**OATMEAL—For Bone and Muscle; or, as Food and Drink for Laborers.**—Liebig has shown that oatmeal is almost as nutritious as the very best English beef, and that it is richer than wheaten bread in the elements that go to form bone and muscle. Prof. Forbes, of Edinburgh, during some 20 years, measured the breadth and height, and also tested the strength of both the arms and loins of the students of the University—a very numerous class, and of various nationalities, drawn to Edinburgh by the fame of his teaching. He found that in height, breadth of chest and shoulders, and strength of arms and loins, the Belgians were at the bottom of the list, a little above them the French, very much higher the English, and highest of all the Scotch and Scotch-Irish, from Ulster, who, like the natives of Scotland, are fed in their early years with at least one meal a day of good milk and good oatmeal porridge.

**As a Drink.**—Speaking of oatmeal an exchange remarks that a very good drink is made by putting about 2 spoonfuls of the meal into a tumbler of water. The western hunters and trappers consider it the best of drinks, as it is at once nourishing, stimulating and satisfying. It is popular in the Brooklyn navy yard, 2½ lbs. of oatmeal being put into a pail of moderately cold water. It is much better than any of the ordinary mixtures of vinegar and molasses with water, which farmers use in the haying and harvest field.—*New York Mail.*

*Remarks.*—I know the value of oatmeal as a food; and I have not a doubt of its value as a drink; putting the meal to common water for the drinking, by laborers, when at work. My son and myself drank of it, as used by the laborers on the Brooklyn bridge, as we visited that structure, passing through there to the Centennial in 1876, and liked it very much; and the superintendent said he should not be willing to even try to do without it; though I think they only put 1 lb. to a pail of water. It would certainly be very nourishing with 2 table-spoonfuls of it to a glass of water, as spoken of by the exchange above, half the amount would meet my own ideas, as sufficient, even when the nourishment was especially needed.

**Oatmeal Porridge, Scotch, and Cracknels, or "Scotch Ban-**

nocks."—An Englishwoman in the Germantown (Pa.) *Telegraph* gives the following instructions to make

**Oatmeal Porridge.**—"Oatmeal porridge is especially suitable for children. It nourishes their bones and other tissues, and supplies them in a greater degree than most foods with the much needed element of phosphorus. If they grow weary of it, they can be tempted back with the bait of golden syrup, jam, or marmalade, to be eaten with the porridge. The Irish and Scotch make their porridge with water, and add cold milk, but the most agreeable and nutritive way is to make it entirely with milk, to use coarse oatmeal, and to see that it is not too thick." The following is a good receipt:

Bring a quart of milk to the boiling point in an enamel-lined sauce-pan, and drop in by degrees 8 oz. of coarse oatmeal; stir till it thickens, and then boil for half an hour. The mixture should not be too thick, and more milk can be added according to the taste.

**For the Cracknels, or Scotch Bannocks, to Keep a Year.**—Take the finest oatmeal and stir in barely enough water to wet it through; add a pinch of salt; let it stand for 10 minutes to swell; then roll it out a quarter of an inch in thickness, first flouring the board and rolling pin with wheaten flour; cut it with a biscuit cutter, and bake in a moderate oven; these cakes will burn quickly and only require to be of the lightest brown. If put in a close jar they will keep for several months. In the Highlands they preserve their bannocks in the barrels of oatmeal and keep them a year or so."

**Oatmeal Mush.**—The true way to make oatmeal mush is in a rice-kettle; but if you have it not, a porcelain lined one is next best; iron will do. If made in the rice or double kettle; simply water enough to cover the meal is enough; then cover the dish and cook till done, without fear of burning. To make in an open kettle, put in water sufficient to make the right quantity, and bring to a boil; adding a little salt; then stir in coarse oatmeal until it is as thick as you wish to eat it; then slip back on the stove to simmer slowly for half an hour, or till done. Eaten with meat, or served with milk, milk or sugar, or cream, as desired.

**Oatmeal to Cook in an Earthen or Stone Jar.**—To one cup of of coarse oatmeal, add 1 qt. of cold water, in a stone jar; set it in a kettle of boiling water and boil 1 hour; do not stir it; serve with sugar and cream.—*Alice Kimball, Winfield, Iowa.*

*Remarks.*—This plan of cooking in an earthen crock in a kettle of water is perfectly safe, and not the least danger of scorching, whether it be oatmeal, hominy, corn, or wheat grits, cracked wheat, corn-starch, sea-moss, farina, or any of the nice breakfast dishes, mixed or cooked in milk. Even in cooking beans there is nothing better to bake them in than a stone jar. I cannot better close this subject than with a quotation from *Cassell's* (Scotch) *Magazine,* which says of oatmeal·

"We have called it the food for bones as well as brain; muscle as well as mind. To the laboring, or artisan class, it commends itself as an article of diet on account of cheapness, the readiness and economy with which it can be cooked, and, while it is easily digested, it contains, as we have seen, a larger proportion than wheaten bread of the elements that go to form bone and muscle. The best Scotch oatmeal costs 2-pence a pound, and this contains far more true nourishment, in the opinion of some medical men, than the same weight of Liebig's extract. It commends itself to literary men, and all workers who earn their bread by the sweat of their brains. There are, as we happen to know, several well-known authors, who, though born and bred this side the Tweed, nevertheless swear by oatmeal porridge as a brain-inspiring compound. Then, as to its palatableness, we ourselves have long held the belief that not only is porridge rich in nutritive matter, but when nicely cooked, and eaten with new milk, is simply delicious, a dainty dish, fit, indeed, to set before any king."

*Remarks.*—The only objection that can possibly be raised against oatmeal in the United States is its cost. With the "Yankee" determination in this country to double our money every time we "turn" it, it costs in this city, Toledo, 1883, 5 cents per lb. which is double what it ought to cost, if millers generally would prepare it; but from the expense of machines to hull it, this will not probably be done very soon. Yet, certainly, everybody can afford to buy enough for the "porritch,' and also to make a mush for breakfast. "So mote it be." Still the fact of having to pay 25 cents for 5 lbs. of oatmeal in free America is simply ridiculous, when oats can be bought for 30 to 50 cents a bushel.

**Cracked Wheat Mush, Very Excellent—The Same Also if Cooked Whole.**—Cracked wheat makes an excellent mush, cooked and eaten the same as oatmeal; and is, no doubt, richer and more palatable to some than oatmeal. The kernel simply needs to be cracked, or broken. If it is done too finely, the flour needs to be sifted out. The author is fond of having wheat cooked whole. It takes longer boiling, but if nicely done and eaten with cream or milk and a little sugar it makes an excellent relish at tea-time, or any time. Can be cooked either cracked or whole, without burning, in a rice-kettle (which see), or by putting into a tin pail and setting into a kettle of water, with sticks or nails under the bottom of the tin pail, so this does not touch the bottom of the kettle.

**Beets, To Bake.**—Beets are sweeter and nicer baked than boiled. The sugar, of which a good beet is full, is retained better by baking than by boiling, which extracts and carries off considerable of their natural sweetness. Turn, if need be, occasionally, to avoid burning. To be washed, but not peeled till after baking. Serve with butter, pepper and salt, the same as if boiled, but they will be found nicer and sweeter than if boiled.

**Stewed Beets with Onions.**—Pare thinly, and slice thinly, and put with some sliced onions, ¼ to ½ as much, according to the fondness of the family for onions, putting into a stew-pan with pepper, salt, and butter rubbed with a little flour; stir into hot water or milk enough to cover them well, and stew till the beets are tender. Young beets will require about an hour, old ones longer. Serve hot at dinner.

**Beets Hashed with Potatoes, a Very Nice Dish.**—The author is very fond of properly boiled or baked beets hashed with an equal amount of cold potatoes, and warmed up by putting in a bit of butter, a little water or milk, as potatoes are often done alone for breakfast. The sweetness of the beets is nicely brought out in this way. Pepper and salt, of course. Don't fail to try it.

**Parsnips, Cakes or Balls.**—Wash and boil in water with a little salt in it until perfectly tender. When cold, scrape off the skin, mash them, and for each cup of the mashed parsnips, put bread crumbs, ½ cup; a beaten egg; salt and pepper, to taste; flour the hands and make into balls, brown in hot butter, and serve hot.

**Parsnips Stewed in Milk.**—Cut cold, boiled parsnips in slices, usually lengthwise; put into milk, with a little butter, pepper and salt, and stew a few minutes; then thicken with a little flour rubbed smoothly in a little water or milk. Parsnips are almost always served hot; but I have been very fond of them cold.

**Fried Parsnips.**—Cut cold, well-boiled parsnips into long, thin slices; apply salt and pepper to taste, dredge or dip in flour, or not, as you prefer, and fry in hot drippings or butter. Drain a moment over a colander before serving.

**Egg Plant, Fried.**—Cut in slices half an inch thick and lay in salt water 1 hour, drain, dip in beaten egg, then in cornmeal, cracker crumbs or flour, and fry until brown and nicely tender. They are good fried after ham. Pick as soon as full grown, not allowing to get ripe.—*Elise, St. Johns, Mich.*

**Tomatoes, To Broil.**—Take ones, not very ripe, cut in thin slices, rub a little butter, salt and pepper together and spread over the slices nicely, and broil on a gridiron or beefsteak broiler,(which see). Serve hot.

*Remarks.*—This is the only way the author cares for them. They are very nice done thus.

**Squash Baked.**—Clean nicely, by cutting open and scraping out the inside with a spoon. Cut in suitable pieces, or, if a fully-ripe Hubbard, break in pieces, and place in the oven flesh side up. Allowing 1 hour for baking. It may be taken out of the shell when done, and seasoned with salt, pepper and butter, before serving; or allow each one to take a piece and season to suit himself. Even those not quite ripe are good thus, baked. Should come to the table "as hot as blazes." Boiled squash are seasoned the same, but the water must be pressed out as much as possible. Summer squash are most frequently boiled, but the water is seldom half pressed out as it ought to be.

**Potatoes—General Remarks.**—Although less than one-tenth of the potato is really nourishing (the rest being water). yet with us Americans, Irish-like, there are but few meals eaten in which potatoes do not form a part. Baking them, it is pretty generally known, is the most healthful way of cooking them, as it drives off much of the water and leaves them more nourishing than by steaming or boiling; steaming is next best, boiling the poorest way of all, as it so often leaves them watery and bad; yet, no one would always like them cooked in the same manner; hence, I shall give a kind of "bill of fare," for a week, differently cooked for dinner, after which I will also give some very choice ways of cooking and serving them. Remember this, however; that the most nutritious part of the potato—the starch—is richest, next to the skin, hence when they are to be peeled, raw, pare as thin as possible. Prof. Blat, the great French cook, says the skinning process, as he calls it, is all wrong. His plan is to dig out the eyes and peel after boiling, etc., claiming that the nourishment from them is not more than 7 or 8 per cent., the balance mainly water, of which there is not a doubt. The following methods of preparing for dinner for each day in the week, will always help one to decide what, in the potato line, shall I have for dinner? And by turning to the actual bill of fare for a week, among the meat dishes, will help to decide the whole question as to what the dinner shall be. These directions, or recipes, are from a writer to the *Housekeeper*, who you will readily see, had an excellent judgment, if not an actual experience in the matter. I am sorry they did not come to me so I can give the writer's name. They were given under the head of:

**"Potatoes in Seven Ways," or for Dinner Each Day of the Week.**—The writer says: "*Editor Housekeeper:*—Let me give you a few little hints in regard to the different methods of cooking potatoes, so that the oft abused boiled potato may be varied during the week at dinner:

I. "SUNDAY.—Mashed potatoes; peel (thin), steam, place in a pan and mash, add milk, butter and salt, and then beat like cake batter, the longer the better, till they are nice and light. This steaming and beating will be found a great improvement.

II. "MONDAY.—Baked potatoes in their jackets. By the way, if any are left over they may be warmed over by not peeling them till cold, and then slicing.

III. "TUESDAY.—Peel and bake them with the roast of beef.

IV. "WEDNESDAY.—Prepare them in the Kentucky style, as follows: The potatoes are sliced thin, as for frying, and allowed to remain in cold water ½ hour. The slices are then put in a pudding dish, with salt, pepper and some milk—about ⅓ pt. to an ordinary pudding dish. They are then put into an oven and baked for an hour. When taken out, a lump of butter the size of a hen's egg is cut into small bits and scattered over the top. Those who have never eaten potatoes cooked thus, do not know all the capabilities of that esculent tuber. The slicing allows the interior of each potato to be examined, hence its value where potatoes are doubtful, though the poor ones are not of necessity required. The soaking in cold water hardens the slices, so that they will hold their shape. The milk serves to cook them through, and to make a nice brown on the top; the quantity can only be learned by experience; if just a little is left as a rich gravy, moistening all the slices, then it is right. In a year of small potatoes, this method of serving them will be very welcome to many a housekeeper.

V. "THURSDAY.—Peel, steam and serve whole.

VI. "FRIDAY.—'Potatoes a la pancake;' peel, cut in thin slices lengthwise, sprinkle with pepper and salt, and fry in butter or beef drippings, turning like griddle cakes.

VII. SATURDAY.—Potatoes boiled in their jackets.

"These are simple ways, but give variety. On Monday and Tuesday always prepare them in some way in the oven, as as to leave top of stove free.

**Fried Potatoes (Saratoga's Secret).**—It is my custom to make my items as short as possible, and have them understood, but " G. B. B." wrote the following in such a spicy manner to the Springfield *Republican*, I think it will give an additional relish to the potatoes to give it in his own words. The nicety or daintiness of the dish more than pays for the labor of preparing it. His words were as follows: "Saratoga Potatoes, the poetry of common life, and costly charm of Delmonico's and Parker's, can be made in perfection in any kitchen by the use of a very simple apparatus, consisting of a large blade set slanting into a wooden trough with a narrow slit in the bottom, two wire screens or sieves, and a common spider   Select 8 large potatoes, pare them and slice very thin with the cutting machine, soak them in cold water for 2 hours, then stir common table salt into the water, 1 tea-spoonful to a quart, and allow them to remain in the brine ½ hour longer. Pour them upon the screen to drain, and put them on a spider with 1 lb. of clear lard over a brisk fire. When the sliced potatoes dry on a towel, wait until the lard is smoking hot, and pour a large plateful into the spider. The result is like a small sea in a white squall, and now the cook shows the artistic soul, which every votary of that noblest of the arts must possess to be worthy of the name. Patient and calm, with steady and incessant motion of the skimmer, she prevents adhesion of any two affectionate slices, and watches carefully for any tender burst of brownness to appear. Slowly it creeps and deepens until it rivals the hue of the fragrant Havana. Haste then takes the place of caution, lest any martyrs burn for the perfection of others; and they must be quickly spread upon another sieve to drain until dry and greaseless enough for the fairest fingers, then served hot to melt away like a kiss on sweet lips, with a dying crackle like the fallen leaves of autumn."

*Remarks.* — Of course, these may be sliced with a knife, cutting them quite thin is the only point requiring special care. Sieves are not absolutely necessary, but help the drying or draining process considerably. A very satisfactory substitute may be made by any intelligent boy of a dozen years old. A frame of wood, about a foot square, on the principle of a picture frame, of soft wood strips, half an inch thick by one inch wide, halved together at the corners and nailed; then small holes every ½ inch and small wires woven across ½ or ¾ inch apart each way, will answer every purpose.

**Home Style.**—Wash, pare, and slice, in the ordinary way, as many potatoes as required for the meal; rinse in cold water, then, having placed a skillet upon the stove, with 2 or 3 spoonfuls of meat drippings, lard, or butter in it, to become hot, put in the sliced potatoes, sprinkling a little salt and pepper upon them, and, as the bottom ones become browned, turn them till all are nicely browned, then take them up at once into a covered dish, to keep hot. This makes a nice dish while hot, but they are not relished after having become cold. Peachblows are not as good for frying as those which do not crack open while boiling—they become softer and more mussy   Raw potatoes are to be taken in both recipes.

**Potato Balls, or Cakes.**—When you have mashed potatoes left over at dinner, which have been seasoned with butter, salt, and milk, or cream, make them, while warm, into cakes ¾ of an inch thick, and set by till morning;

then beat an egg, into which dip the potato cakes, from whence lay them into a frying-pan, having a little butter in it, of the right heat to brown the cakes quickly. Take up in a tureen to keep hot. Potatoes may be cooked and seasoned purposely for making these cakes; but it is best to prepare them and make up the cakes in the afternoon, as they brown better for having dried out over night.

**Saratoga Fried Potatoes, Short Way.**—Wash the potatoes clean, pare, slice with a potato-slicer, very thin, throw into cold water long enough to take out some of the starch, then wipe dry and put into boiling lard, a few pieces at a time. Be sure and keep the lard boiling. As soon as the potatoes are of a clear, golden brown, skim them out, drain them in a colander or sieve, and serve hot.

*Remarks.*—If the potatoes are well covered with water, stirred up two or three times, and the water changed once, they being sliced very thin, an hour will remove much of the starch, which you must understand by the general remarks above, takes away the nourishment; hence I should prefer less soaking than given in No. 8.

**Potatoes Fried With Eggs.**—Slice cold boiled potatoes, and fry in butter till nicely brown, in this time heat 1 or 2 eggs, as below, and stir into the potatoes nicely, and take up at once, so as not to harden the egg, but merely to cook slightly. One egg is enough for 3 or 4 persons who are not especially fond of potatoes; if most of the family are fond of them have plenty, and use additional eggs to correspond. Choice.

**Potatoes "Tip-Top."**—Boil 8 large potatoes in their skins, and let them cool. When cold, peel them and cut them into thick slices. Put into a stewpan 2 oz. of butter, in a thin slice; and when it is melted add 1 tea-spoon of well seasoned stock. or gravy (see gravy below), 1 tea-spoon of finely chopped parsley; chopped lemon, and 1 tea-spoon of mixed pepper and salt. Stir these well together over the fire till hot, add the potatoes, simmer 5 minutes, stir in the juice of a lemon and serve hot.

*Remarks.*—Of course, if you have no parsley, and do not like onions, do without either, and still it will be "tip-top."

**Potatoes en Caisse (In a Case.)**—Wash some large, fine potatoes of a mealy sort and bake them. When done cut a small hole in the top of each and carefully scoop out the whole of the inside; mash this fine, in a saucepan over the fire, mixing with it a large table-spoonful of butter and a generous quantity of cream. Salt and black or white pepper to taste, and stir in the whipped whites of 2 eggs. Fill up the skins of the potatoes with the mixture. Set them into the oven for a few moments and serve hot. These amounts are for 6 large potatoes. Keep the same proportion for any number.

**Potatoes, Duchesse, or Potato Balls, Baked.**—Boil and pass through a sieve 6 fine potatoes. There must be no lumps. Add 1 gill of cream, the yolk of 3 eggs, pepper, salt, a little chopped parsley, and a hint of nutmeg. The mixture must be thoroughly smooth and well mixed. Take a table-spoonful at a time, form into a ball, brush the top slightly with a beaten egg, place in a buttered pan, and set them in the oven till nicely browned.

**Potatoes with and Without Onions for Breakfast.**—Boil pota-toes a little underdone; when cold, peal and chop finely; have an onion or two, if several in the family, also boiled underdone, and finely minced. Put on a saucepan with milk, 1½ cups, and bring to a boil; then add butter, a table-spoonful as lifted from the crock, and when melted, stir| in the potatoes and onion, and cook about 15 minutes, or until creamy. If onions are not tolerated by anyone use the potatoes alone, or with hashed beets, in the same manner.

*Remarks.*—The author takes them one day with onions, the next with beets.

**New Potatoes a la Creme or in Milk.**—Take the small new pota-toes, scrape off the skins when washed, and boil, or better, steam them not quite done, the day before needed for breakfast; in the morning chop or cut fine, with any others left over; salt and pepper to taste. One cup of milk to 2 or 3 of potato. Heat the milk with a table-spoonful of butter, and stir in the potatoes, and warm up nicely.

*Remarks.*—A Mrs. Deacon Warner, for whose husband I worked in hay-ing the first half month I ever worked away from home, over 50 years ago, used to get them up in this way, and I thought them, and still think, they are the nicest I ever ate. Of course old ones may be used in the same manner, and are nice, but the new, it seems to me, at least, richer, and I know, more sweet and tender.

**Potato Fritters.** This receipt was given by one of those persons who more recently have been having schools of instruction in the cities in the art of cookery, Miss Parloa. She says:

One pint of boiled and mashed potato; ½ cup of hot milk; 3 table-spoonfuls of butter; 3 of sugar; 2 eggs; a little nutmeg; 1 tea-spoonful of salt. DIRECTIONS —Add the milk, butter, sugar and seasoning to the mashed potato, and then add the eggs well beaten. Stir until very smooth and light. Spread about ½ an inch deep on a buttered dish, and set away to cool. When cold, cut into squares. Dip in beaten egg and in bread-crumbs, and fry brown, in boiling fat. Serve immediately.

*Remarks.*—I take this to be only another name for potato balls, but they will be a nice thing to have around about mealtime.

**Sliced Potatoes to Bake With Pork.**—Dig out the eyes and pare very thinly, raw potatoes, and slice very thinly also, to nearly fill a 2-quart pudding dish (earthen). Season freely with salt and pepper over the top; then pour over sweet milk ⅔ full, which will carry the seasoning among the slices. Cut 5 or 6 slices of pork and lay over the top, as a covering. Bake about 2 hours. If the pork is likely to get too much browned, cover with thick brown paper till the potatoes are done.

**Escaloped Potatoes, or Potatoes with Cracker Crumbs.**—Slice quite thin, cold boiled potatoes, to the amount of a quart or more, and roll crackers to nearly the same amount. Season the potatoes, about 2 tea-spoonfuls of salt and pepper to taste, and place half of the potatoes in a suitable baking-dish, placing bits of butter upon them: then half of the cracker crumbs, and pour over ½ pint of cream (milk will do, but if milk is used, use butter more freely); then the balance of the potatoes, as the first, and cover with the balance of the crumbs and cream, or milk, as before. with more butter, and bake until richly browned and well heated through. To be eaten with butter or any meat gravies for dinner or tea. The same may be done with sweet potatoes, several other plans of cooking which are given below.

**Potatoes, Gravy for.**—Put a table-spoonful or more of butter, according to the quantity of potatoes you have, into a frying-pan and set over the fire until brown, being careful not to scorch it. Mix a table-spoonful of flour in a cup of thin, sweet cream, or milk, if one has no cream; pour into the browned butter, boil up, season with pepper and a little salt if necessary, and turn over the potatoes.

**Sweet Potatoes, to Bake—Moist and Nice.**—Those with experience in baking sweet potatoes, claim them to be more moist, and sweeter, for having been half boiled, or steamed, before putting into the oven. Very small ones should not be chosen for baking. Bake in a moderate oven.

**Sweet Potatoes, Broiled.**—Thinly pare large, fine sweet potatoes. Cut them lengthwise into thick slices, and broil them, upon a wire griddle, over a clear hot fire. When crisp and brown, put them upon a hot platter, sprinkle pepper and salt over them and add butter cut into small pieces. Serve very hot.

**Sweet Potato Cakes—Very Nice.**—Remove the skin from 2 or 3 medium-sized sweet potatoes, left over, and mash them nicely, and mix in about 3 ozs. (3 small table-spoonfuls) of flour, salt and pepper to taste, a good lump of butter, and warm milk enough to make a good dough. Roll this out on the kneading board, and cut out a cake about the size of your baking tin; butter the tin well, and scatter a little flour over it; then lay in; when you think it is nearly done, turn it over. If the bottom of the oven is very hot, put a grate under the baking-tin to prevent getting too much browned. The danger of burning is lessened if instead of one cake you cut the dough in buscuit-shape about 2 inches thick. If covered while baking, the cakes will be more moist. These can be made of other potatoes as well as of the sweet ones.

*Remarks.*—Either of these plans not only enable one to use up cold or left-over sweet potatoes, but "Irish" potatoes, too, and at the same time make a nice dish for the table—the same as though the potatoes had been cooked purposely for these uses; in fact, it is well to cook some extra ones for either of these purposes, preferred, at the time.

**FRUIT—How and When to be Eaten to Receive the Greatest Benefit.**—*General Remarks.*—We now come to the question of fruit as eaten in its natural state—uncooked—and also in its various forms of cookery. And as apples are used throughout the year, as well as more freely than any other kinds, they will receive the greater attention; but what is said of them will apply, generally, with equal force to most other fruit, in their season. To derive the greatest benefit from the use of almost any kind of fruit, in its natural state, it should be eaten just before the meal, or at its close; then not any "nibbling" of it between meals; for this plan is a very great source, or cause of dyspepsia. When the eating of fruit does harm, it is generally because it is eaten at improper times, in improper quantities, or when imperfectly ripened. An eminent physician recently said: "If my patients would eat a couple of oranges every morning before breakfast, from February to June, my practice would be gone." It is a simple thing to do, but it would be magical in its alterative action upon the system. And to derive the greatest benefit from the use of our common fruits, let only sufficient sugar, cream, seasoning, etc., be used to give a relish, that the pure fruit acids may have their cooling and correcting—alterative—influence upon the system.

**Fruit Cooking, Suitable Vessels for.**—In cooking any acid fruit (and most of them are of an acid nature), tin, brass, or porcelain vessels are the best; never cook them in glazed earthen, on account of the lead in the glazing, nor in copper without especial care to brighten it with brick-dust and flannel, and to pour out as soon as done.

**Fruit as a Medicine.**—Apples, peaches and strawberries, perfectly ripe and juicy, are not only some of our most delicate fruits; but they are a pleasant and alterative medicine (eaten in moderation, as suggested by the physician in speaking of oranges). These fruits, perfectly ripe, digest in 1½ to 2 hours, while boiled cabbage requires 4 to 5 hours. Baked apples and baked peaches (which see) make as healthful a dessert as can be placed upon the table. These, and strawberries uncooked, eaten frequently at breakfast, with Graham bread and nice butter, without meat, will have the effect of removing constipation, correcting acidities, cooling and removing fever tendencies very effectually. This can be done with apples nearly all the year round; and with children, especially, would save many a doctor's bill, as well as meet their craving desires for something of an acid nature, without being obliged to give them food requiring much longer time for digestion. We will first give a receipt for baking peaches, which originated with myself, and carried into effect many times by my dear wife, since passed to her reward in the spirit world.

**Peaches, To Bake for the Table, and for Canning, a Very Choice Dish—Equally Applicable to Apples.**—Wash fully ripe peaches, carefully rubbing off the furze, with a suitable cloth, from the skin, which is needed to hold this lucious fruit together; cut out a little of the skin from the blossom end, to allow sugar to penetrate and the juices to escape; then place a baking tin full of them, stem-end down, pour upon them water to fill half or two-thirds up, and scatter on sugar, according to their tartness, to make them palatable. Place in a moderate oven till entirely tender. Serve hot; but if any are left over they are nice cold. The same plan is equally applicable to apples.

*Remarks.*—My wife, at one time, having some apples baked in the above manner, and there being also a large quantity of peaches that season, and some upon the table at that time, the thought struck me like a flash, to ask her if she ever thought of or saw peaches baked. I never had, nor had she. Then I asked her to try some for the next meal, I think, which she did, with the most perfect satisfaction—the nicest dish of baked fruit that, I think, I ever partook of. It was repeated many, many times, and, finally, when canning-time came, more than half that was put up was done in this way, and also proved entirely satisfactory, and was continued as long as she lived. The author will guarantee satisfaction to all who try it fairly. Many people, of late years, ask: "Will you warrant this to be, or do, as you say?"—I will, hence the guarantee above.

**Peach, Apple, and Berry Fritters.**—Wash, pare, halve or quarter peaches or apples, according to their size, as many as you desire. Make a batter of sweet milk (if you have it, if not, water), flour, and baking powder, at the rate of 2 tea-spoonfuls to 1 qt. of flour, and a little salt, with an egg, if you have it, to each pint of milk used; when of proper consistence, stir in the pieces of fruit, and with a large spoon take up 1 or 2 pieces with some of the batter and drop into hot lard and brown nicely. Serve hot, with cream and sugar. They make an excellent substitute for pies and puddings.

*For Raspberries Blackberries, Strawberries, etc.*—Make the batter the same, but for each cup of berries, sprinkle upon them 1 table-spoonful of sugar; fry the same, but dust them thickly with powdered sugar to serve.

*Remarks.*—Thus, with a little judgment on the part of the cook, an endless variety of dishes or articles of food may be prepared to meet the varied tastes of guests or of the family. English currants, or raisins, both properly stewed in but little water, and the raisins cut into halves to prevent their bursting and scattering the hot fat when put in; or any of the home-dried fruits may be used in this manner, thus extending the variety.

**Apples Dried, Their Wholesomeness as Food, and Manner of Cooking.**—The *Indiana Farmer* recently made a lengthy plea for dried apples, from which I condense the necessary points to a full understanding of the subject. It says:

"Dried apples are not only a cheap article of food, but very wholesome; and if the girls will pay attention, I will tell them how to cook them," etc. These two points being admitted, their cheapness and wholesomeness, I can now condense very much, still retaining everything essential. Cook but few at a time, as they become flat, or stale, by long standing. Take only ⅓ as much bulk as you need when cooked, as they swell very much. Put them into a pan of milk warm water 10 to 15 minutes; then mash thoroughly, and carefully examine every piece to see there are no worms in them, especially so if they were dried upon strings; rinse nicely, and place in a porcelain kettle, or in a tin pan, and cover handsomely with cold water; cover tightly and slowly bring to a boil, having hot water to replenish with if more is needed. When tender, but not mushy, add sugar to taste. If stewed too long they shrink and turn dark. Have plenty of juice, and sugar to make them rich, but not to deaden the flavor of the apples, and you have a dish better than half the canned fruits in use.

**The Juice of Dried Apples a Great Beverage for the Sick.**—The editor closes by saying: "I must not omit to mention that the juice off of nicely stewed dried apples is a delicious beverage for the sick, and possesses a flavor that is peculiarly refreshing and grateful, especially where there is fever."

*Remarks.*—The author fully endorses all the points made by the editor, having always been very fond of sauce made of dried apples, having plenty of juice. For me it is preferable to most other sauces, which are often much more expensive, but not half so palatable. For the beverage for the sick, a dozen quarters will be enough for a quart of water, with simple sugar to taste, as the flavoring needs no doctoring generally. The evaporated apples are still so expensive, that most families having an orchard, should continue their practice of drying for themselves.

**APPLE, PEACH AND OTHER FRUIT BUTTERS—How to Make.**—The *American Grocer*, in giving an account of the manufacture of fruit butters, as a business in the cities, from dried apples, peaches, quinces and pears, using sugar and water in place of the juices of the fruit, closes in the following language, as to making them in the country. It says: "The same purpose that sugar subserves in the manufactories here, may be accomplished there by the use of cider. When apples are ripe make, say 3 barrels, of cider. Then pare, and core, 4 bushels of apples. Then boil down the 3 barrels of cider to 1½ (the author would say boil down the cider first), and set it convenient to the copper kettle, in which place the 4 bushels of apples. Pour on the apples from the cider enough to answer the purpose (to nearly cover them) and fire up. As the cider boils away, add more until it is all used up and the contents of the kettle brought down to a proper consistency, of which one must be judge. A little practice will make one perfect in this process. This is for apples. It will apply equally well to any other kind of fruit from which it is practicable to obtain the juice as one would from apples."

*Remarks.*—Any other fruit may be made with the cider; but the flavor would not be so perfect of the kind used, as it would to use its own juices. Peaches and pears, when fully ripe and juicy, would easily supply the necessary amount of juice, or cider, removing the stones from the peaches before grinding and pressing. And even grape juice has been used to make peach butter.

Of course these ciders should be boiled down the same as apple cider, above. While cooking the butter there must be watchful care and constant stirring, to avoid burning. If cooked down pretty thick, so as to just spread nicely, and then carefully put up in stone jars, and kept in a cool, dry place, it will keep all the year around. Pour into tubs as soon as complete, to avoid creating a verdigris on the copper, by standing, which is poisonous. The cider, in boiling down, needs skimming at each addition, as it is put in. This boiled cider is nice for minced pies, apple sauce, etc.

It is claimed, however, by some, that the best apple butter is made by using sweet apples only; selecting the nicest, both for the cider and for the butter. It may be an advantage to those who have sweet apples in abundance, for, as a general thing, they are not as marketable as tart or sour ones. Most people will be satisfied to have plenty of that made from nice, juicy, tart fruit, at least, I have always been. I have seen apple butter that was flavored with winter-green, but give me the natural flavor only. The following short plans of making peach and apple butters, from a *Blade* writer, may suit some of our readers better than the others, hence I give them a place. Grape juice makes a nice butter with peaches, treated the same as cider, *i. e.*, boiled when just pressed out. Why will it not do as nicely with apples? Those who have plenty of peaches can soon tell by trying it.

**Peach Butter.**—Pare ripe peaches and put them in a kettle with sufficient water to boil them soft, when sift through a colander, removing the stones. To each quart of peaches put 1½ lbs. of sugar and boil very slowly one hour. Stir often so they will not burn. When done season with ground spice and cinnamon to taste.

**Apple Butter.**—Boil down a kettle of cider to ⅔ of the quantity. Pare, core, and slice your apples, and put as many into the cider as you think your kettle will hold without boiling over. Let it boil slowly, stirring often. When done spice with cinnamon, and, if you like it sweet, put in some sugar.

**Pumpkin Butter, as Made in the North Woods.**—Take out the seeds of 1 pumpkin, cut it in small pieces and boil it soft; take 3 other pumpkins, cut them in pieces and boil them soft; put them in a coarse bag and press out the juice; add the juice to the first pumpkin and let it boil 10 hours or more to become the thickness of butter; stir often. If the pumpkins are frozen the juice will come out much easier.

*Remarks.*—All I have to guide me as to the "North Woods" manner of making is that on the back of the slip cut from some newspaper; there was the date of the paper—Feb. 7, 1880,—also "Sleighing fair," and "Loggers feel better," therefore, to know that "loggers felt better," they must have that class of persons among them; and hence it was from some northern paper, where loggers in the winter do congregate. It will make a good butter if boiled carefully to avoid burning. I should say boil the juice at least half away before putting in the nicely cut pieces of the 1 pumpkin, boiling it soft in the juice of the 3 other ones, after its reduction one-half. It makes a very good substitute for cow's butter, and for apple butter, too. But I must say if I used frozen pumpkins to obtain the juice from, I should not want the one frozen that was to be cut up to make the butter of. I think it would not be as good if frozen. If any of these butters are too sour add good brown sugar to make it sweet enough to suit the taste. We return to dishes made with apples.

**Apple Snow.**—Apples, eggs, lemon peel and powdered sugar. Take 10 good-sized apples, peel, core, and cut into quarters; put into a saucepan with the rind of 1 lemon, and water enough to keep them from burning—about ½ a pt. Then the apples are tender, take out the lemon peel, and beat the apples to a pulp; let them cool and stir in the whites of 10 eggs, beaten to a strong froth. Add ½ lb. of powdered sugar, and continue beating until the mixture is quite stiff. Put on a glass dish and serve either with custard made with the yolks of the eggs, or with cream; or garnish with sponge cake or lady-finger cake, as you choose.

*Remarks.*—What is called "pulp" above is often called in these "snow" mixtures *puree*—an East Indian word, meaning gravy, or soft mixture, in connection with their curries or much-spiced dishes. The French call these pulpy mixtures "meringues," but generally bake them into pies, having first baked the crust or pastry upon the plate or pie dish before putting in the meringue; then covering the pie, when just done, with the beaten white of an egg or two, with a table-spoonful of sugar to each egg, and browning nicely before taking from the oven, or returning them to the oven for 2 or 3 minutes for that purpose.

**Apple Snow No. 2, with Roast or Baked Apples.**—The apples may be roasted or nicely baked, then "pulped" or *pureed* through a colander to avoid the skins and cores. Otherwise treated the same as with the above boiled—the latter plan retaining much more of the flavor of the apples.

*Remarks.*—Please tell me why peaches, pears, and, perhaps, berries, will not do the same, except the "snow" part, which would be the color of the fruit used, not so white or snow-like.

**Apple Compote.**—Pare, halve and take out the cores of 6 large fair apples, throwing each piece into cold water to keep it from turning dark. Put loaf sugar, ½ lb., into an enameled stew-pan with sufficient water—about 3 pts. As soon as it boils put in the apples with the juice of 2 lemons, stew gently until the apples are sufficiently cooked but not broken. Then take them out carefully and lay them in the dish in which they are to go to the table. Cut the rinds of the lemons into the thinest possible strips and put them into the syrup; boil till tender, by which time the syrup will be much reduced. When cold pour the syrup about the apples, and also dispose the transparent strips of lemon about them. This dish looks pretty with a bit of quince jelly placed in the hollow of each apple; or with a candied cherry in the hollow, and angelica cut into lozenges and inserted around the top of each apple.—*Evening Post, Grand Rapids, Mich.*

*Remarks.*—The word *compote* is the French for preparing fruit with a syrup for immediate use, as Webster's "Unabridged" puts it. It makes a nice dish.

**Apples, Pears, Peaches, etc., Spiced, or Sweet Pickles.**—For each pound of these fruits, after being pared and cored, or pits removed, nice sugar, about ½ lb., and good vinegar, 1 gill, with unground spices to taste, are boiled together until the fruit is tender; then the fruit taken out and the syrup and spices cooked together until the watery parts coming out of the fruit is evaporated, and then poured over the fruit and securely covered for use. Crab apples or any very sour fruit will require more sugar.

**Cherry Butter.**—Boil the cherries till soft; then rub through a colander, and to each pint of the pulp add a pint of sugar. Boil carefully till thick, like other fruit butters. Can or keep in closely covered jars.

**Lemon Butter.**—Sugar 1½ cups; whites of 3 eggs and yolk of 1 beaten; butter ¼ cup; grate the yellow off of 2 medium sized lemons; then squeeze in the juice and mix all, and cook 20 minutes by setting the basin containing it into a pan of boiling water. Very nice for tarts or as butter upon bread.

**Dulce de Lece, or Spanish Sauce, or Butter.**—Put 1 qt. of nice sweet milk into a porcelain lined dish, with white sifted sugar, 1 lb.; flour and ground cinnamon, each 1 teaspoonful. Simmer, stirring occasionally, 5 or 6 hours, or till of proper consistence when a little is cooled. To be eaten cold, as a pudding sauce, or on bread for children. Valuable for children if at all diarrheal.

**Frosted Figs for Dessert.**—Beat the whites of 2, 3 or more eggs, according to the amount you wish to serve, till so stiff you can almost turn the plate upside down without the egg running off; then stir in powdered sugar, to leave the frosting soft enough to dip the figs into it, to completely cover, if need be, by re-dipping. Dry in the oven or on a shelf above the stove. If done nicely they will be nice.

**Peach Figs, Very Nice.**—Pare, halve and remove the stones from nice ripe peaches; weigh and half the weight in sugar. Heat both carefully without water until the sugar is dissolved in the escaping juices; then boil till the fruit is clear or transparent; then take up with a fork, drawing off all superfluous syrup, placing on plates to dry, as next above, till there will be no more drainage; then sift sugar over them and pack in small boxes, as figs, with plenty of sugar over and between them. It takes labor, but when peaches are plenty they are very nice indeed; eaten same as figs.

**Tomatoes.**—Nice ripe ones treated in the same way, first squeezing out their extra juices, are also nice.

**Honey, Artificial.**—"Polly Anthus," of El Dora, Ill., informs the *Blade* Household to make it as follows:

"Take water, 1½ pts.; heat it till ready to boil; then put in pulverized alum, ⅓ oz., and when that is dissolved pour in white sugar 4 lbs., stirring till dissolved; then continue to boil 2 or 3 minutes. Put 5 drops of rose oil (oil of rose) into alcohol ½ pt., and while the syrup is hot put in 2 tea-spoonfuls of this alcohol and you have 5½ lbs. of nice white honey."

*Remarks.*—The editor asked, "Does 'Polly Anthus' mean 5 drops of the burning fluid known as 'rose oil'?" Of course she did not, it was oil of rose, as I have indicated above, that she meant. For the kind of gasoline known as "rose oil" is not at all fit for such flavoring. That is referred to in Renovating Gloves, etc. The extract of rose, now much used in flavoring dishes, in like amount or a larger amount of rose water, a table-spoonful for a tea-spoonful will do very nicely. Oil of rose is quite expensive, still its flavor comes nearer to that of honey than any other.

**Sour Apples, to Cook so as to Keep Their Shape.**—Some writer upon this subject says: I always cook them in quarters; putting them into boiling water, with sugar to taste; being sure to put on water enough at first, so as not to stir or disturb them until done; then pour into a dish and you have a nice sauce to eat with cream as peaches. I like them better.

*Remarks.*—There is no doubt but what the boiling water sets, or toughens, the surface, and prevents them from coming to pieces; but, it strikes me that I, at least, would like peaches and cream best.

**Apple Charlotte.**—Stew apples quite soft and flavor with lemon or cinnamon; then prepare some nice bread and butter. Line the bottom of your pudding dish with it; then put a layer of the apple, and continue until filled; then pour over it a cold custard, and bake, and when cold turn out and serve with sauce made of cream and sugar.

*Remarks*—Charlotte is the French for a dish made of apple marmalade (a thick sauce), covered with crumbs of toasted bread, while *russe*, which is generally seen in connection with charlotte, is of Russian origination, and refers to cookery—then "Charlotte Russe" signifies a dish of custard inclosed in, or surrounded with sponge cake, etc. With this explanation you can get up either, and understand the whys and wherefores thereof.

**Apple Omelette.**—Take ½ doz. large pippins, or other tart apples; butter, 1 table-spoonful; 3 eggs; a table-spoonful of sugar for each apple; nutmeg and rose water, or other flavor to suit. If rose water is used, but little—a tea-spoonful or two only will be needed. DIRECTIONS—Pare, core and stew as for apple sauce, and beat it into a smooth pulp, while hot, adding the butter, sugar and flavor, and let stand until cold; then the eggs, beaten separately, the whites the last, when ready to pour into a deep, warmed and buttered dish, to be delicately browned in a moderate oven. It is best not eaten too hot. A wholesome dish, especially for children.

**Apple and Peach Preserve for Present Use.**—Peel, halve and core, 6 large apples, selecting those of the same size: make a syrup of 1 lb. of granulated sugar and 1 pt. of water; when it boils drop in the apples with the rind and juice of a lemon. As soon as they are tender, care must be taken that they do not fall in pieces; take the halves out one by one, and arrange, concave side uppermost, in a glass dish. Drop a bit of currant jelly into each piece, boil down the syrup, and when cool pour around the apples. This makes a very nice preserve for tea. Peaches can be substituted for apples, removing the pits carefully; treated in the same manner otherwise.

**Apple Jelly With the Pure Apple Flavor.**—Cut nice tart apples into quarters without paring or coring. Throw each piece into a jar of cold water as quartered; then take out with the hand, when enough is done to fill another stone jar; and place in a moderate oven, with thick paper over the top, till perfectly tender (being in a stone jar they will not burn); then mash and strain off the juice, and boil with 1 lb. of granulated sugar to each pint. The result is the most perfect flavor of the apple which lies near, and in the skin, seeds, etc. Porcelain kettles should be used for boiling.

*Remarks.*—The usual way has been to pare and core, then mash, or grind in a cider mill, boiling the cider, then adding sugar, etc., but the flavor is not nearly so fine. Some use ½ less sugar, and add gelatine (Coxes), or isinglass, about 1 oz. to each 3 large apples used. But the true way of baking, above given, is best.

**Green Apple Jelly.**—Take green apples and boil without paring, until perfectly soft; then rub through a sieve, or colander, and to each pint of the pulp add sugar ¾ lbs., by putting on one-third and letting stand a few hours, then the rest, and to each 3 pts. add the grated peel of 2 lemons, and boil 15 or 20 minutes, or until it begins to look clear, before putting into glasses or molds.

**Apple Short-Cake, Also Applicable to All Fruits.**—Flour, 1 qt.; cream of tartar, 2 tea-spoonfuls; soda, 1 tea-spoonful; salt, 1 tea-spoonful; butter, ½ cup; sweet milk to mix into rather a stiff dough. Roll out and bake nicely and split open; or bake in two thin cakes; and spread with nice butter, and cover with nicely sweetened apple-sauce, grate on some nutmeg; place the other half on this, the crust side down, if it was baked as a whole and split; then butter, etc., the other half the same way. The same if baked in two cakes; but if baked in two cakes it does not soak up so much or the butter and juices; and I think it preferable. Any of the fresh fruits in their season, or stewed properly out of season, are remarkably nice in the same manner; peaches and strawberries, however, are used more often than other kinds; but this is only from their superior delicacy of flavor. If the apple-sauces made by baking and pulping, as for jelly, above, the flavor will be more perfect.

**Apple Dumplings, Baked, Delicious.**—Tart, juicy apples, soda, sour milk, lard, salt and flour. DIRECTIONS—Pare the apples, cut into halves and core. Make the pastry as for biscuit, only using a little more lard or drippings to make it short, as well as light. Take sufficient dough upon the kneading-board to cover one apple. Knead as for biscuit, then roll out large enough to cover the apple, placing one of the halves upon the crust, and putting a tea-spoonful of sugar into the place of the core; then placing another upon the first, folding over the crust and pinching, or crimping, to retain the juices, the same as for boiling. Having buttered a bread-pan, put the dumplings in it as prepared, the same as you would biscuit. Make a little depression upon the top of each and put a bit of butter into it. Bake 1 hour in a moderate oven; but 10 or 15 minutes before taking up take out and sprinkle a good handful of sugar over all and return long enough to brown the top nicely. To be eaten warm, with cream or sugar, or other pudding sauce. Very nice cold; also, by grating a little nutmeg into the sauce.

*Remarks.*—The pastry for these dumplings may be made with sweet milk, or water, and baking powder 2 tea-spoonfuls to 1 qt. of flour, when sour milk is not at hand. Our first trial of them was made with water and baking powder, and gave us entire satisfaction. Milk is the richer, but not always to be had.

**Apple Dumplings, Boiled.**—One of the writers in the *Western Rural* gives the following as her plan of making them. She says: "I make the crust, or dough, as for nice short biscuit, and nothing is better for these than the top of good rich buttermilk. Sift the flour in the bread bowl, making a hole in the center. Put into it 1 tea-spoonful of pulverized saleratus, and mix with it a handful of dry flour; add 1 pt, of rich buttermilk or sour cream and a pinch of salt. Stir briskly until it foams, then stir in the flour until you have a soft dough. Knead but little, and roll out in round pieces as for pie crust, but rather thicker. Put the fruit on one-half of the crust, and dredge over it a little flour, wetting the edges of the crust, as for pies, to make it stick. Lap the crust over the fruit, fastening the edges securely. It now resembles the old-fashioned 'turnover,' and should be pricked with a fork to expel the air, and squeezed in the hand until it assumes a round form about the size of a large tea-cup. When they are all made in this way, drop them into a kettle containing about a gallon of boiling water, previously salted a little, and on the bottom an old plate, to prevent their burning. Keep them boiling briskly for ¾ of an hour, covered closely, when they will be done, which may be determined by trying with a fork. Serve hot with cream and sugar, flavored with lemon or nutmeg. Pieplant is very nice served in this way, as well as strawberries, rasp-berries and other fruits, and they always find a ready market at the dinner table."

**Apple Dumplings, Steamed.**—Pare and punch out the core of nice juicy tart apples that will cook quickly; then take light biscuit dough, roll out ½ inch thick and fold around each apple. Put into the steamer to rise, then steam till done. Eat with cream and sugar, or butter and sugar rubbed together, or, what is very nice, maple syrup.

**Apple Tapioca Pudding.**—Soak 1 cup of tapioca over night in 1 qt. of water; pare, core and slice a sufficient quantity of tart cooking apples, and add sugar as needed, with a little water to prevent burning or sticking to the bottom of the pudding-dish; set in the oven to bake, and when nearly done take out the dish and pour over the tapioca and return to the oven until the tapioca jellies. To be eaten with cream and sugar or other sauce, as preferred.

**Apple Custard.**—Stew some tart, tender apples; sweeten and flavor to taste; then when cold pour over them a boiled custard, made of 4 eggs to 1 qt. of good milk, with sugar and nutmeg as you like. Let it be quite cold before served.

**Apple Custard Pie.**—Stewed apples, green or dried, 3 cups; sugar, 1 cup; 6 eggs; milk, 1 qt. Beat the eggs separately, mix the yolks with the apple and sugar, season with nutmeg, add the milk, and lastly the beaten whites of eggs. Bake like a tart without cover.—*Toledo Post.*

**Apple Bird's-Nest Pudding.**—Alternate layers of thinly sliced bread and butter, and good, tart cooking apples pared, cored and sliced. Sprinkle a little sugar over the apples and dust with cinnamon, nutmeg or allspice, as pre-ferred. When the pudding-dish is filled, grate over the last layer, which should be bread, the yellow rind of a lemon, and squeeze over all the juice of the lemon. Bake 1 hour in a slow oven, taking care to avoid burning the top. It will turn out of the dish if the latter has been well buttered. Serve hot, with or without pudding sauce.—*Toledo Post.*

*Remarks.*—I suppose this takes the name of "Bird's-Nest" from its resem-blance when turned out of the dish to the rough outside of a bird's-nest. But it is delicious, all the same, with cream and sugar or rich milk sauce.

**A Delicious Dish With Sweet Apples.**—Bake sweet apples and slice. Sweeten nice cream, flavor with lemon, vanilla or nutmeg, and pour over the apples.—*Old Housekeeper in Blade.*

*Remarks.*—I think you now have the greatest variety of nice dishes made with apples, that the author has ever seen in one connection; one idea, now, as to prevent the loss of apples by freezing, and I will close the subject. If in the house keep in a closet, or some dark place, and keep covered until thawed out, which it is claimed will save them, by preventing softening and rotting. I think this was first given in the "Household" of the Detroit *Free Press.* And when frozen they may be cooked by putting into a covered dish, and cooked with hardly a perceptible difference.

**TOMATOES—Escaloped.**—Peel and cut the tomatoes in slices ¼ inch thick; make a force-meat of bread crumbs, pepper, salt, butter and a little white sugar; put this in a pudding dish with alternate layers of tomatoes, having the tomatoes for the top layer (except with dry crumbs as below); put a bit of butter upon each slice and dust with salt, pepper and a little sugar; strew with dry bread crumbs and bake, covered, half an hour, then remove the lid and bake brown

**BEANS—Old, to Cook Properly, Baked or Boiled.**—When beans are kept over a year or more they become rather difficult to cook tender. One way to accomplish it is to soak them over night in soft water, and in the morning put them to boil, putting ¼ tea-spoonful of soda into the water (and especially must the soda be used too when you have any time strong water to boil with). The water must be turned off as soon as it boils, and changed two or three times. Have a tea-kettle of boiling water ready to cover them when the other is poured off, as cold water hardens them again. After they begin to crack open they should be put in the oven, with a piece of pork previously freshened, and water enough to keep them from burning, and bake about two hours.

*To Boil.*—The only thing different is to keep them in the kettle with the pork, being a little careful that the amount of water put in is only sufficient to have them only nice and moist when done, as it leaves them richer than if too much water is used; but if there is much water left when the beans are taken up with a skimmer, it will help enrich the porridge or broth next below.

*Remarks.*—Beans are not only a very healthful dish, but they contain more nourishment than any of the other vegetables in use; and as they—properly cooked—are also easy of digestion, they ought to be much more frequently found on every table, for the rich, as well as for the laborer, whom I do not call poor, for if he enjoys his labor as he should, he is the richer of the two. Either baked or boiled beans, warmed up, putting in sufficient hot water to keep them moist, are sweeter and nicer, to the author's taste, than when first cooked—always prepare, then, more than will be eaten at the first meal.

**Bean Porridge or Broth.**—When the beans are skimmed from the kettle leave a tea-cupful or more in the kettle. Set it upon top of the stove where the beans will slowly cook fine. Then season with sufficient salt, pepper, and butter to make it relish, and, with good graham bread and butter, it makes a soup fit for a king or a dyspeptic. With this, also, if more is made than needed at the first meal, it is best, the old saying is, (and it is true, too, if warmed every day), "when nine days old."

**Boston Baked Beans.**—An excellent and favorite dish with every New England family, if carefully prepared: Get a red, earthen jar (I believe the red ones are unglazed and, therefore, preferred). It should be 14 to 16 inches deep, with a wide mouth. Get the beans at a first-class grocery, lest they should be old or poor in quality; pick, wash and soak them over night in plenty of cold water; scald them the next day with a tea-spoonful of soda; they should not boil unless they have been long stored. Drain off the water twice, at least, to remove the taste of the soda, and to each 3 pts. of beans, before soaking, allow 1½ lbs. of good, sweet, salt pork—a rib piece, not too fat, is best. Let the beans cover all but the top of the pork, which must have been freshened if very salty, the rind scraped and scored; adding hot water enough to cover the beans, in which half a small cup of molasses has been dissolved. They should be put in the oven at bed-time, while there is still a moderate fire remaining. They will be ready in the morning. If the pork is not very salt, add a little salt to the water in which the beans are baked.—*Boston Herald.*

**Pork and Beans—Short, or Kansas Plan.**—Pick the beans over carefully, and put into an earthen crock, and fill with cold soft water, and let stand over night; if the pork is too salt parboil it a short time, scrape the rind, and score it; put it, with the beans into a deep baking dish (why not bake them in the crock, the same as the Bostonians above—we know there is much less danger of burning in an earthen jar than in a tin or other metal dish), with hot water cover closely (this is certainly important at first), and set in the oven, and let them bake rather slowly until noon, or from 3 to 4 hours. Do not let them get too dry; if you can not see the water add more hot.—*Kansas City Times.*

*Remarks.*—Although there is, and must be, more or less sameness in all the above plans of cooking beans, yet there is sufficient difference in some things to justify the number I have given. The following will also be found valuable in cooking beans and corn together in winter, warming up, drying string beans, etc.:

**Winter Succotash.**—This may be made with Limas, horticulturals, garden beans, or white field beans. The latter are seldom used for succotash, but they make it very nicely. The method of proceeding in each case is the same. Boil the beans without soaking until three-fourths done. In the meantime put an equal amount (dry) of dried sweet corn with 3 qts. water, and let it steep on the stove for 2 hours without boiling, then add to it the beans, and let them cook together gently until the beans are done. Serve warm and do not break the beans.

**Beans or Succotash, To Warm.**—Put either beans or succotash into shallow dishes and cover with a little hot water. Heat slowly, and do not stir while warming, as that makes them mussy. If they are likely to burn put them back where there is not so much heat. Dish them up with a flat ladle so as to mash them as little as possible. An excellent dish for breakfast. In fact, baked beans, or any dish with beans in it, like bean porridge (which see), is all the better for having been warmed over—the more times the better the dish.

**String Beans for Winter Use.**—Some writer in the "Household" department of the *Blade* informs us, and I have not a doubt of the fact, that string beans can be kept for winter use nicely, in the following manner: "String, but do not break them, scald a few minutes, then dry by fire heat, turning frequently so that they do not sour. When dry enough to rattle, put away in closely-tied paper sacks. To cook them, soak over night and dress the same as fresh. They taste more like green beans than dried corn does like green.

**Corn, To Fry**—Cut corn from the cob till there is about a quart of it, and carefully pick out all bits of stalk or silk. Beat 2 eggs very light, stir them into the corn, with 2 table-spoonfuls of flour, salt and pepper. Have some lard very hot, and drop in the corn a heaping teaspoonful (the author would say a table-spoonful) at a time. Fry a light brown. Canned corn may be used in the same way.

**Corn Oysters.**—Nine ears of corn, 2 eggs, 2 table-spoonfuls of flour, pepper and salt. Cut the rows of corn length-wise, and then scrape it off the cob; beat the eggs light, add the flour, pepper, and salt, and fry the cakes about the size of an oyster in butter.

*Remarks.*—These recipes are much the same, but make a very nice dish for breakfast.

**TOAST—With or Without Milk, and to Use Bread Crusts, Dry Bread. etc.**—A lady writer gives her sisters the following plans of saving bread which has been cut in larger quantities than needed, crusts, etc., which many throw away because they do not know how to use them. Her plans will prove a success, every time when followed with judgment. She says:

"There are times when bread accumulates and is thrown away. We can not make toast, for we have only just a little milk to spare. Let us tell you how to make a good-sized dish of toast with only one cup of milk—or none at all. Toast each slice of bread nicely and brown; have a basin of hot water on the stove; salt the water a little, and dip each slice of toast, 1 at a time, into it. Let it remain a moment. Then lay it on the dish you wish to serve it in. Immediately on taking it from the hot water spread a thin slice of butter on each piece of bread, and so on until your dish is full. It is good just so. But to give it the appearance of milk toast, heat your small quantity of milk, add a little lump of butter, a pinch of salt, and hot water enough to just cover the toast and no more.

**Bread Crusts, for Balls, or Dressing.**—If you have scraps and broken crusts which cannot be toasted, do not throw them away, but soak them until soft, with warm water. Add pepper, salt, and butter, according to taste. Mold into balls like an egg, and lay them in a pan with a roast of beef; turn them when brown and serve with a rich gravy, and you will think it a rich, nutritious dish.

*Remarks.*—You will not only think it a rich nutritious dish, but it will be such, in fact.

**Milk Toast, No. 1.**—First toast the bread and lay it in a deep dish; then put a lump of butter the size of an egg in a frying pan; add 1 heaping table-spoonful of flour, and stir until it begins to brown; then pour in 1 pt. of sweet milk and a little salt, and pour this over the bread. If you like it sweet, add sugar, to your taste.

*Remarks.*—The ground work of this recipe was from a Mrs. S. Bearnes, to the *Blade*, in which she also gave an endorsement of the new plan of using strong soda water on burns (which see, among the recipes for burns), but I will give her plan in her own words. She says: "I want to tell you how I cure a burn. Wet a cloth in strong soda (baking soda) water, and wrap around the burn, or lay a little soda on and dampen it and let it remain a few minutes." If she had given her post-office address, I should have given it too. I have come as near as possible to giving her full credit. The wet cloth is the best plan.

**Milk Toast, No. 2.**—Cut slices of bread very thin, toast quickly to a light brown; butter, while hot, and pile them in a deep dish; then cover them with rich boiling milk. Let it stand a few minutes and serve. A little salt may be added if necessary.

**Milk Toast, No. 3.**—The following is from a writer in the *Rural New Yorker*, and gives a new thought or two, so I give it a place. She says: "A good way to dispose of dry bread is to make it into milk toast. It is very popular with the workingmen and children, and often solves the problem that disturbs the cook when she is thinking what is to be got for supper. Toast the bread a short time before it is wanted. Set a half pan of milk on the stove and let it get scalding hot. Put in a little salt, spread the toasted slices with butter and put them into the hot milk, and in a very few minutes remove to the table. If the toast is put in too soon, the bread will fall in pieces and is not so nice to serve. There should be plenty of milk for the amount of bread."

*Remarks.*—I think it will be popular with everyone. I have made an entire supper of it many times.

**Boston Cream Toast.**—Cut stale bread in slices ¼ inch thick, and toast a nice light chestnut color. Put 1 pt. of milk to heat with ½ cup of butter, a little pepper, and salt to suit the taste. Blend 2 large tea-spoonfuls of flour with cold milk, and when it boils, stir in and let it boil 2 or 3 minutes.—Now have ready a pan of hot water, a little salted, dip each slice quickly in the water, lay in a hot dish and cover with the hot cream. Serve immediately.

II. Another nice dish is made by rolling light bread dough thin, cutting in strips and boiling in hot fat. Break each cake open as it comes from the kettle, and plunge it into the above cream.

*Remarks.*—As Boston claims to be the "hub" upon which the world turns, I have thought to close the toast making with the Bostonian plan of making cream toast, as given by "P." of Toledo. It will be found very nice, and the second dish, or plan, using the same cream, will undoubtedly suit many persons—try them both, if fond of nice dishes.

**Bread to Fry in Batter.**—One table-spoonful of sweet, light dough; make it into a thin batter by 1 cup of sweet milk; add 3 or 4 eggs, 1½ cups of flour, and 1 tea-spoonful of salt. Cut light bread into thin slices, dip into this batter, and fry in hot lard. Sprinkle with powdered sugar and garnish with jelly, if desired.

*Remarks.*—When you have not the light dough on hand to make into a batter, simply beat an egg or two, according to the number of persons to fry for, add a little salt and a very little flour, rubbed smooth in a little cold water; dip in your slices of bread and fry as above, or, I think, butter or drippings is better than lard, as the lady says in " Frying after Ham."

**Fried Bread, After Ham.** — After frying good smoked ham or shoulder, beat 2 eggs and ½ cup sweet milk together, dip slices of stale bread in this, wetting both sides; fry and turn quickly.—*Mrs. M. C. Wanemaker, New-ville, Ind., in Blade.*

**Bread Pudding, Fried.** — When you have bread pudding left over from dinner, it is very nice, next morning, to cut it into slices; then dip each side into cracker crumbs; then into beaten eggs, slightly salted, and again into the crumbs; then fry a nice brown, in hot fat to float them; take out with a skimmer or ladle, and drain a moment; serve hot, with powdered sugar over them.

**French Toast.**—Any meat left over from roast beef, veal, turkey or chicken is to be freed from bone, finely chopped, using the gravy left, or a beaten egg and a little butter, to moisten it; while quite hot, the toast being all ready and nicely buttered, put the mixture over each piece, and send to the table hot.

*Remarks.*—The French people are not only careful to save everything in the line of food, but always re-make it into some nicer dish than at first, and which you would not suppose to have been served before. In this is the secret, not only of their living well, but cheaply.

**Stale Bread, to Fry, or Egg Toast.**—Take 2 eggs, beat well; 1 cup of milk, and flour to make a stiff batter. Cut stale bread into thin slices, and dip into the batter, and fry a nice brown, in sweet butter. Serve hot, with butter, sugar or sauce, as you choose.

*Remarks.*—With coffee alone, or with other articles, this makes a nice dish for breakfast. Well, now, at the risk of being a little out of place with the following plan of cooking eggs, as it is for a breakfast dish, and as these toasts are most generally used at breakfast, I shall give a plan of cooking eggs for breakfast in this place, although it properly belongs with the egg dishes. It will be found very nice, and is as follows:

**Eggs, Fried or Baked, for Breakfast.** — Put a table-spoonful of butter into a tin-plate, upon the top of the stove, and break in 10, or any number of eggs needed for the meal, a little salt and pepper, allowing the eggs to cook until the whites are "set;" then slip the tin-plate into a china, or stone-ware plate, and send to the table hot. If your stove-oven is hot, they will cook in half the time, if put into the oven.

**CUSTARD—How to Make.**—If wanted rich with eggs, some use as many as 8 for 1 qt. of new milk, 1 cup of sugar, a little salt, and grated nutmeg to taste. Some persons use only 3 or 4 eggs to a qt. of milk—suit yourself, therefore, when they are not plenty. Vanilla or lemon extract may take the place of nutmeg for a change. DIRECTIONS—Eggs to be well beaten, and the sugar then beaten in to get it all dissolved; then the milk and seasoning; place in a pudding-dish, or in cups, which is the more tasty way, and bake in a slow oven about ½ hour, or until the custard is firm in the center—when it is done. Some times nutmeg and lemon-peel are grated over the top of a custard, when served, in place of mixing in when made.

**Custard, Frosted.**—Five eggs well beaten (reserving three whites for meringue), 1 qt. of milk, 5 table-spoonfuls of sugar, 2 tea-spoonfuls of vanilla, pinch of salt; put in a pudding-dish, which place in a pan of water in the oven and bake. When nearly baked, put upon the top the meringue made with the 3 whites and 2 table-spoonfuls brown sugar to each white, and any flavoring. Bake a light brown.—*Domestic Monthly.*

**Custard, Without Eggs.**—New milk, 1 qt.; flour, 4 table-spoonfuls; sugar, 2 table-spoonfuls; nutmeg or cinnamon to your liking, and a little salt. DIRECTIONS—Place the milk over a quick fire, and as soon as it boils, having rubbed the flour smooth in a little cold milk, stir it in, and as soon as scalded, add the sugar, spices and salt. Bake, of course.

**St. James Custard.**—Place over the stove 1 pint of milk, in which put one large handful of bitter almonds that have been blanched and broken up. Let it boil until highly flavored with the almonds; then strain and set it aside to cool. Boil 1 qt. of rich milk, and when cold, add the flavored milk, ½ pt. of sugar and 8 eggs, the yolks and whites beaten separately, stirring all well together. Bake in cups, and, when cold, place a macaroon (a cake highly flavored with almonds) on top of each cup.

**French Tapioca Custard.**—Five dessert-spoonfuls of tapioca, 1 qt. of milk; 1 pt. of cold water; three eggs; one heaping cup of sugar; one tea-spoonful of vanilla, and a little salt. DIRECTIONS — Soak the tapioca in the water five hours. Let the milk boil in a farina-kettle or in a kettle set into boiling water; add the tapioca and water, and a little salt. Stir until boiling hot, then add the beaten yolks and sugar. Stir this constantly about five minutes, but do not let it get too thick, or the custard will break. Pour into a bowl, and add the whites of the eggs previously beaten to a stiff froth; stir them in gently. Flavor and set aside in a glass dish till cold. Serve with canned or brandied fruits; it is a very delicious dessert.

*Remarks.*—The French are celebrated for the amount of labor required or the changes to be made, but their dishes are also celebrated for their excellence. The Irish moss or *carrageen,* as called in the next, as well as tapioca, makes a nice dish.

**Carrageen Custard.**—Procure *carrageen* (Irish moss), 1 oz., and divide into 4 parts; 1 part is enough for 1 mess; put the moss into water and let it remain until it swells; then drain it and put it into 2½ pts. of milk and place it over a fire; let it boil 20 minutes, stirring continually; then strain it, sweeten with loaf sugar (any white sugar will do), put into cups, and grate nutmeg over the tops.

*Remarks.*—This is also served cold, of course. Any of the moss that is black, or dark colored, is not fit for this use any more than it is to make a nourishing drink for invalids.

**Apple Custard.**—Pare and punch out the cores of 6 apples (at least 2 for each person to be at dinner); set them in a new tin bread pan with a very little water, and stew them till tender; then put them in a pudding dish without breaking; fill the centers with sugar, and pour over them a custard made of 1 qt. of milk, 5 eggs, 4 ozs. of sugar (1 cup will not be too much), and a very little nutmeg; set the pudding dish in a baking pan half full of water, and bake it ½ hour.   Serve it either hot or cold, at the dinner.

*Remarks.*—For the cold serving, let it be what is left over, as most people like hot dishes for dinner.

**Corn Meal Custard.**—Corn meal, ¼ lb.; sweet milk, 1 pt.; boil together 15 minutes; and add butter, ½ lb.; 6 well beaten eggs; rose water, salt and sugar, to taste.   Bake carefully, not to burn the top.

*Remarks.*—As we have corn meal puddings (which see), why not custard also?  I think for the number of eggs 1 qt. of milk might be used, without detriment to the custard, making more, and still be rich enough for most people.  I know it will be nice, if nicely made.  Custards are generally served cold, at "tea;" but this would be nice hot for dinner, as well as cold at tea-time.

**Snow, or Rock Cream, a Substitute for Custard.**—"Boil a cup of rice in new milk till quite soft, sweeten with powdered sugar and pile upon a dish.   Lay upon it, in different places, bits of currant jelly or preserved fruit of any kind.   Beat the whites of 5 eggs with a little powdered sugar to a stiff paste, flavor with vanilla, and add to this, when beaten very stiff, a table-spoonful of rich cream and drop over the rice roughly, giving it the form of a rock of snow."

*Remarks.*—Ornamental as well as a delicious dish at tea.

**ESSENCES—Lemon and Others.**—As lemon and other essences or flavoring extracts are called for with custards and other dishes, in this connection there can be no better place than here (between the custards and ice-creams) for them.   The following is from a lady writer, no doubt—S. A. C., of Oconee, Ill.—and will be found practical and good.   She says:  "Best alcohol, 1 pt.; lemon oil, 1 oz.; the peel of 2 lemons; put all in a fruit jar; let it stand 1 week, shaking 2 or 3 times daily; remove the peel and bottle for use.   I have used it 2 years and pronounce it much better than any I ever bought.   Nearly all essences are made in the same proportion as lemon."

*Remarks.*—This writer is correct as to the proportions.   The peel gives lemon, orange, etc., an improved flavor.   A fruit jar filled with lemon or orange peel, then filled with alcohol without the oils, makes a nice, highly-flavored extract.   The author has made them for his wife, in her life-time, many times.   Sliced pineapple, no doubt, will do equally well for that most delicious flavor.

**Ice-Creams and Water Ices, Strawberry.**—As the "Widow Bedott," of Nettleton, Mo., gives one to the *Blade*, which is perfectly plain, I will give it first.   She says: "Rub 1 pt. of ripe strawberries through a sieve, add 1 qt. of cream, ¾ lb. of white sugar and freeze."

*Remarks.*—No "foolin'" with this; it is perfect, having the pure flavor of the strawberry and the richness of the cream itself, without alloy. But as some persons will want a more elaborate one, we give the following, although I do not know its originator:

**Parisian Ice-Cream, the Best.**—Rub well together 12 eggs and 1¼ lbs. of white sifted sugar; then add 2 qts. of perfectly fresh and pure cream; flavor as below named and cook in a farina boiler—a tin vessel set in a larger one containing hot water—stirring constantly till it thickens, but it must not curdle. Strain through a fine sieve and put on ice to cool. [The author can see no reason to strain, except it be to get the sugar all dissolved unless some of the egg curdles.] The more slowly the freezing is performed the firmer will be the product. When completed let it remain in the freezer with fresh ice and salt around it for several hours to ripen. [This is the French of it.]

**For Flavors for Ice-Creams.**—For 2 qts. use either 1 table-spoonful of extract of vanilla, 1 table-spoonful of extract of lemon and of lemon juice, or 1 pt. of finely strained strawberry juice with 4 ozs. of sugar, or 3 ozs. of chocolate and 4 ozs. of sugar dissolved in a little water and strained. Or the berries themselves or nice ripe peaches, as in the next recipe.

**Ice Cream with Berries or Peaches.**—Fruit frozen with custard may not be particularly good for the digestion, but as it is a popular dish, it is well to know how to insure success when preparing it. Take 1 qt. of milk and 1 qt. of cream, 6 eggs, 3 cups of sugar. It is a good plan when making any custard to beat the yolks of the eggs and the sugar together; then all the lumps can be crushed without difficulty and there is less danger of the eggs looking stringy. To this quantity of custard one large pint of ripe berries, or peaches cut in small pieces, is the due allowance. To my taste 1 qt. is not too many. Heat the milk and cream, then add slowly the sugar and eggs. Cook it in a farina kettle, or in a pail set in a pan of water. When thick take from the fire, remembering that it will be a good deal thicker when it is cold. When cold stir in the fruit, and freeze as you do any ice cream.

*Remarks.*—This was published in the *London (Ont.) Free Press*, sent me by my daughter, Mrs. Dr. Mills, living there, and I will vouch for it, and support the writer in the use of the quart instead of a pint of the berries. Strawberries, raspberries, red or black; blackberries, either should be perfectly ripe; or perfectly ripe peaches, cut into quite small pieces, may be used with satisfaction without other flavoring. Mix in well just before putting into the freezer.

**Ice Cream Lemon.**—Nice morning's milk, 10 qts.; sugar 10 cups; yolks of 10 eggs; corn starch, 3 table-spoonfuls; extract of lemon, 1 table-spoonful. DIRECTIONS—Pour a quart or two of the milk upon the sugar, and see that the sugar is thoroughly dissolved; rub the corn starch smooth in a little of the milk and stir in with the beaten yolks of the eggs, then the extract, and freeze at once, as but little time can be given to it at hotels or picnics.

*Remarks.*—I have eaten it, and know it is very nice. The following is also made by the same confectionery cook, who gave me the recipes while I was treating a sister of hers, whom she came in often to see, and hence the acquaintance and this information.

**Water Ices, Lemon.**—Fourteen lemons, whites of 18 eggs, sugar, 10 cups; vanilla extract, 1 tea-spoonful; water. DIRECTIONS—Pour over the sugar 3 qts. of boiling water, and boil 10 minutes; add 6 qts. of ice water and the juice of the lemons; then the beaten whites of the eggs, and vanilla, and freeze.

*Remarks.*—Of course, these water ices are simply the juices of any fruit you desire the flavor of, diluted with water, properly sweetened to taste, and frozen the same as ice cream. If you wish to use fruits, as oranges, berries, etc., which contain but little acid, the flavor may be heightened by the addition of the juice of a lemon or two, according to the amount being made, as the following:

**Orange Ice.**—To avoid the seeds, etc., press out and strain the juice of 1 dozen good-sized Florida or other sweet oranges, rubbing off the yellow zest of 4 of them with lump sugar, if obtainable, otherwise grating finely, or using an equivalent of orange tincture or extract, at least 1 or 2 table-spoonfuls; sugar, 3 lbs., upon which pour 1 gal. of boiling water, dissolving by boiling if necessary. Set in a cold place to cool before freezing.

*Remarks.*—It will be noticed in the first, above, vanilla extract was used, but I should use the extract of the fruit used, as the taste will be truer to nature, while the amount there given I should expect to be wholly lost from the large amount of lemons used. A pint of the juice of strawberries to each 3 qts. of water being used, would give their very nice flavor to an ice; the sugar and other treatment the same. The first time I ate of these water ices was at Cape May, where my son and myself had run down from the Centennial, at Philadelphia, to spend the Sabbath. At that time they were made very plain—all there was of the recipe I got by inquiry was "8 lemons to 3½ lbs. powdered sugar, 1 gal. of water and freeze." But it was very nice, even as then made.

**SALADS, RELISHES, ETC.**—There is probably no branch in the line of made-up dishes that will show a woman's skill to better advantage than in the variety of articles to which she can apply a well made salad to give piquancy—*i. e.*, a pricking or sharp stinging, still a pleasant taste—to her salads or relishes for the dinner or tea-table. These may be eaten hot or cold, but I think that, like myself, most people prefer them made in time to get cold before serving. Sometimes the salt, sometimes the sour, and sometimes the mustard, or other spices may be made the most prominent, as she shall choose, or as the nature of the article used for the body of the salad shall require. Salads give a relish to bread and butter, and comes nearer satisfying all tastes than almost all, if not all, dishes; and if not made too piquant (too strongly spiced) are not as unwholesome as they are generally believed to be. Salad oil—pure sweet oil —which the author has a great dislike for on account of its taste, is the richest article used in making salads; but as the place of the oil can be so nicely filled with melted butter, or rich cream (the butter is considered best), in making a "salad dressing," he recommends rather than condemns their use. Any of the salad dressings may be applied, mixed with simply chopped cabbage, chopped

or sliced potates, or any kind of chopped meat, as well as to the more elabor-
ately mixed dishes.

**Salad Dressings, to Make Cold**—Which may be put upon almost
any cold dish left over from dinner, as cold potatoes, beets, string beans, meats,
chicken or fish, and cabbage, or uncooked cabbage or lettuce in its season; any
of which should be chopped rather finely and heaped in the center of a platter
or bowl of sufficient size to allow mixing with it the salad dressing, to be made
as follows: Take an even tea-spoonful of ground mustard and a salt-spoonful
of salt and mix into a paste with good vinegar. It is best to use a fork for this
and to mix in a soup plate. Now add the yolk of 1 egg, being careful not to
allow the white to follow; stir the yolk thoroughly through the mustard and
begin to add the sweet oil or melted butter, as you prefer, in small portions,
not more than a tea-spoonful at a time, but add continually as you mix. If the
dressing becomes too hard, or looks stringy, add a tea-spoonful of vinegar from
time to time, but not often. It should become a light creamy mass, and it will
if it is properly stirred; and you go on adding oil or butter and vinegar until
you have the necessary quantity (using more mustard and salt at the beginning
and the yolk of another egg, if the quantity is known to be for a half-dozen
persons or more), when you taste to see if it is sufficiently salt or sour or piquant
with the mustard; and if not, add either as you wish. Now this dressing is to
be placed upon the chopped cold potatoes, or other chopped cold article or raw
chopped cabbage or lettuce, and properly mixed through it with the fork, or
two forks may be handier, leaving "rough and rocky" in appearance, or
smoothing down with a knife blade, as you choose.

*Remarks*—If this is used upon any cold article, a few fresh lettuce leaves
may be stuck around the edge, or sliced bits of fresh tender radishes; or a few
salt herrings split into fibers, and laid around, or put upon the dish, will meet
with general favor. Many of these ideas I have taken from the *American Grocer*, a very reliable paper upon any class of subjects, to which it calls public
attention. It is usual, when cold chicken is chopped, or other cold meats, for
the ground work of the salad, to chop the white part of the celery, if you have
it, to make an equal amount as there may be of chicken, or meat, and mix
evenly together; then after the dressing is mixed in, garnish with, or stick
around, the green tops of the celery. When cold potatoes are used for the
salad, men will generally like it better; a small onion is also chopped finely,
and mixed with the potatoes, ladies generally prefer it without, so a compro-
mise might be made by using an onion half the time, or occasionally.

**Salad Dressing, to Make With Heat.**—Although this is particularly adapted to raw, chopped cabbage, or lettuce, in its season, it will be found
nice for cold meat, chicken, etc. Cabbage, ½ a small head; or fresh, crisp
lettuce, in equal amount; vinegar, 1 cup; 1 egg; sugar, 1 table-spoonful; made
mustard, 2 teaspoonfuls; butter, 1 tea-spoonful; a little salt and pepper. DIREC-
TIONS—Chop the cabbage or lettuce finely, stirring the salt and pepper into it,
and put into a bowl, or dish to await the dressing. Beat the egg, sugar and
butter together, and add the mustard and vinegar, stirring well; put the mix-

ture into a stew pan upon the stove, stirring all the time, until it comes to a boil, when it is to be poured over the cabbage, or lettuce, or meat, as the case may be. The articles being all mixed cold it does not curdle; and the constant stirring while heating prevents its curdling during this process. The German girl, who first prepared this for us, brought it to the table hot, as her people prepared it; but there being some of it left over, I found that myself and family liked it better cold. So had it prepared, after this, in time to get cold by placing on ice, whether for dinner or tea. It is nice at either meal. I will also give a few others.

**Salad Dressing for Tomatoes.**—The author's preference for cold salads is shown to be the preference of others also, by the following: Take off the skins with a sharp knife, cut into thin slices, and lay in a salad bowl. Make a dressing by working 1 tea-spoonful each of salt and made mustard, ½ tea-spoonful of pepper, the yolks of 2 hard boiled eggs, with 2 table-spoonfuls of melted butter; then whip in with a fork 5 table-spoonfuls of good vinegar. Pour over the tomatoes, and set on ice or where it is cool for an hour before serving.—*Rural New Yorker.*

**Potato Salad.**—A potato salad is easily prepared, and very nice alone; but if you have any cold fish, as called for in this recipe, it gives an additional relish. If you have no cold potatoes, boil or steam a dozen with their jackets on; when done peel and let stand till entirely cold; then slice them ¼ inch thick; mix with some flakes of cold boiled fish (halibut, cod or salmon) and pour over them a salad dressing made with 6 table-spoonfuls of melted butter or salad oil, 6 table-spoonfuls of cream or milk, 1 table-spoonful of salt, ½ the quantity of pepper and 1 tea-spoonful of ground mustard. Into this mix 1 cupful of vinegar. Boil well, then add 3 raw eggs, beaten to a foam; remove directly from the fire and stir for 5 minutes; when thoroughly cold turn over the salad. Garnish with slices of pickled cucumber, cold beet, hard boiled eggs, celery or parsley.

*Remarks.*—It strikes the author that if there is no cold fish on hand that a sprinkling of cold chopped turnips would do remarkably well, for variety's sake, to mix with the potatoes. They make a nice dish mashed with potatoes, for dinner, why not in a salad also.

**Cream Salad Dressing, in Place of Mayonnaise, or Salad Oil.** —Rub the yolks of 2 hard boiled eggs through a sieve, 1 dessert-spoonful of dry mustard, 1 table-spoonful of butter, 1 tea-spoonful of salt, ½ pt. of cream; either juice of 1 lemon or 2 table-spoonfuls of vinegar, and as much cayenne pepper as can be taken up on the blade of a small penknife. This is a good substitute for mayonnaise (given below), for those who like myself, do not like oil, for any dish of vegetables, chicken, or upon meats, at dinner or tea.

**Mayonnaise, Real, or French Dressing for Salads.**—Yolks of 2 or 3 eggs, 1 lemon, salad oil, 1 tea-spoonful each of pepper, salt, and brown or moist sugar. DIRECTIONS—Mix the yolks of the eggs raw with the pepper, salt and sugar (a wooden spoon is said to be best to work it with); then begin to work in, little by little, the salad oil (the author thinks not above 1 table-spoon-ful for each yolk used—the amount was not given by Warne's Model Cookery (English), from which I quote, but left to depend upon its creaming with the lemon juice), mixing so thoroughly that it may appear a perfect cream. Keep by your side the lemon, cut in two. As soon as the oil and eggs begin to mix, squeeze in some of the lemon juice, adding more oil, drop by drop, (little by little, as above mentioned, I think best, as drop by drop, unless you have a helper to drop it, would be too slow for Americans), then more lemon juice, till all is finished. Let it be a perfect cream before you use it, and mix in a cool place.

*Remarks.*—I have no doubt the mixing in a cool place will be an important point in keeping the oil less "greasy," as we say. In case the lemon juice is not acid enough to make all of a creamy consistence, add by degrees stirring all the time, as much good vinegar as will accomplish it. It is generally used for chicken, but may be used on anything used for salad, by those who prefer the oil, in place of butter or cream. It is simple and easily made.

**Lobster Salad.**—Take the inside of a large lobster, boiled and cold; mince it finely; the yolks of 2 hard-boiled eggs, mashed fine, with 4 table-spoon-fuls of sweet oil, or butter softened; pepper, salt, vinegar, and mustard, to taste; mix all well, and add celery or crisp lettuce, also to taste; then garnish with hard-boiled eggs, sliced, when served.

**Chicken Salad.**—Although there are general instructions that ought to enable any one to prepare a salad for a chicken, yet, as there are some people who can only work upon specific or positive directions, I will give one so explicit and plain that none can go amiss: Take a good-sized spring chicken, weighing 2½ or 3 lbs.; boil it till perfectly tender. When perfectly cold, pick the meat from the bones, and if the skin is at all tough remove it, and chop the meat to the size of peas; also, if you have it, chop the white part of 4 or 5 heads of celery to the same fineness, and mix together just before serving, into which the dressing which has been made in the following manner is to be mixed: Rub the yolks of 2 hard-boiled eggs smooth with 1 tea-spoonful each of mustard and salt, 2 tea-spoonfuls of sweet oil or melted butter; 3 tea-spoonfuls of good vinegar, and if you like cayenne, as much as will take up upon half the length of a penknife blade; chop the whites of the eggs finely and mix in; then mix evenly into the chicken an celery mixture, or chicken alone if you have no cel-ery mixture, and garnish with the green leaves of the celery or other sweet herbs, as you like.

**"The Salad Bowl"—The Poetic Effusion of the Rev. Syd-ney Smith; or, A Clerical Salad Adapted to All Dishes, Whether Meats, Fish or Vegetables.**—Our salads would not be com-plete without this one in verse to help rivet the proportions and other points of importance to the memory of all lovers of salad dressings. He says:

"To make this condiment your poet begs
The powdered yellow of two hard-boiled eggs,
Two boiled potatoes passed through kitchen sieve,
Smoothness and softness to the salad give.
Let onion atoms lurk within the bowl,
And half suspected animate the whole.
Of mordant mustard, add a single spoon,
Distrust the condiment that bites too soon.
But deem it not, thou man of herbs, a fault,
To add a double quantity of salt;
Four times the spoon, with oil from Lucan crown,
And twice with vinegar procured from town;
And lastly o'er the flavored compound toss
A magic *soupçon* of anchovy sauce.
O, green and glorious!  O, herbaceous treat!
'Twould tempt the dying anchorite to eat.
Back to the world he'd tempt his fleeting soul,
And plunge his fingers in the salad bowl.
Serenely full, the epicure would say,
Fate cannot harm me, I have dined to-day."

*Remarks.*—You will notice here that a couple of potatoes are brought in, and the smallest proportion of onion also, and a caution against too much mustard or cayenne, if that is used, not to bite too soon, with twice as much vinegar, also of oil, while some use more oil than vinegar; and, lastly, a *soupçon* only of anchovy sauce (*soupçon* being the French for the least bit), a "suspicion" only that a little has been used, as the anchovy sauce is a highly-flavored sauce, the anchovies with which it is made being a small fish of the herring tribe, having a striking flavor of their own.  A bit of that, if obtained, or a small amount of any of the catsups, Worcestershire or any other sauce, may be added to this or any other salad dressing; but the anchovy nor any other need be used unless you choose.

**SAUCES FOR THE TABLE.**—*Worcestershire Sauce.*—The *Druggists' Circular and Chemical Gazette* gives the following recipe for making Lee & Perrin's Worcestershire sauce, which is undoubtedly the most celebrated and popular sauce in the market.  It is made in such large quantities that few, unless it be those manufacturing sauces, would undertake to make it; but it may be reduced (say by 15, or any less number, if one chooses) so as to bring it down to the wants of a family or neighborhood for the year.  It is as follows: "White wine vinegar, 15 gals.; walnut and mushroom catsups, of each 10 gals.; Madeira wine, 5 gals.; Canton soy, 4 gals.; table salt, 25 lbs.; allspice and coriander seed, powdered, of each 1 lb.; mace and cinnamon, powdered, of each ½ lb.; assafœtida, 4 ozs. dissolved in brandy, 1 gal.  Mix together and let stand 2 weeks.  Then boil 20 lbs. of hog's liver in 10 gals. of water for 12 hours, renewing the waste water from time to time; then take out the liver, chop it fine and mix it with the water in which it was boiled, and work it through a sieve and mix it thoroughly with the strained liquor which has been standing two weeks; let settle for 24 hours and carefully pour off the clear liquor and bottle for use.  Prime."

*Remarks.*—I should think the last part, at least, would have to be filtered, or carefully strained again, to get rid of the sediment from the liver. If for sale, it had all better be filtered. And for me, I should prefer that the assafœtida be left out; yet in this amount, about 60 gals., its distinctive taste would not be noticed.

*Canton Soy, to Make.*—Boil 1 gal of haricot (kidney) beans (I think any large bean will do as well) in sufficient water to soften them; add 1 gal. of bruised wheat, and keep in a warm place 24 hours; then add salt, 1 gal., and water, 2 gals. more, and keep for two or three months in a tightly bunged stone jug. After this, press out the liquor, strain and bottle for use. It is chiefly used for fish. It was originally brought from Japan, made there from a bean known as the *Dalichos soya*, hence, for short, *soy*, or Canton soy, as it was shipped largely from Canton, East Indies. Its relish must come chiefly from the salt, which adapts it more particularly, as I should judge, to fresh fish, or, as in this case, making a nice addition to the Worcestershire sauce.

**Celery Sauce.**—Celery, 2 to 4 large heads; veal or chicken broth, 1 or 2 cups, and cream, or rich milk, 1 or 2 cups (*i. e.*, if 2 heads of celery are used, 1 cup; if 4 heads of celery, 2 cups each of broth and milk); salt and a blade of mace, or a bit of nutmeg; flour and butter (as above explained), 1 or 2 tablespoonfuls; water. DIRECTIONS—Wash the celery carefully, cutting out all dark spots; then boil it 15 minutes in salted water; drain away the water, and cut into dice-like pieces; rub the butter and flour together in a sauce pan, adding the veal or chicken broth, cream, or milk, and the blade of mace or bit of nutmeg, and a little salt, stew gently till the celery is tender and pulpy, when it may be poured over the meat or fowl, or served in a gravy boat, or bowl, and let each person suit himself as to a free or less free use of it. Mace and nutmeg are the only spices that seem to agree with the very fine flavor of celery; but they may, or may not be used, as you choose.

**Celery Sauce (or Puree), as Made in India.**—Clean 3 or 4 heads of nice celery, divide and cut into small pieces, using the white part only; boil it in a sufficient amount of white stock. Season with white pepper, salt and nutmeg. When it is tender add a small piece of butter, rolled in flour, and 3 table-spoonfuls of cream. Warm it up again, but do not let it boil. Poured over turkey, chicken or wild duck.—*Indian Domestic Economy and Cookery.*

**Mint Sauce (or Puree), as Made in India.**—Wash nicely half a handful of young, freshly gathered green mint; pick the leaves from the stalks, mince them very fine, and put them into the sauce boat, with a spoonful of sugar, and 4 spoonfuls of vinegar. Served with hot or cold roast lamb, or mutton.—*Indian Domestic Economy and Cookery.*

*Remarks.*—The word *puree* is becoming so common, I will give the following explanation of it:

**Puree, Explanation of.**—The word comes from India, and means a soft, pulpy mass, or sauce, made from either meats or vegetables, fruit, etc., reduced by cooking, beating, mashing and, if necessary, rubbing down to a smooth pulp in a mortar, and then mixing with a sufficient amount of liquid, whether it be stock or broth, for gravies; or milk, cream, etc., for sauces. A puree, then, signifies a sauce, taking its distinguishing name from the meat, vegetables or fruit from which it is prepared, seasoning being added to suit the kind being made. A catsup is really a puree of tomatoes. So whenever you see the word, which has now, even, become quite common in our own country, you will understand, at once, its character and manner of preparation. I have explained in other places that butter they call *ghee*; salt, with them, is *nemuck*.

**Sauce for Beefsteak, or Catsup Improved.**—Black pepper, whole, and salt, of each 1½ ozs.; allspice, whole, horse-radish and small pickled onions, of each 1 oz.; ground mustard, ½ oz.; good catsup, 1 qt. DIRECTIONS—Pound the pepper and allspice finely, then bruise the radish root and onions together, and put all into the catsup, in a jug, cork and shake daily for 2 weeks, and strain through coarse muslin and bottle for use; or moderate heat, applied to all, in a sauce pan, for 2 or 3 hours, then strained, will obtain the full strength of the spices. If too thick for use after the heat, thin suitably with good vinegar.

*Remarks.*—It will be found very nice for any roasted or boiled meats, as well as steak.

**Chili Sauce.**—Large, ripe tomatoes, 20; good sized onions, 6; large green peppers, 3; salt, 3 table-spoonfuls; brown sugar, 6 table-spoonfuls; ground cinnamon, 3 tea-spoonfuls; ground ginger, 2 small tea-spoonfuls; ground cloves, ½ tea-spoonful; good vinegar, 6 cups. DIRECTIONS—Mash the tomatoes, chop or slice the onions and peppers, mix all in a porcelain kettle or large tin pan, and boil till perfectly soft, and when cool rub them through a colander, and cook down to a proper consistency, that of catsup, and bottle for use upon meats, chicken, turkey, etc.

*Remarks.*—To "bottle," means to bottle and cork tightly. And all sauces, catsups, etc., should be kept in a cool cellar, except the one being used from.

**Piccalilli, A Good Substitute for Sauces.**—Green tomatoes, 1 pk.; 1 large cabbage, 1 dozen onions; chop them fine and put on ½ pt. of salt and let them stand over night; then drain off the brine, and scald in weak vinegar and drain off again; and now add 6 good-sized green peppers chopped fine, having removed the seeds before chopping; ½ to 1 pt. (as you like best) of grated horseradish; then season with ground spices to suit the taste, at least 1 table-spoonful of allspice and pepper, and half as much dry mustard; and also ½ table-spoonful of cloves. Now, in packing in a jar, if 6 to 8 or 10 quite small cucumbers (whole), which have stood in salt and water over night, are put upon each layer of an inch or two in thickness, they will be found a valuable addition, putting one in each sauce dish when served at table. Then all being closely packed, just cover with good vinegar, boiling hot, and cover closely, or put up in fruit jars, if plenty, and you will have a dish, as the saying is, "nice enough for a king," the author says nice enough for a better man than a king—nice enough for "an American citizen."

**Chow Chow With Cucumbers.**—Take 6 large cucumbers just before they ripen, peel them, cut in strips, and remove the seed; 4 white onions, 6 good-sized green tomatoes, and ⅛ a head of cabbage. Chop all fine, let them stand in salt water over night, then pour off the water and add vinegar and spices to suit the taste.—*Tribune.*

*Remarks.*—See piccalilli to judge about the amount of spices, the principal difference being that cucumbers are in the lead in place of tomatoes and cabbage. Three or 4 green peppers can be added if desired in any case, seeded and chopped as in the piccalilli.

**Chow Chow Without Cucumbers.**—Take to 1 peck of green tomatoes, 6 large onions, 1 dozen green peppers, 1 large cabbage; slice the tomatoes, sprinkle over them 1 tea-cupful of salt, let them stand over night, drain off the liquor, chop fine, add the onions, cabbage and peppers, also chopped fine; put on the fire to cook, with enough cider vinegar to cover, then add black pepper, cinnamon, cloves and allspice to suit the taste. Cook till tender, then cover closely in jars, but it will keep without sealing.

**Cole Slaw.**—When cabbage is cut fine, seasoned with pepper, salt, vinegar, and a little sugar, it is generally called " Cold Slaw," but our heading is the right one, as it was originally made from the stalk and tops of a species of the cabbage family, but which does not head like the cabbage—kale, probably, the leaves of which curl and wrinkle, but does not head properly. For ½ head of cabbage finely chopped, about 1 table-spoonful of sugar, a pretty free use of pepper and salt, with good vinegar, makes a nice dish with but very little trouble.

**Cole Slaw With Cream.**—For ½ head of cabbage, chopped fine, take ½ cup sweet cream, ½ as much vinegar with a table-spoonful of sugar in it, and mix with the cream; having salted and peppered the cabbage, pour over the mixture when ready to serve. Is also very fine.

**Cole Slaw With a Hot Dressing.**—Slice and chop very fine 1 head (or enough for the family) of cabbage, and season with salt and pepper. Beat 3 eggs well together; mix with it 1 cup of vinegar, 1 tea-spoonful of unmixed mustard, 1 table-spoonful of sugar, and 1 table-spoonful of butter. Bring to the boiling point and pour over the cabbage.

*Remarks.*—If the yolks only are beat and put in at first, and the whites beat and put in after removing from the fire, there will be no danger of curdling —the whites of eggs are very liable to curdle, especially if not stirred all the time while heating with the other ingredients. If not eaten till it gets cold, I should prefer it for my use to leave the butter out, to prevent a kind of greasiness in taste and appearance.

**Hot Slaw.**—Butter the size of an egg, ½ cup of milk, yellow of 2 eggs, 1 tea-spoonful of salt, ¼ tea-spoonful of pepper, small level tea-spoonful of dry mustard, and 3 table-spoonfuls of vinegar. Put the butter into the skillet with the fine cut cabbage and the other ingredients, and stir all the time until the cabbage heats well through.—*Western Rural.*

*Remarks.*—The following will also be found a very nice way to cook cabbage for variety's sake.

**Cabbage Baked, Very Nice.**—Select a firm head of white cabbage, quarter, rinse, and boil 15 minutes; pour off this water, and put on more hot water and continue to boil until tender; drain off the water and set aside till cold; chop fine and season with salt and pepper, and a table-spoonful of butter; beat 2 eggs well, then beat them into 3 table-spoonfuls of rich milk, or cream is better; mix all well together, and bake in a moderate oven till nicely browned. —*Farmer's Wife, in Toledo Blade.*

*Remarks.*—I knew from the nicety of the dish that she was a wife that a farmer ought to be proud of, or, as the saying goes now, might well afford to "tie to." The same of the following:

**Baked Cabbage With Grated Cheese.**—Boil a firm white cabbage for 15 minutes in salted water, then change the water for more that is boiling and boil until tender. Drain and set aside until cool, then chop fine. Butter a baking-dish and lay in the chopped cabbage. Make a sauce in this way: Put 1 table-spoonful of butter in a pan; when it bubbles up well stir in 1 table-spoonful of flour, add ½ pt. of stock and ½ pt. of water, both boiling. Stir until smooth, season to taste with pepper and salt, and mix well with it 4 table-spoonfuls of grated cheese. Pour this over the cabbage, sprinkle rolled cracker over it, dot with lumps of butter and place in a quick oven for 10 minutes. This is almost as good as the more aristocratic cauliflower when cooked in the same manner.

**Currie Powder, as Made in India.**—Take coriander seeds, well roasted, 2 ozs.; tumeric, pounded, 2¼ ozs.; cummin seed, 2 ozs.; fenugreek, ½ oz.; mustard seed, dried and cleaned of husks, ½ oz.; ginger, dried, 2 ozs.; black pepper, 2 ozs.; dried chillies (the pod of the Guinea pepper; we use our common cayenne), 1½ ozs.; poppy-seed, 1½ ozs.; garlic, 1½ ozs.; cardamons, 1 oz.; cinnamon, 1 oz.; all ground finely and mixed well and bottled.

*Remarks.*—As to the roasting of the coriander seeds, I should not, nor should I use the fenugreek. We use it only in horse medicines in this country, so far as I know. The poppy-seed I should not care to use, either; they may do for East Indians who eat so much opium, but should not want them "in mine." I will give a recipe from the Detroit *Tribune* which, I have no doubt, was the kind of currie powder used in making the chicken currie given in another place, of which I partook, and have explained there, as the lady there referred to told me she obtained the powder in Detroit already made. I will only say here I like it extremely well. If the amount given there to make a currie proves too hot of cayenne use less of the powder next time. It is certainly warming and comforting, even to a dyspeptic stomach, and I believe healthful for any one.

**India Currie Powder Americanized.**—Take of ground cinnamon, mace and cloves, each, 1 dr.; coriander seed and fresh yellow tumeric, each, 2 ozs.; black pepper and small cardamon seeds, each, ½ oz.; cayenne, ¼ oz. Put all through a good mill and mix well; put in a closely-stopped bottle.

*Remarks.*—The tumeric is of no particular value, except to give color to the powder. It has slight aromatic and stimulant properties, but they are so slight it is seldom used in medicine except to color ointments, etc. So if the color (yellow) is not desired, it can be left out without detriment to the powder. If this powder is not as hot with cayenne as some may desire increase the amount by ½ dr. or whole dr. at the next making. It is better to add to rather than to get in too much at first to suit those who cannot bear the cayenne if too much is put in. For myself, I should prefer to add ½, or at least ¼, oz. of ginger root to this currie powder and leave out the tumeric altogether, as the ginger is both aromatic and stimulating and a very healthful article, as well as pleasant to the taste, while the tumeric, as mentioned before, is only for its color.

**Catsup, Tomato.** — The editor of the *Journal of Commerce* says the following recipe for tomato catsup has been in use in his family for fifty years. Certainly it is old enough to be a good one. He says: Take 1 bushel of tomatoes, cut them in small pieces, boil until soft, then rub them through a wire sieve, add 2 qts. of the best cider vinegar, 1 pt. of salt, ¼ lb. of whole cloves, ¼ lb. of allspice, 1 table-spoonful of black pepper, 1 good-sized pod of red pepper (whole), and 5 heads of garlic. Mix together and boil until reduced to one-half the quantity. When cold strain through a colander and bottle, sealing the corks. It will keep 2 or 3 years, as fresh as when first made.

*Remarks.*—With the pod of red pepper in place of so much cayenne, as is generally put into catsups, it will be as strong as most people desire it; but if no red peppers are at hand, a small amount of cayenne, say ½ a tea-spoonful, would equal it. More can be used by any one desiring it stronger, and even if 2 or 3 red peppers were put in it would not be too highly seasoned to suit my taste. Let each one suit himself. If I was making this for myself I should not use only half as much cloves as the editor does; but let each one suit his own taste. Cloves, however, as well as red pepper, or cayenne, are rather piquant (sharp and biting) to the taste.

**Mushroom Catsup.**—The editor, or some writer in the London, Ont., *Free Press,* in answer to an inquiry by " R," gave the following recipe for making mushroom catsup, and as it is quite a common thing with the English people, I will give it, believing it to be better than that made by our own people, who so seldom make it; and as it is called for in making the Worcestershire sauce, previously given, I give it a place. When properly made it is a nice thing, for I obtained some at one time of an English butcher, at Ann Arbor, while I was living there, which had been made by another Englishman living near (all English, you see), and it was splendid. This writer says: " Put alternate layers of mushrooms and salt in an earthen jar, using at least ¼ lb. of salt to 2 qts. of mushrooms, and in this proportion for any amount. Let them stand ½ a day; then cut the mushrooms in small pieces and let them stand 3 days longer, stirring them well once a day; then strain them, and to every quart of juice add allspice and ginger, each ground, ½ oz.; powdered mace, ½ tea-spoonful; and cayenne, powdered, 1 tea-spoonful. Put all into a stone jar, set it in a kettle of boiling water, and let it boil for 5 hours, briskly; then let it simmer in a porcelain kettle for ¾ of an hour. Let it stand all night in a cool place; in the morning drain off the clear liquor and bottle it. Cork the bottles and seal tightly. The smaller bottles you use the better, as the catsup will not keep its distinctive flavor long, if exposed to the air, by opening frequently."

**Currant Catsup, for Baked Beans.**—" A. B. C.," in the *Massachu-setts Ploughman*, gives the following plan for an excellent catsup from currants, which needs no comment of mine. He says: I send you a recipe for making currant catsup, as in my mind it cannot be beat, to any lover of baked beans, as a dressing. To 5 pts. of strained currants (the juice from 5 pts. I understand it to mean), add 3 lbs. of sugar (brown will do nicely); 1 pt. of vinegar; 1 table-spoonful, each, of cinnamon, pepper, cloves, and allspice, and ½ table-spoon-ful of salt (I should not be afraid of a whole one). Scald them well ¾ of an hour, then put in bottles and cork tight; it will keep for years; and as farmers generally have a quantity of currants that go to waste, I would like them to try this, and I think they will never be sorry.

*Remarks.*—The author thinks so too, that no one will be sorry for trying it, although it would seem to me that ¾ of an hour only to scald, or more pro-perly, to boil it, would hardly be sufficient, possibly it may, in all cases; but I would sooner risk it on 2 hours moderate boiling. I know it will be nice while it does not sour—the longer boiling will ensure this—still, if it will " keep for years," it is long enough. It will be as nice on other meats as on pork and beans, hence make plenty of it, if you have the currants that go to waste.

**Grape Catsup.**—Pick 5 pts. of catawba grapes from the stem (Concords or Delawares will do, but are not so tart); wash them and let drain; then sim-mer till they are so soft you can rub all but the seeds through a colander (I think grape seeds will go through an ordinary colander, a wire sieve would be better) with care. After this is done add 2 pts. of brown sugar, 1 pt. of vine-gar, 2 tea-spoonfuls each of allspice and cloves, and 1 table-spoonful of cinna-mon, 1½ tea-spoonfuls of mace, 1 of salt, and ½ a tea-spoonful of red pepper. Put all into a porcelain kettle, let them boil slowly until they are as thick as you like catsup to be. Bottle, cork and seal.—*London, Ont., Free Press.*

*Remarks.*—Keep these proportions for any amount desired to make, it will be found good.

**Cucumber Catsup.**—Cucumbers are said to make a nice relish for meat, in winter, treated as follows: Grate about 3 dozen medium sized green cucumbers and sprinkle pepper and salt to your taste (pretty strong I should say) over them, and allow a small sized white onion for each bottle. Heat enough cider vinegar to cover and pour over. Put up in large mouth bottles, and pour melted wax over the corks. If the air is kept from them, when you open a bottle in mid-winter, the odor will be delightful to the lover of the sometimes dangerous cucumber.

*Remarks.*—It seems to the author that if they were scalded in the vinegar, there would be a greater certainty of keeping nicely, although the cucumber flavor might be not quite so natural.

**Fresh Cucumbers, How to Prepare for the Table.**—Slice them into cold water having plenty of salt in it, for an hour before dinner. In this way there is but seldom any bad effects from their being used freely; and if you have not the hour for soaking, slice into a plate and sprinkle on plenty of salt, then turn another plate over them and shake a few minutes, and drain off the salt water and serve as usual, with vinegar and pepper, and a little more salt if needed, which will also avoid the danger of colics, etc.

**Catsup, When Out, How to Make a Supply.**—When your catsup gets low, or is all gone, take some canned tomatoes and add vinegar and spices, as in the Chili sauce, and boil slowly about 30 minutes, and strain if you choose; it will go further without and be nicer too.

*Remarks.*—As we have just been giving a grape catsup, we will also give the plan of preserving grape juice by canning, as I cannot see why it may not be kept in this way sweet and nice for common service, as well as for mince pies, for which a writer says it is "better far than brandy or cider." The writer says:

**Grape Juice to Can for Common Service, etc.**—Prepare the grapes as for jelly, let the juice be boiling hot, and can it in the same way you do fruit. It is excellent for mince pies, better far than brandy or cider.

*Remarks.*—It can be better only in that it is richer in body and flavor than cider made from a poor quality of apples. If I was going to boil it I should be careful to skim off all the scum that would arise, which would remove all pulp of the grapes, that would have a tendency, if left in the juice, to start a fermentation, although if kept air-tight and in a cool cellar I do not see how it can ferment. It will be purer and clearer, however, if the pulp is thus removed by skimming. Should it be too tart on opening for common purposes, a little sugar might be added to make it more palatable, and still it would be far more pure than much that is purchased for this purpose. Only 1 lb. of lump sugar to each gal. might be put in and dissolved by the heat to remove the scum, which would give it more spirit and also help to preserve it, bottling or canning, remember, while hot.

**Canned or Bottled Wild Grape Juice.**—Pick off all bad ones and scald stems and all with a very little water to start the juice, press out and strain, boil and skim, and can or bottle while hot. Makes a nice drink for the sick or well. One lb. of sugar to 1 gal. of the juice will make a nice wine, in kegs or barrels.

**JELLIES—Jelly Bag, Jams and Preserves, How to Make.**—*General Remarks.*—Jellies have, of late years, become very popular, and are much more frequently used than formerly, and, therefore, the housewife who gets hers up the nicest, *i. e.*, the clearest or most transparent, and having the purest flavor of the fruit of which it is made, carries off the premium of the neighborhood in which she lives. We will do our best, so that all may have them equally nice. In the first place, only the choicest, ripe fruit should be used, if plentiful; if not, use such as you have, but cut out bad spots, and do not pare nor core any of the large fruits, as apples, pears, etc., as much of the flavor is contained in these parts; but they should be washed and quartered, or even cut finer if very large, making all pieces as nearly the same size as practicable; then cook perfectly tender and strain through the jelly bag, pressing as little as possible to get all the juices and not to press the pulp through any more than you can help, nor should any more water be put in in the cooking than is absolutely necessary to prevent burning till the juices start by the heat, never more than to barely cover the fruit.

*The Jelly Bag* is usually made of flannel, 10 or 12 inches across the mouth, and tapering to a point, the whole being 18 or 20 inches long, unless large amounts are to be made, in which case make as large as needed; and if only very small amounts are to be made, straining through a piece of flannel will do. If a bag is made there should be a stout cord around the top to suspend it with, over a pole or some other convenience, to drain thoroughly before any pressure is applied; then, if you choose, for clearness' sake, remove this and set another dish, using the first drained off for your choicest friends. Press out then through the bag all you like, which will be more of a jam than a jelly. Jams and marmalades are much the same, thick and containing all the pulp, or substance of the fruit.

*Jams and Marmalades* contain the *puree* (which see for further explanation of), pulp, or substance of the fruit; while jellies contain only the juices, with 1 lb of nice white sugar to every 1 pt. of the juice—jams, about ¾ lb. will do; while preserves contain the whole fruit, and a pound of sugar to a pound of fruit, but brown sugar may be used with the two last, as it is cheaper and they are not transparent to show the difference. Jams and marmalades (for marmalades, see Quince Marmalade,) need boiling or cooking until they are of a proper consistence, like apple butter, or nearly so; while jellies only need sufficient heat at first to raise the scum, which should be removed as it rises, after which to simply boil for a moment, or a few minutes—5 to 20, perhaps,—according to the stiffness desired; longer boiling, of course, with apples or other fruits which are most watery. Pour into jelly glasses, if you have them, which have covers, otherwise cutting white paper to fit the top of the dish used, dipping it in alcohol (some use brandy, but alcohol is purer), and laying on top of the jelly to prevent moulding; then a paper or cloth, wet in the white of an egg, over the top of the tumbler or other dish, to secure it to the top and from the air, will make all as safe as a rubber and screw-top can will do.

**To Preserve Peaches, Very Nice.**—Pare them, and in quartering remove from the stone. Weigh the fruit thus prepared and allow 1 lb. of sugar (white or brown, as you choose,) for each pound of peaches. Put some sugar in the bottom of the kettle, then peaches, and so on till all are in, having a little sugar left for the top. Set the kettle on the back of the stove to heat gently till the sugar is dissolved; then boil until clear and tender, being careful to break the pieces as little as possible. Take off any scum that rises, and when the fruit is clear, *i. e.*, looks transparent, skim it out and put into your jars to fill them about three-fourths full. Continue to boil the syrup until thick enough, skimming when needed; then fill the jars with the syrup while hot; and it is not amiss, even with preserves or jams, to cover the jar with paper soaked in alcohol before covering with cloths—or coarse paper. If they begin to "work," *i. e.*, to ferment, at any time, they were not boiled enough at first, and it must now be done again. Some people think it gives a better flavor to take the meats from perhaps one-fourth, or more, of the stones, cutting them in bits and steeping in as little water as covers them to get their flavor, and putting it in the syrup while cooking. If I did this I should subject the parings to the same process; and this should be done with pears and quinces, putting in the cores also of them, to ensure their highest flavor. This extra water, of course, will be evaporated in cooking the syrup. Treat berries and other fruits in the same manner; but, if you are not particular, continue the cooking without skimming out the fruit, it is more likely. however, to mash it up and make the preserves look mussy and more like jams or marmalades than preserves. Each one can suit herself.

In making jellies, jams or preserves from any kind of berries, currants, grapes, etc., do not do it in a way to mash the seeds, which would injure their otherwise very fine flavor. All fruit should be ripe to make good jellies. As these refer to making jelly with apples, pears, berries of all kinds, grapes, etc., I need not give special kinds, except those made or flavored with other articles, as chocolate, coffee, rice, farina, lemons, etc. Still, I will give two apple jellies from other writers, to show that the instructions above given are borne out or corroborated by others, and to show the old way of using lemons in making apple jelly, which almost, if not wholly, destroyed the fine apple flavor. The first is from a writer in the *People's Ledger*, the second I do not know from whence it came, but both plans are good for their respective ways of making them:

**Apple Jelly.**—Cut your apples in quarters (do not pare or core them), dip each quarter into clear water, and put them into a jar to cook in the oven until quite tender; then strain the juice as usual, and boil with 1 lb. of sugar to 1 pt. of the juice. The most delicious jelly will be the result, with the full, pure flavor of the apple heightened by the cores having been left in, and not spoiled by the objectionable addition of lemon peel and lemon juice.

**Old-Fashioned Apple Jelly.**—Take 20 large, juicy apples, pare and chop; put into a jar with the rind (yellow part) of 4 large lemons, pared thin in bits; cover the jar closely, and set in a pot of boiling water; keep water boiling hard all around it until the apples are dissolved; strain through a jelly bag, and mix with the liquid the juice of the four lemons; to 1 pt. of juice, 1 lb. of sugar; put in a kettle, and when the sugar is melted set it on the fire, and boil and skim about 20 minutes, or until it is a thick, fine jelly.

*Remarks.*—Here you see the apples were pared, and one-fifth as many lemons used as apples, which would make one think of lemons only, when eating it; but if lemon flavor is preferred, it will do very well to make it in this way. Suit yourselves, now you know both ways. Or you may like the next one better.

**Lemon and Apple Jelly.**—Sugar, 2½ cups; apples, 2 large tart ones; lemons, 2 good sized ones; pare the lemons with a sharp knife to get just the thin yellow, and then peel off the white part, which is bitter, and throw away; pare the apples, then grate them and the lemons; put all into a stew pan and cook a few minutes, then strain or not, as you like.

If not strained it will be a kind of marmalade, or jam; but, if to be strained, the apples need not be pared nor cored, but chopped (the spots and specks having been removed), in which case the inside of the lemons may be chopped also, the yellow peeling being put in for chopping too. Either way it is nice; but if not strained it would be for present eating rather than long keeping, unless an equal weight of sugar was used.

**Apple Cider Jelly.**—Boil nice sweet cider until it becomes a firm jelly, when cold. This, says a writer, is done in a large way, in the ordinary sugar evaporators in which maple sap, or sorghum juice, is boiled; but it may be done in ordinary preserving kettles, if copper or brass. Enameled iron pots may be used, but no plain iron ones, as these give a dark color to the jelly.

*Remarks.*—I should think, that unless sugar was used, nearly, at least, in the proportions given for jellies, generally, they would be too sour, or tart, to please most tastes. I see one Mary, of Napa, Cal., has the knack of making the most jelly I ever heard of, or could imagine, with only 1 pint of cider. Hear her: To 1 pt. of clear, sweet cider, allow 1 pt. of cold water; 2 lbs. of sugar; 1 package of gelatine, 1 large pt. of boiling water. Soak the gelatine until it is entirely dissolved in cold water; then add to this the sugar, a spoonful of cinnamon, the juice of 2 lemons, the grated rind of 2, then the gelatine. Add the cider last; then put all in a thick flannel bag, and let it drain. Do not squeeze it at all. Put it in bowls or glasses, and set it away to cool.

*Remarks.*—This is no doubt the place where the saying started, "as big as a pint of cider." It will make more jelly, notwithstanding the additions over-top the foundation, or starting point, and the taste of cider will be lost, that is all.

**Chocolate Jelly.**—Grate 4 table-spoonfuls, heaping, of chocolate, and put into ½ pt. of cold, sweet milk, with ¾ of a lb. of white sugar. Soak a small package of Cox's or other nice gelatine in cold water enough, only, to cover it, and when softened put it into 1 pt. more of milk and dissolve by heat; and when it boils, pour the milk containing the chocolate and sugar into it, stirring briskly; and when it boils again pour into a mold, or cups, and set it in a cold place. Serve with sweetened cream.

*Remarks.*—Although called, and it will be, a jelly, yet, it is much like a blanc mange. Very nice for those who love the flavor of chocolate.

**Coffee Jelly.**—Mrs. W., of Eau Claire, Wis., sends the following way of making coffee jelly to the *Blade*, of Toledo. She says: Soak ½ a box of Cox's gelatine ½ an hour, in ½ a teacup of cold water—as little water as possible—1 qt. of strong coffee, made as if for the table, and sweetened to taste (it will take considerable sugar); add the dissolved gelatine to the hot coffee, stir well, strain in a mold rinsed with cold water just before straining in; set on ice or in a cool place. Serve with whipped cream. This jelly is very pretty formed in a circular mold, with a tube in the center; when turned out fill the space in the center with whipped cream, heaped up a little.

*Remarks.*—The only objection I can find with this lady, none with the recipe, is that there may be other "Mrs. W.'s" there, so her identity is lost.

I have a sister living there now, a Mrs. Wanzer, but I am pretty sure she is not the one.

**Farina Jelly.**—Boil 1 qt. of new milk; whilst boiling, sprinkle in, slowly, ¼ lb. of farina (kept by grocers); continue the boiling from ½ to a whole hour. Season with 5 ozs. of sugar and 1 tea-spoonful of vanilla. When done (this will be known by its jelling when cooled), turn into a mold and place it on ice to stiffen. Serve it with whipped cream.—*Harper's Bazar.*

**Quince Jelly.**—Wash and wipe, then pare and slice them (as the quince is hard and tough, and also being a dry fruit), put into a stone jar, 1 cup of water to every 4 lbs., with the peeling and cores, by which you get the pure flavor; put the jar into a pan or kettle of boiling water and boil until perfectly soft, the jar being covered; then strain through the jelly bag and use a lb. of sugar for 1 pint of juice, as with other jellies, but do not spoil its purity of flavor by adding any other flavoring. [See, also, "Quince Marmalade," following the jellies.]

**Claret Wine Jelly.**—Gelatine, 1 oz., soaked in cold water, ½ pt., till soft; then boil until dissolved and add a tumblerful of currant jelly, ¾ lb. of white sugar and 1 bottle of claret wine, stirring over the fire until the sugar is dissolved; then beat the whites of 3 eggs and stir in briskly for 2 or 3 minutes, removing from the fire and still stirring 2 or 3 minutes longer, then strain through the jelly bag. If nicely done, it will be clear and of a fine red color.

**Port Wine Jelly, for the Sick.**—Gelatine, ½ oz., soaked and dissolved in 1 gill of water, as in the claret above; add a tea-spoonful of thick gum arabic water, a little grated nutmeg and a table-spoonful of granulated sugar, stirring well together in a stew-pan, adding now good port wine, ½ pt., heating to a boiling point, seeing that the sugar is dissolved, then pour into tumblers. Makes a fine jelly for the sick, to eat as a "jell" or to dissolve in a little cold water as a drink. Very nice when wine is admissible, which it generally is.

**Grape Jelly.**—As a more particular guide in making jelly from any of the berries, currants, etc., and to also corroborate my previous instructions, I will give the plan of a writer in the Detroit *Post and Tribune* for making from grapes. She says: "Pick the grapes from the stems (the same should be done with currants) and simmer them till soft in just enough water to cover them, pour into a jelly bag and strain. Measure the clear liquor in pts. and pour back into the kettle (a bell-metal one is best, scoured perfectly bright) and boil gently 20 minutes, skimming constantly. Then add for every pt. as measured 1 lb. of white sugar and boil until it is hard enough when cold. Heat the glasses and pour into them while hot. Cover with egg paper."

*Remarks.*—I would first put alcohol paper, pressed down along on the top of the jelly, as in our general remarks, to prevent a possibility of mold on the top. Treat strawberries and all other small fruits in the same manner. Raspberries are often mixed with half as many currants, when plentiful, to increase the amount of jelly, otherwise made in the same way. I have never seen any cherry jelly, but I should think it would be nice. It might need a little longer boiling, as their juices are very watery; but the flavor and color would be "tip top."

**Grape Jam, Marmalade, etc., Remove the Seeds for.**—To get rid of the seeds of grapes, with thumb and fingers press out the pulp contain. ing the seeds and throw the skins by themselves. Put the pulps in the kettle with very little water and boil till the seeds will separate easily; then run through a sieve, which retains the seeds; then put pulp and the skins together (the skins may be boiled in a little water till quite tender before mixing); then add the sugar, ¾ to 1 lb., as you choose, to each lb. of grapes and cook as fruits till thick enough to suit. Very nice for pies or as a sauce, and if cooked down rather thick makes an excellent marmalade.

**Tomato Jelly as a Meat Sauce.**—Wash them carefully, if of the rough kind, cut them in pieces and stew them in only sufficient water to prevent burning, strain through the jelly bag, sugar pound for pint, as for other jellies, except boil briskly until it jells, depending upon their being very juicy or not.

**Rice Jelly, or Blanc Mange.**—Boil 1 cup of rice in water, 1 qt., (in the rice kettle is the best way). When perfectly tender, rub through a hair or wire sieve, or mash very smoothly, while as hot as you can work it; sweeten to taste, and flavor with vanilla or nutmeg, and put into a mold or cups to cool. Serve with cream and sugar.

**True Rice Jelly.**—Rice flour and white sugar, each, 1 lb.; boil in water, 1 qt., until the whole becomes glutinous; then strain or drain through the jelly bag, and put into cups, mold, or glasses, as you choose. Very light food, either of these, but also very nutritious.

**Lemon Jelly for Jelly Cake.**—Take 6 large lemons, grate the yellow rind and squeeze out the juice. Mix with them thoroughly, 2 lbs. of sugar. Take 12 eggs, retain the whites of 4, and beat the others thoroughly; then put all together into a saucepan, which place in a pan of boiling water, and boil 15 minutes, stirring constantly. This is very nice to lay up jelly cakes with. The whites retained come in for frosting the cakes, using powdered sugar to make pretty thick if you wish it hard. The less sugar the softer the frosting. At least 1 table-spoonful of sugar to the white of each egg.

**Quince Marmalade or Jam.**—Pare, core, slice, and weigh the fruit, stewing the skins and cores in a dish by themselves, with water enough to just cover. When the parings are tender, turn into a cloth bag, and squeeze out every drop of juice; put the quinces into the kettle, pour over the juice, cover, and let cook slowly, stirring and mashing with a wooden spoon (or potato masher, if very tough,) until the pieces have become a smooth paste. Now add ¾ lb. of white sugar to each pound of the fruit, boil 10 minutes longer, stirring constantly. Remove from the fire, turn into jelly jars and tie down.—*Rural New Yorker.*

*Remarks.*—If this was carefully cooked longer, or until quite thick like apple butter, as remarked above, there would be less requirement for absolutely excluding the air.

**Quinces, A Few When Canning Apples.**—When quinces are scarce I have known a lady with whom I have boarded to put a few with her apples in canning, which, for my taste, at least, made both better. Cooking together, of course, till tender, using sugar to suit the tartness of the apples.

**CANNING FRUITS, CORN, ETC.—How to Avoid Breaking the Cans—General Remarks and Directions.**—It is a conceded fact that if fruit is properly put up in air-tight cans and kept in a dry, cool place, it is safe from fermentation; much difficulty, however, has been experienced by breaking cans when putting in the hot fruit. This difficulty has been entirely overcome by a cousin of mine, Mrs. Joseph Sanders, living near Bear Lake, Manistee county, Michigan, by wringing a large towel out of cold water, rinsing or wetting the can with cold water also, then wrapping the can with the cold, wet towel, being also careful to have the can sit on the towel, and every part covered with two or three thicknesses, and immediately filling with the hot fruit. I have seen her doing it; and a recent letter from a daughter of hers assures me that her mother "has put up her fruit in this way for ten years without break-ing a can." Have no fears in adopting it. After the fruit is canned, and stood an hour or two to cool, re-tighten the tops, as the cooling sometimes leaves them loose enough to admit air; then it is well to turn the cans bottom up over night or long enough to see they do not leak, for, if the juice leaks out, air would leak in and spoil it. It is not necessary to put in sugar when canning, unless you choose to do so. Use enough to make it palatable for the table when used. One-fourth to ½ lb. of sugar to 1 lb. of fruit, according to its sourness, will be found plenty to suit most tastes. For apples, pears, etc., which are not juicy, a syrup made with 1 lb. sugar to 1 qt. of water does well to heat them in and to fill the crevices among the fruit. Observe well these points and no trouble will arise. Rhubarb, it will be observed below, can be put up in jugs; tomatoes I have known to be put up in jugs and keep well; so may other things, also, no doubt, when cans can not be obtained in quantities sufficient. Small cans for small families, however, are best, as the fruits do not keep long after being opened. If a dark room is prepared in the cellar for canned fruit, strawberries and some others will not lose so much of their bright colors as they do in a room where the light is not shut out. With these general directions I need give but few recipes for samples of those out of the general lines of fruit.

**Canning Strawberries.**—A lady says she uses ½ lb. of sugar to 1 lb. of the fruit sprinkling it on over night, then brings to a boil in the morning,— in porcelain or brass,—and keeping it in a dark, cool place, as the light discolors them, although it does not hurt the flavor.

*Remarks.*—This corroborates the author in points that she refers to.

**Canning Grapes.**—Take fully ripe and sound grapes (Concords and Isa-bellas are very nice for this purpose), pick from the stems and pulp them, by pressing slightly with thumb and finger upon each one. Put the skins in a sep-arate dish; then heat the pulp and press through a coarse cloth, or sieve, to remove the seeds; then put juice and skins together in your kettle, and when they come to a boil they are ready for the cans (see Mrs. Sanders' plan in the general remarks and directions above, to avoid breaking cans), and secure well from the air; it matters not whether glass cans, or jugs, if properly **corked** and sealed with wax.

*Remarks.*—Familiarize yourselves with the directions to know they will **not** leak the fluid out, nor the air in, before putting away, as above given. Cherries, I cannot see why, if done in the same manner, get rid of the stones, will not be nice for sauce or pies, as well as grapes, the stones, or seeds, are a nuisance, in either case. Currants, berries, or other ordinary fruits need no special instructions; except it may be proper to say that some persons, in canning peaches, boil the stones in a small amount of water to extract the flavor, then heat the peaches in this water, sprinkling in the proper amount of sugar to fit them for the table; and also put a piece of white paper dipped in brandy (alcohol is good, and cheaper) over the top before screwing on the cover.

**Canning Rhubarb Plant, Tomatoes, etc.**—"Pansy," in writing to one of the papers upon this subject, says: Last summer I removed the skin from a quantity of rhubarb, put it over the fire with a very little water, watching it closely to prevent it burning, boiled it 10 minutes, stirring occasionally, and filled and sealed one-gallon jugs, carefully corking them; used common sealing wax; and it is as nice now as the rhubarb we get from the garden in the summer. Grapes are just as nice this way as they are in glass jars. I put away 44 qts. of tomatoes and rhubarb in this way, and never lost 1 pint. I use glass jars, too, for preserves, peaches (canned), and sweet pickles; but I decidedly prefer jugs, for it is no trouble, and everything keeps so well in them.

*Remarks.*—Rhubarb makes as nice a sauce, stewed, and sweetened to taste, as it does pies; and to be able to have it in winter, put up thus cheaply, will add to the variety of side dishes, and life's comforts generally.

**Canning Rhubarb in Cold Water, Without Cooking.**—"S. D.," of Vernon, Mich., directs through one of the papers as follows: Cut the plant, when fully matured, and wash it; put a cup of cold water in the can, fill with the pieces, pressing it full, then fill to running over with cold water. Seal as usual, and set in a cool cellar. When wanted pour the water into the vinegar barrel. Make the pies as usual, except not quite as much sugar is needed as for the fresh plant. I have tested this and know it to be good.

*Remarks.*—I cannot see why this is not a good and reliable way, although it has been deemed necessary to heat everything before canning. This may not be absolutely necessary. The water excludes the air from the crevices, and keeping in a cool place prevents fermentation. Let those who have it plenty try a few cans before going into it heavily. So with everything upon which there is a possible doubt, is the way that our valuable things are found out.

**Canning Sweet Corn.**—It has been generally considered a very difficult thing to can corn, so it would keep well; but a writer at Walled Lake, Mich., to one of the Detroit papers, thinks she has overcome this difficulty, for she says: If these directions are strictly followed, you can enjoy the same pleasure that we have for years, of eating sweet green corn in winter. It will need only to warm when you use it out of the can. DIRECTIONS—Cut the raw corn off the cob and fill your cans (after thoroughly scalding them) with the corn, take a spoon and press very hard so as to fill the can full, put on the cover loosely. Put the cans into your wash boiler after putting something under them to prevent them from breaking. I use the grate from the bottom of the oven. Fill in cold water up to the bulge of the can, put on the boiler cover and boil 4 hours, take off the stove and let stand until cool enough to handle, fasten the covers tight and set in a cool place in the cellar. I usually get mine ready in the forenoon and boil after dinner.

*Remarks.*—There is not a doubt but what if this plan is followed, strictly, being sure that the cans are entirely full, when the cover is screwed down, but what it will keep nicely. Tin cans are used by those who put it up for sale, in large quantities, pressing full, then soldering on the top, boiling for the 4 hours, then piercing a hole to let out the air, and soldering up the hole, at once, which makes all secure. If this long boiling is too much trouble, you must take the old way of packing with salt, as next given.

**Canning or Putting Up Green Corn With Salt.**—Take the corn when just right for the table, which should be the case above as well as in this, and scald it in the ear, as done for drying in the old way; then cut from the cob when cold. Place a layer of salt ½ an inch thick on the bottom of the deep (not the flaring) kind of earthen jar or crock; then a layer of the corn about 2 inches thick, pressing tightly with a potato masher or square-ended stick; next salt again, as at first, or a little thicker, say ¾ of an inch, as you go up; and so alternate till the jar is within an inch of the top, then fill with salt and tie a cloth over all. Set in a cool, dry cellar for winter use. To use, take out as many layers as needed, free from salt as possible, and wash off all the salt sticking to it; then soak in the evening and pour off at bed-time, and renew with fresh water and soak over night; then pour off again, which will generally be sufficient to remove the excess of salt, as the corn will not take up as much salt as supposed. Now taste a kernel, and if freshened enough, stew it for dinner, if not, soak again. Adding a small amount of sugar when cooking is considered an improvement; some do this, even when cooking new corn in summer.

*Remarks.*—A writer says: "I have used the above recipe for three years, and find it to be most excellent, the corn coming out of the jar as good as when first put down. * * * It is such a good thing that every body should know it, and any one who tries it will not regret the experiment." If the canning is too much trouble, or if the canned runs out before the winter is gone, you must take one of the following plans of "Hulling," which is a great favorite with the author, otherwise fill the place with hominy.

**Hulled Corn, Improved Plans of Making.**—The old way was to make a weak lye from hard wood ashes to remove the hulls, but a writer in the *American Agriculturist* gives her plan as follows. She says: "Soak over night by pouring over what you wish to make, hot water. In the morning put it into an iron kettle with warm water enough to just cover it; and for each quart of corn put in baking soda 1 table-spoonful, and boil till the hulls come off readily; then wash in clear water rubbing off the hulls with the hands, soaking and washing to remove the alkaline taste thoroughly; then boil until very ten-

der, salting towards the last to taste.  Turn into a sieve and drain thoroughly.
Eat hot or cold in milk."

*Remarks.*—I cannot see the object of drawing off the water in which it was boiled.  My mother and my wife always designed to have the water pretty well cooked away when done, then lift it together as much of the nourishment would be drained off.  (I see, also, that the following writer does not drain.)  It is very nice warmed up after frying meat, to eat with the same, for breakfast or any other meal, as well as with milk as the above writer only suggests.  The author has often wondered why people did not use more of it, and could only account for it from the objection of the women to work it from the lye with the hands to remove the hulls.  This difficulty has been overcome in the following recipe by using a clean broom for that purpose, which can be done as well with the soda above as with the ashes in the next.  So, now, I trust, all lovers of hulled corn may have it in abundance, as it is a very healthful dish, as well as a very cheap one, and relished by most persons if nicely done, *i. e.*, if it is freed from its alkalinity and cooked until it is perfectly soft.

**Hulled Corn, or Making Hominy Without Putting the Hands Into the Lye.**—Making hominy, or hulling corn, is not a big job nor one that we dread as we did "once upon a time," before we had learned this better way.  This is how we make it:  Take the corn of 1 doz. ears, put it in a kettle with a good bit more cold water than is required to cover it, and down in the center put a stout muslin sack long enough to contain 1 qt. of good ashes.  Let it boil till all the strength is out of the ashes, then remove them and give the corn more room.  Have the tea-kettle on the stove with plenty of boiling water in to pour into the pot as the other boils off,  Do not boil hard, but steadily. When the outside begins to come off the grains they are done enough.  Now remove from the fire, drain off and empty the corn into a tub of cold water. Instead of rinsing with the hands, as our blessed grandmothers did, take a clean broom and swash and sweep the corn about in the tub "like forty," drain off; add 2 or 3 pailfuls of clean, cold water, and go over the cleansing process about 3 or 4 times; then drain off and stand the tub of corn where it may have a chance to freeze all night.  This is as good for it as boiling.  In the morning take a part, or all of it, and put it on to boil in cold water, and cook slowly until done. Never stir hominy; if you begin it you must keep it up, or it will burn fast to the bottom of the pot.  Put a little salt in it.  Have boiling water on the stove ready to replenish.  Instead of stirring, lift the kettle by the bail and give it an occasional twirl, this way and that, to keep it from settling to the bottom.  Let it boil until the grains are swollen and burst and lie up loosely.  Leave in the liquor when you take it off the fire, and cover it up until it is cold.  Cook in meat fryings, with a little of the water in which it was boiled.—*Bonnie Doon, "Doon's Hollow," in Michigan Farmer.*

*Remarks.*—Although the name and place are fictitious, the plan is good and will prove satisfactory, else my name is not Dr. Chase.  The freezing is not absolutely necessary; still in freezing weather it is a help.  I should be glad to know, however, that every family would make it earlier, and later, too, than during the freezing months.

**Hulled Corn, or Hominy, Croquettes.**—To each cup of cold, soft-boiled hominy, or hulled corn, necessary for the family put 1 tea-spoonful of melted butter or drippings, mashing and stirring it well together, then stirring in a cup of milk, or sufficient to make a paste. Now beat an egg with 1 tea-spoonful of sugar to each cup of corn used, mix in and, with floured hands, roll into balls (croquettes) and fry in butter, or after the meat is fried, in the gravy. If made pretty dry, they may be dipped in beaten eggs, then in cracker crumbs and fried in hot lard, as you would doughnuts for tea; and in this case a little finely-chopped ham, veal or chicken mixed in will give them an additional relish. No comments, but simply a trial, is all that is needed.

**Hulled Corn, Hominy, or " Grits," to Bake.**—Milk (always sweet and nice, unless sour is called for), 1 qt.; hominy, hulled corn, "grits" (as kept by grocers), cooked tender and allowed to get cold, 1 cup; 3 eggs and a little salt; sugar, 2 table-spoonfuls. Directions—Bring the milk to a boil and stir in salt and grits, or mashed hominy, or hulled corn, mashed, as the case may be. If uncooked grits are used, continue to boil slowly about 20 minutes, slowly, then remove from the fire, and when cool stir in the beaten eggs and sugar, and bake in a moderate oven, 30 to 40 minutes. The top may be glazed or meringued, with the beaten whites of a couple of eggs and a couple table-spoonfuls of powdered sugar, or not, as you choose. Serve with any pudding sauce, or simple sugar and milk, as you like best.

*Remarks.*—It will be seen by the foregoing recipes that hulled corn, hominy or grits can be got up in different ways, adding to the varieties of the table, which all good housekeepers like to do. Certainly the cheapness of hulled corn, which, when cooked and mashed, is as nice as the hominy, or grits, for these dishes can be no objection to the rich, while it may be a convenience to the laboring classes to use the hulled corn instead of the others, which are more expensive.

**Mush, Rye and Indian, to Make.**—Take rather coarse Indian meal, 2 parts; rye meal or flour, 1 part; stir in Indian first, and cook 15 or 20 minutes; then the rye, mixing thoroughly; then cook slowly for an hour, with the cover upon the kettle. Very nice and healthful with milk, or to fry, as next given.

**Mush, to Fry.**—Beat an egg thoroughly, and roll a few crackers finely; then slice the mush and dip in the egg, then into the cracker crumbs, and fry in drippings, or after frying meat, or if wanted extra nice, in hot lard as you would doughnuts.

**Polenta, or Italian Mush, How to Make and Use.**—A writer says: Boil 1 lb. of yellow Indian meal ("a pint is a pound the world around") for ½ hour, in 2 qts. of pot liquor (water in which meat has been boiled); or boiling water, salted to taste, with 1 oz. of fat in it, stirring occasionally, to prevent burning; then bake ½ an hour in a greased baking dish, and serve it hot; or when cold slice it and fry in smoking hot fat. This favorite Italian dish, she adds, is closely allied to the New England hasty pudding, and to the mush of the south.

*Remarks.*—The difference is in simply leaving the " fat " out of the salted water, using plain water instead of pot liquor. The French make the polenta by boiling the flour of chestnuts, or finely powdered chestnuts, in milk. I think this would be nice occasionally, the Italian frequently.

**Baked Squash.**—Boil and mash a medium sized squash in the usual way, and, when nearly cold, stir in the beaten yolks of 2 eggs; 3 or 4 table-spoonfuls of milk; 1 of butter rubbed in 1 of flour and melted in the milk; pepper and salt to taste as usual, and put into a buttered bake pan and set in a moderate oven until lightly browned; then having beaten the whites, and mixed into them the crumbs of 4 or 5 rolled crackers with a pinch of salt and a tea-spoonful of sugar, if you like, put it over the top and brown again, a few min-utes; serve hot.

*Remarks.*—If summer squash is used, be careful to press out all the water you can, as they are much more watery than the winter varieties.

**Fried Squash.**—Pare the squash and cut into rather thin slices (crook necks are nice for this purpose, other rich winter varieties will do); make a thin batter of flour and water, seasoned highly with pepper and salt; dip the squash into it and fry with hot butter, or drippings, to a nice brown, each side. This may be done in a hot oven, turning in either case.

*Remarks.*—If nicely done, it is very nice, and makes a good substitute for sweet potatoes.

**Bread Balls, or Croquettes.**—Crumble stale bread or bread crusts rather finely and moisten well with warm milk or warm water. If too moist press out with the hand, season with salt and pepper, adding powdered sage or summer savory, parsley or any other sweet herb, as you prefer or have on hand, or a variety of them, as hinted in " Seasoning Fare " below, with a little soft-ened butter and a beaten egg or two, according to quantity, to hold it in balls; make with floured hands. To be fried after meat or put into the dripping-pan in roasting beef, turkey, chicken, etc.

*Remarks.*—I think those who try them will say: "Most noble Festus (author), thou art not mad, but speak the words of truth and soberness," in giv-ing so nice a way to use up stale bread or crusts. These balls will be very nice with the roast turkey and roast pig for Thanksgiving dinner (as below), as well as for common use.

**Thanksgiving Dinner, with Suitable Recipes, Bill of Fare, How to Set the Table, etc.**—And now I don't think I can do better than to close the department of dishes for the table than in giving a bill of fare, with suitable recipes for a Thanksgiving dinner, which was sent to the Detroit *Post and Tribune* with the writer's plan for setting the table, etc., which will cer-tainly be found of great assistance to new beginners and very handy to refer to by every one upon such occasions, or when quite a number of visitors are to be dined upon any occasion. If the writer's name was given I have it not at this writing; but knowing the directions to be reliable, I will let her speak for her-self. She says:

Thanksgiving is almost here, and how shall we celebrate the day? I for ~ne believe in the old-fashioned Thanksgiving dinner. The following bill of ' ~re may be of use to some of your readers:

Oyster Soup.          Celery, Pepper Sauce.

Roast Turkey, with Currant Jelly.

Baked Potatoes.          Mashed Turnips.

Roast Pig.    Carrots with Cream.    Baked Beans.    Chopped Cabbage.

Pumpkin Pie.          Plum Pudding.

Apples.       Nuts.       Cheese.

Tea and Coffee.

For the table I prefer a white cloth with fancy border, and napkins to match. A dash of color livens up the table so, in the bleak November, when flowers cannot be had in profusion. Casters in the center, of course, flanked by tall celery glasses. At each end, glass fruit dishes filled with apples and nuts. A bottle of pepper sauce near the casters, and a mold of jelly by the platter of turkey, and small side dishes of chopped cabbage garnished with rings of cold boiled eggs. The purple cabbage makes the handsomest-looking dishes. Serve the soup from tureens into soup dishes, handing around to the guests. After this comes the *pièce de resistance*, "Thanksgiving turkey." A piece of dark meat with a spoonful of gravy, and one of white with a bit of jelly and a baked potato (I should prefer a spoonful of mashed) should be served on each plate, leaving the other vegetables to be passed afterward with the roast pig. After this the salad, and then the plates should be taken away and the dessert served. Then come the apples and nuts, the tea and coffee, well seasoned with grandpa's old-time stories, grandma's quaint sayings and kind words and merry repartees from all.

Below I give some recipes for these old-fashioned dishes, hoping they may be of use to some young housekeeper, preparing, perhaps, her first Thanksgiving dinner:

*Oyster Soup.*—Pour the liquor from 1 qt. of oysters, set over the fire with 1 pt. of boiling water; skim when it boils up, and add 1 qt. of sweet milk; when it again boils up, stir in 2 tea-spoonfuls of butter rubbed in 1 of flour; then add the oysters, and salt and pepper to your taste; let it boil only a minute or two, and serve in a hot tureen. See, also, that the soup dishes are well warmed before sending to table.

*Roast Turkey.*—Make a stuffing of moistened bread-crumbs, rubbed smooth, with salt, pepper and powdered sage. Fill the breast and body, and sew it up with a needle and coarse thread. Put in the oven in a pan with a little water, basting it often. A turkey weighing 12 lbs. should roast at least 3 hours. Having washed the heart, liver and gizzard, boil them an hour or so in a saucepan; to make the gravy chop the giblets fine; put them back in the water in which they were boiled; add flour, rubbed smooth, in a little water; boil a minute or two, and serve in a gravy boat.

*Roast Pig.*—Sprinkle inside with fine salt an hour before it is put into the oven; cut off the feet at the first joint; fill it very full of stuffing, with plenty of sage in it; tie the legs; rub it all over with butter to keep it from blistering; baste very often while roasting. It will require about 2½ hours to roast. Make gravy as for other roasts.

*Carrots with Cream.*—Boil very tender with plenty of water; when done slice into a saucepan with a gill of cream; let them boil up once; salt and pepper to taste, and serve in hot nappies (side dishes).

*Boston Baked Beans.*—Take 1 qt. of white beans, wash and soak over night in 2 or 3 qts. of water; in the morning pick them over and boil until they begin to crack open; put them in a brown pan; pour over them enough of the water in which they have been boiled to nearly cover them. Cut the rind of a pound of salt pork into narrow strips; lay the pork upon the top of the beans and press down nearly even with them; bake some 4 or 5 hours.

*Pumpkin Pie.*—Stew a kettle full of pumpkin and press it through a colander. For a quart of the stewed pumpkin use about a pint or a little more of sweet milk, 2 cups of sugar, 3 eggs and a tea-spoonful of ginger· bake in a crust in a deep pie plate.

*Remarks.*—The plum pudding will be found in another part of the book; also salads, sauces or any other thing that may be desired upon Thanksgiving, or most other important occasions. "Always room for one more" in an omnibus or street car, so I give one on

**Seasoning Food, Sweet Herbs for—How to Raise, When to Cut and Dry, and How to Preserve their Flavor, etc.**—It is a mistaken idea that nicely flavored dishes are expensive. If purchased the herbs cost but a trifle per oz., and if raised at home it costs only a trifle to buy the seeds for them. The principal kinds used are sage, summer savory, thyme, parsley, sweet basil and sweet marjoram, tarragon, mint, mace, cloves, celery seed and onions. The mints grow readily along small streams and the others may be raised in boxes, even in the window or garden, wherever the sun will shine upon them. Sage need not be gathered till the last of September or first of October; summer savory, thyme and marjoram in July and August; basil in August and September; tarragon and parsley in June or July, or just before flowering; mints for winter use, when fully matured, in June and July. All should be gathered on a dry, sunny day and dried in the shade, and best if carefully dried in an open, moderate oven, or else hung up close by a stove to dry quickly. And when very dry is the time to powder and sift them, and then to bottle and cork tightly or keep in air-tight cans, which saves their flavor perfectly.

*Remarks.*—The reason why French dishes are superior to other cooking is that they are seasoned with a variety of herbs or spices, or both; and the flavor, although indistinct (*i. e.*, no one thing overbalancing another) from the variety used in a single dish; yet they are remarkably fine in themselves. Do the same if you wish an equally nice dish. [See, also, "Value of Sweet Herbs for Stews." Vinegars, pickles and some of the more common dishes, for the table will be found in the Miscellaneous Department.]

**Roast Goose.**—A goose should not be more than eight months old, and the fatter the more tender and juicy the meat. Stuff with the following mixture: 3 pts. of bread crumbs, 6 oz. of butter, or part butter and part salt pork, 1 tea-spoonful each of sage, black pepper, and salt, 1 chopped onion; do not stuff very full, and stitch the openings firmly together to keep the flavor in and the fat out. Place in a baking-pan with a little water, and baste frequently with salt and water (some add vinegar); turn often, so that the sides and back may be nicely browned. Bake 2 hours or more. When done, take from the pan, pour off the fat, and to the brown gravy left, add the chopped giblets, which have previously been stewed until tender, together with the water they were boiled in; thicken with a little flour and butter rubbed together, bring to a boil and serve. English style.

# MISCELLANEOUS RECIPES.

**1. WASHING FLUID.—Labor-Saving and Not Injurious—** Concentrated lye, 1 lb., muriate of ammonia, and salts of tartar, each 2 ozs.; rain water, 2 gals. DIRECTIONS—Dissolve the lye (here is a *lie*, indeed, as lye proper is a fluid, but this *concentrated* lye is a solid potash) in 1 gal. of the water and the salts of tartar, and muriate of ammonia in the other gal. of water, and put all into a 2 gallon stone jug, cork and shake, when it is ready for use. Put a suitable amount of water into your boiler for boiling your clothes; and when it is of a proper heat to put in the clothes, if they are very dirty, stir in 1 small teacup of the fluid, stirring well before putting in the clothes; if not very dirty, ½ cup will be plenty; add half as much more to each additional boiler, if more than one is to be used at the same time.

*Remarks.*—To soak clothes over night in cold water, use half as much of the fluid, stirred well into the water before putting the clothes into the tub this saves very much in the labor of the washing, as it neutralizes the grease, or sweat, and loosens the dirt, or rots its face; but remember, no soap should be put upon the clothes, nor into the soaking water, unless you use our bar Stanley soap given below. If they cannot be soaked over night, soaking them from early-rising till after breakfast, will help considerably, putting in some of the fluid, the same as directed for over night. Then run through the wringer, soap dirty places, and they are ready for the boiler, as in the directions above, boiling 10 to 20 minutes, after which but very little rubbing on the board will be needed, rinse well in the bluing water, as usual.

Mrs. Hardy, who gave me this receipt, and the foregoing instructions, is my sister-in-law, who has spent most of her life in a hotel, or a large boarding house, where much washing was to be done, and this is her favorite receipt after trying many others, and hence, from her practical knowledge and my own knowledge of the nature of the articles, I have every confidence it will prove satisfactory to all; still, as there are those who have tried other receipts, and think so much of them, I will give a few more.

**2. Washing Fluid or Powder.**—Sal-soda, 2 lbs.; borax, 1 lb.; salts of tartar, 2 ozs.; muriate of ammonia, 1½ ozs.

DIRECTIONS. I. *For the Powder.*—If it is to be used as a powder, pulverize all, and mix thoroughly, put into a large mouthed bottle and cork for use, and use one rounding tablespoonful in each boiler of clothes, and half as much for each additional boiler, and this same amount to a tub of clothes for soaking, to be well stirred in, in either case.

II. *For the Fluid.*—If to be used as a fluid, dissolve the sal-soda and borax in 1 gal. of water, and the other articles in another gal. of water, mix and

515

put into a 2 gal. jug and keep corked for use. To be used in the same quantity
and in the same way as No. I.

**3. Washing Fluid.**—Sal-soda, 1 lb.; potash (or concentrated lye), 1 lb.;
each dissolved in 1 gal. water respectively, then mix together and bottle.—"Josie,"
of New York City, in *Blade*.

*Remarks.*—She does not tell how, nor how much to use; but the author
says, use the same as No. 1, and a two gal. jug will do to hold it in. It will be
found good and no trouble to make.

**4. New Mode of Washing, Saving Time, Labor and Fuel.**—
"The ill effects of soda on linen have given rise to a new method of washing,
which has been extensively adopted in Germany, and introduced into Belgium.
The operation consists in dissolving 2 lbs. of soap in about 3 gals. of water as
hot as the hand can bear, and adding to this 1 teaspoon of turpentine and 3 of
liquid ammonia; the mixture must be then well stirred, and the linen steeped in
it for 2 or 3 hours, taking care to cover up the vessel containing them as closely
as possible. The clothes are afterward washed out and rinsed in the usual way.
The soap and water may be reheated and used a second time, but in that case
½ teaspoonful of turpentine and 1 teaspoonful of ammonia must be added. The
process is said to cause a great economy of time, labor and fuel. The linen
scarcely suffers at all, as there is little necsssity for rubbing, and its cleanliness
and color are perfect. The ammonia and turpentine, although their detersive
(cleansing) action is great, have no injurious effect upon the linen; and while
the former evaporates immediately, the smell of the latter disappears entirely,
during the drying of the clothes.—*Rural New Yorker.*

*Remarks.*—This writer speaks of the "ill effect of soda on linen," etc.; but
the author must claim if soda is properly used in washing, it will not injure
clothes, *i. e.*, if it is combined with potash or lime, which give it its causticity,
detergent or cleansing powers. For, during the past 20 years or more, I think,
of my wife's life, she always kept a washing fluid ready for use, made of sal-
soda and stone-lime, some of which was always put into the water to soak the
clothes in, and also into the water to boil them in, and I never saw a yellow
shirt, nor heard of any discoloring nor rotting of the clothing. I will guarantee that by none of the processes here given will they be injured, nor become
yellow. Borax, which is particularly the thing used in the next, I know to be
an excellent article to cleanse clothing, as well as to cleanse the scalp from
dandruff. A teaspoonful of powdered borax, to water enough, washing the
head daily, will soon remove the dandruff, and leave the scalp in a smooth and
healthy condition.

**5. Washing—The Use of Borax in Washing Linen, Flannels,
etc.,**—The following suggestions as to the use of borax in washing is from a
correspondent of the *Western Rural* who had tested them. She says:

"For an ordinary washing, use 1 teaspoonful (the author would say 2, for
borax is a neutral salt and it has no excess of alkali, nor acid, and therefore
does not injure clothing) of borax to 5 gals. of water and 2 ozs. of soap (it
would have to be soft soap, else dissolved); soak the clothes in this over night;
give them a thorough boiling, without wringing before the boiling. When the
clothes are very much soiled, see that the water is made soft with borax.
[Made to feel soapy.] 2 tablespoonfuls to a pail. Clothes thus washed will
not turn yellow."

In washing flannels, use 1 table-spoonful of borax to 5 gals. of water, without soap. It will not shrink them. For starching linen, use 1 tea-spoonful of borax to 1 pt. of boiling starch. For washing and bleaching laces, put 1 tea-spoonful of borax to 1 pt. of boiling water, leave your articles to soak in the solution for 24 hours, then wash with a little soap. For cleansing black cashmeres, wash in hot suds with a little borax in the water; rinse in bluing water —very blue—and iron on the wrong side while damp."

*Remarks.*—For its use in removing dandruff, see the close of the remarks last above. A drachm of powdered borax dissolved in 2 table-spoonfuls of vinegar is said to be an excellent lotion for ringworm of the scalp; and its powder dusted about pantries, libraries, etc., is also said to be effectual in driving away roaches and other insects.—*King.*

The author does not have to say "said to be," about its driving away roaches, as he has done it with great satisfaction, in drawers where they congregated so it could be got upon them; they left on the "double-quick."

**6. Borax, as Used By the Washer-Women of Holland and Belgium.**—"The washer-women of Holland and Belgium, so proverbially clean, and who get up their linen so beautifully white, do it by the use of refined borax (kept by druggists) as a washing powder, instead of soda, in the proportion of a large handful of borax powder to 10 gals. of boiling water, saving in soap nearly half. All of the large washing establishments adopt the same plan.

"For laces, cambrics and lawns an extra quantity of the powder is used, and for crinolines (skirts) requiring to be made stiff, a stronger solution is necessary. Borax being a neutral salt does not in the slightest degree injure the texture of the linen. Its effect is to soften the hardest water."—*Youman's Dictionary of Every-Day Wants.*

**7. Washing Fluid, Requiring but Little Boiling or Rubbing.** —"Camphor gum, ½ oz., dissolved in alcohol, ½ pt.; borax, ½ lb.; sal soda, 1 lb.; dissolve the borax and sal soda in hot rain water, 1 gal., and stir in the others, and put into a 2 gallon jug, having 1 gal. of cold rain water in it, cork and shake, when it is ready for use. DIRECTIONS—Put ½ cup of this to 1 pt. of soft soap, and apply to the dirty parts of the clothing, and soak in warm water ½ an hour, or while breakfast is passing; need not then boil over 5 minutes. Washing will be done in half the ordinary time. Does not rot clothing, but makes it white. Table-cloths stained with tea, coffee, or fruit, throw into boiling water a few minutes, when they will be free from stains (I have seen statements to pour hot water through such spots would free them from the stain), while soap or suds when the clothes are dry will set the stains permanently."—*Germantown, (Pa.) Telegraph.*

*Remarks.*—I take this to be a very good fluid, as it has neither turpentine nor ammonia in it, and the quantity of camphor and alcohol is so small it will not be liable to open the pores of the skin, by which means colds are so easily taken by exposure while hanging out clothes after being over the hot suds in washing. The Bark Shanty Soap, below, will be just the kind to use with this fluid; but the common soft soap, such as is usually made from ashes and grease of your own saving, is, no doubt, the kind this Pennsylvanian refers to. I trust that all of our lady readers will be able to find something among these washing fluids or powders that shall fully meet their wants. Bluings are kept so generally now by the grocers and druggists they can be bought for less than they can be made.

**8. Flannels, To Wash and Dry, Without Shrinking.**—Flannels should be washed with as little rubbing as possible; or, better still, pounding without any rubbing at all, and drying rapidly, and pulling freely, both length-wise and across the goods, if you would avoid shrinkage.

**9. Washing Muslins, Cambrics, and Calicoes.**—Stir some of the starch, after it is prepared for use, into the water in which any of these goods are to be washed.

**10.** Or, soak them a while in water in which you have put 1 or 2 table-spoonfuls of salt to a pail of water.

**11. For Black and White Calicoes.**—A cup or two of weak lye to a pail of water is best for soaking in.

**12. For Pink or Green.**—One or 2 table-spoonfuls of good vinegar to the pail of water is best.

**13. For Purple or Blue.**—Use sal soda, or borax, in powder, 1 or 2 table-spoonfuls to a pail of water; but, now, if you use the washing fluid, above, soak them a little in that, and wash out, as usual, it saves all these troubles with the different colors.

**14. Ribbons, to Wash.**—Wash ribbons in cold suds—not very strong, and do not rinse.

**15. Silk, Cashmere and Black Alpaca Dresses, to Cleanse.** —Dissolve a table-spoonful of powdered borax in 1 qt. of warm water (soft water), and after dusting thoroughly brush such parts as need it, or the whole, if much worn, and iron on the wrong side.

**16. Black Silk, Alpaca, Serge and Lawn Dresses, to Do Over.**—The following on the care and manner of doing over black silk, cashmere, alpaca, serge and lawn dresses, which I take from *Harper's Bazar*, is well worth a place here, and will be found worthy of consideration by every woman into whose hands this book shall come. It says:

"No lady should ever don her alpaca, cashmere or serge without giving it a thorough dusting with broom or brush. Dust permitted to settle in the folds of pleat or shirring will soon be impossible to remove entirely, and give the whole gown that untidy air so much to be deprecated in everything pertaining to a lady's person.

"But after constant use for months, or maybe a year, the most carefully kept black dress will begin to show the effects of use, in a certain rustiness of hue and general dinginess of aspect, if no place actually rubbed or worn. Now is the time to expend a little skill and ingenuity in its renovation, when the economist may be rewarded by coming out in an old dress made new, sure of eliciting the admiration of at least all those who are in the secret. For the undertaking provide yourself with ten cents' worth of soap bark, procurable at an herb or drug store, and boil it in 1 qt. of hot water. Let it steep a while, and then strain into a basin for use. If the job is to be a perfect and thorough one, take the body and sleeves apart and to pieces; rip off the trimming from skirt and over-skirt. Brush off all loose dust first, and then, with a sponge dipped in the soap bark decoction, wipe over each piece thoroughly, folding up as you proceed. Have ready a ladies' skirt board, for pressing, and well heated irons. Smooth every piece on the wrong side, including even silk trimmings; and when you have once more put it together you will be amazed to see the results of the simple process. One advantage in taking the whole dress apart is that, by putting the trimming on in some style a little different from what it was at first, the attraction of novelty is added to make the effect more pleasing. If one has not time, however, to go through the whole process, a dress may be greatly improved by being wiped over with this mixture (or the borax water above), and pressed on the wrong side while damp—indeed, for a time, it will look quite as good as new. The process may be repeated from time to time, as shall seem advisable. I have seen a cashmere, which had been worn two whole winters, taken apart and treated in this way, and the closest observer would have supposed the dress to have been put on for the first time, such was its soft, fresh look, and the vividness of its black. Grenadine may be submitted to the same sort of cleaning with fine results.

" When a black lawn has become limp, tumbled, and generally forlorn-looking, the best mode of treatment to subject it to is, first a submersion in a pan of warm water, colored highly with indigo; then exposure to the air until just dampness enough is left to enable one to press it to advantage with a hot iron; and if this is carefully done, always on the wrong side, the lawn will come forth quite fresh, stiff, and renovated from its blue bath, and again do good service for another while.

"Every particle of dust should be removed from a black silk or poplin every time it is worn, for nothing cuts either out so soon as these often imperceptible little gritty motes with which the air of a city is filled where coal is in such universal use."

**17. Washing or Cleansing Woolen Blankets.**—It is quite as important to have the woolen blankets on our beds clean, as to have our sheets pure and white. For the emination from our bodies are more quickly absorbed by them than by the muslin sheets; and as the women look upon the washing of a pair of blankets as a great undertaking, I will give them the easy way, recommended by the Boston *Journal of Chemistry*, which is about the same as practiced by my wife, in her lifetime. It is as follows: Put 2 heaping table-spoonfuls of powdered borax and 1 pt. of soft soap (or its equivalent of dissolved bar soap), into a tub of cold soft water. Stir well to dissolve and mix; then put in the blankets, thoroughly wetting, and let them soak over night. Next day rub (the author says pound), and drain them out, and rinse thoroughly in two waters, and hang them to dry. Do not wring them by hand, but press out the water. They may be put through a wringer.

*Remarks.*—This makes light work of washing blankets. It will not be amiss, however, to say the washing water and the rinsing water should always be as nearly as possible the same temperature, but only to take the chill off, so as to avoid taking cold by having the hands in cold water—no soap should ever be rubbed on the flannels, but sudsing be used; and do not hang out on a very cold day, nor hang close to a hot fire or stove; and iron with a moderately cool iron—not very hot—while damp, and there will be but little, if any, shrinkage, after moderate pulling even of skirts or other woolen goods. Under-skirts, etc., of wool can be washed in the fluid water, as above given, otherwise as nearly like blankets are done as you can.

**18. Borax, Its Value Corroborated.**—In the same connection the *Journal* goes on to say, further, of borax:

**19. Borax is the Best Roach Exterminator Yet Discovered.**—This troublesome insect has a peculiar aversion to borax, and will never return where it has once been scattered. And, as this salt (chemists know all these things as a "salt") is perfectly harmless to human beings, it is much to be preferred for this purpose to the poisonous substances commonly used.

"Borax is also valuable for laundry use, instead of soda. Add a handful of it, powdered, to about ten gallons of boiling water, and you need use only half the ordinary allowance of soap. For laces, cambrics, etc., use an extra quantity of the powder. It will not injure the texture of the cloth in the least.

"For cleansing the hair, nothing is better than a solution of borax water. Wash afterward with pure water, if it leaves the hair too stiff. Borax dissolved in water is also an excellent dentrifice, or tooth wash."

*Remarks.*—See how well this plan agrees with the Holland and Belgium washerwomen above, as to the use of borax for laundry, or washing purposes. This writer says, also: "Dissolved in water, it is also an excellent dentrifice, or tooth wash, as scientists think it destroys the parasitic mite, or insect that exists in the fermenting food between the teeth."

**Borax as a Tooth Powder, or for Washing the Teeth.**—I use borax in powder every morning, to cleanse my teeth. Borax in powder, ½ oz., with precipitated chalk, 3 ozs., with a few drops of oil of winter-green, which keeps my teeth clean and white, by rubbing the brush first on soap, then into the powder. Soap is essential once a day in cleaning teeth. Borax is, indeed, one of the most valuable salts we have for washing and cleaning purposes; but as we have now had a pretty thorough course of instruction in the various methods of washing, we will take up the question of soaps, for domestic purposes. Our first one, however, claims also, to make washing easy, which I very well know it will do. If you use any of the white bar soaps, your soft soap will be white—if any of the rosin-colored or yellow soaps, to make it with, such will be the color when done.

**1. Bark Shanty Soap, or Washing Made Easy.**—Good bar soap, 4lbs.; washing (sal) soda, 3 lbs.; freshly burned stone-lime (which is also called "quick-lime"), 1lb.; salt, 2 ozs.; soft water, 5 gals. DIRECTIONS—First, put the stone-lime into one gal. of the water, which is boiling hot; and, after stirring it a few times within an hour or two, let it settle, then pour off the clear liquid into a suitable sized kettle to hold all, and add the balance of the water; cut the bar soap into thin slices, and put it with the soda, into the kettle, and boil until the soda and soap are fully dissolved, then stir in the salt, and pour when a little cool, into suitable jars (a pine half-barrel will do very nicely), and keep covered for use.

*Remarks.*—This soap will save much of the rubbing of the clothing if a cup or two of it, according to the size of the washing, is dissolved by stirring it into cold water enough to cover the clothes, and they are soaked over night in it; then dirty places are soaped with this before boiling; 15 or 20 minutes will, be long enough to boil them, and slight rubbing of soiled places will be all that is needed, rinsing, bluing, etc., as usual. This amount of soap will do four times as much washing as the bar soap would have done by itself, and that, even if the money paid for the soda and the lime, which ought not to be above 15 or 20 cents, at most, had been added to the purchase of bar soap. The lime, especially, costs a mere nothing, but adds greatly, as well as the soda, to the detergent or cleansing properties of the soap. I call this " Bark Shanty Soap," from the name of the place where we lived one season, and where I obtained this recipe. It is on the shore of Lake Huron, 31 miles above Port Huron, where the timber is chiefly pine, and hence the ashes were not good for making soap; we, therefore, had to get the best substitute we could, and this being in use there, we soon learned its value, and will only add that although it will be found a great help and saving to those living in shanties, yet it will also be just as satisfactory to those living in cities, if they will give it a trial. It makes a half-solid soap very convenient to use.

**2. Soft Soap for Washing and House Cleaning.** — There are many other ways of making soap, nearly all of which contain some of the improvements or newer articles which have been introduced within the last few years in soap making, such as sal soda, lime, borax, etc.; but few of them contain more than one or two of these. The next, although it has only one— the sal soda—yet you will at once see that Mrs. J. Lute, of Liberty, O., who sends it to the *Blade*, thinks very highly of it; and I give it to show the value of the sal soda mixed with soap which, in my own as well as in Mrs. Lute's opinion, will be a great help in washing clothes or house cleaning, as the case may be. She says:

"Take 4 lbs. of white, bar soap, cut it fine, and dissolve by heating in 5 gals. of soft water, adding 2 lbs. of sal soda. When all is dissolved and well mixed, it is done. Yellow soap does very well, but I think the white is the best. This makes a very nice, white soft soap. You will think it a fraud when you first take it off the fire, but when it gets cool you will change your mind, and after one trial of it you will have no other. I have used it for three years, and am not afraid to recommend it to your readers."

*Remarks.*—If this is thus good, where the lime can be got, will not the following be considerably better?—I think so.

**3. Hard Soap, Fifteen or Twenty Pounds from Seven.**—Take 7 lbs. of good hard soap; cut it in thin slices; sal soda, 2 lbs.; unslacked (that is stone) lime, 1 lb.; alum, 1 oz.; borax, 2 ozs.; benzine, 1 oz.; soft water, 2 gals. DIRECTIONS—Put the sal soda and lime into a dish and pour over them the water, boiling hot, (what is better, is to use a kettle which you can boil these in till the soda is dissolved and the lime all slacked), stirring well a few times, and let settle; then (or in the morning, if done over night,) pour off the clear solution into the kettle containing the slices of soap, put on the fire and let it remain until the soap is dissolved; then, having dissolved the alum and borax in a little water, pour them in just as the soap comes off of the fire; and when a little cool put in the benzine, stirring well, and when it gets perfectly cold it will be hard, and can be cut in pieces to dry.

*Remarks.*—I have this from a Mrs. Baldwin, who has done a great deal of washing in her life, at Put-in-Bay, Ohio, and who has used this soap and knows its value, and hence recommends it very highly. And this recipe, I am well satisfied, has had a wide range, for I found, when I come to look over the items on hand for this department, I had the same recipe from a friend who lived in the southern part of the state, and his family prized it highly. Of course, this could be made into a soft soap by adding 5 to 10 gals. more of water, according to whether you would have it quite firm, or more easily taken up with the hand, and I will say here, too, I think if ½ to 1 cup of salt was put in with the alum and borax, it would be a little firmer, as a hard soap, and also dry a little quicker. Rosin is also put into hard soap for the purpose of making it tougher, so it will not rub off quite so fast when rubbing it upon the clothing. Some persons think the rosin is detergent, that is it helps to cleanse away the dirt, but this is a mistake, if not wholly, it certainly has but very little power to do this. A table-spoonful of spirits of turpentine, has more of this cleansing power than a pound of rosin, but it does make the soap wear or last longer. See next recipe for using rosin.

**4. Hard Soap with Concentrated Lye.**—"Take 2 boxes (2 lbs.) of concentrated lye; soft water, 5 gals.; grease, 9 lbs.; rosin and borax, each, ½ lb.; salt as below. DIRECTIONS—Dissolve the lye in the water, and add the rosin, broken finely, and boil till dissolved, stirring well; then add the grease and the borax, in small pieces, and boil about 2 hours, or till the grease is taken up, and it becomes soapy. If the grease was salty, stir in ½ tumbler of salt; if it was not salty, a full tumbler of salt, dissolved in ½ gal. of warm water, and stir in, and continue the boiling ½ an hour longer. Soak a tub well in cold water, and pour in the soap, and let it stand till cold. Cut out in cakes and put in a cool dry place to dry. You may leave out the rosin, if you desire, I do not always use it."—*Keystone, Cannonsburg, Pa.*

*Remarks.*—As I said in last recipe, above, the rosin makes the soap wear longer, when rubbing upon the clothes, if it rubs off too slow, so you have to rub too long to get on soap enough, use less rosin, or none at all, as you prefer.

**5. Hard Soap with Soda, Lime and Accumulating Grease, etc.**—Mrs. C W. Phillips, of Glencoe, Minn., informs us through the *Blade,* how to use the accumulating grease, by making a "hard soap which is excellent and economical." She says:

"Nearly every family accumulates, through the winter, drippings from beef, mutton, ham, etc. These can all be utilized by boiling the grease in water, allowing it to cool, then removing it from the water, and boiling by itself again till all the water is expelled. Of course, the whiter the grease, the nicer will be the soap."

Then take 6 lbs. of this grease, 6 lbs. of sal-soda, and 3½ lbs. of newly burned or good stone-lime, with 4 gals. of soft water, and ½ lb. of borax; or in these proportions. Put soda, lime and water into an iron kettle and boil;

stir till the soda is dissolved, and the lime is all slacked; then, when it is well settled; pour off the clear liquid; wash out the kettle and put in the liquid, grease and borax, and boil till it comes to soap, and pour into a well-soaked tub to cool, and when sufficiently hard, cut into bars and put on boards to dry. It is very nice, even for washing white flannels and calicoes; and, if a little perfume is put in it is nice enough for the toilet."

*Remarks.*—The old Windsor soap, as it used to be made, was flavored with oil of caraway, but more recently the oil of sassafras, which is cheap, has been used for perfuming soaps; ½ to 1 oz. would be enough for a "batch of soap" of 5 to 10 gals., according to whether a little or a considerably strong perfume is preferred. It should not be put in until the soap is pretty cool, then stirred in thoroughly.

The *Rural Home*, under the head of "Home-Made Soap," gives the same recipe as this last, except it used only 3 lbs. of lime and no borax—otherwise just the same—and makes these remarks about it: "Were the good qualities of this inexpensive soap more generally known no family would go without it. It is valuable for washing clothes, making them very clean and white, without in the least injuring them, and is excellent for flannels and petticoats. It is good, also, for the hands, making them soft and smooth." Could any higher encomiums or better recommendation be asked or given? I think not. And the only reason I give them is that the people may have confidence enough in these soaps to give them a fair trial, as they positively do not injure the clothing, but save much labor and expense, as compared with using only bar soap kept by grocers. I had also another recipe from the *Inter Ocean*, but it was just like this, except a caution to "be very careful not to get any sediment in from the lime." Simply be careful to pour off the liquid clear of sediment in any recipe using the stone lime, as the lime will not dissolve, but simply slacks, yielding up its caustic power, for which purpose only it is used, except for the hand-washing soap below, and there it is used only upon the hands; for clothing it is best not to get in any lime lest it spot some colored goods. I will give you one more of these hard soaps from soda, lime and grease, as the amount is smaller, and is from a lady who is not afraid to give her name, and address also. It is as follows:

**6. Hard Soap, With Soda, Lime and Grease Only.**—Soft water, 1½ gals.; sal soda, 3 lbs.; unslacked lime, 1 lb.; clean grease, 3 lbs. Directions—Put the three first articles together and boil to dissolve the soda and slack the lime; then let settle and pour off the clear liquid and put on the fire again with the grease and boil to proper consistence. One oz. of any flavored oil may be added, if desired.—*Mrs. W. W. Morse, of Lann, D. T., in Inter Ocean.*

*Remarks.*—As named in another place, any of these hard soaps may be made soft by using the proper amount of water to give the right consistence.

**7. "Why is Lime Used in Making Soap?"**—*Explanation.*—People seem to be so afraid of using lime in making soaps, like the foregoing; the question is often asked: "Why is the lime used?" and hence I will take the

Yankee way of answering it: "Why does everybody that makes soap **from** ashes put lime in the bottom of the leach?" Simply because if he does **not** he will have great trouble, even if he can make it at all, unless he does put **the** lime in, is about all the reason they can give. But lime causes the absorption of carbonic acid in the lye from the ashes, and also gives the lye a caustic property that enables it to combine with the grease, and thereby makes the soap, which it could not do, or at least not well do, except for the lime. The lime, then, does not hurt soap, but makes a better soap than can be made without it. Well, then, if it is good to assist in making soap from ashes, or potash, which comes from the ashes, why should it be thought injurious to combine it with sal soda for the same purpose? The one question answers the other, and ought to satisfy every reasonable person that lime is good and not injurious, as some suppose, for soap-making purposes. The manufacturers make soap by the use of potash, or soda, in the form or what is known as soda-ash, which is caustic, by means of its process of manufacture; but this article (soda-ash) cannot always be obtained, while the sal soda, which is a carbonate, can always be got; then we combine the lime with it, which gives it the same causticity that soda-ash has, and we thereby get just as good a soap. So have no fears in using them.

**8. Soft Soap From Concentrated Lye.**—To make soft soap with concentrated lye, take 1 lb. of it and dissolve it in 2 gallons of soft water; and, when it boils, add tallow, or clear grease, 4 lbs. Let it boil till it becomes clear; then add 2 gallons more of rain water. Mix well and set it by to cool; then take a cup of it, and add as much cold water as it will take, and still be as thick and ropy as you wish it, then add water in the same proportions to the whole.—*Prairie Farmer.*

**9. Soft Soap for House Cleaning, Washing Clothes, etc.**—It is well to have two or three strings to one's bow; hence I give one or two more soft soap recipes. This one I take from the *Medical Brief*, of St. Louis: Hard soap, 3 lbs.; sal soda, 1 lb.; aqua ammonia and spirits of turpentine, each 1 oz.; soft water, 3 gallons. Boil the water and dissolve in it the soap and soda; remove from the fire and stir in the others.

*Remarks.*—Oil of sassafras, $\frac{1}{2}$ to 1 oz., may be used for flavoring, **if** desired, in this amount of any soaps.

A lady editress of one of the "Household Departments" of an agricultural paper makes it as follows, using less soda, and no ammonia nor turpentine, still it will be found excellent for the purposes named

**10. Soft Soap, for Removing Grease from Floors, Shelves, etc.**—Sal soda, $\frac{3}{4}$ lb.; bar soap, 1 lb.; cut into small pieces; put them into a stone jar on the back of the stove, or range, when not very hot, and pour over it a pailful of cold water; stir it once in a while, and after some hours, when thoroughly dissolved, put it away to cool. It forms a sort of jelly, and is excellent to remove grease on floors or shelves.

*Remarks.*—The author will say good for cleaning all wood-work, and for general washing too.

**11. Soap from Refuse Grease.**—Another lady says: The best way to use up small lots of refuse grease, is to buy a box of concentrated lye (for sale by all grocers) and follow the directions on the box. Nothing can be simpler, and we have never failed in getting the soap to come.

*Remarks.*—This lady's instruction is sound common sense, and confirms what I have said heretofore. A little judgment will enable any one to succeed, by simply modifying, or changing, sometimes, to meet different conditions which may arise, in not always being able to get just what is called for in one recipe, by taking up another, the articles for which can be obtained.

**12. Pearline, Soapine, etc., to Make.**—The *Scientific American*, which is one of our most reliable papers, informs us that these articles are made of powdered soap, and powdered sal soda, equal, or about equal parts of each. Thus you see for a few cents you can make what they ask much more for; and it shows, too, what is thought by scientific men of sal soda as an aid in washing.

**13. Soap for Machine-Shop Men, Blacksmiths, Engineers, Printers, Scouring. etc.**—Take 10 lbs. of hard, yellow soap; sal soda, 3 lbs.; borax and tallow, each 1 lb.; fresh slacked lime, as below; soft water, 3 gals. DIRECTIONS—Put the water, soda and borax into the kettle, and when dissolved add the tallow and the soap, shaved fine; and when these are dissolved stir in as much freshly slacked, sifted lime as you can stir in well. The lime is to be sifted through a common kitchen sieve to avoid coarse lumps.

*Remarks.*—The lime thus stirred in greatly helps its scouring and cleansing properties; its roughness also helps greatly in washing hands covered with grease, ink, etc. It makes a good washing soap without the lime, but that adds more than half to its power of removing grease, ink, tar, etc., from the hands of machinists, where iron is worn into the grease on journals and by filing, etc. Without the lime it would make about 10 gals of splendid soft soap, if preferred in place of the hard; and in this case the tallow need not be put in.

**14. Medicated, or Sulphur and Tar Soaps, To Make.**—So much is being said about sulphur soap, in skin diseases and for toilet purposes, it will be a satisfaction to many people, no doubt, to know that if you take a 1 lb. bar of any good, hard white soap, cut it fine and put it into a small jar and set that into a basin or pan of water and set on the stove till the soap is melted, then stir in, thoroughly, 1 oz. of the flour of sulphur and pour into a paper or wooden box to cool, after which you can cut it into squares and dry it, and your sulphur soap will be as good as any you buy. For the tar soap, do the same as above, except stir in $\frac{1}{4}$ oz, of creosote, which is the same in action as tar—contains the active principle of tar. No harm in combining them in one soap; the combination would work very mildly on any irritable skin.

*Remarks.*—Renovation, or general cleansing of clothes of all kinds, gloves, boots, shoes, etc., very properly follows the foregoing soaps, washing fluids, etc.

**Renovation, Clothes Cleaning, etc., Explanation of.**—Renovation is the art of making new after injury or partial decay—re-making, from the Latin *re,* again, and *novare,* to make new. This word, then, may very properly be applied to the cleansing of wearing apparel of all kinds, gloves, boots and shoes, paint and grease about the house; ink, paint, tar and grease spots upon clothing; also re-coloring faded and worn garments—in fact, everything in the line of cleaning or renewal may come under this head. It will be my purpose, then, to so explain as I proceed, the art of renovation that those who desire to do so may restore their faded or injured or soiled garments to be nearly equal to new. In the cities there are those who follow the various branches of this art with great success and profit. The following recipes and instructions will give the people the secrets of doing it at home just as well as to pay for doing it away from home, and, no doubt, also give some of the professional renovators some things new to themselves. The following compound or soap will, probably, clean a greater variety of colored garments, without injuring the cloth, than any preparation in use. Of course, I have not practiced this art myself, but I obtained these recipes from a woman who lived for a year or two in a house owned by me at the time, and who practiced the art, and had renovated clothing for myself and other members of the family, so I know their reliability. And I may be excused for saying I paid more for these recipes alone ($5) than I get for the book.

1. **Renovating Soap.**—Marseilles (French) or Parker's best soap, such as used by barbers (I have seen Babbitt's common soap used, but the above was the original recipe), ¼ lb.; alcohol, 1 oz.; beef's gall, 2 ozs.; saltpeter, borax, honey, sulphuric ether and spirits of turpentine, of each, ¼ oz.; camphor gum, 3 drs.; pipe clay, 1 dr.; common salt, 1 small tea-spoonful. DIRECTIONS—Put the camphor into the alcohol, the powdered pipe clay into the beef's gall, pulverize the saltpeter and borax and put them and the salt into the honey. After 2 or 3 hours slice the soap into a porcelain kettle, with the gall mixture, and place over a slow fire, stirring till melted; take off and let stand until a little cool; then add all the other articles, stir well together and put into a glass fruit jar as soon as possible, as it soon hardens; then screw on the top, to prevent the evaporation of the strength, keeping in a dark closet, ready for use, as light decomposes or injures it.

*Remarks.*—Those desiring to engage in the business permanently can take double or four times these quantities, according to the amount of work they may expect to do.

2. **Clothes Cleaning.**—GENERAL DIRECTIONS—To clean a pair of pants or coat (any color) that has been considerably soiled, open the jar, and with a stiff spoon loosen up some of the renovating soap and take out ½ an oz. (a rounding table-spoonful) and dissolve it in 1 qt. of boiling soft water in a porcelain kettle, so as to keep it hot. Now whip and brush the article to be cleaned thoroughly, to remove all the dust; then, with a scouring brush (a partly worn, consequently stiff, broom brush will do very well), saturate, or wet the soiled spots thoroughly with the hot solution from the kettle; and, as a general thing, it will be best to saturate the whole garment, else a part will look new (that which is renovated) and the rest will look old or dirty, except in cases of getting spots upon new clothing. After thoroughly wetting the garment with

the solution, dry as thoroughly, in the open air is best. This wetting of the garment is best done by drawing it on a press-board, if you have one, as described below, also by spreading on a table or counter to be handy. After being dried, press the garment well, using what is called a "sponge-cloth," of stout unbleached muslin or drilling. If this is to be followed for a business, buy 2 yds. and tear it in two, lengthwise, keeping one for light shades of cloth-ing, the other for dark. When ready to begin to press the garment take a basin of soft water and put into it some aqua ammonia, at the rate of 1 table-spoon-ful to 1 qt. of water, and, with the ammonia water, keep your sponge-cloth wet while pressing.

*Remarks.*—For those following the business, a press-board, which can be got up by any good joiner, so that a pant's leg may be drawn upon it, and a smaller one suitable in size to enter a coat-sleeve, will be found more than suffi-ciently handy to pay their cost, as they will be found almost absolutely neces-sary in applying dye to black clothing where the color has been spotted or faded, as explained under that head further on. The press-board referred to has two parts, a base, or bottom piece, then the pressing-board proper is supported by two standards about 5 or 6 inches from the bottom piece, with one end running out free to allow the leg or sleeve to be drawn upon it 15 to 18 inches for con-venience of pressing the single thickness of cloth, instead of double, if the leg or sleeve is simply spread out on a table or counter.

3. **Alpaca Dresses—To Remove Wrinkles and Brighten their Luster.**—Dust them nicely with a brush and spread them upon an ironing-board, or press-board, as referred to above, then, having wet the sponge-cloth with the ammonia water, as directed for pressing clothing above, pass a moder-ately warm iron over them quickly a few times, and the work is complete.

4. **Renovating Dye for Black Clothing, to be Applied Only on the Outside—Cheap Ink, etc.**—Logwood chips, 1 lb.; soft water, 1 gal.; bichromate of potash, 24 grs.; prussiate of potash, 12 grs. Put the log-wood into the water and let stand 12 hours, then boil ½ hour, strain while warm, and having dissolved the potashes in a little boiling water, add them to the dye. Bottle, cork, and keep in a dark place. This is to be applied to spots on black clothing, coat collars, etc., where the color has been injured or faded out, the spots having been renovated and dried as given under the head of renovation; then, first having sponged the spots with suds, or the whole gar-ment, if it is to be applied to the whole, applying the dye with a brush, and dry again before the pressing is done. This dye may be used also to color worn or injured spots upon black kid gloves, black kid boots, etc., in place of ink, spoken of under those heads; in fact, this makes a very good, cheap ink for school children.

**Paint, Tar, Pitch, Ink, Grease Spots, etc., To Remove from Clothing.**—Take a little of the renovating soap, above, without water, and rub it into the soiled spots; let it remain a few minutes, then scrape off and cleanse with the ammonia water, also given for pressing clothing, under the head of renovation. If this does not fully accomplish it, use the renovating soap with the ammonia water. The drying, coloring, if needed, pressing, etc., to be the same. Tailors, it is claimed, use equal parts of ammonia and alcohol for cleaning coat collars, grease spots on pants, etc., and that nothing is better; but for very nice articles chloroform is better than anything else, removes grease of all kinds, also paints, varnish, etc.

**Paint, Pitch, Oil, and Grease, To Remove from Silk, Linen, etc.**—Benzine (purified), also called benzole, 2 ozs.; oil of lemon, ¼ oz. Mix and keep corked. DIRECTIONS—Apply with a cloth or sponge to any spots upon any of the above named kind of goods, rubbing with the fingers until removed. The colors will not be injured.—*Indian Domestic Economy.*

*Remarks.*—For sake of safety in using benzine, or benzole, as one kind is called, see note after Kid Glove Cleaning. The lemon is only for flavor, or to hide the odor of the benzine.

**Fruit Stains, To Remove from Clothing, etc.**—To remove fruit stains, hold them so you can pour boiling water through them; and if this fails in any case to remove the stain, then dip the table-cloth or other article into hot water, and place it over burning brimstone, as for bleaching flannels, below.

**Bleaching Flannels.**—Wet them and place upon a stick over the top of a barrel, in the bottom of which is an old pan with some burning coals, and sprinkle on the fire a little, broken bits of brimstone and cover over with a piece of carpet to retain the smoke. Particularly applicable to children's flannels which have become yellowish, and which you do not like to wash for fear of shrinkage.

**Silks, To Remove Spots, etc.**—Fuller's earth, 1 oz.; saleratus, 1 even tea-spoonful, (if saleratus is not obtainable, get bi-carbonate of potash of a druggist, the same amount); lemon juice. DIRECTIONS—Dry the earth thoroughly, and mix in the saleratus evenly; then moisten with the lemon juice sufficiently to form it into a roll or stick; dry in the sun. Wet the spots with hot water and rub it with the prepared earth. Dry in the sun; then cleanse with clear water.

**Ink Spots, To Remove From Clothing.**—Wet the spots with milk —sour milk is best—if you have no milk, wet with water, and rub a piece of lemon on some salt, then upon the spot, a few times will always remove it. If you have no lemon, a little oxalic acid in water, rinsed out with clear water, will do it—except the cheap school inks made with chromates of potash, even oxalic acid will not dissolve them; but the better inks, which are set with iron, the above will dissolve out.

*Remarks.*—Remember, if oxalic acid is used, to keep it away from children, as it is poisonous, or corrosive upon the flesh, so upon clothing if left without rinsing. A drachm will be enough for any ordinary spot, the size of the hand. If rinsed out as soon as the spot disappears it will hurt no clothing.

**Ink—Printer's, To Remove From Clothing.**—Saturate with turpentine, let alone for 2 or 3 hours; then rub well with the hands and dust out. Saturate means to wet thoroughly. It may be necessary to use some of the renovating soap, or erasive compound, or some of the soap for the machine-shop men to wash away the discoloration.

**Tar Spots, To Remove.**—Tar spots may be removed by putting butter upon them for a few hours; then cleanse with soap and water to remove the grease, using the renovating soap if needed.

**1. Kid Gloves, To Clean.**—Take purified benzine, in a bowl or suitable dish, sufficient to cover the gloves. Put the gloves into the benzine and saturate or soak to wet thoroughly; then having placed one upon a clean, smooth board, with a soft brush or soft sponge rub one way only, from the wrist towards the fingers, wherever there is any dirt, or all over is best, to make all look alike—clean, dipping them or the brush into the benzine as often as necessary to get out all the dirt; and if this can not be done with the first lot, throw it away and pour in fresh, and rinse and squeeze out in the benzine till perfectly clean. White gloves you will suppose, while cleaning, to be spoiled, as it gives them a dingy appearance. Tinted or light shades will not look quite so dingy; but, never mind, partially dry them in the sun. Now, having previously prepared a stick, a foot or more in length, carefully tapered, and rounded at one end to resemble a finger, insert it into each finger, carefully pulling the glove on by the wrist until smooth, then rubbing dry with fine soft muslin. When all is dry, polish with French powder (white), using soft white flannel in polishing. Use care on the stick, and in all the processes, to keep the gloves smooth, for if wrinkled the surface would be broken. Keep them from shrinking by putting upon the hands occasionlly when nearly dry; but if you are cleaning a smaller glove, for others, than will go upon your own hand, carefully pull them as needed to prevent shrinkage.

*Benzine, Benzole, Rose Oil, Naptha, etc.—Explanation.*—Naptha, which is a preparation made by the destructive distillation of wood, but now better known as "wood alcohol," was formerly used for this purpose; but as this is now worth 50 cents a quart, at least, and as the purified benzine, which is made from coal oil or petroleum, does this work just as nicely, and cost not more than 10 or 15 cents a quart, it is now almost wholly used for these purposes. This purified benzine is also known as "rose oil." Druggists understand all these names. Gasoline, even, will do the same work, but it has more of the odor, not being so thoroughly purified. Remember, it is the purified benzine that should be obtained; and, remember, too, all these articles are not only inflammable, but also explosive, if fire gets to them or the vapor arising from them. So do not use them near a fire, lamp, or gaslight, to insure safety.

*Remarks.*—The gentleman from whom I obtained this recipe—using naptha —told me he paid $15 for it, after he had carried on clothes cleaning for eight years, and he considered it a good investment at that price. It will do the work nicely, but the benzine is now the cheapest.

**2.** Or if the gloves are not much soiled, set a saucer of sweet milk, and a piece of white soap upon the table. Fold a clean towel, 3 or 4 thicknesses, upon the table, or upon your lap, and spread the glove smoothly upon it. Take a piece of clean white flannel and dip it in the milk; then rub it upon the soap, then upon the glove, from wrist to fingers, continuing the process until the dirt is removed, when, if a white glove it will have a yellowish tint, dark shades of gloves will be darker still. Be careful to clean every part of the glove thoroughly, else there will be spots when done. Let dry, or nearly so, then put on your hands and work soft, and polish as in No. 1 above, and the result will be very satisfactory.

**3.** Or, take a pan of white corn meal, sifted; put on the gloves and make believe washing hands in the meal, carefully, for 10 or 15 minutes, according to the extent of soiling. Fold in a clean towel, and put a weight upon them for a time. (See also white furs to clean, for the propriety of using corn meal in removing dirt.)

**Kid Gloves, Black, Worn Spots, to Restore.**—When black kid gloves are soiled, or turned white, in spots, from wear, wet the spots with black ink—a little poured into a sauce-plate, and apply by means of a bit of flannel, upon the end of a small stick, is a good way—then, leaving a few drops of the ink in the plate, pour in a tea-spoonful of salad oil or sweet oil, and with the flannel rub the mixture over the whole gloves, and dry in the sun—polish on the hand with soft flannel.

**Ladies' Kid Boots—Black, to Re-Color Soiled, or Worn Spots.** —First brush off all dirt, then color the spots with ink, or with the renovating dye, then with a little of the ink, or dye, in a little oil, as with black gloves, polish the whole uppers, so all will look alike.

*Remarks*—Jettine, or liquid blacking, is much used, of late years, instead of ink and oil; suit yourself.

**Woolen Hoods (White), Nubias, etc., to Cleanse, or Renovate, Without Washing.**—Dry nice wheat flour in a clean pan in the oven and rub it thoroughly into the hood, or nubia, until thoroughly cleaned, adding a very little bluing powder, if you have it, to the last rubbing—cleans them nicely and saves the shrinkage from washing; although our plans of washing woolens are excellent, and may be followed with these articles, if preferred.

**Paint Spots Upon Windows, to Remove.**—Dissolve sal soda, 1 oz., in soft water, 1 pt.—in this proportion for as much as needed. Use it hot, with a piece of flannel, or sponge, on a stick, not to affect the fingers. Wash off with hot water, as soon as the paint spots are softened.

**Kid Boots, or Shoes, White and Light Shades, to Clean.**— Use the purified benzine and sponge as for gloves, drying and polishing the same. If they are too small to admit the hand, stuff them to keep them full size.

White kid boots, or shoes, can be cleaned by dipping a perfectly clean piece of white flannel in a little ammonia, and rubbing the cloth over a cake of white soap; after which gently rub the kid diligently, until the soiled places are white again. As the flannel becomes soiled change for a clean one, or a clean place.

**White Furs, to Clean or Renovate.**—Half fill a stone jar with white corn meal (for a child's muff and tippet, a 2 gallon jar will be suitable), place it on the stove and heat the meal as hot as the hand can be borne in it, stirring to prevent the meal from scorching. Put one piece, at a time, in this, and rub until thoroughly clean; then beat out the meal with a stick. Heat further, if needed, for other pieces—the meal must be hot.

**Finger Marks Upon Doors—To Remove.**—Dissolve sal-soda, 1 oz.; in soft water, 1 pt., and go over the soiled doors or other painted wood-work with it, using a sponge or cloth, following with a wiping cloth, slightly wrung out of hot, clean water.

**Erasive Compound, or, Soap for Cleaning Clothes.**—Sal-soda, ¼ lb.; castile soap, 2 ozs.; starch 1 oz.; borax, ½ oz.; soft water, 1 qt. DIREC-ʟɪONS.—Boil the soap in the water till dissolved, then add the other ingredients, all pulverized, and stir till all is dissolved, and pour into a square pan or box, to cool, when it can be cut into bars, of suitable pieces to wrap up for sale, if that is the purpose. Used for removing grease spots, paint, tar, etc., apply with a wet sponge by rubbing on the soap first, then on the spot till clean.

*Remarks.*—The friend who sent me this for insertion in my "Third and Last Receipt Book," says: "It is equal to the "Lightning Eradicators," which are generally sold for 25 cents a cake, and as you will know, is much cheaper."

These cakes of soap sold on the street corners for 25 cents, are only about 1 or 1¼ inches long by ¾ wide and ½ inch thick. The same friend also sent me the following ink, and the remarks connected with it are his also, but they can be depended upon, except the one I have modified, as to its not being equal to the best writing fluids.

**Ink—Black for School Purposes—A Quart for a Dime.**—Extract of logwood, ½ oz.; bi-chromate of potash, 10 grs.; dissolve in a quart of hot rain water. When cold, put into a bottle and leave uncorked for one week, when it is ready for use. At first it is a steel-blue, but becomes quite black. I used this ink for a long time while in an office, and considered it equal to the best writing fluid. [This last remark, is all in which I disagree with him. It does, however, make a good school ink.] Moderate freezing does not hurt it.

**Brocade or Broche Shawls—To Clean the White Center— Also Applicable to Fine, White Lace.**—Spread a clean, white cloth upon the table and sift over it, dry, white corn-meal, as large a spot as the shawl center, and lay the shawl upon it, and cover the center also, with the meal; then roll it up closely and put it away for a week, when, by dusting out the meal, the shawl will be nice and clean," so says " Valentia," of Brockwood, Ill., in the *Blade*, or, she says:

**2. Another and Quicker Way.**—Is to take the same kind of corn meal, ½ pt. and coarse salt, ½ pt.; mixing well, then with a brush, all being dry, scour, or rather rub well, both sides, this does the work quicker; but the first is the best because it saves the rubbing, which frets out the texture. Of course the lace would not stand the rubbing of this last plan. Understand no water is to be used, it is all done by the dry process.

**HINTS FOR THE LAUNDRY.—Washing All Colors of Cali-cos, Percales, Muslins, Brown Linen, etc., and to Remove Paint and Wine Stains From Silks, Woolen and Cotton Goods.**—Besides the foregoing receipts on general washings, etc., I deem it best to put in a few items, or "hints," as the above heading has it, from various sources, which are generally short, and right to the point for quick work. These first are from Mrs. E. S. Barrett, of Sing Sing, New York, July 1882, in the *New York Examiner*, wherein she says: "Every housekeeper knows how vexatious it is to have colored fabrics ruined in the process of cleansing. A few practical hints about washing calicoes, percales and muslins will therefore be of real service to the readers of the *Examiner*.

1. **For Washing Black and White, Stone, Slate, or Maroon Colored Cotton Goods.**—Before washing black and white, stone, slate, or maroon colored cotton goods; dip them in a solution of salt and water, made by dissolving two cupfuls of salt in 10 quarts of cold water, and hang them in a shady place to dry. The salt sets the colors. When dry, wash in a light suds in the usual way. Calicoes and muslins do not require a hot suds; water moderately warm is best. Never allow them to soak in the water. Wash quickly, turn the wrong side out, and dry in the shade. A little salt in the rinsing water is an improvement. Another way is to mix two cupfuls of wheat bran in cold water, making a smooth paste; then stir it into 1 qt. of soft boiling water. Let it boil 1 hour, then strain into 5 or 6 qts. of soft warm water. No soap is necessary, for bran has cleansing properties of its own. If there is black in the dress, or any other color that is liable to "run," add a tablespoonful of salt. Rinse thoroughly in one water. For starch, use a little white glue-water, cool and clean. Always iron on the wrong side with a moderately hot iron.

2. **How to Fix the Above Colors Permanently.**—Blue, stone, and slate-colored articles may be made to retain their color perfectly by adding sugar of lead to the water in which they are to be washed for the first time. Dissolve 1 oz. of sugar of lead in a pailful of hot water; stir carefully until it is thoroughly dissolved, and let the mixture cool. When about milk-warm, put in the articles and let them remain an hour. Hang up to dry before washing. When dry, wash as directed in bran water. The sugar of lead fixes the color permanently, so that this treatment with it will not need to be repeated. Use this preparation with caution; sugar of lead is poisonous, but no danger in this way of using it.

3. **To Wash Brown Linen.**—Take enough good timothy hay to fill a 10-quart kettle two-thirds' full when pressed down; cover it with soft water, and let it boil until the water assumes a dark greenish color. Make flour starch in the usual way, and strain the hay water into it after it becomes cool or tepid; let the linen soak ten or fifteen minutes—not longer—then wash without soap. I divide the preparation into two parts, using one for rinsing. Linen dresses and dusters washed in this way will look new as long as they last

4. **Fruit or Wine Stains, to Remove from Silk, Woolen, or Cotton Goods.**—Fruit or wine stains can be removed from silk, woolen or cotton goods by sponging them gently with ammonia and alcohol— a teaspoonful of ammonia to a wineglass of alcohol. Finish with clear alcohol. The fumes of a lighted match will remove remnants of stains.

**Washing Fine Under Clothing.**—The *Germantown Telegraph* says that a leading firm of that city, importers and retailers of hosiery goods, gives the following directions for washing the above named line of goods, and also says their own experience enables them to testify to its excellence. Dissolve 1 lb. of nice soap in 4 gallons of warm soft water in which well rinse the articles to be washed, drawing them repeatedly through the hand; press them as dry as possible, to remove the soap; rinse them again briskly in clean, lukewarm water; press out or put through a wringer, if you have one, and stretch them to their proper shape, and dry in the open air if possible. The only effects of rubbing are to shrink and destroy the material; it should therefore never be resorted to with these kinds of goods. The material used in manufacturing silk underwear being an animal product, it is absolutely necessary that nothing but the best quality of soap and warm water should be used.

**Washing Flannels of Any Kind, so they Shall Not Turn Yellow or Shrink.**—A lady signing herself " Michigan," says she wants to tell the ladies of the *Blade* how to wash flannels of any kind, so they won't turn yellow, nor shrink up, and that sort of thing. Wash in cold water, using soap in both suds. Of course you can take the chill off if you are afraid of taking cold, but not have it a bit hot. Now don't laugh at such an idea and not give it a trial, but this spring you wash your flannel blankets, woolen stockings, baby's flannel and then report. I learned of a Scotch lady years ago and never think of using hot water; use soft water of course.

*Remarks.*—Certainly the water being made a little warm will not cause shrinkage. The suds should be made before putting in the flannels, and not by rubbing the soap on them.

**For Washing Scarlet Flannels, etc., Without Fading or Shrinking.**—To prevent scarlet flannels or worsted goods of any kind of this color, from fading by washing, it is claimed by some washer-women that the following plan is perfectly safe: Mix flour, ½ cup, little by little, with cold water, 1 qt.; then boiling 10 or 15 minutes and mixing with the lukewarm suds, pressing and rinsing, up and down, a number of times, then passing through the wringer, the goods will not be faded or thickened, as there is to be no rubbing.

*Remarks.*—Hatters make wool, or felt hats, as they are called, by plaiting out a layer of wool upon a piece of cloth, at first, and dipping it into hot water, then rolling it with a little roller, re-dipping and rolling till they get the desired thickness, by the little hooks that are seen by the microscope only, which are upon the fibers of all good wool, to so take hold upon each other, as to make as heavy a body as desired. The same is done, to a certain extent, every time woolen goods is washed in hot water, by rubbing. Now any one can see to avoid thickening, "shrinking," as it is called, in washing flannels, simply avoid hot suds, and do not rub them. (See Washing Fine Under Clothing, etc., above.) Sudsing by an up and down motion, in first and second suds, is the safest method.

**Colored Silk Handkerchiefs, To Wash.**—To wash colored silk handkerchiefs make a good suds in lukewarm water, in which a little bit of carbonate of ammonia has been dissolved; rub the handkerchiefs lightly in the hands till all the spots have disappeared.    Then rinse them in lukewarm water, and squeeze them as dry as possible.    Take hold of the two corners and shake and snap each one for a few minutes.    Roll in a soft towel lightly, laying the handkerchief flat on the towel at first, squeeze tightly, and iron at once.— *Detroit Free Press.*

**Old Silk Dresses, etc.—To Renovate to Look Like New.**—A writer says: "A most satisfactory way to renovate old silks is to boil an old kid glove in 1 pt. of soft water until the glove shrinks to the size of a 4-years-old child's hand; the liquor will then be glutinous: when cold, having brushed out every particle of dust, sponge the silk thoroughly and smooth wtth a hot iron upon the wrong side."

*Remarks.*—If a dress, it may be well to take it to pieces, if much soiled, as recommended with "Silk Cashmere, etc., to Clean," which see.

**Washing Carpets Without Taking Up.**—Put a table-spoonful of ammonia in 1 gal. of moderately warm water, and with sponge or soft broom go all over the carpet, and you will be astonished to see how brightly it will look for the little labor and expense.    [See "Spirits of Ammonia—Some of Its Uses, etc."]

**Washing Windows.**—A writer says: "Have a pail partly filled with water a little warm and dissolve in it a tea-spoonful of borax [the author thinks it would be better to use a table-spoonful of powdered borax, or else the same amount of spirits of ammonia to 1 gal. of water, as above for washing carpets]; have one chamois (a cloth will do nicely) dipped into the water to wash the windows with, then with a dry chamois rub the window dry and polish.    [A chamois skin is best to polish with, as it leaves no lint as a cloth will.]    In this way windows may be cleaned in a very few moments and not wet the carpets nor tire the person."

**Lace Veils and Other Laces—To Wash or Renovate.**—Wash veils carefully in alcohol and soft water, equal parts, simply squeezing in the hands in and out of the mixture; then lay a towel on a table and smooth out the veil and pin the edges to the towel to dry, when, if carefully done, it will look as good as new.    Borax water is also used for the same purpose, drying the same way.

**For Other Nice Laces.**—Naomi King, in *Farm and Fireside*, says: "When you have some nice laces to wash put a little borax in warm soap suds and allow them to soak 1 hour; then shake about in it well and rinse in 2 or 3 clear waters, as you see necessary, and to the last water add a little white sugar; never use starch.    Pull out well, and place between white cloths in an old book until dry."

*Remarks.*—She says a "little" borax and a "little" sugar, which is very indefinite.    A rounding tea-spoonful of powdered borax and the same amount of sugar would be plenty for 1 pt. of water.    The borax would do good in washing veils, and I think the sugar would also be good there, as with white or other laces.

Softening Hard Water for Washing Clothes, Dishes, or House Cleaning.—A writer says: "Take 2 lbs. of washing soda (sal soda), and 1 lb. of common stone lime, and boil in 5 gals. of water for 2 or 3 hours; then stand away to settle, and· dip off the clear water from the top and put into a jug (pouring off carefully is better). Can be used for washing dishes or cleaning, and 1 teacup in a boiler of clothes, put in after the water is hot, will whiten the clothes, and soften the water, without injury to the hands, or clothes. I use an old iron pot to make it in."

*Remarks.*—Some of these newspaper writers get some most excellent things, but again, some of them make poor describers as to the best plan of using; for instance, this woman (for it is undoubtedly a woman), says: "Boil in 5 gals. of water," then further on, "put into a jug. Now, would it not take a big jug, or two or three small ones? and again, it cannot be to be used even in 5 gals. of water, without further dilution, for she says: "1 tea-cupful in a boiler of clothes, put in after the water is hot," etc., then why not boil it in say 2 gals. of water? then a 2 gal. jug will hold it, and use a little less to a boiler of clothes, stirred well into ·the water when hot, before putting in the clothes; and half as much more for each additional boiler at the same washing will be plenty; in fact it does make a splendid washing fluid as I have above suggested, and a table-spoon of it in a dish-pan of water for washing dishes will help much in cleaning the dishes; and a little of it in a pan of water for house-cleaning is, or will be, "just splendid," as the girls say. · A spoonful of it in a pt. or a qt. of water for cleaning finger-marks off of doors or other wood-work, is good, and if kept ready-made, is always handy, although the spirits of ammonia (which see) in like quantities, is good for general house-cleaning, window-washing, etc. I do not know who this writer was, as it was a slip sent to me having no name attached, but I know enough to know it is a grand good thing. A little of this, say 2 table-spoonfuls of it in 2 qts. of hot water, is just the thing to soak feet in, to soften corns and to soften the dead skin about the heels, and to make a thorough work of cleaning the feet, generally.

Softening Water—Clark's Method.—By adding burnt quick-lime (quick-lime is freshly burned or unslacked lime), to hard water, which contains lime (all hard water contains lime, 'tis the lime that makes it hard), it will become soft. The added lime seizes the carbonic acid gas which held the carbonate of lime in solution, and so both the original carbonate of lime and that formed in the process, fall together as a white sediment. This method is truly homœopathic.

*Remarks.*—This writer is right as to the way it softens, but is tame in not giving the proper amount for a bbl. or some other measure. About 2 or 3 table-spoonfuls of this stone-lime, just slacked with a little hot water, will be enough for a barrel, just drawn from the well. Rummage it in thoroughly, that is stir it with a stick that will reach the bottom till well mixed, and let it settle over night, or 2 or 3 hours.

Ammonia, its Various Uses in House Cleaning, Washing, etc. —"A Farmer's Wife," in the *Country Gentleman*, says of it: There is no telling what a thing will do till you try it. I knew ammonia, diluted in water, could restore rusty silks and clean coat collars, but when I got a green spot on the carpet, I tried half a dozen other things before I thought of that, and that is just what did the work effectually. I put a tea-spoonful into about a tea-cup of hot water, took a cloth and wet the spot thoroughly, just rubbing it slightly, and the ugly spot was gone. It is splendid for cleaning your silver; it makes things as bright as new without any expenditure of strength; and for looking glasses and windows it is best of all; and one day when I was tired and my dish cloths looked rather gray, I turned a few drops of the ammonia into the water and rubbed them out, and I found it acted like a charm, and I shall be sure to do so again some day. I suppose housewives have a perfect right to experiment and see what results they can produce; and if they are not on as large a scale as the farmers try, they are just as important to us, and they make our work light and brighter too. Now, I do not believe in luxuriating in a good thing all alone, and I hope all the housekeepers will send and get a 10 cent bottle of spirits of ammonia and commence a series of chemical experiments and see what they can accomplish with it. Take the boys' jackets, the girls' dresses, and when you have cleaned everything else, put a few drops in some soft water and wash the little folks' heads, and report results.

*Remarks.*—These items are valuable in giving new thoughts to those who have few opportunities for observation, or reading the literature of the day; but they would be more valuable if they gave the proportions for each class of work to be done. This lady speaks of restoring rusty silk, how strong? For cleaning greasy clothing, use it strong, say a table-spoonful to 1 cup of warm, soft water, washing off with pure water directly; for silks, alpacas, etc., the same strength ammonia will be strong enough, brushing off soon with pure water; for looking glasses a little put on a cloth, clear, and folding some of the dry cloth on the back of the wet part, to keep it off the fingers, is best, as it takes but a moment to take off fly specks, or dirt; for windows a table-spoonful of it in 1 pt. of water will be plenty, wiping off nicely with a dry newspaper, as it leaves no lint like a cloth does; one-fourth ammonia for cleaning boys' coat collars, and greasy clothing; for cleaning silver, 1 table-spoonful to 1 pt., or a little less of water, is enough, and, as she says, it is splendid for this and all other similar work; and as it is cheap, it makes a great saving.

**For Bee and Wasp Stings.**—A little ammonia put upon bee and wasp stings, bites of spiders and all other poisonous insect bites, will neutralize the poison, preventing soreness and swelling. But mind, it only needs a very little put on, and wash off soon, to prevent its making a sore.

**Borax, for Roaches, Washing, and as a Dentifrice and Catarrh Snuff.**—Although I have given an item on its uses, yet as I have another short item upon it, I will give it, to corroborate the other, and to show in a few words, what some people know of its value. This writer says: One-half pound of it powdered, and sprinkled around their haunts, will drive the roaches out of any house. A large handful of the powder to 10 gallons of water will effect a saving of 50 per cent. (one-half) in soap. It is an excellent dentifrice, and the best material for cleaning the scalp. (See the author's remarks upon it, following the other recipe.) A recent medical writer also claims powdered borax to be valuable as a catarrh snuff.

**Iron Rust, to Remove from Clothing.**—Get ½ oz. of oxalic acid, in small pieces, in a vial and keep corked. When a spot of iron rust shows on white table cloths, or other white clothing, dissolve ½ tea-spoonful of the acid by pouring upon it 2 or 3 table-spoonfuls of hot water, and dip the spot in or wet it with a sponge, or bit of rag, and as soon as the rust is bleached out wash right out with clean water, so the acid will not hurt the goods. Lemon juice and a little salt is also good for the same purpose, laying out in the sun to bleach; if one application does not wholly remove it, do the same again. Or, instead of putting out in the sun, wet with lemon juice, and hold the spot over a steaming hot tea-kettle will do it very quickly. Or, the cream of tartar plan, as given below, for removing fruit stains, will also remove rust.

**Fruit Stains, Recent, or Old, to Remove.**—"Aunt Sophia," in the *Blade*, tells us recent fruit stains may be removed by holding the linen tightly across the tub and pouring hot water through them, before any soap is put on; if old, tie up a little cream of tartar in the places, put into cold water and bring to a boil. If got upon table linen, rub on some salt, at once, then pour on the hot water.

**Bleaching Muslin.**—Mrs. "S. M. B." sends the *Blade* the following directions, which she has practiced for 12 years without injuring the cloth. She says: "Into 8 qts. of warm soft water put 1 lb. of chloride of lime; stir with a stick a few minutes, then strain through a bag of coarse muslin, working it with the hands [the author says with the stick] to dissolve thoroughly. Add to this, in a tub, 5 buckets of warm water, stir in the chloride water thoroughly and put in the muslin. [The muslin ought to be thoroughly wet first in plain water, so it shall take the lime water evenly.] Let it remain in 1 hour, turning it over occasionally, that every part may get thoroughly bleached. When taken out, wash well in two waters, to remove the lime, rinse and dry. This quantity will bleach 25 yds. of yard-wide muslin. The muslin will bleach more evenly and quickly if it has been thoroughly wet and dried before bleaching."

*Remarks.*—This lady makes a "mighty sight" of work, more than is necessary. She wants it wet and dried before putting into the bleaching water, when simply wetting is sufficient, and one good washing and rinsing after the bleaching is enough—all you want is to get rid of specks of the lime, and this has been done largely by straining off the water from the lime sediment at the beginning. Spreading on the grass is a good way to dry it.

**Mildew, to Remove from Clothing.**—Take common soft soap and stir in quite a bit of salt, so the soap crumbles or grains, as it were, and rub on the spot and lay out over night, and if not effaced by morning wet it occasionally during the day. The chloride solution above is also good to remove mildew. Or, to put about ½ a cup of chloride of lime into 2 qts. of hot water, wetting the mildewed articles first in cold water, then put into the lime water until the mildew is bleached out, then rinse well in plenty of water to remove the lime.

1. **GLOSSY LINEN—How it is Done.**—To give starched linen the appearance so much desired put a small bit of paraffine (size of a small pea for each bosom, or its equivalent of cuffs) into the hot starch, and when it comes to ironing use a small iron having a rounded point that is very smooth, and rub with great pressure and for a considerable time. A great deal of "elbow-grease" is absolutely necessary.

2. **Scorched Linen in Ironing, To Whiten.**—If a linen shirt bosom, or any other article, has been scorched in ironing lay it in the bright sunshine, which will remove it entirely.

**Flat-Irons, To Clean from Rust or Starch.**—Flat-irons often have starch stick to them, and occasionally a spot of rust from a drop of water shows upon them, and I have often seen directions for cleaning them with salt, but the following plan is the only sensible way of doing it that I have seen: Have a piece of yellow beeswax in a coarse cloth; when the iron is almost hot enough to use, but not quite, rub it quickly with the beeswax cloth and then with a coarse cloth.

**Oil-Cloth—To Keep Bright.**—Oil-cloths should never be scrubbed with suds, but carefully swept with a soft hair brush and washed with a cloth dipped into milk and water, half-and-half, but no soap, and dry and polish with an old soft cloth. In this way they will keep their original color a long time.

**Color of Plants and Flowers, to Retain, in Drying for Herbariums.**—Botanists who are grieved at the rapid loss of color in the plants and flowers of their herbariums will be pleased to learn, says a Vienna journal, that if plants or flowers be dipped in a warm mixture of 1 part of hydrochloric acid to 600 of alcohol before being placed between the driers they will not only retain their natural colors, but will also dry with greater quickness.—*Harper's Weekly.*

*Remarks.*—This is in the proportion of 1 dr. of the acid to 9 ozs. and 3 drs. of alcohol, and must prove very satisfactory.

2. **Another Way.**—Another new way for preserving the color of autumn leaves is given as follows: "Iron them fresh with a warm (not hot) iron, on which some spermaceti has been lightly rubbed. This method preserves perfectly their lovely tints, and gives a wavy gloss which no other one secures. The process is very rapid and very agreeable, and no lady who has ever tried the tedious and uncertain experiment of pressing will ever again resort to it after trying this new and better way."

*Remarks.*—The iron must be kept hot enough to keep the spermaceti soft, else it will not spread on the leaves.

**Tomatoes, To Ripen in December.**—A Massachusetts gardener sells ripe tomatoes in December, by sowing the seeds in July, then potting the plants in a 9-inch jar, and maturing in a green-house with artificial heat as soon as needed. An infusion of tomato leaves has been recently found to not only destroy plant lice, but from its peculiar odor prevent their return for a long time. See these destroyers.

**Plant Jars, To Paint and Bronze for House Use.**—Plant jars for out-door use ought, to look well, be painted with bright colors, as red or blue—the foliage gives the contrast with its green; but for house use paint them over with plain, cheap varnish, then with a bit of pad, or piece of broadcloth upon a thin, small bit of board, apply common bronze powder all over; or, to make them nicer, paint the bodies, some red and some blue, then bronze the rim, which gives them a gold-like appearance, contrasting prettily with the painted body. The bronze on a varnish will not stand the rains and exposure out of doors.

**Cracked Hands, To Cure.**—A laboring man who had been troubled with cracked hands, and tried many other remedies without success, was finally told to put common copal varnish into the cracks which, in 48 hours, entirely cured them. Others came, but the same remedy always cured. He had given it to others with the same success before making it public. He bought a 10-cent bottte, kept it corked, and applied when needed with a bit of sliver from the fire wood. It is simple and efficient. Most all painters and paint dealers keep it.

**CARROTS.—Their Value as Food for Man and Domestic Animals.**—A writer, with whom the author agrees—except that he thinks parsnips preferable to carrots for horses—says: "The carrot is one of the most healthful and nutritious of our garden roots, and deserves to be much more extensively used for culinary purposes, and we urge our readers to give some of the early table sorts a trial. As an agricultural root, the carrot is not surpassed for feeding horses and milch cows, and every farmer should plant a few for this purpose. The carrot succeeds best on light, sandy loam, made rich by manuring the previous year. In freshly manured land, the roots often grow awkward and ill shaped. It is better to sow as early in the spring as the ground can be made ready, but if planting is necessarily delayed until late in the season, soak the seed 24 hours in tepid water, dry by mixing in sifted ashes or plaster, and sow on freshly prepared soil."

*Remarks.*—In drills would be best, the author thinks, as explained in the item referred to.

**Pickled Carrots for Table Use.**—A recent writer in the *Rural New Yorker* says, under this head: "Wash and scrape, boil until tender, cut into quarters of convenient length, and cover with vinegar. It is the best way to prepare carrots for the table."

*Remarks.*—If the vinegar is properly spiced, this plan makes them very palatable.

**Beans Should Always be Cooked in Soft Water.**—A. C. Arnold, of Stamford, Conn., says: "I notice those who tell how to cook beans omit to say that soft water must always be used in beans, otherwise some of them will remain hard—a fact that I learned in the army."

*Remarks.*—It is undoubtedly better to use soft water for cooking generally, when it can be done. The same man sends the next item also, through the *Blade*, and as it is a thing needed in every household that ever cooks apples, I will give it a place. His measurements are correct to make a suitable-sized corer.

**Apple Corer, to Make—Size to Cut the Tin, Etc.**—Cut the tin 3 by 4 inches and roll it up to be 4 inches long, and ¾ inch in diameter, at the smallest end, as it should be a very little larger at the other end, to withdraw easily.

*Remarks.*—If a small wire is put into the large end before rolling up, it will not hurt the hand to push it through the apple, without which, it would soon injure the hand.

**1. Silverware, to Brighten with Little Labor.**—When it is desirable to brighten silverware without a formal scouring, prepare some pieces of silver cloth, as follows: Obtain hartshorn (carbonate of ammonia), 2 ozs., powdered or broken up finely, and boil it in 1 pt. of soft water. Dip suitable pieces of muslin in the liquor and hang up to dry without wringing. When dry, fold closely and put away for use. Simply rubbing the silver with one of these pieces will surprise you by its improved appearance. Never put soap on silverware, if you wish to keep its original lustre.

**2. Frosted Silverware, How to Clean.**—Frosted ornamentation on silverware should never be cleaned with powder, but only with a soft brush and strong lye (from wood ashes, strained, or from concentrated lye or potash), accompanied by rinsings with soft water. After the frosted parts are properly dry, the smooth parts should be rubbed carefully with powder.—*Harper's Bazar.*

*Remarks.*—The silver-cloth in next recipe above, will do nicely for the smooth part.

**3. Polish for Silverware.**—In place of using Paris white for a dry powder to polish the smooth parts of silverware, the following will be found better: Put 4 ozs. of Paris white into soft water, 1 pt., and boil it; when cool, bottle it, and add one oz. of aqua ammonia. Rub with a cloth wet with this mixture, shaken, and polish with chamois.

**Stains from Nitrate of Silver, to Remove.**—Wet nitrate of silver stains with discolored tincture of iodine in as much water as tincture. Then rub the stained spot with a piece of cyanide of potassa. It fades out, or changes at once (or the hyposulphite of soda will do, and is not poison), then wash immediately with water. Always use soft water if you can. This is from a photographer, and reliable.

**Cabbage, to Destroy the Cut-worm of, and to Prevent Club-feet.**—Sprinkle a table-spoonful of salt around each plant as set out, and mix slightly with the soil. Thus, you "kill two birds with one stone," besides it is a good fertilizer. I have seen more than half the plants set out in a garden patch, which were cut off the first night. This little trouble saves the loss, and makes them grow faster, too. [See also, cut worms to destroy.

**Crickets, to Drive Away or Destroy.**—Put Scotch snuff into their holes. It is too much for them, and I think it would be more than roaches could stand the presence of. Put into crevices with a feather.

**1. Chimneys, How to Build to Avoid Burning Out.**—When

building chimneys, keep a mortar-board of mortar for the purpose of plastering them upon the inside as the work goes on, tempered up by adding one-fourth as much common salt as of mortar, which forms a glaze that soot can not stick to, and hence there is none to burn. " Prevention is better than cure."

**2. Chimneys, to Build to Avoid Smoking.**—A builder of long experience says: " To build a chimney that shall not smoke, give a large space immediately above the throat, which will cause a draft. It may then be narrowed, if desirable." This is good logic.

**3. Chimneys, Sky-lights, etc., to Stop Leaks.**—Take fine, white sand, 20 measures; litharge, 2; freshly slacked lime, 1; mix evenly together, dry; then wet to the consistence of soft putty with boiled linseed oil. It sets quickly, and forms a hard and durable cement.

**1. Moths in Carpets, to Prevent.**—Wet the floor around the edge of the room thoroughly with spirits of turpentine before laying the carpet, apply with a brush as you would paint; it kills the nits or eggs under the base, and also prevents further nesting. Salt sprinkled freely about the edge and over the whole carpet, while sweeping, is not only a preventive, but it also helps to remove dirt, and if damp, prevents dust from rising while sweeping.

**2. Moths in Carpets, To Destroy, Without Taking Up.**—On parts of a carpet where moths are suspected lay a coarse towel, slightly wrung out of clear water, spreading out smoothly; then place a piece of firm wrapping paper upon the wet towel to keep in the steam, and iron it thoroughly with a hot iron. If thoroughly done, the heat and steam kills them. Repeat at any time if satisfied more have hatched and come out from under the base or other hiding places. It does not injure the carpet, nor fade the colors, and does not need hard pressure, as it is the heat and steam that kills them.—*The Household.*

**3. Moths in Upholstered Furniture, Certain Remedy, Also Good for Furs, Flannels, etc.**—A writer in one of the Grand Rapids' (Mich.) papers says, upon these subjects: "A sort of trade secret among upholsterers for ridding upholstered furniture of moths, is the following"; and gives an example: " A set of furniture that seemed to be alive with the larvæ (the insect moth in its first stage of development,) from the time it came new, and from which hundreds of these pest. nad been picked and brushed, was set in a room by itself. Three gallons of benzine were purchased at 30 cents a gallon, retail. Using a small watering pot with a fine rose sprinkler, the whole upholstery was saturated through and through with the benzine. Result— Every moth, larvæ and egg were killed. The benzine dried out in a few hours, and its entire odor disappeared in 3 or 4 days. Not the slightest harm happened to the varnish, or wood, or fabrics, or hair stuffing. That was months ago, and not a sign of a moth has since appeared. The carpets were also well sprinkled all round the sides of the room, with equally good effect. For furs, flannels, indeed, all woolen articles containing moths, benzine is most valuable. Put them in a box; sprinkle with benzine, close the box tightly, and in a day or **two** the pests will be exterminated, and the benzine will evaporate on opening."

*Remarks.*—In using benzine, as stated in connection with cleaning gloves, remember there must be no fire nor lamp burning, as the vapor of it carries the fire to the stuff itself, which is very inflammable, and explosive. With this care it is safe.

**4. Moth Powder, To Put Away Furs, Woolens, etc.**—Lupulin (flour of hops), 1 dr.; Scotch snuff, 2 ozs.; powdered gum camphor and black pepper, each, 1 oz.; cedar sawdust, 4 ozs. Mix thoroughly, and strew (or put in small paper bags) among the furs or woolen goods (after they have been thoroughly whipped with small rods) which are being put away. This powder contains some of all the best-known preventives. But if moth eggs have already been laid in them, unless the whipping takes them out, they will hatch and start their destructive work, unless the benzine or some other "killer" is used; hence it is best to keep an eye on them occasionally, and whip thoroughly again if any are seen. This whipping the moth and their eggs out, then sealing up in boxes or paper bags, is from the *Boston Transcript*, which adds: "If you shut moths out, and shut none in, you are perfectly safe." Not a doubt of it.

**Cracks and Small Holes in Walls, To Fill.**—Mix plaster of Paris to the consistency of soft putty, and apply immediately and smooth with a case-knife, will make it as nice as a mason would do it. Mix but little at a time as it sets quickly, unless you work it over every minute or two; but after it "sets" or becomes hard it is not good even to work over after that. If you have a nice, white sand, a little of it may be mixed in, but it does very well without it.

**ONIONS—Medicinal Effects Against Worms in Children and Colds in the Chest.**—A mother writes to *Hant's* (*Eng.*) *Advertiser* upon these matters (which, also in my own judgment, may be relied upon) as follows: "Twice a week invariably—and it was generally when we had cold meat minced—I gave the children a dinner which was hailed with delight and looked forward to; this was a dish of boiled onions. The little things know not that they were taking the best of medicine for expelling what most children suffer from—worms. Mine were kept free with this remedy alone. Not only boiled onions for dinner, but chives also they were encouraged to eat with their bread and butter, and for this purpose they had tufts of chives in their gardens. It was a medical man who taught me to eat boiled onions as a specific (positive cure) for a cold in the chest. He did not know at the time, until I told him, that they were good for anything else." The editor adds: "A case is now under our own observation in which a rheumatic patient, an extreme sufferer, finds great relief from eating onions freely, either cooked or raw. He insists that it is by no means a fancy, and he says so after having persistently tried Turkish baths, galvanism, and nearly all the potions and plasters that are advertised as certain alleviates or cures."

*Remarks.*—For the author's opinion, and that of others, as to the value of onions as an alterative, see Medical Department upon them as an alterative.

**Onion Culture—The Newest Way.**—The following item was

recently published in the *Evening Post*, of Toledo, and I give it a place that my readers may judge for themselves whether they will continue to drill their rows only about a foot apart and cultivate wholly by hand or drill at least two feet apart and use the horse hoes or cultivator, which will, of course, require more land to raise a certain amount of bushels. This must, or ought to, be governed by the amount of land one has, and also more particularly upon the amount of help which one has to aid in the hand part of the culture; for the thinning out the plants, as well as pulling the weeds within an inch or two of the row, must, in all cases, be done by hand. The writer says: "Onions will thrive in any soil, with proper fertilizers and good cultivation, yet they produce more profitably on old onion land, annually fertilized. Drilling in the seed and cultivating with horse power is a great improvement upon the old method. The rows should be far enough apart to cultivate with a horse hoe. This takes more land but pays best, where not very large onions are desired. Thinning onions so that only 1 is left to 3 or 4 inches of ground is being abandoned by onion culturists, as medium-sized bulbs demand better prices in most city markets. Everything which can promote rapid growth is essential in onion culture. It is better to sow the seed too thick than too thin. A drill set to drop 2 or 3 seeds to each inch of a row answers the purpose best."

*Remarks.*—Unless my ground was very rich and had been previously cultivated with onions, to have the weeds "well in hand," I should certainly prefer not to have more than one seed to an inch at the very most.

**3. Onions, How Many Can be Raised to the Acre.**—This question being often asked, should be judiciously answered, lest some person may be led into the business too extensively for his knowledge of how it must be done, as the *Ohio Farmer* speaks of, from a report that D. M. Ferry, of Detroit, Mich., grew 600 bushels of onions on an acre, and for which he was offered $2.50 a bushel, or $1,500 from an acre; and this, says the *Farmer*, led a farmer who heard of it, and knew no more of onion growing than he did of Sanskrit, to plant 5 acres of common corn land in onions, the next season, the seed costing him $100. He didn't grow a bushel of marketable onions. Had he studied up the subject and planted the first season ⅛ or ¼ of an acre, he might now be a successful onion grower, whereas he indulges in profanity at the smell of an onion.

*Remarks.*—But over 700 bushels have been raised to the acre, on a field of 7 acres, as the *Congregationalist*, of Boston, shows by the following in answer to an inquiry of a correspondent, who asked: "How many onions can be raised to the acre?" To which the editor makes this statement: "In answer to the above, we give a letter received recently from Deer Island, Boston Harbor, where one of the public institutions of Boston is located. 'In reply to yours of this date, I would say that in the year 1869, we raised, on 7 acres of land, 5,000 bushels of onions, good measure. I selected and had measured off ½ an acre of land where the crop was the best, and measured from this ½ acre 486 bushels of onions. The onions grew very large. I sent 1 bushel to the fair that averaged 1 pound each.'"

*Remarks.*—But now, it is not to be understood that this was done on poorly prepared soil, but rather soil adapted to them (a sandy loam is considered best), and previously, no doubt, cultivated to onions, having been well manured and well worked.

**4. Onions, How to Avoid Scullions.**—Notwithstanding some people think that scullions will be scullions, the following from "D," of Fenton, Mich, through the *Post and Tribune,* of Detroit, in answer to a query of L. C. Zarbell, on avoiding scullions, says: " I will tell him what an old gardener says, and that is to draw the earth away gradually from the bulbs until they are quite uncovered and only the fibrous roots are in the earth, and you will never have scullions, but very large, sound onions. The seed should be sown very early to have the benefit of the coolness and moisture of early spring."

**5. Onion Raising, Value of Wood Ashes as a Manure for.**—A writer in one of the agricultural papers upon this subject says: Farmers who are so fortunate as to have an open fire-place, should place, as an offset to the cost of the wood, the value of the ashes produced. For onions there is no fertilizer equal to wood ashes, as they require a great deal of potash. Market gardeners and others who make a specialty of growing onions will understand that to succeed with the crop they need larger supplies of potash than they will ordinarily receive from barn-yard manures.

*Remarks.*—I am unable to see why ashes from a stove are not better than from an open fire-place, as above named, as those from a stove are certainly more thoroughly burned, and hence must be stronger and better. Although wood ashes are undoubtedly an excellent manure for onions, yet well rotted stable manure must be the principal dependence, except with those who have plenty of hog manure, which has long been considered the best, but chiefly, no doubt, because it is more free from weed, and grass seeds, than stable manure; yet, where much corn and corn meal are fed to hogs, their manure is more than ordinarily rich. The following is a summing up of the whole matter of raising onions.

**6. An Acre in Onions.**—Under this head recently, the Chicago *Times* gave such minute instructions upon the whole question of onion raising, I will close the subject by giving it entire; as I deem the subject to be of such importance as to justify all that has been said, and that this item will add to it; for there is not a doubt but what onions are the most healthful vegetable grown, being a valuable alterative, as well as nourishing, and also an article for which there will always be a reasonable demand in the cities. The *Times* says:

"Few farmers seem to realize the fact that as much money may be obtained from an acre of land in onions as from a 40 acre farm devoted to the usual crops. At present prime onions are worth $4.00 per barrel by the car-load, and 250 barrels may be, and not unfrequently are, produced from an acre of land. Let no one, however, expect to realize $1,000 from an acre in onions who does not pay the best attention to the crop. To begin with, land naturally adapted to producing the crop should be selected. Experiments made in the eastern states, where large quantities of onions are raised for the southern market, show that there is no better soil for onions than that of a reclaimed bog. [Equivalent to our western marshes, which have been drained and well cultivated.] Of course the land must be well drained and the surface soil decomposed by exposure to the action of the atmosphere. Most of our black prairie soils are suitable to the production of onions if they are rightly treated. The turf must become entirely rotted and mixed with the earth below. Land that has been in pasture for several years is easily prepared for a crop of onions, as the turf is comparatively thin, while the soil is quite free from weeds. That portion of a pasture on which cattle and sheep lie at night may be converted into an onion-patch to excellent advantage.

"A field for onions should be very nearly level. If there are elevations in it, the soil on them will be likely to wash away, carrying off the seed before it germinates, or leaving part of the onions exposed to the sun. A piece of land intended for onions should be entirely free from the seeds of weeds in the start, and there should be a determination on the part of the grower to allow none to attain any considerable size. Absolutely clean culture is essential to producing a paying crop. Neglect in this matter will cause a vast amount of work, which will not, after all, insure a good crop. A field of onions cannot be neglected on account of a demand for labor on other parts of a farm. Unless a farmer has help that can attend to his field of onions during the season of plowing corn, cutting grass and harvesting grains, it will be better not to attempt to raise the crop at all. The care of onions, however, calls for light work, which may be chiefly performed by old men, partial invalids, women and children. Persons who cannot perform heavy work on the farm may engage in onion-raising to excellent advantage.

"It is useless to undertake to raise a paying crop of onions on land that is not very highly manured. From 30 to 50 loads of manure should be applied to an acre of land designed for producing this crop. It should be well rotted and free from the seed of grass and weeds. Unleached ashes form a valuable addition to composted stable manure. After a piece of land has been prepared for onions it is best to continue the crop for a series of years. As onions are gross feeders, it will, of course, be necessary to apply a coating of manure every season. The soil of an onion-field should be well pulverized and the manure thoroughly incorporated with it. After it is plowed and harrowed a roller should be employed for crushing the lumps.

"Many growers employ a hand-rake for fining the soil before the seed is sown. About 4 lbs. of seed are required for an acre. It should be the product of the previous season. [I would never use old seed.] The seed may be tested by counting out a certain number and placing them on some moist cotton laid in a saucer. If good, it will germinate in 3 or 4 days. The seed should be sown as early in the spring as it is possible to prepare the land. Growers who aim to get the largest yield from a given amount of land allow only the space of a foot between the rows. There is a drill which plants two rows of onion seed at once. If sown by hand one seed should be dropped every inch. In order to mark the rows it is well to drop a radish seed every 5 or 6 inches [merely to point out the row so you can cultivate varieties]. The radishes will grow very rapidly, and will be large enough to pull before the onions attain sufficient size to be injured by their presence. If there is no market for radishes in the vicinity, cabbage plants may be raised in their place. When of sufficient size they may be pulled and transplanted.

"The cultivation of onions must be chiefly performed by means of hand tools. [See No. 2.] The shuffle hoe is the best implement for doing most of the work. It should be of the best quality, and great pains should be taken to keep it clean and sharp. After the plants are about four inches high they must be thinned so that each has a space of about three inches in which to grow. Some growers who seek to raise very large crops allow three onions to grow in the space of six inches. Of course, they crowd each other after they have become of nearly full size, but this thick setting is necessary to secure the maximum yield. After they are thinned to the proper distance nothing is required by way of cultivation except to keep the soil light and free from weeds."

*Remarks.*—I hardly suppose it would "pay big" if every person in the land should engage in raising onions, or even to put out and properly cultivate "an acre;" but of this there is no probable danger. But if those who do go into it from what has been here said upon the subject do not do it well, it will not be the fault of the author. [See, also, "Cucumbers, a Paying Crop."]

**CEMENTS.—Dr. Choris' Magic Mender, or "Boss" Cement.** —Acetic acid, 4 Fs—the strongest—2 lbs.; French isinglass, 1 lb. Boil in a porcelain kettle.

*Remarks.*—I paid $5 for this recipe, and the above is all there was of it. The man, however, was selling it upon the street corners of this city (Toledo), and seeing what it would do, I paid the money, but was allowed to go with him and see it made. He bought the isinglass in a 1 lb. package for $1.25, and the acid, 2 lbs. for 50 cents, including the bottle, and he had a 1 gal. porcelain kettle with him, and first put the acid in and placed it on the stove in the hotel, kitchen where he was stopping, and when it was about boiling hot he took the package of isinglass by the end and stirring the acid with it it soon dissolved down near his fingers; then he dropped all in, and with a sliver from the wood, stirred it around a little all the time till it was dissolved; then commenced bottling it directly, by pouring some into a milk pitcher and then into the bottles, keeping the rest hot until all was poured in. He charged not to allow it to burn; and I afterwards found it would burn easily, hence he was careful of this, as it blackens and destroys it. He said the isinglass generally cost him $1.25 per lb.; the acid, 15 to 25 cents per lb.; ½ oz., square, flint glass bottles, $1.25 per gross, in 6 gross lots, in Pittsburgh; and the corks, 12 cents per gross, in Cleveland, in 5 gross lots. I have made it in those quantities and placed it on sale in the stores and know its value. It was first shown at the Centennial in Philadelphia, under the name of "English Stratena," and the following rhyming, as given on some of the hand-bills wrapped around the bottles, will show

**What it is Good for.—**

> For the carpenter putting his frame together,
> For the shoemaker working on fancy leather,
> For putting patches on boots so nice,
> And it holds them on as tight as a vice;
> For splicing belts and mending harness,
> Lamps, chimneys, or looking-glasses;
> For the clerk at his desk pronounces it safer
> Than any description of wax or wafer;

For mending sugar bowls or ladles,
For mending canes, clocks, or babies' cradles;
For mending all dishes with ease,
On which you can put bread, butter, and cheese;
And every housewife, too, declares
It beats the world on broken chairs;
For fancy boxes, chessboards, stands;
For picture frames and ivory fans;
For broken tables, writing cases;
For fractured lamps, Bohemian vases.

All articles of glass or bone;
For marble, porcelain, or stone.
For fancy figures, busts of plaster;
For images in alabaster.
For meerschaum pipes it can't be beat—
It's all the better for the heat.
In billiard halls it's largely used
For putting tips upon the cues.
For hobby-horses, wood of skates,
Dolls, hoops, and broken slates;
For parasol handles, tips, and hooks;
For fastening loosened leaves in books.
In fact, 'twould take too long to mention
All uses of this new invention;
Whatever else there is about it,
Whoever tries it ne'er does without it.

*Remarks.*—Where glue will answer the purpose, it will, of course, be found much cheaper (see No. 3); but for all nice work, if carefully made, without bunring, it will be found to beat it, as it takes considerable heat to dissolve isinglass, hence its value for dishes. I sealed the bottles with No. 2 sealing wax, red, for bottling medicines.

**2. Cement for Tin Cans.**—Into a small saucepan—block-tin is best—put 1 lb. of rosin, ¼ lb. of gum-shellac and 2 ozs. of beeswax. Melt this and mix well with an old iron spoon—both spoon and saucepan must be devoted to the purpose, for they will be useless for all others. When the cans are ready for sealing, pour a fine stream of hot cement from the spoon into the groove as directed. It is better to fill it only half full, and when all the cans are finished, give each one an additional coating. Stick labels on the can with this wax while it is hot. In opening them, crack the wax, and with a pair of scissors or claw, loosen a portion of it. Brush off the dust; pry up the lid, and the balance of the wax will come off easily. Be careful that none of it falls into the fruit. Put the scraps of wax into the saucepan, and it will help towards sealing next season's cans.—*Mrs. L. V. M. A., Morrisonville, Ill., in Prairie Farm.*

**3. Cement, White and Cheap, with Glue, for General Purposes.**—Best white glue, 1 lb.; gum-shellac, 1 oz.; alcohol, 4 ozs.; aqua ammonia, 1 oz.; soft water, 2½ pts.; dry, pulverized white lead, 4 ozs. DIRECTIONS—Dissolve the shellac in the alcohol, to have it ready; then put the glue in the water, in a basin which can be set in a pan of water upon the stove so as to dissolve the glue without burning it; when the glue is dissolved, but still hot, stir in the powdered lead and the dissolved shellac; then add the ammonia, to keep it in liquid form, and bottle.

*Remarks.*—It is valuable for everything except materials where its whiteness would be an objection. Glue is always best to be applied hot, and to hot edges when practicable, but with this it is not necessary. Everything, however, must be kept in place till dry. Leather belts or cloth must be weighted till dry.

**4. China and Glass Cement.**—A writer says: "To 1 pt. of milk add 1 pt. of vinegar; separate the curds from the whey, and mix the whey with the whites of five eggs; beat it well together, sifting into it a sufficient quantity of quicklime to convert it into a thick paste. Broken china or glass mended with this cement will not again separate, and will resist the action of fire and water."

*Remarks.*—The curd is not used, and quicklime means the unslacked lime, but pulverized very finely before sifting in. I cannot see, however, why, if the lime is only recently burned, and good, it may not be slacked, and the finest powder of it used. Oyster shells burned make an excellent lime for cementing with white of eggs. I have used it. A lime of these may be used in the above if very finely pulverized.

**5. Cement for Marble and Alabaster.**—Portland Cement, 12 parts; slacked lime and fine white sand, each 6 parts; infusorial earth, 1 part. Make into a thick paste, with silicate of soda. Needs no heat; sets in 24 hours; crack is not readily found.—*Druggists' Circular.*

*Remarks.*—As stated in other places, where "parts" are mentioned, it matters not what sized measure is used, whether a spoon, pint or peck, or if weights, whether it be drs., ozs. or lbs. Simply 12, 6 and 1, in this case, would be the number to use, or the proportions to keep.

**6. Japanese Cement, To Make—Strong and Colorless—For Fancy Paper Work, Etc.**—Mix the best powdered rice with a little cold water; then gradually add boiling water till a proper consistency is acquired, being careful to keep it well stirred all the time; lastly, it must be boiled for one minute in a clean saucepan. This paste is beautifully white, almost transparent, and well adapted for fancy paper work, or other things requiring a strong and colorless cement.

**Coffee-Pots, Tea-Pots, Tin Saucepans, Etc., To Clean Inside.**—When the inside of a coffee or tea-pot has become black from long use, fill it with soft water; throw in a small piece of hard soap, and boil it from ½ to 1 hour; and it will be as "bright as a new button," without labor or expense. When tin sauce-pans become "grimmy" or dark from use, do the same with them, and you will be pleased with the result. Cover while boiling. Then scald out well and all is complete.

**Rust, to Remove from Stovepipe.**—Rub a very little raw linseed oil upon it, which stops its further eating; then dry it with a moderate fire, after which polish may be used if desired; but polish does not stop the deeper corrosion, or eating into the pipe; hence, after a little, it will again show through the polish, unless the oil is first used.

**Barrels and Other Wooden Vessels, to Cleanse.**—Barrels for wine, or cider, also vessels for culinary purposes, holding food, etc., are rendered fit for immediate use by a solution of sal-soda, says the *Journal of Chemistry*, thus: "An ordinary barrel should be filled half full of water, and a solution of about 2 lbs. of the soda in as much water as will dissolve it, poured in, and the liquids thoroughly mixed by shaking the barrel, which should then be filled to the bung with water, and allowed to remain from 12 to 14 hours; then, after withdrawing the discolored liquid, it should be well rinsed and filled with pure water, and should remain a few hours more, when it will be fit for use. Other wooden utensils may be similarly treated.

*Remarks.*—The soda should be fully dissolved in 3 or 4 qts. of water, by heat, before putting in. If not much musty, 1 lb. of soda will do.

**Cauliflowers, to Raise Successfully.**—To raise this delicious species of cabbage, successfully, it is necessary to plow very deep, and upon a good or well manured soil; for the roots of the cauliflower, by the middle of August have been known to penetrate to the depth of 3 feet. The main, or upper roots, however, extend horizontally, and are more numerous than the penetrating ones. The seed should be sown in rich soil, heavily fertilized and well pulverized, in frames, or hot houses, and should be transplanted while small; and, at first, like cabbages, the plants ought to be frequently hoed and the dirt well loosened about them. Every morning was my rule with cabbage, and I always had good ones; but after they are well established, they do not need so much care.

**1. EGGS—How to Preserve Them, Four Plans.**—Whatever excludes the air prevents the decay of the egg. What I have found to be the most successful method of doing so, is to place a small quantity of salt butter in the palm of the left hand and turn the egg around in it, so that every pore of the shell is closed; then dry a sufficient quantity of bran in an oven (be sure you have the bran well dried). Then pack them with the small ends down in a layer of bran and another of eggs until your box is full; then place in a cold, dry place. If done when newly-laid, they will retain the sweet milk and curd of a new laid egg for at least 8 or 10 months. Any oil will do, but salt butter never becomes rancid, and a very small quantity of butter will do a very large quantity of eggs. To insure freshness, I rub them when gathered in from the nests; then pack when there is a sufficient quantity.—*E. Alexander.*

**2. Eggs, to Keep from September to May.**—This receipt is from Mrs. Wm. Church, who says: "The best way she finds is to take a pot or pail, or anything convenient, put about an inch or two of bran of any kind—I generally take shorts from flour—being a farmer's wife I generally have it on hand—in it, put a layer of eggs, either end down, close together; then cover with meal, another layer of eggs, and so on until the box is full, occasionally giving it a shake to fill well between the eggs. This plan I have adopted for years with success, and the last when used—which is often the last of April and the beginning of May—are as good as the first. I commence to pack in September. The whole secret lies in carefully selecting fresh eggs, packing on end and keeping the air from them. Keep in a dry, cool place."

**3. Eggs, to Keep from September to April, as Good as Fresh.**—This is from J. B. Strathnairn, who says: "I take a tub of any size and put a layer of common salt about an inch deep in the bottom; then grease the eggs with butter (of course salted butter), and place them in the salt with the small end down, so that they will not touch the wood of the tub near each other; then fill the vacancies with salt, and cover them again about an inch deep as before; then place another layer of eggs as before; then salt alternately till the tub is filled; then cover the top with salt, and put them where they will not freeze. I have kept eggs in this manner from September until April as good as fresh. The grease on the shell keeps the salt from penetrating, thereby keeping the eggs fresh, while the saving qualities of the salt keep them from becoming putrid. This recipe is both cheap and good, as the salt can be fed to cattle afterward.

**4. Eggs—To Keep Two Years Perfectly Good.**—This is from Emily Audinwood, Stanstead Plains, P. Q.: "I have tried several experiments, but find none to answer so well as the following: I have kept eggs for two years, and found them perfectly good when used. Two pounds of coarse salt boiled 10 minutes in 1 gal. of rain water; pour off into an earthen jar. When nearly cool, stir in 5 table-spoonfuls of quick lime; let it stand till next day; then put in the eggs and keep them tightly covered until wanted for use."

*Remarks.*—I formerly understood "quick lime" to signify slacked lime, but it is more generally conceded to mean unslacked, which has been powdered so it can be measured, about three times the strength of slacked, as by slacking it increases nearly, if not quite, this much in bulk. To be certain of having good lime, I should always obtain it unslacked and slack it only when I was ready to use it. The above, and the next item, I have quoted as reported in the *Free Press*, of London, Ont. It was sent to me by my oldest daughter, Mrs. Dr. Mills, who lives there, and knowing they must be valuable I give them. The *Free Press* closed by saying:

**5. Eggs—To Keep Nine Months.**—"Wright, in his poultry book, recommends the following method for preserving eggs: To 4 gals. of boiling water add ½ a peck of new lime, stirring it some little time. When cold, remove any hard lumps there may be with a sieve, add 10 ozs. of salt, 3 ozs. of cream of tartar, and mix thoroughly. The mixture should stand a fortnight before using. The eggs to be packed as closely as possible, and to be closely covered up. If put in when new laid, he says they will keep nine months."

*Remarks.*—This is something of the character of the old English patented recipe, except in that it recommends the mixture to stand a fortnight (two weeks) before using, which will temper it nicely, as the plasterer says of his mortar. Were it not that Mr. Wright says "remove any hard lumps," etc., I should suppose he meant slacked lime, but this would have no lumps in it which need be put in, hence he, too, means "quick," or unslacked lime, which is pretty certain to have lumps, and which, if left in, is liable to break the eggs that might settle upon them, if not removed.

**6. Eggs, Preserving Six Months, Equal to Fresh.**—A writer in the *English Mechanic* says: "In the year 1871–2, I preserved eggs so perfectly that after six months they were mistaken when brought to the table for fresh laid eggs, and I believe they would have kept equally good for a twelve-month. My mode of preservation was to varnish the eggs as soon after they were laid as possible with a thin coat of varnish, taking care that the whole of the shell was covered with the varnish. I afterwards found that by painting the eggs with fresh albumen (whites of eggs), beaten up with a little salt, they were preserved equally well, and for a long period. After varnishing with albumen I lay the eggs on soft blotting-paper, as I found that when allowed to rest till dry upon the table the albumen or varnish stuck so fast to the table as to take a chip out of the shell. This is entirely prevented by the use of the blotting-paper. I pack the eggs in dry bran."

**7.** The following is from a lady writer who does not boil salt, as in No. 4, nor cream of tartar as in No. 5. I can see no special advantages from the cream of tartar, only to make it look a little more formidable to obtain a patent upon in England, where first obtained some 75 years ago. She does not give her name, but says:

**8. Eggs, To Preserve Two Years.**—To each patent pail (the common wooden pail), add 1 pt. freshly slacked lime and 1 pt. of common salt; mix well. Fill your barrel half full with fluid of this strength; put your eggs down in it any time after June, and they will keep two years if desired.

**9. Eggs, To Keep all the Year—Never Failing.**—Put perfectly fresh eggs into a net, willow or wire basket; and hold them in boiling water while you count 20; then pack in jars, little end down, in dry salt, and keep from frost. Put up in the fall for winter use.—*Mrs. Tillie Wales, Detroit, Mich.*

*Remarks.*—The author is well acquainted with this lady, and knows her to be practical and reliable. An Iowa lady pursues the same plan, except that she dissolves sugar in the water and packs them in charcoal and bran, as follows:

**10. Eggs, To Preserve.**—Select perfectly fresh eggs (this must always be done, as old eggs or those exposed to heat or cold can not be preserved), put them, a dozen or more, into a small basket and dip for 5 seconds (20, as above, I consider not too long a time,) into boiling water, having 5 lbs. of sugar to 1 gal. of water. Next place them immediately on trays to dry. The scalding water causes the formation of a thin skin of albumen next the inner surface of the shell, the sugar effectually closing the pores of the latter. The cold eggs are then packed, small end down, in a mixture of 1 part charcoal finely powdered and 2 parts of dry bran. Eggs so treated have been found perfectly fresh and unaltered after six months.—*Mrs. A. Noyes, Volga County, Iowa, in Blade.*

**11. Egg Preservatives, from Experiments at the Agricultural College of Iowa.**—Eggs packed in dry, pulverized charcoal at the college, June 25th, were all bad November 20th.  Eggs packed in finely pulverized gypsum in June were good in December.  Eggs kept in a refrigerator at 54 degrees remained fresh and sweet from July to November, seeming to prove that unaided cold air is a good preservative.

*Remarks.*—Thus, it seems that dry gypsum (plaster of Paris), is an excellent preservative.  I should expect it would so prove for it is, when dried in a kettle over the fire, a very fine powder, perfectly excluding the air, and if kept in a cool place no evaporation of the moisture of the eggs would escape.

**12.**  Eggs packed in boxes or barrels in dry oats, little end down, and the covers nailed if boxes are used, and headed up if barrels are used, then the boxes or barrels turned bottom up every week or 10 days, has proved successful; and the eggs were ready for shipment.  Salt has been used in the same way, and the plaster of Paris might be, except from its being so fine it will run out of very small cracks or holes.

**13.  Preserving Eggs Two Years, The Swiss Plan.**—Prof. Sace, of Switzerland, reports having kept eggs two years by the following method.  He says: "Cover the eggs—fresh ones—with a coat of paraffine, 2 lbs., 3 ozs., avoirdupois, to 3,000 eggs.  They do not lose weight or freshness.  Has kept them two years.  Stops the pores, but if not fresh and decomposition has commenced, it does not stop it."—*Druggists' Circular.*

*Remarks.*—I have seen a report in some of the papers that this plan failed; but I honestly believe that it was not the fault of the plan, but from not having fresh eggs; because it not only fills the pores, but moisture can not go out through the coat of paraffine.  Still, some of the other methods may be equally good; for family use, the boiling in sugar water of No. 10, or the gypsum (plaster of Paris) of No. 11, would be less trouble, packing away and keeping cool, as in a refrigerator or cold room, also mentioned in No. 11.  Any of these plans properly done will not fail.

**14.  Eggs—To Determine the Sex of—Tested.**—In "Navin's Work on Poultry" he gives a test made by A. T. Newell, of Philadelphia, Pa., who says: "Pullet eggs, or those which will produce pullets, are smooth on the ends; while those which produce the roosters have a zig-zag mark or quirl on one end.  In selecting 200 for roosters, only 1 produced a pullet; and out of 50 for pullets he got 50 pullets."

*Remarks.*—See "Positive Remedy for Hog Cholera" for further knowledge of Navin's reliability.  I have no doubt of the facts stated in that, as well as in this case.

**1.  GRAFTING WAX—To Make.**—Rosin, 4 lbs.; tallow and beeswax, each, 1 lb.  Melt, mix well and work, after cooling a little in cold water, until pliable.  May be used at once, or will keep for years.—*Blade.*

**2.  Grafting Wax.**—A cousin of mine, Jerry Lawrence, of Strykersville, N. Y., who has followed grafting over 25 years, uses rosin, 1 lb.; beeswax, 6 ozs., and mutton tallow 4 ozs., claiming that, with the mutton tallow, it is a good salve for cuts and bruises, which are often received in climbing and sawing among the trees.  Using these proportions, and keeping a ball or two of the wax in a covered pail with blood-warm water during the coldest part of the spring, when the wax would otherwise crack in spreading, saves the trouble of making two kinds.   He keeps a little lard on the back of the hand to use occasionally to prevent the wax from sticking to the fingers.   Make into balls of ½ to ¾ lbs., pouring from the kettle into the water only so much of the wax mixture as can be worked at a time, keeping the balance warm until all is worked, or pulled to whiteness.   Melt the rosin first, then add the others.   No. 1, it will be seen, is softer, and if anyone chooses they can make both kinds, the first for the coldest weather and this for the warmer, as the season advances.

**3.  Sealingwax, Red, for Bottling Medicine.**—Rosin, 1¼ lbs.; tallow, lard and beeswax, each, 1 oz.  Melt together and add American vermilion, 1 oz.

*Remarks.*—Dip while hot.  It is nice for druggists, who dip their vial corks, to have ready for use, or for bottles after the cork is cut off closely.

**4.  Sealingwax for Fruit Jars.**—Best orange (gum) shellac and beeswax, each, 1 lb.; rosin, 4 lbs.  Melt and dip or paint the corks with a brush. 'Tis a red shade, but may be colored more if desired, any color.  [See No. 3 for a bright red.—*Druggists' Circular.*

**1.  DOGS—Mange Upon—Sure Remedy.**—Powdered aloes, ½ oz.; flour of sulphur, 1 oz.  Mix to a consistence of porridge, with spirits of turpentine, and apply with a brush or swab.

*Remarks.*—" Cures every time," said a citizen of Ann Arbor to me, who had tested it.  The word "mange" undoubtedly comes from the French *demanger*, to itch, as it causes such a degree of itching as to cause dogs and other animals to rub themselves almost constantly against whatever they can find.  What will cure it in one animal will do the same with others.  Probably arises from the *acarus scabies*, or itch mite, affecting children, and is, therefore, "catching," or contagious.

**2.  Dogs Poisoned by Strychnia, Antidote for.**—Salad oil (which is pure sweet or olive oil), ½ pt., has saved them; so, also, has lard.—*Journal of Applied Chemistry.*

*Remarks.*—The lard was used by the late James F. Reed, of San Jose, Cal., as they use strychnia there largely to kill gophers; hence the dogs are often poisoned.  And as my books have always sold as readily in California as in the East, I deem it an important recipe, and add: 'Tis very important to give the oil when a person is thus poisoned, or warm lard if no oil is at hand—½ pt. at least—strong coffee, etc., as directed under that head.

**3.  Dogs, Cats, Hogs and Horses, To Drive Off Fleas on.**—The *Scientific American* gives us the following for this purpose.  The pennyroyal flavor is very strong and offensive to these "gentry," although many people, of which I am one, are very fond of it.  The herb makes an effective tea, drank hot, to break-up colds, by starting perspiration.  It says, under the head of " Pennyroyal for Fleas:"  " The oil of pennyroyal will drive these insects off; but a cheaper method, where the herb flourishes, is to throw your dogs and cats into a decoction of it once a week.  Mow the herb, and scatter it in beds of pigs once a month. I have seen this done for many years in succession. Where the herb cannot be got, the oil may be procured. In this case, saturate strings with it, and tie them around the necks of dogs and cats; pour a little on the back and about the ears of hogs troubled with fleas, which you can do while they are feeding, without touching them. By repeating this application every 12 or 15 days the fleas will flee from every quadruped, to their relief and improvement, and your relief and comfort in the house. Strings saturated with the oil of pennyroyal, and tied around the necks and tails of horses, will drive off lice; the string should be saturated once a day."

**Bread, Why We Butter It.**—The layers of the wheat berry, as we proceed towards the center, become more and more completely starchy, and at the center but little else is found, and this portion makes our finest flour (super-fine). The finer the flour the less fit it is for nutrition. In its natural state, the wheat, with all its components present, is not fitted for perfect human development. There is a deficiency in the potential heat-producing materials, especially for cooler climates, there being only 2 per cent. of fat in wheat. We instinctively supply this deficiency by the addition of fatty bodies. We spread butter upon bread, we mingle lard or butter with our biscuits or cake, and the fat meat and bread are taken alternatively or coincidentally. The starch, being a carbon hydrate, can afford, comparatively, but little heat in consumption, and the fats (butter) are demanded by the wants of the system.—*United States Miller*.

*Remarks.*—This is perfectly philosophical; we need fat in some form to keep up the heat of the body, and now-a-days so few persons will eat fat meats we must have butter; and it is only from eating too large an amount of it, or eating that which has become rancid or "strong," and therefore almost abso-lutely indigestible, that harm may arise from its use. A little nice butter is as necessary as it is desirable to almost every person.

**1. FENCE POSTS, TELEGRAPH AND TELEPHONE POLES, ETC.—To Prevent Decay.**—Among the various methods here-tofore practiced for preserving the ends of fence posts, telegraph poles, ties and other timber to be placed in the ground, has been charring, or coating with coal tar, but it is said that while neither of these modes is sufficient alone, the two combined answers every purpose. The tar filling the pores of the charred surface, which in itself is indestructible, prevents absorption of moisture from the ground into the interior unaltered portion of the wood. In time the tar is converted into a kind of rosin, which is very durable.—*Harpers' Weekly*.

**2. The Science, Best and Cheapest Way of Preserving Wood.**—The *Journal of Forestry* thus explains what is necessary to preserve wood: "The primary cause of decay in wood is the fermentation and the decomposi-tion of the sap that is within the pores. Wood, pure and by itself, is not easily destroyed by the ordinary agencies of nature, namely, wet and dry weather, heat and cold, etc. If the sap within the pores can either be removed or ren-dered inactive, the wood may be preserved. There are several methods of doing this, such as saturating the wood with mineral salts, creosote, etc. The cheapest, easiest and therefore the best method seems to be to charge the wood with crude petroleum. Pine (if seasoned), for example, is made almost waterproof by saturating it with this simple material, and, therefore, made much more lasting. Crude petroleum is very cheap, and may be applied with a brush until the wood will soak up no more. In the application care should be taken to avoid accidents by fire, and not approach the work with a flame until it is dry. An application of petroleum is especially valuable to much exposed woodwork."

*Remarks.*—For fence posts, it is well known to be important to place the butt end of the timber upwards, from the greater difficulty that water finds in ascending against the natural course of sap, in the pores. This done, then, and the posts painted with the crude petroleum, or by the charring and painting with the coal tar, it would appear they should become almost everlasting; and why our railroad men do not try this on sections of their ties, is almost unaccountable. With the great destruction of our forests, yearly, for this and all other purposes for which timber is used, must soon compel them to resort to this practice, else to be compelled to use iron or steel ties, at a much greater expense. Of course this is a free country, and they have a right to use unpainted and unprotected timber, so long as they can buy it; still, the painting with the petroleum would be far cheaper than such constant changing, as is now the necessary custom. Were not only the whole of the posts, but also fence boards, petroleumed thoroughly, it would pay big. Try it a few times, as the fellow said about cedar rails, they would last a thousand years, for he had tried it several times! Of course this man's disregard to truth was very great; but not so great as these railroad men and timber speculators disregard to the destruction of our forests. In some parts of Europe, iron ties have already been tested, hence correct information could easily be obtained upon this important subject. Probably, in the United States, with the improvements in the manufacture of steel, this would take the place of iron for ties; but the importance of protecting fence posts is too great to be so generally neglected as it is.

**3. Fence Posts, the Importance of Seasoning, etc.**—An experimental writer upon this subject very sensibly says: "To have a fence that will last we must have good posts, for that is the part that gives out first by rotting off at the surface of the soil. Then the fence has to come down, new posts be set, and the boards replaced. Sixteen years ago I experimented with fences, and find seasoned oak posts, oiled and then tarred with boiling coal tar, last the longest. I took green posts that were sawed 5 inches square at one end and 2 by 5 inches at the other, and 7 feet long. I tarred half as many as would build my fence, and the other half I put into the ground green with nothing done to them. In 5 years after, the tarred posts were nothing but a shell under the ground, all the inside being decayed. Some of the other posts were rotted off, and some were about half rotten. Two years after, I built another fence, with seasoned oak posts, same size as the first, giving them all a good coat of oil, and in a few days after tarred them, as I did before, with coal tar, heated in a can made for the purpose, 4 feet deep and large enough to hold 4 posts set on end. I left them in the boiling tar for about 10 minutes, then took them out and ended them up to dry. And now, after 14 years, not 1 in 10 needs replacing. I shall never build another fence for myself requiring posts without first thoroughly seasoning, then oiling, and then tarring them. If they are tarred when green, the tar does not penetrate the wood, and in a short time will all scale off. When the wood is seasoned the oil penetrates the wood, and the coating of coal tar keeps out the moisture, thereby preserving the wood from decay."

**4. Fence Posts, Importance of Tamping, etc.**—A correspondent of the *Country Gentleman* gives the following as his plan, which the author fully endorses, of setting fence posts, except that when the hole is dug 2 feet deep to be tamped with stone I should not cut back ·in sharpening more than 6 inches, while he cuts back 12 to 15. If only to ·be driven 1 foot, or even 18 inches, 6 is enough in gravelly or any soil except hard-pan or hard clay. He says:

I. "I first sharpen my posts, cutting back from 12 to 15 inches, according to the size. I then dig good sized holes, say 15 inches across and 2 feet deep; then take a crowbar and punch a hole in the bottom 10 or 12 inches deeper, making it large at the top by working the bar back and forth. I then drive the post with a heavy iron maul until the post is fully 3 feet in the ground. [The author can not think he means 3 feet below the hole dug for the stones; if he does it would require a 9 foot post—not at all probable.] I then fill the hole with small stones well tamped with the head of the bar. Posts set in this way will be sound and serviceable when those set at the same time in the ordinary way and tamped with earth will be decayed and useless. A neighbor tells me that he made a piece of board fence over 30 years ago, in part of which he set the posts with stones, and the rest were tamped with earth. Those set with stone remained sound when the others had rotted away.

II. *Straight Post and Rail Fence.*—He continues: "The best and most economical fence I can make is a straight fence of posts and rails. I set the posts in a line, 11 feet apart, using 12 foot rails, nailed on alternate sides of the posts, which gives them a small lap. I drive a good stake by the side of each post, held to the post by a wire placed above the bottom rails and a second wire below the top rails. Fence built in this manner is firm and strong, taking much less room than an ordinary rail fence, and is more serviceable in restraining unruly stock than board fence. One strand of barbed wire across the top of the posts, 8 or 10 inches above the top rail, will cause unruly stock to keep at a respectful distance after one trial."

*Remarks.*—There is not a doubt but what rails, properly nailed upon the posts, are more economical than boards, yet, I think, more expensive, especially on our western prairies, and there, too, almost absolutely impossible to get the rails at any price. There is no doubt, either, but what the barbed wire along the top would be respected, even by unruly stock, after a single trial. Now, if the seasoned, oiled, and tarred oak posts of No. 3 are preferred, then set by tamping stones around them, as in this last recipe, and no dirt put on top of the stones, you will have a post that will last much longer than any other way, and well worth adopting especially where timber is scarce.

**1. ADVICE—Poetical, to Boys, but Equally Applicable to Young Men.**—The following item, from the poetic writer, Eben E. Rexford, covers so much good in such a small compass, I am glad to lay it before my young readers. It is true in every point, and should be adopted as the rule of life, by not only every boy, but every young man coming upon the stage of action, for himself. The two next items I do not know who their author's are, still, as they teach us all a lesson of fact, they very appropriately follow the first. Rexford says:

> My boy, you're soon to be a man;
>   Get ready for a man's work now;
> And learn to do the best you can,
>   When sweat is brought to arm and brow.
> Don't be afraid, my boy, to work;
>   You've got to, if you mean to win!
> He is a coward who will shirk;
>   "Roll up your sleeves, and then 'go in!'"
>
> Don't wait for chances; look about!
>   There's always something you can do,
> He who will manfully strike out,
>   Finds labor; plenty of it, too!
> But he who folds his hands and waits
>   For "something to turn up," will find
> The toiler passes Fortune's gates,
>   While he, alas, is left behind!
>
> Be honest as the day is long;
>   Don't grind the poor man for his cent,
> In helping others, you grow strong,
>   And kind deeds done are only lent;
> And this remember: if you're wise,
>   To your own business be confined,
> He is a fool, and fails, who tries
>   His fellow-men's affairs to mind.
>
> Don't be discouraged and get the blues
>   If things don't go to suit you quite;
> Work on! Perhaps it rests with you
>   To set the wrong that worries, right.
> Don't lean on others! Be a man!
>   Stand on a footing of your own!
> Be independent, if you can,
>   And cultivate a sound backbone!
>
> Be brave and steadfast, kind and true,
>   With faith in God and fellow-man,
> And win from them a faith in you,
>   By doing just the best you can!

**2. It Never Pays to Fret and Growl.**—This writer has concentrated the whole plan of life's work into a nut-shell, as follows:

It never pays to fret and growl
  When fortune seems our foe;
The better bred will push ahead,
  And strike the braver blow.
    For luck is work,
    And those who shirk
Should not lament their doom,
    But yield the play,
    And clear the way,
That better men have room.

*Remarks.*—It is only those who are determined to shirk, that need clear the way, for those who are alike determined to labor, as the first writer says, can find plenty of it, hence there is no need for any such to be left behind. It has been more recently taught that luck is simply pluck, and as experience shows this to be a fact, and also that pluck means for every one to be at work, this writer is correct. And now, with a temperance pledge, written for little boys, being equally applicable to men, I will close these subjects, with the very best wishes that all shall succeed, as I know they will, if they adhere to the principles here taught, so plainly that even a little child cannot misunderstand them.

### 3. A Temperance Pledge.

A pledge I make, no wine to take;
Nor brandy red, that turns the head;
Nor whisky hot, that makes the sot;
Nor fiery rum, that ruins the home.
Nor will I sin, by drinking gin;
Hard cider, too, will never do;
Nor lager beer, my heart to cheer;
Nor sparkling ale, my face to pale.
To quench my thirst I'll always bring,
Cold water from the well or spring;
So here I pledge perpetual hate,
To all that can intoxicate.

*Remarks.*—It is certain that these writers had the welfare of the rising generation deeply at heart, as well as the ability to clothe their thoughts with words calculated to make a lasting impression upon the minds of those for whose sake they were writing; and I should have been glad to have found their names connected with their articles; but as I did not, I can only ask that they be committed to memory by the youth of every household, and that they form the governing principles of their lives, so shall peace and prosperity be doubly assured.

Now the foregoing advice, or, more properly, suggestions, to young men and boys, would seem to be incomplete, without a word to young women; hence we will give them an item, written for the *Blade*, by W. S. Frazier, under the head of "Beware." I shall head it as follows:

### YOUNG LADIES—"BEWARE."

Beware, young lady, beware!
A serpent lies coiled in the lees of that cup,
Which your handsome "young man" has so gaily caught up
And drained to the dregs. He may laugh at your fears,
But if you would shun the disgrace and the tears
Of the helpless, despairing, disconsolate wife
Of a drunkard who has driven all hope from your life;
When the years have flown by and the fiend has control
Of that handsome young man, mind, body and soul—
                              Beware!

Beware, young lady, beware!
This life has enough of pain, trouble and care
For those who act wisely. Then turn from the snare
Of the deadly drink demon; that promise, fair-spoken,
Of reform after marriage, is sure to be broken.
Oh, heed thou the counsels of wisdom and truth,
That thy age be not cursed with the choice of thy youth.
There are many young men, brave, noble and strong,
Then choose not from Satan's Bacchanalian throng—
                              Beware!

*Remarks.*—All the counsel above given as to young men's success, if they heed or are governed by the "advice" given, is as applicable here to young women as to them; and I need only add that I have known several young women in my lifetime who, if they had heeded the advice of their friends and not married young men already addicted to drink, would have saved themselves from a life of suffering and wretchedness. Those who begin early in life to drink seldom reform; and, if they try to do so, more "seldom" hold out but a very short time. It does seem as though they might, but they do not look high enough for support. Christ has said: "My grace shall be sufficient for thee." It must be to all who trust it fully, for He never spoke only what He knew to be facts.

**A Mortgage, Its Staying and Destructive Properties.**—In the whole range of sacred and profane literature, perhaps there is nothing recorded which has such staying properties as a mortgage. A mortgage can be depended upon to stick closer than a brother. It has a mission to perform, which never lets up. Day after day it is right there, nor does the slightest tendency to slumber impair its vigor in the night. Night and day, on the Sabbath and at holiday times, without a moment's time for rest or recreation, the biting offspring of its existence—interest—goes on. The season may change, days run into weeks, weeks into months, to be swallowed up in the gray man of advancing years, but the mortgage stands up in sleepless vigilance, with the interest a perennial stream, ceaselessly running on. Like a huge nightmare eating out the sleep of some restless slumberer, the unpaid mortgage rears up its gaunt front in perpetual torment to the miserable wight who is held in its pitiless clutch. It holds the poor victim in the relentless grasp of a giant; not one hour of recreation; not a moment's evasion of its hideous presence. A genial savage of mollifying aspect while the interest is paid; the very devil of destruction when the payments fail. [Beware of them.—AUTHOR.]

**1. Feather Beds, Old, to Renovate Without Steam.**—Old feather beds may be renovated or cleaned very satisfactorily by putting them out during a heavy shower, turning, to give both sides a good soaking. [And the author can't see, if it does not rain when and as hard or as long as it is desired for this purpose, why a woman can't get up a good "heavy shower" of her own by means of plenty of warm water and the ordinary house or garden sprinkler; she certainly could, and I think be better than the natural cold shower.] Dry thoroughly in the sun, beating with a stick to loosen up the feathers, as you do a carpet to get out the dust. The bed may lay upon the ground to receive the water, but should be placed upon slats or sticks across chairs, or something of this character, while drying.

*Remarks.*—On boards or poles, one end on the fence sloping towards the sun, is the better way. If there are stains on the tick they can be cleaned at the same time in the following manner:

**2. Feather Bed Tick, To Remove the Stains.**—Pulverize some starch and stir it into sufficient soft soap to make quite a thick paste, enough to cover the spots caused by children's wetting it. When dry, brush off and wash with clean water by means of a wash-cloth or sponge. Dry again in the sun, and whip to lighten up the feathers.

**Corn Crib, Rat Proof.**—A correspondent of the *Practical Farmer* gives the following directions for making that most necessary of farm buildings—a rat proof corn crib. He says: "Build a good substantial house, 12 feet wide, 8 feet high and as long as you want it. This will give you 2 cribs, 1 on either side. Put your building on stone pillars, 1 foot, or more, above ground (mind, the pillars must not be wider than the sill, else the rats will stand on them). Side up with lath 2½x1 inches of hard wood—I used oak—putting them on up and down, being careful to have them just ½ inch apart. The gables and any part of the building that does not come in contact with the corn can be sided up with common pine boards; for bottoms of cribs, laths lengthwise, ½ inch apart; balance of floor between cribs lay tight, of pine boards. My building has a string of ties between the sill and plate to nail to and cross ties to hold the building together. Every 8 feet of these ties spike a good strong scantling, or plank across them lengthwise of the building as far in from the plate as you want the width of top of crib, then set up studding from floor, as many as will be sufficiently strong for crib; mortice the end in floor, gain the top into the horizontal scantling about ¾ of an inch, then lath the inside of the crib with any kind of lath (I would keep up the hard wood), just close enough to keep in the corn, commencing 10 inches from the floor, to leave room for the corn to come down into the trough, putting these lath on lengthwise. Then put a common sized door in the end, between the cribs. You can put a lock on the door, and all is secure—I did not lock mine and gained something by it, as I found a stray mitten in the crib on a cold morning. To get the corn in the crib make doors above the plate the size you want them, the same as dormer windows, and hang the doors on and it will be completed. If any one wishes, to have a granary, they can use one side of the building for that purpose and the other for a crib. The size of my cribs is 3 feet in the clear at the bottom and 5 feet at the top, but I am well satisfied they might be much wider and still the corn would cure well. I have used this crib for about 10 years, and I can recommend it as an entire success. The secret of this crib is putting the lath on up and down; this gives no place for the rats to stand on to cut holes, and the building being 1 foot above ground they cannot reach the bottom. We are infested with swarms of gray rats, and there is not a building on the farm from which we can keep them out except the corn crib. We keep corn over a year until the new crop is gathered in perfect safety."

*Remarks.*—The 10 inches at the bottom, up to where the lath begins, may have a board of that width, or better still, 3 laths nailed on end cleats, to slip down behind cleats nailed on the studs. By taking one of these up, you have a nice opening to pass the scoop shovel under for corn, when desired. Having worked at carpentering and joining work for 20 years, before I began to read medicine, I know this will prove every way satisfactory, if done by a good common sense man.

**Bushel Boxes, How to Make.**—In gathering potatoes, apples and other things, quite a saving in time and trouble can be brought about by making enough bushel boxes to fill the wagon-bed. If the inside of the wagon-box is 36 inches, the length of the boxes should be 17½ inches (which gives 1 inch play to get them in and out). An ordinary wagon-box will hold 32 to 36 of them. With these boxes one has no use for baskets, and the trouble of shoveling out the load is saved. In handling apples and potatoes they are much less bruised and marred than when no boxes are used. Where one has a supply of these boxes, a large number of them, after being filled with apples, etc., can be piled up and emptied at leisure. In this case the time on stormy days can be devoted to assorting the products. They are also quite convenient, being square, for shipping on the cars. The ends are made of common pine boards, 12 inches wide, planed on both sides, sawed to the exact width of 12 inches, and then cut into lengths of 14 inches. In these, holes are cut for the hands, as cleats would take up too much space and they would not pack well. To make, take an inch bit, bore 3 holes and trim with knife. The sides and bottoms are made of lath, cut just 17½ inches in length. Six pieces are required for the bottom and 5 for each side. One lath will make 2 lengths for sides or bottom. For 100 boxes 800 lath and 200 feet of common lumber will be required. Two 4-penny nails in each end of the lath is sufficient to make a permanent box. Get them ready in the rainy days of summer for fall use, and you will never be sorry.

**Dio Lewis' "Breakfast for Two Cents"—Good for Light Laborers.**—Notwithstanding a large amount of sport was made over Dr. Lewis' publication upon the "Two-cent Breakfast," still for persons of a sedentary life and only light labor to perform, or perhaps no labor at all, his plan is most excellent for those who desire to enjoy good health and long lives.

Let this class of persons try it, and they will soon realize a feeling of enjoyment and hilarity of spirit never before experienced. He says, "My experience and observation has been that meat is a large item in the cost of living.
By using less meat and more oatmeal, beans, peas, etc., the same amount of
nourishment may be obtained. Get a good article of Scotch or Canada oatmeal,
and to 1 qt. of boiling water slowly stir in 1 tea-cupful of oatmeal, to which
add a little salt; let it cook slowly for half an hour, when it may be served
with milk or cream and sugar. Three cents worth of oatmeal, 3 cents worth
of milk, and 6 cents worth of sugar will make a good meal for a family of 6
persons. Some of the most healthy people I have ever seen had oatmeal morning and night, and had fresh meat with vegetables at noon. By this method of
living we make the morning and evening meal so inexpensive that the cost of
our food will be reduced at least one-half. Beans and peas are cheap and
nutritious."

*Remarks.*—If I could say anything more to induce people to pay a greater
attention to what the great hygienic doctor has said upon this subject I would
most cheerfully do so, but I will only add that it is of the most vital importance
to all who do not work at hard manual labor for a living; they must have the
meat, if they can get it; but even with them the supper may, or ought, to be
only a light meal, if continuous health and long life are any object.

**Pea Vine Hay, To Cure.**—Those who raise peas to any extent will be
surprised to see how stock will relish the vines in winter, if properly cured, and
the best way to do it is to build a pen 3 rails high; then floor it over with rails
and build up 3 or 4 rails more, according to how green the vines are, and fill in
the vines; floor again, build up and fill in until 10 or 12 feet high; then cover
to shed the rain perfectly. Like bean straw, they will not bear deep packing, but still they are too valuable a feed for stock to be thrown away. And
when oats are sown with them, as they generally should be, the oat straw gives
an additional relish and object to save them.

**Hogs, Fall Care of, for Early Slaughter.**—Although considerable
has been said in that department as to the care of hogs, as well as the treatment
of hog cholera, etc., yet as I find an item upon this subject among my miscellaneous matter I have thought best to give it here, hoping it may receive greater
attention standing alone. It is best, when possible, to let swine have the range
of a newly cleared field, where logs and brush have just been burned off, as
they instinctively eat the coals that are left, which, it is well known, does them
great good; but when this can not be done the next best thing is to place a mixture of salt, ashes (unleached), and charcoal (pulverized), and, the author thinks,
sulphur, also, equal quantities, except the sulphur, perhaps, only one-half as
much as of either of the others, under shelter, but where they can have daily
access to it; and also to begin to feed early with peas, pumpkins, potatoes, etc.,
the potatoes and pumpkins properly cooked and thickened with pea meal, if
plenty, else with shorts, or a little cornmeal when no cheaper article is at hand
to be worked off; so that by November 15th, or 20th, at farthest, they may be
ready for slaughter. The charcoal is of vital importance to hogs, unless the

stove coal, as mentioned in the other connection, proves to fill its place; and there is no danger of their eating too much ashes or salt. Running water ought always, if possible, to pass through their pasture; and when not possible fresh water should be pumped daily for their use, as well as for all other stock, even to the chickens.

**1. CODLING MOTH, Remedy.**—Dr. Hull, a leading horticulturist of Illinois, says that his lime remedy for the codling moth has proved completely effectual. The freshly slacked lime is thrown into the trees when the dew is on, or just after a rain, and after the fruit is set. A dipper or a large spoon may be used; but best of all, is a bellows made for the purpose (the author would say, with a long nose or nozzle to reach well up into the trees). The insects will not go where the lime is scattered; he says, "they go away."

*Remarks.*—The author has not a doubt but what the lime will prove effective, for the item given in his first recipe book, for destroying the curculio on plum trees, wherein sulphur and gunpowder with the lime was effectual; but it seems that lime alone does equally well, and is much less expensive. "Codling' means an immature or small apple, but so far as the moth is concerned, it is applied to plums or any other fruit. But the curculio, a species of weevil, is most destructive to the plum, as you will see by referring to them.

**2. Codling Moth Effectually Disposed of.**—A writer who signs himself "H," of Fenton, Mich., sends a plan to the Detroit *Tribune*, which he says effectually disposes of the codling moth. He says: " I take a piece of old woolen cloth, 5 or 6 inches wide, and long enough to go around the apple tree and lap an inch or two, and place this around the tree midway between the lower branches and the ground, and fasten it there with a tack driven in just far enough to hold. The moth will go under this cloth and deposit her egg, which matures in 12 days. Every 10 days I go through the orchard, draw the tacks carefully, unwind the cloth and mash every worm and moth I find, sometimes as many as 40 under a single cloth. This followed up will utterly destroy them."

*Remarks.*—It is said that the most successful fruit growers, east and west, have decided that there is no better remedy for the codling moth than to pasture hogs in the orchard to eat the wormy apples and the moths or worms therein. Chickens running in the orchard are also very destructive to moths, by eating all the worms or bugs they see; and I have seen it stated that 2 or 3 pigs put into a pen of one length of boards around apple, peach, or plum trees will destroy all these depredators. (See Borers, Remedy for, Curculio on Plums, Description of and how get rid of them, next below.)

**Borers in Peach and Apple Trees, Remedy for, and for Bark Lice on the Trees.**—Mr. M. B. Batchman, of Ohio (residence not given), writing to the *Fruit Recorder*, of Palmyra, N. Y., gives the following valuable remedy to prevent the borers getting into the peach and apple trees. He says: "Take a tight barrel and put in 4 or 5 gallons of soft-soap with as much hot water to thin it, then stir in 1 pt. of crude carbolic acid and let stand over night, or longer, to combine. Then add 12 gallons of rain-water, and stir well; apply to the base of the tree with a short broom or old paint brush, taking pains to wet inside of all crevices. This will prevent both peach and apple borers. It should be applied the latter part of June in this climate, when the moths and beetles usually appear. The odor is so pungent and lasting that no eggs will be deposited where it has been applied, and the effect will continue till after the insects have done flying. If the crude acid cannot be obtained, ⅓ of the pure will answer, but it is more expensive." [Crude carbolic acid is a black and dirty looking fluid, and if not kept by small druggists they can obtain it in the cities; but, mind you, it is a strong acid, and it will destroy the skin or clothing if you get it on them by breaking the bottle or otherwise, so be careful. The crude is what is used in washes for lice about poultry, horses, etc.]

*Remarks.*—To the above, the editor of the *Recorder* added: "We believe the above remedy for borers would also exterminate grubs from strawberry, raspberry and blackberry roots—only that for strawberries dilute it with double the amount of water." To this I may add: I think 6 or 8 qts. of fine soot dissolved in a barrel of water and thoroughly sprinkled about the roots of these berry plants will kill the borers or grubs that trouble them, and probably 2 lbs. of potash in the same water would also destroy them, sprinkled on in the same way.

**Forcing Plants.**—For forcing plants that you wish to hurry forward for any reason, 6 or 8 qts. of fine soot dissolved in a hogshead of water and sprinkled upon them and about the roots freely, is said, by the *American Gardener*, to do as well for plants as for bulbs, flowering plants, shrubs, etc.

**Bark Lice, or Scale Bugs on Trees, Shrubs, Plants, etc.—Positive Remedies.**—Prof. J. H. Comstock says that in fighting scale insects (scale bugs, bark lice) on trees and shrubs that poisonous fumes nor powdered substances have done any good, and that "they cannot be destroyed otherwise than by actual contact. Lye and solutions of soap have been eminently successful. Common or whale oil soap, ¾ lb., to water, 1 gal. (dissolve by heat); or lye (concentrated, in lb. cans), 1 lb. to 1 gal. of water, applied when the trees are dormant (not growing—fall or very early spring), has been found to work equally well. Apply with a stiff brush, which reaches the scale under the bark and sweeps off others, but cannot be used on the small branches, and on these Whitman's fountain pump syringe may be employed for spraying."

*Remarks.*—Charles Downing, through the *Rural New Yorker*, says he uses "1 lb. of the lye to 6 qts. of water, just as the buds begin to swell in the spring. This is undoubtedly strong enough to kill every one it touches.

**For Lice on Plants.**—Prof. A. J. Cook, in the New York *Tribune*, says that one application of the following mixture is a complete cure for lice on plants: Soft-soap, 1 qt.; water, 1 gal., and kerosene, 1 pt. The soap and water are heated to the boiling point, the kerosene added and all well stirred. The mixture is thus made permanent. It is also used on trees, killing the lice and restoring the vigor of the trees.

**Curculios on Plum Trees—Description of and How to Destroy Them.**—Mr. A. R. Markham, of Mayville, wrote to Prof. A. J. Cook, of the

Agricultural College, Lansing, asking as follows: "Will you kindly describe, through the columns of the *Post and Tribune*, or otherwise, the plum curculio so that an amateur grower can find him? There are many among our farmers who don't know the pest. I have hunted with great care but have not yet found a sufficient description for me or my friends to identify him. Please make the description sharp and decisive so we can find the terror."

To this Prof. Cook made the following answer through the *Post and Tribune:* "The plum curculio, which has now for more than a week been making its destructive punctures and characteristic crescents in our plums, and which will continue its ruinous work for a month to come, is a little weevil—that is a beetle, with a prolonged snout or proboscis—not more than $\frac{8}{16}$ths of an inch long. It is dark in color, marked with indistinct gray and buff. When at rest its snout or trunk is bent under the body. To surely find it at this season place a white sheet or table spread under a plum tree which is bearing plums, and then give the trunk of the tree or the branches, if the tree is large, a sharp blow. The curculios will fall to the sheet. If early in the morning or late in the afternoon they will remain in their humped up condition, by which they feign death, and in which they resemble small dried buds so closely that they must be carefully inspected to remove the deception. If in the hot sunshine, in the middle of the day, they will soon crawl, or often at once take wing. In this way any one will be able to identify the pests. Very soon their appearance is learned, and one has no trouble to see them at once, when they may be grasped between the thumb and finger and crushed. I have four plum trees. It takes me about 10 minutes each day to catch and destroy the curculios, and by this slight trouble we shall have a fine quantity of beautiful fruit. If we should neglect to fight the "little Turk" we would get not a plum."

*Remarks.*—On May 25th Prof. Cook had given, in answer to a Mrs. O. L Morgan, of Hillsdale, Mich., a more full direction as to the sheet, which should cover all the space under the tree, or such part of the tree as was being jarred; and also of the mallet, etc., which should have a handle at least 6 or 8 feet long, and the ends of the mallet to be well padded with cloth, so as not to bark the tree, nor the large limbs, which must be hit quite hard to fetch them down. But I think a strip of board, 2 or 3 inches wide, 6 to 10 feet long, one end padded, will do as well, and white sheets enough laid down to cover the ground under the tree; and the curculios are then, of course, to be mashed, or destroyed, as you like, and all green and other worms, which also eat into apples, pears, cherries, plums, etc., which, when they shake down should also be destroyed. The shaking, or jarring down should be done just at dusk of the evening, and at early dawn, as long as they are found. It is said that corn cobs saturated with kerosene, and hung by strings to the branches, keeps the curculios away from the trees. This lady also made the following inquiry in relation to

**1. CURRANT WORMS.**—"Is London purple as good a remedy for currant worms as white hellebore, and in what proportion is it to be used in small quantities?"

To which Prof. Cook gave this answer: "I should prefer white hellebore to London purple in fighting the currant worms, as it is just as effectual and not so poisonous. If it is thought best to use London purple, and it is safe with the requisite precautions, use 1 oz. of the purple to 5 or 6 gals. of water." Knowing the ability of this gentleman to answer all such questions correctly, I have given them most cheerfully. (For the strength of the hellebore water for this purpose, see how to use it, below.)

**2. Currant Worms, to Avoid.**—A writer of experience in the *Fruit Recorder* says: "There is no necessity of breeding currant worms; which is done by leaving bushes untrimmed, the worms always attacking the new growth first." He continues: "My plan is this: In starting a currant patch I confine the bush not to exceed from 1 to 3 main stems, and give all the strength of the root to their support. As hinted above, sprouts will start from the roots each spring, but they must be rubbed off when small. All currant-growers are aware that worms first make their appearance on a new growth and then spread over the bush. Consequently, no sprouts, no worms. This is just as plain as that 2 and 2 make 4. I have followed this plan for the past 2 years to my sat-isfaction, and have barely seen the effects of worms on 1 or 2 bushes where my plan was not fully carried out. But such currants I never saw grow, the common red Dutch being nearly twice as large as the cherry currant and a bet-ter bearer. I had a few bushes that actually broke down from their load of fruit."

*Remarks.*—The plan of making a kind of tree of the currant gives so much better chance of cultivating around them, I have often wondered it was not adopted generally; and if any one will adopt this plan, he will see how much easier it will be to adopt the use of soot, as the Scotch do, to eradicate the worm, and at the same time to fertilize; as given in the next item.

**3. Currant Worms to Destroy, and to Fertilize the Ground.** —Instead of the powdered hellebore, as heretofore used, copperas water, at the rate of 1 lb. to water, 6 gals., not only destroys the worm, by pulling over the top of the bush to sprinkle it upon the under side of the leaves, but also fer-tilizes the soil. But possibly the Scotch method of dusting fine soot upon them after a shower, or when the dew is on, and also working small quantities of it into the soil around the bushes, is the best way after all, as it is claimed this latter plan in a year or two will eradicate them from the garden altogether.

**4. Lime, Another Certain Remedy.**—A horticulturist near this city, Toledo, O., says in the *Post* recently: "The only remedy for the currant worm known to us, is to begin early in the season to scatter air-slacked lime on the leaves. This work must be frequently and thoroughly done, always after sun-down. Throw the lime from below upwards, or pull the bushes over, in order to let it catch on the under side of the leaves, and also from above. This will save the currants if done thoroughly and often."

*Remarks.*—I know the lime will prevent the *conotrachelus nenuphar* (a big name for the plum weevil), or curculio, from stinging, and thus destroying plums, if thrown on freely, while in blossom, and for a few days thereafter; then why may it not also destroy or prevent the currant worm from putting in his work upon currants? I have not a doubt of it. The same writer says also that cultivators of small fruits recommend Fay's Prolific currant as a healthy and vigorous grower, productive and easily picked from the bush, and as a rule making fruit-buds under cover of every leaf. Then it must be a good one to raise. I think the best plan of applying the lime, or any powder, upon currant bushes, more especially upon fruit trees, would be to have a bellows like painters use to put sand upon their painted work, putting the powder in the hopper, the wind carries it out freely. The nose must be quite long for fruit trees.

**5. Currant Worms, New Way of Destroying.**—The Kalamazoo (Mich.) *Telegraph* gives a plan of destroying the currant worm, or caterpillar, as some call them, discovered accidentally by a piece of woolen rag having been blown into a currant bush by the wind, which was found to be covered with these leaf-destroying pests. Pieces of woolen cloth were then placed in every bush, and the next day the worms had almost wholly taken to them for shelter. In this way every morning they were taken out and destroyed, and the rag replaced for a new crop, until completely used up. If this fails to reach all, use the lime dust, or some of the solutions with the syringe or atomizer. See "Currants and Gooseberries, Setting Out, etc.

**6. Currant Worms and Rose Slug, How to Destroy with Hellebore.**—I. *For the Currant Worm.*—There are many persons who from the certainty of hellebore to destroy them, claim it the best remedy yet known. If to be used, the *American Agriculturist* tells us how to do it. It claims, also, that if used in this manner it is perfectly safe. As to the way of using it it says: " Place a table-spoonful of the powdered hellebore in a bowl; pour upon it a little boiling hot water; stir so as to wet every particle, then add more water, stir well and pour into a pail; then rinse the bowl and pour the washings into the pail, which is then to be filled with cold water. Thus prepared, the mixture is to be syringed over the bushes. Two, or at most three, applications will finish the worms, and it would be difficult to find a safer or more effective remedy. Success with this, as with all similar things, depends upon applying the remedy early. Those who will take the pains, and where there are but few bushes it is advisable to do so, can avoid much of the necessity of poisoning by destroying the eggs of the caterpillar. These are laid upon the underside of the lower leaves of the bushes, and the leaves themselves may be plucked and burned, or the eggs crushed between the thumb and finger."

*Remarks.*—This would be about at the rate of 1 lb. of the hellebore to 25 gals. of water; and if this much is needed, and it is put into a barrel containing this much water a day or two before it is to be applied, first pouring boiling water upon it in a pail, etc., as if the bowl was used, then stirring it 2 or 3 times daily, it will be ready for use; but cover up carefully, that nothing may drink of it and be thus also destroyed.

II. *For the Rose Slug.*—The same strength of the solution of the hellebore will also destroy the rose slug, generally, by a single application, if thoroughly done; but if one application fails apply again more thoroughly.

Chloride of lime dusted on both sides of the leaves has also destroyed the currant worm; but this soon absorbs dampness from the air, hence must be kept in an air-tight can, only when being used.

**7. Dust of Coal Ashes, Destructive to Currant, Cucumber and Cabbage Worms.**—The *Fruit Recorder* says it has for 3 or 4 years saved their currants by dusting on the fine sifted ashes the same as the lime above, and adds: "They are as effective to keep the striped bug off the cucumber vines," and it thinks also effective against the cabbage worm. Certainly coal ashes is an excellent fertilizer for currants and all other small fruits, as given next below, and I have not a doubt, equally valuable for the orchard generally.

**Coal Ashes as a Fertilizer for the Soils; Also Valuable for Cherry and Other Fruit Trees, etc.**—I. *For the Currants.*—Common coal ashes, well distributed about roots of currants, is one of their best promoters. This should be done by loosening the soil about their roots and placing the ashes near them, cover firmly with earth above, and the bushes will bear such clusters as will speak the beneficial effects of this application of material too commonly thrown aside as of no use.

II. Cherry and other fruit trees also greatly accept this renovator, and if carefully bedded about the roots with coal ashes in the fall the yield of fruit the following year will surprise the cultivator. Especially is this effect produced in the black loam of Illinois. We have in our mind one fruit garden there where all the small fruit was treated in this way, and have never seen their yield excelled.—*National Farmer.*

*Remarks.*—Vick, the florist, says that "coal soot is one of the most valuable substances the gardener can apply, either as an insecticide (insect killer) or fertilizer. It will kill insects on cabbage and other young plants. In liquid form, of about a peck to a hogshead of water, sprinkled over strawberries and roses from the watering pot, it acts as a fertilizer and insect destroyer."

**9. Currants and Gooseberries, Setting Out for Trees or Bushes.**—Both the currant and gooseberry do better to grow from cuttings than from the roots. The wood of the last year's growth must be taken, cut it into pieces from 8 to 10 inches in length, and insert about half the length in the usual prepared garden soil, press the ground firmly with the foot, mulch, and there will be no danger of not growing. Set them where they are desired to remain permanently. If a small tree and not a bush is preferred, cut out all the eyes entering the ground. If a bush, let the eyes remain. We prefer the bush for two reasons: the first is, more fruit is obtained; the second, it is longer lived. In fact, the bush will live half a century, only requiring thinning out of the wood once in a while. As to the variety of currants, we prefer decidedly the old Dutch Red. It is not quite so large as some others, but it bears as abundantly and is less acid and of better quality. Of gooseberries we prefer the Downing. It is of good quality, an excellent bearer, and has never mildewed upon our premises.—*Germantown Telegraph.*

**10. Grafting Currants—To Avoid the Borer and Mildew.** The *Rural New Yorker* says: "Lovers of the currant and gooseberry have reason to feel jolly over the success which seems to attend grafting them upon the Missouri currant (*Ribes aureum*), which is not liable to the attacks of the borer. Besides they are exempt from mildew. And thus by a single, happy hit the two great drawbacks to currant and gooseberry cultivation have been overcome. The beauty of these little trees when loaded with their pretty berries, as displayed at the Centennial, is of itself enough to insure their general cultivation. It would be well for those who intend experimenting with grafting currants to bear in mind that there is a great difference in the variety of the Missouri currant, some making better stocks than others."

*Remarks.*—I will add, here, that there is no fruit that will show more speedily than the currant the effects of high manuring. If large and luscious berries are expected, thin out the bushes, and cover the surface with good rich manure, after having poked some into the ground around them as far out as the roots extend.

**Gooseberries, to prevent Mildew.**—Edward Martin, of Freehold, N. J., says he prevents mildew on his gooseberries by raising the English variety, and applying soapsuds with a garden syringe, costing only $1.50, beginning its application as soon as the fruit begins to form, twice a week for 3 or 4 weeks, has never failed him, saving the suds on wash-days, for this purpose.

**1. CABBAGE WORM—Successful Remedy.**—A correspondent of the New York *Tribune* makes the following statement as to the destruction of this late pest of the garden, not in the least injuring the cabbage, as anyone can judge. He says: "I have used salt for the cabbage worm—at the rate of a large tea-cupful to a pail of water—for the last two years with perfect success. Two applications have been all that were needed. It killed the worms (or at least they died) without hurting the cabbage at all."

*Remarks.*—The cabbage worm being a soft-skinned thing, I think the salt will destroy them; if it does not in any case, try the copperas water, as given for destroying the currant worm above. The copperas will not injure the cabbage, and, I think, either might be used double the strength given, if needed.

**2. Cabbage Worm, the Best Remedy, as Shown by the New York Experiment Station.**—Common yellow hard soap, 1 oz.; kerosene, 1 pt.; water, 1½ gals.; well mixed and stirred and applied by means of a watering-pot, proved the best of anything tried at the above station in 1883. They state that "it kills all the worms it thoroughly wets, and does not injure the plant." They say "it must be kept thoroughly stirred while applying. Several applications may be needed."

*Remarks.*—But if they will bring the soap and water to the boiling point, then stir in the kerosene, it will make a permanent mixture, like Prof. Cook's in reference to nearly the same for lice or scale bugs on trees.

**3. Cabbage Plants, Best Manner of Setting Out.**—In setting out cabbage plants it has been found best to pull off the largest leaves, leaving only the center, as they are then more certain to live and to do better, from the fact that the large leaves often wither and die for want of a ready support from the transplanting.

**1. ANTS, ROACHES, LITTLE SPIDERS, ETC.—To Destroy.** —"Hot alum water," says a recent practical woman writer, "is the latest suggestion as an insecticide (insect killer). It will destroy red ants, black ants, roaches, spiders, chintz bugs and all other crawling pests which infest our houses."

*Remarks.*—This writer does not say how much alum to use. I should say ½ lb to 1 pail of water, sprinkled about their haunts boiling hot, would do the work well.

**2.** Another writer, after being pestered with red ants a year or two, drove them away by placing raw sliced onions about the closets.

**3.** Another by putting tar, 1 pt., into water, 2 qts., and placing in shallow dishes in the closets.

**4.** Another by wetting sponges in sweetened water and placing where they enter the house, if that can be found, else in the closets, and after an hour or two dipping into boiling water.

**5. Another.**—Destroys roaches by distributing the freshly dug roots of the black hellebore, bruised or strewed around the floor, or places where they frequent at nights, claiming it to be as infallible as it is poisonous, and they eat it with avidity. It grows in marshy places, and it is kept by druggists—these being dry however, would have to be soaked or steeped a little to allow it to be mashed. The water then might also be placed in shallow dishes, with bits of shingle laid on the edge to allow them to go up to it. See 8, 9 and 10, etc.

**6. Ants, to drive from Lawns or other Grounds.**—Carbolic Acid, crude, 1 part to the water 40 parts, (ounces, pounds, or pints); mix and sprinkle upon their mounds. Why not good then, about the houses where they infest? Standing the legs of safes for victuals in dishes of water will beat them all badly as to getting their dinner from that quarter.

**7. Roaches.**—Have been driven off, or killed, as I suppose by laying red wafers around for them to eat; the red being the result of the use of red lead, which is poisonous and destructive. Lozenges made with red lead would do the same thing; a mixture of red lead, say one oz., with corn meal, ½ pt. moistened with molasses to a consistence of batter, and spread on the bottom of plates turned up, or on thin pieces of boards, will also destroy them, as they eat it greedily.

**8. Roaches.**—I have seen it stated that a lb. of powdered borax scattered around their haunts would clear any house of roaches. I have scattered it upon them where they nested in drawers, etc., and have seen them scatter with the dust upon them, like leaves before an autumn wind—like the leaves, never to return. Yet I have heard others say it did no good; but with some of these plans, perseverance must conquer.

**9. Roaches, Ants, Spiders, Chintz Bugs, etc., to Destroy.—** The *Journal of Chemistry* publishes the following, as efficacious for all these pests. It says: "Hot alum water is a recent suggestion as an insecticide, (insect killer). It will destroy red and black ants, roaches, spiders, chintz (striped or spotted) bugs, and all crawling pests which infest our houses. Dissolve alum, 2 lbs. in 3 or 4 qts. of boiling water; then apply it with a brush, while nearly boiling hot, to every joint and crevice in your closets, bedsteads, pantry shelves and the like. Brush the crevices in the floor of the skirting or mop boards, if you suspect that they harbor vermin. If, in whitewashing a ceiling, plenty of alum is added to the lime, it will also serve to keep insects at a distance, and also cause the white-wash to stick better; 2 lbs. to a pail is enough. Roaches will flee the paint which has been washed in cool alum water of this strength.

*Remarks.*—This is confirmed by the *Cincinnati Times*, only the *Times* recommended it as strong as 2 lbs. to 2 qts. of water, put on hot with a whitewash brush. It also recommends carbolic acid diluted with water, and applied with a brush of feathers for the destruction of red ants; and says: "If they do not leave the first time, apply again stronger," but it does not give the proper strength. The crude, or black, dirty acid, which the crude is, could not be used on shelves in the cupboard or closets, but the pure, which is clean and transparent would have to be used, such as druggists sell, of about 50 per cent. strength, for about 25 cts. an oz. This strength would kill them certainly, and I think if as much water is added, it would still be strong enough.

Roaches may be driven away by putting Scotch, or other highly dried snuff into their haunts, or crevices, and about the shelves, etc.

**10. Roaches Utterly Destroyed.**—A correspondent of the *Country Gentleman* says: " I give a recipe to your correspondent who wishes to know how to get rid of the insects he calls the cockroaches, although I think he misnames them. Let his wife finish making peach preserves late at night in a smooth, bright, brass kettle; then persuade her it is too late to clean the kettle till morning, but set it against the wall where the insects are thickest and retire to rest. In the morning he will find the sides of the kettle bright as a new dollar, but he will find every insect that was hungry in the bottom of the kettle, when, if he uses the recipe I did, he will treat them to a sufficient quantity of boiling water to render them perfectly harmless. As I thought molasses cheaper than peach preserve juice, I ever afterward baited the same trap with molasses, and I caught the last one of millions. I pity any person troubled with them. I have lived 30 years since making the discovery (accidental), and have never had to repeat it."

*Remarks.*—There is no mistake about the name, as Webster's Unabridged calls them cockroaches; but, for short, I have called them roaches, which everybody understands just as well; as it is only because they are so very troublesome, and hard to get rid of, that I have given so many plans by which they can be driven away or destroyed.

**1. BED BUGS—To Destroy.**—Take a quart bottle and fill it with equal parts of best alcohol and spirits of turpentine, and add camphor gum, 1 oz. Shake well when used, and with a small brush wet the crevices, foldings of the curtains, etc., if there is the least sign of the bugs having been about them. This is harmless, and safe, except by candle light. If any doubt of its success, touch a bug with the least bit of it you can put on him. Use it freely, as it is inexpensive, but positive, in its destructive powers; and does not stain bed clothing. Still I must give some more, which are poisonous. Though the next is not poisonous, but more likely to inflame, or explode, than this; but, no matter what may be used, look over the bedstead in a week or two to meet any new ones, from nits not touched at first.

**2.** Naptha alone, or even gasoline, will destroy bed bugs utterly and quickly. Put on as No. 1, freely.

**3. Bed Bug Poison.**—Beat the whites of 4 fresh eggs well, and then put in 1 oz. of quicksilver; or in this proportion, for as much as needed, and apply with a brush, or feather, as most convenient—keep it out of the way of children, as it is very poisonous. Corrosive sublimate pulverized, ¼ oz., beat in, in the same way, will do the same thing. Or it can be used in liquid form, as in the next recipe.

**4. Bed Bugs, to Get Rid of.**—Spirits of turpentine, ½ pt.; corrosive sublimate, ¼ oz. When dissolved apply with brush or feather to every crevice. Go over every 2 weeks till all nits are hatched out and killed—2 or 3 times will do it every time. It is poisonous. These poisonous things are more certain to prevent a return than the others.

**5.** Another and better plan is to use carbolic acid, 2 drs., to water, ½ pt., and apply as the others.

**6.** And finally, the grease cooked out of salt pork, or bacon, applied hot, by keeping over a dish of coals, is said to be everlasting in its effects of killing and keeping them away. The reporter of the plan had been 30 years without their return. I should only fear the everlasting squeak of the bedstead, if applied in the joints, just where the bugs most do congregate.

**7. Bed Bugs, to Clear from Old Cracked Walls, etc.**—Tear off the old paper and wash the walls with pretty strong boiling hot lye, made from wood ashes, or the concentrated lye, of which soap is made. Two ozs. of this would be enough for a pail of water. Put it freely to every crack, and about the base, at the floor joint, as well as next the plaster; then repaper and you are safe. If the wall is rough, and danger of nits, wash the whole wall with the hot lye.

**Caterpillars on Fruit Trees, To Destroy.**—If for no other reason than for the looks of an orchard every bunch of caterpillars should be destroyed as soon as seen; but if left alone they multiply and soon extend from tree to tree so quickly, to the destruction of the orchard, it should be done to eradicate them entirely from the grounds, as nothing is so unsightly as an orchard or tree infested with these pests. The most positively destructive way of ridding the trees of them is to have a sheet-iron dish made about 6 inches deep and 4 inches in diameter, with a tube-like piece, 5 or 6 inches long, standing at an angle of 45° (quarterly pitch) from the perpendicular, at the bottom, into which put the end of a slender pole, fitted to enter the tube 2 or 3 inches; the tube, say, ¼ inch in diameter, having 2 or 3 small holes near its attachment to the main dish, to allow the circulation of air to prevent its heating and burning the pole; and near the bottom of the dish 3 or 4 holes of $\frac{1}{2}$ or $\frac{3}{4}$ inch diameter are to be made to allow a draft of air to make the charcoal burn, which is to be put into the dish and set burning; then an extra person besides the one managing the pole with the chafing-dish upon it, drops in a few pieces of broken up roll brimstone, when it is to be at once elevated to the nest; the fumes of the brimstone and the heat soon causes a stampede that is effectual. If you don't believe it, please burn a match under your nose, and you can soon tell what the result would be, if long continued. To give the caterpillars a chance to drop out, pass the apparatus up through their nest. No living thing can stand the fumes of burning sulphur; but brimstone in small pieces is best for this as it does not burn out so quickly as the fine sulphur. As soon as a nest is seen go for it, and you will soon eradicate them. The plan of of burning kerosene destroys the limbs too quickly. A day without wind is best, lest it drive the fumes away, rather than allow them to go directly upward through the nest.

**Weeds, To Destroy, in Gravel Walks.**—To destroy weeds in gravel walks sprinkle them with carbolic acid, about the strength of 1 of acid to 40 of water. I have found it successful, but the process must be repeated at least once a year.—*London Journal.*

*Remarks.*—There is no doubt of its success, but 1 lb. of stone lime boiled to each gallon of water, stirring a few times while boiling, then the clear water sprinkled on, or poured along the cracks of plank walks, will kill them just as surely, and not cost one-quarter as much.

**1. CISTERN—How to Build.**—I see that a subscriber wishes to know the best way to build a cistern. I have had the care of building quite a number, and would say to him, build two instead of one so large; dig the holes and put on two good coats of cement on the bank, and arch with good hard brick. One of my neighbors has one that I built for him 16 years ago, in this way, and it has been in use ever since. I had one built for myself 6 years ago; the masons put brick all round, the brick settled and it leaked. I had another built 2 years ago, which was 8 feet across in the clear after finished, and 9 feet deep. This was plastered on the bank and arched with brick, and has been full of water ever since, and has not leaked a drop that I know of. I could mention more made in this way, but this is enough. I would not have brick or stone in the sides of a cistern if they were put in for nothing; they are simply thrown away.—*Mentor, in Country Gentleman.*

*Remarks.*—If the Portland cement, which is the best water-lime, I think, in use, is obtained, or the best water-lime which can be got is used, there can be no doubt of the success in soil that does not cave; but in clay soil, they claim, nothing but tubs built of plank will keep out the surface water. This may be so, but it seems to me, even on clay, 2 coats of a mortar made with the best Portland cement would keep the surface water out as well as it would keep in what comes in by the spout. It would save much expense if successful, which I fully believe it would be. Any plasterer would know the proper amount of clean sand to use with it.

**2. Cisterns, How to Build Square or Round—The Difference in Capacity with the Same Number of Brick.**—But few persons are aware that a square cistern holds considerably less than a round one, the walls containing the same number of brick. But it is a fact, nevertheless. For instance: about 2,800, or at most, 3,000, brick will make a cistern 10 feet square and 10 feet deep, having an inside surface of 400 square feet, and will contain 1,000 square or cubic feet of water, equal to about 7,500 gallons, while the same number of brick will make a round cistern of about 12¾ feet in diameter and 10 feet deep, which will contain about 1,270 cubic feet, or 9,225 gallons, a gain of about 27 per cent. in capacity, with no more cost, either in brick, mortar, or laying the walls. Calculate about 7 brick to lay a 4-inch wall, for each square foot of wall desired, whether larger or smaller, deeper or less depth, it matters not. For the size above given, about 2 barrels of cement will be required, as the bottom ought to be about 2 inches thick. In laying the wall great care should be taken to ram or pack the dirt down very firmly behind it, so as to resist the pressure of water. The roof should be arched 2 feet below the top of the ground.

**ICE-HOUSE.—To Build Good but Cheap.**—A year or two ago I had my attention called to an ice-house built by a farmer near me, which was simply a bin, made of rough boards, 16 feet square, and roofed over, leaving a large opening in the front and sides. He said his ice kept perfectly until the next winter. He put a layer of sawdust, about a foot thick, on the ground, and then stacked the ice snugly in the center, 18 or 20 inches from the walls, and then filled in with sawdust, and up over the top a foot or more thick. Last winter, before filling my ice-house, I determined to try this method. I accordingly tore out all the inside wall, and shoveled out the sawdust; then filled by stacking it snugly in the center, 15 or 20 inches from the wall. This space I filled in with pine sawdust, and covered the whole over the top a foot thick or more. I left out the window and took down my door and left it all open, so that the sun could shine in every day. Now for results. At the present time I have an abundance of ice, and the cakes seem to come out as square and perfect as when they went in, seemingly nothing lacking except what is used out. I am satisfied how to build an ice-house.—*Cor. N. Y. Farmers' Club, in Rural New Yorker.*

*Remarks*—I see this writer speaks twice of a "foot or more," *i. e.*, of the sawdust over the ice. I should "go" for more, say as least 18 or 20 inches, and it strikes me as more correct also to keep out the sun; but have a window in each gable to allow the wind to pass through to carry off the moisture arising from the ice I am honest in the opinion that a simple wall with 18 or 20 inches of sawdust between the wall and ice is better than a double wall. Tramp the sawdust down well as filled in.

This is confirmed by J. S. Stephens, of Moore's Hill, Ind., writing to the Cincinnati *Gazette,* with a slight difference, in that he built his only 12 feet square, keeping 18 inches of sawdust between the ice and boards, giving him a block of ice 9x9 feet, and digging six inches into the ground at the bottom, then putting in sawdust enough to give him 1 foot when settled with the ice upon it, so he had 6 inches drainage above the ground; he says, too, "the space above the ice to be open and free for circulation and for the sun to shine in." I would keep the sun out, except by windows, to let the air go through. The *Gazette* added the following comment: "We regard the above as one of the best plans for a cheap ice-house ever published. Many ice-houses costing three times what the above would cost, have proved failures, the ice all melting by mid-summer.

**SHINGLES.—To Make Fire-Proof and More Durable.—**The *Scientific American* says: "Take a potash kettle or large tub, and put into it 1 barrel of wood-ashes lye; 5 lbs. white vitriol, 5 lbs. alum, and as much salt as will dissolve in the mixture. Make the liquor quite warm, and put as many shingles into it as can be conveniently wetted at once. Stir them up, and when well soaked (say 2 hours) take them out and put in more, renewing the liquor as necessary. Then lay the shingles in the usual manner. After they are laid, take the liquor out that is left, put lime enough into it to make whitewash, and if any coloring is desirable, add ochre, Spanish brown, etc., and apply to the roof with a brush or an old broom. This wash may be renewed from time to time. Salt and lye are excellent preservatives of wood. It is well known that leach tubs, troughs, and other articles used in the manufacture of potash, never rot. They become saturated with the alkali, turn yellowish inside, and remain impervious to the weather."

*Remarks.*—Where no wood-ashes are to be had, potash, or the concentrated lye for soap-making, 5 lbs. would be equal, or probably half stronger than the wood-ashes lye, as above given. Of course, putting the shingles loose into the mixture, takes up twice as much fluid as to put the butts in up to the hand, as sometimes done, and does not increase their fire-proof. nor lasting qualities. The dryer the shingles the better will they absorb the mixture.

**1. CLOTH.—Fire-Proof.—**For clothing to be starched, put ¼ as much tungstate of soda as you use of starch; starching as usual, and ironing, which does not affect its fire-proof qualities. The tungstate of soda is often used as a mordant in dyeing, which, of course, makes them much less inflammable. There is so much life lost by dresses taking fire now-a-days it seems that advantage ought to be taken of this plan of fire-proofing them when starched.

**2.** For goods not needing to be starched, make a solution of ½ lb. of the tungstate to each gal. of water, wet thoroughly, and dry, twice, if to be absolutely sure against blazing. Soft water always. May be ironed.

**Cloths, to Water-Proof.—**Dissolve sugar of lead, 10 ozs., in a common wooden pail of water; do the same with the same amount of powdered alum in another pail of water, and then pour together, and thoroughly wet the cloth therein, and dry, better without wringing. If weighted and allowed to soak awhile, all the better.

**Water Proof Solution, or Paint, for Awnings, etc.**—Put 1 oz. each of rosin and beeswax, to each pint of linseed oil needed. Apply 1 to 3 coats, as you desire.

**Oiled Cloth for Hot Beds; Boxes for Hills, for Early and Safe Culture from Bugs, etc.**—Linseed oil, 4 ozs.; lime water, 2 ozs.; white of eggs, 1 oz.; yolks of eggs, 2 ozs. DIRECTIONS—Mix the oil and lime water with a very gentle heat; beat the eggs, separately, then mix all together. Keep these proportions for any amount wanted. Take stout, white, cotton cloth, of a close texture; stretch and tack it closely upon frames, or boxes, of any size you wish; then, with a paint brush, spread 2 or 3 coats of the mixture, as each coat dries, till the cloth is water proof.

*Its Advantages Over Glass.*—It does not cost one-fourth as much; repairs are easily made; the boxes or frames are light to handle; and there is plenty light for healthy growth; and the moisture rising from the earth condenses on the under side of the cloth, and drips back; while glass becomes hot, and hence calls for more sprinkling,—*Fruit Record.*

*Remarks.*—A box a foot square, placed over the cucumber or squash hills, and the dirt packed a little at the bottom ensures against bugs, as well as to hasten their growth. Tomatoes, melons, etc., and garden seeds of any kind will be hastened by their use; and if packed away carefully when done with them, they will last several years, by a new coat yearly. This covering is a certain protection also against late spring frosts.

**Greenhouse, or Hot Beds, Best Shading for the Glass.**—Peter Henderson says the best shading he has ever used for the glass in greenhouses or hot-beds is naptha, mixed with a little white lead, so as to give it the appearance of thin milk. This can be put on the glass with a syringe, very quickly, at a cost not exceeding 25 cents per 100 square feet. It holds on the entire season, until loosened by the fall frosts. There is no better authority than Mr. Henderson.

**1. CANDIES—Everton Taffy, with Brown Sugar.**—Put butter, ¼ lb., into a suitable dish, with brown sugar, 1 lb.; stir over the fire for 15 minutes, or until the mixture becomes brittle when dropped in cold water; add lemon or vanilla flavoring after the cooking is completed; cool on flat buttered tins and mark in squares, before cold, so it can be easily broken. This is a cheap confection, and it is safe to say that no kind of candy brings in so large a revenue to the small manufacturers and dealers from the school children of New York as Everton taffy.

**2. Everton Taffy, with White Sugar.**—Put loaf sugar, 1 lb., into a brass pan (any sauce-pan will do) with a cup of water; beat ¼ lb. of butter to a cream; when the sugar is dissolved add the butter, and keep stirring the mixture over the fire until it sets, when a little is poured on a buttered dish. Just as it is done add 6 drops of essence of lemon. Butter a tin, pour on the mixture, ¼ to ½ inch thick, and when cool it will easily separate from the dish. Mark off in squares, if you wish it to break easily.

*Remarks.*—If this was not called Everton taffy, after its first maker, I should consider it butter scotch, but under its new name, it will taste all the sweeter.

**3. Molasses Taffy.**—Molasses, 2 cups (Porto Rico is best); sugar, 1 cup; butter, size of a Guinea hen's egg; nuts, a cup or two, if you like; soda, ½ tea-spoonful. DIRECTIONS—Put molasses, sugar and butter together, and boil to nearly the brittle point; add the nuts, if used, then the soda and if not brittle when dropped into cold water, boil until it is. Pour into buttered plates to cool.

**Chocolate Creams and Caramels.**—These Creams and Caramels were sent to the New York *Examiner*, by "Nula" of Clyde, Wayne co., N. Y., with the following explanation, also vouching for their reliability. It says: "Candies made at home are so much purer than those made by confectioners that reliable recipes for making them are really valuable. We have used the following ones long enough to know that they can be depended upon."

*Chocolate Creams.*—Take 2 cups of granulated sugar, and ½ cup of sweet cream, and boil them together for just 5 minutes from the time they begin to boil. Remove from the stove, add a tea-spoonful of vanilla, and stir constantly until cool enough to work with the hands. Roll into little balls, and lay on buttered papers to cool. Put ¼ of a cake of Baker's chocolate in a bowl, and set the bowl in hot water to melt. Do not add water. When the chocolate is melted, roll the balls in the melted chocolate with a fork, and replace them on the buttered papers. I never ate richer or more delicious chocolate creams. When the white mixture has partly cooled, it may be dropped on buttered papers, and nut meats be put on top, making it a pleasing variety.

*Chocolate Caramels.*—Molasses 1 cup, 2 cups sugar, 1 cup rich milk or cream, and ½ a cake of Baker's chocolate. Boil 20 minutes and turn into buttered tins. Cut into squares when partly cool. Flavor with vanilla as you remove it from the stove. The flavoring for any candy ought not to be put in until it is a little cool, to save evaporation of the fine aroma or flavor.

**Cocoanut Candy.**—Put into a suitable kettle pulverized white sugar, 4 lbs.; the beaten whites of 2 eggs, and the milk of 2 cocoanuts. Stir together, and place over the fire until you see it is thickening; then, having the meats nicely grated, put in, and watch and stir carefully, till it hardens quickly when dropped into cold water; then pour on buttered tins or marble slabs. Spread out to thickness desired, and before cold mark off to suit.

*Remarks*—If done with judgment and care, it is very nice. A gentleman or his wife, in the house where I room at this writing, Jan., '85, makes a batch of this nearly every evening, and sells it the next day to the school children. They sometimes cook it till it takes rather a yellow or brown shade, as some of the children like it better than if left entirely white.

**Putty (Old), To Remove Easily.**—It is quite difficult to remove the old putty from the sash when a glass is broken; but if you apply a hot soldering iron to the putty and pass it slowly over all that you desire to remove it softens it quickly so it can be removed nearly as readily as if just put on. Any iron that is of such shape as to allow its close contact with the putty will do as well as a regular soldering iron, but one of these would be very convenient in every family—especially in the country—for purposes of soldering tinware, to save taking it to town to get it done, or otherwise stuffing a rag into the hole. Soft soap will do the same, but takes much longer.

**Flavoring Extracts, Lemon and Orange, Home-Made.**—Whenever either of these fruits are being used cut the rinds rather finely and put into fruit jars or large-mouthed bottles and cover with alcohol; fill and press in from time to time until full, keeping covered with the alcohol. After a couple of weeks the flavor will be nearly or quite equal to the extracts kept on sale, especially so, if the bottle or jar is pressed full of the rinds and the crevices only filled with the alcohol. Use the same as the extract.

**Elevator from Cellar to Pantry.**—Elevators from kitchen to dining-room are very common, but not any more important than one from cellar to pantry. It can be made with 3 or 4 shelves, using plank for end pieces, and will be better if made with a back of wire cloth, with doors in front, having the same covering in the place of panels, the same as safes for victuals; then the woman can place her victuals therein and lower to the cellar without going down at all, and raise when wanted for the next meal. If a wife is worth saving, have one put in at once, and she will bless you, as well as the day you had it done. Make as light as possible to be stout enough for the purpose. Any good mechanic can do it.

**1. VINEGAR—from Sugar.**—Good brown sugar, ¼ lb.; soft warm water, 1 gal. Keep same proportions for any amount you desire to make. Yeast, good brewer's, ½ pt. or hop, home-made, 1 pt. strained for each 10 gals. DIRECTIONS—Dissolve the sugar in a pail by pouring hot water upon it and stirring, or else put into the keg and shake thoroughly to dissolve it; then add the balance of water for the amount to be made, and add the yeast when the water is only warm. To scald yeast kills it. The kegs or bbls. should never be more than ⅔ or ¾ filled, as vinegar to make quickly must have a large surface to allow warm air to come in contact with the fluid. Put mosquito netting or coarse cheese cloth over the bung to keep out the flies and let the air in. If shaken daily it makes quicker—in from 2 to 4 weeks, according to the heat of the sun or the warmth of the room in which it is placed. A pt. to 1 qt. of shelled corn will do very well in place of yeast, as it has a great fermenting power; but after 3 weeks at most, if corn is used, the vinegar must be drawn off to get rid of the corn. If you have 1 gal. of good vinegar to put into each 5 being made, no yeast or corn need be used.

**2. Vinegar, from Molasses.**—Good molasses, 1 qt. to each gal. of warm, soft water. Make every way the same as No. 1.

**3. Vinegar, from Sugar or Molasses, Hop Yeast and Corn.**—Mrs. R. J. Simpson of Hedgeman, Kan., in answer to an inquiry in the *Blade*, "how to make vinegar," says: "To 10 gal. of water take 10 lbs. of sugar, 1 gal. of hop yeast sponge, set and let get light as for bread, boil 1 gal. of corn till tender, when cool pour in an open keg or jar all together, and in 2 or 3

**weeks** you will have the best of vinegar. Shaking or moving around does not **injure** it at all; it never dies; keep covered."

*Remarks*—Here you see an open keg or jar is called for, knowing that air must come in contact with a large surface of the fluid to make quickly; but a keg or bbl. only ⅔ full, or a little more, gives a larger surface to the air, of course, laying on its side, and the bung only covered with open cloth or mosquito netting, keeps out the flies and dirt and allows the daily shaking, which also hastens its oxygenation, souring, by giving a new surface to the air at each shaking. It is also more cleanly, because less likely to have anything get into it. But remember where sponge yeast and corn are used, when the fluid has worked clear, in about 3 weeks, it should be poured off, the dregs and corn strained out, or otherwise got rid of, and the fluid returned and shaken daily till the vinegar is as sharp as desired. Another lady signing herself "M. A. M." —Mama, I suppose it means—gives the following plan of making:

**Corn Vinegar.**—"Cut off of the cob 1 pt. of corn, then take 1 pt. of brown sugar or molasses to 1 gal. of rain water; add the corn, put into a jar, cover with a cloth, set in the sun, and in 3 weeks you will have good vinegar. I have made it 5 years, and know it is good. Have cider vinegar, but like the corn vinegar best."

**Cider Vinegar.**—Pure cider vinegar is acknowledged to be the best that can be made. To make it quickly, a writer gives us the following plan. He says: "Expose a large surface of the cider to the action of the atmosphere; it will turn rapidly to vinegar; for instance, if the cider is put into buckets or tubs in the sun, and a mosquito netting is laid over the top of it so that the flies will not touch it, and shield it also from rain by boards, in 3 or 4 weeks you will have strong vinegar. The larger the surface exposed to the air, the sooner the fermentation will take place and vinegar be formed. Place a bucket of cider behind a cooking stove constantly in use, and you will soon have vinegar. Warmth and air are all that are needful."

*Remarks*—This would be impracticable except in small quantities, and in warm summer weather. If this writer had said warmth, air and time are all that are needful to make vinegar out of cider, he would have covered the whole ground, for 'tis rather a slow process. Not much use to try to do anything more with cider the season it is made only, only to leave the bungs out of the bbl. to allow its first fermentation to proceed, or it is best to leave the bung out all the time, if the cider is to be made into vinegar. And those who desire to make it in quantities for sale, will do best, no doubt, to follow the French plan below described by the *Maine Farmer*, as follows:

" Old cider or vinegar barrels, if sound, are preferred to new ones, but if new they are washed with scalding water; boiling vinegar is next poured in and the bung closed and the barrel allowed to stand until its sides become thoroughly saturated with the vinegar. This requires from 1 to 3 days, according to the material of which the barrel is made. After this preparation it is filled about one-third with strong and pure cider vinegar and 2 gallons of cider. Every eighth day thereafter, 2 gallons of cider are added until the barrel is two-thirds full. In 14 days after the last two gallons are added the whole will have turned into vinegar; one-half of which is drawn off and the process of filling with cider begun again. In summer the oxygenation will go on in the sun, but in cool weather the liquid is kept where the heat can be maintained at about 80 degrees. By this process it takes a little more than two months to produce vinegar."

*Remarks.*—You will understand this 16 gals. is produced in each bbl., so if a man is working 100 bbls. he makes 1,600 gals., or about 50 bbls. of 32 gals. each (which is a legal bbl.), every two months of the summer season; and if he is going to carry it on for a business, as a man does in this city (Toledo, O.), and has a suitable building, he can work 500 bbls. as well as 100. In summer, free air is admitted by lowering and raising windows, and if he chooses, can make considerable in the colder months by keeping his room warm with stoves or furnace, if the demand justifies it. This gentleman tells me that some old, pure cider vinegar, to mix with the newer cider, is far preferable to yeast or any other ferment, which will be found to be a great aid, as mentioned in the close of the directions of No. 1; and if a larger amount than there named is used, even 1 to 3, or the bbl. filled one-third full, as in the French plan above, it will make all the quicker. Quite an important point for those who may wish to manufacture vinegar of pure cider, in the cities or for city trade, is to have one or more large casks in the building, holding 1,000 gals. (Mr. Hine, of this city, before referred to, has two such), into which it is all placed, before sold, as it insures a greater uniformity of taste, from the large amounts always kept in these large tanks or casks. Mr. Hine's 1,000 gal. casks, in cheap times, cost him only $50 each, but he thinks they pay in giving this uniformity of taste; as without them the taste depends upon the kind and quality of the apples from which the cider is made. A 3-story building is none too high, as, after the first working of the cider is over in the lower story or basement, it is pumped to the third, and after 6 months or so it is run into barrels in the next story below by means of rubber tube siphons, and then again into the large casks, when properly worked or having become vinegar fit for sale— it is the true way of making pure cider vinegar in large quantities.

**Vinegar From Tomatoes.**—It is claimed that ripe tomatoes furnish a juice, or cider, if you wish to call it such, that makes an excellent vinegar without the addition of sugar; but my own idea would be, that from $\frac{1}{4}$ to $\frac{1}{2}$ lb. of sugar would be required to each gal. to make excellent vinegar. With this addition, no doubt, it will make good vinegar, for with 3 or 4 lbs. to each gal. it will make a good wine, if a slight taste of the tomato, which it retains, is not objectionable.

**Vinegar From Alcohol, or Proof Spirit, Strength Required.**— It is recently claimed that to make vinegar with alcohol, or proof spirit, which is the cheapest—either should contain 80 per cent. of alcohol. It is necessary to use from 17 to 25 per cent. of it, *i. e.*, 17 gals. of proof spirit with water to make 100 gals. makes good vinegar—this is about 1 to 6, while 25 per cent., or 1 to 4, makes extra strong. This can be made in the sun, or a warm place, by working with yeast, as other vinegars are made, or by putting it through what is called the German process of filtering it through beech shavings, described in the U. S Dispensatory. But the plan of using any of the mineral acids in making vinegar is deleterious to health, and ought not to be done.

**VINEGAR, SPICED—For Table Use, Mixed Pickles, etc.—** People of late years have got into the habit of spicing vinegar highly for table use, as well as for various kinds of mixed pickles, and even for the common or cucumber pickles, and as it gives an extra relish, if nicely done, I will give one of the best; then one with plain celery, and one of currie flavor, which can be prepared and bottled or jugged, always ready for use. For a highly spiced vinegar make as follows; but, if in any case the onions, garlics, or any of the spices are not desired from not liking their peculiarities, leave them out; or you may add half as much more of any spice you prefer to be most prominent in the vinegar:

For each gallon of good cider vinegar, slice small garlics, 6; and small onions, 1 doz.; horse radish, 2 good sized roots, also sliced; bruised ginger root, 4 ozs.; black pepper and allspice, unground, each 2 ozs.; cloves, 20; cayenne peppers, 1 doz., or 3 or 4 medium sized red peppers; and mustard seed, 4 ozs.; and if a yellow shade or color is desired, put in tumeric root, bruised, 1 oz.; but as this is only to color, I prefer it without. DIRECTIONS—Put all into a stone jar, place on the back of the stove, cover, and let steep, or keep hot 6 to 10 hours; then strain and bottle for use; or set away in the jar, closely covered, as you prefer. Suitable for cauliflower, cabbage, cucumbers, or any mixed pickle; or to use on the table, in place of common, plain vinegar, for which I like it very much.

**Celery Vinegar.**—Put 3 ozs. of celery seed into a quart bottle, and fill with good cider vinegar, or white wine vinegar. After a few days it is nice to flavor soups, or gravies, or to use in place of celery salt, upon meats, etc. The more seed used, up to 4 ozs., makes the stronger flavor. Diluted alcohol, or brandy, will suit some persons better than the vinegar. Let them use either, as they like best.

**Currie Vinegar.**—Put currie powder (which see), 3 ozs. to each quart of good cider vinegar, and steep as spiced vinegar, above, then bottle, and add, as you like, of it to meat gravies, or sour pickles, etc.

**PICKLES—Very Fine for Present Use and Keeping Over.** —Emma, of Hancock, N. Y., in the *Blade*, gives the following plans, and as I know they are good, I adopt them:

I. *For Present Use.*—I will give them in her own words; she says: "I want to give the best recipe for pickles I ever used. I found it 2 years ago in an old book, and I do wish you could all have one of the pickles, now about a year old Pick the cucumbers, being careful to leave on the stems. Small cucumbers make the nicest pickles. [I always prefer a medium sized pickle.] Wash them, sprinkle on enough salt to nearly cover, then pour boiling water over them. Let them stand till cold, or over night. Drain off the salt and water, and put them into cold, spiced vinegar. Repeat this whenever the cucumbers are picked, or until you have made pickles enough."

II. *To Keep Over Winter.*—"Now for those wanted to keep all winter; take them out of the first vinegar, and cover them with some more, in which put spices to suit the taste. Be sure to have it scalding hot, and put a piece of alum in; also, a dozen slices of horse radish. A piece of alum the size of a large hickory nut for every 3 gallons of pickles. If you try this recipe, I don't believe you will make them any other way. I do hope this will be published before it is time to pickle. Every one that has ever eaten any of mine say, 'How do you make them? I never ate such pickles before.'"

*Remarks.*—The putting on salt, and the water boiling hot, causes the cucumbers to shrink, *i. e.,* they part with their own superabundance of water, so they do not reduce the strength of the vinegar; not only this, but it also extracts a gummy, or resinous juice, making them more palatable, and more healthful. Still if it is seen at any time the vinegar is not as strong as it should be, re scald, or throw away if very weak and flat, and put on new spiced vinegar, or good plain vinegar, as you choose. The alum sets, or helps to retain, the green color; and in the amount she uses, it will be no objection. Of course pickles, or cucumbers for making them, can be put up with salt, covering fairly, each well placed layer, with salt, as filled in, and weighted to keep them close, and thus they part with water enough to cover them, without any being added; then freshened, and treated as fresh, when desired to prepare them. No danger of getting on too much salt, if soaked about 3 days, changing the water daily, when put into vinegar.

**French Pickles, Delicious.**—Mrs. E. S. Swartsy, in the *Housekeeper*, of Minneapolis, Minn., gives us her recipe, which she says is delicious. "One colander of sliced, green tomatoes; 1 qt. sliced onions; 1 colander of pared and sliced cucumbers; 2 handfuls of salt; let stand 24 hours. (I should think over night was long enough.) Then drain and add celery seed and allspice, each ½ oz.; 1 tea-spoonful of pepper; 1 table-spoonful of tumeric (this is only for color—a yellow shade); 1 lb. of brown sugar; 2 table-spoonfuls of mustard, and 1 gallon of vinegar.

*Remarks.*—I should think a small head of cabbage, and 1 of cauliflower might be added also, with satisfaction; and it would be more Yankeefied, if all were chopped, and the vinegar put on hot. The currie vinegar, above, would be nice on some, of any kind of pickles, for a change.

**1. APPLES—Dried and Evaporated, How to Cook.**—A lady in one of the *Rurals* becomes enthusiastic over dried apples, and tells us how to cook them, with which the author so fully agrees that he gladly gives it a place. She also covers the ground of cooking the evaporated apples prepared by the manufactories, but they sell so high I am glad to be able to give a plan, in the next recipe, of drying at home so they shall be nearly if not quite equal to those of the manufactories. This lady says: "After the apples are well washed and rinsed in at least two waters, place them in a porcelain kettle or tin pan; fill the vessel nearly full of cold water; this, however, must depend on the size of the vessel and the quality of the apples. Let them very gradually come to boiling, keeping them covered tightly. As soon as they are boiling put in as much sugar as you think will be required. I generally use a tea-cupful to 1 qt. of apples, measured before being washed. Keep a tea-kettle full of boiling water always ready when you are cooking, and while the apples are stewing add boiling water from time to time, as it is needed. Boil them slowly and steadily until tender, but not until they seem to shrink up and turn dark. If you use white or brown sugar, and don't add spices, and don't mash the apples into an unsightly mass, and have plenty of juice, with sugar enough to make it rich, but not to deaden its taste of the apple, and serve up while fresh, you can have a dish good enough for anybody to eat, and something better than half the canned fruit in use.

"The evaporated apples are better than the dried. They should be covered with cold water and only let simmer 10 minutes. They are not in general use, and are of high price. I must not omit to mention that the juice of nicely stewed dried apples is a delicious beverage for the sick, and possesses a flavor peculiarly refreshing and grateful, especially where there is fever."

*Remarks.*—This lady is perfectly correct in the idea that plenty of juice is the important part of cooking dried apples. They should also be covered, as she says, while cooking, and although they ought to be cooked tender, yet they should not be done to pieces nor mashed. In this manner, as the girls say now-a-days, "They are just splendid,"—no better sauce made, for me.

**2. Drying Fruit at the Manufactories, and Home-Drying.—** At a recent meeting of the Ohio State Horticultural Society, at Canton, Mr. James Edgerton read a paper upon the modern methods of drying or evaporating fruits. Mr. S. B. Mann, of Adrian, Mich., in response to requests from the members, gave an account of a fruit-drying establishment in his town, in which five large Alden machines were used. It had cost $10,000, and had paid for itself in five years. Its capacity was 400 bushels every 24 hours. It gave employment to 50 or 60 hands, chiefly girls, working in 2 sets, day and night, paring and cutting the fruit. The benefit to the community from the establishment was great, and the neighboring farmers would be sorry to lose it from among them. Mr. Mann said, for the benefit of the ladies, that if they would slice fruit across, in thin slices, place it on trays in the sun, covered with thin muslin cloth, they could dry fruit which would closely resemble that prepared by the Alden process. Mosquito netting was not so good for covering as thin cloth. In the Alden process, the white color was obtained by driving the fumes of sulphur through the dryer. (See "Evaporated Fruit.")

These thin sliced apples ought to be dried on wooden trays, not on old tin, by any means. Wooden trays might be easily made about 2 feet long and 15 to 20 inches wide, by nailing pieces of lath, slit up to ¼ or ⅜ square, nailed on end cleats, with a lath of full width on the ends of the cleats running the whole length, to form sides, to prevent the apples from slipping off—the square bits of lath forming the bottom, nailed about ¼ inch apart, to allow air to pass up through; the side lath going down a little, say ¼ inch below the bottom ones, which would thus allow the free passage of air under and up through the bottom. The thin, or cheap muslin covering preventing the sun from turning the fruit dark colored, and the wood has no tendency, either, to darken the shade of the apples, or other fruit. When once made they last for years, with proper care.

**Canning Fruit.**—The Manchester *Mirror* gives the following tables for time to boil, and the amount of sugar to each quart jar:

|  |  | Minutes. |  |  | Ounces. |
|---|---|---|---|---|---|
| Boil | cherries moderately. | 5 | For | cherries | 6 |
| " | raspberries " | 6 | " | raspberries | 4 |
| " | blackberries " | 6 | " | Lawton blackberries | 6 |
| " | plums " | 10 | " | field blackberries | 6 |
| " | strawberries " | 8 | " | strawberries | 8 |
| " | whortleberries " | 5 | " | whortleberries | 4 |
| " | pie plant, sliced | 10 | " | quince | 10 |
| " | small sour pears, whole | 30 | " | small sour pears, whole | 8 |
| " | Bartlett pears, in halves | 20 | " | wild grapes | 8 |
| " | peaches | 8 | " | peaches | 4 |
| " | peaches, whole | 15 | " | Bartlett pears | 6 |
| " | pineapple, sliced ½ in. thick | 15 | " | pineapples | 6 |
| " | Siberian crab-apple, whole | 25 | " | crab-apples | 8 |
| " | sour apples, quartered | 10 | " | plums | 8 |
| " | ripe currants | 6 | " | pie plant | 10 |
| " | wild grapes | 10 | " | sour apples, quartered | 6 |
| " | tomatoes | 20 | " | ripe currants | 8 |

*Remarks.*—The plan of preparing fruit for canning is so well understood, generally, it is not deemed necessary to give any more instruction than is found in the tables. The sugar and the juices are calculated to make syrup enough to fill the crevices. If there is no juice, in any case, a very little water must be put in to start the juice and prevent the sugar from burning at the first.

**1. RATS—To Destroy or Drive Away.**—Arsenic, bread, butter, and sugar. DIRECTIONS—If arsenic is to be used, get ¼ or ½ oz., and label poison, and keep it away from children. To use it, first spread some slices of bread lightly with butter; then sprinkle on rather freely of the arsenic, and over this with a little sugar, and with a case-knife press the sugar and arsenic well into the butter, so they will not fall off. Now, cut the slices of bread into squares of half an inch or so, and drop into the rat-holes, out of the way of children, chickens, and other animals which you do not wish to kill.

*Remarks.*—The rats will eat enough of it to kill some of them, and as soon as they begin to die the others will go away and remain a long time; but as soon as they begin to show again repeat the dose, and this generally makes a clear riddance of them.

**2. Rats, To Get Rid of Without Poison, German Method.**—A German paper gives the following plan of doing this: "Having first for some days placed pieces of cheese in a part of the premises, so as to induce the rats to come in great numbers to their accustomed feeding-place, a piece of cheese is fixed on a fish-hook about a foot above the floor. One rat leaps at this, and of course remains suspended. Hereat all the other rats take sudden flight, and at once quit the house in a body."

*Remarks.*—Possibly our Yankee rats may be too smart for this, but it would make some amusement for the boys to try it, and it may prove satisfactory, especially if the hair of the one caught was singed enough to give a smell, not to burn the rat, then allowed to run into the hole, has driven them away many times.

**3. Rats and Mice, Simple Exterminator.**—Another German newspaper gives the following simple method for exterminating rats and mice, which, it states, has been successfully tried by one Baron Von Backbofen and others for some time past: "A mixture of 2 parts of well-bruised common squills and 3 parts of finely chopped bacon is made into a stiff mass, with as much meal as may be required, and then baked into small cakes which are put around for the rats to eat."

*Remarks.*—Several correspondents of the same paper afterwards wrote to confirm the experience of the noble baron, as they call him, in the extermination of rats and mice by this simple remedy. It must arise from the action of the squills.

**4. Another Simple Remedy.**—A writer in the *Scientific American* says: "We clean our premises of rats by making whitewash yellow with copperas and covering the stones in the cellar with it. In every crevice or hole in which a rat may tread we put crystals of the copperas and scatter the same in the corners of the floor. The result was a perfect stampede of rats and mice. Since that time not a footfall of either has been heard about the house. Every spring a coat of the yellow wash is given the cellar as a purifier and rat exterminator, and no typhoid, dysentery or fever attacks the family. Many persons deliberately attract all the rats in the neighborhood by leaving fruits and vegetables uncovered in the cellar, and sometimes even the soap is left open for their regalement. Cover up everything eatable in the cellar and pantry, and you will soon starve them out. These precautions, joined to the services of a good cat, will prove as good an exterminator as the chemist can provide. We never allow rats to be poisoned in our dwelling, they are so liable to die between the walls and produce much annoyance."

**5. Another very Simple Remedy—Not Poisonous.**—Take equal quantities of rye meal, and unslacked, finely powdered lime, mix well, dry, but water in flat dishes may be set near. Put this on pieces of dry boards, in places which they infest. They will eat it readily, and soon become thirsty, and go for the water which slacks the lime, and the gas destroys them quickly.

**6. Chloride of Lime**—Put into their holes and scattered around the cellar, or wherever they trouble you, will absorb moisture, and then throw off chlorine gas, which they do not like, and they generally leave on the double quick.

**7. Tar**—Daubed into and around their holes they very much dislike, and will not stay unless they can keep their feet clean; they are a very cleanly animal, and cannot bear to get daubed with any sticky stuff.

**8. Rats, Mice, Roaches, Bugs and other Vermin—to Destroy**—Phosphorus, 6 oz.; flower of sulphur, 1 oz.; cold water, 16 oz., (1 pt.); flower of mustard, 2 ozs.; brown sugar, 8 ozs.; rye flower, 12 ozs.

DIRECTIONS—First, rub the phosphorus and sulphur together, by adding from time to time 6 ozs. of the water, then the mustard, the balance of the water, sugar, and lastly rye flour, and stir to the consistence of rather a soft paste. Put up in closely covered boxes or jars. Persons desiring to make only small quantities for home use, will take drachms — ⅛ of the amounts. It is to be spread freely upon slices of bread, and sugar sprinkled over it, and pressed down with the knife; then the bread cut into small squares and several of them put in different places where the vermin will easily find them. Tumerac or red saunders may be used for coloring by steeping some of the water, if it is being made for sale.

*Remarks*—King says, in his Am. Dispensatory, that the above paste is considered the best for the above purposes. It was first published by the Am. Journal of Pharmacy, and may be relied upon. The phosphorus has a tendency, of itself, to turn the paste to a reddish shade, in a little time after being mixed. Any of the foregoing plans will give satisfaction. Dr. King's Dispensatory, I have had nearly 20 years, and always find it correct.

**RATS, ROACHES, ANTS AND MOSQUITOES**—Penny-royal, Potash and Cayenne too much for them.—The *Scientific American* says:

**1. Against Mosquitoes.**—If mosquitoes or other bloodsuckers infest our sleeping rooms at night, we uncork a bottle of the oil of pennyroyal, and these animals leave in great haste, nor will they return so long as the room is loaded with the fumes of that aromatic herb.

**2. Rats, to Drive Away.**—If rats enter the cellar, a little powdered potash thrown in their holes, or mixed with meal and scattered in their runways, never fails to drive them away.

**3. Roaches, Ants, etc., to keep from the Buttery.**—Cayenne pepper will keep the buttery and store room free from ants and cockroaches. If a mouse makes an entrance into any part of your dwelling, saturate a rag with cayenne, in solution, and stuff it into the hole, which can then be repaired with either wood or mortar. No mouse or rat will cut that rag for the purpose of opening communication with a depot of supplies.

**1. ROSE, OR SCALE BUGS—A New and Successful Remedy for.**—At a recent meeting of the California Academy of Sciences, Dr. Gibbons exhibited a large bunch of beautiful roses of exceeding fragrance, and in full bloom, which he gathered from a bush in his garden that 2 months before was overrun with scale, or rose bugs, and nearly dead. He applied to it a mixture of crude petroleum and castor oil, daubing it slightly on the leaves and stem, with a small brush, not allowing any to fall to the ground or reach the roots. Rain followed, and the plants were then throwing out their first growth of leaves, to which the scale bugs had been directing their attention. No sign of any scale insect could be seen in the garden.

*Remarks.*—He does not give the proportions; but equal parts might be used. I see no use for castor oil at all. I believe the crude petroleum to be the destroyer. See the next receipt for using kerosene to destroy Lice on Plants. I think the kerosene would do as well, or perhaps better, on the rose-bugs than the crude oil, and it can be put on handier with the atomizer than the thicker oil with a brush. These bugs being on the under side of the leaf, the bush must be bent over, or the atomizer carried under the leaves, as tobacco smoke is done, or as the tobocco solution in No. 3.

**2. Lice on Plants—Successful Destroyer.**—A correspondent of the California *Horticulturist*, having exhausted all the known remedies for destroying plant lice and other minute forms of insect life which play upon plants, resorted to coal oil (kerosene) which proved a complete exterminator. He says: "I procured from a druggist an atomizer, and filling the bottle with kerosene, sprayed over a camelia to be experimented upon. It was a very dirty plant, branches and leaves covered not only with scale; but with black fungus; a very small quantity sufficed to vaporize and cover the entire plant. After the fluid had evaporated and the plant was dry, the scales were found dead, shriveled, and partly detached, and with the slightest touch fell off; the black fungus, also, which everybody knows is so tenacious on the leaf, was dried up into a loose powder, which a shake sent to the ground."

**3. Green Lice on Plants, To Destroy.**—A writer says: "Steep tobacco in water, and when the liquid is lukewarm, sprinkle the plants thoroughly with it. Two or three applications will cause them to hasten their going, and generally prove sufficient to rid the plants entirely of them. If it does not, repeat until the plants are free. The natural dried leaf is best, in the proportion of one leaf to a quart of water, but any tobacco will do. The above will not injure the most delicate plant, and is better than smoke, so often recommended

*Remarks.*—This can be applied much the handiest with an atomizer or garden syringe, and if either of these are thoroughly used success is certain.

**4. Rose-Bugs Killed by the Pyrethrum Powder, if Properly Applied.**—The *Rural New Yorker*, among its brieflets, says; "The increase of the rose-bug is killed by pure pyrethrum powder, if blown upon it through a bellows.

*Remarks.*—There is not a doubt of this fact, when it is properly applied, *i. e.*, actually brought into contact with the bug, as it is a soft skinned mite, and the poison is thus absorbed which must kill it. The only trouble is in not being thorough and careful enough to reach all the bugs. The pyrethrum is also known as the Caucasian or Persian insect powder. It is imported from there under these names, and is very effectual in the destruction of insects upon which it is freely blown, except those like squash-bugs, which have a hard shell to protect them, allowing no absorption of the poisonous substances. The technical name of the plant is pyrethrum roseum, from rosa, the rose, arising, probably, from the fact of its destructive power over the rose-bug; at least I so reason, unless its own flames resemble the rose, which is not as likely to have originated its name as the fact of its destructive powers over this insect.

**5. Rose-Bugs Killed in Air-Slacked Lime.**—Air-slacked lime S. M. P. in the *Rural New Yorker*, says will kill rose-bugs on grape-vines, blown on in the same way as the pyrethrum powder; then why not kill them when at home, on the rose? I know it must, if applied thoroughly to reach them all. I should, however not want the lime to lose its strength by very long standing before using If, however, put on too freely, it may turn the leaves yellow, which is the only objection to its use.

**6. Insecticide, or Insects on Plants, to Kill with the Juice of the Tomato Plant.**—A writer in the *Deutsche-Zeitung* states that he had an opportunity of trying a remedy for destroying green fly and other insects which infest plants. It was not his own discovery, but he found it among other receipts in some provincial paper. The stems and leaves of the tomato are well boiled in hot water, and when the liquor is cold it is syringed over the plants attacked by insects. It destroys black or green fly, caterpillars, etc.; and it leaves behind a peculiar odor which prevents insects from coming again for a time. He states that he found this remedy more effectual than fumigating, washing, etc. Through neglect a house of camelias had become almost hopelessly infested with black lice, but two syringings with tomato plant decoction thoroughly cleansed them.—*Gardeners' Chronicle.*

**7. Insects on Hot-House Plants, as Destroyed in Paris, France.**—Baron Rothschild's gardener, at Paris, France, says he destroys all the troublesome insects that may be in the hot-house, by vaporizing 2 qts. of tobacco juice in the hot-house; and he considers the remedy infallible, and also says it rarely injures the tenderest plants.

*Remarks.*—He does not give the strength, but I should say 4 ozs. of tobacco would be plenty for the 2 qts. of the juice, as he calls it; and I should expect the doors ought to be closed also while being done. The vaporizing being done by setting the dish over a charcoal fire, on the plan of a tinman's heater used for heating his soldering irons.

**7. Bugs on Squash and Cucumber Vines, To Destroy with Saltpeter.**—The following appeared in the *Southern Husbandman*: "To destroy bugs on squashes and cucumber vines, dissolve a table-spoonful of saltpeter in a pail of water, put a pint of this around each hill, shaping the earth so that it will not spread much, and the thing is done. The more saltpeter, if you can afford it—it is good for vegetable but death to animal life. The bugs burrow in the earth at night and fail to rise in the morning. It is also good to kill grub in peach trees—only use twice as much, say a quart to each tree. There was not a yellow or blistered leaf on 12 or 15 trees to which it was applied last season. No danger of killing any vegetable with it. A concentrated solution applied to beans makes them grow wonderfully."

*Remarks.*—This same thing has been recommended also by the *Wisconsin State Journal*, and I have seen an inquiry about the proportion to use, in another paper, which answered 1 tea-spoonful to 1 gallon of water, or 1 table-spoonful to a pail. I do not believe that a ¼ lb. to a pail of water would hurt the plants, as saltpeter is nitre, and this is naturally in the soil and is brought to the surface by shading the soil with clover or even with a board.

**8 Bugs on Cucumber and Melon Vines, etc., Simple Remedy.**—"For the last five years," says a writer to the Chicago *Times*, "I have not lost a cucumber or melon vine or cabbage plant. Get a barrel with a few gallons of gas tar in it; pour water on the tar, always have it ready when needed; and when the bugs appear, give them a liberal drink of the tar-water from a garden sprinkler or otherwise, and if the rain washes it off and they return repeat the dose. It will also destroy the Colorado potato beetle, and frighten the old·long potato bug worse than a thrashing with a brush. Five years ago this summer both kinds appeared on my late potatoes, and I watered with the tar-water. The next day all Colorados that had not been well protected from the sprinkling were dead, and the others, though their name was legion, were all gone, and I have never seen one of them on the farm since. I am aware that many will look upon this with indifference because it is so cheap and simple a remedy. Such should always feed both their own and their neighbors' bugs, as they frequently do."

*Remarks.*—The gentleman does not say how many gals. of tar to a bbl. of water. · I should say 4 or 5 would be plenty. See oiled-cloth for hot beds; boxes for hills, etc., which protects from bugs.

**9. Hubbard Squash, the Black Bug upon.—To Destroy.**—A writer,—"M. A. M.,"—to the Detroit *Post and Tribune*, from Mt. Morris, says he destroys these black bugs by putting a shingle on the ground as near the hills as possible, at night, and in the morning scraps the bugs off the shingle into a bucket of hot water. If very thick, repeat 2 or 3 times a day as long as they last. Don't forget; it is a sure remedy.

*Remarks.*—I should hardly expect many would crawl under the shingles in the day time, unless the sun was very hot, as the day is their time of depredation; but that in the night they would harbor under the shingle.

**10. Bugs, on Squash, Cucumber and Melon Vines—Kept off with Cayenne; also the Worm from Cabbage.**—A farmer by the name of Lynn, writes to one of the papers, that he has succeeded for many years in driving away cucumber and squash bugs from his vines, by dusting cayenne pepper upon them while wet with dew in the morning. He repeats the operation once a week, and finds 5 cents worth sufficient to keep his cucumber, melon and squash vines free during the season. He recently tried it upon the cabbage worm with success. I have no doubt a few tastes of the cayenne would be enough for them. See remarks, also about boxes, after No. 8 above.

**11. Striped Bugs, to Destroy.**—Another farmer says: "Saturating ashes with kerosene, and applying a handful in a hill will keep the striped bugs from cucumbers. It is not the bugs that recommend the recipe, but the people who have tried it. It is said to be more effective than a legislative enactment."

*Remarks.*—If it is good for cucumbers, I will also warrant it as good for melons and squashes.

**FUNGUS—In Cellars, to Destroy.**—The use of sulphur to destroy fungoid growths in greenhouses and vineries is well known to horticulturists. The same remedy may be applied to destroy fungus and mould in cellars, in many of which it exists to such an extent as to damage produce stored there. Take some stick sulphur, generally called brimstone, but 'tis only sulphur in stick form, and place in a pan and set fire to it, on a pan or kettle of coals is the best plan; close the doors, making the cellar as nearly air-tight as possible for a few hours, when the fungi will be destroyed and the mould dried up. Repeat this simple and inexpensive operation every 2 or 3 months, and the cellar will be free from all parasitical growth.

*Remarks.*—I do not know the writer of this item, but I know the plan will accomplish the work. Fungus is a parasitical growth of living bits of animal life, meaning one only of the animals of which fungi is the plural, and means the mass of these actual living growths.

**1. PASTE.—Cement or Mucilage for Labels, Postage and Revenue Stamps, etc.**—Soak good glue, 5 oz., in water, 20 oz., for one day; after which add rock candy or loaf sugar, 9 oz., and gum arabic, 3 oz.; and when these are dissolved, it is ready to be spread on paper. It keeps well; does not get brittle nor wrinkled, and does not make the sheets stick when they are piled upon each other.—*Dingler's Polytechnic Journal.*

*Remarks.*—This paper said "parts" instead of oz. The author has made it plain for any one to understand; drachms or pounds can be substituted for ozs. just as well, according to the amount needed. It will be found reliable. The next receipt is from the same journal, and will be found equally reliable for labeling letters, or bottles in damp cellars, as this gum stickum is for stamps and common labeling.

**2. Paste, for Labels for Letters, Newspapers (Used by Printers), for Soda-Water Bottles, etc., for Damp Cellars.**—"Stir into 1 lb. of paste of glue and ryemeal, spirits of turpentine ½ oz. Labels attached with this paste do not get loose in damp cellars. But if for convenience sake it is desired to gum the labels before using them, add oil-varnish ½ oz, and magnesia ¼ oz. to each lb. of the paste, then gum them."

*Remarks.*—See remarks with No. 1. Make a good thick paste, with rye flour, with 2 ozs. glue, first dissolved in the water will be about right.

**3. Mucilage, Simple and Good.**—Put nice gum Arabic, ¼ lb. into a ½-pt. bottle, then fill it with soft water, and cork. Turn it bottom upwards and shake occasionally for a day or two, or until dissolved, and it is ready to use for putting paper together of any kind.

*Remarks.*—I made a quart of it using 1 lb. of the gum some 2 years ago, for use when I had a quotation to put on in writing this book, and although it is sour, still it is just as good as when made. It is said 3 or 4 drops of oil of cloves prevents it souring or moulding. It may prevent mould, but I doubt its preventing it from souring. The souring does not hurt it, nor has mine moulded. Some persons use as much gum tragacanth as they do of Arabic, say 2 ozs. each to ½ pt. of water. The tragacanth is a little harder to dissolve, and, of course, is a little stronger also (see the next recipe), but the Arabic is good enough for me. This might be called "scrap-book paste," or mucilage, as you choose. I use it upon my little photos which I have for years attached to my letters—putting it upon the sheets, before I cut them apart—and when dry they never have stuck together, although a book is laid upon them to keep them flat. It is an excellent mucilage.

**Mucilage, for Fancy Work.**—Gum tragacanth, 1 oz., corrosive sublimate, a thimbleful, and soft water, 1½ pts. Put into a bottle and let dissolve, corking tightly. Stir occasionally with a stick. As it is poisonous, it should be kept out of the reach of children. The mucilage will keep for months.—*Toledo Post.*

*Remarks.*—The sublimate being poisonous prevents insects from eating the fancy work put together with it. If it is too thin to suit any one, which I should think it would be, add more powdered tragacanth to suit.

**CEMENT, OR PASTE—New and Strong, That Sticks to Leather, Wood, Stone, Glass, Porcelain, Ivory, Parchment, Paper, Feathers, Wool, Cotton, Linen, and Even to Varnish.**—A new cement which is well spoken of is made by melting in an iron vessel equal parts of common pitch and gutta-percha; it is not attacked by water, and adheres firmly to leather, wood, stone, glass, porcelain, ivory, parchment, paper, feathers, wool, cotton, linen, and even to varnish.—*Pansy, Stryker, Ohio, in Blade.*

**1. Glue, Liquid, and Moth Glue.**—Take any sized bottle, and half fill it with whisky, and put in nice bits of glue to make it, when dissolved, which it will do in two or three days, as thick as molasses. It remains liquid, and is good for any purpose that glue is used for.

**2.** For the moth glue, dissolve any amount of glue in as little water as possible, by putting it in another dish of water to prevent burning, then add only one-fourth as much nice white sugar, by weight as you use of glue, and when melted pour upon a slightly greased slab, or tin. Used by wetting the glue in the mouth, and touching the parts to be united and holding together a moment.

**3. Glue, Water-Proof.**—Best clear glue, ¼ lb.; new milk, 1 pint. DIRECTIONS—Soak the glue in the milk 8 to 10 hours; then boil, by setting the basin in a pan of water, with nails under the bottom of the basin, to prevent burning. Use as other glue. The casein of the milk aids in resisting dampness.

See 4 and 5 which come from "D. B. M." of Oconomomoc, Wis., to one of the papers.

**4. Glue, to Resist the Action of Water.**—"A glue which will resist the action of water is made by boiling best glue, 1 lb. in skim milk, 2 qts."

**5. Glue, Very Strong for Veneering and Inlaying.**—"Take the best light brown glue, free from clouds and streaks; dissolve in water to the consistence of well-made glue, and to each pt. add half gill (2 ozs.) of the best vinegar, and 1½ ozs. of isinglass."

**5. Glues, Liquid.**—"H.," of Mt. Clemens, Mich., in writing to one of the papers, says: "Liquid glue can be made by adding to the ordinary solution of glue, for each lb. of glue used, 1 fl. oz. of strong nitric acid."

**6.** "Or, take 1 part (oz.) of dry glue, powdered, and 3 parts (ozs.) of commercial acetic acid, which will dissolve the glue without heat."

*Remarks*—See "Dr. Chase's Magic Mender," among the cements, which is made with isinglass dissolved in acetic acid, and is very strong. Glass or porcelain dishes only, can be used with any acid, without dissolving the glues. See also mucilages, cements, etc., for fancy or other work, above.

**7. Glue, Liquid, Simple, and Easily Made.**—An excellent glue is made as follows : White glue, 2 ozs.; good vinegar, 1 gill (4 ozs.) Put into a wide-mouthed bottle, and set the bottle in cold water, letting it come to a boil gradually, and boiling until the glue is dissolved; then add alcohol, 1 oz.; and after this keep corked, for use.—*Toledo Post.* Good.

**1. WIRE-WORMS—Protection Against for Corn.**—I give you my experience with the wire-worm. Being troubled with the little pests one year, I was advised to soak my seed corn in a solution of copperas and saltpeter, using ¼ lb. each to a bushel of ears of common eight-rowed corn. The result was that my seed all grew, and I lost none by the wire-worms, and I never saw corn have so dark and vigorous a color before. Since then I have always soaked my corn 12 hours after being shelled. I do not know as it would affect the cut-worm, but I have never been troubled with them since I used the solution of copperas and saltpeter. Neither was I ever troubled with them when I plowed my corn ground in the fall, which I would invariably do on old sod. Some farmers exterminate them by hunting them out in the hill and killing them by hand, but this is slow and tedious, and is liable to be slighted by hired help. An ounce of prevention is worth a pound of cure is a proverb true in this case.— *J. B.., in Country Gentleman.*

**2. Wire-Worms, Protection Against, as Done near London, Eng., where Soot is Plentiful.**—An agricultural writer in the London *Land and Water*, under the head of "Soot vs. Wire-Worms," says: "I found the wire-worm so abundant in every part of the garden I was set to cultivate that I could scarely grow a potato or a carrot without its being rendered useless by it; and, among the various things I was led to adopt as preventives, soot appeared to be the only effectual remedy. This I applied to potato crops in the following manner: The drills were got ready in their usual way and the sets laid in at the bottom of each drill. The soot was then put down upon them in quantity sufficient to cause the drills to assume quite a black appearance. This being done, the drills were closed in the ordinary manner to the natural level, and the work was finished. Wherever soot was applied the crops turned out clean and good; scarcely a trace of the wire-worms' ravages was to be seen, while those from rows not dressed with soot were quite the reverse, the potatoes being pierced through in every direction and fit only for feeding pigs."

*Remarks.*—This, of course, would be as good in America as in England. The chimney-sweeps of London make the soot plenty there; but this is not followed in our country as closely, notwithstanding its great importance in preventing the start of fires. Where the soot can be obtained it is worthy of a trial.

3. Wire-worms among strawberry vines may be destroyed by a liberal use of wood ashes, or some other form of potash.

**4. Wire-Worms, to Starve, or Destroy, When the Ground is Full by Summer-Fallow and Salt.**—A Michigan farmer writes to the New York *Tribune*, desiring information in relation to the treatment of low river-bottom land, on which he has failed to get a catch of cultivated grass. He says the original sod of wild grass was turned over and a fair crop of buckwheat grown; but the seeding of a cultivated grass was a failure, at least in spots. That the next season the land was well prepared and planted to corn, which wire-worms destroyed. To this the agricultural editor of that journal replies: "The corn crop being destroyed by wire-worms is evidence that the same insect destroyed the grass seeding. I have never known any crop to grow uninjured, except buckwheat, on land infested with wire-worms. Weeds and some wild grasses, having a hard and tough root, like the buckwheat, will grow; but the more delicate grasses and grain crops are destroyed. The best means of getting rid of the worms is to starve them, or they may be otherwise destroyed by the liberal use of salt, say at the rate of two barrels per acre; or sowing two crops of buckwheat in succession, keeping the land well cultivated during the time the crops do not occupy it, so that the worms can find nothing to feed upon, will starve them, as they cannot feed on the buckwheat root, it being too hard.

"I have in two instances destroyed this insect by a thorough summer-fallow. A field of some ten acres of flat and mucky land was so full of worms that no crop could be successfully grown. This I desired to cultivate. The land was plowed late in the fall, and the following season plowed four or five times, at intervals, so that nothing was allowed to grow, since which time, some 20 years, no worms have been seen or their work. In another case a field of about 20 acres had been much damaged by them. It was summer-fallowed and plowed but three times, with intermediate cultivation with harrow and cultivator, so that nothing grew and no signs of the worm have appeared since, which was some six years ago, a crop of grain or grass having been grown annually since. I would advise the inquirer to summer-fallow his land one season in this thorough manner, allowing nothing to grow to feed the worms; then seed, first of October, to grass, of such variety as he desires to raise, without any grain crop with it, and I think he will gain his object of a good seeding."

*Remarks.*—Although this edition does not speak of applying salt, the season of summer-fallowing, yet, I should certainly do so; and by the way, it has been found the refuse salt, which can be obtained at salt-boiling houses, can be got much cheaper than good salt, while it also contains chemical properties which make it much better than common salt as a fertilizer. This has been proved at the Saginaw. Two birds again killed with one stone, where this can be attained; and where it cannot, the dirty and refuse salt from pork-packing houses, is much cheaper than barrel salt.

**5. Cut Worms, to Destroy.**—By accident I have discovered a means and time by which to destroy the great garden pest, the cut or collard worm. On picking up a piece of board that lay in my walk-way, a few days ago, I discovered several worms. Curiosity led me to turn other boards that lay near. To my great astonishment, when I had turned nearly a dozen, in different parts of the garden, I found that I had killed 76 worms and destroyed scores of eggs, which look like little bits of lint cotton rolled up. The next day I searched the same boards, which I had carefully replaced, and killed 78 worms. The third search I found a small collar-head (small cabbage) that had been cut for cows and left by being overlooked. On examining it, there were found under it and on it 26 worms. My suggestion is to lay boards (pine is the best) about for traps, in the spring, and watch them closely; the saving in young vegetables will be immense.—*Southern Plantation.*

*Remarks.*—Let this destruction of these worms commence as early as the spring opens, and you may consider your cucumbers, cabbages, etc., quite safe.

**6. Cut-Worms and Birds, to Prevent From Cutting or Pulling Corn and Other Grain, by Preparing the Seed Before Planting.**—The *Ohio Farmer* tells us that a horticulturist "prevents all kinds of grain from the ravages of the cut-worm, birds, etc., by dissolving sulphate of iron (copperas) 1 lb. and aloes 1 oz. in water heated to 90 or 95 and sufficient to soak 1 bushel of seed grain in, before planting." The iron and the aloes are too much for them. I think also this would be too much for bugs on cucumbers, squashes, melon vines, etc.

**1. CUCUMBERS—Fresh for Townspeople, who have only a Small Yard.**—A Wisconsin gardener, on the strength of experience, recommends townspeople who want fresh cucumbers, to grow them in a barrel half sunk in the back yard, half filled with manure, and the remainder with soil; the seeds planted on the surface, and vines drooping over the sides.

*Remarks.*—They do well, I know, by supporting the vines on bushes, although planted in the ordinary way in a garden. One writer says they will grow on a trellis as readily as grape-vines. In small gardens this is an object.

**2. Cucumbers, Melons, Cabbage, Tomatoes, etc.—To prevent Bugs from destroying the Plant.**—I. *For Cucumbers.*—Experience has shown that if a box or frame about 12 inches square, and 5 or 6 inches deep, having neither top nor bottom, is put over each hill of cucumbers when planted, and banked up around the bottom so that the striped bug cannot crawl under, they will never light down in the boxes, and hence, any plants thus protected are safe from their depredations. Boxes may be removed before the plants begin to run over them, and be saved for another year. Half-inch stuff is heavy enough for them, if well nailed. See also Oiled Cloth for Hot-Beds; Boxes for Hills; Safe Culture from Bugs, etc., which is only a little more expensive.

II. *For Cabbage, Tomatoes, etc.*—In place of boxes, other persons have recommended the peeling of ash, bass wood, or other saplings of about 4 inches in diameter, that will peel, be cut off in lengths of about 4 or 5 inches, and the rings placed over cabbage, tomatoes, or other plants as a perfect protection, securing well at the bottom to prevent their crawling under. When the bark of any suitable tree cannot be got, pasteboard rings, I think, would answer all purposes, tied together to prevent them from opening out. The same as the barks would be.

III. *For Melons*, or other plants in hills, use the bark of larger trees. This, the writer claimed to be better than paper, which I had recommended in one of my former books, as the bark does not soften down by the rains. Boxes will do just as well, if any less trouble to obtain. Either must be pressed a little into the ground so the bugs cannot crawl under. See also insecticide, and other things to destroy insects, bugs, etc. upon plants.

**4.** Another plan, and claimed to be safe, is to sprinkle a little fine soot upon cucumber vines, squash, etc., which are liable to be attacked by any insects. If good against wire-worms (which see), why not good against these pests, too? It no doubt is.

**5.** Another writer says: "Last season I kept the striped bugs from my cucumber vines by saturating (making perfectly wet) ashes with kerosene and applying a handful to a hill." He does not say, but I think he means to the ground, as they burrow in the ground at night, and, as a writer says in some other place, "they don't come up, or out, in the morning." They are killed by it.

**6. Cucumbers a Paying Crop.**—A correspondent of the *Country Gentleman* tells us how he makes cucumbers a paying crop. He says:

"I find cucumbers a paying crop when grown for pickles, and sold either before or after salting—price per hundered the same in either case. I plow as deep as 2 horses can pull the plow, then mark one way 4 feet apart, letting the plow run as deep as the ground was plowed. I then put a large shovelful of good barnyard manure where each hill is wanted, say 4 feet apart, and then thoroughly mix with the soil, making the hills about 2 inches higher than the general surface of the ground. I plant about the middle of June.

"As soon as the plants get large enough to be out of the way of the striped bug, I thin out to 4 plants to each hill. I cultivate them frequently, and hand-hoe them 2 or 3 times before the vines commence to run. In this vicinity the price ranges from 50 cents to $1 per hundred, and the product of an acre sells from $400 to $800."

On the same subject a correspondent of the Portland (Me.) *Transcript* says:

"In my opinion there is nothing that a farmer can realize so much money from as he can from raising cucumbers. If they are pickled the right size and well preserved in strong salt pickle, there is always a market for them. Some farmers have already commenced raising cucumbers for the picklers, and are well pleased with the undertaking. The average crop for 1 acre of ground is about 50 barrels, which will bring about $5 a barrel at the factories. Perhaps it will be well to state to the farmers of Maine that on account of the scarcity of cucumbers here hundreds of thousands of dollars go out of this state annually for pickles. Even in Massachusetts and New York the supply does not meet the demand and they are compelled to go west for their pickles.    This state is well adapted to the growing of cucumbers, and they are preferable to those raised in warmer climates."

*Remarks.*—Although cucumbers are a paying crop near the cities, yet it is not expected that the general farmer throughont the country would find it so, unless he can make previous arrangements with some of the city dealers, or factories which put up pickles, to buy what he may raise, put up in brine, or salt pickle as above called, which may then prove profitable, after a little experience at first, in a small way.    See also the profitableness of onion culture.

**TURNIPS, BEETS, ETC.—To Keep Nicely in Cellars for Winter Use.  Applicable to all Kinds of Roots and Large Fruits.** —All kinds of roots keep better in the cellar by throwing fresh dirt over them; but turnips and beets especially keep much better for this, as they soon wilt and lose their freshness without it.    Put in barrels, if it is too unhandy to thus cover them on the floor, by putting dirt in the bottom, and a layer every few inches, the roots not to come out to the sides by an inch at least, and then 5 or 6 inches of dirt on top.    Large casks or boxes will do as well, and be less trouble.    Some people do not put any earth in until the barrel is filled to within 6 inches of the top, then shake in dry sand, or dry road-dust, and cover with the same, or fresh earth.    Only such as are wanted for winter use are treated in this way, the others stand in root-pits, ventilated as seen under that head.

" A cellar," says a writer, " that is cool dry, dark and well ventilated, is the best place for preserving potatoes in large quantities.    When smaller quan- tities are to be preserved there is nothing like dry sand.    The same may be said of fruits and roots of all sorts."    See below.

This is fully confirmed by the next item, so far as lemons and oranges are concerned, from a California paper.

**2.  Fruit Packing, Lemons, Oranges, Sweet Potatoes, etc., by Sand, Effectual for, as Done at Los Angeles, Cal.**—"The citrus, or lemon men, of Los Angeles," says the correspondent, "have made a discovery of great value to Florida."    [Then why not to every place, or man who desired to keep fruit, sweet potatoes, etc., any considerable time, for any purpose?] "dry sand," he goes on to say, " is the best packing for lemons and oranges. The fruit must touch the sand.    Experience (is our best teacher) warrants keeping for 5 months at least.    The dry sand has absorbing power that appar- ently takes up all exudations subject to decomposition, the rind being very por- ous.    Naturally the thoughtful mind suggests that, on the same principle, dry sand must have similar preservative effect on other fruits, such as pears, plums, nectarines, apples, and other smooth-skinned varieties."

*Remarks.*—Yes, that is just what the principle does teach.    If dry sand will keep lemons and oranges for 5 months, it will do the same with apples and the other fruits he names, and sweet potatoes as well, and every other fruit which perishes from the outside from natural dampness or from dampness arising from the rotting of the skin, which is the way most fruits, sweet potatoes, etc., do decay, as well as from slight bruising, which everyone must be careful not to do.

**Root Pits, To Ventilate.**—A gentleman of Oswego county, New York, "J. T.," writes to *Farm and Fireside*, of Springfield, O., of the importance of ventilating root pits. He says: "I have found, by costly experience, that it is not safe to pile a great quantity of roots together and cover with earth, unless some means of ventilation is provided, such as by carrying one or more pipes, made of drain tile set on end, or narrow boards nailed together, from the center of the heap to the surface. These pipes may be loosely plugged with straw, which will prevent the entrance of frost. I once lost several wagon loads of beets, during a December thaw, by neglecting this precaution."

*Remarks.*—This accounts for many "holes" of potatoes and other roots I have seen rotted, undoubtedly, for want of ventilation. I should prefer the small board box, in place of pipes, to run down well into the heap and have holes bored into the sides, to carry off the moisture clear up to the top of the heap, because if there is moisture at the top, the rotting will begin, and thus run downwards, by dripping from the rotting ones, and spoil all.

**1. CONCRETE—Proportions of Cement, Sand and Granite Used in Foundations in the United States and England.**—A gentleman of Kansas made inquiry of the *Blade* for the process of making concrete, or artificial stone; to which the answer was: "There are various processes. The immense masses of concrete that form the foundations of the great East River bridge, between New York and Brooklyn, are composed of Rosendale cement, 1 part (say bushels), 2 of sharp, clean sand, and coarse beach gravel, 4 parts. The gravel was from 1 inch to $2\frac{1}{2}$ in diameter. The cement and sand were first mixed with water in a mill, and afterwards mixed with the gravel by means of shovels used by hand. This concrete, it is expected, will last for centuries."

**2. Concrete, Proportions as Used in England.**—Cooley, in his Practical Receipts (English), says: "Concrete, proper, is a compact mass, composed of pebbles, lime, and sand, employed in the foundations of buildings. The best proportions are 60 parts (bushels or any other measure) of coarse pebbles, 25 parts of rough sand (meaning clean, sharp sand), and 5 parts of lime."

*Remarks.*—Of course, he means water-lime, or, as we call it here, cement; the Rosendale, I think, being considered the best. Still, any good article will do. But many houses are built of it in the United States, and in doing so, generally, the pebbles or gravel are not used as coarse as above given, but finer, and make up for it by putting in coarser stone, from the size of the first, upward; and often flat stone are put in; but care should be observed in placing these in the frames of plank in which the house is carried up, that these stone are all well imbedded in the mortar or cement, else they weaken, rather than strengthen, the concrete walls. I like the proportions as used in No. 1 best, as it makes a stronger cement, and, especially, should greatly prefer it if I was going to use common stone lime in building a house or other concrete building. Good common lime may do well for stables and other small out-buildings; but I should prefer the water-lime or cement for houses in which I expected to live.

**FRUIT, EGGS, Etc.—Kept well by Cold Storage.**—The *Scientific American* gives us the following practical fact upon this important point. It says the increasing use of cold storage for perishable food stuffs, which are apt to be scarce at certain seasons, is one of the characteristics of the time. Last summer when fresh eggs were plentiful and cheap, a gentleman in Chenango county, N. Y., stored in a mammoth cooler some 5,000 barrels of eggs. Now they sell in this city as "fresh laid" eggs, at a large profit. As the eggs are removed, the cooler is filled up with ducks and other fowl to be sold next spring.

*Remarks.*—This plan is certainly practicable, and has been done for some time past. It is done by means of ice. I think there is a patent on some forms of the coolers, but I have no doubt a good mechanic can get up a plan with an ice house that would be effectual, and not be an infringement. See other Plans of Preserving Eggs also.

**STAMMERING—to Cure.**—A gentleman who had stammered from childhood to nearly manhood, gives the plan that cured him, as follows: He says, go into a room where you will be quiet and alone, get some books that will interest but not excite you, and sit down and read 2 hours aloud to yourself, keeping your teeth together. Do the same thing every 2 or 3 days, or once a week if very tiresome, always taking care to read slowly and distinctly, moving the lips but not the teeth. Then, when conversing with others, try to speak as slowly and distinctly as possible, and making up your mind you will not stammer. Well, I tried this remedy, not having much faith in it, I must confess, but willing to do most anything to cure myself of such an annoying difficulty. I read for 2 hours aloud with my teeth together. The first result was to make my tongue and jaws ache, that is while I was reading, and the next to make me feel as if something had loosened my talking apparatus, for I could speak with less difficulty immediately. The change was so great that every one who knew me remarked it. I repeated the remedy every 5 or 6 days for a month, and then at longer intervals until cured.

*Remarks.*—It will be found tiresome at first, but, no doubt effectual if faithfully done, observing the rules, to speak slowly and distinctly in after conversation as well as while reading; and I should think it important also, for some time at least, to keep the teeth shut while talking, as it gives something new to engage the mind in place of the old habit of hesitation which started the habit of stammering. 'Tis worthy of a fair, and if need be a long trial.

**PAPERING.—Making the Paste, etc.**—As many people desire to do their own papering, a few hints will not be amiss:

I. Walls that have been white-washed may be papered by first wetting the walls well with alum water, 1 lb. to 2 gals. of water, and letting dry before papering.

II. Trim one edge off with the shears, and match the pattern as you cut off the lengths.

III. Make the paste the day befor it is wanted to have it cold when applied to the paper. A gal. or 5 qts. will be needed for a room requiring 12 to 14 rolls. Mix a little over 1 pt. of flour into a thin dough, and thin down to to avoid lumps; put then 1 gal. of water into a kettle, and when it boils, pour in the thin, hot batter and stir to avoid burning until it boils again; then pour into a tin pail or pan, and let stand till next day, and if lumpy, strain and press through a coarse muslin, and proceed with the papering. Rub out carefully with a towel all wind puffs, to avoid wrinkles when dry.

**PLANTAINS, Etc.—To Destroy on the Lawns.**—The country gentleman tells us to destroy these pests by dropping carefully a simple drop of sulphuric acid into the center of the plant. One drop will do the business; more will be likely to do harm.

*Remarks.*—The harm would be in its spreading to kill grass. The best way to do it carefully is to get what druggists call a "dropper." A small glass tube, having one end small and bent, while at the other end is a small rubber bulb; but you must be careful, also, not to take up acid enough to reach the bulb, as it would destroy that as well as the plants; and your clothes or fingers too, if you get it upon them. I like to see the dandelions in blossom; but they spread so fast 'tis well to destroy them. It must be done as soon after they come up as possible, lest they get too large for a single drop.

**Toothache Drops, Japanese, Magical.**—To quiet the pains in an aching tooth nothing can excel Japanese Drops. The formula (recipe) is: "Put together equal parts of creosote, chloroform, carbolic acid (liquid), oil of peppermint, oil of cloves, and oil of camphor (camphorated oil, kept by druggists). The result is a liquid that will give almost instant relief, if applied on a bit of cotton to the cavity of an aching tooth, and yet is no more fiery in the mouth than oil of cloves would be. The drops smell most strongly of creosote, while peppermint predominates in the taste. It is best to swallow as little as possible of the mixture."—*Country Gentleman.*

*Remarks.*—This properly belongs to the Medical Department, but it is too good to lose, and hence I put it here. A little of it might be rubbed on the gum, but if you get too much about the mouth it will irritate it and make it sore. So only wet a small bit of cotton to put in the tooth, not to have an overplus to run out. See also "Headache Cure, Magical." I have found it the most magical of anything I ever tried for the headache.

**Rum Sherbert.**—Rub loaf sugar over the rinds of 3 fresh oranges. To 3 qts. of water, add the juice of 1 doz. large oranges; sweeten to taste with loaf sugar (any white sugar will do), using also the sugar rubbed over the oranges; flavor highly with rum, and freeze. Grated pineapple may be added when it is partly frozen, if liked.

*Remarks.*—I should like it better as a drink, rather than to freeze and eat.

**1. SCARE-CROWS—How to Make.**—Take two small, cheap mirrors, fasten them back to back, attach a cord to and hang them to a pole. When the glass swings the sun's rays are reflected all over the field, even if it be a large one, and even the oldest a d bravest crow will depart precipitately should one of its lightning flashes fall on him. [Good only while the sun shines.]

II. The second plan, although a terror to the crow, is especially well suited to fields subject to the inroads of small birds, and even chickens. It involves the artificial hawk, made from a large potato and long goose or turkey feathers. The maker can exercise his imitative skill in sticking the feathers into the potato so that they resemble the spread tail and wings of a hawk. It is astonishing what a ferocious looking bird of prey can be constructed from the above simple material. It only remains to hang the object from a tall, bent pole, and the wind will do the rest. The bird will make swoops and dashes in the most threatening manner. Even the most inquisitive of venerable hens have been known to hurry rapidly from its dangerous vicinity, while to small birds it carries unmixed dismay.—*Scientific American.*

*Remarks.*—Take a long potato, and if the boy takes a little pains, he can get up a good representation of a hawk; and the longer the string, the more flopping around there will be to frighten the hens from scratching up the corn. Crows, I hardly think, would be much frightened by this last plan. A stuffed coat and pants would be better for them.

**2.** Another plan is to string a few kernels of corn on long horsehairs, and place about the corn fields. The crows will swallow some of them and make such a noise of alarm as to drive the others away, while he will continue to scratch his throat to get rid of the corn, or rather the hair, which is said to rid the field of them for the season. It is easily tried.

**3. Hawks and Owls, Best Way to Catch.**—Set a pole, 15 feet high, or thereabouts, in a place near where the chickens are kept, and fasten a steel trap on the top and set it, so that when they light on it which they will do, it takes them, "sure pop," every time.

**STORING CELERY—For Spring Use.**—The *Germantown Telegraph* says: "We have tried most ways, but prefer this one, followed for many years. A trench is dug from 12 to 15 inches in depth and as long as may be suitable. Place the roots in this singly, side by side, at an angle—that is, leaning somewhat; three inches of soil are packed against them; then another line of stalks, until the bed is as large as may be convenient for covering, when another, if required, can be made. The soil should be added until within 6 inches of the top of the stalks; then a layer of straw, then a layer of dry leaves; the whole to have a good board covering, to keep out water. Of course, rather high ground for the bed, or beds, should be selected, and a trench dug around the bed deeper than the bottom of the celery trenches, so made as to be sure to carry off all the water. If this plan is followed strictly, all others may be abandoned, as the celery will keep not only till spring, but as long in spring as may be desired, if it is not all eaten beforehand."

**FLY POISON.**—Arsenate of potassa, 1 oz.; red lead, ¼ oz.; sugar, 5 ozs. Mix well together, bottle and cork for use, and label *Poison.*

DIRECTIONS—Put a suitable quantity on plates, moisten with water and place where they are thickest. It is very destructive because very poisonous, yet so pleasant to the taste of the fly, they "go for it" quickly.

**FLY STICKUMFAST—Not Poisonous.**—Melt rosin, 6 ozs., in a tin cup, then put in lard, 1 rounding table-spoonful, as a woman takes it up for shortening, or about 2 ozs., which should make it like very thick molasses when cold. Spread upon rather stiff paper with a little flat piece of wood or a knife, and place about the shelves, rooms, etc. If a knife is used to spread it, heat the knife over the fire when it will all wipe off with a piece of newspaper or cloth. It will hold all that light upon it, and the more that light the more will come, thinking something good has been found. It holds them fast. Place a paper over the cup to keep flies out when it is set away.

**LEGITIMATE BUSINESS—To be Stuck to if You Would Avoid Failure.**—There so very many failures, I desire to say a word, if possible, to those who mean to do the right thing, to enable them to be success-ful, hence with some modification by myself on some points, I give the follow-ing sensible article of some writer, I know not who, but I do well know if business men will be guided by it, *i. e.*, stick to their legitimate business, keeping all their capital in it, necessary to carry it on, there will not be one failure where there is now a score.

"Well-directed energy and enterprise are the life of American progress; but if there is one lesson taught more plainly than others by the great failures of late, it is that safety lies in a legitimate business. No manufacturer, trader, or banker has any right to be so energetic and enterprising as to take from his legitimate business the capital which it requires to meet any emergency which may arise.

"Apologies are sometimes made for firms, or persons, who have failed, by referring to the important experiments they have aided, and the unnumbered fields of enterprise where they have freely scattered their money. We are told that individual losses, sustained by those failures, will be as nothing compared with the benefits conferred on the community by their liberality in contributing to every public work. There is little force in such reasoning. A man's rela-tions to a creditor are vastly different from his relations to what is called the public. The demands of the one are definite, the claims of the other are just what the ambition and legitimate means of the man may make them.

"The histories of honorable, successful business men unite to exalt the im-portance of sticking to one legitimate business, and it is most instructive to see that, in the greater portion of the failures, the real cause of disaster was the branching out beyond his legitimate business, in the taking hold of this and that tempting offer, and, for the sake of some hoped-for gain, venturing where they did not know the ground, and could not know the pit-fall until in it."

**Wages—Table Showing the Rate, from $2 to $25 a Week, 10 Hours Per Day, Also Rate Per Day and Hour.**—This table is so care-fully worked out a mere glance shows the desired amount:

| Per Week. | Five Days. | Four Days. | Three Days. | Two Days. | One Day. | Half Day. | Fourth Day. | One Hour. |
|---|---|---|---|---|---|---|---|---|
| $ 2.00 | $1.66⅔ | $1.33⅓ | $1.00 | $ .66⅔ | $ .33⅓ | $ .16⅔ | $ .8⅓ | $ .3⅓ |
| 2.50 | 2.08⅓ | 1.66⅔ | 1.25 | .83⅓ | .41⅔ | .21 | .10½ | .4 |
| 3.50 | 2.91⅔ | 2.33⅓ | 1.75 | 1.16⅔ | .58⅓ | .29 | .14½ | .6 |
| 4.00 | 3.33⅓ | 2.66⅔ | 2.00 | 1.33⅓ | .66⅔ | .33⅓ | .16½ | .6⅔ |
| 4.50 | 3.75 | 3.00 | 2.25 | 1.50 | .75 | .37½ | .18¾ | .7½ |
| 5.00 | 4.16⅔ | 3.33⅓ | 2.50 | 1.66⅔ | .83⅓ | .41⅔ | .21 | .8⅓ |
| 5.50 | 4.58⅓ | 3.66⅔ | 2.75 | 1.83⅓ | .91⅔ | .46 | .23 | .9 |
| 6.50 | 5.41⅔ | 4.33⅓ | 3.25 | 2.16⅔ | 1.08⅓ | .54 | .27 | .11 |
| 7.00 | 5.83⅓ | 4.66⅔ | 3.50 | 2.33⅓ | 1.16⅔ | .58⅓ | .27 | .11⅔ |
| 7.50 | 6.25 | 5.00 | 3.75 | 2.50 | 1.25 | .62½ | .31 | .12½ |
| 8.00 | 6.66⅔ | 5.33⅓ | 4.00 | 2.66⅔ | 1.33⅓ | .66⅔ | .33⅓ | .13⅓ |
| 9.00 | 7.50 | 6.00 | 4.50 | 3.00 | 1.50 | .75 | .37½ | .15 |
| 10.00 | 8.33⅓ | 6.66⅔ | 5.00 | 3.33⅓ | 1.66⅔ | .83⅓ | .41⅔ | .16⅔ |
| 11.00 | 9.16⅔ | 7.33⅓ | 5.50 | 3.66⅔ | 1.83⅓ | .91⅔ | .46 | .18⅓ |
| 13.00 | 10.83⅓ | 8.66⅔ | 6.50 | 4.33⅓ | 2.16⅔ | 1.08⅓ | .54 | .21⅔ |
| 14.00 | 11.66⅔ | 9.33⅓ | 7.00 | 4.66⅔ | 2.33⅓ | 1.16⅔ | .58⅓ | .23½ |
| 16.00 | 13.33⅓ | 10.66⅔ | 8.00 | 5.33⅓ | 2.66⅔ | 1.33⅓ | .66⅔ | .26⅔ |
| 17.00 | 14.16⅔ | 11.33⅓ | 8.50 | 5.66⅔ | 2.83⅓ | 1.41⅔ | .71 | .28⅓ |
| 19.00 | 15.83⅓ | 12.66⅔ | 9.50 | 6.33⅓ | 3.16⅔ | 1.58⅓ | .79 | .31⅔ |
| 20.00 | 16.66⅔ | 13.33⅓ | 10.00 | 6.66⅔ | 3.33⅓ | 1.66⅔ | .83⅓ | .33⅓ |
| 21.00 | 17.50 | 14.00 | 10.50 | 7.00 | 3.50 | 1.75 | .87½ | .35 |
| 22.00 | 18.33⅓ | 14.66⅔ | 11.00 | 7.33⅓ | 3.66⅔ | 1.83⅓ | .91⅔ | .36⅔ |
| 23.00 | 19.16⅔ | 15.33⅓ | 11.50 | 7.66⅔ | 3.83⅓ | 1.91⅔ | .96 | .38⅓ |
| 25.00 | 20.83⅓ | 16.66⅔ | 12.50 | 8.33⅓ | 4.16⅔ | 2.08⅓ | 1.04 | .41⅔ |

**INTEREST—Simple and Easy Rules to Compute.—**For finding the interest on any principal for any number of days. [The answer in each case being in cents, separate the two right-hand figures of answer to express in dollars and cents]: Four per cent.—multiply—the principal in all cases—by the number of days, and divide by 90; 5 per cent.—multiply by number of days, and divide by 72; 6 per cent.—multiply by number of days, and divide by 60; 7 per cent.—multiply by number of days, and divide by 50; 8 per cent.—multiply by number of days, and divide by 45; 9 per cent.—multiply by number of days, and divide by 40; 10 per cent.—multiply by number of days, and divide by 36; 12 per cent.—multiply by number of days, and divide by 30; 15 per cent.—multiply by number of days, and divide by 24; 18 per cent.—multiply by number of days, and divide by 20; 20 per cent.—multiply by number of days, and divide by 18; 24 per cent.—multiply by number of days, and divide by 15; without regard to fraction or remainder in any case; may add, however, the interest to the amount found for any fractional part of a dollar, if any such is found in the note or principal.

**1. STRAWBERRIES.—To Raise Large and Abundant.—**We have known strawberry growers to have the soil for strawberry plantations spaded 2 feet deep, and to apply 100 two-horse wagon loads of good stable manure per acre, before a plant was put out. Then during the first season the soil between the rows was stirred at least every 2 weeks, and in the fall the entire ground and plants were entirely covered with bog hay, which protects them in winter, and this mulch was left on the following season, not only to keep the berries clean but also to keep the soil moist underneath. Slaughter house manure of the rankest kind is also used for this purpose, and the growth of vine which follows, and the size of fruit would certainly astonish any man who was not in the secret as to how the thing was done. This is the way in which new sorts are treated by professionals who expect to make a show of their pets at exhibitions or elsewhere.—*Phonograph*, Colby, Wis.

*Remarks.*—If this is the plan to show off their pets, it is the plan to raise them on generally. The deeper working of the soil, (see No. 3), and heavy manuring pay, also the covering or mulching with cheap hay, to avoid the soil getting upon the berries, and also the keeping of the ground moist, and weeds from growing.

**2. Strawberry Growers—a Hint—Kind's to Plant with Wilson's Albany.**—A correspondent of the *Fruit Recorder*, (see No. 4), complaining that Wilson's Albany toward the last part of the season run small in the size of the berry, and that rich soil and good cultivation do not change this habit, is told [to plant amongst the Wilsons every third or fourth plant of Charles Downing, Colonel Cheney or Jucunda, all of which are in their prime toward the last run of the Wilsons. This proportion of these large sorts mixed in with the Wilsons will give a fine appearance to the fruit, and make them sell well to the last.

**3. Strawberry Culture—Kinds, and How to Grow Them.**—A correspondent of the *Post and Tribune* says: "Any one can raise strawberries who can grow corn or garden vegetables; yet few attain to perfection in strawberry growing.

I. The first requisite is a deep, rich bed.

II. The second requisite is good plants, and of kinds which will bear fruit without some other variety to fertilize them. If the Col. Cheney is planted alone very little fruit will be had, because this is a pistillate variety; so is the Green Prolific, and these varieties require the presence of some staminate sort to fertilize them. The Wilson's Albany is a good staminate sort, and bears fruit without the aid of any other variety, except to get larger berries the last of the season as in No. 2. It is the best kind for general planting. A good variety to plant beside the Wilson is the Green Prolific.

III. *Thirdly*, after the plants are done bearing, the tops should be mown off close, or cropped with a sharp knife. This prevents the plants throwing out runners so freely, and thus avoids the tendency to become matted together; it causes a strong growth of roots, and gives new, fresh and healthy foliage. It is almost equal to renewing the bed, because the plants are not taxed to support a new generation.

IV. *Lastly*, strawberries need the earliest culture possible in the spring. The beds ought then to be covered with manure or hay, to keep the soil cool aud damp, and to prevent the growing of weeds. With these points attended to, large crops will reward the grower.

*Remarks.*—The author agrees with this gentleman, except in the spring culture. I believe it is a conceded fact, generally, that the culture, manuring and putting on hay, or straw, or sawdust, should be done in the fall. The manure spaded or forked in, and the straw or other covering put on, so the fall rains and the melting of the snow in the spring will carry the virtue of the manure well among the roots, and, consequently, give a better crop. In such a case as given in the next, where no time could be given in the fall to do as these did, I would take time to put on a good covering of straw, or marsh hay, if plenty, which is no doubt best, as it is not so likely to blow off, after being wet by the rains.

4. **Strawberries, Killing Weeds Among.**—The Palmyra (N. Y.) *Fruit Recorder*, upon this subject says: "One of the finest yields of strawberries we ever saw was years ago on an old bed of Early Scarlet, grown on the farm of a brother-in-law. It had been kept clean up to July, when the press of farm work prevented any further attention to it, and the vines run helter-skelter and weeds grew freely, so that by December it was a complete mat of vines and weeds. We recommended setting fire to it, which was done, and quickly burned over. In the spring the vines started freely, and soon covered the surface with their green leaves, and from about one-third of an acre, nearly 50 bushels of splendid fruit was gathered. You can do this, and if the weeds are not sufficiently scattered over it to burn over the entire surface, scatter a little straw or hay over the vacant places. The fire destroys the seeds of weeds but does no harm to plants."

**Strawberries, Liquid Manure for, While Growing.**—I filled a half-hogshead with rainwater, and put into it a ¼ lb. aqua ammonia and ¼ lb. common niter (saltpeter). When the strawberry plants were blossoming out I gave them a sprinkling of the solution at evening twice a week until the fruit was nearly full size. The result was double the amount of fruit on those where the liquid was applied to what was obtained from those right alongside upon which none of the liquid was applied.—*Fruit Record.*

*Remarks.*—With all these points, I think any one can raise strawberries, as No. 3 puts it, if they will pay reasonable attention; and if extra attention, they will get extra crops.

**RASPBERRY CULTURE—How to Prepare The Ground.—** The richer the soil naturally, that can be given to them the better, then, one writer says, "The ground is prepared as you would for a crop of sugar beets (that is, deep ploughing and plenty of manure), using plenty of old manure and plowing deeply as possible: Shallow culture will not do for raspberries as the roots require coolness and moisture. Without these conditions, in dry seasons the crop will not perfect itself. The plants are usually set 4 feet apart each way, though some cultivators prefer 6 feet one way and 3 feet the other."

2. **Keeping Clear of Weeds the Two First Seasons, then Mulching or Covering.**—C. Engle of Paw Paw, Mich. says: "Rasp-

berries should be hoed and kept well cleaned from weeds the first two seasons after setting. After that, a very good and easy way to tend them is to cover the surface, between the vines, with some kind of coarse litter, (straw or marsh hay is first rate), 5 or 6 inches in depth. That will prevent the weeds from growing, and keep the ground cool and moist. I have treated a patch in that way for 7 years past, (adding an additional light coating every spring), and see no dimunition in quantity or quality of the fruit. They do equally as well in the dryest season. I do not know that it would be practicable on a large plantation, but for a small patch it is just the thing."

*Remarks.*—If it is just the thing for a small patch, 'tis just the thing for a large one, if you desire to have it pay big. Undertake no larger field than you can do well, then you may reasonably expect it to do well. If you have not mulch enough to cover all the ground, let the hills be well mulched with manure; and if considerable straw is in it, 'tis so much the better, for the roots must be covered, if you expect large yields.

3. **The Kind to Raise.**—The McCormick, also called the Mammoth Cluster Raspberries, is becoming one of the leading varieties among the black caps. T. T. Lyon says it is the largest, most vigorous and productive of them all. Charles Downing says: "It has stronger and more vigorous canes, has fewer spines, and is the largest, best and most productive Black Cap we have seen."

*Remarks.*—There may from time to time be varieties brought out that will eclipse the McCormick. Let everyone engaged in the business look well to this in obtaining plants or canes, as everyone wants the best.

Even now, 1884, the *Rural New Yorker* in its brieflets suggests Shaffer's Colossal as a large berry, combining a pleasant acidity with the true raspberry flavor among the black caps; and the Crimson Beauty or Hansell as the earliest red· and the Sneider among blackberries to take the place of a part, at least, of the Kittatinny's, being more fruitful, and far more hardy; certainly good qualities to recommend it. And so may improvements go on.

4. **Pinching Off, or Cutting Back the Leaves, the Best Way** —Those that understand the cultivation of the raspberry consider it the best way to pinch off when 3 or 4 feet high, according to the richness of the soil, else to cut back as soon as they reach 5 or 6 feet high, which certainly tends to make them more stocky, and to produce much stronger, lateral or side branches, which should also be pinched off or cut back, to insure a larger berry, and a larger yield of fruit.

5. **Blackberries**— And red raspberries need much the same treatment as the black caps.

**Gardening in a Hogshead.**—Sometime ago Mr. G. L. Record, of this city bored holes in rows around a hogshead, at a regular intervals, 6 inches apart, filling the hogshead with earth, and set a strawberry plant in each one of the holes, beside putting a number of plants on top. There are 100 plants growing from the sides of this novel Garden, which are now in full beauty and bloom, having a prolific growth of berries, and looking remarkably thriving and healthy. Some of the berries are ripe, and have attained great size, one measuring 3 inches in circumference.—*New Orleans Times-Democrat.*

*Remarks.*—I have seen cucumbers growing in, or rather on top of kegs filled with rich earth, so I know the thing is practicable for those who have only a small yard and no garden.

**Finger Marks Quickly Removed from Mirrors, Windows, etc.**—Putting a few drops of ammonia on a cloth will do the work admirably. The same also from doors about the locks and latches. Take the cloth in such a way as not to irritate the fingers with the strong ammonia. See "Ammonia—Its Uses, etc."

**BRIMSTONE—A Disinfectant After Deaths from Cholera, Also an Exterminator of Bed Bugs, Roaches, etc.**—L. H. Spear, in the *Rural New Yorker*, makes the following statement upon this subject, which will be found reliable. He says: "The 'Epidemic of Cleanliness,' as the present effort to prevent cholera has been called by those who have the sanitary condition of our great cities in charge, mentions, among numerous preventives of malarial poison, the burning of brimstone in houses, and I doubt if any who hastily read the various directions for fumigating dwellings, know half the merits of this agent. A distinguished chemist once said of it: 'While other disinfectants act for a time, so as to seem to destroy bad odors, they chiefly *cover them up*, but brimstone kills them.' All housekeepers should also know that by burning brimstone in a room infested with bugs, it will kill them. Put burning charcoal into a kettle and sprinkle a ¼ lb. of powdered brimstone over it. Close all windows and doors for an hour or more, when they can be re-opened.

*Remarks.*—Let any one who thinks this will not kill the bed bugs, roaches, etc., even in the cracks and crevices of the walls, pass a lighted sulphur match under his nose, and then judge if he could stand it an hour? If the cholera visits your neighborhood, which it is almost certain to do at some time, this should be done to every room in which a cholera patient dies; and may be done at any time in rooms where these pests have got a lodgement in the cracks of old walls. It is recently claimed that even cholera is caused by a living mite or "microbe," as they call them, and, therefore, the burning of the powdered brimstone, is sure death to them, and that no further spreading of the disease is possible.

**Cess Pools Disinfected Instantly.**—Prof. Thos. Taylor reports that 1 table-spoonful of spirits of turpentine in 1 pail of water will disinfect an ordinary cess pool instantly, and that in the sick chamber it will prove a powerful auxiliary against germs and bad odors.

*Remarks.*—Then, I think, 2 or 3 spoonfuls to the pail of water would be equally effective for a water-closet—privy.

**Oil on the Water has Enabled Vessels to Outride Storms at Sea.**—The schooner George Sherman was reported, May 30, 1884, by the Chicago papers, to have ridden out the gale on Lake Michigan that week by pouring on the water 12 gallons of linseed oil, which calmed the waves for a distance of half a mile from the ship. This is, no doubt, true, but wonderful all the same—one of the mysteries of nature—Nature's God.

*Remarks.*—If sailors do not have opportunity to read this, their friends may, and communicate it to them.

**INKS, Black.**—Inks of late years are mostly made from the analine colors, which have been brought to such perfection as to make good ink, by putting the right amount of powder to the certain amount of soft water.   John B. Wade, No. 40 Murray street, New York, deals in them, but druggists can furnish them anywhere, and others will of course soon deal in all these colors.

I.   The black is made by using what is called "nigrosine" or black analine, 1 oz. to water 1 gal.

II.   Violet, which is a very popular color, is made by using Hoffman's violet, 3 B., 1 oz., water 1 gal.   DIRECTIONS—Dissolve the powder with a little alcohol or boiling water; and if desired to use as a copying ink, sugar and gum Arabic, in the proportions given in the black ink from nut galls and logwood below.

III.   Blue is made by using Lieman soluble blue, ½ oz, to water 3 gals.

*Remarks.*—I have these receipts from a nephew of mine, and have not personally tested them, but I have others (see below as to 3 of these colors).   Still it looks to me this would be rather pale, then try ½ gal. of water only to the ½ oz. of the soluble blue, and if this is darker than needed take a tea-spoonful of it and add a tea-spoonful of water, this would be equivalent to 1 gal., and so if it takes 3 tea-spoonfuls of water to make the desired shade, it will take the full 3 gals.   This will be better than if I had tested it myself, as it puts so many upon a plan to experiment for themselves.

*Bluing for Clothes.* — And by the way now this soluble blue is just the thing to make bluing for clothes being washed.   But where the common soluble blue or Chinese blue is kept and used by painters, we put 1 oz. to 1 qt. of water, then a table-spoonful or two is enough for a tub of clothes, the woman judging for herself the depth of shade, putting in more or less to suit.

IV.   Red ink is made with eosine T. extra, or J. yellowish shade, ½ oz. to water 1 gal.

V.   Green is made very nice, by using methyl green, B. bluish dark shade, ½ to 1 oz. to water 1 gal.

*Remarks.*—I think all the powder should be dissolved in a little alcohol, else boiling water as with the violet No. 2.   These are all analine inks, or colors, although they have different names to distinguish them.   The nephew that sent me these recipes also sent writing done with the red, black, and the violet. They were as nice shades as could be desired.   Any one can make as dark, deep shade as they may choose by first using only half the water, then adding more as they prefer.

**2.   Black Ink, With Nut Galls and Logwood for Writing and Copying.**—Inks made from the nut galls alone as the coloring agent are not as good a black as those made with the addition of logwood chips; hence we say:   Logwood chips, 1 oz.; nut galls in coarse powder which have not been eaten by moths or worms, ¾ lbs.; purified copperas, 3 ozs.; acetate of copper (verdigris), ½ oz.; pulverized sugar, 3 ozs., and gum Arabic, 4 ozs.; soft water 1 gal. If not to be used as a copying ink no sugar need be used and only 2 or 3 ozs. of the gum Arabic to hold the colors suspended in the ink else they settle. DIRECTIONS—Boil the logwood chips in the water for an hour or two, or as long as a woman would boil it for coloring; when cool, strain, making up for evaporation with more hot water; bruise the best blue galls, coarsely and put over the fire again till it begins to boil, adding the other articles and set away until it acquires the desired blackness, strain and bottle for use.

*Remarks.*—If properly made it is a black ink, at once, and all the time, does not fade, and is therefore suitable for all records. The others are cheaper, and a little less trouble to make, but do not give permanent satisfaction.

**3. Black Copying Ink, Cheap.**—Ex. of logwood, ¾ oz.; alum, powdered, 160 grs.; bi-chromate of potash, 48 grs.; soft water, 1 pt. DIRECTIONS—Dissolve the ex. and other drugs in half of the water, and percolate the rest of the water through the drugs.

*Remarks.*—This percolation is the same as straining, only it is done through filtering paper in a glass funnel or tunnel, by druggists, the paper can be got of the druggist, and put into a common tin tunnel, such as used in almost every family in the country, the puckering of the paper as it is pressed down into the tunnel lets the fluid run down readily. This receipt is the same as one of the best druggists in Ann Arbor, Mich., uses.¶ If not wanted for copying, add water to give the desired shade, and to make it flow more freely as a general writing ink. It is cheap and good. See also an ink for school children, also cheap, and flows easily.

**Ticket Writer's Glossy Ink.**—To any good ink, 4 ozs., add gum Arabic, ½ oz. Let stand in a warm place, and shake frequently. When dissolved, if too thick, add more ink, if too thin, more gum. It will produce a fine glossy letter; blue, red or other colors work with equal satisfaction.— *Oracle*, Ont.

**INDELIBLE INK—For Marking Clothing, To Write With a Pen.**—I. *Ink*, into an ounce bottle, put nitrate of silver, (lunar caustic), 1 dr.; gum Arabic, clean and white, 3 or 4 pieces the size of a common pea; then fill ⅔ full with soft water. This ought to be in a dark-colored, glass-stoppered bottle. Else it must be kept in a dark place when not in use. This is the ink proper; but to make it permanent, we have to first use a pounce, which also prevents the ink from spreading in the cloth, as follows:

II. *Pounce*—Into a 4 oz. bottle put sub-carbonate of soda, 2 drs.; fill with water. DIRECTIONS.—Wet the places to be written upon with the pounce, and iron smooth with a properly heated iron; then rub hard over the same spot with the end of a tooth brush handle, to polish, that the writing may be done nicely with the ink, using only a quill pen; then pass the hot iron over the writing to dry, and set the ink, else dry in the sun. This, if properly done makes it perfectly indelible.—*Indian Domestic Economy.*

**Indelible Ink, Quickly and Cheaply Made.**—A correspondent of the Detroit *Free Press Household*, gives us the following very simple home made way of making the ink and doing the work, and I will guarantee it will prove satisfactory. She says:

I. Rain water, 1 table-spoonful; vinegar, ½ tea-spoonful lunar caustic, druggists keep this in small sticks, a piece 3 inches long; put all in an ounce bottle, and shake occasionally till dissolved. Keep in a dark place.

II. DIRECTIONS.—To each tea-spoonful of milk—needed to wet the places upon which the name is to be written—dissolve a piece of baking soda as large as a grain of corn; iron it smoothly, and write the name with a quill pen with the ink immediately.

*Remarks.*—Dry with the hot iron or in the sun, as in No. 1. In the same communication the lady said: Common soda, (the same as baking soda), in powder, with a damp cloth, and a brisk rubbing, is the best thing to clean tin-ware, rubbing it dry.

**INK, INDELIBLE—To Mark with a Plate.**—Dissolve pure sulphate of iron, (pure copperas), 1 lb. in acetic acid, 1¼ lbs., and add precipitated carbonate of iron, (sesquioxide), 1 lb., and stir till they combine. This should be done in an iron kettle over a slow fire. Then put in printer's varnish, 3 lbs., and fine book ink, 2 lbs., and stir till well mixed; and to complete it add æthiops-mineral (black sulphuret of mercury), finely pulverized and sifted, 1 lb. mixed in thoroughly.

*Remarks*—This I obtained from an old stencil plate cutter, who had made and sold it many years. He said this would fill nearly 1,000 1 dr. bottles which he sold for 25 cts. each. The sulphuret of mercury gives it its indelibility. If you use ozs. in place of lbs. it will make about 60 bottles. If drs. are used instead of ozs. you will have only 7 or 8 bottles. Now suit yourself as to the amount you will make. Of course, to be kept corked.

**COLORING FOR DOMESTIC USES.**—As the "Diamond," dyes, analine and other colors are being so considerably used in coloring, at the time of writing this book, I shall only give a few recipes for those purposes, which are vouched for mostly by ladies who have used them, some of them yearly for 20 years, suitable for woolen, silk, cotton, carpet rags, dresses, etc.

**Black on Dress Goods.**—From a lady who has used it yearly for 20 years. In an iron kettle put warm water enough to cover 15 yards dress goods. In this dissolve ex. of logwood, 4 ozs.; blue vitriol, 2 ozs.; copperas, 1 oz. Be careful to have the ex. well dissolved. Of course everything should be dissolved, but the ex. dissolves slowly. Wet the goods thoroughly, then put into the dye, and let simmer slowly, stirring and handling often, till dark enough; then wash in strong soap suds 2 or 3 times, and rinse until the water is clear. Press while damp. If the goods look rusty, the dye is too strong, put in more water. Cashmeres may be colored by this dye, and make up as good as new.

**Black, on Wool or Cotton.**—And let me say right here, what will color wool nicely will also color silk. This is from Mary Zaring to one of the papers. She says: "I have seen so many recipes to color black, but I think none as good as mine, as it leaves the yarn or wool soft as blue dye does. **To** 10 lbs. of wool or cotton take 1 lb. of logwood (ex.) and 3 ozs., bichromate pot- ash, cost 10 cents; simmer your goods or wool 1 hour in the potash, then take the goods out in a tub and put in your logwood (ex.) and melt; wring out your goods and put in the logwood dye and let simmer 1 hour; then put back in the potash in the tub and let stand a little while; then wring out. This will not fade nor rub out as other black. I have colored fine pants this way three years ago and they are nice yet."

**Another Black.**—For 10 lbs. of wool or other goods take 10 ozs. of bichromate of potash and 6 ozs. of crude tartar, or cream of tartar; dissolve together in an iron pot in 10 gals. of water, enter the wool or goods and boil 1½ hours, stirring occasionally; empty the pot and boil 3½ lbs. of logwood or its equivalent, say 1½ lbs. of extract of logwood, in enough water to cover the goods well (better to have too much than too little); enter the goods and boil 1 hour; take it off and wash the goods in clean cold water, thoroughly, using 2 or 3 waters. If too much of a blue black, add a little more logwood and boil again.—*The Cultivator.*

*Remarks.*—The 8 next recipes are from *Reidout's Magazine,* adapted to small amounts of goods, and will be found very satisfactory:

**Black for Worsted or Woolen Dress Goods, etc.**—Dissolve ¾ oz. bichromate of potash in 3 gals. of water. Boil the goods in this 40 min- utes; then wash in cold water. Then take 3 gals. water, add 9 ozs. logwood, 3 ozs. fustic, and 1 or 2 drops D. O. V., or double oil of vitriol; boil the goods 40 minutes, and wash out in cold water. This will dye from 1 to 2 lbs. of cloth, or a lady's dress, if of a dark color, as brown, claret, etc. All colored dresses with cotton warps should be previously steeped 1 hour in sumach liquor; and then soaked for 30 minutes in 3 gals. of clean water, with 1 cup of nitrate of iron; then it must be well washed, and dyed as first stated.

**Black for Silk.**—Dye the same as black for worsted, but previously steep the silk in the following liquor: scald 4 ozs. logwood and ¼ oz. tumeric in 1 pt. boiling water; then add 7 pts. cold water. Steep 30 or 40 minutes; take out and add 1 oz. sulphate of iron (copperas), dissolved in hot water; steep the silk 30 minutes longer.

**Brown for Worsted or Wool.**—Water, 3 gals.; bichromate of pot ash, ¾ oz. Boil the goods in this 40 minutes; wash out in cold water. Then take 3 gals. water, 6 ozs. peachwood, and 2 ozs. tumeric. Boil the goods in this 40 minutes; wash out.

**Imperial Blue for Silk, Wool and Worsted.**—Water, 1 gal., sulphuric acid, a wine-glassful; imperial blue, 1 table-spoonful or more, accord ing to the shade required. Put in the silk, worsted, or wool, and boil 10 min utes; wash in a weak solution of soap lather.

**Sky Blue for Worsted and Woolen.**—Water, 1 gal.; sulphuric acid, a wine-glassful; glauber salts in crystals, 2 table-spoonfuls; liquid extract of indigo, 1 tea-spoonful. Boil the goods about 15 minutes; rinse in cold water.

**Claret for Wool or Worsted—A Short Way of Dyeing the Same.**—Water, 3 gals.; cudbear, 12 ozs.; logwood, 4 ozs.; old fustic, 4 ozs.; alum, ½ oz. Boil the goods in it 1 hour. Wash. This will dye from 1 to 2 lbs of material.

**Crimson for Worsted or Wool.**—Water, 3 gals.; paste cochineal, 1 oz.; cream of tartar, 1 oz.; nitrate of tin (tin dissolved in nitric acid, I think, —it used to be dissolved in a mixture of sulphuric and muriatic acids, and called "muriate of tin,") a wine-glassful. Boil your goods in this 1 hour. Wash first in cold water, then in another vessel with 3 gals. warm water with a cup of ammonia, the whole well mixed. Put in the goods and work well 15 minutes. For a bluer shade add more ammonia. Then wash out.

**Fawn Drab for Silk.**—Hot water, 1 gal.; annotto liquor, 1 wine-glassful; 2 ozs. each of sumach and fustic. Add copperas liquor according to the required shade. Wash out. It is best to use the copperas liquor in another vessel, diluted according to the shade desired.

**Blue on Cotton Rags—Does Not Fade.**—For 3 lbs. of rags: prussiate of potash, 1 oz.; oil of vitriol, 1 oz.; and 2 large table-spoonfuls of copperas. Put all the ingredients together in an iron kettle, with a sufficient quantity of water, and when well dissolved put in the rags, stir well, and when they are of the desired color take them out and rinse well. It will probably take from ½ to ¾ of an hour to color. Be sure and rinse thoroughly.

**"True Blue" for One Pound of Rags that will Not Fade.**—A lady in writing to the *Blade* says: "I see Mrs. Gloyd wants a recipe for coloring blue on cotton, that will not fade, so I come in with one that I know to be good, as I have used it for 2 carpets and it has proved itself 'true blue' every time. One oz. Prussian blue, ½ oz. oxalic acid; pulverize together, and dissolve in hot water sufficient to cover the goods. Dip the goods in this dye until they are the desired shade; then wring out and thoroughly rinse in alum water."

**Blue for Carpet Rags—Better than with Prussian Blue.**—To the same inquiry " Perseverance Ann," of Pleasant Lake, Ind., says: "I must tell Mrs. E. G. Gloyd of a better way to color carpet rags blue than with Prussian blue and oxalic acid. Take 4 ozs. prussiate of potash, 2 ozs. copperas, and 2 ozs. nitric acid, and dissolve in warm soft water, enough to cover the rags. This will color from 3 to 5 lbs., according to the shade you want. If you color part of them at a time you will have different shades. Wash the rags in the dye, wring out and air, and wash again till the color sets, which ought to be within half an hour; then rinse thoroughly and dry slowly in the shade. This colors woolen as well as cotton."

*Remarks.*—Take your choice of plans, now, you have both. See her drab, below.

**Copperas Color for Carpet Rags, with Lye.**—Mrs. M. M. Stark, of Nankin, Mich., to an inquirer in the Detroit *Tribune*, for coloring with copperas, says : " I have a good one, which I send. Dissolve ½ pound copperas in a pail full of hot water, also have a pail full of white lye prepared. **First**

dip the rags in the lye, then hang them in the sun and let dry, then dip in the copperas water and let dry, then in the lye, drying each time after dipping until you have the desired color."

*Remarks.*—I notice that some others use as much as 1 lb. to a pail of water, and do not dry the rags between the dippings, but drain well, choosing a sunny day to do it out of doors. Certainly the stronger ˌthe dye the deeper will be the color, and the less times of dipping would be necessary. None of them speak of putting water into the lye, perhaps the strength as run off from the ashes is intended, but it looks to me to be rather strong, if the ashes are from good hard wood. If more than one pail of copperas water is needed keep the same proportions. I should say 1 lb. to each pail needed. Dissolve in an iron kettle, as copperas is the sulphate of iron. One lady speaks of a strong lye, and she also used 1 lb. to a pail of water.

**Drab, with Tea, Pretty and Cheap, for Rags, Alpaca Dresses, etc. For Five Pounds of Goods.**—The same Perseverance Ann, of Pleasant Lake, Ind., that gave the blue above, comes in with a drab. These persevering old maids are the ones to have around the home; they do things well and keep all in order. She says: "To the old lady who wanted my recipe for coloring drab, I send the following: To 5 lbs. of goods take ¼ of a pound of the cheapest green tea, and 2 table-spoonfuls of copperas. Tie the tea in a cloth and steep in a brass kettle, then add the copperas and skim thoroughly. Put in the goods, and stir and air till colored enough, which will be in a few minutes. If this is not dark enough take out the goods and add more dye-stuff (tea). This is very cheap and pretty for carpet rags and a weak dye will restore a faded drab alpaca to your complete satisfaction."

**Drab, with Nut Galls, for Rags or Yarn.**—To make a very pretty light drab for a carpet, take 1 pound of nut galls, and after breaking them up, put in an iron kettle with a sufficient quantity of water to dip 16 lbs. of rags or yarn. Boil 1 hour, then add 1 ounce of blue vitriol. When this is thoroughly dissolved, put in the yarn or whatever material you desire to color, and let it simmer for 1 hour. If not as dark as required add a small quantity of extract of logwood and dip again.—*Mrs. Helen Wood.*

**Drab, with Sumach for Rags or Yarn. Lovely and Dark.**—Another writer, name nor place given, says: "I like drab in a carpet so well, and I heard the other day that sumach bobs make a lovely dark drab, just boil them up and put in the rags, it needs no setting or preparation whatever; our neighbor girls had splendid luck in this way, and it is so easy."

*Remarks.*—The only inconsistency I can see here is that no mordant to set the color is directed. I think without copperas or vitriol, as in the next ones above, it would soon fade. I leave that part to those, however, who have more experience in coloring than the doctor has, but merely suggest its necessity from the nature or things.

**Seal Brown, for 10 Pounds of Goods.**—For 10 lbs. of goods, take 3 lbs. of catechu, and put it in about as much water as you need to cover the goods well. Boil it until dissolved, then add 4 ozs. of blue vitriol, and stir until every particle dissolves. After wetting the goods thoroughly, put them in the dye, and lift, and stir, and turn, and air, until there is no danger of spots; then let them remain in the dye until morning. Wring or drain. Then make another dye, by dissolving in hot water, 4 ozs. of bichromate of potash, 3 ozs. of copperas, and 2 ozs. of ex. of logwood, in water enough to cover the goods. Allow them to remain in this dye 15 or 20 minutes, or until they are of the desired shade; but if they were some dark color when you first commenced, it would be well enough to leave out the logwood and copperas, and add them gradually, until the required shade be obtained.

*Remarks.*—I am sorry I cannot give credit for this recipe, as I am well satisfied it is a nice one. It was an answer to an inquiry, and she begged pardon for not answering sooner, and in closing said: " This will dye cotton or wool, and as said ex. of logwood dissolves so slowly, I always begin that part a day or two before hand by keeping it soaking, stirring occasionally."

**Brown, with Japonica, for Seven Pounds of Rags.**—In answer to an inquiry for coloring brown with japonica, I send the following, which I know is good : Take 6 ozs. bichromate of potash, 5 ozs. alum, 1 lb. japonica. Soak the japonica over night, dissolve the alum, wring the rags through the alum-water, then put them in the japonica and let them come to a boil; dissolve the bichromate of potash, wring them through the potash twice and wash them in soap-suds.—*Mrs. M. C. Lawton, of Coopersville, Mich., in Detroit Free Press Household.*

**Dark Brown, with Catechu, for Woolen, Cotton Not So Dark.** To 5 lbs. of goods take catechu, $\frac{1}{2}$ lb., bichromate of potash and blue vitriol, each 2 ozs. Make a dye of the catechu and vitriol, in which boil the goods (of course, always water enough to cover nicely) slowly $1\frac{1}{2}$ hours, handling properly, wring out; made a dye of the bichromate of potash, and dip in it 15 minutes or till the shade suits. It is inexpensive and durable, says "Emma S. H.," of Nashport, O., in answer to "Black Eyes," inquiry in *Blade*. Tested.

**Butternut Brown, for Four Pounds of Goods.**—A writer in the *Maine Farmer* gives the following : "Steep hot, but not boil, $\frac{1}{2}$ bushel butternut bark, until the strength is out. Then steep the goods 1 hour and air; then put in and steep $\frac{1}{2}$ hour and let them cool. Add 1 oz. copperas to the liquor and bring it to a boil. If not dark enough use more copperas. Various shades may be produced in this dye by varying the bark and copperas. One part butternut and one part walnut bark answers well for a brown."

*Remarks.*—Butternut is white walnut then what this writer means by " walnut," of course, is black walnut bark, each in equal amounts. It will make a darker shade, using the same amount of copperas.

**Brown, from the Scaly Moss of Rocks, Permanent.**—After giving the last, the same paper added: The scaly moss from rocks and ledges is a good material for coloring brown. Gather the moss and place it in a brass kettle or tin dish, upon which pour cold water, then let it boil on the stove 3 or 4 hours. Then skim out the moss, put in the goods, and boil until you have the requisite color. It will never fade.

*Remarks.*—Thus you have a variety of excellent browns to meet all reason-able demands, and some of the articles can be obtained everywhere.

**London Brown.**—Goods, 3 lbs.; camwood, ¾ lbs.; logwood, ½ lb.; quercitron bark, 1 oz.; copperas, 2 ozs. DIRECTIONS—Boil the dye-woods for 1 hour, add the copperas, and handle, at boiling heat for ½ hour. Rinse in cold water.

**Blue, Permanent.**—For 3 lbs. of goods, take alum, 5 ozs.; tartar, 3 ozs., chemic. DIRECTIONS.—Boil the goods with the alum and tartar, in brass, in water to cover well for 1 hour; remove the goods to warm water, in which you have put a little chemic, and if not as deep a blue as desired, take out and add a little more chemic 'till the shade suits.

**Yellow On Cotton.**—For 10 lbs. of goods, take acetate of lead, and nitrate of lead in solution each, 1 lb. in a tub of cold water sufficient to work well. Work 15 minutes and wring out; into another tub of cold water, put bichromate of potash, 6 ozs. in solution, and work 15 minutes through this, and wring out; again work 10 minutes in the lead solution, wash and dry.

**Green**—First color blue then color yellow, and you have a beautiful green. I know these receipts, (this plan, and the yellow above) to be excellent, for I have used them, says Leo, of Ft. Collins, Col.

**Scarlet on Cotton or Silk.**—Warm water, 3 gals.; cream of tartar and cochineal, 1 oz. each; solution of tin, 2 ozs. Wet the goods in warm water, and when the dye boils, put in the goods and boil 1 hour, frequently stirring, them (I say always stirring handling back and forth to air, and make the shade even); then take out the goods and rinse in cold water.—*San Francisco Cook.*

**Pink on Cotton—Beautiful, That Does not Fade**—Trailing Arbutus, of Steuben Co., N. Y., in writing to the *Free Press* (Det.) Household upon another subject, concludes as follows:

"I am fearful of being too lengthy, but please have patience, for I want you to know how we color a beautiful pink that will not fade. After 3 years constant wear, ours is as good as new. To 4 lbs. cotton goods, put in a brass kettle enough soft water to cover them well; put in a bag 2 ozs, cochineal, and let it lie in the water ½ or ¾ of an hour, heating to a scalding heat. Get all the strength from the bag of color, then put in 2 oz. of cream of tartar, and 4 ozs. muriate of tin—taking care not to get it on the hands. Put in the goods, stirring well, till the desired shade is obtained. If you wish more than one shade, put in part of the goods at a time—for the darkest first, and so on. It is a fine, light rose color for silks."

**Dark Tan for Cloth or Rags.**—To 5 lbs. of cloth, 1 lb. japonica, 8 oz. bichromate of potash, 2 table-spoonfuls alum. Dissolve the japonica and alum in soft water, enough to cover the goods. Wash the goods in suds and put them in the dye; let them stand 2 hours at scalding heat; then set them aside in the dye till next morning. In the morning take them from the kettle, and after having put on as much soft water as before, dissolve in it the bichromate of potash, into this put the goods and let them remain an hour at scalding heat. Wash in soft water suds and dry. It will color twice as much dark enough for rags. It does not make the rags tender.—*Jean, Lockhaven, Pa.*

**Bright Red for Rags.**—For 6 or 7 lbs.: Take redwood chips, 2½ lbs.; soak over night in a brass kettle; next morning put in alum, powdered, ½ lb., and boil to obtain the strength of the chips, leaving them in; put in the rags, or yarn, as the case may be, and simmer, airing occasionally, until bright enough to suit. It makes a color nearly resembling the flannel we buy.

**Nankeen, to Color.**—Fill a five-pail brass kettle with small pieces of white birch bark and water, let steep twenty-four hours and not boil, then skim out the bark, wet the cloth in soapsuds, then put it in the dye, stir well and air often; when dark enough, dry; then wash in suds. It will never fade.—*The Household.*

**1. CIDER, GRAPE JUICE, ETC.—To Keep from Fermentation.**—I. A writer in the *Prairie Farmer* says "that M. Pasteur, the great French scientist, has discovered that any fruit juice which is liable to ferment, can be kept any length of time by heating to 140° F., and then sealing it up, while hot, in air-tight vessels," and continues:

II. "This is nothing new. Cider brought to a boil, skimmed, and then put into tight 10-gallon kegs will keep as long as wanted in cool cellars. Those who are fond of sweet cider can in this way provide to have it at all times. If a slight fermentation is desired, a gallon or two may be drawn into a common jug and exposed to the air for a day or two, to give it a slight sparkle on the tongue. Cider should be boiled in brass, copper or iron, not in tin or galvanized iron pans."

III. This is confirmed by the following, by bottling while hot, by a writer to the Elmira (N. Y.) *Farmers' Club*, who says: "Cider may be kept by heating to the boiling point when sweet, just from the press; skim and bottle while hot. Also that apples may be kept fresh until new fruit comes again by packing in hemlock sawdust. They should be first put into piles to sweat."

IV. Another writer claims that "there is no benefit from any of the bung-hole additions," but "to make cider keep sweet have it made late in the fall, from sound, ripe fruit, and put the casks in a cool place till spring; then bottle, cork tight and tie the corks down. Lay the bottles on their sides in a cool dry cellar and you will be able to give your harvest hands a sip of cider at dinner any year."

*Remarks*—Unless the cider is racked off, so as to get rid of the pomace (which is got rid of by the heating, or boiling, and skimming in the other cases), as soon as it has become clear by working or fermentation and settled, I ascertain it must become quite sharp before spring. Some persons, however, prefer it sharp; but as the sharpness comes from fermentation, which produces alcohol, if no alcohol is desired in it, the fermentation must be avoided; and that is done by the heating to 140 degrees and bottling, as M. Pasteur, in I., above, or by boiling and skimming, as in II., which removes the pomace, as it rises on being boiled, then bunging up in small, or 10-gal. kegs, though I think barrels will do as well.   The skimming should be done as it rises, before it really boils, adding a little cold cider, if need be, till all is well removed, else, as they say, the pomice will " boil in," become firm and settle, which, if it does, must be avoided in pouring off for bottles or kegs.

V.   Grape Juice, or that of other fruits treated in the same way as M. Pasteur and others recommend, bottling or canning while hot, and placing in a cool cellar, before any fermentation has begun, the result has been, and therefore will be the same.   Thus heating and canning, or bottling grape juice you have an unfermented wine for communions, which does not intoxicate; but it never does, until after fermentation has taken place, which cannot occur without the presence of air.   See unfermented wines below, where water and sugar are added.

**2.**   At a cider-makers' convention recently, a Mr. Cane, of Lenawee Co., Mich., claimed that sugar, 2 lb., and alcohol, 2 qts. to each lb., was better than lime and all other compounds to keep cider sweet   I think it is a fact, even with 20 times 2 lbs. to a bbl.   With that I will guarantee it, even without racking off till spring.

**3.   Bottling Cider, to Keep for Years.**—A writer in the *New England Farmer* gives his plan of bottling cider that will keep for years; and its excellence was endorsed by the editor.   He says:   Leach and filter the cider through pure sand, after it has worked and fermented, and before it has soured. Put no alcohol or other substances with it.   Be sure that the vessels you put it in are perfectly clean and sweet.   After it is leached or filtered, put it in barrels or casks filled, leaving no room for air; bung them tight, and keep it where it won't freeze till February or March, then put it into champagne bottles filled; drive the corks and wire them.   It should be done in a cellar or room that is comfortable for work.   The best cider is late made, or made when it is as cold as can be and not freeze."

*Remarks.*—The leaching or filtering through sand, takes out the pomace, as the heating above does; but know ye, you cannot filter it until after it has worked, and the pomace settled, as the pomace clogs the sand.   I wish to say here, I see it stated that 1 bu. of blood beets to every 7 bu. of apples makes a cider richer, and of superior flavor to that made of apples alone.   I think, too, it would give it a fine color like wine.

**4.   Boiled Cider—How to Do It, and Its Uses.**—This is prepared by boiling sweet cider down in the proportion of 4 gals. to 1 (I have always bottled only 3 to 1).   Skim it well during boiling, and at the last take especial care that it does not scorch.   A brass kettle, well cleansed with salt and vinegar, and washed with clear water, is the best thing to boil it in.   For tart pies for summer use it is excellent; and for mince pies it is superior to brandy or any distilled liquor, and in fruit cake it is preferable to brandy, and also nice to stew dried apples in for sauce.   It is a very convenient article in a family.— *Country Gentleman.*

**1.   WINE—Wild Grape, to Make.**—I had occasion at one time, in Ann Arbor, to use some wine, and a neighbor woman told me she had some very nice of her own make. I obtained some, and proved it to be as she said, I found it was made of wild grape juice—half-and-half—with water. First having mashed the grapes and let it stand 2 or 3 days, then press out and strain, adding the water and white sugar, 16 lbs. to each 5 gallon keg, and let work 2 weeks, filling up full with more of the same, and bung tight. In February, when I obtained it, it was very nice indeed. Almost, if not quite, equal to port —better than half the port we buy.

2. **Blackberry Wine, to Make Properly.**—Take, of course, clean kegs or casks; let the berries be ripe; extract the juice with a small wine or cider press, or it can be done through coarse cotton cloths; then pass the juice through a strainer; let the juice stand for 2 or 3 days in the tub until the first fermentation is over, then skim off the top carefully, and add to every quart of juice 3 lbs. of the best yellow sugar, and water enough to make 1 gallon. Put all in a kettle and let it come to a boil, and then skim again. When cool put in a keg, fill up to the bung, place in the cellar and let it remain there with the bung off until after the second fermentation, which will be in 4 or 5 days. Meantime keep the cask full by pouring in wine that has been reserved for the purpose. After the second fermentation put in the bung tight and let it remain in the cask several months, say to the following February or March, when it should be carefully drawn off and put in bottles, or, what is better, demijohns of from 1 to 5 gallons. It will keep for any length of time without the addition of a drop of whiskey or brandy, and will prove a very agreeable and wholesome drink.—*"Sophia B," in Germantown Telegraph.*

*Remarks.*—Mostly used as a medicine in looseness of the bowels, debility, etc.; taken immediately after meals, as a tonic, in quantities of a wineglassful or more, as needed.

3. **Unfermented Wines, to Make.**—The juice of grapes, blackberries, raspberries, etc., pressed out without mashing the seeds, adding water, 1 pt., and sugar, ½ lb. for each pint of the juice; then boil a few minutes, skimming if any sediment or scum rises, and bottling while hot, corking tightly, cutting off the corks, and dipping the tops into wax, and keeping in a dry, cool place, gives a wine that no one would object to, if iced when drank. They are nourishing, satisfying to the thirst, and not intoxicating, because there has been no fermentation. Made of grapes, this wine is in every way suitable for communion, but might be preferred as first mentioned in V., under Cider, Grape Juice, etc., to Keep, above, where no water nor sugar are used.

1. **BEERS—Ginger, English.**—Loaf sugar, 2¼ lbs.; cream of tartar, 1½ ozs.; ginger root, 1½ ozs.; 2 lemons; fresh brewer's yeast, 2 tablespoonfuls; water, 3 gals. DIRECTIONS—Bruise the ginger, and put into a large earthenware pan, with the sugar and cream of tartar; peel the lemons, squeeze out the juice, strain it, and add, with the peel, to the other ingredients; then pour over the water boiling hot. When it has stood until it is only just warm, add the yeast, stir the contents of the pan, cover with a cloth, and let it remain near the fire for 12 hours. Then skim off the yeast and pour the liquor off into

another vessel, taking care not to shake it, so as to leave the sediment; bottle it immediately, cork it tightly; in 3 or 4 days it will be fit for use.

**2. Ginger Pop.**—White sugar, ¾ lb; cream of tartar and ginger root, bruised, each, ¾ oz.; juice and grated yellow of 1 lemon; water, 1 gal.; fresh yeast, 1 table-spoonful; ess. of winter green or sassafras as you prefer, or half as much of each, if a mixed flavor is liked. DIRECTIONS—Put all into a jar, except the yeast and ess.; and pour out over the water, boiling hot; cover, and let stand until it is only luke-warm, and add the yeast and ess., and let stand in a cool place 24 hours, strain and bottle, securing the corks tightly. It will be ready in about 3 days. More or less flavor may be used to suit different tastes.

**3. Cream Beer or Soda, any Flavor.**—Sugar, 2¼ lbs.; citric acid, 2 ozs.; juice of 1 lemon; water, 3 pts. DIRECTIONS—Dissolve by heat, and boil 5 minutes; when cold add the beaten whites of 3 eggs, beaten into a small cup of flour; and then stir in the ex. of lemon, or the ex. of any other flavor you desire; bottle and keep cool; put 2 table-spoonfuls more or less as you prefer into a tumbler, of cold water, and stir in ⅓ to ½ tea-spoonful of soda, and drink at your leisure, as the eggs and flavor holds a cream on top.

**Summer Drink, Pleasant for Sick or Well Persons.**—Mash a few currants, and pour on them a little water, strain, sweeten, and add sufficient cold water to suit the taste, though it is best to use the currants pretty freely, and sugar accordingly, as the acid of the currant makes this drink peculiarly grateful to the sick as well as those in health, satisfying the thirst of either. Currant jelly in cold water makes a good substitute for currants; and is next to that of tamarinds, which is undoubtedly the best to allay the thirst of fever patients of anything known. Lemons do very well. See next receipt.

**Lemon Syrup, to Prepare, When Lemons are Cheap.**—A very handy way of supplying summer drinks, or even for winter, when lemons are at a low figure, is to take any quantity, press the hand upon each, and roll it back and forth briskly, to break the cells, and make the juice press out more easily into the bowl, never into tin, as it gives a bad taste from the action of the acid upon the tin. Remove all the pulp from the peels, leaving the rind thin, cut them up, and boil a few minutes in water, 1 pt. to a doz. peels; strain the water, and add the juice to it by measure, and put nice white sugar, 1 lb. to each pt, there was of the juice; leave in boil for 10 to 20 minutes to form the syrup, then bottle and cork tightly. One to 2 table-spoonfuls to a glass of cold water gives you a cool, very healthful and very pleasant drink, for sick or well, at any time of the year; and a currant syrup may be made in the same way, using about half as much more sugar to each pint.

**Lemon, and Other Syrups, for Fountains, Home Use, or the Sick.**—Put in 4 ozs. of citric acid in a bottle with soft water, ½ pt. To make lemon, pine apple, orange, or any of the acid berry syrups, put ½ oz. of the above solution into 1 pt. bottle, add 2 drs. of ex. of lemon, or any of the others named, and fill with simple syrup, shake, and 'tis ready for use. One table-spoonful of this syrup to a glass of water makes a very satisfactory drink for the sick or well. When made in a glass, if effervescence is desired, stir in ½ tea-spoonful, or a little less, soda.

**For Sarsaparilla, Vanilla, Etc.** That have no acids in their composition no acids should be put in—still they will not effervesce with soda unless the acid is used.

*Remarks.*—I have used the lemon syrup made as above, 1 tea-spoonful, and 1 tea-spoonful of sugar put in ¾ pt. of hot water, which makes it very palatable. When taken an hour before meals it has no injurious effect upon the stomach or other parts of the system. See Hot Water for Dyspepsia for example.

**Lemonade—Portable, Convenient and Excellent.**—Powdered tartaric, or citric acid (the latter is preferable), 1 oz.; powdered sugar, 6 ozs.; extract of lemon, 2 drs. DIRECTIONS—Mix thoroughly and let dry in the sun. Rub thoroughly together after drying, divide into 23 powders. One makes a glass of good sweet lemonade. Handy to have when going hunting or picnicing.—*San Francisco Cook.*

**1. SUMMER DRINKS—For the Field or Workshop, Nourishing as well as Allaying Thirst.**—Make oatmeal into a thin gruel; then add a little salt, and sugar to taste, with a little grated nutmeg and one well-beaten egg to each gallon, well stirred in while yet warm. This was first suggested by the Church of England leaflets put out among the farmers and others to discourage them from carrying whiskey into the field.

**2.** If the above plan is too much trouble, although it is, indeed, very nourishing and satisfactory, take the Scotch plan of stirring raw oatmeal into the bucket of cold water and stir when dipped up to drink. I drank of this at the building of the New York and Brooklyn bridge, which I visited with my son while in New York in the Centennial year of 1876, on our way from Philadelphia, and we were highly pleased with it. As near as I could judge, ½ to 1 pint was stirred into a common 12-quart pail. The workmen drank of it freely, preferring it to plain water very much.

**Home-Made Filter, Cheap and Very Satisfactory.**—Take a large flower-pot, put a piece of sponge over the hole in the bottom, fill ¾ full of equal parts of clean sand and charcoal the size of a pea; over this lay a woolen cloth large enough to hang over the sides of the pot. Pour water into the cloth and it will come out pure after the dust from the coal has been run off by a few fillings. When it works too slow take off the woolen cloth and wash it thoroughly and replace it again is all that will be required for a long time.

**Interest, Rates of the Western States and Territories, New York and Canada, and Consequences of Taking Usurious Rates.**—The following rates of interest and consequences of taking usury, was collected by the *Ledger*, of Philadelphia, a very reliable source, and will show any one at a glance where they can obtain the largest interest for money they wish to invest in any considerable amounts :

*California*—Ten per cent after a debt becomes due, but parties may agree upon any interest whatever, simple or compound.

*Colorado*—Ten per cent on money loaned.

*Dakota*—Seven per cent. Parties may contract for a rate of interest not exceeding 12. Usury (illegal or exhorbitant interest) forfeits all the interest taken.

*Idaho Territory*—Ten per cent. Parties may agree in writing for any rate not exceeding 2 per cent per month. Penalty for greater rate is 3 times the amount paid, fine of $360, or 6 months' imprisonment, or both.

*Illinois*—Six per cent, but parties may agree in writing for 10. Penalty for usury forfeits the entire interest.

*Indiana*—Six per cent. Parties may agree in writing for any rate not exceeding 10. Beyond that rate is illegal as to the excess only.

*Iowa*—Six per cent. Parties may agree in writing for 10. A higher rate works a forfeiture of 10 per cent.

*Kansas*—Seven per cent. Parties may agree for 12. Usury forfeits the excess.

*Michigan*—Seven per cent. Parties may contract for any rate not exceeding 10.

*Minnesota*—Seven per cent. Parties may contract to pay as high as 12, in writing but contract for higher rate is void as to the excess.

*Missouri*—Six per cent. Contract in writing may be made for 10. The penalty of usury is forfeiture of the interest at 10 per cent.

*Montana*—Parties may stipulate for any rate of interest.

*Nebraska*—Ten per cent, or any rate on express contract not greater than 12. Usury prohibits the recovery of any interest on the principal.

*Nevada*—Ten per cent. Contract in writing may be paid for the payment of any other rate.

*New Mexico Territory*—Six per cent, but parties may agree upon any rate.

*New York*—Seven per cent. Usury is a misdemeanor, punishable by a fine of $1,000 or 6 months' imprisonment, or both, and forfeits the principal, even in the hands of third parties.

*Ohio*—Six per cent. Contract in writing may be for 8. No penalty attached for violation of law. If contract is for a higher rate than 8 it is void as to interest, and recovery is limited to principal and 6 per cent.

*Oregon*—Ten per cent. Parties may agree on 12.

*Utah Territory*—Ten per cent. No usury laws. Any rate may be agreed on.

*Washington Territory*—Ten per cent. Any rate agreed upon in writing is valid.

*Wisconsin*—Seven per cent. Parties may contract in writing for 10. No interest can be computed on interest. Usury forfeits all the interest paid.

*Wyoming Territory*—Twelve per cent, but any rate may be agreed upon in writing.

*Ontario*—Six per cent, but parties may agree upon any rate

*Quebec*—Six per cent, but any rate may be stipulated for.

**BOOTS AND SHOES**—Cement for **Patching Without Sewing.**—Pure gutta percha, eschewed or cut fine, ¼ oz., sulphide of carbon, 1½ ozs. is about the right proportions. It should be the consistence of thick molasses. Keep corked when not in use, as the sulphide is very evaporative. DIRECTIONS—Cut the patch the right shape, pare the edge thin, remove all dirt and grease from the place to be mended. Apply 2 or 3 coats of the cement to boot and patch,, with a suitable spatula or flat stick, as a brush soon dries up; heat each and press on the patch with a warm burnishing iron, as shoemakers understand.

*Remarks*—The sulphide of carbon, has proved the best solvent for the gutta percha. If well done, it will prove permanent and satisfactory. I have had them thus applied, and they kept their position for many months.

**Boots—To Make Water-Proof.**—Farmers and others whose business calls them into wind, snow, etc., ought to have their boots made purposely for them, not of thick, heavy cowhide, but kip or some soft and pliable leather, a kind the shoemakers know as a "runner," is good, and the soles should be double the whole length, and of firm and well tanned leather, and before wearing the soles should be well filled with tallow, heated and dried in; then oil the uppers with **castor** oil, also heated in, at least, a tablespoonful of it to each boot; then, if out in muddy or damp weather, or snow, or if you are compelled to stand or work in water during the day, wash off the boots clean at night, warming them by the fire while wet, and rub in the castor oil, a teaspoonful at least to each boot, and there will be no shrinkage, nor hard boots to get on in the morning. Do this twice to thrice a week all winter, as the snow or mud demands.

*Remarks.*—I have condensed this from a report of one Delos Wood, address not given, to the *Indiana Farmer*, retaining all that is essential to understand it. He says, "I have stood in mud and water 2 or 3 inches deep, for 10 hours a day for a week, without feeling any dampness or having any difficulty in getting my boots on or off, by this heating every night." He had previously tried one of the water proof receipts containing rosin, tallow, etc., but found this the best plan. I will, however, give one of this kind, that any one may suit himself as to plans. The compounds containing rosin, however, must have a tendency to harden the leather, but kerosene, as mentioned below, is now said to soften them as soft as when new, so suit yourselves as to which shall be used. The oil dressing and blacking for leather, carriage tops, etc., below, must, from the nature of its ingredients, prove a good dressing for boots; but if I was making it expressly for boots, I'd leave out the Prussian blue. Neat's foot-oil, and castor oil are both very softening for all kinds of leather. Still, it is considered that rosin, and Burgundy pitch both have a tendency to harden leather; but, as seen below, it has recently been discovered that kerosene will soften old boots equal to new.

**Boots—Water-Proofing for.**—D. S. Root, of Grand Rapids, Mich., a traveling man, whom I met at Eaton Rapids, after learning that I was the author of the Receipt Books bearing my name, and that I am preparing my Third and Last, desired to give me the following receipt, hoping it might thereby do others as much good as it had him when tramping in snow and wet:

I. "Linseed oil, 1 pt.; spirits of turpentine, ¼ pt.; beeswax and Burgundy pitch, each, 4 ozs.; ivory black, ¼ oz. Make, or simply heat together over a slow fire."

*Remarks.*—He kept it with him in winter, and applied as needed. I should prefer neat's foot oil or castor oil, as they are not so drying in their nature as linseed.

II. Mutton tallow with twice as much beeswax, makes a valuable water-proofing for boots, and they will soon take blacking after its application. One-fourth as much Burgundy pitch as tallow, might be put in.

**Farmer Boy's Water-Proofing for Boots.**—"Farmer Boy," of Buchanan, Mich., gave one of the papers the following water-proofing for boots, which will be found good. He says: "Melt together beef tallow, 4 ozs.; rosin and beeswax, each, 1 oz., and when nearly cooled add as much neat's foot oil as the above mixture measures (6 ozs. will be near enough). It is to be applied with a soft rag, both to the soles and uppers. The leather should be warmed meanwhile before the fire, and the application well rubbed in. It requires two applications to make the leather thoroughly water-proof."

**Rubber Water-Proofing for Boots.**—Neat's-foot oil, 1 pt.; old rubber boots, 2 lb.; rosin, 1 oz. DIRECTIONS—Melt slowly, and then pour off from or take out the cloth of the old boots, and apply warm. The boots will be water and snow-proof.—"*C. E. G.*" *in Scientific American.*

**Jettine, or Liquid Shoe Blacking—Water-Proof, and Does Not Soil Ladies' White Dresses.**—Alcohol, 1 qt.; gum shellac, ½ lb.; camphor gum, size of a hen's egg; lamp black, 1 oz. DIRECTIONS—Break up the shellac finely and put into a bottle with the alcohol, keeping in a warm place and shaking a dozen times daily till dissolved; then break up the gum camphor and put in, and when dissolved add the lamp black, when it is ready for use. Apply with a sponge fastened with wire to the cork. The camphor prevents the cracking of the varnish. It may be applied to anything requiring a black finish.

**Boots and Shoes, Jet Polish for.**—Nice clear glue, ¼ lb.; logwood chips, ½ lb.; powdered indigo, isinglass and soft soap, each, 2 tea-spoonfuls; best cider vinegar, 1 qt.; soft water, 1 pt. DIRECTIONS—Put all together and boil 10 minutes, after it begins to boil. When cool, strain. Remove all dirt from the boots or shoes and apply with sponge or swab.

**Boots, Hard, to Soften.**—The latest discovery as to the uses of kerosene is that it softens boots or shoes which have become hard from water-soaking, making them as pliable as new; but they should then have a coat or two of one of the castor oil or Neat's-foot oil dressings to prevent a like condition again. If you doubt it, try it on a piece of old leather, as I did first.

**Oil Dressing and Blacking for All Kinds of Leather, Carriage Tops, etc.**—For 1 gal., take Neat's-foot oil or fish oil (Neat's-foot is the best), 3 qts.; mutton tallow, 2 lbs.; castor oil, 1 pt.; ivory black, very fine, 1½ lbs.;

Prussian blue, ¼ ℔.; beeswax, ½ lb.; rosin, ¼ ℔.; Burgundy pitch, 1 oz. DIRECTIONS—Put all together in an iron kettle over the fire; boil and stir ½ an hour; then set off and let settle 15 minutes, and pour off, free of all sediment. When cold it is ready for use,

*Remarks.*—Valuable as a water-proof for boots and shoes, harness, carriage tops, etc. The dirt in all cases to be cleaned off or washed off and allowed to dry, as the case demands. For this recipe, and the one for "Excelsior Axle Grease," an old farmer friend of mine and myself joined, paid $1 for them to a man who lived near Ann Arbor and was selling them on the streets, and had been doing so for some time, the articles giving satisfaction  As the two seem to belong together, I will give the axle grease here,  He called it

**Allen's Excelsior Axle Grease.**—Castor oil and linseed oil, each, 1 qt.; tallow and rosin, each, 2 lbs.; beeswax, 1 lb.  DIRECTIONS—Heat all well together, stirring to incorporate, and stir till cool.

*Remarks.*—"If either of these are too hard," he said, "add a little Neat's foot oil; if too soft, a little more tallow." They will prove valuable.

**Boot, Shoe and Harness Edge Blacking, Cheap.**—Soft water, 1 pt.; alcohol, ½ pt.; tinct. muriate of iron and ex. of logwood, each, 2 ozs.; best blue nutgalls, 1½ ozs.  DIRECTIONS—Pulverize the galls and put into a bottle, adding the others; let it stand a few days, shaking several times daily, until the extract of logwood is dissolved, when it is ready for use and will give great satisfaction.

*Remarks.*—It has been customary to use all alcohol, but a shoemaker, considering the use of all water in inks, concluded, and proved by test, that for summer, water is just as good; and for winter the above amount of alcohol is sufficient.

**Rubber Boots, To Mend.**—In a recent *Blade* a request was made for the publication of a recipe to mend rubber boots and shoes, to which they gave the following: "Cut 1 lb. of caoutchouc into thin, small slices; heat in a suitable vessel over a moderate coal fire, until the caoutchouc becomes fluid; then add ½ lb. of powdered rosin, and melt both materials at a moderate heat. When these are perfectly fluid, gradually add 3 or 4 lbs. spirits of turpentine in small portions, and stir well. By the addition of the last, the rapid thickening and hardening of the compound will be prevented, and a mixture obtained fully answering the purpose of gluing together rubber surfaces, etc.

*Remarks.*—A coal fire is called for merely to avoid the blaze of a wood fire, which is liable to set the turpentine on fire while pouring in. Avoid a blaze, and let there be only a moderate fire, makes it safe with wood. Over a stove will be most safe. One-fourth or ¼ the amount can be made as well, keeping the same proportions; and, if I was making it, I should put all together in the vessel, as there would be less danger of burning the caoutchouc. Keep covered when not in use, to prevent its drying up. The rosin makes it very tenacious.

**Tanning Skins with the Hair or Wool On.**—Alum, 3 lbs.; rock salt (good hard salt will do), ¼ lb.  DIRECTIONS — Soak the skin in water for one day; then remove all the meat, fat, etc. Dissolve, by boiling, the alum and salt in sufficient water to cover the skin—this amount for a deer, dog, wolf, or sheep skin—pour into a tub, and when only lukewarm, put in the skin and let it soak for 4 days, working it with a pounder or square-ended stick of wood every day; then dry in the shade—a warm shed is a good place to dry in. Then heat up the tan liquor again, and re-soak as before, after which wash out well and beat it with a wooden mallet till quite soft; dry again in the shade, rubbing it well from time to time with the hands. If this is properly done, you will have a very soft and pliable skin, suitable for any purpose for which such skins are used.—*Indian Domestic Economy.*

*Remarks.*—The following, which is somewhat different, I take from the Toronto *Globe*, as it suggests the plan of coloring or dyeing, making them equal to those on sale in the stores. It was given under the following head:

**To Make Mats from Sheepskins.**—"Take a fresh skin and wash the wool in strong soap-suds only slightly warm to the hand. Pick out all the dirt from the wool, and scrub it well on a washboard. A table-spoonful of kerosene added to 3 gallons of warm soap-suds will greatly help the cleaning. Wash in another suds, or until the wool looks white and clean. Then put the skin into cold water, enough to cover it, and dissolve ½ lb. of salt and the same quantity of alum in 3 pts. of boiling water; pour the mixture over the skin, and rinse it up and down in the water. Let it soak in this water 12 hours, then hang it over a fence or line to drain. When well drained stretch it on a board to dry, or nail it on the wall of the wood-house or barn, wool side toward the boards. When nearly dry, rub into the skin 1 oz. each of powdered alum and saltpeter (if the skin is large, double the quantity); rub this in for an hour or so. To do this readily, the skin must be taken down and spread on a flat surface. Fold the skin sides together and hang the mat away; rub it every day for 3 days, or till perfectly dry. Scrape off the skin with a stick or blunt knife till cleared of all impurities, then rub it with pumice-stone or rotten-stone. Trim it to a good shape, and you have an excellent mat. Dye it green, blue, or scarlet, and you have as elegant a mat as those bought in the stores. Lambskins may be prepared in the same way and made into caps and mittens. Dyed a handsome brown or black they are equal to the best imported skins. Still-born lambs, or those that die very young, furnish very soft skins, which, if properly prepared, would make as handsome sacques, muffs, and tippets as the far-famed Astrakhan. In dyeing these skins shallow vessels are used, which permit the skin to be placed in them wool-side down, so that the skin itself is not injured by the hot dye."

*Remarks.*—The coloring can be done with any of the recipes for coloring woolen goods, being careful that the skin itself is not allowed to touch the hot dye.

**1. RECIPES FOR BAKING POWDER.**—Tartaric acid, 1 oz.; cream of tartar, 10 ozs.; bicarbonate of soda, 5 ozs. Mix thoroughly. This is improved by the addition of 4 ozs. of flour.

**2.** Cream of tartar, 6 ozs.; bicarbonate of soda, 2⅔ ozs.; flour, 4½ ozs.

*Remarks.*—This receipt was procured from a chemist, and is a receipt for one of the best brands of baking powder sold by the trade.

# HOUSEHOLD MEMORANDA.

I once heard a prominent merchant say: "I have saved a good many dollars, and added a good deal to the comforts of life, by carefully preserving valuable receipts, that I have from time to time come across in the papers and from friends. I presume I have two or three hundred pasted and written in a scrap book, and would give $50 if I had them in book-form." Knowing the value of preserving valuable receipts, etc., I give here a few pages of blank leaves, that the patrons of this, my last book, may continue this subject of "Miscellaneous Receipts," and thus have in convenient form whatever they may deem worthy of preserving.

# HOUSEHOLD MEMORANDA.

## HOUSEHOLD MEMORANDA.

## HOUSEHOLD MEMORANDA.

# HOUSEHOLD MEMORANDA.

## HOUSEHOLD MEMORANDA.

## HOUSEHOLD MEMORANDA.

## HOUSEHOLD MEMORANDA.

# THE TOILET.

## BARBERS' AND DOMESTIC.

1. **HAIR DYE.—Black—Eley's Best.—I.** Pyrogalic acid, 1 dr.; distilled, pure rain-water, 6 oz.

II. Nitrate of silver, crystals, 2 drs.; strong aqua ammonia, 1 oz.; gum arabic, dissolved in a little water, 1 dr.; mix all.

DIRECTIONS.—First apply No I, and let it dry; then No. II, and let dry. And if by carelessness there are any spots on the face, take them off with No. I of the "Brown." Alcohol will take them off, but not as nicely as the sulphuret of the next dye.

2. **Hair Dye—Brown, or a Lighter Shade.—I.** Sulphuret of potash, 1 oz.; distilled or pure rain water, ½ pt.

II. Use the No. II of the "Black,"—in other words, the dyes are the same.

DIRECTIONS.—Apply No. I, the sulphuret, and let it dry; then apply No. II of the "Black" until you get a little darker shade than you desire; then re-apply the No. I, sulphuret, which leaves the desired shade by making it a little lighter than it was.

*Remarks.*—With care in this, you can make the beard or hair a very light brown, or quite a dark one; for if you get it darker than you wish, wash right off with the luster below. These dyes and the 1st luster below are from my friend C. S. Eley, a practical barber, and are very reliable; but it needs care and a little experience to work well with hair dyes.

1. **LUSTRAL OIL.—Hair Tonic, or Sea Foam—Eley's.—** Alcohol, 1 pt.; glycerine, 1 oz.; tinct. cantharides, 2 drs.; aqua ammonia, 1 oz.; rain water, 5 ozs.; mix. DIRECTIONS—Pour upon the head, or into the hand and apply to the head, rubbing well until the foam subsides. Apply more or less, freely at first, as the condition of the scalp demands. It dissolves the dandruff; is good for a sore scalp, chapped hands, etc. For sore scalp apply once daily; for chapped hands, night and morning. See remarks above as to its reliability. I keep it in the office, and have used it many times.

2. **Barbers' Luster, or Hair Tonic—Bowers'.—**Alcohol, 1 qt.; distilled or pure rain water, 1¼ pts.; glycerine, 1 oz.; aqua ammonia, ¾ oz., or just enough, when shaken together, to make it look milky or a little white. This receipt is from Henry Bowers, with whom I have shaved about 2 years. It is not quite as strong as Eley's, but cleans the scalp nicely. He has used it on my head with satisfaction.

1. **BOB HEATER'S SHAMPOO—Hair Tonic—Very Strong.** —First put oil of sweet almonds, 4 ozs., into alcohol, 1 pt., and put in oil of

bergamot, 2 drs., or 1 dr., with oil citronella, 1 dr., when it can be had; then add aqua ammonia, 4 ozs.; rye whiskey 8 ozs.; gum camphor, ½ oz.; mix. Shake before applying, and rub in thoroughly.

*Remarks.*—"Bob" Heater, a barber of Dresden, Ohio, where I married, and afterwards lived 14 yrs., obtained the first part of this receipt from a Mr. Squires, and put to it what we call the *addenda* or added portion, which makes it a strong and efficient tonic, to be used in cases where there is much falling out of the hair, or if considerable dandruff is present. He used it upon my own hair during the winter of '74, which myself, wife, and son spent in the "old home." It eradicated the dandruff and stopped the falling hair, and I still have an excellent head of hair at nearly 68 years of age, while at that time I thought it was all going. He had equal success with some others in a similar condition.

**1. HAIR OIL, OR DRESSING—Very Fine.**—Castor oil and cologne alcohol, each ½ pt.; oil of lemon-grass, 1 dr.; oil of bergamot, ½ dr.; mix.

*Remarks.* When in Detroit a year or two ago, a barber applied some oil to my hair, after asking, "some oil, sir?" and the perfume being superior to what my home barber used, I inquired its composition; and being referred to his druggist, the above was the result. I have never smelled a nicer perfume. Barbers often use 2 ozs. of castor oil to 1 oz. of alcohol, when they desire an oil to help keep the hair in position. Even 2 to 1, like this, it is not gummy or sticky. But for ladies to keep their hair crimped, see "Crimps in damp weather." The next has 2 to 1 of castor oil.

**2. Hair Dressing—Striking in its Perfume.**— Castor oil, 1 pt.; cologne alcohol, ½ pt.; oil of lavender (English is claimed to be the best), 2 drs.; oil of bergamot, 3 drs. oil of citronella, 4 drs.; mix.

**3. Hair Dressing that Turns Gray Hair to a Dark Shade, Without Lead—Cheap and Very Nice.**—Glycerine and rose-water, equal parts; say 1 or 2 ozs. each. Work well into the roots of the hair at each morning's dressing.

*Remarks.* It is remarkable what a change in the shade of gray hair will soon take place by the use of this simple, but very nice dressing. I speak from personal experience and knowledge.

**4. Hair and Hand Dressing—Home Made Perfume—Very Fine.**—Put rose petals (leaves of the flowers), or geranium leaves, or the flowers or leaves of any other perfume plants (the mignonette and heliotrope would be fine), that you desire into a bottle, pressing the bottle pretty full, then put in glycerine, all the bottle will hold; cork, or if a glass-stoppered bottle all the better. In 3 or 4 weeks the aroma (perfume) will all be extracted by the glycerine, when it may be stained or not, as you choose. Alcohol will do the same, but it is not equal to the glycerine. DIRECTIONS: Pour a few drops of this perfumed glycerine into a bowl of water, and wash the face, hands and hair. Bay rum or a little spirits of camphor, poured into the water for the same purpose is cleansing and fine. My wife always used spirits of camphor for these purposes, with entire satisfaction. Washing the scalp once or twice a

**week** with a weak solution of salt, in water, strengthens the hair follicles and skin, rubbing well in, after drying the hair with a brush as well as the ends of the fingers.

**SHAMPOO OR WASH—To Cleanse the Hair and Scalp.—** Salts of tartar, powdered borax, aqua ammonia, each 1 oz.; rain water, 1 qt.; mix. DIRECTIONS—Rub well into the roots of the hair once a week. Good for a tettered spot on any part of the body. Applying freely, (after using the hair dressing above) of glycerine and rose water.

A wash of sage tea and borax, say 1 or 2 ozs., powdered to 1 qt. of the tea, is claimed to cleanse the scalp, make the hair grow nicely and keep it soft.

**1. HAIR DRESSING WITH BAY RUM NICER THAN ALCOHOL.—**"Dr. Cap," of New London, Conn., gives "Angeline," of the *Detroit Free Press* Household, the following:

"Bay rum, imported, 6 ozs.; castor oil 2 ozs.; tinct. of cantharides, ½ oz. Perfume with anything you wish; will not only be good but harmless,"

*Remarks.*—Oil of bergamot, 1 dr., will give it a nice flavor, or oil of lemon-grass, or of heliotrope, 1 dr., would be "just splendid," as the girls say.

**1. HAIR RESTORATIVE — Which has Raised a Thick Head of Hair on a Bald Scalp.—**Notwithstanding there are those who claim it cannot be done, there are those also who claim it can. The following is claimed by a physician to have done it upon his own head. It will do no harm, and on some heads it will, no doubt, produce a head of hair "where the hair ought to grow," but does not, while in some cases it may not. It is owing to the condition of the hair follicles. If inflammation has destroyed them there is no hopes; while if the work is only in progress it will; so it is no harm to try it. It is:

"Castor oil and alcohol, each 2 ozs.; tinct. cantharides and rain water, each 1 oz.; oil of bergamot, 1 dr.; mix, and use with a stiff brush."

*Remarks.*—He does not say how often to apply. I should say twice a week; but I do not like a stiff brush, but rather the finger ends to rub it in thoroughly. If it excites any inflammation on the scalp use it only once a week. It will be noticed it is quite strong, so keep an eye to its action, so as not to inflame the scalp.

**2. Hair Wash or Restorative—Italian.—**I will give one more wash or dressing, easily made, and very satisfactory. I have used it. It is:

Syrup of rosemary, 2 qts.; liquid potassa, ½ oz.; aqua ammonia, 1 oz.; oil of sweet almonds, 2½ ozs.; castor oil, 1 oz.; good whiskey, 1½ pts.

*Remarks*—It looks a little milky at first, but soon clears up. Shake when used. This is good for dandruff and to clean the scalp.

**3. Hair Restorative—To Turn Gray Hair to a Dark Color —Said to be Hall & King's.—** Lac sulphur, sugar of lead, each 1 dr. muriate of soda (common salt), 2 drs.; glycerine 2 ozs.; bay rum, 8 ozs.; Jamaica rum. 4 ozs.; soft water. 1 pt. Shake well before using and keep in a dark place.

*Remarks.*—Preparations containing lead sometimes effects the muscles of the eye-lids causing them to droop. I think if only used once a week, even wetting the scalp will not do this; but if the hair only is moistened, it is all sufficient, not wetting the head or scalp, I believe it will change the hair to a dark color, even without the sugar of lead; then there would be no possible danger. I obtained this of my cousin, Dr. A. B. Mason.

**1. COLOGNE—Exceedingly Fine.**—Oils of bergamot and lemon, (oil of lemon-grass would be nicer), each 2 drs.; orange, 1 dr.; rosemary ½ dr.; neroli, ¾ dr.: essence ambergris and musk, each 4 drops; cologne alcohol, 1 pt, Shaken occasionally.

*Remarks.*—Cologne alcohol has been purified to remove all of the flavor of the corn spirits, and should always be used for all purposes where a fine perfume is desired, the difference in expense should be very trifling only. I could give more colognes, but if the oil of lemon-grass is used in this there can be none nicer. I will give a cheaper one which will be quite fine in flavor.

**2. Cologne—Cheap.**—Cologne alcohol, 1 pt.; oils of English lavender and bergamot, each 1½ drs.; oil of rosemary, ½ dr.; oil of cinnamon, 2 drops; essence of lemon, 1½ drs.; mix.

**1. PERFUME BAGS—To be Put in Among Clothing— Also a Preventive Against Moths.**—Cloves, nutmegs, mace, carraway seeds, cinnamon, and Tanguine leaves, each ½ oz.; Florentine orris root, 3 ozs. DIRECTIONS.—Have all ground to a fine powder, nicely mixed, and put up in small bags to place among clothing. It gives them a fine perfume which the moths protest against, and hence the clothing is saved from their destruction.

**1. BANDOLINE—For the Hair—As Used in India.**—Quince seed (which, in India, is called behdana), ½ oz.; essence of bitter almonds, or any perfuming oil, a few drops only; water 1 pt.; alcohol 3 ozs. DIRECTIONS. —Pour the water, hot, upon the behdana, and let stand over night; strain; put the essence of perfuming oil in the alcohol, and add; then bottle, and keep corked.

The ladies know that the miscellaneous properties of the behdana (quince seed) enables them to maintain any desired position of the hair, by first wetting with it and keeping the hair as desired until dry; but probably are not so well aware that the alcohol prevents it from spoiling by keeping it corked.

*Remarks.*—The word, bandoline, comes from the French word *bande* or *bandeau,* meaning a band or belt, because the hair has to be kept in position by a band of thin cloth, or better, a bit of old lace, to allow the air to come in contact with the hair until dry. When quince seed are not obtainable, the following makes a good substitute:

**2. Crimps in Damp Weather—To Keep in Place.**—A very good bandoline is made by the use of gum Arabic or gum tragacanth (the Arabic is most use while the tragacanth is the best), say ½ oz. powdered, pouring on just enough boiling water to dissolve it; then adding alcohol enough to make it rather thin, (about 1 oz.). Let stand open all night, then bottle for use. DIRECTIONS—Wet the bangs with this mixture at bed time, and twist or curl the bangs upon the forehead, as desired; then put over a bit of lace, or a gauze band (French *bandeau*), to keep it in position till dry, or rather, till morning; then remove the *bandeau*, and pull the crimps out with the fingers until they are soft and fluffy." It does not injure the hair, nor will the bandoline of quince seeds above. It will not come out, even in damp weather. If there is any gum on the hair, rub it off with the fingers, and if it looks dull, touch the fingers to a little of the glycerine and rose-water dressing above, and pass them lightly over the hair to give it a shiny appearance.

**Hair Curling Liquid.**—Salt of tartar (which is carbonate of potassa), ¼ oz., aqua ammonia and cologne, each, 1 dr.; glycerine, ¼ oz.; alcohol, 1 ½ ozs., distilled or pure soft water, 1 pt. If you wish it to have color, add ½ dr. of powdered cochineal. Shake daily for a week, and filter, or strain. DIRECTIONS—To use it, moisten the hair with it and adjust it loosely, as it dries it shows its tendency to curl; then run the fingers through it to lighten it up, as you desire.

**1. COSMETICS FOR THE FACE.**—For a very fine one, (see face wash), Mrs. Chase's following treatment of pimpled face, etc.: Put flake white, ½ oz., in bay rum and water, each 2 ozs., and applied after shaking, to the face, with a piece of soft flannel, and when dry, wiped or rubbed off where too much white shows, is excellent. But I have much faith in the old lady's only cosmetic, given next below:

**2. An Old Lady's Only Cosmetic.**—"The only cosmetic I have used," said an old lady, "is a flannel wash-cloth. For forty years I have bathed my face every night and morning with clear water as hot as I can bear it, using for the purpose a small square of flannel, renewed as often as it grows thick and felt-like. My mother taught me to do this, as her mother had done before her. No soap nor powder, nor glycerine even, has touched my face, and this is what my skin is at 60," she finished, touching with pardonable pride a cheek whose peachy bloom and fine soft texture gave effective emphasis to the recipe. —*Harper's Bazar.*

*Remarks.*—This bathing of the face and neck with the hot water every night and morning, with a good rubbing with the flannel, certainly brings the blood to the surface, and what is there so nice as the beautiful carnation of a lady's cheek and lips, who has never spoiled God's beautiful arrangement for this beauty with pinky powders, or the swarthy liquids, in her attempt to outdo nature's handiwork. The pale and sickly may be excused for trying to imitate it, but the healthy and naturally beautiful, cannot be excused in their attempts to beat it. It cannot be done, no matter how skillfully it may be tried.

**Hair to Bleach, or Color a Blonde.**—"A. L. B." of Paragon, Ind., says to the *Blade:* Please give a recipe for coloring the hair a blonde. I have tried a good many things and have not succeeded; to which they gave the following: Mix in 10 ozs. of distilled water (pure rain water will do; but druggists keep distilled water, and it costs but little), acetate of iron and nitrate of silver, each 1 oz., with nitrate of bismuth, 2 ozs. Moisten the hair with this mixture and, 1 hour after, touch it with a mixture of equal parts of sulphide of potassium and distilled water.

*Remarks.*—From my knowledge of the nature of the articles, I haven't a doubt of its success; but not wishing to change my white locks to a beautiful blonde, I have not tried it. To give the hair a glossiness after its use, apply some of the dressings before mentioned.

**1. POMADE—For the Hair, Lips, Chapped Hands, etc.—Oil** of sweet almonds, 4 ozs.; spermaceti, 1 oz.; oil of lemon-grass, or oil of neroli (which is oil of orange flowers), ½ dr. DIRECTIONS—Use sufficient heat to melt the spermaceti in the oil of almonds, and when cool stir in the perfuming oil, and put into a large mouthed bottle, to reach it with the finger. Of course, all flavored, or perfumed, or alcoholic mixtures, should be kept corked.

**2. Pomade, Very Fine.**—White wax, 1½ ozs.; pure glycerine, 2 fl. ozs.; castor oil, 12 fl. ozs.; oil of lemon (I would say lemon-grass), 5 drops; oil of bergamot, 2 drops; oil of lavender, 1 drop; oil of cloves, 10 drops; annatto, 10 grs.; alcohol and water as below. DIRECTIONS—Dissolve the wax in ¼ of the castor oil, with as little heat as possible, then titurate, or rub in the balance of the castor oil and glycerine, and stir till cool, and add the perfuming oils. Rub the annatto in 1 dr. (tea-spoonful) of water until smoothly mixed, then add the same amount of alcohol to it, and stir it into the pomade. Do not use too much heat, and use the bandest (nicest) castor oil.—*American Journal of Pharmacy.*

*Remarks.*—This makes a very fine pomade. The annatto is only to give it color. The same amount of cochineal would give it a reddish shade, instead of a yellowish, with the annatto. Tumeric would give a yellowish shade, and carmine a carnation, all fine in themselves, to choose from. But it is just as good without either.

**1. DEPILATORY—To Remove Superfluous Hair, Boudets, or the Best French.**—Crystallized sulphide of sodium, 3 drs.; quick (unslacked) lime, 10 drs.; starch, 11 drs. DIRECTIONS—Reduce each, separately, to a fine powder. Mix and keep in well stoppered bottles. When to be used, moisten to a paste, with a little water, spread on the part to be denuded (from the Latin *de*, and *nudare*, to make naked), and leave on only 2 to 4 minutes. Lift it off with a dull knife, which fetches the hair with it.—*Druggists' Circular.*

**2. Depilatory, Our Own Druggist's.**—Powdered, unslacked lime, 8 drs.; carbonate of potash (which is salts of tartar), and sulphuret of potassium, each 1 dr. Mix and keep dry, as the first above. DIRECTIONS—Mix only to cover a small space at a time, leaving on only 5 to 10 minutes; then scrape off, which fetches the hair.

*Remarks.*—I have had this prepared and sent to various persons, on their application to me for such a preparation. I tell all, however, better let the hair grow, than to try to destroy the follicles, as this would require to keep on the mixture till it would make a sore, equal to a bad burn. If in any case this is done by accident, or to destroy the hair follicles, treat the sore the same as a burn.

**3. Superfluous Hair, To Destroy.**—Under this head some writer gives the following, which is so near like what I have proposed for others, I will copy it, as he has a plan of washing off with vinegar, which would be good if either of the above depilatories (this is a depilatory) are used: "Take fresh stone lime, 1 oz.; pure potash, 1 dr.; sulphuret of arsenic, 1 dr. DIRECTIONS—Reduce them to a fine powder in an earthen or glass mortar, and add enough soft water to make a thin paste. Then wash the hair in warm water, and apply the paste, by rubbing gently a little on the spot where you wish to remove the hair. As soon as the skin is much reddened, wash it off with strong vinegar. Do not let it remain on more than 3 to 5 minutes. Wash the place with a flannel cloth, and the hair will be removed. The skin will be softened and improved in appearance.

*Remarks.*—This, of course, can be kept in the dry powder in closely stoppered bottles, as well as the others, but wet up only as much as you need to put on at a time, It should be put on as thick as a case-knife blade, either of them.

**Camphor Ice, for Rough Face, Lips, Chapped Hands, etc.**—Benzoated suet, ½ lb.; white wax, 2 ozs.; powdered camphor, 1 oz.; English oil lavender, 1 dr. DIRECTIONS—To make the benzoated suet, it is rendered and strained and 2 drs. of powdered benzoin, or benzoic acid, stirred in; the wax is melted in it by gentle heat; the camphor gum has to be powdered by putting a few drops of alcohol upon it (best let the druggist do this), then stirred into the wax and suet mixture, and when quite cool, the lavender added, and poured into boxes or large mouthed bottles. Apply as often as needed to keep soft.

*Remarks.*—I think vaseline, as now kept by druggists, equal, if not better, than the suet (lamb suet is used).

**1. Bay Rum, Barbers'.**—Magnesia and powdered borax, each, 30 grs.; oil of bay, ½ to 1 dr., alcohol, 2 ozs.; dilute alcohol, 1 qt. DIRECTIONS—First, rub the magnesia, borax, and oil of bay in the 2 ozs. of strong alcohol, in a mortar; then put into a filter and gradually pour on the dilute alcohol to percolate through the magnesia.—*Mt. Vernon (O.) Barber.*

*Remarks.*—The more oil of bay the more it is like bay rum, It will prove very satisfactory for the hair or to use about the person when sick, by washing with a sponge and putting on the handkerchief, the same as cologne may be used, then passing over the face, smelling, etc. It is a grateful relief to the sick, thus used as freely as they desire.

**Wash for Ladies' Hands.**—This very appropriately comes in here, as it is really a toilet wash. Put powdered borax, 5 ozs., into a bottle with water, 1 pt. If this all dissolves, put in enough to always keep some borax, undissolved, at the bottom. When the garden work is done for the day, put enough into the water in which the hands are to be washed to make it soft or slippery as suds. "It is very cleansing," says Prof. Beal, of the Michigan Agricultural College, Lansing, "and by this use of it the hands will be kept in excellent condition, smooth and soft and white." Of course, a little of this in water to wash the head will cleanse the scalp as nicely as the hands.

**Wash for the Hands When Roughened by Cold or Labor.**— Wash the hands in vinegar in which a handful of Indian meal is put, rubbing thoroughly, then wash off and apply some of the hair dressing, made of equal parts of glycerine and rose water, which will soften and heal them, and be found· very grateful to their irritated, or even chapped condition, in the cold wintry winds.

2. Wheat bran, in the water, is also considered excellent, so is oatmeal also good for the same purpose, but the following, perhaps, is a better way to use the last.

3. **Oatmeal Soap to Keep the Hands Soft in Winter.**—Take the white castile soap (the white is the mildest), ¼ lb., and melt it with very gentle heat, in sweet almond oil, 1 oz.; then remove from the fire and stir in oatmeal. 1½ ozs.

*Remarks.*—"Rosemary" says this is the only soap ladies should use in the winter; I will add if 1 dr. of Rosemary's oil were put in, it would make them think of her peculiar flavor, every time they used the soap.

1. **DANDRUFF—To Remove.**—Cleanse the scalp thoroughly. Take as much boracic acid as you can dissolve in a cup or pint of water, and apply the solution 3 times a day.

*Remarks.*—There is nothing better than the white of an egg, well beaten, to cleanse the scalp.

2. Mr. E. Wilson recommends the following wash for dandruff: Take of caustic potash, in solution, 2 drs.; rose water, 8 ozs. Mix, and apply.

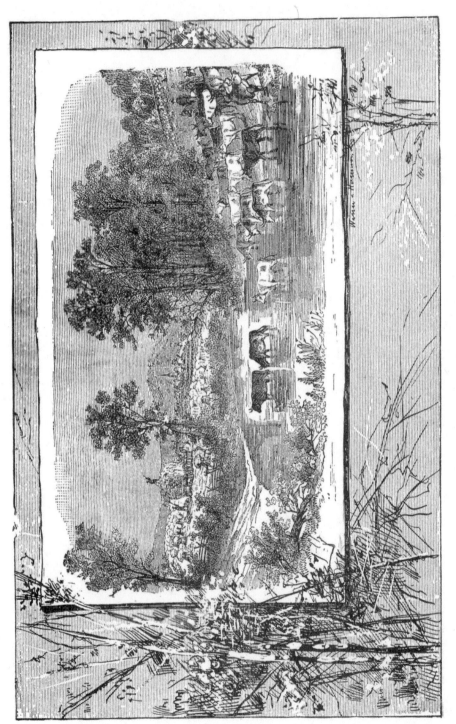

A MODERN DAIRY SCENE.

# RECIPES FOR THE DAIRY.

## BUTTER.

**BUTTER MAKING—A** "New Departure," or New Discovery in Setting Milk, Claimed to be of Swedish Origin but really a Yankee Invention.—The Rev. Dr. Prime published in the New York *Observer* what he understood to be, and consequently gave, as a recent Swedish discovery. He said:

"A discovery has recently been made by M. Swartz, which promises to be most important to the dairy farmer. In the ordinary method of cream-setting, the milk is placed in very shallow pans, and stands for 24 hours or more while the cream is rising. The milk, during that time usually turns sour, and the cream becomes contaminated with free fatty-acids, with partially decomposed albuminous bodies, and with other products injurious to the flavor or keeping qualities of the butter. In Swartz's plan the milk, as soon as it reaches the dairy, is placed in deep metal pails standing in a vessel full of ice. Not only does the low temperature reduce the process of change to a minimum, but, quite unexpectedly, it also greatly facilitates the rising of the cream; so that in pails having sixteen inches depth of milk, the cream is nearly all obtained in twelve hours. The butter churned from the product is not only pure in flavor, but has remarkable keeping qualities. The plan is spreading rapidly."

To the above I give the following explanation by a gentlemen signing himself Ivenans, which shows that if the discovery was not actually made by Mr. Starr, of Litchfield, Conn., it had been used by him three or four years, at least, before it was made public in Sweden. This writer and traveler says:

"I find the above in a newspaper of Paris, France, showing that the discovery is considered to be something new and wonderful. Some three or four years ago I wrote a notice, which was published in the New York *Observer*, of the splendid dairy of my friend, Mr. Starr, at Litchfield, Connecticut. In that notice I stated distinctly, with great particularity, Mr. Starr's method of *setting* his milk for cream; not in shallow pans, as the women of old were wont to do, but in narrow vessels about twenty inches deep, standing in ice-cold water, or a very cold place. This is the identical process now boasted of as the new discovery in Sweden, and spreading rapidly. It is a Yankee invention, and, how long it has been in use I do not know. But they are smart in Sweden, as I know from observation, and will make use of every good invention or valuable discovery in butter making or anything else."

*Remarks.* There are those who claim that to heat the milk after straining into the pans, by setting upon the stove until the film upon the top of the milk begins to wrinkle will cause the cream to rise quicker and better than without the scalding, which experience will soon determine; but I am well satisfied that those who are situated so they can have cold spring water to run through their milk house, by which they can reduce the temperature of the milk quickly; or those who are near large streams of water or lakes, so that they can cheaply supply

641

themselves with ice for the same purpose, will find the cooling process not only the best but a very necessary plan to pursue, if they wish to make the most out of their opportunities.

**Butter—Gilt-Edged—How to Make.**—At an exhibition of the Chester County Agricultural Society, Pa., Isaac Acker received the first prize on butter making, managing as follows:

He feeds 10 qts. of corn meal and bran (mixed half and half, no doubt) to each cow per day, with hay, but does not think that corn fodder makes good butter. The temperature of the cream at churning was fifty-seven degrees, and it was churned from 12 to 20 minutes. Use 6 ozs. of salt and 3 ozs. of white sugar to 20 lbs. of butter.

**Butter Churning, or "Getting on Time."**—There are many people who complain that "butter will not come." To such I would say that "Aunt Ellen," of Oxford, Pa., has found a remedy, given through the *Blade*. She says:

"I have had a similar experience, and found the remedy by appealing to my sisters through the press. There came many replies, but I tried the advice of but one, and have never since had any difficulty about getting the butter on time. My adviser said never to let the milk stand longer than 24 hours, or 36 at most, before skimming. That plan I have followed letting the night's milk stand 36 hours, and the mornings milk 24 hours. Most butter makers claim that the quality of the butter is better than if the milk is allowed to stand a longer time. In cold weather, I think the temperature of the cream, when churned, will bear to be higher than in summer. Sixty-six degrees is about right."

**Butter Coloring From Ten Years Experience.**—Upon the subject of artificial coloring for butter, I will give you the experience of Mrs. "S. E. H.," of Circleville, O., also given in the *Blade*. Her remarks are as follows:

In answer to an inquiry how to color butter, I would say that I have used *annatto* for ten years, and find that it gives entire satisfaction. I buy it by the ounce. Take a lump about the size of a hickory nut and dissolve it in a cup of water. This will do several churnings. When you have the cream in the churn, stir up and add one tablespoonful, which will color 5 lbs. I expect to catch a "blowing up" from some of the sisters, but we cannot make yellow butter in the winter without it. If you make good, sweet butter the *annatto* will not injure, but improves the taste, for if an article doesn't look good and appetizing, what is it good for? I am a farmer's wife, but I have good bread and butter the year around, and sell an average of 10 lbs. of butter a week, receiving the highest market price."

*Remarks.*—I can hardly understand why there should be any objection to the use of *annatto*. I know that my mother used it for coloring cheese when, from any cause, she thought the cheese would look better with it. Webster says it is "a species of red, or yellowish-red dyeing material, prepared from the seeds of a tree (Bixa orellana) belonging to the tropical regions of America. It is used for coloring cheese and butter." So whatever fault there is in its use must be charged to Webster. But I agree fully with the Circleville lady's opinion, that the *annatto* will not injure the butter nor those who use it, although for home consumption it need not be colored, but for what is to be sold, will sell better, *i. e.*, it will bring a higher price, and will give better satisfaction to the consumer, if it is properly colored; then, as it will not injure, why should it not be used, especially in winter? But I would recommend those who do color their butter, to use the annatto, preparing it themselves, as above, for you know not what the preparations may contain which are offered for sale, for this purpose, the annatto alone is all that is necessary; and in winter, I do think it is necessary.

But there may be some persons who will prefer the following plan of coloring with carrots, such can take their choice. I take the item from the *Germantown Telegraph*, in which it seems to have first been published, quite a number of years ago, by which means the *Telegraph* thinks the "Farmer's Wife" obtained it, reporting, or republishing, through the *Western Rural*, from which the *Telegraph* takes it up again, and endorses, and tells how it came by it, at the first. With this explanation, and the addition of my own endorsement, I will let the *Telegraph* tell its own story. Have no fears in trying either the annatto or the carrots, as your convenience of obtaining the one or the other may demand. It says under the head of coloring butter:

We notice in the *Western Rural* a brief communication from a "Farmer's Wife," describing her mode of coloring butter, which does not at all injure, but adds to the flavor of the butter, It is simply using the juice of the orange carrot, as follows: "For about 3 gals. of cream take 6 or more good sized carrots, wash them and grate them on a coarse grater; when grated pour on boiling water, which will extract the color. Put the cream into the churn; strain the carrot juice through coarse muslin into the cream, and churn. Should the cream be warm enough, the carrot juice must be cool before using. Aside from the coloring the carrots give the butter a sweet taste, similar to grass butter."

This is the statement, and we wish to add our endorsement to its correctness in every respect. Some 15 years ago a neighbor asked us to buy her butter, and after trying it, and finding it unusually good, we engaged all she had to spare. Although it was in the midst of winter when we commenced to take it, we found it not only to be equal to grass butter, but to be similar to it in taste, and we decided that it was equally as delicious. Being unable to discover the secret of its excellence, we called upon our neighbor for information. She smiled and said it was the way she always made butter in winter, as did her mother and grandmother; and then went on to describe the way it was done, which was exactly in accordance with that of the "Farmer's Wife" aforesaid—that is to say, grated orange carrot, boiling water, straining it out, pouring into the churn, etc. We published the recipe at the time, which was republished in a number of other papers, and it is quite probable that this was the source whence the "Farmer's Wife" derived her information.

Now this recipe is easy enough for any one to adopt. It is as plain as to make a cup of tea, and is equal to any so-called "gilt-edged butter" that was ever made in the absence of pasturage. From this it will be seen that there is no excuse for making the poor butter in winter that we see so much of. The only expense is a few carrots at a churning, and a few minutes of labor, which are overcome a half score of times by the increased price of the butter sold.

**Butter Making, Good in Winter.**—As there are a good many persons who think they can not make good butter in winter because the yellow color of summer is not imparted to that made in the winter, and hence that it is not of so good a quality. But, to such persons, the above will enable them to give their butter the proper color, and the following from an old butter maker, S. F. Adams, will, no doubt, be found very interesting, because practical and certainly, satisfactory. To the inquiry of the editor of the *Farmer*, he makes the following full and very instructive answer:

"At your request, I herewith give you our method of making butter in winter. We keep 10 cows, part of them are natives, and part are Jerseys. The feed is nice, early-cut hay, given twice a day, regularly; I water them immediately after eating, when they will usually drink. Feed cornmeal, wheat bran, 1 qt. each, scalded, adding 2 qts. of sweet skimmed milk, to each cow, twice a day. Bed freely with sawdust and leaves. Give them all the salt they wish. We always milk before feeding them, and always clean the stable before sitting down to milk. We strain the milk through a cloth, then heat it to a temperature of 130°, then set in small pans, in which it never stands over 36 hours, before skimming. The cream is kept in as cool a place as possible, without freezing. The room we keep the milk in has an even temperature by using a soap-stone stove. The milk is set on circular racks attached to upright posts, 6 inches by 6, and 8 feet long, slats nailed across 8 inches apart; a pivot in each post allows the racks to swing around convenient for skimming or removing the milk. The racks made thus will hold 64 pans. I skim twice a day, and churn twice a week; the cream stands 12 hours after the last skimming, to ripen, before we churn it. It is warmed by sweet, skimmed milk in the churn, temperature 62°. The butter is washed in 3 waters, then weighed, allowing ½ oz. of salt to a pound of butter. I use the best salt I can find in Boston. I use no tray, do not like them, but use a butter-box with tight cover, instead. I want my butter, after it has been salted, kept air-tight till lumped, then sent air-tight to market. The hand is not allowed to touch it at all. We use a butter-worker; would not make butter a week without one. The butter is put in square, pound lumps, stamped, and sent twice a week to Boston. Farmers who make a business of selling milk, do it the year round. Why should not butter makers do the same? Some may say, 'I can find no market for it,' but if they will make a nice article, they can find a market. Why is it that seven-eighths of the butter that is sent to market sells for only about 30 cents, when, if made as it ought to be, it would bring about 40 cents, or more? Butter making, like other work, is a trade, and how many dairymen have yet to learn the trade? If a few men and a few women can make good butter and get a good price for it, why can not a large number do it, other things being equal? I hear some one say, 'It is too hard work for the women; let the men do it.' A man can make as good butter as a woman if he tries, and he should do it when there is a large amount to be made."

*Remarks.*—If dairymen or farmers who wish to make good butter in winter will follow the instructions of this old butter maker, I have not the slightest doubt but what they will succeed; but I wish to call especial attention to the importance of sending to market twice a week, for it matters not what pains may be taken to keep butter from becoming rancid, it never tastes so fresh and nice as when just made. I speak, as it were, from a double experience upon this point, *i. e.*, by dealing in it and in eating it. I say, therefore, both in summer and winter, what butter is to be sold, send it to market as soon as made, if you wish to obtain the best prices.

**Butter Not to be Gathered in the Churn, Nor Washed in Water, but Brine.**—At a meeting of the Ohio Dairyman's Association, Mr. Hawley, of Syracuse, N. Y., said: "Butter should not be gathered in the churn, nor should it be washed with water, but with brine. If the butter is gathered in the churn it is spoiled by breaking and tearing down the grain and making it salvy, whereas it should stand in the grain like particles of steel. Brine will dissolve or cut the skins of the pellicles, and they will then be washed out with the buttermilk, instead of being left to putrefy and spoil the aroma of the butter.

**Butter Not to be Worked Too Fast Nor Too Much.—**The *Journal of Chemistry,* in relation to the working of butter, says: "Do not work butter too much nor too fast. Work slowly until all salt is thoroughly and evenly absorbed. Otherwise the butter will not be of uniform color. Working it too fast will destroy the grain, and the butter becomes salvy and lard-like in the texture. Let it stand or put it away in the tray for 24 hours. Then work it enough to remove all the buttermilk or surplus brine, so that the butter may become dry or like a piece of cheese. Mold into rolls and set them away for 24 hours, or until they become hard and firm. The cloth should now be put on, so as to cover one end, while the other is left open for the stamp. The cloth should be cut in pieces of exact size and dipped in brine and the butter rolled when the cloth is dripping wet. Butter should never come in contact with the bare hand. When in bulk it can be easily handled with a ladle and flat paddle."

**To Make Butter Firm and Solid in Hot Weather.—**An exchange gives information concerning a method in practice among the best English butter-makers for rendering butter firm and solid during hot weather: Carbonate of soda, 1 tea-spoonful; powdered alum, 1 tea-spoonful, are mixed, and at the time of churning put into such a quantity of cream as will make about 20 lbs. of butter. The effect of this powder is to cause the butter to become firm and solid and sweet flavored. Its action is upon the cream and passes off with the buttermilk. The ingredients of the powder should not be mixed until the time when it is used.—*Harper's Weekly.*

**Prize Butter, First and Second—How They Were Made.—** Charles S. Sargent, of Brookline, who took the first prize at a recent fair at Greenfield, Conn., reported his plan as follows: "The accompanying sample of butter is made from a small herd of registered Jersey cows. The cows are fed 1 qt. Indian meal, 2 qts. shorts, ¼ bus. carrots and about 10 lbs. English hay each per day. The milk, which is set in shallow pans, stands 24 hours before being skimmed, the temperature of the milk being as near 62° Fahrenheit as it is possible to keep it. In working this butter two rules are observed: 1. No water is ever allowed to touch it; 2. The hands of the operators are never allowed to touch it, wooden paddles being used to work it with. It is salted with the best quality of table salt and is not colored. It sells at the present time at $1 per lb." The Farmington (Ct.) Creamery Company, which took the second premium, explains as follows: "This butter was made from the milk of four imported Guernsey cows, which were fed on hay, sweet corn stalks and 2 or 3 qts. daily of bran. It was made at the Farmington Creamery, and set 24 hours in water in deep coolers. The cream stood 24 hours before churning. The butter was salted at the rate of ¾ oz. of salt to the pound.

*Remarks.*—You see the importance of not washing the butter with water, but with brine; and also that it must not be handled with the hands, but paddles or spatulas only.

**Butter to Keep During Hot Weather.—**Butter to be kept into hot weather ought to be packed in jars, pressed in firmly, and a pickle made by using common salt, 2 lbs.; saltpeter, ½ oz.; lump sugar, 2 ozs. to each qt of

not water needed. Pour the hot water upon the salt, etc., and stir until dissolved, and let stand till cold; then pour over the butter, at least 2 inches in
depth, it will keep it nicely. New ash or oak firkins will do, but are not as good
as stone jars.

II. A new flower-pot, washed clean, and wrapped with 2 or 3 thicknesses
of wet cloth, is said, by turning it over a dish of butter, to keep it as hard as if
placed in an ice-box. The same with a dish of milk. The cloth must be kept
wet.

**Creamery, the Management and Advantage of in Butter-
Making.**—The management of a small creamery differs in no respect from
that of a well-appointed private dairy. The only respect in which a creamery
is different from a dairy is that it does the work of several dairies, and in doing
this work it greatly reduces the cost of making the butter. If we follow up
the season's work of a small creamery of, let us say, 200 cows, we shall find
that one person, with the partial help of another, will be able to do all the work
for this number of cows, which would probably be otherwise done in 20 separate dairies. The advantage is obvious. In place of 20 sets of pans, the use
of 20 milk-rooms, 20 churns and 20 pairs of hands in cleansing milk-pans and
other utensils, there is but one, and the labor and time of 18 or 19 persons are
saved. Besides, the product is all alike, of even quality, packed similarly and
marketed through one agent; so that all through the work there is saving of
labor and economy of expense. This, of course, reduces the cost of making
the butter to the least possible amount, and at the same time raises the income
to the highest possible point. Instead of all the butter from these 20 small
small dairies being sold at a village grocery, and put up in the old-fashioned
rolls, and being disposed of in trade, as was formerly the custom, at a very low
price, the aggregate product is sent off at short intervals, and while fresh, in
refrigerator cars, and along with the product of other creameries packed in a
similar manner in the same kind of packages, and reaches the market in such a
condition as to realize the highest price. This is an advantage which is equal
in value to the saving of the cost, so that the patron of a creamery enjoys the
double benefit of the lessened cost and the increased value. If dairymen lived
before, it is not surprising that they can make money now, under these considerable advantages.—*N. Y. Times.*

**Milking Shed—Care and Kind of Milk-Pails, etc.**—For summer
dairying an open shed in which the cows can be tied and given a few mouthfuls
of fresh green fodder after they are milked, and which should be cleanly
scraped after each milking, is a very great advantage, which can also be utilized in winter for sheep or other stock. Then the milk can be drawn free from
dust and dirt "flicked" by the switching of the cows' tails; as will happen
with cows loose in a barn-yard. Moreover, the milk-pails should be of tin and
not of wood. An old wooden milk-pail can not be made clean by dint of any
amount of scouring. Nor should the milk-pail be used for any other purpose,
but, as soon as the milk is strained, the pail should be washed with cold water,
scalded and turned bottom upward upon a bench or on a stand.

# CHEESE.

**HOME-MADE AND FANCY FACTORY — MADE FOR SHIPPING.—I. Home-made.**—Even those keeping only 5 or 6 cows will find it very convenient to know how to make good home-made cheese after the butter season is over; and as I always draw upon those who do "know how" for points upon which I have not personal experience, I will first give an item from an experienced man, L. B. Arnold, as given in the N. Y. *Tribune,* upon this subject; then a shorter explanation obtained from a cousin of mine, David Sanders, of Strykersville, N. Y., who used to keep about 12 to 20 cows, and for several years made his own cheese at home, and sold it to the village retailers around him, whose demand, you will see in his statements, he could never fully supply, for the reason, I will add (for I have many times eaten of his cheese), that his cheese was better than that made by others around him, for the home market. Mr. Arnold says:

"As rennet is the principal agent in making cheese, that should be provided first. If rennet extract can be obtained, that will be the best, because it is always pure and sweet, and uniform in strength, and comes with directions for using. But if it cannot be had, rennet may be prepared by steeping a good clean and sweet rennet in a weak brine at least two days in advance, and giving it a half dozen or so good rubbings before using. The next thing will be a tub large enough to hold two milkings of the dairy, with a little room to spare; for 4 or 5 cows a new wash-tub will do. It should be accompanied with a perforated division board about 10 inches wide, and just long enough to set down in the middle of the tub with a good fit; also a half-round perforated board just the size of one-half of the bottom of the tub, with the round part beveled to an edge on one side, both one-half inch thick. The tub should also have 2 spiggots, or faucets, at the bottom and placed on opposite sides.

"A thermometer will be wanted. Some convenience for heating one mess of milk so it will not get scorched must be devised. For a few cows this may be done on the kitchen stove or range, with a tin pan large enough to hold the mess to be heated set in, or over, a pan or kettle containing water, or by some similar means. Then something must be provided for cutting the curd. If but little cheese is to be made, a carving knife or a thin spatula with sharp edges will do. If much is to be made, it will pay to get a five-bladed curd-knife. There must also be provided hoops of the right size, form, and number, which may be of wood or tin, with wooden followers and cloths for pressing, and a press sufficient to give a pressure of 15 or 20 hundred weight. Lastly, a place to cure the cheese without much variation from seventy degrees, and where it will not be very damp or very dry. Exclusive of a place to set the milk and cure the cheese, the whole apparatus for making cheese from three to six cows need not cost more than $10.

"With this preparation we are ready to begin. I assume that the milk is furnished by the hand of the dairymaid clean and sweet. When the night's milk comes in, it will be strained into pans and set away where it will keep cool and sweet through the night. In the morning the cream should be dipped off and the milk emptied into the tub. The morning's milk will be heated, not

647

enough to warm the night's mess, from 90 to 94 degrees. Our grand-dames warmed the night's milk, but we prefer to warm the new milk. The new milk will be improved by heating, the night's milk will not. It would facilitate the work to heat the cold milk, but a good cheese is preferable to one quickly made. The cream should be put into a clean strainer, and after the hot and cold milk have been mixed, the cream may be washed through the strainer by pouring warm milk upon it; and thus the cream is returned to the cheese. This done, rennet enough should be thoroughly stirred in to make coagulation begin in 12 to 15 minutes, and the tub well covered to prevent cooling.

"When the curd has become hard enough to split with a clean fracture before the finger as it is passed along, the curd may be cut or carefully broken into half-inch cubes and left a while to settle, when a portion of the whey may be dipped off, and the curd again gently worked to prevent it becoming a solid mass again, and from the bottom, so that no part shall be missed. Repeat the stirring and dipping till the bulk of the whey is well reduced, as it will be in about an hour after the first stirring, and then turn in water enough at 140 to 150 degrees to raise the contents of the tub 3 or 4 degrees, stirring carefully in the meantime, that no part shall heat faster than the rest. When the bits of curd have had time enough to warm through, apply more water, and so repeat till the whole comes up to 98 or 100 degrees. Then stir enough to prevent the curd from adhering till it will begin to squeak between the teeth, or spring apart when pressed in the hand, when stirring may cease and the curd be allowed to settle together, and left in this condition as long as it can be, and not have the whey begin to turn sour.

"Whey has generally been heated to raise the temperature of the curd. The only advantage in raising it is to prevent diluting the whey. But water is preferable, because the whey, which is heated to warm the rest, has its souring hastened. Water, too, is better for the curd than whey. When the whey is suspected of approaching change, it should be dipped off close, the division board put into the tub, and the curd all put on one side of it, and the tub tipped so it will drain. After a few minutes the tub may be tipped the other way, the division board removed, the curd turned back from the middle of the tub, the half-round board slid under it and raised a little from the bottom of the tub, the division board replaced and tub tipped back as it was at first, when the curd will be in a condition to drain from the side and bottom. In this condition it should be left until the curd becomes so fibrous that it will pull apart and split with the appearance of well-boiled lean beef.

"While lying in this condition to drain and ripen, it should be turned occasionally to keep all parts warm alike, and prevent an accumulation of escaping whey in any part of it, and kept covered to prevent cooling. The ripening of the curd is done by the influence of the rennet, and it goes on best at 98 degrees. If the temperature falls below that, the tub should be tipped back and the curd covered with water at 100 degrees, till it is well warmed up. When the curd has assumed the condition described it may be considered done. It will then be in a tough, solid mass, and must be made so fine that salt will strike through it in a short time and evenly. A small mess of curd may, in a few minutes, be hashed into inch cubes or less with a chopping-knife. For larger messes a curd-mill should be prepared with a concave and cylinder filled with spikes, something like those in threshing machines, with a hopper over them to hold the curd for grinding, the cylinder being rotated by hand.

"If the cheese is wanted for immediate use, salt at the rate of ½ lb to 25 lbs of curd should be evenly mingled with the curd. If to be kept long, ½ lb of salt to 15 or 16 of curd may be used. The pressing, bandaging and care in the dairy room may be left to the taste and skill of the dairy-maid. If it is desired to make cheese larger than the milk of one day will make, the curd should be made and pressed as described, and the pressed curd of one day may be chopped fine (or ground) and after being warmed by lying in water at 100 degrees, may be mixed with the curd of the next day and both pressed together, a little extra salt being added for what may have been taken up by the warm water. It was the practice of our ancestors in making dairy cheese, to drain, cool, salt, and press the curd as soon as it was out of the whey. This was their supreme error. The most essential improvement in modern cheese making consists in keeping the curd warm and as clear as possible of whey, and without salting, for 2 or 3 hours or more, after separating it from the sweet whey, and after our forefathers thought it necessary to hurry it into the press.

"The treatment between the time of dipping and pressing is the most important part of the process of manufacture. It is only while lengthening out this time, under proper conditions, that the curd ripens so rapidly and vigorously as to overcome accompanying defects. It will cure as much in 1 hour, under proper treatment at this time, as it will in a week in the curing room. It is then more than at any other time that it is made to acquire a full and pleasant cheesy flavor, and a solid, yet rich and plastic texture. It is also at this time more than at any other that the digestibility of the resulting cheese is promoted, and its healthfulness and value as food determined, rendering certain a cheese which is at the same time palatable to all lovers of cheese, and wholesome even to invalids, and more nutritious than any other animal food, and this is more than I dare say of the old modes of making. By dipping and pressing at once these benefits were, and still are to a large extent, missed. Formerly it seemed to be an important point to get through with the work quickly. He was the best maker who could get through at the earliest hour. This is now reversed; time has become an element of importance in cheese making when quality is the object, and the best workmen are those who make haste slowly."

*Remarks.*—I think his instructions are so plain that none need fail to make a good home-made cheese. And I think every farmer ought to make the cheese used at his own table.

II. For making cheese from a dozen cows, or more, and it would be all the better if for any number above 5 or 6, to have what is called a vat, which would hold nicely all the milk for making the cheese. Such vats are made to be surrounded with water; or, at any rate, water under the vat, to prevent a possibility of scorching the milk; as they are placed upon a furnace to allow a fire under them, for warming the milk and whey at the proper time; and also to allow cold water to be put into the outer shell which surrounds the milk vat proper, to aid in cooling down the night's milk, as you will notice my friend, Mr. Sanders, mentions in his explanations below. I had written to him in 1879, when I first began writing upon this, my " Third and Last Receipt Book," now well on to six years ago (this writing is done Feb. 17, 1885, and I have written faithfully upon it all the time I could command, ever since, and, thank the Lord, it is now nearly completed, and I hope, and trust it shall do a great good to the people, for whom I have done my best).

In writing to my cousin Sanders about sacking, or putting the cloth around the cheese, as we see it comes from the factories, amount of rennet to be used, best form of press, and several other points, as you will see in his answer, which I did not see given in the published items. I mention this that his answer may be the better understood. His letter is as follows:

"HOLLAND, N. Y., April 14, 1879.

"DEAR COUSIN, A. W. CHASE, M. D.—Yours of April 4th duly received.

1. "In answer about sacking cheese: After the cheese has been in the press, say, 2 hours, take out, put on the sack snugly, turn the cheese, and

return it to the press for 24 hours, or till next morning. Commence with light weight, and heavier towards the last, that will press the bandage firmly into the cheese, and prevent flies from getting in. I think the lever press the true principle of pressing.

II. "In regard to skim-milk cheese, you can keep the milk just as long as it will keep perfectly sweet, although in quite cool weather it will frequently get bitter, and that would spoil the flavor of the cheese.

III. "I can tell no exact rule for the amount of rennet, for there is so much difference in the strength of them. Must use judgment and practice.

IV. "I will try to tell how we make our cheese. We strain the night's milk into the vat and put cold water around the milk (that is, in the outer shell under and around the milk, by which the milk is also heat, when desired, by a fire in the furnace,) to keep the milk from souring. In the morning, skim, put the cream in the strainer, and strain the morning's milk, which is warm, through it to dissolve the cream (so you see, the cream is not to be taken away for butter, if you wish good rich cheese); then heat to 80 or 85 degrees, when we add the rennet. It should coagulate in from 30 to 35 minutes; then stand 40 minutes, and cut the curd; then stand about the same length of time before heating up the whey; when the heat has been raising about 10 minutes, commence working gradually, till it gets to 100 degrees. Work it up with clean hands to keep the curd from sticking together, until it will cleave apart; then let the fire go down, and let it stand till the whey becomes a sickish sweet, then drain off the whey, add salt (see Mr. Arnold's plan for the right amount), put into hoops, press 2 hours, sack, turn, and put back and press till next morning.

"Last season we sent our milk to the factory, for the reason wife's health was not good enough to see to it (his wife made the cheese generally, which I always thought was too hard work for a weakly woman, and still think the same); but it did not net more than two-thirds as much as when made it ourselves. The lowest I have sold our own make of cheese for, since the war, is 12½ cts. per lb. It is lower now; but my customers last spring offered me 10 cts. if I would supply them; but I have never been able to supply the adjacent villagers with what they wanted. I have not kept my dairying accounts so as to give you figures of the amount of milk for a certain amount of cheese, nor of the profits of the business. Suffice it to say, I think it the best business for a farmer here, he can follow; and I agree with you, that every farmer should make his cheese for his own table.

"Our best respects to yourself and family.       DAVID SANDERS."

*Remarks.*—I think between this gentleman's explanations and those of Mr. Arnold, any man, or woman, who is stout and healthy enough to do the work, will be able to master all the intricacies there are in the business of cheese making, whether it be with few or many cows, as the plan is the same; and those who keep a large number of cows, and wish to make cheese for the London (England) market, will be able to do so, by the following item, from the *Rural New Yorker*, which was given under the following head:

2. **Fancy Shipping Cheese.**—The following is the process for "gilt-edge" fancy cheese for the London market, at one of the most noted factories in Herkimer county, N. Y.;

"In warm weather, during summer, the milk is cooled by running water under the vats to a temperature of 70° Fahr. The water is then turned off for the night, and the agitator kept moving very slowly until morning. If the weather is cool, in summer, the water is turned off when the milk has fallen to a temperature of 74°. In the morning the temperature of the milk ranges about 64° Fahr. Mr. Fairchild, the manager, says he does not want the temperature of the milk to have fallen below 64° in the morning because, when this is the case, the milk is too sweet, or has not sufficiently ripened for his method of cheese making. In summer the milk is raised to a temperature of 82° Fahr., and a sufficient quantity of good, sweet rennet added to produce coagulation so it will be fit to cut in 1 hour. The coagulation should be carried so far as to have the mass break smooth and clear, on introducing the finger and raising it.

"Then the curds are cut lengthwise of the vat with a gang of steel knives, and allowed to remain at rest for a space of ten minutes. They are now cut crosswise, and immediately after this operation the horizontal knives are used to divide the perpendicular columns of curd, and when this is completed no more cutting is allowed. Heat is now immediately applied to the mass, and its temperature is raised slowly, or gradually, until it reaches 98 deg. In the meantime, the curds are very carefully moved with the hands and the particles of curd are about ¾ths of an inch through. Water is used under the vats for heating, and this is regarded as better than dry steam. When the mass has reached a temperature of 98 deg., heat is shut off; but in equalizing the temperature of the water under the vats and the curds, the latter will run up to about 100 deg. The curds are now stirred for from 10 to 15 minutes, and very slowly, or until the heat is all equalized through the mass. Then the curds are left at rest—the cheese maker's office being to watch and stir the curds occasionally until the acid begins to develop. It generally takes about an hour for the acid to develop sufficiently during hot weather, and when this point is reached which is indicated by the odor, or if the hot iron is employed the curds should only spin threads about ⅜ths of an inch long. At this point, which must be determined correctly by the cheese maker, the whey is immediately drawn, and the curds dipped into the sink. They are here stirred until the whey is all out, when salt is applied at the rate of 3 lbs. salt to 1,000 lbs. of milk.

"A proportion of annattoine is used during summer in the milk, as the London dealer to whom the cheese goes, on orders, require a colored cheese. The annattoine proportion is after Whitman & Burrell's recipe, and takes one teacupful for 1,000 lbs. of milk. This gives the desired shade and suits the London trade exactly.

"In spring and fall, when the patrons are allowed to skim a portion of the milk, the process of manufacture is varied, and is as follows: The milk is set at a temperature of 84 deg., and a quantity of rennet added sufficient to produce coagulation completely in 40 minutes. It is then cut in the same way as for whole milk-cheese and the mass raised to a temperature of 96 deg., which ultimately runs to 98 deg. in equalizing the temperature of the water and curds. The late fall cheese is salted at the rate of 2¼ to 2½ lbs. salt to 1,000 lbs of. milk and the winter cheese gets only 2 lbs. For this character of cheese he does not want so much development of acid as for the summer make. When under the hot iron test the acid is far enough developed when you can just perceive the strings to start on withdrawing the lumps of curd from the iron. In winter he regards it important to draw the whey as quickly as possible and get the curds in the hoop rapidly.

*Remarks.*—Thus we have the home-made cheese, on a small and on a large scale, and the very tip-top fancy cheese of the factories, so that all can be pleased. The factory plan, without the coloring, would be just the thing, for home market or home use.

**3. Buttermilk Cheese, Plain and Spiced, if Desired—German Plan—Excellent.**—According to a German agricultural journal excellent cheese may be made of buttermilk by the following process: "The buttermilk, after being boiled and allowed to stand until cool, is placed in a cheese-form (loop) or heavy linen bag until the whey is drained off, when it is salted, not too heavily, and spiced according to taste, and thoroughly mixed. About a spoonful of alcohol is then added for each pound, and the mass is thoroughly kneaded, and formed into cheeses of any desired size or form, which are dried in the air, and then wrapped in clean linen cloths that have previously been moistened with hot whey, and packed in a well-covered cask, and stowed in a warm place. Four days suffice to render them fit for use, but they improve by age. The small hand-cheeses, which especially become very dry in winter, may be rendered palatable by simply wrapping them, when dry, in horse-radish leaves, and packing them closely in a cask. They will be found of a very agreeable flavor in from 3 to 4 weeks."

*Remarks.*—Many persons are very fond of buttermilk cheese, and those who do not desire to spice them will simply use a little salt.

**Cheese Factory—What it Costs to Fit Up, Articles Needed, With Price of Each.**—I cannot settle this point better than by giving an explanation in a recent number of the Fostoria *Review* by E. A. Davidson, of Gilroy, Cal., who reported the fitting up of his factory there for using the milk of 500 cows, which is probably as small a number as will pay to prepare for. It is probable that to buy in the cities of the Middle or Eastern States the cost would be somewhat less than in California. He says:

* * I have recently fitted out a factory for about that number of cows, the cost of which forms the basis of the figures I give. The following will be found reliable. It will be observed that in my list no provision has been made for engine or force pump for forcing water into tanks, which in some localities may be necessary. It will be found much more desirable to have running water, either from spring or artesian well, where it can be procured without too great expense, as it will materially lessen the running expense of the factory as well as prove at all times a safeguard from tainted or sour milk, both of which are very liable to occur where there is a lack of good, pure running water. There are also cases of defect sometimes in the working of either pump or engine, and this causes much inconvenience, and many times actual cost in handling the milk. The following is a list of necessary apparatus, with present cost of each item:

| | |
|---|---:|
| Three 600-gallon vats, $80 each, . . . . . | $240 00 |
| One press with capacity for thirty 60-pound cheese, . | 25 00 |
| Ten press screws, . . . . . . . . | 70 00 |
| Thirty telescope hoops, . . . . . . | 90 00 |
| One 80-gallon weighing can, . . . . . . | 15 00 |
| One milk conductor, . . . . . . . | 5 00 |
| One curd sink, with perforated bottom, . . . | 20 00 |
| One 6-horse-power boiler, with injector and pipes complete, to connect with vats, . . . . . | 275 00 |
| Two bandagers, or curd fillers, . . . . . | 5 00 |
| Two curd knives, one horizontal and one perpendicular. | 15 00 |
| One pair of scales, 900 pounds capacity, . . . | 45 00 |
| One pair of scales for weighing salt, etc., . . . | 10 00 |
| Two rennet jars, . . . . . . . . | 5 00 |
| Two jars for coloring, . . . . . . | 2 50 |
| One curd mill, . . . . . . . . | 30 00 |
| One sink for washing and scalding dairy fixtures, . | 10 00 |
| One set of testing instruments, . . . . . | 5 00 |
| Pails, dippers, curd scoop, etc., . . . . | 6 00 |
| Total, . . . . . . . . . | $873 50 |

*Remarks.*—Although our items, or recipes, for making and managing butter and cheese are few, yet we think they are plain and perfectly reliable.

# DOMESTIC ANIMALS.

## HORSES.

**General Remarks Upon Their Dispositions, Etc.**—It is an admitted fact that " kind and gentle treatment makes a kind and gentle horse." Again, " a balky man makes a balky horse." " Bad drivers," too, " make bad horses." It is only in a few exceptional cases that a horse is naturally vicious, or even stubborn. Let good sense be shown, then, on the part of those who have the raising and care of horses, and they will show theirs by their kind and willing submission to all reasonable requirements which they understand. Kindly teach them, and they will as kindly learn. But curse and scream at them, and you excite their fears and injure their disposition to be kind, by every such want of judgment on the part of the driver, or the one who has the care of them in the stable. Then, if you want a kind and gentle horse, be kind and gentle towards them, and they will not fail you in more than one case in a hundred. But a pet to-day and a kick to-morrow will destroy their confidence in you, and leads them to expect abuse rather than kindness. The Arabs are accredited with being the most successful horse-trainers in the world; and they so appreciate the value of kindness that they take them into their tents with them, and bestow upon them as much love as they give to their children; and the children, in turn, make playfellows of the colts; and thus, although the Arabian horse is considered the most spirited of any in the world, yet with their intelligence gained by this constant and kind companionship, they are the most easily controlled of any. Beware of the impatience of boys and hired help, who are likely to think there is no way of showing their power over a horse but by jerking at the reins, and yelling or cursing at him. Treat horses with uniform and unvarying kindness and they will soon learn to have confidence in their master, and there will be but few "tricky" horses. It is well even to be on friendly terms with cows and sheep as well as the horse family, giving them salt, or a little sugar, pieces of apple, or any palatable thing, as bits of carrots, beets, etc., and especially so with the younger stock, and thus teach every animal to allow itself to be handled in the yard. And if, when a colt or a calf is seen for the first time, it is handled kindly, and so petted every time it is seen afterwards, it will soon love to see you for the sake of the feeding, handling, etc., and never more be afraid of you, as it soon will be unless this kind course is introduced and constantly pursued. That the disposition of

653

the horse is, generally, kind, no one can doubt; therefore, if he receives kindness, and only kindness, in return, he will become more, and still more kind to his master and associate, which the master thus becomes, rather than an austere, rough, harsh and abusive one, which the naturally kind animal will soon learn to fear, and the next thing is to hate, and consequently kick or bite, or both, in self defense or to prevent your coming near enough to abuse him, when this is the custom of the master; and no one can honestly blame them for it, either. Learn then, to give the kindness you expect in return, and there will soon be a lasting friendship established that will end only with the life of one or the other.

**How Long a Horse Ought to Work.**—It is now claimed by our best horsemen, that, with our many labor-saving machines, a horse ought not to be worked over 9 hours a day; at any rate he should have two hours at noon for eating, and to allow the digestion of his food, by which his strength will be greatly aided in his afternoon's work. See the digestion of the horse compared with that of the ox, showing how each should be fed.

**Raising and Breaking Colts.**—A correspondent of the *Practical Farmer*, who says he has had considerable experience in handling colts, gives his views and practice upon this subject, also such examples of docility, after his manner of handling them, which are so consistent with what I consider the right thing to do in raising and breaking colts that I believe it will carry more force, or be more likely to be followed, than what I might be able to say, without corresponding examples, which I could not give. He says:

"I have adopted the rule of haltering my colts at 10 days old, and lead it at its mother's side whenever I drive her. I have never found any trouble in teaching a colt to lead in this way, and long before it is weaned it will be perfectly halter-broken. I have just brought up from the pasture a colt that was 2 years old in April, to give it a little training. This colt was halter-broken and led at the side of its mother when sucking, and it is now as docile as any horse on the farm. A boy 16 years old, who is living with me, harnessed it a few days ago, and, after driving it round the yard for a short time, hitched it to a spring wagon and went off alone with it. I should not have allowed it had I known what he was about, but he came back with the colt as gentle as my old carriage horse. This has been about my experience with colts that have been taught to lead and handle when young. It is easy to accustom a colt to have the harness thrown on it, and chains wrapped around its legs, or to have something fall from its back, without its being frightened, and if these things are ever learned it must be when the animal is young. I believe that it is easy to so train a colt that if the hold-backs come loose on a hill, and let the buggy against it, instead of being frightened and running away, it will brace itself and stop the buggy. I remember twice being placed in a position of great danger, with a spirited mare that I had trained from a colt, and if I had not accustomed her to just such treatment as I recommend, I should undoubtedly have been severely injured or killed. The instances were these: I was approaching the Miami river, on a turnpike, and had just started down a long, winding hill, over a fourth of a mile long, when one of the bolts by which the shafts were attached to the buggy, dropped out. That side of the shafts dropped on to the mare's heels, and whenever I attempted to rein her in to stop her, the buggy would run against her. I went fully 300 yards down the hill before I could get her checked so that it was safe for me to jump out and catch the wheel and stop the buggy, but the mare made no attempt to kick or run. The other case was this: I had stopped at the top of a long hill with a load of wood, and when I stepped on to the doubletree to climb on to the load, the stick I took hold of to pull myself up by, pulled out, and I fell with my head between the mare's heels, and the stick came rattling down over the chains on top of me. If she had started at all the wagon would have run over me, for I was exactly in front of the wheel. Now, I do not say that every horse can be trained to do as mine did, but I do say that if it is ever done it must be while it is young, and that what the colt is taught young it never forgets. I have no faith in the theory that a colt should never be put to work until it is 4 years old. Of course, we must exercise judgment and not strain our young horses by pulling them hard, but I see no more reason why a colt should do nothing until it is full grown, than a boy, and every boy works from the time he is 12 or 14 years old. A well grown colt can be used for light work from the time it is 30 months old and made to pay its keeping, and if good judgment is exercised it will be all the better for it. One thing is indispensable in training a colt, and that is that you control your temper. The man who will get angry, and jerk and whip a colt, is not fit to have charge of it, and need not expect to render it docile and obedient.

*Remarks.*—As this gentleman says, every horse may not be as docile as his was, even if trained the same; but the author fully believes that 9 out of every 10 would be equally docile under just such circumstances. But most positively would not without this early training.

**Bitting the Colt and Training to Harness.**—In the warm days of spring, when the colt is 1 year old, let the bitting process be commenced; and if the colt has been handled from its birth, as above suggested, it will usually submit to the bitting process as quietly as he will to any other training. After putting on the bitting fixtures, turn him loose in a safe yard, *i. e.*, with no obstructions, as wagons, sheep racks, etc., with which he might come in contact, allowing him an hour or so to become familiar with the harness, being careful to check him up but little the first time above what he carries his head naturally, but checking higher and higher each day until the proper carriage of the head is attained. I dislike an over-high carriage of the head in any horse. After a day or two, a cord 12 to 15 feet in length may be tied to the bits and the colt allowed or trained, if need be, to exercise in a circle or around you, but never carrying it so far as to tire or worry him, gently patting and petting him from time to time to show that no harm is intended. This should be gone over again and again through the summer and winter following, and when it is 2 years old it may be harnessed and hitched beside its mother, if she be gentle and kind, else beside an old, gentle horse, and driven quietly about, at first with only the harness on, then to a light carriage, with never more than two therein, and accustomed to driving until it becomes second nature to do as its companion does, but never upon long and exhaustive journeys; but simply enough to harden its flesh and aid its muscular development. And even from 3 until 4 years old a colt should be driven with exceeding care, never over-loaded, as this is the critical age of the colt, or its period of second dentition, and it can not, therefore, masticate hard food, as it can after its teething is completed. Indeed, all young horses should be used with care, and never put to steady exhaustive work until they are 6 years old, after which, with this early care, they will become stouter and increase in power and speed until 10 or even 12 years old while if put to the hardest work at 4 or 5, they will not improve beyond 8 or 9.

**Weaning and Wintering Colts.**—If the mare is allowed a few oats while in pasture, which is a very proper thing to allow, the colt will soon learn to eat with her, and as soon as this is observed, it should have a handful or two daily, where the mother cannot get in to eat them from it; by which means you increase its development and growth, and save the trouble of having to teach it to eat them at time of weaning. And as cool nights approach, it is best to take the mare to the stable over night, tying the colt near her; if a double stall, by her side; but not to allow suckling, which will take away half, at least, of the trouble of weaning without their knowing it; and if the mare will eat roots, give such as beets, carrots, turnips, apples, pumpkins, etc., all properly cut into small pieces to prevent choking; and some persons think all breeding mares should be taught to eat roots to ensure a better condition of health. The colt will also soon learn to eat them, but should not be allowed so much as to produce loose-ness of the bowels; enough, only, to aid digestion. Some persons allow their colts to run with the dam till winter sets in; but it is not good for either the colt or the mother, especially if she is again breeding. The colt should be weaned, or shut off from the mother, about the end of the sixth month; but should be well cared for the first winter — in fact, all winters; should have either a warm stall, or at least a warm, dry place, with plenty of bedding, and a good brushing every day, being very careful and kind about the legs, to accustom it to after grooming; give a quart of good, sound oats daily, with sweet, clean hay, and its little feed of roots, if you have them; but coarse cut food is not proper for a colt, as it packs too closely for the easy digestion of young animals. If the fall is particularly dry, when a colt is being weaned, a few bits of carrots, beets, or turnips will more especially be called for as aids to digestion, on account of the shriveled condition of the grass. With these aids it will not miss the mother's milk near as much as it otherwise would; and if it has already been accustomed to them, so much less trouble will now be exper-ienced. If 3 or 4 colts can be shut off together in an adjoining field from the dams, there will be still less trouble than with one alone.

**Profit of Raising Colts.**—A colt may be raised for about the same cost as a cow; but, at three years old, is generally worth as much as three or four cows. Not only must the right kind of mares be kept, and the right kind of colts be raised, but the mother must have the proper care, as indicated under the head of Brood-mares, Proper Care of, etc. She must also have ample stable accommodations, when needed. And as the profit of raising good colts is so large, as before remarked, and the demand for them is becoming so great, let the farmer keep the mares, which are just as kind and good to work on the farm as the geldings, and let the latter go to the town-people who care not to engage in the breeding business.

**Colts of Ordinary Training—To Cure of Halter-Pulling.—** Colts which have not been broken young to lead by the side of the mother, as previously instructed, often annoy their trainer by pulling at the halter. For such, place a spring-pole, a pretty stiff one, on the opposite side of the manger so he shall not see it; then pass the halter-strap, or what is better, a rope halter, that may pass through a hole in the partition or boards, put up for the purpose, passing to the pole, which shall give him at least 3 or 4 feet of play, and he will soon try his full strength upon it; but if properly done it will still hold him, and he will finally walk up to the manger—"the captain's office"—and consider his passage paid for life on not a very large number of pulls either, if it is skillfully arranged. I have seen this done effectually and satisfactorily by taking the colt to the woods and trimming a sapling of such a size as to have the right spring to it, then cut off the top at a proper height, bending down and tying a long rope to the top and to the halter, then letting it up gently, when the contest would begin, but always with victory to the sapling, with only a few trials, although it is believed to be best to have the sapling hidden from his sight, yet he hardly suspects the sapling of being his opponent.

Colts, to Teach How to Back.—When a colt has been somewhat accustomed to the harness, after our method of training and breaking, it will be well also to teach him how to back in the following manner: Having put on a bridle, lead him to the top of rather sloping ground, not very steep, placing the hind feet down the slope; then facing him, taking hold of the reins, close to the bits, with a hand on each side, press him gently backward, at the same time saying "Back, back," while you follow him, guiding him as he backs, to keep him descending the hill or slope, and not allowing him to turn sideways, stopping occasionally to caress him, but under no circumstances allow yourself to strike him, and he will very soon learn what is wanted of him and will will-ingly do it at the word being spoken every time, if done with patience and gen-tleness. After he has learned it fairly on the descending ground, do the same upon the level, after which harness him to a light empty buggy or wagon and do the same thing, first upon descending ground, then upon the level; and finally, if upon a road where the ground is solid, you may get into the vehicle, and with the reins gently pull upon him, always repeating the words, "Back, back," until he perfectly understands what is desired of him, when he will do it as readily as any other thing. It is only that horses do not know what is wanted of them, or that they are at first required to back greater loads than they are able to do, that there is so much trouble in backing them. If the colt is taught, the horse will know how to do it. And this plan is as applicable to horses as it is to colts; but for horses which have not had the advantage of training and breaking while a colt, as above indicated, it will require more time, as well as more patience, and a greater amount of gentleness, to accomplish the undertaking. Observe the three things above indicated and you will never fail:

I. To place the colt or the horse with his back down hill.

II. When harnessed, let it be only to a light empty wagon.

III. Always be perfectly kind and gentle, teaching him what you desire him to know. Take only one at first, and after he is learned, if you have a mate for him, do the same with him; and finally, harness them together and carefully do the same with the span. It will more than pay in the after usefulness of the horses for all the labor and pains of teaching.

**Brood Mares, Proper Care of, Before and at the Time of Foaling.**—The author is indebted to the "Veterinary" of the New York *Spirit* and a correspondent of the *Michigan Farmer* for the following sensible instructions as to the proper food and care of brood mares at this critical period of their lives; and especially will it be found necessary to have an eye to the mother's conduct towards the foal or colt, if it is her first, as she may be kind to it and she may not; still, watchful care is very important in all cases until the colt is up and doing well. The writers speak very much alike, as though one had copied from the other, in parts at least, but which is the copyist I do not know; but as each is more full in some points than the other, I shall use all important points without giving both in full, as that would only be a repetition, my credit being given jointly, as above. The combination is sensible and worthy of consideration. It is as follows:

"The best feed for the brood mare is corn stalks or good timothy hay, with from 4 to 6 qts. of ground oats and wheat bran (equal parts) each day. The ground oats and wheat bran not only enable the dam to make all necessary preparations to supply the coming foal with nourishment at the time when most needed, but it keeps her healthy and strong, and enables her to furnish the growing fœtus (colt in uterus) with the best kind of material to make the best bone and muscle. The dam should also have moderate exercise, but it should be regular. If she be used in a team, she should not be driven faster than a walk, nor loaded too heavily, for in either case there is danger of injuring the dam and ruining the foal. She should be housed or sheltered nights and in all stormy weather. As foaling time approaches, she particularly needs the practiced eye of the careful and experienced breeder. For she should be watched both day and night, as many a valuable colt has been lost that two minutes' labor at the particular time would have saved. As soon as the colt is dropped, the attendant should see that its head is free from the membrane or sac with which it is enveloped, as the colt will otherwise soon smother. The next thing is to sever the umbilical cord about 5 inches from the foal and tie the end next to the colt to prevent bleeding, etc. This, if possible, should be done before the dam rises, as many a colt has been ruptured at the navel by the dam rising before the string was severed. After the above has been promptly attended to, leave the dam alone with the foal for half an hour and carefully watch her actions. Now, in case she seems disposed to injure, or in any way abuse the foal, it should be taken away from her and covered with a blanket until dry. at the end of a few hours, the attendant with whom the mare is most familiar should endeavor to assist the foal to suckle. If necessary the mare must be placed under more or less restraint. The twitch, strapping up one foot, or the side line must be resorted to, while the assistant renders the necessary assistance by holding the colt at the side and by putting the nose to the teat of the mare. After the colt is able to draw its nourishment from the dam without the aid of its attendant, little need be done but furnish a shed, if the weather be inclement, and a liberal supply of good hay or stalks, and a peck of ground oats and bran per day until there is a full growth of green, spring grass."

*Remarks.*—The author can see nothing to add to these instructions, except, should it ever occur that from storms, or from the mare's "coming in" out of the ordinary season, she should have a double stall or a barn floor, well bedded, entirely to herself at such time, together with the same watchful care to avoid accidents, that is above recommended, with which no danger generally need be apprehended.

**How to Choose or Buy a Horse.**—The following simple rules will be found useful to all parties about to buy a horse:

I.  Never take the seller's word; if dishonest he will be sure to cheat you; if disposed to be fair, he may have been the dupe of another, and will deceive you through representations which cannot be relied upon.

II.  If you trust the horse's mouth for his age, observe well the rules given below, for that purpose.

III.  Never buy a horse while in motion; watch him while he stands at rest, and you will discover his weak points.  If sound he will stand squarely on his limbs without moving any of them, the feet planted flat upon the ground, with legs plump and naturally poised.  If one foot is thrown forward with the toe pointing to the ground and the heel raised; or if the foot is lifted from the ground and the weight taken from it, disease of the navicular bone may be suspected, or at least, tenderness, which is precursor of disease.  If the foot is thrown out, the toe raised and the heel brought down, the horse has suffered from laminitis, founder or fever in the feet, or the back sinews have been sprained, and he is of little future value.  When the feet are all drawn together beneath the horse, if there has been no disease there is a misplacement of the limbs, at least, and a weak disposition of the muscles.  If the horse stands with his feet spread out, or straddles with the hind legs, there is weakness of the loins, and the kidneys are disordered.

IV.  Never buy a horse with a bluish or milkish cast in the eyes.  They indicate a constitutional tendency to ophthalmia (soreness or weak eyes) moon blindness, etc.

V.  Never have anything to do with a horse who keeps his ears thrown back.  It is an invariable indication of bad temper.

VI.  If a horse's hind legs are scarred the fact denotes that he is a kicker.

VII.  If the knees are blemished the horse is apt to stumble.

VIII.  When the skin is rough and harsh, and does not move easily and smoothly to the touch, the horse is a heavy eater, and his digestion is bad.

IX.  Avoid a horse whose respiratory organs are at all impaired,  If the ear is placed at the side of the heart, and a whizzing sound is heard, it is an indication of trouble.  Let him go.

**How to Judge the Age of a Horse.**—The age of a horse, up to a certain period, is generally determined by his teeth.  There are no two opinions alike on this point.  But as almost every writer on this subject has some pet theory of his own, there are probably no two writers whose opinions agree as to the exact manner of arriving at a horse's age after it has attained the age of 5 years.  For the edification of our readers, we give from "Kendall's Treatise on the Horse," the following concise rules, which will be found generally correct:

I.  Eight to fourteen days after birth the first middle nippers of the set of milk teeth are cut; four to six weeks afterward, the pair next to them, and finally, after six or eight months, the last.  All these milk teeth have a well defined body, neck and shoulder fang, and on their front surface grooves—or furrows, which disappear from the middle nippers at the end of one year; from the next pair in two years, and from the incisive teeth (cutters) in three years.

II.  At the age of two the nippers become loose and fall out, in their places appear two permanent teeth, with deep, black cavities, and full, sharp edges. At the age of three the next pair fall out.  At four years old the corner teeth fall out.  At five years old the horse has his permanent set of teeth.

III.  The teeth grow in length as the horse advances in years, but at the same time his teeth are worn away by use, about one-twelfth of an inch every year, so that the black cavities of the nippers below disappear in the sixth year; those of the next pair in the seventh year, and those of the corner teeth in the eight year; also the outer corner teeth of the upper and lower jaws just meet at eight years of age.  At nine years old cups leave the two center nippers above, and each of the two upper corner teeth have a little sharp protrusion at the extreme outer corner.  At the age of ten the cups disappear from the adjoining teeth; at the age of eleven the cups disappear from the corner teeth above, and are only indicated by brownish spots.

IV.  The oval form becomes broader, and changes, from the twelfth to the sixteenth year, more and more into a triangular form, and teeth lose, finally, with the 20th year, all regularity.  There is nothing remaining in the teeth that can afterward clearly show the age of the horse or justify the most experienced examiner in giving a positive opinion.

V.  The tushes or canine teeth, conical in shape, with a sharp point and curved, are cut between the third and fourth year, their points become more and more rounded, until the ninth year, and after that more and more dull in the course of years, and lose, finally, all regular shape.  Mares have frequently no tusks, or only faintly indicated.

**What Makes a Horse Shy, and How to Avoid it.**—A correspondent of the *Michigan Farmer*, says: "There never was a shying horse that was not near-sighted.  Such horses do not see the object until getting right near it.  Nothing will break the horse of this habit unless the blinders are discarded and an open head-stall used.  Treat the horse kindly.  Never whip him, but try to coax him up to the object, that he may smell of it.  One of the worst shyers was broken by leading, riding and driving in a meadow among stone, stumps, boxes and buffalo robes in different positions every day, the horse being led up to them and allowed to eat a few oats off of the object.  Let any one examine a well-behaved horse's eye and then a "shyer's" eye, and note the difference.

**Managing and Shoeing Fractious Horses.**—The following valuable information is from the *Live Stock Journal:* "A beautiful and high-spirited horse would never allow a shoe to be put on his feet or any person to handle his feet.  In attempting to shoe such a horse, recently, he resisted all efforts, kicked aside everything but an anvil, and came near killing himself against that, and finally was brought back to his stable unshod. This defect was just on the eve of consigning him to the plow, where he might walk barefoot, when an officer in our service, lately returned from Mexico, took a cord about the size of a common bed-cord, put it in the mouth of the horse like a bit, and tied it tightly on the animal's head, passing his left ear under the string, not painfully tight, but tight enough to keep the ear down and the cord in place. This done, he patted the horse gently on the side of the head and commanded him to follow, and instantly the horse obeyed, perfectly subdued, and as gentle and obedient as a dog, suffering his feet to be lifted with entire impunity, and acting in all respects like an old stager. The gentleman who thus furnished this exceedingly simple means of subduing a very dangerous propensity, intimated that it is practiced in Mexico and South America in the management of wild horses."

**Vicious Horses, Efficient Method of Subduing.**—A new and very simple method of subduing or training vicious horses was recently exhibited at West Philadelphia, Pa., where the manner in which the very wildest horses were subdued so quickly, caused the *Record* of that city, in making the following report, to call it "astonishing." It says: "The first trial was that of a kicking or 'bucking' mare, which her owner said had allowed no rider on her back for a period of at least five years. She became tame in about as many minutes, and allowed herself to be ridden about without a sign of her former wildness. The means by which the result was accomplished was by a piece of light rope which was passed around the front of the jaw of the mare just above the upper teeth, crossed in her mouth, thence secured back of her neck. It was claimed that no horse will kick or jump when thus secured, and that the horse, after receiving the treatment a few times, will abandon his vicious ways forever.

*"Method for Shoeing.*—The method for shoeing was equally simple. It consisted in connecting the animal's head and tail by means of a rope fastened to the tail and then to the bit, and then drawn tightly enough to incline the animal's head to one side. This, it is claimed, makes it absolutely impossible for the horse to kick on the side of the rope. At the same exhibition a horse, which for many years had to be bound on the ground to be shod, suffered the blacksmith to operate on him without attempting to kick, while secured in the manner described."

*Remarks.*—Much less trouble than the old Rarey plan; and the more simple the plan the easier it is to use it. If this ever fails, put under an ear, as they do in Mexico.

**White Feet in Horses or Spots on the Forehead—How to Produce a Match.**—Take a piece of Osnaburg (coarse linen cloth originally made in Osnaburg, Germany) the size of the white on the corresponding foot; spread it with warm pitch and apply it around the foot, tying it afterward to keep it on in the right position; let it remain on three days, by which time it will bring off the hair clean and make the skin a little tender; then take of elixir of vitriol a small quantity, anoint the parts 2 or 3 times; or use a common weed called arse-smart, a small handful, bruise it, and add to it about a half pint of water; use it as a wash until the soreness is removed, when the hair will grow entirely white.—*Cricket on the Hearth.*

*Remarks.*—If this will do the work on the feet, of which I have not a doubt, it will do the same upon the forehead, and in either case will do the horse no harm.

**Kicking and Runaway Horses—How to Cure of the Habit.—** *The Kicking.*—If you have a horse which is accustomed to knocking out the dash-board with his heels, when things do not work to please him, proceed as follows: "Place around his neck a band like that used for riding with a martingale. Then take two light straps (made for the purpose) and buckle them to the bits, on each side, and pass them through the neck-band, and also inside the girth, and buckle them securely to each fetlock of the hind feet, taking care, in the making, to have them of the proper length. When a horse is rigged in this manner, if he attempts to 'kick up behind,' each effort will jerk his head down in such a way as to astonish him, perhaps throw him over his head. He will make but a few attempts to kick when he finds his head thus tied to his heels, and two or three lessons will cure him altogether."

*For the Runaway.*—The method for the runaway is equally simple and effectual: "First of all, fasten some thick pads upon your horse's knees, then buckle a strap, about the size of a rein, upon each fetlock forward, and pass the straps through the hame rings or some part of harness near the shoulder on each side and lead the straps back to the driver's hand as he sits in the buggy. He has thus four reins in hand. Start the animal without fear; don't worry him with a strong pull upon the bit, but talk to him friendly. When he attempts to run, he must, of course, bend his forward legs. Now pull sharply one of the foot reins, and the effect will be to raise one of his forward feet to his shoulder. He is a three-legged horse now, and when he has gone on in that way a little distance drop the constrained foot and jerk up the other. He can not run faster on three legs than you can ride, and when you have tired him on both sides pretty thoroughly, or if he refuses to take his trot kindly and obey your voice and a moderate pull on the bit, you can raise both his fore feet, drop him upon his knees, and let him make a few bounds in that position. The animal will soon find that he can not run away; that he is completely in your power, and by soothing words you will also be able to convince him that you are his friend. He will soon obey your commands, and will be afraid to extend himself for a run. Within a week or two some horses that were quite valuable animals in respect to everything but their bad habits of kicking and running in harness, were cured by methods described above."—*Boston Herald.*

*Remarks.*—These plans, if managed skillfully, must prove effectual and satisfactory; and they ought to be generally known, for there are many horses given to one or both of these viciously evil habits.

**Digestion of the Horse Compared with that of the Ox, Showing How Each Should be Fed.—**The study of the physiology of the horse, as compared with that of the ox and other animals, is calculated to give such a knowledge to stockmen and farmers, that shall enable them to feed them in such manner as to obtain the strength needed at once by the digestion of the more concentrated articles of food, as oats or other grain, which for this purpose must be retained in the horse's stomach, while the hay or other coarser food may have passed on into the intestines. The horse's stomach has a capacity, generally, of only about 16 qts., while that of the ox has about $15\frac{1}{2}$ times as much, or about 250 qts. But the intestines are somewhat reversed, the horse having a capacity of 190 qts., or thereabouts, while the ox has only 100. And, again, the ox has the advantage of a gall bladder for the retention and continuous distribution of bile during the digestive process, while the horse has none, and depends upon the saliva being properly mixed with his food by slower mastication, the bile flowing into the intestines at once, as it is secreted. "This construction," says Colvin, "of the digestive apparatus indicates that the horse was formed to eat slowly and to digest continuously the more bulky and innutritious food." Then, when fed on hay, it passes very rapidly through the stomach into the intestine. The horse can eat but about 5 lbs. of hay in an hour, which is charged, during mastication, with four times its weight of saliva. Now, the stomach, to digest it well, will contain but about 10 qts., and when the animal eats $\frac{1}{3}$ of his daily ration, or 7 lbs., in $1\frac{1}{2}$ hours, at least, 2 stomachfuls of hay and saliva, one of which must have passed on into the intestines. And, as observation has shown that food is passed into the intestines in the order in which it is received (first come, first served), we find that if we feed a horse 6 qts. of oats, it, with the saliva and swelling of the grain by mastication (chewing), will just fill his stomach; and then, of course, if, as soon as he finishes his oats, we feed him his ration of hay, he will eat sufficient in $\frac{3}{4}$ of an hour to force the oats entirely out of the stomach into the intestines, while but slightly digested. Then as it is more particularly the office or function—duty or natural work—of the stomach to digest the nitrogenous parts of the food — as oats or other grain — while it is believed the duty of the intestines is to digest the less nitrogeneous and more bulky parts of the food, as hay, etc., by the continuous pouring upon it of the bile, as above indicated (the probable reason why a horse has no gall bladder), and as oats contain four or five times as much nitrogen or nourishment as the same bulk of hay, it stands to reason that the stomach must either secrete the gastric juice five times faster than usual, which is impossible, else it must retain the oats sufficiently long for digestion, or otherwise very much of their strength-giving properties are lost. Therefore, this knowledge says to the horseman, if you are going to feed hay, give it first and let the oats be given last, so that they drive the hay into the intestines, while they remain in the stomach for a more full and complete digestion. With the large stomach capacity, and the reserve of bile in the gall-bladder to be poured out, as required with the ox, it matters not so much as to which class of food may be first given; still, I think there will be less colic and gaseous disturbances in either case when the hay is fed first, if it is to be given at all, especially at the mid-day meal. But, as the ox is a ruminating animal (chews over again), he ought to be fed differently from the horse; having a large stomach capacity, as above explained, he needs coarse food to fill it; hence if working oxen are to be fed meal of any kind, at noon, let it be mixed with cut hay, or other coarse food, and he will be much more strengthened and refreshed for his afternoon work than if fed meal alone; and, as mentioned for the horse, let two hours be given them to eat, and ruminate, or re-chew, their food, by which means they obtain their strength for the balance of the day's work. Then, again, as the ox does not sweat like the horse, he cannot stand the mid-day heat as well as the horse can—a double reason for this rest at noon. [See also How Long the Horse Ought to Work.]

**Cribbing of Horses, What It Is and How to Cure It.**—The subject of cribbing is such a distressing thing to see a horse continuously doing when hitched to anything upon which he can press his teeth; and which must be more distressing to the horse, to be compelled, either from necessity or habit, to do it; and, as it is a subject which I never heard anyone give a plausible reason as to why horses get into the habit of it, and as I never saw anything printed upon the subject which appeared to throw any light upon this mystery, until Dr. Tuttle, of Clinton, Mich., Feb. 28, 1880, sent a communication to the *Post and Tribune*, of Detroit, which seems to give such a rational explanation as to its cause, and also a rational treatment, or cure, for it, I have felt constrained to give his ideas, although I shall feel compelled to condense his letter considerably; yet, I will give that which will enable anyone to avoid the difficulty with colts, and to treat horses upon his rational plan, that have become diseased, as he claims, which has addicted them to this terribly distressing habit. I am aware that most people claim it to be wind sucking, and hence call them wind suckers, but it never seemed to me to be the fact; and Dr. Tuttle's idea that it is to get wind out of the stomach rather than to suck it in, as you will see below, I fully agree with, and believe his theory to be the correct one, hence I give it the more cheerfully. In answer to "What is Cribbing?" he says: "Belch of wind from the stomach. This is absolutely true in the first stage of every case." He admits the possibility "that horses which have followed the habit for years, may suck in and swallow wind, though I doubt it," he continues, " for by carefully watching 'an old stager' go through the motions of cribbing, you will observe that the shape of the neck, along the line of the gullet, indicates something coming up out of the stomach, but which is swallowed back again. As to its cause, he claims it to be indigestion —dyspepsia, which in man, by fermentation, or souring of the food, produces gas, and therefore belching of wind, as it is called—does the same with the colt, for he claims that it generally begins with the colt and the cribbing, at first, so far relieves the distress from the distention of the stomach, the habit is formed, and he ever afterwards follows it; unless the cause, indigestion, is cured. As to the cause of the indigestion, he thinks that it arises mostly with fall colts, which have been too early put upon dry feed, grain, etc., which it was not properly able to masticate, or chew sufficiently fine to make it digestible, " for remember," he says, " if you please, that a colt doesn't have a full colt mouth (full set of milk teeth) until 2 years old; so don't feed them on dry, hard, old corn, to 'keep 'em thriving,' any more than you would feed a 3 months' old babe on corned beef and boiled cabbage and expect it to thrive."

The last would be as sensible a thing to do as the first. Raising spring colts is his remedy, so as to avoid putting them so quickly upon other feed than grass-made milk, with grass to eat, if they want it, and warm weather in which to grow and develop. Then when winter comes, if grain seems necessary, give boiled oats, or oatmeal in limited quantities, just enough to keep the colt growing, and in condition. Early cut hay, a warm shed for stormy weather; feed regularly, water regularly before feeding, never after," etc. If after the foregoing care, signs of dyspepsia and cribbing appear, he claims there is somet' ing wrong in the diet, or handling, which must be corrected, and hot bran mashes must be given, and continued, to keep the bowels continuously free, never allowing the movements to be hard and difficult. And the further treatment to be the following, as for horses, in proportion to the age. To cure the disease when developed, " Bear in mind," he says, " you are treating dyspepsia, not cribbing, for the latter is only a symptom, a result of the former, and the treatment must be thorough and persistent" (continued). The following is his treatment for a horse of five years or older:

I. Tinct. of nux vomica, 20 drops, in a swallow of water, before each feed, continued for months, if need be. "The effect of a small dose is all you need." It may be given by putting into a small bottle with a long neck and with about a gill of water, and given by putting into the mouth, as a drench, or by putting into a small amount of water in a bucket and drank before giving his full drink before the feeding.

II. *Condition Powder.*—A heaping dessert-spoonful (small-sized table-spoon) of the following tonic powder (condition powder), thoroughly mixed with the feed at every meal: Powdered gentian, powdered Peruvian bark (always get the best red, unground Peruvian bark, and have the druggist grind or powder it fine), of each, 1 lb., and powdered Jamaica ginger root, ½ lb., mixed thoroughly. [And the author would say, keep it in a closely-covered tin box.]

III. *Graduated Dose According to Age.*—He has graduated the dose to the age, as follows: For a horse 5 years or older, full dose, as above (20 drops); 4 years old, ⅞ (17 or 18 drops); 3 years old, ¾ (15 drops); 2 years old, ½ (10 drops); yearlings, ⅓ (6 or 7 drops); sucking colts, ⅛ to ¼ (2 to 3 drops, according to the robustness of the colt). That in parenthesis is the author's, and will save every one the trouble of calculating at each time of giving the medicine. I will give Dr. Tuttle's closing paragraph in full. He says:

" In closing, I would say I am not a horse doctor, nor do I wish to be, but a regular physician of nine years' experience; that in the first years of my practice, by hard, irregular work and unwise handling, I made a cribber of one of the finest horses ever owned in Michigan or driven by any man. Since then I have tried to study carefully and scientifically his very intelligent efforts to obtain relief, and likewise the effects of treatment, hygienic and therapeutic (*i. e.*, care as to proper feed and medicine. And with my knowledge of disease and remedies in man I have, by analogy and experience, arrived at the above conclusions, which I give to the public, hoping to assist horse-loving men to a better understanding of a hitherto unscientifically-treated disease, which is distressing to both horse and owner. And I am confident that if this advice is carefully followed it will be found to result in cures far beyond that ever produced by the choke-strap, to say nothing of the peace of mind which follows the humane treatment adopted for the relief of a distressing disease of the much-abused, unappreciated, though intelligent horse."

*Remarks.*—That but very few old horses which have long been in the habit of cribbing will be cured, is not probable, even with this treatment, which the author believes is most excellent; but that it will cure many colts of the dyspeptic tendency, and consequently prevent the establishment of the habit he as fully believes, if done with care and persevered in, as Dr. Tuttle above describes, for months, or as long as needed; for his plan is in accordance with the principles of treating persons, which is reliable. And what is good for a man is good for a horse.

**1. Big Head or Big Jaw of Horses—Preventive and Curative Treatment.**—Big head or big jaw proper is an enlargement and often a diseased and ulcerated condition of the bones, and treatment, unless taken early in the disease, seldom does much good; but for swellings of any of the fleshy parts proper treatment will cure, and may, if taken in time, prevent the bone difficulty.

I. Then as soon as swelling of any fleshy part of the head appears apply the following volatile liniment freely: Olive oil, 8 ozs.; hartshorn, 4 ozs.; mix, and shake when used. It is very stimulating and valuable for man or beast. Keep it well corked.

II. Apply a bran poultice, re-applying as long as necessary, always applying the liniment at each dressing.

III. If the difficulty has long existed, and there is considerable constitutional disturbance, as swellings or lumps in other parts, apply some good blistering liniment under the belly, well forward, to establish and maintain a running sore as long as the swellings or lumps continue, giving, also, one of the alterative condition powders daily in his feed, with such other treatment and care in his diet or feed as may be necessary to re-establish good general health.

IV. *The Eyes.*—The eyes in this disease, as well as other parts of the body, often become sore or swollen, or both. In such cases, make and use the following:

**Cooling Eye Water for Big Head, Swellings, Sprains, etc.**—Take a quart bottle and put into it pulverized, purified niter, ¼ lb.; and soft water, ½ pt.; and shake till dissolved; then fill with more soft water and cork for use. For the eye, dilute a little of this mixture with three times as much water, and wash the eyes two or three times daily. For swellings, sprains, etc., apply it as often, full strength.

V. *For Weak Eyes*, shown by their watering more or less freely apply the following:

**Eye Water.**—Acetate of lead, sulphate of zinc, and laudanum, each, ¼ oz.; soft water, 1 pt. If the eye is very weak, reduce some of this with an equal amount of water, and apply as the mixture above. A tea-spoonful of this put into a 1 oz. vial and filled with soft water, will be an excellent remedy for sore or weak eyes of persons. Either of these are as good for cattle as for horses.

**2. Big Jaw in Horses and Cattle, and Its Remedy.** — The *Live Stock Journal* speaks of this disease as follows: "This is more properly called 'dilation of the jaw bones.' In horses it is sometimes called 'big head;' it is a bony tumor, in which the interior of the bone is absorbed, sometimes leaving a mere shell of bone divided into cells containing purulent or thick matter. This is supposed to be caused by a deficiency of phosphate of lime in food, rendering the bones deficient in this most important element, and the following prescription is often given with good result:

"*Phosphate Powder.*—Phosphate of lime, 6 ozs.; powdered golden seal, 2 ozs.; powdered sassafrass, 3 ozs.; powdered ginger, 2 ozs.; oatmeal, 4 lbs.; mix. This will be divided into 16 parts, one given in the food every night.

"This will have a tendency to restore the missing elements in the bone. And the general diet should be food rich in phosphates. You may get your phosphate of lime by boiling beef bones in lye of wood ashes, and after it is reduced fine, wash with water and give a small quantity daily in food. The first thing to do surgically is to open it and let out any matter that it contains. Having removed the matter, inject the cavity with weak pyroligneous acid or weak carbolic acid. This will cleanse it and render healing possible."

*Remarks.*—I should prefer the pyroligneous acid to the carbolic, and 1 part of the acid to 3 of soft water would be weak enough to use at first; and afterwards 1 to 2, or even equal parts, to speed its healing. Both of these acids are disinfectant, *i. e.*, remove bad smells, as well as cleanse and heal, when used of proper strengths as above.

**3. Big Head in a Colt, and the Remedy**—"L. P. J.," of Benzonia, Benzie county, Michigan, May 27, 1880, wrote to the *Post and Tribune*, of Detroit, as to the condition of his colt, as follows:

"What ails the colt? In December I discovered a small lump or bunch coming on the left side of the face of my colt half way between the eye and the nostril. This grew larger until about the size of a man's fist. I then opened it with a knife. I had been using Centaur liniment and iodine and it had softened a little, but when opened it did not discharge and bled but little. I had also used beef brine. Almost immediately another bunch began to grow below this or back of it, and now the side of the face is badly swollen and the colt is falling away in flesh. He is 3 years old this spring."

To this their veterinarian, H. W. Doney, of Jackson, who had this department in charge, made the following answer:

"Big head. The disease is located on a line between the eye and the nostril. Its first appearance is a small lump on the side of the head, which continues to enlarge until the whole side of the face becomes swollen. It is on both sides sometimes. If your colt is very valuable, it will pay you to try a cure; if not, get what you can for it and do not bother with it.

"*Remedy.*—Take white arsenic the size of a common field pea, or 6 or 8 grs.; wrap it in fine paper as close as possible, make an incision in the skin over the hard tumor, insert the arsenic, or the paper containing it, take one stitch, tie the ends in a hard knot, bleed the horse, and turn him out. In a short time the horse will swell, and this will continue until the effects of the arsenic are exhausted. In a short time the effects of the arsenic will be seen. A circular piece of skin and the porous bone of the face will begin to slough off. In the course of time the diseased portion will drop out. leaving a healthy sore, which may be healed by an ointment made of elder and bittersweet fried in lard, with 1 oz. of turpentine."

*Remarks.*—A good-sized handful of each of these herbs to ½ lb. of lard and the 1 oz. of turpentine put in when taken from the fire, would be about the right proportion, and it will make a very healing ointment for any sore whatever. I now leave every one to adopt the plan of treatment in their stock, horses or cattle, here given, according to their condition, each judging for himself which plan or medicines will be the best to meet their respective cases, being careful to look well to the general health in every case. In connection with the arsenic treatment, given in this receipt, I should also use the Phosphate Powder, in the next above, as it is both alterative and tonic.

**1. Bots in Horses, A New Remedy Worth its weight in Gold.**—The department of agriculture publishes the following experiments, which a gentleman from Georgia tried and found effective in dispelling serious trouble in horses. He says: "About 30 years ago a friend lost, by bots, a very fine horse. He took from the stomach of the dead horse about a gill of bots and brought them to my office to experiment upon. He made preparations of every remedy he heard of, and put some of them into each. Most had no effect, a few effected them slightly, but sage tea, more than anything else; that killed them in fifteen hours.

He concluded that he would kill them by putting them into nitric acid, but it had no more effect on them than water; the third day they were as lively as when put in. A bunch of tansy was growing by my office. He took a handful of that, bruised it, added a little water, squeezed out the juice and put some bots into it. They were dead in one minute! Since then I have had it given to every horse. I have never known it to fail of giving entire relief. My friend had another horse affected with the bots, cured by this remedy.—*Grange Visitor.* Springfield, O., Nov. 1875.

*Remarks.*—I have had no opportunity of testing this, but I give it, believing it is reliable. Is it not possible that it was because tansy would kill worms, that tansy bitters were once so common and popular? I believe it was.

Drenching a horse with sweetened milk following it, half hour later, with strong sage tea then working it off with currier's oil, has been, heretofore, considered the best known remedy for bots; but it is probable that a strong tea of tansy may be found a much better remedy than the sage, used similarly, 1 pt. each, in the order above named, a half hour apart, only.

**Tansy Tea for Bots.**—There is undoubtedly more in the virtues of tansy for bots, than appears upon the face of it; for the following item has been more recently going the rounds of the papers: "Tansy tea is said to be a sure remedy for bots in horses. Experiments tried upon bots show that while they resist the action of almost every other substance, they are quickly killed by tansy. It is an easy matter to test it, by those who keep horses, when some of the bots have been passed, by putting them into some of the extracted juice of the tansy leaves.

**Bots, their Manner of Production and How to Avoid them.**—It will not be amiss to state here, that bots do not, as many suppose, breed in the stomach of the horse, but simply grow there from the egg which is deposited on the flanks and legs by the bot-fly, in their season, which is from July to October, during which time if an oiled rag is kept in the stables, and used upon the legs and sides of horses, as regularly as they are fed, with much rubbing, also with straw, which takes the nits off better than a brush; these nits or eggs will be mostly rubbed off, and consequently the horse will get but few, if any, into his mouth by licking or biting these parts, to be swallowed into the stomach, in which, if they reach it in this way, and this is the only way they do, or can reach it, the bot will be produced, and fully grown by spring, at which time also, they begin to let go their hold on the stomach. They hang to the stomach by little hooks upon their feet, and are carried on by the food passed off; and again develop, as the butterfly is produced from a grub, as it were, another gad-fly; and so on from year to year.

Be careful, then, to use the oiled rag freely, and scrape off, if need be, as many as possible of these nits, or bot seeds, every day, as they are deposited, and you will have but little trouble with bots; and in fact bots never make trouble, except there be indigestion or other disease, which first disturbs them.

During the fly season, also, if not at all times, the hair on the back part of the legs should be kept closely trimmed, as the rubbing off is easier upon short hair than that which is long and loose; and the shorter the hair the less deposits upon it can be made.

**1. COLIC, OR BOTS, IN HORSES—To Cure.**—A friend of mine near Ann Arbor, makes the following his dependence. He says: Steep 1 doz. good sized red peppers in 1 qt. of water; strain and give the whole, while warm. Work off, in an hour, with 1 pt. of currier's oil.

*Remarks.*—He said it can be depended upon—neither colic nor bots can stand before it, and it will not hurt the horse nor cattle either. This gentleman assured me he had used it, and knew its exceeding value, but did not wish to have his name connected with it—contrary to the desire of most people. I have every confidence in it, for I knew him well—being a very quiet and diffident, or bashful man; and hence I promised him not to publish his name. Red or cayenne pepper is the purest stimulant we have, and hence I have not a doubt it will do as he assured me it would. As it will warm up the stomach to do its work, and prevent the further accumulation of gas, or wind, from the indigestion, and thus cure colic and give bots a legal notice to vacate the premises.

**2. Colic in Horses—Its Cause and What is Needed to Cure It.** As colic is caused by the indigestion of the food, a sour or gaseous stomach, as we say of persons, all that is needed to cure it is something to correct the acidity and to warm up the stomach, so that the digestion can proceed again; but as the indigestion and consequent acidity may have progressed so far it cannot be corrected, making it necessary to give an active cathartic to hasten the fermenting food out of the system, it is well at first to give a full table-spoonful of saleratus dissolved in warm water, ½ pt.; then, if you are where the pepper tea can be steeped at once, give it; but 'tis well to have something of an anodyne nature to help allay the pain, as well as to stimulate, which can be kept in the stable, always ready for use, like the following: Laudanum, sulphuric ether, chloroform, tinct. of cayenne pepper and ess. of peppermint, each, 1 oz.: tinct. of belladonna, ½ oz. Mix. Dose—For a full-sized horse, give 1 table-spoonful in warm water, ½ pt., and repeat in 30 minutes, if not before relieved; or, put the pepper to steeping at once on giving the first dose of this, and if not relieved in 30 minutes give the pepper tea, as in No. 1, above, instead of repeating this, would be preferable. But, if no peppers are at hand, repeat this as above without fear of injury. For I know that a dozen drops of chloroform in a spoonful of water has relieved gaseous dyspepsia of persons, while this mixture has several other things in it making it more reliable in colic of horses and would be good for persons in doses of ½ tea-spoonful, repeated once or twice only, if not relieved in the ½ hour.

II. In the meantime, if there is great distention of the bowels by gas, which is almost always the case in colic, do not overlook the importance of giving, or having given, the table-spoonful of saleratus dissolved in water, ½ pt., to stop the fermentation of the food, which causes this gaseous condition; and also to have got ready a physic containing ½ to ¾ oz. of aloes dissolved in ½ pt. of water, in which you have put another table-spoonful of saleratus to make it dissolve, so it shall be quicker in its operation to carry off this fermenting food.

III. If very great pain still exists, or does exist at any time, even as much as 2 ozs of laudanum has been given, so also has 2 ozs. of ess. of pepperment, or 1 oz. of sulphuric ether, or ½ oz. of chloroform, or ½ oz. of hartshorn, in ½ pt. or 1 pt. of warm water, has and may be given; the laudanum to stop the pain, the others more to stop the fermentation, and consequent distention of the stomach and bowels by the gas. Sometimes this gas is aided to pass off by the rectum by giving warm water injections, turning the horse's head down hill and pumping in freely all the bowels will retain, even if it is a bucketful will do no harm, but by its wetting and softening influence aids the escape of gas and also the quicker action of the physic, if one has been given. If the gas is once started freely by the rectum consider your horse safe.

IV. But, lastly, in no case allow the cruel custom of taking the horse out and running him, nor even trotting him, nor "rub his belly with a chestnut rail," nor the wicked and cruel custom of laying him on his side and getting a big heavy man with coarse boots to walk back and forth upon him. Some of the mixtures to relieve pain and stop the accumulation of the gas, then physic, and injections, if needed, to start the gas off, must be the main dependence. And, I will only add, if you now allow your horses to die with colic it is not the author's fault, but will be chargeable to yourselves by neglecting to have a supply on hand of what is liable to be needed any day.

**Corns, or Shoe Boil of Horses' Feet, Explanation of and Remedy.**—Corns, also called shoe boils, are generally the result of bad shoeing, *i. e.*, allowing the heel of the shoe to rest too far in, upon the sole of the horse's foot. They should have their bearing upon the shell, or solid, outer part of the hoof; then there will be but few corns. But when they exist, the soft and diseased part of the sole must be cut away, to allow the application of the following remedy: Sulphuric acid, 1 oz.; nitro-muriatic acid, ½ oz.; corrosive sublimate, 1 dr. DIRECTIONS—Add, little by little, of one acid to the other, in an earthen bowl, in the open air, to avoid breathing the fumes arising from them in mixing. Mash the corrosive sublimate finely and add it to the acids. Then, having pared and trimmed down to the sore, apply the remedy with a swab, or pledget of lint and bind on till the corrosion or destruction of the hoof is stopped; then apply a soft healing ointment.

*Remarks.*—This is from my old friend Wallington, a farrier of long practice, which ought to be an assurance of its value; but knowing the nature of the preparation, I can assure anyone it will be found just the thing desired. Do not get it or either of the acids on hands or clothing.

**CONDITION POWDERS—Tonic and Purifying to the Blood.** —Sulphur, 6 ozs.; gentian root, sassafras, bark of the root, elecampane root, ginger root, saltpeter and rosin, each 2 ozs.; digitalis leaves, buchu leaves, blood root, skunk cabbage root, cream of tartar, epsom salts, black antimony, fenugreek seed, and rust, or carbonate of iron, each 1 oz. DIRECTIONS—Pulverize finely, mix thoroughly, and keep in air-tight boxes. DOSE—give 1 tablespoonful in feed, as below.

*Remarks.*—In spring and fall use with all stock, as well as horses, 1 tablespoonful daily, in a bran-mash, until you see its beneficial action, or for 2 weeks; but in case of a horse, cow or ox, being in bad health, at any time of year, the same dose twice daily, in a bran-mash, may be given for a couple of weeks, or until the desired result—good health—is obtained. Some horses will not, however, eat bran-mashes, then stir it in wetted oats. This is especially valuable in all the chronic diseases, as mange, distemper, grease-heel, big-head, big-leg, poll evil, fistulas, yellow water, etc. It will show its beneficial effects very quickly.

**2. Condition Powder, Relaxing, for Use in Scratches, Grease Heel, etc.**—The following was published in the *Post and Tribune*, by H. W. Doney, of Jackson, Mich., in answer to an inquiry of "J. W.," of Paw Paw, for a condition powder to cleanse the blood, in spring, adding, "I have got 1 horse that has had scratches most of the time for 3 years, and I have doctored her most of the time." Mr. Doney, in answering, says:

I. "You have a number of them already given, but here is one for the special purpose: Mandrake, aloes, epsom salts, gentian, blood root, skunk cabbage, gum myrrh, golden seal, stillingia, each 2 ozs.: sulphur, licorice root, ginger root and coriander seeds, each 4 ozs.; nitre and lobelia, each 3 ozs.; camphor gum and copperas, each 1 oz. Powder and mix thoroughly. DOSE—One-half ounce (about 1 table-spoonful) once a day, in feed or drench. To aid the operation and produce better results, give 1 pt. of sassafras tea (daily). If fever is present, give 15 drops of aconite (tinct. or fl. ex.), once a day. If paralysis in any form exists, give 15 drops of belladonna (tinct. or fl. oz.) once a day; or if nerve power is lacking, give 15 drops nux vomica (tinct. or fl. ex.), once a day." [These last medicines are poisonous, if used too much, or too often.]

II.  *Physic, or Purge.*—Mr. Doney continues:  "Give a good purge made of fluid extract of mandrake, blood root, liquorice, each 1 oz.  Dose, 1 dr. Adding to each dose 1 oz. of aloes and 2 ozs. of epsom salts until the bowels respond freely; then lessen the dose.

"II.  *Wash.*—One oz. of white vitriol, 1 oz. of alum, 1 oz. gum catechu, 1 qt. of oak bark solution, 1 oz. turpentine.  Mix and use as a wash twice a day. Take the water in which you boil potatoes, 1 qt.  Wash the limb with it before using the other.  If it will not cleanse the limb thoroughly use oat meal soap. Rub the limb until the sore looks a bright pink, and the surrounding portions of the leg white.  Keep the stable well cleaned.  Use a brush on the leg often."

**3.  Condition Powder for a Stallion.**—White rosin and madder, each, 4 ozs.;  black antimony gentian root, fenugreek seed, sulphur and ginger root, each, 3 ozs.;  anise seed, 2 ozs.;  Spanish flies, 1 oz.  All made very fine and intimately mixed.  DOSE—A table-spoonful, a little rounding, in the morning's feed, as he begins to drag toward the last of the season.  This is from Robt. Hudson, Winfield, Kansas.  No one need fear to use it.  And without the Spanish flies, it is a good alterative and tonic powder for any other horse.

**Distemper in Colts—Treatment.**—Distemper in a colt has about 3 weeks to run its course; all the medicine required is a light dose of Epsom salts, say 4 to 6 ozs., and good nursing.  Give warm bran mashes, linseed or oatmeal gruel; keep the animal warm, and rub the legs with cloths dipped in hot water; a table-spoonful of mustard in the water would be beneficial if the legs seem to be weak and numb, or cold.—*N. Y. Times.*

**Epizootic, the Most Successful Treatment.**—Wm. Horne, a veterinary, in the *Country Gentleman,* says:  "In the treatment of the epizootic in horses, in 1872, no treatment in my own practice was so effectual, and none brought speedier or more permanent relief than a powerful stimulant applied to the throat outside, and tincture of lobelia, 1 oz.; gelsemium, ½ oz.  Mix and place on the roots of the tongue, 30 to 40 drops, 3 times a day.  Plenty of pure air and general warmth, and comfort, make good nursing; not too much pampering and medication.

*Remarks.*—The Sweeny Cure, which is a powerful liniment, and without the alcohol, will be as powerful a stimulant as anyone will need in these cases.  It is not necessary to blister, however, if it is likely to do that; rub over with sweet oil to prevent the blistering.  Or, if made without the cantharides, it will not blister.  The lobelia helps the cough, and the gelsemium keeps down the fever by lessening the pulse.  This is claimed to be a bad disease; then use the condition powder No. 1, in connection with the other treatment.

**Galled Shoulders and Saddle Galls, To Prevent and Cure.**— I.  To prevent shoulder galls for horses easily galled, have a collar shield of firm, smooth-surfaced leather, upon which the collar will move or slip easily, and thus not abrade or chafe off the surface hair, skin, etc.; and have the saddle lined with hard, smooth-surfaced leather—rawhide is best—like the military saddle, but never have one lined with any woolen stuff.

II. *To Cure.*—Wash with soap suds, and apply the following solution: Copperas, 1 dr., and blue vitrol, ½ dr., in water, 1 pt., which will reduce inflammation, harden the surface, and aid the growth of new skin, if broken. Never put on the saddle nor the harness while the place is wet from the application.

**Grease Heel.**—[See Scratches, Grease, etc.]

**Heaves or "Windbroken,"—Necessary Caution in Feeding, and Cure for Many.**—"Heaves and windbroken are one and the same disease, the first being used to designate its mildest form; and the latter when it reaches its severest stages. It is in reality a kind of asthma caused by over-feeding on clover hay, chaff, and other coarse, bulky and dusty fodder. The disease is seldom known where horses are pastured all the year, and clover in some of its species does not enter into the hay crop. If the horse has not had the heaves so long as to be wholly beyond help, try feeding on corn stalks, cut moist hay, with carrots, beets, turnips, potatoes, and other well known nutritious roots. Keep the bowels open by laxative medicines, and for a tonic give arsenic in 3 gr. doses for 2 or 3 weeks. Give the animal no dry hay, except a little handful at night; and if you have good, well cured corn stalks, these will suffice, with plenty of roots and cut hay (wet), with grain 3 times a day."—*New York Sun.*

*Remarks.*—There are some veterinarians who claim that the air cells, or some of them, are ruptured; when this is actually the case, there is probably no cure; but before this has occurred, it has been claimed by M. Hew, a French veterinarian, I think, that 15 grs. of arsenic, daily, for 2 or 3 weeks, as McClure and Harvey, in their work on the horse, inform us, "with green food or straw, and in some cases bleeding, was perfectly successful," in ten reported cases. In one it returned after 3 months, which "speedily yielded to a repetition of the same treatment." The way to give it would be to sprinkle it in fine powder on a few thoroughly chopped roots, 5 grs., morning, noon and night. There would be no danger in its use, stopping at the end of 2 or 3 weeks, or when the difficulty has been fairly overcome.

**INFLAMMATION OF THE BLADDER—Cause, Symptoms and Treatment.**—*Cause.*—A correspondent of the *Blade*, of Watertown, N. Y., says: "It is often caused by the abuse of diuretics, and the frequent use of rosin, with the idea that it loosens the skin and improves the appetite, too often results in this trouble.

*Symptoms.*—"The symptoms are the passage of the urine in small quantities, and frequently, with evident pain. The animal turns and looks at the flank; the hind legs are restless, and the tail is switched about violently, but chiefly downward. The horse moves stiffly, and with a straddling gait of the hind legs.

*Treatment.*—"No diuretics should be given, but soft, mucilaginous food, such as linseed (flaxseed) and oats boiled (½ pt. to 1 pt. would be enough to boil in a feed of oats), and given with cut hay and slippery elm bark tea. This will relieve the organ better than medicines. After the inflammation has subsided and the symptoms have been relieved, 1 dr. of chlorate of potash may be given daily for 2 weeks in the food, which should be continued as before for a few days."

*Remarks.*—The author would prefer the use of acetate of potash, rather than the chlorate, in like amount. The chlorate can be powdered and put in the feed; 1 oz. of acetate would have to be put in a bottle with 8 table-spoonfuls of water, as it softens very quickly in the air; then 1 table-spoonful contains 1 dr. Put it in the food or drink. as you choose.

**Liniments, Oils, Salves, etc., for Horses.**—I. *California Liniment.*—"Opodeldoc, spirits of turpentine, oil of origanum and black oil, each, 2 ozs.; gum camphor and red pepper, each, ½ oz.; aqua ammonia, 1 oz.; best alcohol, 1 qt. Mix and keep well corked. Good in all acute pain, rheumatism, sprains, and swellings in man or beast."

*Remarks.*—This, with the Black Oil, White Oil, Gargling Oil, and the Green Salve following, and the Condition Powders for Stallions, were obtained from the diary of Robert Hudson, of Winfield, Kans., who had spent considerable time in California, where he obtained them from practical horsemen; and from my own knowledge of the nature of the articles used, I am free to say one will search a long time to find others equal to them:

II. *New York Sun's Liniment.*—The New York *Sun* says: "Of liniments there are as many different compounds as of condition powders; but a good one for horses and other animals may be made of 2 ozs. each of oils of spike, origanum and wormwood, spirits of ammonia and spirits of turpentine; then sweet oil, 4 ozs., and best alcohol, 1 qt. Mixed and kept in a bottle, corked when not in use."

*Remarks.*—It is a good one for general purposes. See, also, "Sweeny Cure," which is a liniment.

III. *Black Oil.*—British oil, oil of spike (balsam of fir), tanners' oil, tamarack balsam and oil of vitriol, each, 1 oz.; spirits of turpentine, 2 ozs. Mix in the order named, putting in the oil of vitriol slowly, and when cool the spirits of turpentine. Better be in a quart bottte. Very healing, and to reduce inflammations by rubbing in or laying on with wet cloths or soft paper on either man or other animal.

IV. *White Oil, English.*—Spirits of turpentine and alcohol, ½ pt.; olive oil, 1 pt.; hartshorn, 4 ozs.; camphor gum, 4 ozs. Mix. Used especially in wounds and upon old sores.

V. *Gargling Oil.*—White wine vinegar (good cider vinegar will do), 1 pt.; spirits of turpentine and sweet oil, each, ½ pt.; oil of vitriol, 1 oz.; castile soap and saltpeter, each, 2 ozs. DIRECTIONS—Shave the soap fine, pulverize the saltpeter and shake occasionally till dissolved, when it is ready to use upon swellings, wounds, frostbites, etc., on horses or cattle, and it has been used extensively on persons.

VI. *Green Salve.*—Spirits of turpentine, 4 ozs.; beeswax, rosin and honey, each, 2 ozs.; lard, 12 ozs.; finely pulverized verdigris, 1 oz. DIRECTIONS—Heat all gently together, except the verdigris, then remove from the fire and stir that in as it begins to cool, and stir till cold. Put in tix boxes for use.

*Remarks.*—Used upon old sores, cuts and wounds, and Mr. Hudson, named under the California Liniment, says it was considered there "the best salve known."

**Mange in Horses, Remedy.**—Wilkes' *Spirit of the Times* published the following as a safe and effectual remedy: "Whale (sperm) oil, 6 ozs.; oil of tar, 3 ozs.; lac-sulphur, 2 ozs.; mix thoroughly and apply with a hair brush, first washing the skin thoroughly. And at the end of the second or third day, the animal is to be again washed, and the remedy re-applied; as it is very probable that all the ova (eggs) of the mange (or itch) insect are not killed by the first application.

*Remarks.*—As mange is as contagious with animals as itch is with children, keep them from others; and be careful also to purify the stalls, or places where they may rub; and the harness, or saddles, or such parts of them as come in contact with the diseased parts of the animal, should be washed with strong soap suds having 1 part of carbolic acid (liquid) to 6 or 7 of the suds, and care-fully dried and aired, and the blanket, if any has been worn, should be boiled in soap suds, with 1 oz. of the carbolic acid, at least, to 1 pail of suds; and the curry comb, brush, etc., washed in the same while hot; and afterwards wet with a solution of arsenic, or corrosive sublimate, 10 grs., to each ounce of water needed, to wet them thoroughly; for it is very difficult to kill all the itch or mange-mites which cause the disease. Rub well with sulphur, also, the saddle, and inside the harness, before again putting upon the horses. With these cautions you may feel safe. See also the preparation for mange in dogs. It is certain there, why not with horses? I think it would be. If there are any scabs on harness, or saddle, be careful to first remove them. And I think it advisable not to let the mites upon one's hands, lest he, too, get the itch. Remember the sublimate is poison, as well as the arsenic, so keep either out of the way of children.

**1. Poll-Evil, Fistula, etc., Successful Remedies.**—Poll-evil simply means a disease of the head, as the word "poll" comes from the Low Dutch polle, the head, and as the word evil, in connection with disease, signifies one causing suffering, we get poll-evil, a disease of the horse's head from which there is much suffering. As to *fistula*, it is a Latin word and signifies a hollow seed, or pipe; hence, where we have a hollow pipe, running down into a sore, it matters not whether upon the head or the withers (highest part of the shoulders), of a horse it is really a fistula or a fistulous sore; and, as what will destroy the pipe which runs down to the bone, in one case, will destroy it in the other, we couple them together.

When either has become a running sore, you will find the following recipe from the *Germantown Telegraph*, very satisfactory, as I have always observed the reliability of its recommendations. It says: "First, clean the sore with warm, soft water, and dry with soft, warm cloths; then drop on 8 or 10 drops of muriatic acid twice daily, till it looks like a fresh wound; after this, wash with suds of castile soap, and leave it to heal, which it will speedily do, if enough acid has been used.

*Remarks.*—If a pipe or pipes have already formed, be sure to drop a few drops of the acid into each pipe, else it will be sure to break out again if the pipe is not destroyed.  Do not touch the acid with the fingers, nor get it upon any place outside of the sore, for if you do, it will make a sore of itself, destroy clothing, etc.  An alkali, as a lye made of wood ashes, or sweet-oil would be the antidote, and would need to be used quickly, if got upon the person or clothing.  Any of the healing ointments or liniments may be used to heal with, keeping the sore properly covered to avoid dust and dirt getting into it.

A bit of concentrated lye, which is used for soap-making, the size of a bean or pea, wrapped in a couple of thicknesses of tissue paper (white) and pushed to the bottom of the pipe, or each pipe, if there is more than one, will destroy the life of the pipe, and, hence, cause it to come out, and give a chance to cure it from the bottom.  Keep a piece of cotton saturated with a good liniment or healing ointment, pushed to the depth of the sore, it causes it to heal from the bottom, otherwise it will break out again.  The concentrated lye is better than arsenic or corrosive sublimate which are poisonous, and cause inflammation of themselves, while the concentrated lye does not cause inflammation of the parts, only to kill the unnatural growth.  The *Telegraph* claimed to have known the successful use of the acid plan for a number of years.  The acid on the sore, and the lye in the pipes, if there are any, with cathartics and general tonic treatment with some of the condition powders, will cure every case, the author has not a doubt.

**Pawing in the Stable, to Cure Horses of the Habit.**—Fasten a short piece of log chain—say five or six links—by means of a light strap to his leg, just above the knee—in the stable, of course—so the chain stays on the front of the leg, and see how quick the pawing horse will leave off the habit. In most cases a few days will be sufficient to effect a cure.—*New York Weekly,*

**Pawing, Cure for.**—It is said that this annoying habit can be cured in the following manner:  Bore a hole on each side of the stall a little in front of where the foreleg stands.  Insert a raw-hide, wedge tightly in, and allow the ends to reach well out toward the center of the stall.  When the horse paws he will catch the rawhide with the foot with which he paws, and in fetching back the foot the cord of the rawhide hits him on the other foot.  A few experiments will convince the horse that pawing with one foot always causes punishment on the other, and soon the annoying habit is cured.

**1.  Ringbone, Spavins, etc.—Certain Remedies.**—*Ringbone.*—Ringbone and spavins, poll-evil and fistulas are the most annoying diseases with which our domestic animals are afflicted; but with careful observation of the recipes the author has gathered during ten years of close scrutiny of everything published in our most reliable farm journals, will, we have not a doubt, enable our patrons to not only cure the lameness, but also to remove or cause the absorption of the bony enlargements in most ringbones and spavins, and to also cure the unsightly sores of poll-evil and fistulas.  The first recipe I shall give for ringbone is from a correspondent (" J.H.M., of Wyoming, O.) in *Farm and Fireside*, of Springfield, O., in answer to " S. F. W." in the same, desiring a cure for this disease, which, if followed, he says, will never fail: "Take cantharides (of course, powdered), 2 ozs.; mercurial ointment or spirits of turpentine, each, 4 ozs.; tinct. of iodine, 5 ozs.; corrosive sublimate (powdered), 5 drs. Mix well with lard, 2 lbs. DIRECTIONS—Cut off the hair from the lump and grease with and rub in well the above preparation. In two days after grease with fresh lard, and in 4 days wash off with soap suds. Repeat every 4 days until the lump disappears. I have cured two cases of ten years' standing."

2. **Ringbone and Spavin Cure.**—In the same issue of the *Farm and Fireside* "O. H. L.," which I afterwards learned, by correspondence with the editor, to be the initials of O. H. Loomis, of Kewanee, Ill., says:

"MR. EDITOR:—I see in your excellent paper now before me an inquiry about 'ringbone' on colts. Allow me to say that over thirty years since, having a horse with bone spavin, I obtained, from an English farrier, this recipe, which he said would stop the growing of the spavin and also cure ringbone. I tried it on my horse with success. I afterwards gave it to a friend with a colt which had a ringbone, and it cured it, and within the last year I had a young horse with ringbone growing so badly as to render him useless. I had the medicine applied and it checked the growth, removed the lameness, and the horse has done a fine summer's work, apparently cured of ringbone. The recipe is this: Equal parts oil origanum, tinct. myrrh and corrosive sublimate. Used as a liniment, carefully, as it is severe but effective."

*Remarks.*—The amount of corrosive sublimate not being given in this recipe, only to be equal with the origanum oil and tinct. of myrrh, led to the correspondence, which I shall give below, after having given what I consider to be a proper amount of the corrosive sublimate, not only in my own judgment, but I have also consulted one of our most reliable chemists and druggists in the city of Toledo of over 25 years practical experience, and he thinks with me that to dissolve 1 dr. of the corrosive sublimate in 1 oz. of best alcohol will be the right amount, and mix with 1 oz. each of the oil of origanum and tinct. of myrrh. But if the best re-sublimed iodine, 1 dr., is added to the oz. of alcohol with the corrosive sublimate it will be all the better and more certain for it. To apply, follow the same plan as directed in No. 1 above, and remember it is as good for spavins as for ringbones. Label it "Poison," and keep it out of the way of children. This recipe, as first published, led some of the subscribers of the *Farm and Fireside* to inquire of the editor to obtain further instruction as to the amount of the corrosive sublimate intended, and this led the editor to write "O. H. L." (Mr. Loomis, as above explained), and he said in answer: "The last time the druggist had the tincture already prepared, It is very strong—will take the hair off when applied—but it does the work. I have just returned from Kansas, where the horse is that I had it used upon last. He is well. The ringbone does not show only to a careful observer; has been worked hard all summer When the remedy was first applied he could not trot —could hardly walk, and was pronounced worthless by horsemen. I do not think there is any danger in using the remedy, if careful." So it will be seen that our plan of the tinct., 1 dr. of the corrosive sublimate to 1 oz. of alcohol, is the true plan; adding, also, 1 dr. of iodine, in crystal, to the same will improve it and cure without a doubt. Still, I cannot see why a man who desires to do good to his fellow-men should give only his initials instead of his full name; for everybody knows that the name carries more than double weight that any man's initials will do. I trust I shall not offend Mr. Loomis by having given his name without asking his permission. If I have, I beg his pardon, my excuse being a desire to do the greatest good by giving the greater faith or confidence in his recipe, which I know is good.

**4. Spavin, to Cure the Lameness.**— Iodide of mercury, 2 drs.; lard, 2 ozs. Rub well upon the enlargement; repeat in 2 weeks, or when the new hair has started out; and so continue till the lameness is cured.—*Dr. Horne, in Michigan Farmer.*

*Remarks.*—He does not claim that it will remove the bony enlargement; but I think upon a recent case and a young horse, it will cause its final absorption. (See Fleshy Tumors on Cows and Calves). It is from the same veterinarian. If the same amount of corrosive sublimate were put in, it will be likely to cause the absorption of the bony enlargement, as well as to cure the lameness.

**5. Ringbone and Spavin Cure.**—Powdered cantharides, powdered or finely shaved castile soap, rosin broken up finely, tinct. of iodine, and laudanum, each, 2 ozs.; mercurial ointment, 5 ozs.; pulverized white vitriol (sulphate of zinc), $\frac{1}{2}$ oz.; oil of origanum, camphor gum, and Venice turpentine, each, 1 oz.; pulverized corrosive sublimate, $\frac{1}{2}$ oz.; lard, 2 lbs. DIRECTIONS— Melt the lard and stir in the mercurial ointment and rosin, stirring until these are also melted; then add the powders, mixing well; then add the others, and stir till cold. For ringbone or spavin, clip off the hair, and rub in the ointment well with a wooden spatula, or the heel of the hand; after two days, oil the place with sweet oil (lard will do), and in two days more wash the place with soap and water, and rub in the ointment again, as at first, and so repeat till the bone enlargement is all gone.

*Remarks.*—A nephew of mine, Wm. J. Call, of Gaylord, Mich., of whom I obtained this recipe, told me he had cured ringbones with it satisfactorily. If it will cure ringbones, it will also cure spavins. Keep the same proportions if you wish to make less. Remembering it will be better if the tincture of iodine is made double the usual strength by adding $\frac{1}{2}$ dr. more to each ounce used. With the foregoing variety of ringbone and spavin cures, with the following one for wind-galls or bag-spavins, no one need long keep a horse with these blemishes upon him.

**6. Ringbones and Spavins, Ointment for.**—A farrier living near Toledo uses the following ointment for these purposes, which will be found good, used the same as the other applications, cutting off the hair, greasing, washing off, re-applying, etc., with care. "Bin-iodide of mercury, iodine, corrosive sublimate, and cantharides, all powdered, and mixed into cosmoline 4 ozs."

*Remarks.*—None of these preparations should be applied in winter, unless the animal can remain in stable, and be secured so his mouth can not reach the place, and to avoid cold, snow, etc.

**7. Ringbone, California Cure.**—In February, 1883, I received a letter from a Mr. W. J. McClane, of Oakland, Cal., who said: "I am, and have been for the past 21 years, engaged in stock raising on an extremely large scale," etc. The correspondence arising from the fact of his having recently purchased a copy of my "Second Receipt Book," of which he spoke very highly, especially on the subject of making and keeping butter; and he continues: "Hoping to hear of a third volume, in the course of time, I herewith send you a few recipes, which we Californians have used and greatly rely upon.

I. "*To Cure Ringbone.*—Take a piece of soft lead pipe, or round bar about ½ inch in diameter (a common bar of lead, the author is sure, will do as well as anything, putting the round side next to the foot), and long enough to extend around the fetlock, above the enlargement. Bind the ends well with copper wire, sufficiently tight to let the lead bear upon the upper part of the ringbone quite loosely. The weight of the lead and the healing qualities therein will in a few weeks remove any ringbone. I have removed two from a horse in six weeks which were of two years' growth."

*Remarks.*—I had heard of such a proceeding before, but not so distinctively as to feel assured in giving it. Now I have not a doubt of its practicability.

II. "*Warts on Stock, to Remove.*—This gentleman's cure for warts was to saturate every morning with the milk of a milk-thistle, found in grain fields; or saturate a few times with a solution of corrosive sublimate."

*Remarks.*—Proper strength of this would be ½ dr. to 1 oz. of alcohol. He added, "This is very poisonous," which is correct. The author has seen it stated by a stock-keeper that for many years he had cured warts on horses and cattle by putting on a good daub of tar such as wagons are greased with.

III. "*Hair on Galls, to Restore.*—Make the spot or part sore if not already so, and heal it by rubbing it every morning with smoked bacon in the raw state.

IV. "*Branding, to Deface.*—Create a sore, and apply the raw bacon grease, as above."

*Remarks.*—A sore may be made with any of the blistering liniments. See Horseman's Hope Liniment, among the Sweeny cures, and the pain killer with the pennyroyal in it. They are both from the same gentleman, and will be found very valuable. He will please accept the author's thanks for his interest in the welfare of man and the animal kind, by his contribution to the doctor's "Third and Last Receipt Book."

**8. Spavins, Blood or Bag (Wind Galls), Thoroughpins, Splints, etc., Permanent Cure for.**—Very strong vinegar, 1 pt.; aqua fortis (nitric acid), spirits of turpentine, and best alcohol, each 1 oz.; mix. DIRECTIONS—Bathe freely, rubbing hard. Rub downward until you cause quite a heat in the leg. It will not cause any blister, whatever, and before you realize it, it will disappear. It has been over 2 years since I cured my mare, referred to below, and she is as good as ever to-day. Bathe 3 or 4 times a day, rubbing hard every time. It seems a very simple recipe, but I can warrant it a good one.—*B. F. Chamberlin, of Rich, Lapeer county, Mich., in Detroit Post and Tribune, Dec. 1880;* to which he added:

"It effects a permanent cure. I have tested it on my own horse, also on others. I have a mare which had 2 spavins, 1 on each hind leg; also 2 thoroughpins came with them. I tried several kinds of medicine with no effect, until I got this recipe. The spavins (wind galls) were as large as a pint bowl. I considered her almost worthless, she being a very small horse; but I not only cured her lameness, but caused the enlargement to disappear entirely in 3 weeks. You would not know to-day that she ever had a spavin."

*Remarks.*—Certainly testimony as large as a pint bowl is all that may be demanded, for I never saw one of these wind-galls, or puffy lumps, larger than half a hen's egg—this was an extreme case—and so much the more satisfactory for those who may need to try it, so I give his own words of assurance. A thoroughpin is the same as a bag-spavin, or wind-gall, as they are also called, except it extends along a tendon up and down the leg, rather than in a lump, or puff—treatment the same. If it is ever found necessary to blister any of these wind-galls, as they are more often called, use No. 3, above, which contains all that is required for the longest standing cases, even for curbs, on the back of the leg, or splints. If not applied too long, and well greased with raw, fat bacon, the hair will come out again. (See Hair on Galls, to Restore, above.)

**9. Splints, Ointment for.**—Bin-iodide of mercury, 1 dr.; powdered cantharides, 2 drs.; and lard, ½ oz.; mix evenly into an ointment. DIREC-TIONS—Shear off the hair from the enlargement, and rub in the ointment 15 minutes. The third day after apply sweet oil, lard oil, or lard, to soften and aid in removing the scab. The horse, or colt, must not be allowed to get at the sore with his mouth. Continue until cured.

*Remarks.*—The bin-iodide and cantharides in this case, and all the blistering, and applications of strong liniments, act as a counter-irritant to the *periosteum* (the membrane covering all bones), or the membraneous sheath of the tendons, which are inflamed, in these diseases, and also stimulates the parts to an increased healthy action, by which the cure is effected. The cutting off of the hair is to prevent too thick a scab, which cannot be removed so easily.

**SWEENY—Liniment, Oils, and Other Cures for.**—Webster gives us no such word; but it is well understood by horsemen, to refer to a shrinkage of the muscles over the shoulder-blade of the horse, with a tightening down of the skin to the shrunken condition of the muscles. If it was upon a person, physicians would say the muscles were *atrophied*, from lack of nourishment; then what will stimulate them to a healthy action, so that they shall receive their proper share of nutrition, will soon cure the difficulty; hence, the propriety of using some of the following liniments, or oils, upon the affected shoulder. And first I will give one from a Kansas stage driver, which he called:

**1. Sweeny Cure.**—Oil of origanum, 4 ozs.; oil of spike, 2 ozs.; oil of hemlock, tinct. of cantharides, spirits of turpentine and camphor gum, each 1 oz,; mix and keep corked. DIRECTIONS—Rub on well, once daily, lifting the skin well at first. Two to three weeks will cure bad cases. It will blister. But if it gets too sore miss a few applications, or rub over with sweet oil (lard will do), after applying.

*Remarks.*—This was given me by a stage driver, over whose route I passed, April 20, 1876, from Wichita (Wich-e-taw) to Winfield, Kan., assuring me he had cured many bad cases with it. The above, without cantharides, put into 1 qt. of alcohol, will make a splendid liniment for man or beast, for general pur-poses. Next I will give you the one spoken of in No. 7, of ringbones, Califor-nia cure, which see.

**2. Horseman's Hope Liniment—A Cure for Sweeny ("Cali-fornian").**—I will give it in his own words: "Ninety-eight per cent. alcohol, 1 qt.; 4 ozs. origanum oil, of best quality; 2 ozs. hemlock oil, pure; 2 ozs. sas-safras oil, pure; add the oils and stand till cut (they will cut, or dissolve, by shaking, immediately); then add the following: 8 ozs. aqua ammonia, strong; 4 ozs. gum camphor; 4 ozs. castile soap, shaved and dissolved in a little hot water; then add the whole to the alcohol and it is fit for use. I have cured Sweenys on 3 or 4 occasions with the above by applying and immediately cover-ing the parts with a heavy woolen blanket."

*Remarks.*—I do not think Mr. McClane [see No. 7 of Ringbones for expla-nation] intends to be understood that one application would cure, but that to continue its use a reasonable time daily would do it, of which I have not a doubt. Still, I think it a good plan in all cases to lift up the skin, by means of the thumbs and fingers, to break it loose, as it were, from its attachments to the muscles for the first few applications. Some persons, you will see in the next recipe, claim this "lifting up of the skin" and allowing it to fill with air will cure the disease. I cannot say that it will, but I know the breaking up of the attachment will help the cure by its stimulating the muscles and blood vessels of the shoulder to increased action, and the admission of the air will undoubt-edly cause an irritation, and thus help the stimulation.

**Sweeny, Simple and Certain Cure for.**—A. W. Baird, of Gibson, Ill., writes to one of the papers in answer to an inquiry for a cure for this dis-ease, saying: "The cure is short, easy, sure and simple. It is this: With the forefinger and thumb of the left hand pull up the skin on the shoulder, pretty well up on the shrunk place; then with the small blade of a penknife make an incision through one side of the skin that is pulled up. Then with both hands raise up the skin around the incision, and it will fill with air. Fill the shrunk place full; let your horse stand a few days, or run on pasture; he will soon be well; it is a certain cure."

*Remarks.*—It strikes me that there would be more certainty of filling with air if a goosequill was passed just through the orifice in the skin and then inflated to its full extent by blowing. I will give one more, the oil, made with angle-worms, taken from the veterinary department of the *Post and Tribune*, and will also remark that angle-worm oil has been considered valuable also for stiff joints, rheumatism, etc. The additions to this will make it so much better than without them. It is as follows:

**4. "Oil for Sweeny.**—Dig and wash clean angle worms to make 1 pt, and put them into a suitable bottle, adding salt, by weight, 1 oz.; spirits of tur-pentine and sassafras oil, each, 1 oz. Hang in the sun until the worms are dis-solved, then strain and add oils of spike, hemlock and cedar and gum camphor, each, 2 ozs.; best alcohol, 1 pt. Shake and bathe the shoulder night and morn-ing. If it blisters, or gives too much pain, rub on a little lard oil (or lard)."

*Remarks.*—I think this will prove a very valuable oil for sweeny, and for the general purposes of a liniment. In the same issue was the following treat ment for

**Strains, Swelled Legs, etc.—Lotion and Liniment for.—I** *Lotion.*—Steep wormwood herb, 4 ozs., in sharp vinegar, 2 qts., and add salt, 2 lbs. Bathe the limb thoroughly with this, then use the following:

II. *Liniment.*—Oil of spike, 1 oz.; oils of hemlock, cedar, and camphor gum, turpentine and sweet oil, each 2 ozs., in 1 qt. of arnica. Shake before applying.

*Remarks.*—The author not being much of an arnica man, would say, that in his estimation, this would be a far better liniment to put these into 1 qt. of alcohol.

**1. SCRATCHES, GREASE HEEL, ETC.—To Avoid and to Cure.**—To avoid, keep the horse in good health, and in the wet and muddy season—fall, winter and spring—keep the naturally long hair of the fetlocks, especially of the hind legs, which are much the more liable to this disease, cut rather closely, so that by proper grooming, these parts soon dry, and thus avoid this difficulty—I say this, for as a general thing, it begins with slight inflam- mation of the skin, when it is scratches, proper; but which, if allowed to pro- ceed to deeper and more extensive inflammation, causing the cracking of the skin, and the escape of a greasy and purulent, or foul matter, to exude from the cracks, which also excoriates and extends the inflammation to all parts which it touches, when "grease" may be considered to have taken full pos- session; and if not now met with proper treatment, the exudation assumes a foul smell, and finally a fungus growth may arise in lumps—grape-like—to cover the whole of the diseased parts, leaving a red and angry appearance. Of course this is not common; for proper constitutional treatment, by condi- tion powders, combining cathartics and diuretics, as well as tonics, with some of the following local applications, will prevent, or cure, this disease. (See Con- dition Powders, Nos. 1, 2 and 3, and also the one given in connection with Cribbing.)

**2. Grease Heels, National Live Stock Journal's Cure.—** Attend to cleanliness. Apply during 2 days poultices of equal parts of bran, flaxseed meal, and powdered charcoal. Thereafter apply twice or thrice daily a portion of oxide of zinc ointment (this is made with oxide of zinc, 1 oz., to benzoated lard, 6 ozs.), previously removing all secretions of matter as well as dry scabs and crusts. [This must be done with warm water and castile soap, washing carefully and drying perfectly.] If, after a week or 10 days, the case does not improve satisfactorily, apply instead of the ointment twice or thrice daily a portion of a mixture of 1 oz. of Goulard's extract and ½ oz. of car- bolic acid to ½ pt. of water. Give loosening food, among which may be mixed 2 drs. of nitrate of potash, morning and evening, during 1 week.

*Remarks.*—This poultice may be considered one of the best that can be made, which I know from personal experience, except the bran, to which I have no particular objections. Although I have never had the scratches proper, yet I had something much worse some 50 years ago. I had a foot mashed in a threshing machine, and mortification set in upon two of the toes, but the young physician was equal to the occasion with a poultice of flaxseed (properly boiled, as there was no flaxseed meal then kept by druggists), and thickened with powdered charcoal, the mortification was stopped from extending, and the mortified parts separated from the healthy parts; when the tendons only had to be clipped to remove them wholly from the foot; hence no one need be afraid to tie to this poultice, and the whole treatment will be found good, not forgetting the constitutional or condition powder part of it, in all cases.

**3. Scratches, Canadian Remedy.**—A Canadian correspondent of the *Scientific American* gives the following simple remedy for scratches in horses. He says: "Having tried many lotions, etc., only to obtain temporary relief for my horse, I concluded to try a mixture of flowers of sulphur and glycerine, which I mixed into a paste using sufficient glycerine to give it a glossy appearance, and the results I obtained in a short time were truly wonderful. I apply this paste at night, and in the morning before going out I apply plain glycerine."

*Remarks.*—This is undoubtedly very valuable, for in McClure and Harvey's edition of Stonehenge's English work on the horse, in speaking upon the subject of grease, says: "The skin must be kept supple (soft and pliant), and at the same time suitable to a healthy action. For the former purpose, glycerine is the most valuable, being far more efficacious than any greasy dressing, such as we were obliged to employ before the discovery of this substance, etc."

He uses it in all stages of the disease, to keep the skin soft. To stimulate to a healthy action, he uses: "Chloride of zinc, 30 grs., to soft water, 1 pt., and thorough cleansing with soap and warm water, and thorough drying, applying this with a brush, only sufficient to dampen the parts, and 15 minutes after, applying glycerine, and if not improved in a few days, he increases the strength of the zinc solution to 40 or 50 grs. to the pt.—repeating night and morning with, of course, constitutional treatment.

**4. Scratches, Simple Remedy for.**—A correspondent of the *Western Rural* sent this, as he calls it, "Simple Remedy for Scratches," which he also said has been thoroughly tested and proved highly successful: "Wash the sores thoroughly with warm, soft water and castile soap; then rinse them off with clear water, after which rub them dry with a cloth. Now grate up some carrots and bind them on the sores. This should be repeated every day, for 4 or 5 days, when the scratches will be cured.

*Remarks.*—I know that carrot poultice is very good; but I would suggest here, that it should be repeated twice daily, night and morning, instead of only daily, as the writer directs; but, if no carrots are to be had, take the following, unless you prefer the first one, or some other of the recipes here given. Boiled and mashed turnips, thickened with powdered charcoal, are undoubtedly good, whether they will prove as good as the bran and flaxseed meal of No. 1 or not, I leave for each one to judge for himself, when either can be had; or to use the one he can get the materials for, when the other cannot be obtained, this is the object of giving several recipes for any disease. There is, however, a different dressing in the next, to follow the poulticing, which is undoubtedly valuable, especially when the white lead is mixed with tanner's or currier's oil, as there recommended.

**5. Scratches or Grease Heel in Horses, Simple and Cheap Remedy.**—The following which is the last I shall give upon this subject, was from one signing himself "A Subscriber," of Hillsdale, Mich., to the Detroit *Tribune,* in answer to an inquiry of H. E. Lyon, concerning the treatment of scratches; but to which he says: "I will state that I think it a case of grease heel, which is far worse than common scratches. The remedy prescribed in the *Tribune* is a good one, but I have a simple and cheap remedy. Cleanliness in the stable has much to do in the case, keeping the stable well cleaned and littered with clean, dry straw.

I. "Give the following condition powder: Jamaica ginger, 8 ozs.; gentian root, 2 ozs.; niter, blood root, and arnica, each, 1 oz.; crude antimony (black), ¼ oz. Directions—All to be finely powdered and thoroughly mixed together, then give 1 large table-spoonful in bran mash once each day for 6 days; then omit 3 days, and again repeat 2 or 3 days. This is equally good for any horse that is out of condition, or wants an appetite.

II. "For the sore heels: Cleanse the parts affected thoroughly with castile soap and soft water, and when thoroughly dry, boil turnips (have boiled and mashed and already mixed,) and mash, and to this add finely pulverized charcoal. Poultice with this for 3 days, changing the poultice twice each day; then cleanse thoroughly again with castile soap and soft water, and when the parts are thoroughly dry, mix (have already mixed) together tanner's oil and white lead to the consistency of paint; apply thoroughly with a brush to the affected parts once each day. A few applications will generally suffice. Cleanliness in the case has much to do in effecting a cure. The white lead is of the greatest importance in the case, but works best when incorporated with tanner's oil. Hoping this may prove beneficial to Mr. Lyon, I submit it to your consideration if you think proper to publish."

*Remarks.*—Of course they published it, and it will be found good treatment, although I must say that our condition powders will have a more general action upon all the secretions than "Subscriber's"; but his turnip poultice with the charcoal thickening and the white lead in tanner's oil, will no doubt prove very satisfactory to all who try them. I have known common white-lead paint to act nicely upon galled shoulders, while this, with the tanner's oil in place of linseed oil, will prove more softening and, I think, also more healing.

**Surfeit in Horses, Cause and Cure.**—Surfeit is a disease more particularly affecting the skin, in which at first there will be found hard lumps, and if not soon cured, will finally become sore and a sticky matter exude, forming scales or scabs, and the treatment become more difficult. It is believed to arise from the horse having been overworked or overdriven, by which the blood has become heated; then, by drinking cold water, or standing in the cold, they become chilled, which shows itself in the skin, more particularly because the kidneys fail to depurate the blood, *i. e.*, to take up and carry off the effete or worn out portions of the system, which are, therefore, thrown upon the skin in too great quantities to obtain free escape, and hence, diuretics, such as niter, ½ oz., dissolved in a little water, and given in its drink night and morning, or an ounce daily of sweet spirits of niter in the same way for a few days, will if taken in hand soon, generally correct the difficulty; but if the horse is not in general good health, a general constitutional treatment, with some of the condition powders, care in his feed and grooming, as well as to see he is not again over-heated, will be necessary. Cathartics, however, are not considered as essential in this disease as diuretics. I do not see that any writer upon this subject directs any application to the skin; but I should most positively recommend the daily, or twice daily, application of a good stimulating liniment to be well rubbed into the diseased parts of the skin, for I know it will expedite the cure as much as an itch ointment helps to more quickly cure the itch.

*Remarks.*—Many is the horse that has been spoiled by hitching into a buggy or wagon and being driven quickly to town, then allowed to stand for hours, often I have seen it till eleven o'clock at night, in a cold, dreary wind, while the driver " gossiped " and " guzzled" in a warm, comfortable room. If this must be done, for humanity's sake put the horse into a comfortable stable.

**1. WARTS ON HORSES OR OTHER STOCK—To Cure.—** A farmer writing to one of the papers says: " I had a mare some years ago that had a large wart on her side, where the harness rubbed and kept it sore. In the summer the flies made it worse. To prevent this I put on a good daub of tar, and in a few weeks the wart was killed and disappeared. I have frequently tried it since on cattle and horses, and seldom had occasion to make a second application. The remedy is simple and effectual."

*Remarks.*—I am not able to see any chemical property in the tar to effect a cure; yet I have not a doubt of the fact, as above given. If this fails in any case apply the following:

**2. Warts, Effectual Cure for, on Horses or Persons.—Take** full strength acetic acid, and with a 3-cent camel's hair pencil (brush) just fairly wet the wart all over. A few applications will cure them on man or beast. Don't put on enough to run off the wart upon the skin, to make a sore.

**3.** Put 1 oz. of powdered sal-soda (washing soda) in a 2 oz. vial and fill with water, and wet the warts thoroughly with this, is also effectual, by a few applications, in all cases, as with No. 2. A little of this soda in water to soak the feet in, for those who have corns, (which see) will soften up the dead part, and make its removal easy.

**1. WORMS—Successful Remedies.—**For the long worm which inhabits the small intestines of the horse, and sometimes find their way into the stomach, a Mr. Rhodes, a farmer near Ann Arbor, Mich., gave me the following as a certain cure: Burn black ash bark, and give the ashes, in 1 table-spoonful doses, in his feed every morning for 3 mornings, then skip 3, till 9 doses are given.

*Remarks.*—Believing that the alkali arising from these ashes coming in contact with the linings of the stomach, and intestines, will correct the mucus condition of these parts, in which the worms find themselves, I give it, expecting it to cleanse the parts and eradicate the worms. If this fails in any case, however, give a drench of linseed oil, 1 pt., with ¼ oz. of spirits of turpentine in it, and repeat it the third morning after, if the first dose does not carry them off freely. The same you will see is used as an injection for pin-worms, below. It is safe in either method of using.

**2. For the Pin-Worms that Infest the Rectum.**—I cannot see why a solution, weak lye, made with these ashes, and injected, for a few times, will not also eradicate them. Some of these, however, almost always go higher up, to get out of the reach of injections, and after a week or 10 days return to the rectum, when the same shall be repeated, to clear them out entirely, no matter whether you use this, or inject the usual remedy; which is linseed oil, 1 pt., with ¼ oz. spirits of turpentine in it, injecting every morning for a week, with the repetition, as above. It is well also, after either of these treatments, to tone up the system with the tonic condition powders, which never come amiss, spring and fall, although no special disease may manifest itself.

**Heaves, a Claimed Cure.**—Although this is out of its alphabetical place, as I have tried to arrange the horse recipes, yet as it was given by the same man who gave the ash plan, above, for worms, I will give it here, and although I can hardly expect it to cure the worst heaves, as he claims, it may prove better than I have dared to hope, as the article, blood root, is known to be valuable in coughs and throat difficulties of persons. He says: Get blood root, ½ lb., pulverized, and give 1 table-spoonful in the feed, the same as the ashes were to be given for the worms, above, (on the old plan of take 3 and skip 3, till nine are taken), will cure the worst heaves: He says, however, follow it up till cured.

**Feeding Stock Horses, and Also Best Rations for Winter Feeding on the Farm.**—Although considerable has already been said as to proper care in feeding work-horses especially to avoid colics, etc.; yet stock horses, nor the plans of general feeding, and especially the winter care of horses, when but little is being done with them, have not been fully considered; and as such matters are known to be better understood by stockmen, I will quote from E. W. Stewart, in the *Rural New Yorker*, one of the most prominent men of that class in our country. See, also, an item taken from his prize essay on "Fattening Cattle," found under that head. Every word from such a man may be considered perfectly reliable and the best thing to "tie to" that can be found upon the subject upon which he is speaking. Upon the importance of the horse as the motive power on the farm, and also the importance of keeping him in full condition and strength in winter, he says:

I. "The horse is the principal motive power on the farm, and therefore needs the best attention. This class of stock is kept wholly for its muscle, and the working and culture of the farm must depend greatly upon the character and condition of the horses. The winter season is one of comparative leisure for horses, as farms are usually managed, and farmers appear to think horses require little attention when they are not in hard labor. They are quite in the habit of keeping them upon poor hay and straw at this season, reserving all grain for spring feeding. But this is very bad policy. Horses generally come to winter quarters in thin condition from their summer's labor, and require judicious feeding and good care to recover their full working capacity; and farmers should remember that it is much cheaper to put horses in condition when work is very light, and that all the extra flesh put on in winter represents so much extra labor available in spring. Besides, it should always be the aim of team-owners to keep their horses in good working condition, for it takes less food to keep up condition than to recover it when lost."

II. *To avoid colics and aid in digestion* he says: "Let us examine a few rations for work-horses in winter. Horses are often subject to colic from improper feeding. When fed upon cornmeal alone, its large percentage of starch renders it too heating, and, besides, it is a very concentrated food, and being just moistened with saliva so as to be swallowed, it goes into the stomach in the compact form of dough, and the gastric juice cannot circulate through it so as properly to perform its office, and internal heat, fever and colic often occur from want of proper digestion. All such concentrated food should be mixed with cut hay, the hay being just moistened so that the meal will adhere to it. This mixes the concentrated with the bulky food, and the hay separates the particles of meal so as to render the mixture porous and the gastric juice now circulates freely through the mass and operates upon the whole contents of the stomach at once. The best way to use cornmeal as a single grain food is to mix it with moistened (cut) clover hay. If the clover is of good quality it contains a larger percentage of albuminoids (muscle-forming food) than cornmeal, and thus helps to balance the constituents."

[Possibly it may not be amiss to call attention here to the subject of scalding meal by pouring on boiling water, as mentioned under the head of "Meal and Hay for Fattening Stock." If scalding it for fattening purposes makes it more digestible, why not in general feeding? Still, as it is to be mixed with cut hay here it is not so absolutely necessary.—AUTHOR.]

III. *On the Best Feed or Rations for Work-Horses* he says: "But one of the best rations for work-horses is corn, oats and flaxseed, ground together—the corn and oats in equal weight, and to 19 bushels of the mixture of corn and oats add 1 bushel of flaxseed, and grind fine, all together. The corn and oats make a well-balanced ration, and the flaxseed is rich in oil, muscle-forming and bone-building elements; but its oil is its greatest sanitary element. This small proportion of oil is just sufficient to keep the bowels in excellent condition, the coat sleek, and every part of the system in well-balanced activity. And then by feeding this ground mixture with twice its bulk of moistened cut hay you have as perfect a ration for work-horses as can be compounded. All regular grist-mills now have an apparatus for mixing different grains together, so that the farmer has only to carry the oats, corn or flaxseed in proper quantity to mill and they will all be mixed without hand labor. If the farmer has no straw-cutter he may use oats or wheat chaff to mix with the meal to render it porous."

[The author would hardly risk the mixture of so small a proportion of flaxseed with the other. I should prefer it to be ground alone and put in the proper amount with each feed; but possibly the machinery Mr. Stewart refers to may do it better than I should expect.]

IV. *For Wintering Horses Doing but Little Work—Amount and Kinds of Feed Necessary.*—Upon this subject he closes by saying: "In wintering horses that are doing but little work, straw may be fed with the last ration and the horses will do well. From 8 to 10 lbs. of this meal to each horse daily will bring them through finely, even on good straw. When oats are too expensive cornmeal and wheat bran mixed in equal weights, with 1 pt. of oatmeal to each horse, will give a good result. If hay is scarce, 2 lbs. of decorticated (hulled) cotton-seed meal, 4 lbs. of cornmeal, 4 lbs. of bran and cut straw will winter horses well. But there should always be a variety in the food. If the farmer has clover hay and straw, these should be mixed together—better if both be cut before mixing, but they may be mixed in the manger without cutting."

**Amount of Food Necessary for a Horse at Work.**—The English railway (or, as we call them here, street car) companies, feed their horses a mixed feed, about as follows, for 6 horses: Hay, 376 lbs., and straw, 84 lbs., both cut into chaff; oats, 336 lbs.; Indian corn, 252 lbs.; beans, 84 lbs.; bran, 14 lbs. All mixed evenly together and ground; then, I should judge, mixed proportionally, with the moistened cut hay and straw. This makes an average of 11 lbs. of the mixed hay and 16 lbs. of the mixed grain for each horse daily. A fair feed, if not overworked, as many of them do in our cities.

A Pennsylvania farmer says: Two quarts of meal per day is not enough for a horse that is working; but an excellent mixture of grain is cracked corn, 1 bushel, and oats, 2 bushels. [The author would say better if ground together in equal proportions. See Mr. Stewart's Best Feed, or Rations for Work Horses.] Of this, he goes on to say, a small horse that is driven, or worked, should have 2 qts. at a feed, given 3 times a day, with 5 lbs. of hay (cut), night and morning. And a horse that is not working, but will be, soon, would be the better for a daily feed of 2 qts of grain (oats) given at noon.

*Remarks.*—This undoubtedly refers to a horse which is not being fed upon the meal mixture, but simply hay, or other coarse food.

**For Old Horses.**—For old horses the oats should most certainly be ground, and their coarse food also cut, dampened and the ground oats mixed with it, as their teeth are not in condition to grind for themselves; and if they are left to do it, they do not get half the value of the grain. It is worthy of attention. Younger horses may do tolerably well grinding for themselves; but they will do much better if it is ground for them.

**Apples Valuable for Horses.**—Remarks have been made in connection with the subject of carrots, parsnips and other roots of valuable food for cattle, etc., in which apples are shown to possess, largely, the power of dis solving other coarse food for them, why not then good for horses? (See this pectine, or dissolving power, described in connection with carrots and other roots for cattle. Apples possess it in greater abundance than almost any other article known.) Of course it is only sour apples that have this power, and hence it is only them that should be fed. One writer says: I have occasionally fed sour apples to my horses, with excellent results. They are a certain cure for worms. I feed half to a whole pailful once a week. Another one says: I am in the habit of turning my horses into the orchard in the fall, where they can eat as many apples as they like. I find they derive much benefit from them, and gain flesh much more rapidly than others which did not receive an apple feed.

**Parsnips Valuable as Food for Horses.**—In the article above referred to, parsnips were spoken of as having been fed in France, by a horse breeder, there, for 20 years, with better success than when he used to feed carrots, from the larger amount of pectine, or pectic acid, which they contain. It is from the presence of this dissolving power, in apples, as well as parsnips, carrots, beets, rutabagas, etc., which make them so valuable as food, when properly cut and mixed with other coarse food, as hay, cornstalks, straw, etc., all properly cut, both for horses and cattle.

**Turnips Valuable as an Occasional Feed for Horses.**—Turnips are healthful for horses, when sliced, or what is better, pulped finely and mixed with a little salt and corn meal. Of course rutabagas are richer than the flat, or field turnip.

**Bran, its Value for Reducing Inflammation, and as a Laxative.**—Bran mashes are cooling and laxative, and valuable after inflammations, and for giving various medicines in, but should not be given in a dry state; for if fed to any considerable extent dry, it is liable to form into lumpy secretions, which become almost, if not wholly, impossible to pass the bowels, and hence death has been known to occur from this cause.

**Halter Pulling, Sensible Remedy.**—The *Country Gentleman*, in response to a request from a correspondent for a cure for horses which have contracted the habit of halter pulling, says: " Take a sufficiently long piece of ½ inch rope, put the center of it under the tail like a crupper, cross the rope on the back and tie the two ends together in front of the breast snugly, so there is no slack, otherwise it would drop down on the tail. Put an ordinary halter on—a good one—and run the halter strap or rope through a ring in the manger or from the stall and tie fast in the rope on the front of the breast, and then slap his face and let him fly back. He will not choke nor need telling to stop pulling back. Let him wear it awhile, and twice or thrice daily scare him back as suddenly and forcibly as possible. After one or two trials you will see that he cannot be induced to pull back."

**Lice Upon Colts, Cattle and Other Animals—Easy and Safe Remedy.**—J. M. Johnson says in the *Iowa Homestead* that aloes, in fine powder, is a specific for the destruction of lice on all animals. It has no poisonous properties, its intense bitterness being what kills. It can be freely applied, and as it is to be used in a dry state, its application is as safe in cold as in warm weather, consequently it is free from all objections urged against other remedies. Use with fine pepper-box, dusting and rubbing it in all over, then curry out inside of a week; repeat if necessary.

**Ointment for Grease-heel in Horses.** — Honey and lard, of each ½ lb.; tar, ½ lb.; white vitriol, and sugar of lead, of each 1 oz.; alum, ¾ lb. The first 4 articles are to be melted together, and the others finely powdered and mixed in by stirring, and stirring until cold to keep them evenly mixed. This, in grease-heel, must be put on cloth and thoroughly bound on, and kept on for 36 hours; wash with casteel soap, and repeat the whole as needed. No case is known where 3 applications did not effect a perfect cure

*Remarks.*—When cleaning or rubbing with fingers to remove scabs, always use flat of fingers and *never* the finger-nails. The parts must be dried by rubbing, after cleansing with casteel soap, before applying the ointment.

If a man has a horse with grease-heel, this ointment is worth as much as his horse.

# CATTLE.

**Working Oxen, etc.—Digestion—How to Feed.—**See "Horses —Digestion of," compared with the ox, how they should be fed, etc. I will simply say here, that an ox having a larger stomach, or rather four stomachs, while the horse has but one, is not refreshed and strengthened as the horse is by a feed of meal alone, but needs it to be mixed with cut hay or cut straw, for a noon feed, and at least two hours for feeding and ruminating, *i. e.*, "chewing his cud," to get the full benefit of his dinner.

**As to Cows.—**Although they ought to have the best of feed and care all the time, if rich milk, good butter or good cheese are expected from them; yet, the time when they need more especial care, is for a couple of weeks before, and at the time of calving, for if they pass this period without accident, and do not have milk-fever following it, there is generally but little trouble with them. This disease is not as prevalent in the Western States as in the Eastern, especially Rhode Island, Massachusetts, and Connecticut, and it is believed to be more prevalent on account of their higher feeding to obtain all the milk possible from them, and also that of a rich butter, or cheese producing quality, and hence meal enters largely into their feed, which alone, is of a heating nature, and has a tendency, at this particular period, it is believed, to make the cow more likely to have milk-fever. A Mr. Ansel W. Putnam, of Danvers, Mass., gives his experience to his fellow dairy-men through the *New York Tribune*, to enable them to avoid having this disease, which is far better than to be able to cure even after it has once set in, but the fact is few are cured. Let me say then, that as I fully believe Mr. Putnam's plan of giving cold water enough to satisfy thirst, is better than the giving only a little warm water, as heretofore recommended. I the more cheerfully recommend every one to follow all his directions, and thus avoid the disease. He says:

**Milk-Fever, To Avoid.—**"I am in the habit of giving water to cows, as soon as they drop their calves, and I have never known a case of milk-fever when the cow had all the water she wanted soon after calving, and the want was kept supplied at short intervals, giving a pailful at a time, fresh from the well. In all cases of milk-fever that I have known anything about, the cows went without water for a long time, and then were allowed to drink a large quantity, and the re-action was too great for the system.

"Cows which are fat," Mr. Putnam says, "should have no heating food for two weeks before calving. And, first, to milk the cow as soon as she calves, then to give her a bucket of water, fresh from the well, such as a thirsty man would relish. In half an hour after give her another, and so on until she is satisfied. Very few," he continues, "understand how necessary it is to supply the cow's system with water soon after calving, but it should be done gradually, as above directed." Mr. Putnam concludes as follows: "If the bag and teats are full before calving, the milk should be drawn out, and when great milkers are on pasture, it is a good plan to take them up two weeks before calving, and put them on dry food so as to check the flow of milk, for, when a cow is fed on dry hay only, before calving (the calf is ready for the milk as soon as it is ready), there is no danger of inflammation or fever."

*Remarks.* Having become fully satisfied of the necessity of giving fresh, cold water to persons in fevers, as shown by the remarks following Typhoid Fever, and reasoning from analogy (the likeness or agreement between things, although the circumstances may be quite different), I see, at a glance, that the cool water to satisfy the cows, this within a reasonable short time, a (pailful every half hour, as Mr. Putnam has found, as above given), is the true way to prevent a cow from having milk fever, at all; for no person, animal, or thing can long continue hot (and all fever is heat) if filled or covered with cold water. Nothing further need be said in favor of Mr. Putnam's plan. It will be safe to follow it.

## MILK, TO INCREASE THE FLOW IN DAIRY COWS. AND THE BEST FOOD TO INSURE IT.

**1. Milk to Increase.**— The agricultural editor of the *Bee-Keepers Journal* vouches for the following, handed him by one who had tried the plan to increase the flow of milk, and I have seen the same thing given in various other sources, and from the nature of the mixture I have every reason to believe it good. He says:

"If you desire to get a large yield of milk, give your cow, three times a day, water, slightly warm, slightly salted, in which bran has been stirred at the rate of 1 qt. to 2 gals. of water. You will find that your cow will gain 25 per cent. immediately under the effects of it, and she will become so attached to the drink as to refuse clear water, unless very thirsty; but this mess she will drink almost at any time, and ask for more. The amount of this drink is an ordinary water pailful at each time—morning, noon and night. Your animal will then do her best at discounting the lacteal (*lac*, the Latin work for milk, hence "lacteal," milky) fluid.

**2. The Best Food for Increasing the Flow of Milk.**—In the Eastern States, as before stated, milch cows are fed largely on corn meal, but I have the statement of a well-informed dairyman, that equal parts by measure, of corn meal, ground oats and wheat bran, well mixed, makes the best and most profitable feed for increasing the flow of milk, being much less heating than corn meal alone, and still very nourishing and satisfactory to the animal as well as to the dairyman by saving considerable expense, while at the same time he gets his increased flow of milk, and the cow is not too fat for comfort and health, as they often become on corn meal alone. There are those, also, who claim that milch cows will be greatly benefited by mixing their feed with warm or hot water, if this can be done without too much trouble, at each milking. It is well-known that to give a family cow a warm mess in the mornings increases the flow of milk perceptably. Why should it not, then, do the same with any number of dairy cows? Cut the hay and pour hot water over it, and mix it so it is all wetted, then add the meal, or the mixed feed, referred to above, mixing thoroughly and feeding while warm. In a dairy of 20 cows the extra milk will more than half pay for the extra labor. (For the value of meal daily, to a cow giving milk, see next receipt.)

**Meal, the Value of, for Dairy Cows.**—The editor of the *Farmer and Mirror* gives the following item, coming, he says, from one of the best dairymen in Vermont. He says:

"I have come to the conclusion, after seven years' experience in the feeding of meal every day to such of my cows as were giving milk, that in the future I would feed more meal instead of less. I believe that when the cows have been properly selected, and are of a breed that is reliable as to butter qualities, it amounts to a certainty that all we feed them above what is required to sustain their bodies, will be returned to us in butter with a large profit on the investment. At the same time care should be taken not to overfeed. Gilt-edged butter cannot be made from cows thin in flesh or poorly fed."

*Remarks.*—This idea of feeding meal is correct, but the mixed feed in the receipt above is the most profitable. To judge about the "breed that is reliable," as this writer puts it, see Jersey Cows, or the Best Cow for Small Farms, for I think it is now generally conceded that the Jerseys, also called Alderneys, are the best, although the Durhams are good as you will see under that head.

**To "Dry off" Cows and other Animals.**—I. As we have given the plan above, for increasing the flow of milk, it may not be amiss to also give a good plan here for drying-off, which is occasionally important, and as it is just as applicable to mares, when weaning the colt; and with slight modification, also valuable for caked-breasts, it is worthy of a place in this connection. It is as follows: Tar and good vinegar, each ½ pt.; spirits of turpentine, 6 ozs.; beeswax and camphor gum, 2 ozs.; tallow, 4 ozs. DIRECTIONS—Boil all together for 15 minutes, except the turpentine and camphor gum, the latter of which should be broken up very fine or pulverized by the druggist, by dropping upon it a few drops of alcohol, then these added when removed from the fire, and stirred until cold.

The cow or the mare is to be milked dry night and morning, and the ointment rubbed into the udder and along the milk-veins for 3 or 4 days, or until the milk ceases to flow.

For Caked-Breasts make it without the tar and rub it in well as long as needed to remove the soreness, then cease unless you desire to dry up the milk as the camphor has a great tendency to do.

*Remarks.*—The camphor was not in the recipe as the author obtained it; but knowing its value upon the female breast, I have added it to the recipe, knowing it will prove so much the more reliable. The only objection to the tar upon the breast is, it stains the clothing, and is also more sticky.

II. Another writer says a cow may be dried off in a short time by not milking her quite out, leaving some in the udder each milking, and by feeding 4 qts. of dry corn meal in the course of the day, which, if she is to be fatted, will help to lay on fat, and gradually dry her off. This is no doubt the fact.

if toward the close of her milking season. Still I can see no objection to the dry meal, even if the ointment is used.

**Ointment for Swelled Bags, or Udders of Cows.**—Sweet oil, 4 ozs.; pulverized camphor gum, 1 oz. Dissolve over a slow fire, and rub in well 2 or 3 times daily. The author thinks the ointment for drying off cows, above, fully equal, if not even better, than this camphorated-oil, although only swelling is to be remedied here, which generally arrives from colds.

**Choked Cattle, Sure Remedy.**—J. B. J. in *Country Gentleman* speaking of choked cattle, says: "The following recipe ought to be printed twice every year, as it is a sure remedy: Take of fine-cut chewing tobacco enough to make a ball the size of a hen's egg, dampen it with molasses so it adheres closely; elevate the animal's head, pull out the tongue and crowd the ball as far down the throat as possible. In 15 minutes it will cause sickness and vomiting, relaxing the muscles, so that the potatoe or whatever may be choking it will be thrown up."

*Remarks.*—It is an almost absolute certainty that the tobacco will cause the relaxing of the muscles and consequent throwing up of the contents of the stomach, and a cure is just as certain as a relaxation. The laying of moistened tobacco upon a person's stomach with lock-jaw, has relaxed them, and saved the patient. It must not be kept on so long, however, as to cause deathly sickness.

**To Cure Foul Flesh or Sores Upon Stock.**—C. Becker, of Bloomville, N. Y., writes one of the *Rural's:* "I have been in the habit for 35 years of using oil of vitriol (sulphuric acid) and water in all cases of bad flesh, and never knew failure. Put 1 teaspoonful of the vitriol in ½ teacupful of water, cleanse out the sore with a soft rope, or otherwise make a swab by tying a piece of cloth on the end of a stick, saturate the afflicted part well with the wash and I never knew it to fail by two washings."

*Remarks.*—It would, most undoubtedly, prove as valuable for foot-rot in sheep, as for foul sores.

**To Cure Fleshy Tumors Upon Cows or Calves.**—Bin-iodide of mercury, 1 dr.; cosmoline, or vaseline, 2 ozs.; thoroughly mixed and well rubbed upon the tumors."—*Dr. Horne in Michigan Farmer.*

*Remarks.*—For directions how to continue it [see Spavin to Cure Lameness]. It is from the same veterinarian, but he prefers the bin-iodide here, to the iodide as used on spavins.

**Hoven or Bloat in Stock—Prevention and Cure.**—O. J. L. of Modest Town (a very appropriate name for a place where the men are so modest they dare not give their name when reporting for an agricultural paper on the above disease), Va., made a report of the death of a cow and calf to one of the the farm papers, I think the *Farm and Fireside,* to which the veterinary surgeon A. T. Wilson, made the following sensible answer: "Your cow and calf both died from hoven or bloat, a very common result of injudiciously turning cattle into a rich clover patch. To prevent bloat, turn them in for an hour or so every day for a week until they get used to it. To cure bloat, when seen in

time, use 2 ounces each of hyposulphite of soda and tincture of ginger added
to a quart of cold water. But in extreme cases, make an opening with a pocket
knife, in lieu of a trochar, in the most prominent swelling or point on the left
flank, and insert any small tube—a funnel. A quill or pencil case might
answer."

*Remarks.*—Saleratus used to be given to try to prevent the continued accumulation of gas in these cases, but of late ½ cup of freshly powdered charcoal
in a drench of water, is considered better treatment, as it aids the future digestion, as well as the present difficulty. This may be repeated morning and evening for a day or two, if the animal continues to show any signs of indigestion.
But the hyposulphite of soda and tincture of ginger, if on hand, is reliable;
even baking soda, double the quantity, will do well, with the tincture of ginger,
or even without, if none is by you; but there is not much time to wait. Do
quickly what is to be done.

1. **Hollow Horn, to Cure.**—Alcohol, ½ pt.; camphor gum, 1 oz.
DIRECTIONS—When the gum is dissolved, put half of it into one ear of the animal, and as soon as it has done snorting and blowing, put the other half into
the other ear. Once cures every time.

*Remarks.*—This is from a Mr. Bradly, living 2 miles below Ann Arbor,
Mich. He said a druggist told him, at first, it would kill the cow. "It did
not," he continued, "but cured her," and he said he had tried it several times
with like success.

2. **Old Treatment of Hollow Horn.**—The old treatment was to
bore into the horn with a gimlet and inject vinegar, pepper, salt and water; and
after this was injected into the horn, a couple of pieces of fat, salt pork, the
size of one's two forefingers, with a tea-spoonful of cayenne put in a slit in
each slice, was placed between the animal's grinders, and the head elevated
until it chewed and swallowed them; and next day repeat without the pepper
if dumpishness is still manifested. This would be good, too, for any animal
which is, as they say, "off its feed," or dull and heavy in appearance—ick, in
other words. Let one piece be chewed and swallowed before the other is introduced.

**Scours and Diarrhœa in Cattle, Colts, etc., to Cure.**—For scours
in cattle, change the food and water. Give first 1 qt. of lard oil, with laudanum,
2 ozs. After 3 to 4 hours, give powdered gum catechu, ginger, and gentian
root, each, 2 ozs., in flaxseed tea, 1 pt., to any animal over 2 years old; half this
to those under 2 years, and over 9 months, and one-fourth to one-third the
amount to younger stock; repeating the dose twice daily, and withholding it as
soon as the discharges diminish. Give nourishing food, and flaxseed tea to
drink. In chronic (long standing) diarrhœa, give, morning and evening, 1 dr. of
ammoniated sulphate of copper, dissolved in cold water, ½ pt.— *Western Rural.*

*Remarks.*—While spending a couple of months at Eaton Rapids, Mich., I
became acquainted with a gentleman there, Mr. A. Button, quite a "family
doctor," by the way, who told me he once expected to lose a colt with the
scours, as the veterinarians failed to cure it; but some one told him to dissolve

a piece of alum the size of a hen's egg in a bucket of water, which would cure it. He tried it, and it did cure it. Why should it not again, and cattle as well as colts? I would try it, if the above ever failed, or one of the following:

**Diarrhœa of Cattle, Remedy.**—Another writer says: "Three pecks of boiled potatoes, fed in the day, in 3 messes, warm, is an excellent remedy for diarrhœa in cattle."

**Scours in Cattle, Remedy.**—Mr. James Door, of Dorchester, Mass., recommends fine wheat flour as a cure for scours in cattle. He says, "Take 1 qt. of the finest flour, mix smoothly with water, making it just thick enough to run, and administer at one dose. A second dose may be necessary, but one is generally sufficient for a cure."

*Remarks.*—The author knows a rather thick milk porridge, given warm, is good for "looseness" of persons. Why not good for cattle? I should prefer it warm to cold, as this gentleman uses it, as I understand him. It may be good enough cold, but warmth will not make it less valuable, I am sure.

1. **Kicking Cows, to Make Stand Quiet.**—A dairyman who has been troubled with the kicking of young cows, and who has found a plan to prevent it while milking, makes it public through the New York *Tribune*, and seeing at a glance that it must be a success, I give it a place. He says:

"If cows kick, tie their legs together, I find it much better for myself and for the discipline of the cows to let the rope hold them than it is to try to hold them myself. They soon learn that the rope can hold them; they also soon learn that man cannot hold them without a rope. The rope I use is 6 or 7 feet long, and has a loop on one end. I put it around the right leg above the gambrel, through the loop, and draw it tight enough to keep it from dropping down, then behind the left leg and take a turn once around it (like a figure 8), then around both legs, then between the legs, around the rope that crosses in front and back of the legs, in such a way as to draw them as near together as desirable, then make fast. It is not necessary to draw the rope tight enough to hurt the cow if she stands still. It matters not how hard or how long she tries to get away from the rope; it will stay there and it will hold her legs very near to each other so she cannot kick, and however hard she may pull on the rope, the part that is on the inside of one leg being on with a slip-noose, that on the other with a round turn, as soon as she stops struggling and the rope is slack they do not stop the circulation of the blood. I am particular in telling how I put the rope on when I need to tie a kicking cow, because it is the only way I have ever seen that will hold every time and not get tight enough to stop the circulation."

II. Another dairyman takes the following plan to prevent cows from kicking when being milked. He says: "Before sitting down to milk I put a 'snap' attached to the end of a small rope into her nose and tie the rope to a pin put into the scaffold girt over the manger, slightly elevating her nose, and she stands as quietly while she is milked as the most gentle cow in the stable."—*American Cultivator.*

*Remarks.*—I have not a doubt but what either of these plans will secure the cow against kicking—they have something else to think of. On the same principle that the cord in the mouth of a vicious horse carried up over the head and enclosing an ear tightly enables the blacksmith to shoe him without trouble, which see.

**Lice, To Kill, on Cows, Calves, Dogs and Poultry.**—The New York *Times* informs its readers that "any oily or greasy substance kills them on any of the animals named; that sulphur is also fatal to them; that Persian insect powder, which is kept by all druggists, is the best of all remedies. Linseed oil and sulphur, well mixed, is an effective remedy when it is thoroughly applied. But it is useless to kill the lice all over the back of an animal and leave a colony alive on the brisket or under the thighs, where they usually abound, as in this case they soon spread all over again.

I.   "Sulphur, 1 oz.; fresh lard, 4 ozs., well mixed, makes the right proportions.

II.   "Raw linseed oil, 4 ozs.; kerosene, 1 oz., or sulphur, 1 oz.

III.   "Persian insect powder, 1 oz.; fresh lard, 4 ozs."

*Remarks.*—Any of these thoroughly mixed and thoroughly rubbed in about the ears and all along the spine to the tail, briskets, between the thighs, where the skin is thin, about twice a week will soon eradicate them effectually on any animal; but with poultry they must also be reached in the cracks and crevices of their roosts. You will find to put these parasitic animals (lice) into any of the above greasy mixtures they soon die. It is believed the grease stops up the pores in their skins or surface, and thus kills them, as a man would soon die if covered with an impenetrable varnish. But if the above ever fails, try the following:

IV.   *Death for Lice on Animals or Plants.*—Pour boiling water (1 gal.) on 1 lb. of tobacco leaves; in 20 minutes strain and use it judiciously (simply wetting the parts with a sponge) on animals; on plants more extensively.

*Remarks.*—It is believed that the reason why this may have failed in some cases, both on animals and plants, is because stems and not leaves have been used. Double the quantity of stems and longer steeping may answer the purpose; but the leaves are undoubtedly the most certain.

V.   *Lice on Stock, Simple Remedy for.*—A Mr. D. K. Shaver, in a letter to the Iowa *Homestead*, says: "A simple, sure and easily applied cure for lice on animals is to give a few slices of onions in their feed. They eat them readily, and one or two feeds does the business effectually."

*Remarks.*—Certainly easy to try, and I have not a doubt but what all stock, as he says, will eat them readily.

**SALT—Its Importance for Milch Cows and Other Stock—Amount Daily Necessary.**—I. *Its Importance.*—An American, traveling in Switzerland, writes that "Here the milch cows are salted early every morning, and if fed in the stable, as they usually are, the salt is given before feeding. And they claim that by salting in this way their appetite is improved, they drink with more regularity, keep in better health, and give more milk, than when salted in the usual way, as practiced by dairymen in America. The Swiss dairymen think it very injurious to salt milch cows only once or twice a week, as they would lick too much salt at one time, and drink too much water for the day; they consider that stock in order to do well must be fed with regularity every day alike, and never given too much of anything at one time."

II. *Amount Necessary..*—One of our own stockmen says: "Salt should be furnished to all animals regularly. A cow, an ox, or a horse, according to size, needs 2 to 4 ozs. daily. Salt increases the butter in milk, helps the digestion and nutritive processes, and gives a good appetite.

*Remarks.*—What more can be asked of any one thing which costs so little? I have seen dairymen who keep salt, in some covered place, where all the stock can lick it at their pleasure, and claim great advantage by it. The Swiss plan, for milch. cows, is, no doubt, the best one; for twice a week, the custom of Americans, is not often enough to insure all the advantages to be derived from it, if given daily, or at least every other day. But the daily plan is undoubtedly the best, as the Swiss put it, lest they drink too much water for the day.

III. *Salt, Amount Necessary for Different Kinds of Stock.*—The French government, according to their custom of testing all such points scientifically, appointed a commission to examine into, and experiment if necessary, which reported upon the amount proper for different kinds of stock, in ordinary condition, as follows: "For a working ox or a milch cow, 2 ozs. daily; for fattening stall-fed oxen, 2½ to 4½ ozs., according to size and fatness; for fattening hogs, 1 to 2 ozs.. for store sheep, ½ to ⅔ of an oz.; fattening sheep, double the amount; for horses and mules, 1 oz."

And a private dairyman found, after many trials, that with 2 ozs. of salt daily, his cows gave the most milk. And the noted French farmer and chemist, Boussingault, to test it thoroughly, "Fed 6 steers for 13 months, in 2 lots, the food being the same for each lot; but to one lot he gave 1⅛ ozs. of salt daily, to an animal, and to the other lot none. A remarkable difference was at once manifest. The first lot were all sleek, smooth-coated and in perfect condition. The other became rough, mangy, and ill-conditioned, and weighed at the end of the test 150 lbs. less than those that had been supplied with salt."

"Many other similar results," says the *Michigan Farmer*, which gave the above facts, "might be cited; but there ought to be sufficient to induce those who still doubt the value of salt for all kinds of farm stock, to test it for themselves." It closed as follows:

"Not only is salt an agreeable and needful article of food, but is in some diseases almost a specific remedy. For those parasitic diseases to which sheep are subject—such as the liver-rot (flukes in the liver), verminous bronchitis, (worms in the bronchial tubes),and worms in the stomach and intestines—salt is an unfailing remedy, as well as an effectual preventive. The irritating worms, which sometimes infest the rectum, of horses are removed at once by an injection of a solution of 1 oz. of salt in 1 qt. of water. But it is as a constant addition to the food that it is most useful as a preservative of the health of our domestic animals."

**2. Salt and Ashes for Stock off Their Feed**. — The *Maine Farmer*, says that one of their substantial subscribers recommends with neat stock (young, growing stock),—then why not good for cows when they get-off their feed?—chewing wood, bones, etc., to mix leached ashes, 1 qt., with the same amount of salt, and feed to a dozen head once a week, especially in the spring of the year, as it improves their appetite and agrees with them wonderfully. I should try it under such conditions whenever theyoccur.

**3. Salt as a Vermifuge, its Value for Cattle, Horses, Sheep and Hogs.**—The New York *World*, speaking of salt for stock, says: "If you want to keep your cattle, horses, sheep and hogs healthy, give them salt regularly. There is no better vermifuge than salt. Much of the so-called hog-cholera is due to intestinal worms. Plenty of salt would prevent the accumulation of these worms. All animals desire salt, showing that it is a want of their nature, and undoubtedly for wise purposes."

*Remarks.*—Who can fail to see the value of salt for all stock, and that it should also be given regularly? None, certainly.

**Cows, Accidentally Over-Eating Meal, What to do.**—When a cow has accidentally eaten her fill of meal, do not allow her to drink; and as soon as discovered, according to the size of the animal, give a drink of from 1 to 2 lbs. of Epsom salts, dissolved in warm water, and repeat the dose in 6 hours if it has not operated; in 6 hours more, if has not yet worked a hole through, repeat half as much more, and so continue until a movement is obtained.

**Jersey Cows, the Best, Large Amounts of Butter from them Yearly, etc.**—The *Live Stock Record* says: "Our opinion, and also that of the principal dairymen of the country, is that the Jersey, commonly called Alderney, is above all others the best cow. They are easily kept, very docile—a point not to be overlooked—and beautiful; give milk of superior richness, from which is produced finely-colored, solid butter, having an equal texture and flavor. Butter made from such milk has been known to keep when placed in a dry (not cold) cellar without the use of ice, and when taken out was in a hard, firm condition, and was then sold 12 to 15 cents per pound higher than best ordinary butter. The cost for Jerseys is not much more than for scrub, and they will more than make up the difference in price in a few months."

Mr. R. Goodman, in the *Rural New Yorker*, makes the following statement as to the superiority of the Jersey over all others. He says: "The Jerseys of the present day, all over the United States, are not small or ill formed, but larger and much more symmetrical than was the average Jersey of 20 years since, the production of milk also being greater, and the yield of butter surprising. In the latter respect the breeders of all other classes of stock, and even the ordinary farmers, who have continued to swear by their native cows, are forced to admit that the Jerseys are superior to all others."

Mr. Goodman, after speaking of some very large yields of milk, one herd of 65 cows averaging 295 lbs. of butter each per year, one of 17 head, averaging 225 lbs. each., and one of 15, averaging 281 lbs. each; and of the great Jersey cow, "Flora," owned by Mr. Motley, making 511 lbs., 2 ozs., in one year, "Pansy," 572 lbs., etc., closes as follows: "It is not always the Jerseys of the largest yield of milk which make proportionately the greatest amount of butter. Those more moderate in quantity are apt to be richer in quality, and a cow giving 12 to 14 qts. of milk per day is usually a more profitable buttermaker than one giving 20 qts. We have in our herd Jerseys which produce, when flush, over 40 lbs. of milk per day, but we set a higher value on others which yield less, but whose butter average for the year is greater."

*Remarks.*—There may be an occasional cow of other breeds, or possibly, a native, which gives an excellent yield, but the best general average belongs, undoubtedly, to the Jerseys. Only think of it, many Jersey cows have an average of from 9,000 to 10,000 lbs. of milk in a year. The well known Jersey cow, "Belle," owned by Mr. Elms, of Scituate, Mass., through the summer averaged 1 lb. of butter to 5 qts. of milk, and in December 4 qts. made 1 lb. of butter; but, suppose it took 5 qts., and she gave even only the 9,000 lbs., and as "a pint is a pound the world round," Belle's yield of butter for a year would be 900 lbs. Is there any wonder, then, that Mr. Elms should have refused $3,000 for her? The Board of Agriculture of the State (Mass.), speaking of this celebrated Jersey in their report for 1876-7, say, that, "in March she made 19½ lbs. of butter per week; 16 in June, 14 in September, and in December, 10 months from calving, and due to calve again in 2 months, made 1 lb. of butter daily." I have mentioned these facts that our readers may see the possibilities of the Jerseys, and that they may strive to reach the same point of excellence, by always saving the best calves for dairy and breeding purposes, and to breed from the best bulls that can be obtained, if it is expected to ever have a herd of cows that will pay any considerable sum over and above the expense and care of keeping. What has been done can be done again; but if we do not know what has been done we have no particular point to strive for. Yet it is only proper and right that all shall have an opportunity to judge for themselves, so I will mention what some writer has recently said upon the Durham, claiming superior milking qualities, and also an advantage for "beefing," as they see it in Ontario, for they, like the English, are great on beef, and fat at that. After giving an item from the Toledo *Post*, of what the Canadians think of the Durhams, I will also speak of one formerly owned by myself. The item was given under the head of

**Durham Cows, Their Value for Milk and Beef.**—"In Ontario, Canada, considerable attention is being paid to raising Durham cows, on account of their superior milking qualities, and for their good beefing. It is claimed that a 9 year old Durham, fed on ground grain, with bran and grass, will give 30 lbs of milk at a morning's milking, and from 15 to 16 lbs. of butter is made weekly from her milk: The mixture of the Durham breed with the pure Canadian improves the beefing power of the animals, but decreases the quantity of milk. In regard to beefing, however, the Durham is far more profitable than the Alderney—Jersey."

*Remarks.*—Just at the close of the late war I owned a remarkably fine Durham cow. She was not only an excellent milker, but was an easy keeper, and above all was remarkably kind; almost affectionate, if I may be allowed the expression, in relation to a cow. She would follow me, not only from place to place, about the lot, but if she saw me going to town, while she was at liberty, she would follow me, and even into a store, if I had occasion to go in, unless I set a clerk to stand by the door to keep her out. I had to do this several times, when she would see me start off, and I not see her in time to shut her into the yard. No person could be more kind than she was, in her way. And if all Durhams are as good as she was to give milk, and as easily kept, the author would be a Durham man every time. (See Fattening Cattle, how a Yankee Farmer Makes it Pay in Massachusetts; also see What Durhams are for Milk, and for Beef, above.)

**Calves, Raising by Hand—Hay, Tea, etc., for Them.**—With good pasture for calves to run in, early cut and properly cured hay, of which to make the hay tea; oil-cake, or home-ground oatmeal, and the milk of one cow, three calves, after they are 10 days old, have been successfully kept, and all the cream from the cow made into butter after the calves were 4 weeks old. The plan was as follows: DIRECTIONS—Boil good timothy hay, 1 lb. (better cut in a cutter, if you have one) and boil in water, 6 qts., for an hour, keeping covered, and make up for what may evaporate; then strain and let cool. While cooling, stir 3 table-spoonfuls of oil-cake, made fine, or pretty finely ground meal from oats, into 1 qt. of boiling water, slowly, as if making "hasty pudding," and when properly cooked stir this and the milk of the cow, with a very little salt, into the hay tea, and give equally to the three calves. At the first feed while warm, but after a week or two it does not matter if given cold, but with each two weeks increase the oil-cake meal or the oatmeal, 1 table-spoonful for each calf. And it was claimed that at three months old calves raised in this way looked as well as those fed on milk entirely. They began to feed on grass at a month old, and increased their feeding on the grass until they depended upon it almost entirely at 3 months. The trifle of salt must not be forgotten; and if they begin to scour, the milk was boiled and 1 table-spoonful of flour stirred in before it was added to the tea. But I should stir the flour into the milk while scalding. After the first week there was no trouble of this kind, unless over-fed.

*Remarks.*—I have condensed the above from some agricultural writer who was not willing to put his name to his recommendations; but as I see it must be good and was endorsed by the following, I have given it. I would say also, in case of much scouring, 15 to 20 drops of laudanum to each calf which may scour may be added until relieved. For further instructions upon this point, if any bad cases, see "Calves, Indigestion of," etc.

II. *Hay Tea, Also for Calves, Without Other Help.*—The "Young Farmer" who does the agricultural writing for the Boston *Journal*, under the above head, gives his experience, which goes to show plainly that calves can be raised upon hay tea, without milk or other help. Whether this one swallow (contrary to the general rule, that one swallow does not make a summer), shall be considered a sufficient ground of reason for others to try it, I leave each one to judge for himself. I should have no fears in trying it, if I had calves to raise; still I cannot see why a little thickening of the hay tea might not be made, with a proper amount of the finely ground oatmeal, although the milk, it seems, can be left out without detriment. He says:

"Being obliged to buy another cow a short time ago, to keep along my supply of milk, I picked one out with a calf 5 weeks old at her side. The calf was by a Dutch or Holstein bull out of a ⅝ths Jersey cow, and was a very promising heifer, in every way well formed. I could not bear to devote it to the butcher; and I was in a bit of a quandry as I had not a bit of milk, new or skimmed, to give it. At last a neighbor suggested hay tea. And hay tea it has had. Not a quart of milk or a spoonful of meal since I got it, and it is doing as well as any calf I ever raised; grows finely, is fat enough, and seems to like its hay tea, and to be just as well satisfied with a full meal of that as it would be if it had taken its fill right from the cow. I never tried hay tea before, and never saw it made or fed out. I should have given a few roots or a little meal, but for a desire to see how the tea went, without any other food, that I might know whether the calf thrived on that, or on other food. Thus far, I am very well pleased with the result. It is not as much trouble to make the hay tea as to make porridge, and the cost is nothing. I cut my hay, the best and finest I have, about 4 inches long, and pour boiling water over it. Let it stand until about the heat of milk from the cow, then take the hay out and give it to the cow and the tea to the calf. One of my neighbors says I am making the hay worth more for the cow, and so getting a profit, besides raising the calf. At any rate, she eats it greedily. The longer the hay steeps before it gets cool, the more strength there is in it."

*Remarks.*—It will be seen in No. 1 that 1 lb. of hay was used for 3 calves. This "Young Farmer" does not give any weight, nor the amount of water, but I should suppose that at least 2 qts. should be left after what is absorbed by the hay, *i. e.*, for one calf, and that if only the hay tea was to be given, I should use at least $\frac{1}{2}$ or $\frac{3}{4}$ of a pound of hay for 1 calf. Still, the author must advise, or think, it better to use a couple of table-spoonfuls of the oat-meal, made into mush, or hasty pudding, as No. 1 has it, than to depend on the hay tea alone. I think it will prove the most healthful in this way for the calf. That the hay tea is a grand invention, in raising calves, I have not a doubt.

**Feeding Calves in Winter.**—A person signing himself "Experience," of Muir, Mich., in answer to the inquiry of "Breeder," in the Detroit *Tribune*, that some of its many readers would tell him the best feed for calves in winter, says: "If he will give his calves wheat bran for their morning meal, and turnips for their evening meal, with what good clover hay they want, and give them a warm, clean stable, never let them out doors in the cold; water them in their stalls once a day—in the evening—he will have no trouble to raise good calves and keep them fat and growing. But under no circumstances should they be turned out of doors until spring, and if they are kept in the stalls on bran and turnips until feed is good, they are better for it. The bran should be fed dry with a small quantity of salt twice a week.

*Remarks.*—The author cannot see why good, warm, dry sheds, with plenty of bedding or littering daily, will not do very nicely when stable room is not plenty.

**Indigestion of Calves, Remedies for.**—Calves that are fed on milk principally, and carelessly managed, are liable to indigestion; becoming "pot-bellied," dull and thriftless, appetite varied, sometimes voracious, then not caring for their food at all; bowels irregular, or else regularly loose, and their passages offensive, which, if not soon remedied, the diarrhœa becomes chronic and troublesome to cure. The trouble is believed to arise from an accumulation of curdled milk in the fourth stomach (which is the one used until they begin to ruminate—chew the cud—); hence laxatives are first called for, such as castor-oil or linseed oil, with bicarbonate of soda (baking soda) and ginger, and if really scouring, 15 or 20 drops of laudanum should be added. The dose for a calf of 3 months, of castor-oil, would be 2 ozs., with ½ oz. each of the soda and pulverized ginger, with the laudanum, as above, if scouring. And for a few days, or until the condition is greatly improved or health established, give morning and evening, salt, soda, and pulverized ginger, ½ oz. each, in a little milk; or if the calf is flatulent (windy) dull and weak, add 1 oz. of sulphate of soda (glauber salts), to the salt, soda and ginger, twice daily till corrected.

The diet in all such cases, must be carefully attended to. If unweaned the calf should have its milk fresh and sound thrice daily. A daily allowance of linseed or gruel or bruised linseed cake will further be serviceable. Comfortable shelter, a dry bed and plenty of room are also essential. When protracted indigestion appears to result from weakness, and the mucous membrane has become irritable and relaxed, advantage usually follows the use of 8 or 10 drops each of muriatic acid and creosote, given every morning until it abates.

**Scoures, in Cattle, Horses, Calves and Cholera, or Diarrhœa of Persons.**—Lewis Boynton, of Farmingdale, Bledsoe Co., Tenn., in answer to an inquiry about scours in cattle, in one of the papers, says: " Frequently a handful of salt will relieve cattle and horses of scours. It does not afford relief in 12 hours, I have recourse to a remedy for cholera that never fails: Spirits of camphor, tinct. of rhubarb, and laudanum, equal parts of each Mix. Dose—For an adult, 30 drops; for a horse or cow, a dessert-spoonful; for a calf, 1 tea-spoonful. If not relieved in 3 hours, repeat the dose.

*Remarks.*—For a child I would add 8 to 10 drops, according to age, and repeat on persons half to an hour, if needed. Give in a little sweetened water to children. For stock, in ½ pt. drench. It will be found very valuable.

**Dairying—Its Profit if Well Managed.**—To show the profits of a well managed dairy, I cannot do better than condense a report made by Jeremiah Pierce, of Hamburgh, N. Y., to the *Live Stock Journal*, in 1873. Hamburgh is in a great dairy section, and its cheese is celebrated all over the country. Mr. Pierce milked 18 cows, and from April 14th to Nov. 15th—215 days, sent to the cheese factory 80,708 lbs of milk; kept at home to feed calves up to July 1st, 9,625 lbs., making a total of 90,333 lbs., in the 215 days, Sold 837½ lbs. of butter made before sending to factory. He allows 23 lbs. of milk for 1 lb. of butter, I think rather a large allowance [see Jersey cows the best, etc.] which would regain 19,262 lbs. of milk to make the butter sold, or a total of 109,595 lbs. of milk from the 18 cows—an average of 6,088 lbs. of milk to each cow for the season. Jerseys, it will be remembered under that head, have given 9,000 to 10,000 lbs. per cow, in a year.

He received for cheese, $886.14; for butter, $293.13; for calves, sold while young, $43.00; value of 5 calves raised on milk, $60 00; pork made, 500 lbs., $30.00, making a total of $1,310.27. Gross receipts for each cow for the season, $72.79. The season being a very dry one, he fed, to make up for short pasturage, barley sprouts and bran costing $161.08, being $8.94 to each cow, reducing the proceeds to $63.85 for each cow, which I still think is a pretty good average.

Notice the point, however, that he feeds extra, as recommended in the next item, and by all dairymen, so far as I know, to make up for short pasture. He claims too, that he got more from his extra feed, than simply making up for the shortage of the grass, besides keeping his cows in good condition, and good heart, for the full supply of grass after the fall rains set in. Mr. Pierce says in his communication: "I raise my own cows," claiming that cows may be purchased for less money than it will cost to raise them, but many of these will be dear at any price. Then raise them, and raise the best you can. In this report Mr. Pierce made another remark which I consider of the utmost importance, *i. e.*, that "cows which do not come in until they are 3 years old, make much better milkers, than those that come in at 2." He closes with this important exhortation: "Brother farmers, don't be afraid of feeding your cows too well. I hope to do better next year."

**Dairy Cows, to Feed Liberally.**—The importance of feeding dairy cows liberally, more especially when pasture is short, was recently shown so satisfactorily by the *National Live Stock Journal*, I will give all its principal points, although largely condensed. The editor starts out with the idea that dairymen should study to produce all the food necessary for his cows upon the farm, using his most intelligent foresight to this end; but that he should never suffer them to go with deficient food, even for 1 week; for this he cannot afford to do. Hence, he says, when pasture is short, and he has no extra green feed for them, let us compare the cost of nutriment in some by-product, such as bran, cotton seed meal, linseed meal, corn meal, etc., some of which he can always find near at hand, with pasture grass. Pasture grass, he continues, has about 80 per cent. of water; and the nutriment of 100 lbs. of it is supposed to be worth 21 cents. The nutriment of 19 lbs. of fine bran, or 19 lbs. of corn meal, is just equal to 100 lbs. of grass. Cotton seed meal, 10 lbs.; linseed meal, 12 lbs., have just the same nutriment. Then, as 100 lbs. of grass are considered a ration for an ordinary sized cow, per day, it is easy to get at the proper amount of substitute; for if ⅓ or ½ short, in the bite of grass, take the proportionate amount of the kind of feed, in pounds, daily, to make up the deficiency; which any dairyman can calculate for himself, knowing how much short the grass is. Let us suppose the dairyman is feeding 7 lbs. of fine bran; this, at $8 per ton, would cost 2⅘ cents per day, or 19⅗ cents per week. Now, the extra milk per week, would more than pay the cost. Besides, he might have added, it keeps the cow from falling off in flesh, and losing heart, or vital activity. But, he continues, if he should feed, instead of bran, 4 lbs. of linseed meal, daily, it would cost him 28 cts. per week; or if 3⅓ lbs. of cotton seed meal, it would cost 22 cts. per week, or 6⅓ lbs. of corn meal, it would cost from 20 to 35 cts. per cow a week. If he has a command of all these, let him make up a ration nearly as follows: 4 lbs. of bran, ½ lb. linseed meal, and 1½ lbs. corn meal, to each cow per day, which will, in most cases, cost only 20 cents per week; and will keep up a generous flow of milk till the fall rains renew the pasture, and then the extra food (the author would say only ¾ths of it) can be discontinued. He closes as follows: We have known many who have used an extra ration similar to this during short pasture, and never found one who reported it unprofitable. The ration may be varied to suit all circum- stances. Corn meal will be found cheap in some localities; but it is always best to mix some bran with it; and in most parts of all our broad dairy belt bran will be found the cheapest extra food to make up for short pasture.

*Remarks.*—Of course, any other class of feed can be chosen according to what is found in the market of the different sections of our great country —coarse middlings, shorts, etc. Then some millers mix all grades together, and in the Eastern States it is known as "mill stuffs," while the Westerner and Southerner know this mixture as "ship stuffs," "mill feed," etc. But I should prefer to buy them separate, then you know exactly what you are feeding. See "Milk—To Increase the Flow in Cows," and the remarks following it, for what many claim to be the best mixture for this purpose. The importance of the various roots, more especially as winter feed, will be seen below; also, for the value of parsnips for milch cows see close of remarks after "Carrots, Parsnips, Beets, etc.," below. I must be allowed to state here that Mr. O. W. Wanger, a dairyman of Illinois, says: "For ground feed for milch cows an effort is made to combine the elements that will produce the largest flow of milk and at the same time keep the cow in good condition, but not too fat. And it is found one part (equal parts) each of corn meal, ground oats and bran will bring the best results." [This is the "Best Food" referred to above, and hence is confirmatory of that recipe.] "And," he adds, "with these con- veniences, good hay, this ground feed, good water and good care a cow yields as much milk during 6 months in winter as in summer, when the cow feeds on grass." And he recommends a little grain all summer. This, I suppose, refers to the ground feed above, for he adds: "When the milker is to milk a cow he first feeds her and then sits down to milk. The result is, the cow stands quiet, gives her milk at once and the flow is increased." He also recommends sowed corn to help the cows in dry times of the summer. Very important points, I know, from what I have seen done by others. He does not say whether his parts are to be by weight or measure, but I think he means by measure, as that is the common way unless weight is mentioned.

**Winter Feeding of Cows, Horses and All Other Stock—The Importance of Roots or Oil Meal, etc., for.**—It is a great change for cattle, horses, sheep, etc., from a pasture where there is plenty of grass, and also plenty of exercise, to the stable or even a barn-yard, where comparatively there is neither grass nor exercise; but the milch cows will show it the quickest by the shortness in quantity of milk given, unless some of the succulent roots or oil meal are given at once to make up for the change from grass to dry hay. Then, again, dry hay, oats, corn or cornmeal have a tendency to produce cost- iveness, and hence the importance of some of the roots or oil meal to be given directly to avoid the probability of costiveness becoming thoroughly established. People eat oatmeal or cornmeal mush, corn bread, apples, peaches, berries, etc., for this very purpose; why should it, then, not be as necessary for stock as for persons? It is, and should receive the same care and attention, if we would keep them in a continuous healthy condition, so that the cows shall give the largest flow of milk, and that other stock shall continue to thrive instead of the hair becoming rough and staring and the animals losing flesh as well as heart and appetite. Even poultry should have something of a succulent or juicy character to make up for the loss of green feed, insects, etc.

**Extra Value of Oatmeal or Flaxseed, Roots, etc., in Winter for Cows and Breeding Ewes.**—The editor of the *National Live Stock Journal* makes a very important suggestion in speaking upon the subject of roots or oil meal to make up for the absence of green food, that for cows or breeding ewes the oil meal or flaxseed, for these animals especially, have another and important value, enabling them to produce their young without trouble. We have such medicines of value in this respect for our own race, why not for stock? He says: "Every dairyman, so far as he can, should supply himself with 1 pt. of oil meal for each cow per day, or ½ pt. of flaxseed, which should be boiled to a jelly and given with her other food. Oil meal is worth all it costs for food, besides being an excellent preventive of disease; and, also, has this further property, that when a small quantity of it is fed to cows during the winter we have never had any trouble with them at calving; and the small quantity of oil left in it seems to perform the same office as a little grass or carrots and beets would, to cleanse the bowels as well as an emollient, or some such property or effect, upon the reproductive organs; and to this end some persons feed a small amount of flaxseed to their breeding ewes in winter with a like success." Sensible and well put, and the author knows them to be of extra value for all these purposes.

**Carrots, Beets, etc., their Value as Food for Stock.**—It has been heretofore claimed that the chief reason why the above named articles were valuable for stock was to avoid costiveness, and that carrots alone possessed this property—pectine, or pectic acid—which has the power of dissolving or gelatinizing—turning to jelly—other kinds of food, which not only gave health and vigor, but also gave brightness to the eye, and a smooth, glossy coat to the animal. But a horse-breeder, in France reports having fed his horses for 20 years on parsnips, instead of carrots and oats as formerly, with a remarkable success, his stock showing a greater vivacity of spirit and a sleekness of coat than when fed on carrots. And Yeomans, the celebrated veterinarian, informs us that this beneficial result, from feeding these roots, arises not so much from their nutritive properties as from their effects in gelatinizing and dissolving other foods, thereby rendering them more easy of digestion. Portions of other coarse food, otherwise almost indigestible, when acted upon by this principle in these roots, are easily dissolved by the gastric juices, and a thorough and perfect digestion is obtained.

*Remarks.*—It has been well known that apples contain this principle—pectine, or pectic acid—in a great degree; hence, we can account for both horses and cattle thriving so well, as many have reported, while being fed a peck of apples morning and night, or when allowed to run for a time in the orchard, where they ate of them at pleasure. (See Apples for Horses, etc.) But

Yeomans also says it is found in pears, quinces, currants, raspberries, and many other kinds of fruit, and also in various roots, such as turnips, beets, parsnips, etc.; hence their great value as a food, or as auxiliary to the food both of man and beast. Closing with this important sentence: "A small quantity of roots or fruit mixed with other food, especially with dry food, has a wonderful effect upon the flesh, health and spirits of animals." Thus it may be seen, and I have given this item chiefly that it might be seen, that it does not matter so very much which kind of roots for animals, nor which kind of fruit or roots for man are raised and eaten; but that it is very important that some of them should be raised and used, if the best health of man and beast is worth looking after and working for.

Then let every dairyman or farmer look at the matter in a common sense way, and raise the kind of roots that his land is seen to be the best adapted to—the longer and larger roots require the deepest and richest soil, and all require close and careful culture to obtain the best results; then, for winter-feeding, to have them carefully housed, and properly cut when fed, so that each animal shall get its proper share, remembering that while you thus aid the digestion of the coarser food, as hay, stalks and straw, by this admixture of roots, you also avoid costiveness, which was originally supposed to be the chief object to be gained by feeding roots. In other words, "two birds are killed with one stone," and really, the bird last found is of the greater importance of the two —the aid to digestion. (See Comparative Value, as Generally Understood, and also Nutritive Value, with table by which the difference is more easily seen.)

I will only add here that of later years parsnips have been found more valuable than formerly supposed, and they are now commended by many dairymen as excellent for milch cows, increasing the flow of milk one-half, besides keeping them in a good healthy condition. Try them, thoroughly, by all means.

**Variety of Food for Stock—Very Important.**—It is a well established fact that a single kind of food is not enough for the best growth, health or comfort of animals. Like ourselves, the stock which we keep, does relish a change of diet—thrives better with a change of pasture so to speak—and gives fuller returns for the trouble of providing the variety of foods. Coarse fodder should be mixed with that which is of a finer nature; and the highly nitrogenous, fed with substances weak in nitrogen. Some farmers will feed their sheep corn one morning, add barley or oats the next, and thus keep up a continual surprise, heightened by a lick of salt now and then. It is the same love of change which makes the colt, cow, and even the oldest horse feel glad when turned into a new field. What man would like living on bread, or potatoes, or meat, alone? Then feed your stock meal, or shorts, or roots—sometimes one, then the other, is the better way—as remarked about the sheep above being sure to have a supply of roots for every winter.

**The Comparative Value of Roots for Winter Feeding as Generally Understood.**—A writer in the *Rural Home* places the comparative value of roots in the following order: Carrots, parsnips, sugar-beets, mangelwurzels, rutabagas, Swedish turnips, and lastly, English or common field turnips, which are lighter, but do well for early feeding, before beginning on the richer roots, which also keep better. This writer did not mention potatoes, but another writer who had been experimenting upon the subject under the head of "Potatoes for Stock," says: "Potatoes for stock are worth 30 cents per bushel to feed to stock. They are not only nutritious, but excellent appetizers, and promoters of digestion. My experiments go to show that a peck of potatoes will produce as much milk as a bushel of carrots, beets or turnips."

*Remarks.*—Although potatoes are well known to contain much more general nutritive and fat-producing properties than the other roots named, yet, as the others can be raised in so much larger quantities to the acre, and with so much less labor also, it is not probable that they will become the best for general winter feeding. And I must say here that I think this writer is in error as to carrots, and I might say parsnips, too (he does not mention the latter), but as to beets and turnips, they are not as valuable as potatoes. I will, however, give a table below, showing the proportionate nutritive, flesh-producing, and fat-producing properties of 22 different kinds of food for farm stock. I am sorry, however, that the sugar-beet is not shown among them. The table was made up from the experiments and analysis of the most eminent agricultural chemists and English feeders; and are undoubtedly the most reliable and trustworthy that can be gathered at the time of this writing; and believing that they will prove of real value to farmers, dairymen, etc., I give the table a place. The calculation is based upon equal weights of each article, and is as follows:

## Nutritive Value of 22 Different Kinds of Food for Farm Stock:

| Food. | Flesh producing. | Fat producing. | Total. |
|---|---|---|---|
| Turnips, | 1 | 5 | 7 |
| Rutabagas, | 1 | 7 | 9 |
| Carrots, | 1 | 7 | 10 |
| Mangels, | 2 | 8 | 12 |
| Straw, | 3 | 16 | 22 |
| Potatoes, | 2 | 17 | 22 |
| Brewer's grains, | 6½ | 18 | 25 |
| Hay (early cut), | 8 | 51 | 64 |
| Millet (seed), | 8 | 76 | 85 |
| Buckwheat, | 9 | 61 | 69 |
| Malt, | 9 | 76 | 81 |
| Rye, | 11 | 74 | 88 |
| Oats, | 12 | 63 | 70 |
| Corn, | 12 | 53 | 80 |
| Wheat and barley, | 12 | 66 | 32 |
| Dried brewer's grains, | 16 | 67 | 82 |
| Beans (English field), | 22 | 46 | 74 |
| Peas, | 22 | 61 | 79 |
| Linseed, | 23 | 112 | 82 |
| Cotton seed cake, | 24 | 46½ | 61 |
| Linseed cake, | 28 | 56 | 73 |
| Bran and coarse millstuff, | 31 | 54 | 76 |

*Remarks.*—By this table, if you want simply to lay on flesh, you see the food for it; if fat for butchering purposes, it is equally plain, while the general value for keeping stock in the most healthy and growing condition is shown in the total column. Milk being of the nature of fat, it can also be seen which will be the best food for milch cows, that which produces most fat. I will simply mention here that there is quite a doubt amongst dairymen as to whether sugar beets do, or do not, lessen the flow of milk, and it is perhaps from this fact that they were not considered in the table. Although the sugar beet may not be equal to some of the other roots for milk, yet, for other stock they are good; and as they can be raised in such large quantities to the acre, many, no doubt, will raise them for general use. The mangel-wurzels and rutabagas can, with a rich and properly cultivated soil, be made to yield from 1,000 to 1,500, and, in a few cases, even 2,000 bushels to the acre; and with any of these roots, if the ground is properly worked, it will be left in excellent condition for succeeding crops. It would not be advisable, however, to feed roots too exclusively. It is better to feed part roots and part grain. Nor is it advisable to feed one kind of roots only. It is better to have a variety, both on account of the health and condition of the stock, and for the better results in milk which will be produced by a variety over any single kind.

**Roots, Culture of, for Stock.**—As above remarked, the culture of roots needs a rich soil; and if it is not rich naturally, it must be made so with manures, fertilizers, etc., and also by deep plowing and thorough harrowing. Plow deeply, and harrow; then re-plow and harrow, until as fine as possible, leaving no stones or turf to obstruct cultivation. The mangel-wurzel, it is claimed, is a great lover of salt; and as high as 30 bushels to the acre, Dr. Loring says, has been used with profit. Fifteen two-horse wagon loads of good, solid manure to the acre, is not too much, if you expect 1,500 to 2,000 bushels of mangels (which has been raised) to the acre. The fertilizer when used, must, as well as the manure, be well worked into the surface of the soil. Sow in drills, beets, mangels, rutabagas, and parsnips, 30 inches apart; carrots, 24. If possible, have a drill which completes the work of covering evenly as it goes. Begin to cultivate them as soon as the rows can be seen; keep clear of weeds, and thin carrots and parsnips to 4 inches; beets, rutabagas or mangels, 6 to 10 inches, as you think the richness of the soil will demand. Of course, let all be done with horse-hoes, or such conveniences as you have, so that the rows simply need to be done by hand, remembering this, if the weeds get the start of you, you will pay dearly for it. Some claim that 5 lbs. of mangel seed is not too much for an acre; but if sowed with a drill, get it to scatter them properly as you go; then have enough to go over the piece is all you want for any kind. Absolute amounts can hardly be given, as no two men would think exactly alike about it; better pull out a good many, however, rather than not to get in seed enough.

**Field Turnips, How to Feed to Cows Without Flavoring the Milk.**—A writer in the *Maine Farmer*, says he raised 800 bushels, and fed all to his 16 to 20 cows—1 pk. twice a day—by trimming off the rootlets and feeding only the solid turnip, after milking, no bad flavor was imparted to the milk.

*Remarks.*—That the whole flavol of turnips is in the rootlets, I should hardly expect to be the fact, but that feeding them only after milking is the more probable reason why the flavor is not retained. The plan is worthy of a trial, and if the reasoning is not correct, the turnips can be fed to other stock, while the milch cows can be supplied with something that has no partic· ular flavor as parsnips and turnips have, making either an unsuitable feed for cows while giving milk, unless the removal of the rootlets, as above, is found to be of general application.

**Growing Stock, Pea and Bean Meal Better than Corn for.**— Much has been said of late years, as to feeding pea and bean meal to stock, as though they were equally valuable for all stock which the author does not think is correct, and seeing an item, in the *Philadelphia Record*, giving them the preference over corn for growing stock, which so nearly agrees with what I know to be the fact, I will give the item in full. It is as follows: " Growing stock should not be kept in a fat condition, for the demand of the system is chiefly for muscle producing matter. There is no concentrated material on the farm that supplies the desideratum in full, and though nature has furnished farmers with splendid agents for this purpose in the shape of peas and beans, the opportunity is not improved. For early pasture or soiling after rye, a piece of land broadcasted to tall-growing green peas mixed with oats, is invalu- able. The writer of this once kept a cow up to a flow of ˙milk till late in the season by a succession of such crops, and that, too, on a piece of white sand land. It is not known by some that if these vines are cut and nicely cured, when just about to bloom, they will furnish a good crop of nutritious hay, but if not cut at flowering time the leaves will crumble away. Ground peas or beans are economical for feeding, owing to the great saving they effect. Farmers are tempted to part with them at $2.10 a bu., and they often bring more than that sum; but if we will stop and reflect that this meal, mixed half and half with corn meal, will enable us to dispense with one-third the quantity of hay, a great saving is made through the winter. For young calves nothing can equal it. If the farmer has no convenience for grinding them, the peas and beans can be cooked into a "mash" in the ordinary way, and if thus given liberally to stock, especially the younger portion, will push them rapidly for- ward. Pigs will grow fatter on it than on anything else. Young heifers become matured several months sooner. By the use of pea or bean meal, wheat straw (cut) can be used in the place of hay, and, taken as a whole, it is almost a necessity on well-regulated farms. Bear in mind, as stated above, peas and beans will not fatten stock as readily as corn, nor will the corn make the stock grow as quickly as these. Hence in winter we should feed these arti· cles together in order to get the best results."

*Remarks.*—The author having been raised on the hard-pan hills in the town· ship of Holland, Erie county, N. Y., where corn even was not a paying crop, something that could be more easily raised and in better paying quantities had to be sought out; and it was found in peas and oats sown broad-cast, as the above writer suggests, for the especial purpose of feeding to hogs, cutting up— mowing—and throwing to them as soon as the peas were well filled, at which time they would not only eat the peas with avidity, or greedily, but also chew the pods and vines with like relish, and at once begin to show their value which was continued until they were ripe, after which they were ground together and the meal used to thicken potatoes and pumpkins which were boiled together for the purpose of fattening the hogs until within a few weeks of killing time, when cornmeal was used in its place, or else corn alone fed to harden the pork. And when any horses, cattle, or sheep, happened to be running in the pasture with the hogs they would eat the pea vines and oat straw with the same eagerness and relish that the hogs did the peas and oats. So I can vouch for the pea and oat mixture; and I have not a doubt of the value of beans, or bean meal, as a food for growing stock, although, generally, the trouble and labor of raising them will be much greater than that of raising peas, hence the advantage would be in favor of peas, the oats being sown with them for the purpose of holding up the peas, rather than for the oats themselves, although they are good. It is remarkable how much faster young pigs will grow as soon as the peas and oats are full and are thrown to them regularly. It only needs a trial to be adopted by those who have not seen them used.

**Soiling Cows.**—It undoubtedly pays to judiciously soil cows, as there is no other way by which so much milk can be obtained from a small number of acres. When the land is in proper condition, a cow can be kept upon one-half acre for summer and one acre for winter. Even better than this has been done. In starting, prepare the ground well—one-eighth of an acre of oats, thickly, for each cow, as early in the season as you can; two or three weeks after this sow the same amount of land to oats again for later cutting. Then prepare the ground and sow one-fourth of an acre to corn for each cow, which will probably leave a surplus towards the winter feeding.

**Sweet Cornstalks for Cows.**—When the ears have been gathered the stalks of sweet corn make the very best of fodder. It is not only very sweet and nutritious, but as the ears are gathered before maturity the stalks, if cut at once, as they should be, are in the very best condition for use as fodder. There is some difficulty in curing the stalks; but in several years' experience with them in a rather large way we have had no trouble in keeping the fodder in excellent condition. The great point and need is to thoroughly dry the stalks out of doors. They should be first well wilted and partly dried upon the ground, laid down as they are cut in small bundles, which, when bound afterward, will make easily handled sheaves. After 24 hours or more of exposure the bundles may be bound with a straw band or an osier stalk, and the sheaves so made set up in stocks, loosely placed, so as to admit the air freely among them. The stock or small stack should be well bound at the top to exclude rain, and left out of doors until completely dried and cured. The fodder may then be safely housed in the barn or under the roof of an open shed near the barn, where it can be reached conveniently for use. Fodder so cured is equal to the best hay, and will be eaten with avidity and without waste or loss. Of more than 17 acres grown last season and fed to cows in our dairy the past winter there was scarce a particle to be found in the manure, every fragment excepting some few pieces of some of the coarser butts having been consumed. This, of course, is due in a great measure to the fact that the fodder was finely cut and wetted, and the meal given mixed with it. The economy of such a practice and such a crop so used is too obvious to need comment.—*Farmer's Magazine.*

**Sweet Cornstalks with the Corn for Milch Cows.**—The stalks above, when cured as in the foregoing recipe, are excellent even as winter food; but the following plan of feeding the corn upon the stalk while green as a summer food, as practiced by Dwight Judd, of South Hadley, Mass., for two years past, in the New York *Herald,* has the advantage largely in its favor. When asked what he considered the feeding value of sweet corn for milch cows, he said: " It is invaluable. Cornmeal is not to be compared with it as a feed for producing milk." He keeps, says the *Herald,* a herd of 20 as nice cows as can be found in this vicinity, and says: " When my cows fail a little in milk and I want for my trade a couple of extra cows, I tell my man to cut an extra row or two of corn, and in two or three days I have the amount of milk desired." He plants with a corn-planter, the rows $3\frac{1}{2}$ feet apart, and 22 inches apart in the hills, dropping only 2 or 3 kernels in a hill; and commences feeding it as soon as the corn is fit for table use.

**Dry Cornstalks, the Best Way to Feed Them.**—When hay is scarce, but cornstalks and straw are plentiful, the best way is to cut both finely and mix in proportions of 2 baskets of stalks to 1 of straw, and mix dry for several days' feeding, as it will not heat, but improve, by standing together. Of course, hay is better than straw treated the same way, and all classes of stock will relish it, and especially so if, when to be fed, it is first slightly wet, then a good sprinkling of meal or bran mixed in, nothing except occasionally, perhaps, a large butt may be rejected, but seldom that much is left; nor will any part of them be seen in the manure if a proper amount of roots are also fed to help dissolve and gelatinize this coarser food, as previously explained. A correspondent of the *Country Gentleman* says he had rather have this fine cutting of coarse food than to have it steamed, if it was done even for the same expense. The cutting is certainly very desirable, no matter what stock is to be fed with it.

**Corn Fodder vs. Hay, Comparative Value of.**—Professor J. W. Sanborn, of the Missouri Agricultural College, claims that he has proved, through a long practice and many experiments, that corn fodder has a practical feeding value of two-thirds to three-fourths that of good hay. [Our own experience fully justifies the above estimate.—*Editors, Farm and Fireside.*]

**Hungarian Grass for Milch Cows, Claimed better than Hay.** A correspondent of the *New York Sun* claims that Hungarian grass, when sown thick enough to make fine stalks, is better than even good hay. He sows 3 pecks of seed to the acre, on fine soil, and finely worked with harrow and roller, both before and after sowing; and sowing any time from the 15th of May to the 10th of June. Fit to cut in 9 weeks. Another writer thinks it valuable for horses, after having fed it two winters. Changing only occasionally with cut oats; and he adds: " nothing better for calves and milch cows." He sows even a bushel to the acre, and thinks it very valuable as a top-finish to stacks of wheat, clover, etc., as it is impervious to water, and very little injured, even that which is exposed on the outside of the stack remaining sound. Two to four tons have been raised to the acre, with 12 to 15 bu. of seed, worth $1 to $1.50 per bu., and the straw valuable for feed after threshing, and a never failing crop, if sown on good mellow land. So, let all try it who think their hay crop is going to be short.

**Fattening Cattle.**—A few words now upon the subject of fattening cattle, hogs, etc., would seem to the author as very proper; then, to close the cattle department with the consideration of silos, which, of late years, has been almost continually before the mind of the agriculturist, through this class of papers, until, finally, the government, through the agricultural department, has taken it in hand in such a way it would seem, at least, there can be but little chance for further doubt upon the subject of which however, it is our intention to leave each one to judge for himself, after he has any matter properly laid before him for examination, as we have done in all parts of this, our "Third and Last Effort," to benefit the people. Other people write items for their agricultural papers, I get them together, condense, and often re-write, to make a continuous whole, such parts as will enable any sensible man to profit by the hints, suggestions, and practice of their fellow farmers. First, then:

**Meal and Hay for Fattening Stock — Scalding the Meal a Great Saving.**—An old farmer, whose custom has been to fatten a few animals, gives his experience as to scalding his meal, merely, instead of cooking it, as has been the custom of many. He says: "My practice in fattening sheep and swine, as well as for feeding milch cows, has been to pour boiling water on as much meal as would not make the animals bowels move too freely, both at night and morning, and when the mush is cool, give it to the cow or pig. In covering the meal with boiling water in this way, the starch of the grain is dissolved, and the latent nutritive properties extracted, and the animal receives the entire nutriment of the grain. I have for 2 years past fatted 2 ordinary sized cows, feeding only hay, and only 300 lbs. each of meal, and yielded upwards of 40 lbs. of rough tallow. Salt was given once a week, and occasionally a table-spoonful of wood ashes. In my experience 100 lbs. scalded and fed as above, is equal to 200 lbs. fed dry."

*Remarks.*—This is an undoubted fact—a great saving in the question of meal—as he speaks of knowing others who had fed from 700 to 1,000 lbs. of meal, without scalding, who got no more benefit than he did with his 300 lbs. Facts like these are "worth their weight in meal," if not "in gold." It saves others the labor and trouble of experimenting for themselves.

**2. Fattening Cattle, How a Yankee Farmer Makes it Pay in Massachusetts.**—We take the following from the Springfield (Mass.) *Republican*, not so much to show how it was done, but to show that it can be done; for what has been done, can be done again, and if not done better than at first, it is because careful attention is not paid as to how others have made improvements upon the common ways of doing things. It says: "Franklin county has long been famous for its fat cattle, but the 47 head now standing in the stables of Geo. W. Jones, at Deerfield, Mass., go a little ahead of anything yet seen in the county. They are all Durhams (see mention made of them, following what is said of the Jerseys, as the Best Cows. The question may be considered yet, as an open one—awaiting further discussion, and to be somewhat governed by circumstances, after all that may be said upon the subject); great fellows, so large they can hardly move themselves, the heaviest yoke weighing 4,600 lbs., the next 4,400, and the whole averaging over 4,000 per yoke. They are fed 8 qts. a day each of meal and bran, and all the hay they want; water is supplied to their mangers in pipes. Those now in stall will be taken to Boston about Christmas, when Mr. Jones will stock up for the winter, his usual supply being 80 to 90 cattle, 600 to 700 sheep, and about a dozen horses. Last year he cut about 350 tons of hay, all of which, and about 75 tons more, he fed out. The cattle are kept in a sub-basement of the barn which has to be well ventilated during the winter, else it would become oppressively warm from the number of cattle confined there. Jones puts upon his own land, which lies along the west bank of the Connecticut river for half a mile, all the manure from his stock, raising 12 or 14 acres of heavy tobacco every year, for which he gets prices considerably above that paid for tobacco grown by patent fertilizers. In fact, he is one farmer who has found out how to make farming pay."

*Remarks.* — Now, then, suppose Mr. Jones did this without cutting his hay (having machines for that purpose), and without scalding his meal (which, of course, he did not, otherwise it would have been mentioned), and, again, without the addition of the molasses, as given in the next item, whereby time, and consequently that much of the feed would have been also saved, any one can see, at a glance, how much better it would have paid if all these plans had been known and adopted, as every one can do, hereafter, thanks to Dr. Chase.

**3. Fattening Cattle, to Give Appetite.**—The following item, with which we shall close the question of fattening cattle, is a quotation from *Stewart's Prize Essay* upon feeding and fattening stock, which is so unique, *i. e.*, so unlike anything else I have ever seen upon the subject, and yet, is so apparently reasonable, to say the least, I cannot do better than to quote what he says in his essay, as to the use of molasses in fattening stock, by which he claims a great saving in time, and consequently a saving of the additional food that would be required for the longer period required to fatten them, if the molasses was not used. It is intended to be understood, no doubt, that by using molasses with 8 or 10 times as much water with it, to moisten the dry food, they will eat more of it, and consequently fatten in less time than if the molasses was not given. His ideas about cooking food is also worthy of consideration, especially in fattening stock. The item is as follows:

" In fattening animals time is often a matter of importance to the feeder. Sometimes a month gained is equal to 20 per cent. greater weight at a later period. Cooking food renders its constituents more soluble and digestible, therefore more rapidly entering on flesh an fat. As a condiment and appetizer for fattening animals, molasses has no equal. A small quantity of sweet, upon hay, will cause a larger quantity to be eaten with a relish. We have often tried molasses upon poor animals with great satisfaction. A poor horse will show a change in condition in a few days. The molasses is not only an excellent condiment, but an excellent food; and being so soluble and assimilable that it produces an immediate effect upon the condition of the animal. Three pints may be fed to fattening animals per day, but to cows and breeding stock it must be fed sparingly, and not more than 1 pint per day to a cow, as too much sweet will prevent their breeding. When necessary to use straw for fattening stock, the use of molasses diluted with 8 to 10 proportions of water to wet the straw before steaming, will be found to render it very palatable, and cause it to be eaten, incorporated with other fattening food, as readily as hay. Some noted chemists have supposed all starchy food to be converted into sugar by the action of the stomach, before it becomes assimilated as food. Perhaps this will account for the remarkable effect of sweet food upon animals.

*Remarks.*—The word condiment really means something to give an increased appetite, and a relish for other articles of food; and there is no doubt but what this plan of wetting the cut hay, corn stalks, or other articles of dry food, with sweetened water, as we will call it, does have this remarkable effect, as Mr. Stewart says, in fattening, and no doubt would also have the same effect in feeding generally; unless the question of silos and ensilage shall mark a general revolution in the whole subject of feeding. Of course that we must leave each one to judge for himself, after duly considering the whole matter, which we shall now lay before him. Bear this in mind, however, the food is found to be sweeter for having been put into silos—this molasses plan, to a certain extent, will, no doubt, help those who have not a silo, as yet, ready for use.

**SILOS AND ENSILAGE—Full Explanation to Build—What Crops are Best Adapted—Twenty-Six Questions and Answers.** —Probably there has been no subject of more interest to the farmers which has been discussed more fully, and yet, upon which there was so much doubt as to whether it was really valuable or not, as that of silos and ensilage; and that doubt might not even yet have been made very clear, had not the government, through the agricultural department, taken it up, and through Mr. D. M. Nesbit, proceeded to make an investigation into it, by addressing letters to well-known specialists, living in different states, and also in Canada, putting no less than twenty-six questions, which embraced all the vital points, and asking a free discussion upon all the points, which could be of general use, in understanding the whole subject. The questions were all numbered, and were all answered satisfactorily, and in such a manner, that each answer related to the number of the question, and could thus be readily understood, by referring back to the number of the question; but to put it in book form, it will be better to put first, the question, and the answer immediately following, hence I shall adopt this plan, for the better understanding of the matter by our readers. The subject was published in the Toledo *Blade*, September 22d, 1882. Of course it was not possible to publish the whole of the letters received, in the newspapers, so a summary was prepared by the Department of Agriculture, which will give a fair idea to those interested, as to the value and profitableness of giving a fair trial, by those who have not already done so, of the silo. The question will first be given then the summary or condensed answer, immediately following :

I.  Q. What is the best location of silo, with reference to feeding-rooms ?

A. A few have been built at a distance from the stables, but generally the silos are located with reference to convenience in feeding, in, under or adjacent to the feeding-rooms. Local considerations will determine whether the silos should be below the surface or above, or partly above or partly below. This is not essential. Where the stables are in the basement of a bank barn, the bottom of the silo may be on the same level, or a few feet below, and the top even with the upper floor. This arrangement combines the greatest facilities for filling, weighing, and feeding.

II. Q. What form, or shape, is best for the silos?

A. With rare exceptions the silos described show a rectangular (longer than wide) horizontal section, a few have the corners cut off, and one is octagonal (8 square). The cylindrical (round) form seems to have obvious advantages. If under ground, a cylindrical wall is self-supporting against outside pressure, and may be much lighter than would be safe in any other form. If of wood and above ground, the walls may be stayed with iron bands. In any case, for a given capacity, the cylindrical form requires the least possible amount of wall. A given weight of ensilage in a deep silo requires less extraneous pressure, and esposes less surface to the air than it would in a shallow silo. For these reasons depth is important. If too deep there is danger of expressing juice from the ensilage at the bottom. Where the ensilage is cut down in a vertical sec. tion for feeding, a narrow silo has the advantage of exposing little surface to the air.

III. Q. What dimensions, or how large, ought the silos to be?

A. The silos reported vary in capacity from 364 to 19,200 cubic feet. It entirely full of compressed ensilage the smallest would hold 9.1 tons, and the largest 480 tons, estimating 50 lbs. to the cubic foot. Practically, the capacity of a silo is less to the extent that the ensilage settles under pressure. This should not exceed ¼th, though in shallow silos, or those filled rapidly and with little treading, it is likely to be much more. A temporary curb is sometimes added to the silo proper, so that the latter may be full when the settling ceases.

IV. Q. Of what should the walls be built—material and construction?

A. For walls under ground, stone, brick and concrete are used, The choice in any case may safely depend on the cost. In firm soils that do not become saturated with water, walls are not essential to the preservation of ensilage. Above ground, two thicknesses of inch boards, with sheathing paper between (the latter said, by some, to be unnecessary), seem to be sufficient, if supported against lateral (side) pressure from the ensilage.

V. Q. With what, and how, should the silo be covered?

A. A layer of straw or hay will serve in some measure to exclude air, but it is not necessary. Generally boards or planks are placed directly on the ensilage. The cover is sometimes made in sections of 2 feet or more wide; oftener each plank is separate. The cover is generally put on transversely, having in view the uncovering of a part of the silo while the weight remains on the rest. Rough boards, with no attempt at matching, have been used successfully. A little space should be allowed between the walls and cover, that there may be no interference as the settling progresses.

**VI.** Q. Weighting down, what materials are used, amount required and how applied?

A. Any heavy material may be used. The amount required depends on various conditions. It will be noticed that practice and opinions differ widely. The object is always to make the ensilage compact, and thereby leave little room for air, on which depend fermentation and decay. In a deep silo the greater part is sufficiently compressed by a few feet of ensilage at the top, so that there is small percentage of waste, even when no weight is applied above the ensilage. Screws are used by some instead of weights. The objection to them is that they are not self-acting like gravity.

VII. What is the cost of a silo?

A. The cost of silos, per ton of capacity, varies from $4 to $5, for walls of heavy masonry and superstructures of elaborate finish, and 50 cents or less for the simplest wooden silos. Earth silos, without wall, can be excavated with plow and scraper. when other work is not pressing, at a trifling cost.

VIII. Q. What crops are used for ensilage?

A. Corn takes the lead of ensilage crops. Rye is grown by many in connection with corn—the same ground producing a crop of each in a season. Oats, sorghum, Hungarian grass, field peas, clover—in fact almost every crop used in soiling has been stored in silos and taken out in good condition. There are indications that some materials have their value enhanced by the fermentation of the silo, while in others there is loss. The regular values for ensilage, of the different soiling crops, can only be determined through careful tests, often repeated, by practical men. All thoughtful farmers would be glad to get more value from the bulky fodder of their corn crops than is found in any of the common methods. There are accounts of plucking the ears when the ker- nels were well glazed, and putting the fodder into the silo. The value of such ensilage, and the loss, if any, to the grain are not sufficiently ascertained to warrant positive statements.

IX. Q. What is the best method of planting and cultivation?

A. Thorough preparation before planting is essential. Corn, sorghum, and similar crops should be planted in rows. The quantity of seed corn varies from 8 quarts to a bushel and one-half for an acre. A smoothing harrow does the work of cultivating perfectly, and with little expense, while the corn is small.

X. Q. At what state of development is the fodder the most valuable for ensilage?

A. The common practice is to put crops into the silo when their full growth has been reached, and before ripening begins. Manifestly one rule will not answer all purposes. The stock to be fed and the object in feeding must be considered in determining when the crop should be cut On this point must depend much of the value of ensilage.

XI. Q. What weight of fodder is generally produced to the acre?

A. Corn produces more fodder per acre than any other crop mentioned. The average for corn is not far from 20 tons—which speaks well for land and culture. The largest yield from a single acre was 58 tons, the average of a large area on the same farm was only 12½ tons.

XII. Q. What kind of corn is best for ensilage?

A. The largest is generally preferred; hence seed grown in a warmer climate is in demand.

XIII. Q. What is the value of sweet corn as compared with other varieties?

A. It is conceded by many that the fodder of sweet corn is worth more, pound for pound. than that of larger kinds, for soiling. Some hold that the same superiority is retained in the ensilage, while others think that the advantage after fermentation is on the other side. The sweet varieties generally do not yield large crops.

XIV. Q. Preparation of fodder for silo; what machinery, etc., is used?

A. The mowing machine is sometimes used for cutting corn in the field—oftener the work is done by hand. Various cutters having carriers attached for elevated silos, are in use and are generally driven by horse, steam or water power. Fine cutting, a half-inch or less, is in favor. It packs closer, and for this reason is likely to keep better than the coarse ensilage. Fodder of any kind may be put in whole, and, if as closely compressed as cut fodder, will keep as well, if not better; but it requires much greater pressure. [And the author would say he should think it would be much more troublesome to get out, and not half so convenient to feed.]

XV. Q. What is the best manner of filling the silo?

A. During the process of filling, the ensilage should be kept level and well-trodden. A horse may be used very effectively for the latter. Some attach much importance to rapid filling, while others make it more a matter of convenience. With the packing equally thorough, rapid filling is probably the best.

XVI. Q. What is the cost, per ton, of putting the fodder into the silo?

A. The cost, from field to silo, is variously reported, from 35 cents—and in a single instance 10 or 12 cents—for labor alone, to $2.00 and upwards per ton, though the higher amounts include the entire cost of the crop, not the harvesting alone. There is a general expectation that experience will bring a considerable reduction in the cost of filling.

It is probable that with a more general adoption of ensilage, the best machinery will be provided by men who will make a business of filling silos. This could hardly fail to lessen the cost and bring the benefits of the system within the reach of many who otherwise would not begin.

XVII. Q. What length of time before the silo should be opened?

A. The ensilage should remain under pressure at least until cool, and be uncovered after that when wanted. [This point seems to be the most vague, i. e., the most indefinite of any of them. To "keep under pressure until cool," —how long is that? It is understood, of course, that the ensilage goes through a process of fermentation and becomes pretty hot, but how long it will be can only be told by the subsidence of the heat, after which, it seems, they can be opened when needed; but I should suppose it necessary to keep them tolerably well covered all the time until fed out—not necessarily weighted, but, still, properly covered to exclude the air as much as possible. See next answer.]

XVIII. Q. What is the condition of ensilage when opened?

A. In nearly all cases the loss by decay was very slight, and confined to the top and sides where there was more or less exposure to air.

XIX. Q. What deterioration, if any, after opening?

A. Generally the ensilage has kept perfectly for several months, showing no deterioration while any remained in the silo, excepting where exposed for a considerable time. It is better to uncover the whole silo, or compartment of a silo, at once, and thus expose a new surface each day, than to cut down sections.

XX. Q. What value has ensilage for milch cows?

A. Ensilage has been fed to milch cows more generally than to any other class of stock, and no unfavorable results are reported. There can be little doubt that its greatest value will always be found in this connection. Several readers consider it equal in value to one-third of its weight of the best hay, and some rate it higher.

XXI. Q. What effect has ensilage on dairy products?

A. There is a marked increase in quantity and improvement in quality of milk and butter after changing from dry feed to ensilage, corresponding to a similar change to fresh pasture. A few seeming exceptions are noted, which will probably find explanation in defects easily remedied, rather than such as are inherent.

XXII. Q. What value has ensilage on other stock?

A. Ensilage has been fed to all classes of farm stock, including swine and poultry, with results almost uniformly favorable. Exceptions are noted in the statements of Messrs. Coe Bros. and C. B. Henderson, where it appears that horses were injuriously affected. It should be borne in mind in this connection that ensilage is simply forage preserved in a silo, and may vary as much in quality as hay. The ensilage that is best for a milch cow may be injurious to a horse, and that on which a horse would thrive might render a poor return in the milk-pail.

XXIII. Q. What quantity is consumed per head, daily ?

A. Cows giving milk are commonly fed 50 to 60 lbs., with some dry fodder and grain.

XXIV. Q. What is the method of feeding—alone or with other food?

A. Experiments have been made in feeding ensilage exclusively, and results have varied with the quality of ensilage and the stock fed. It is certain that ensilage of corn cut while in blossom, or earlier, is not alone sufficient for milch cows. It is best to feed hay once a day, and some grain or other rich food, unless the latter is supplied in the ensilage, as it is when corn has reached or passed the roasting-ear stage before cutting. Ensilage, as it is commonly under-stood, is a substitute only for hay and coarse fodder generally, and does not take the place of grain.

XXV. Q. What is the condition of stock fed on ensilage, both as to gain, or loss, of weight and health.

A. The condition of stock fed on ensilage, both as to health and gain in weight has been uniformly favorable.

XXVI. Q. What is the profitableness of ensilage, all things considered?

A. There is hardly a doubt expressed on the profitableness of ensilage—certainly not a dissenting opinion.

*Remarks.*—What more could be asked as to whether the silo, and consequently ensilage, was profitable, or not, when out of all these many inquiries of those who have fairly tested the matter, in eighteen different states and Canada, not one gives an unfavorable opinion. It is remarkable indeed, and should give encouragement to those who have not already tested it, to begin at once, with an expectation of final success. After having prepared the above, on the subject of silos, ensilage, etc., I saw the following items upon these subjects as they see them in England, and as a few practice them in America, and as there are a few points in them of a more practical character, showing an increase of nutrition, and making it easier of digestion by ensilage, and also giving more particularly the manner of building silos, etc., I will give them a place, as follows:

**Ensilage (in England) Claimed to Increase the Nutritive Powers of Green Forage.**—The *Chemist and Druggist* (English) in the winter of 1884, referring to previous notices of the subject of ensilage, says: " Since then two most encouraging statements have been published with regard to its value. Professor Thorne Rogers reports that ensilage increases the nutritive powers of green forage; that the process obviates waste, saves time and increases the productive powers of the soil. The forage is made more digestible, and the farmer is enabled to get a double yearly crop. The silos should not be too shallow; not less than 20 to 25 feet deep. [This, the author thinks, should depend wholly upon the amount to be put up—if this amount of room is necessary, for the amount of stock kept, then the deeper the better, perhaps.] Had silos been common in England, millions of pounds worth of fodder would have been saved last summer. This is not the time, remarks the professor, when British agriculture can afford to neglect economies, whether large or small. [If English agriculture can't afford to neglect economies, can American?] Mr. F. Sutton confirms this view by comparing the relative value of hay and ensilage from a poor quality of grass. The hay was coarse and poor, destitute of sweet taste and odor, and contained a trace of ready-made sugar. Distilled with water, no essential oils were yielded, nor was there any flavor, save that of decaying grass. The specimens obtained by ensilage were highly odorous from the essential oils, and had a vinous fragrance, accompanied by a slight acidity. No ready-made sugar could be detected. It is argued, then, that a manifest improvement had been effected. That which was tasteless had been rendered appetizing and succulent (full of juice). A much larger proportion of soluble albuminoids (like albumen—white of eggs), soluble extractive matter, and digestible fiber was found in the dry ensilage as compared with dry hay, leading to the inference that a partial digestion had taken place in the silo. It seems a question which fairly invites discussion, as to whether ensilage could not be employed advantageously in the storage of medicinal plants. The question has already been advanced; recent experiments might claim further attention to the subject."

*Remarks.*—It is not expected that farmers will feel any particular interest in the last clause, as to ensilage benefiting medicinal plants; but the other parts are so much to the point, as to the value of ensilage for feeding stock, I deemed the item well worth a place in this connection.

**Silos and Ensilage—What They Are, How It is Done, and What They Think of It in Vermont.**—T. H. Hoskins, M. D., reports the following in one of the agricultural papers as to the value of ensilage, and also the most substantial and a cheaper way of carrying out the work. Under date of February 13, 1881, writing from his home, Newport, Vt., he says:

"Gen. Thomas, of Montpelier, Gen. Grout, of Barton, and Capt Morton, of Essex, are the only persons in Vermont, within my knowledge, who have made public the results of their experiments with the new method of preserving forage in the moist state by strong compression in air-tight pits. All three report entire success, and express enthusiastic confidence in the future of this new departure in farming.

I. *"What Ensilage and Silos Are, and How to Make and Feed Them.*— 'Silo' is French for 'pit,' and 'ensilage' the French equivalent of the English word 'pitting.' It is applied in this case to the pitting of green forage in such manner that it shall be preserved, by the exclusion more or less perfect, of the air from the contents of the pit. This is effected by lining the bottom and sides of the pit with concrete or masonry (brick or stone), the surfaces of which are plastered with water-lime cement. The lines and right angles of such a pit must be straight and true, so that no hinderance shall be offered to the settling of its contents under the pressure which is applied to them after filling. So far, green maize, taken about the time when the grain is 'in the milk,' has been used for ensilage almost exclusively; but all green forage may be equally well preserved in the same way. The preparation of ensilage is simply the cutting of the forage, by a suitable machine driven by horse or steam power, into small bits, not exceeding half an inch in length. These are dropped into the pit or silo, and rapidly levelled and trod down by men or horses. This levelling and treading should be as exact and thorough as possible. To facilitate the former, horizontal lines about a foot apart may be drawn around on the walls of the silo. The treading must be especially well done at the corners, and some silos are built with curved in place of square corners, to facilitate this work.

II. *" How to Build a Substantial Silo and to Fill Further Described.*—In constructing the pits (making the silos) there is opportunity for the display of ingenuity and calculation, and upon the degree in which these enter into the work the cost in a general measure depends. Gen. Thomas enclosed his silo with a heavy stone wall laid in cement, at a cost which he did not like to state, but which he afterwards thought entirely unnecessary. Its size was 40 by 15 feet, and 15 feet deep. The corn from 5 acres did not nearly fill it. He used a Baldwin cutter, propelled by horse-power, cutting a two-horse load every eight minutes. The whole cost of getting the ensilage from the field into the pit was less than the cost of cutting and stocking the same even in the field would have been. The work was completed in October. The ensilage was covered closely with planks, and heavily weighted with stone. When opened in December the preservation was found to be perfect, and the ensilage was greedily eaten by all kinds of stock. To his cows he feeds a ration of 50 lbs. of ensilage daily. With this, and a moderate ration of cotton-seed meal, as good and as much butter is made as on the best pasturage. Referring to the construction of the silo, Gen. Thomas said it could be equally as well lined with brick or concrete as with stone, and much cheaper, one brick in thickness being sufficient when earth or sand was firmly rammed in behind the walls. [The author would say never less than an 8-inch wall.] The main point was to have the walls perfectly true and smooth, and the corners square, so as not in any way to interfere with the settling of the contents under pressure. The variety of the corn planted was the common Southern horse-tooth, which he thought the best. His crop was 20 tons to the acre, but he thought this might be doubled by high manuring. He estimated the feeding value of ensilage equal to twice the weight of average hay."

III. *Two Cheaper Methods of Building Silos.*—The doctor goes on to say: "Captain Morton's silo was much more cheaply made. He dug a trench 12 feet wide and 60 feet long, and only 3 feet deep. He walled this with stone, making the wall 9 feet high, and banking it up on the outside to within 3 feet of the top. It was pointed with mortar and cemented with water-lime on the inside, the whole cost being $100. This silo was divided by a cross wall in the middle, and only ½ was used, in which the corn from 2 acres was placed, being cut in ½ inch lengths, firmly trodden down, covered with boards and heavily weighted. The preservation was excellent, and all kinds of stock eat it freely. The whole cost of getting the fodder into the silo was under $10. He is now feeding it in combination with fine-cut hay and meal to 27 head of stock, young and old, including 7 cows in milk. The daily feed for the whole is made by mixing 250 lbs. of the ensilage, 180 lbs of cut hay, and 75 lbs. each of corn-meal and wheat bran, the whole well shoveled together, and fed to each animal in proportion to its size. They are all thriving, and his butter sells for 35 cents a lb. His ensilage (which was exhibited at the meeting he addressed) was slightly acid, but he said that with a perfectly tight silo and sufficient pressure, he thought it could be preserved almost perfectly sweet. This was also Gen. Thomas' opinion. Captain Morton agreed with Gen. Thomas in preferring southern corn for ensilage. He planted in drills 2 feet apart, using 1 bushel of seed to the acre, and tilling entirely by machinery.

Gen. Grout built his silos with concrete walls, loose stones being puddled in with mortar, and the inside coated with water-lime cement. The fodder was badly frosted when ensilaged, but kept perfectly. He used 300 lbs of stone to the square foot of surface to compress the ensilage, and would never use less. He is feeding it to 72 head of cattle, and 100 sheep. The daily cattle ration is 30 lbs. of ensilage in the morning, and a mixture composed of 15 lbs. of finely-cut and moistened straw, upon which 2 lbs. of shorts are sprinkled; which is fed in two feeds, noon and night. All the stock are gaining on this feed. The sheep were fed almost exclusively on ensilage, and had much improved on it.

The entire cost of the crop in the silo was slightly less than $2 a ton, which Gen. Grout believes can be considerably reduced. Like the other gentlemen named, he thinks the feeding value of corn ensilage equal to twice its weight of average hay. I fear this will prove an over-estimate.

"We, in Vermont, are gratified to find that there is not going to be so much difficulty from the freezing of ensilage as we feared. When the whole of the silo is below the surface no frost enters. The slight fermentation which goes on in the mass keeps the temperature well above freezing. This fermentation is very slight, and when the face of the mass is cut down in feeding that which remains undisturbed is unaffected; but that which is cut out, if left exposed to the air in a place where the temperature is not very low, will ferment so as to be decidedly warm in 12 hours. In this condition it is greedily eaten by the stock. It has then a slightly alcoholic odor, and a more or less acid taste. The better the preservation the less there will be of the latter."

*Remarks.*—This item was so distinct and covered so much of importance for one to know who is contemplating a beginning with ensilage, I could not satisfy myself without giving it. The next and last item is upon the question of feeding ensilage to dairy cows and fattening steers, very plain and distinct, and of much importance to those who have no experience in its use for these purposes.

**Ensilage for Dairy Cows and Fattening Steers, How to Feed.**—The following is from a correspondent of the *Country Gentleman,* who says: "Such grave uncertainties seem to pervade the minds of many farmers as to the use of ensilage as food for milch cows; such doubts as to a possible peculiar taste of the milk, cream, or butter made from this food, that with your permission I will give my experience of last season, hoping it may lead some doubters to the right track. Last year I built a silo of 200 tons capacity, wholly of stone and Rosendale cement, with a frame and roof for cover. It is a good one (I believe in no other), no water can get in, no sap from the corn can get out, as so many complain of when their silos are not half built, or made from stale cement or any poor material. On account of the long-extended drouth in this part of New Jersey, I was able to scrape together of good, bad and indifferent, half-dried, wilted, grown and half-grown corn, some 30 tons of ensilage after cured. This, however, was enough to satisfy my mind on this subject, if there ever had been any doubts. I used it as food for cows 110 days continuously, until all was fed out. Within a week from the time we began feeding hay, and though with an addition of grain, the cows lost at least 25 per cent. of milk, the cream did not make as much butter, and the butter was not of as good color or flavor. During the time of feeding ensilage we were unable to discover any other than the most satisfactory taste to milk, cream, or butter. The cows were in the most perfect state of health, and kept in fine condition.

*Fattening Steers.*—I fed for 90 days 8 western steers, which averaged a gain of over 1½ lbs. per day. The ration for cows and oxen was 22 lbs. of ensilage morning and night, and 15 lbs. of cut cornstalks at noon. The cows had 3 qts. of cornmeal and 2 qts. of wheat bran per day, and the steers had 4 qts. of cornmeal for 45 days and 5 qts. for the last 45 days. Our success with the steers astonished my neighbors, who feed in the old way. The butcher says the cattle slaughtered well, and the meat was remarkably fine and gave every satisfaction. The use of poor ensilage, made from corn half ripe or frost bitten, like mine was, I have reason for believing, would not give such satisfactory results, as if I had had more perfect material. I am one who believes that to make good ensilage the corn should be cut at the right time, cut the right length, put away in a good silo and covered over nicely, and then well and thoroughly weighted down. The seed planted should be the Southern gourdseed, drilled in rows 30 to 40 inches apart, and the ground cultivated the same as any corn. The ensilage should be cut $\frac{3}{8}$ to $\frac{3}{4}$ of an inch long. It is important to have a good, water-tight silo and heavy weighting—300 to 350 lbs. to the square foot of surface. I believe in giving the animals all they will eat up clean, be it more or less. Contentment means fat in the bovine tribe, as well as riches in the human.

*Remarks.*—The author agrees with this man in New Jersey, that "what is worth doing is worth doing well," if you can; if you have not the means to build the best silo, build a small one till you can do better, but don't fail to try it according to your means and ability, by which you will get more means. That is the object of the author in writing this book. What it may pay me is nothing as to what it will pay others, if they heed its teachings. I would never have written it for what it will pay me, but the belief in what good it will do others has made it a delight, and the labor endurable.

**Ensilage Congress, Report of in 1886, Held in New York.—** We will say, in closing the ensilage question with the following report, that we are indebted to a Frenchman by the name of August Goffart, for the discovery of this plan of preserving fodder in its green state, some 20 years ago, which, for economy or saving financially, for the farming community, probably, has not its superiority in the whole century, or for the past 100 years; and it is now admitted that he who does not make use of it, now, stands in his own light. The following facts were stated by those members of the Congress or convention, who had given it a fair trial:

"Alfred Reid, of Providence, gave the result of his experiments at feeding ensilage to twenty-eight head of cattle. He gave them three times a day all they could eat. He had put into his silos, corn, rye, grass, clover, Hungarian grass and sorghum. He gave the details of his expenditures on four acres of corn. The total cost in the field was $159.51 to raise 66 tons and 427 pounds of corn fodder. The cost of getting from the field to the silos was $69.37 for the 66 tons. The total cost of raising, carting and packing was $3.45 per ton.

"A Mr. Roberts, of Poughkeepsie, asserted that with ensilage he had kept twenty-six cows, where without it he had kept but six. Probably this was under highly favorable circumstances, though fresh, green fodder undoubtedly yields more than double the nourishment of dry. Cattle eat ensilage food ravenously, and it fattens, and increases the production of milk.

"Some silos, or pits, are built 50 by 20 feet in size and bricked up. Others are made of boards, tongued and grooved and lined with tar paper. When built in barns they are said to work excellently, as the frost is more eas-fly kept off—although cattle eat ensilage food when frozen, though it is less healthful.

"Mr. Percy, of Chatham, N. Y., estimates the cost of a wooden pit lined with the paper, 24 x 30 feet, at $125. Another member of the Congress made the astonishing statement that with ensilage food he had kept a cow on two and a half cents per day. Ensilage food requires much pressing to properly preserve it, sixty-two pounds to the square inch being deemed about the right weight. A Pennsylvania farmer declared that with ensilage he had made butter at six cents per pound and sold it for fifty cents, asserting that old and toothless cows would thrive on it. Some dairymen mix it with meal.

"All present at the Congress gave testimony to its great value, in increasing the quality and quantity of milk, in creating flesh, keeping cattle in a healthy condition, and in its cheapness in comparison to dry fodder. Cheap pits or silos were pronounced just as good as expensive ones, and having the green fodder cut by means of a cutting machine, proved more efficacious than placing the fodder uncut into the pits. Ensilage food is said to smell like New England rum, and some joking rendered the Ensilage Congress lively, regarding the effect of fermented food in producing drunkenness among cattle."

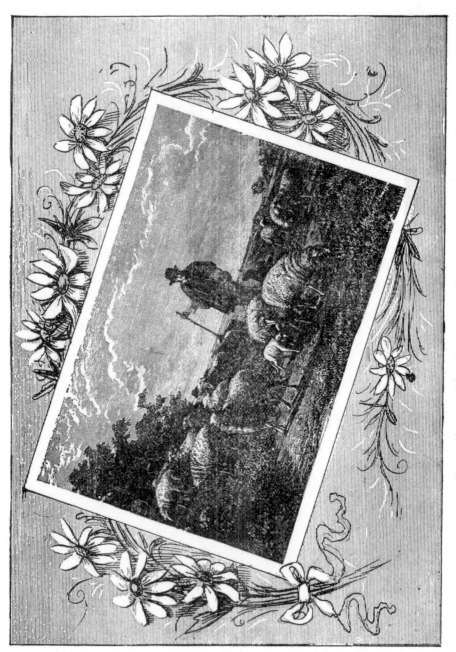

TWENTY-EIGHT YEARS IN SHEEP HUSBANDRY.

# SHEEP.

**TWENTY-EIGHT YEARS IN SHEEP HUSBANDRY.—As** the raising of sheep has become so common on almost every farm, we have thought we could not do better than to devote a few pages to this important subject. First, we will give a paper read before the Farmers' Institute, at Hudson, Mich., Jan. 10, 1880, by Sidney Green, the well known farmer of Pittsford, Hillsdale County, whose experience of 28 years will give valuable hints, to say the least, upon almost all the important points of sheep husbandry, so that new beginners may avoid the mishaps which Mr. Green and others have fallen into for the want of this very experience in their beginning. He says:

**I. Introduction.**—"Ladies and gentlemen, I want to say right here that what I have to say will be largely in the line of my experience, and the way that I have managed my own flock of sheep during the past 28 years.

"A year ago last July, a friend of mine living in Missouri, wishing to engage in the business of sheep raising on a large scale, and knowing that I had been somewhat successful on the small scale in the same business, wrote to me asking advice, and, in fact, asked of me just what this Institute now asks. I complied with his request, and my whole essay was comprised of but one word, and that was "Care." If every man, woman and child that owns a sheep, or even ever expects to, will take that one word and make it the key note of every move they make, guided by their best judgment and discretion, I will guarantee success in this important branch of farming.

**II. Care—What it Will Do.**—"Care will make carcass; care will make constitution, care will save fodder; care will ward off disease; care will make fat, and fat will make wool and grease, and wool and grease will make money, and that is what we are after. Yes, care will do one other thing, care will make blood.

"Were it not for the promise I have already made that I would relate my 28 years experience with sheep, what I have already said, carried out, would accomplish a better purpose than anything I could add, and this paper would be complete. It is true that we are guided to some extent by the experience of others.

**III. When and How He Began.**—"In the fall of 1852 I bought in Oakland county, this State, 53 ewes of common stock for $1 per head, and one ewe, said to have been a pure cross between the Spanish and French Merino, for which I paid $25. I drove them to this county (Hillsdale) in the winter of 1853.

725

**IV. Shearing—Average Weight of Fleece.**—"The first shearing the lot averaged a little less than 4 lbs. per head. I raised 24 lambs the first season; I had the good fortune to raise from my pure-blooded ewe an extra buck lamb, which was the foundation for great improvement of my flock for those days. For the first few years the flock showed a greater improvement per year than they have since they have been brought to a greater degree of perfection. This, in fact, is my experience with crossing full bloods with natives. It requires greater skill to improve really good sheep than it does to improve an inferior grade. The second shearing showed an improvement of nearly 1¼ lb. per head. In the course of 5 or 6 years the average of the flock, numbering from 80 to 100, was a trifle over 6 lbs. per head. With good luck in the selection of rams, in 10 years from the start, my flock averaged 7 lbs.

**V. Drawbacks in the Business.**—"Sheep business, like any other business, has its drawbacks. The use of what I supposed to be a full-blooded Spanish ram from Webster's flock of Vermont, set my flock backward on an average for 2 years ½ lb. per head. This is the only real set-back that I ever have experienced. I soon recovered that loss, and have made steady gain since. So I estimate my average this coming spring at 9 lbs. per head, with the prospects of a little more.

**VI. Increase of Wool per Head by Using Blooded Rams.**—"I have thus far shown simply the increase of wool per head during this time with the use of what we might call blooded rams, with the single exception of one blooded ewe. Here occurred an incident which was curious in its effects, and in after years proved to be an adulteration of blood.

**VII. Danger of a Grade Buck upon a Blooded Ewe.**—"My eyes have been wide open ever since to prevent the repetition of the mishap. The blooded ewe, which was pure gold in my eyes at the time, was, through carelessness, mated with a grade buck, and her second lamb was a nice grade; but the curious part of the affair was that that high and pure blooded ewe never afterwards raised a pure blooded lamb from mating with the purest blood I could find. Her breeding qualities were destroyed and her progeny was not reliable. I kept the ewe till she died—15 years of age.

**VIII. Buck, Selection of, Suitable for the Flock.**—"In selecting a buck that is suitable for the flock lies the secret of success. If a man has not the judgment for himself, he had better borrow it from some one that has, until he is acquainted with the business sufficiently to prevent mistakes and set-backs. In choosing a ram for myself, I want a low, heavy body, straight on the back, clear to the roots of the tail, broad and level over the shoulders, deep and heavy in the brisket, thick neck with heavy gullet; in short, constitution is the first strong point that will receive my attention. I want the wool of medium length, smooth on the surface, the thicker the better. The staple rather stiff and stubbed, with plenty of oil distributed evenly from the roots to the end. I like heavy folds, but do not want them to run over the back, nor do I like to see them too heavy over the neck. Horns, if any, set well from the head, fore-top as long as the rest of the fleece, down even with the eyes, then stop. Smooth, clear pink face and nose, short, thick velvety ears, wool full length, well down on the legs, and full heavy fleece on the belly. The foregoing is something of my ideal of a ram.

**IX. Time of Washing and Shearing and Putting Ewes and Lambs by Themselves.**—"My flock is well washed and sheared from the 15th to the 20th of June. They are turned on the largest range that I can spare. The ewes and lambs by themselves, the bucks by themselves; the rest, counted as store sheep, by themselves, making three flocks. From that time till after harvest all the attention they get is salt once a week (twice or three times I believe better), and all carefully counted. About the 20th of August I wean the lambs, taking them as far from their mothers as I can. Generally saving a piece of clover stubble for them, and giving them the best chance that I can. About the first of October I commence giving them about a gill ($\frac{1}{4}$ pt.) of oats apiece daily. This is kept up until cold weather sets in, and then their grain is increased about $\frac{1}{2}$ more and kept up until grass grows the next spring. They have a good shelter if they choose to occupy it. During storms they are forced to their shelter. I feed clover hay twice a day, and water once a day, and feed them grain at night. With this treatment my lambs are kept thrifty all winter. I claim that the grain fed early in the fall is the secret of wintering successfully.

**X. Time to Sort Out Breeding Ewes.**—"About the first of October I sort my breeding ewes. In doing this important work, I have diverged from the well established rules of breeders and made one of my own. Here I would call the attention of the Institute to a statement made before the Institute one year ago, by our worthy president. He made this statement I think: 'He raised all the lambs he could.' Now if he meant that he tried to raise all that was born, then we do not differ, but if he meant that he tried to increase his flock as fast as he could, then his line of policy and mine lie in a different direction.

**XI. His Rule.**—"My rule is, in sorting for the breeding band, that none shall be less than $2\frac{1}{2}$ years old, and none that are inferior as to size, constitution or thinness of wool. My year-old ewes are turned with the wethers; and the older ones that have been excluded from the breeders are marked for sale.

**XII. The Result.**—"The result of this policy is a large and uniform flock, with strong constitutions and heavy sheerers.

**XIII. Average Weight.**—"I have just weighed three of my breeders, which is the fair average weight of the lot of 30. The heaviest weighed 140 lbs., the lightest 100 lbs., a pick of the average 116 lbs.

**XIV. Land Too Valuable to Keep Inferior Sheep.**—"Our lands are too valuable to keep inferior sheep, or to try to increase in numbers at the expense of size and quality.

**XV. Time to Divide in the Fall.**—"My flock of 80 are divided from October, until they are brought into the yard in three lots, breeders, store sheep and lambs. Then the breeders and store sheep are turned together fo the winter. I feed stocks twice a day. At noon they are fed light, with wheat, oats or pea straw. At night they are all fed about 1 gill of corn each. All have shelter, and are compelled to use it during storms. Your essayist last year made one remark that was worth its weight in gold as to the care of sheep, that was, 'to be quiet among them.' I treat my sheep so they think I am in their way, instead of their being in mine when I am among them. I feed a very little sulphur mixed with salt during the winter. I think it a preventive for pulling their wool. The first of March I take the breeders and keep by themselves till nearly shearing time. In connection with their grain, I prefer to feed a few roots or a little bran, but do not always find it convenient.

**XVI. Time for Lambs to Appear.**—"The lambs begin to make their appearance about the 20th of April. Great pains are taken at this time with this part of the flock. Let the weather be what it may, the ewes and the lambs are all driven to their shelter every night, and the little ones are carefully cared for. This precaution is used until the weather gets warm and settled.

**XVII. Time for Trimming, Care of Fleeces, etc.**—"My whole flock is carefully trimmed and examined about the first of April. The wool is washed and put in the fleeces at shearing time, so there is no waste. The theory that sheep will not do well for a long term of years on the same farm I take no stock in. For 28 years my stock has been kept on the same farm and the one adjoining. You see that I have reported a continued progress. This, I can assure you, has not been accomplished in a haphazard way. Nothing has been left undone for their thrift and comfort that is reasonably in my power to do."

*Remarks.*—There is one point, however, that I desire to call especial attention to, shown by Mr. Green's carelessness, as he admits, after having given a whole essay in the one word "care," which would do everything he claimed in sheep culture—*i. e.*, never allow a blooded breeding ewe to run with a lower grade buck, as his experience shows that it destroys, for some unaccountable reason, her power to afterwards produce full-blooded lambs, although mated with a full-blooded ram. By his carelessness he lost, as a breeder, the value of his $25 ewe, therefore have a care to his dearly bought experience in this particular. This gentleman's experience was with the Merinos; but as there are those who consider the Cotswold as superior in several respects, I will give a short item upon them from the *Country Gentleman*, a part of which was from a catalogue of Mr. Harris, of Rochester, N. Y., whose opinion is considered reliable. The editor gives it under the head of

**Cotswolds and Cotswold Crosses, the Coming Sheep of America, Furnishing the Largest Fleeces and the Largest Carcass.**— Mr. Joseph Harris, of Rochester, has lately published a catalogue in which he gives his views of Cotswold sheep in the following terms: "The sheep are thoroughly acclimated. They have not been forced; they are kept for use—for real value and not for show. They are housed in winter; they have sheds to run under, but spend most of the time in the open air. If well fed, and provided with dry quarters under foot, there are no sheep that will stand exposure to our severe winters better than the Cotswolds. The ewes are good breeders and good nurses. They frequently have two strong lambs, and occasionally three at a birth. I have never had a pure-bred Cotswold ewe in the flock that would not breed. We let the ewes have their first lambs when two years old, and they frequently continue to be good breeders till 10 years old. The Cotswolds are the hardiest of all the English breeds of sheep. Of all well-established breeds, the Cotswolds are the largest. The celebrated experiments of Lawes & Gilbert proved beyond all question that the Cotswolds produced more mutton and more wool than any other breed. In other words, they gained more rapidly, both in fleece and carcass, than any other breed. And not only this, but they gained more in proportion to the food consumed than any other breed." Mr. Harris' experience in crossing Cotswold rams on ordinary Merino ewes has heretofore been frequently referred to in these columns, especially in connection with notices of the cross-breeds exhibited by him at several shows of the State Agricultural Society. On this subject he remarks: "I am decidedly of the opinion that the 'coming sheep' of this country will be what I will take the liberty to call 'American Cotswolds.' I have hitherto called these sheep 'Cotswold Merinos.' This designates their origin. But the time has now arrived when the name loses its significance. For instance, I have Cotswold Merino lambs with three or four crosses of pure Cotswold blood in them. In other words, these lambs have $93\frac{1}{4}$ per cent. of pure Cotswold blood in them and only $6\frac{1}{2}$ per cent. of the native or Merino sheep. The next cross will have only $3\frac{1}{4}$ per cent. of the native or Merino blood, and the next only a little over $1\frac{1}{2}$ per cent. A few years hence American Cotswold sheep will be shipped by thousands and tens of thousands every week to the English markets. There is no reason why they are not now shipped in large numbers, except—the fact that they cannot be found. We do not raise enough of them or feed them well enough. Our beef cattle are better than our mutton sheep. The intelligence and skill of the American sheep-breeder has been largely directed to the perfection of the Merino. Wool and bulk have been the objects aimed at, and great success has attended their efforts. There are no better fine-wooled sheep in the world to-day than can be found in the United States. There are many sections where Merinos are the most profitable breeds of sheep to keep. But railroads and steamboats lead to rapid and wonderful changes. There was a time when I thought Cotswold or mutton sheep could not be raised with profit in the far West. I thought it was too far from market; but, if cattle can be raised and shipped with profit to England, long-wooled mutton sheep can be raised and shipped with still greater profit."

*Remarks.*—Notwithstanding the superiority of the Cotswolds in some particulars, the Merino will still form the majority of our flocks, I have not a doubt, for many years to come, except it may be in favorable points for shipping to England or our largest cities, as our American people do not, as yet, eat half as much mutton as would be best for their health. Pork, I am sorry to say, except in the cities, is more frequently found upon our tables than any other meat.

**Sheep, Value of on a Poor Farm.**—" Some farmers of our acquaintance," says the *American Agriculturist*, "feel an antipathy to sheep for the
reason that they 'bite close.' We consider this their chief recommendation.
They can only bite close where the pasture is short, and the pasture is short only
on a poor farm. A poor farm will necessarily be encumbered with briers,
weeds, and brush in the fence corners. Under such circumstances we should
say to a farmer who has $20 or upward in cash, or credit for it, let him borrow
the amount if he has to pay 1 per cent. a month for the use of it, invest it in as
many ewes, not older than 3 years, as you can get for that money. Put them
in such a field as we have described, and give them, in addition to what they can
pick up, a pint of wheat bran and oatmeal each daily, with free access to water
and salt. They will first go for the briers and clean them out; every portion of
that field will be trodden over and over again, and the weeds will have no
chance. Fold them on that field during winter, and carry them feed sufficient
to keep them thriving. Get the use of a good buck in season—Southdown
would be preferable—and in the spring, if you have luck, that means if you
give them proper attention and feed regularly, you will raise more lambs than
you have ewes. The money will be more than doubled, and the wool and
manure will pay for their feed and interest. In the spring you may put that
field in corn with the certainty of getting 50 per cent. increase of crop.

*Remarks.*—The author considers this perfectly sound advice to any farmer
under the circumstances; and sound to every farmer who has not already got
sheep on his farm, to obtain a few as soon as possible; for he will undoubtedly
find them the most profitable for the amount invested in them of anything on
the place. Confirmatory of this see the next two or three items.

**Sheep Better Than Neat Cattle.**—A competent and experienced
writer on this subject says: "One great advantage sheep have over other stock
is, they never die of the contagious diseases which they contract. They get the
scab, or foot rot, or something else, and if unchecked it gets them in bad condition, and would ultimately, perhaps, kill them. But the very worst contagious
diseases to which sheep are subject give the owner ample time to treat the
affected animals, and the diseases are generally of a character which yield rapidly to treatment. But a man may have a lot of hogs and feed them on hundreds of bushels of corn, and about the time the bottoms of his cribs are neared
and he is thinking of selling, some disease breaks out among them—no one
knows what it is or what to do for it—one animal after another, following in
rapid succession, is affected, and the greater portion die. I have known farmers to be well nigh ruined by the appearance of a contagious disease of this
character. Sheep are, happily, exempt from such rapid and fearful mortality.
Besides, when a sheep dies—and they do die, sometimes,—its pelt is sufficient
to pay for its keeping from the last shearing to its death. It makes no difference
when it dies, or what kills it, the sheep never dies in debt."

**Sheep, More Made on Them than Upon Horses.**—The Iowa
*State Register* says that an old and careful farmer of Indiana, after 33 years'
experience, informs them that he has made most on sheep, for the money

nvested, and the least on horses. The following will show what an English farmer thought upon the subject as early as 1523, and also be quite a curiosity to compare the spelling of those days with the present. "Boke," was book, and "cattell," cattle; "shepe," sheep, etc. But it will explain itself:

**Sheep the Most Profitable—Any Man Can Have Cattle (1523)** —The "Book of Husbandry," published in the year above named, by Sir Anthony Fitzherbert, who styles himself "a farmer of 40 years' standing," in this work says: "A houseband can not thryve by his corne without cattell; nor by his cattell without corne." And adds: "Shepe, in my opinion, is the most profitablest cattell any man can have."

*Remarks*—Certainly no higher authority nor older testimony need be sought to establish the fact that sheep husbandry is profitable—only use care, as Mr. Green tells us in the first item above, and success is certain.

**Sheep vs. Cows—Comparative Profit of.**—This subject having been under considerable discussion of late, as to whether there was more profit in keeping sheep than cattle, or cows, I will give an item or two upon this subject. The first is from F. D. Curtis, in *Rural New Yorker*, compared with cows. He says: "Five coarse-wooled sheep will produce lambs at the rate of 1 and ½ to the sheep, but quite often they will double their number. Medium-wooled sheep may be safely relied upon to increase their numbers one and ½, while fine-wooled sheep will return a lamb for a sheep. The value of the lambs depends upon their quality when kept for breeding; or on their earliness and condition, when fitted for market. The price of lambs for these various breeds will range from $3 upwards. Wool was worth the past season from 35 to 45 cents per lb. Six lbs. of wool per head is not an extra average for a well kept flock. They may be made to average more than that by extra care. A flock of combing wool sheep, with the same care and feeding which a good dairyman would give his cows, will average per sheep at least $10. This would afford an income of $50 on a flock of five in the place of one cow. The proportion of income would not be so great in a large flock, as the average yield of wool would be less. The percentage of increase is likewise reduced, owing to the fact that the ewes receive less care and to their increased liability to accidents. If the flocks should be separated and kept a few in a place, not exceeding 12, a month before weaning time, the losses would be very few."

*Remarks.*—Mr. Curtis being well-known in agriculture, there can be no doubt in his reasoning, and, therefore, his thoughts are valuable. The next item is from the *Practical Farmer*, in relation to general stock, or steers, more particularly.

**Sheep vs. Cattle—Which Pays Best?**—The *Practical Farmer* gives us the following upon this subject: "How often do we hear farmers ask this question: 'Which will pay me best, cattle or sheep?'" Now there is much difference of opinion on this question. Those that keep cattle claim that they are the most profitable, and those that keep sheep think the same of their flocks. I claim that sheep are the most profitable, and I will try and prove it. Take, for instance, a 2-year-old steer, weighing 1,000 lbs., worth 4 cents per lb., or $40.

What is the cost of raising to that age? First year to milk, grain and hay, $12; one summer's pasture, $4; six months' feeding hay or grain, $16; making a total cost of $32    This is a very low estimate; everything is down to the lowest notch.    Now you see that it has cost $32 to raise this calf.    Subtract his keeping from what he sold for, and you have the profit of $8.    This is counting for your trouble, allowing the manure to balance that.    Now for the sheep.    It will cost to keep and raise 8 lambs until they are 1 year old, for pasture, hay and grain $12; for 1 year more for hay and grain, $20; making their total cost from birth to 2 years old, $32.    Now, for the 8 head of sheep, weighing 125 lbs. per head, making 1,000 lbs. at 4 cents per lb., is $40.    Two clips of wool, 16 fleeces, weighing 5 lbs. per fleece, makes 80 lbs. of wool; at 32 cents per lb., $25.60.    Now take the $40 that the sheep sold for, and you have $65.60 as total receipts.    Subtract cost from this and you have $33.60 profit on 8 sheep against $8 profit on 1 steer, both weighing the same at same age, and both costing the same for keep, leaving a balance of $25.60 in favor of sheep, showing clearly that it is better to keep sheep than cattle, especially where we have small farms.    I think that this estimate is correct, taking prices in this neighborhood as a basis.

*Remarks.*—This shows very clearly, for all ordinary cases, that there is more real profit in sheep than cattle; still every farmer must consider his situation as to the adaptation of his farm to one or the other, and perhaps keep both, if his farm is large and adapted to either; otherwise he must keep the kind of stock best adapted to the circumstances around him; but it is always an advantage to be well posted in everything in which he may engage.    But I do think that every farmer should keep a few sheep, under all circumstances.

**Sheep, a Few Short Rules for the Care of.**—The American Emigrant Company's circular says: 1. Keep sheep dry under foot, with litter. This is even more important than roofing them.    But never let them stand, or lie, in the mud or snow.

II. Drop or take out the lowest bars as the sheep enter or leave a yard, thus saving broken limbs.

III. Begin graining with the greatest care, and use the smallest quantity at first.

IV. If a ewe loses her lamb, milk her daily for a few days, and mix a little alum with her salt.

V. Give the lambs a little mill feed in time of weaning.

VI. Never frighten the sheep if it is possible to avoid it.

VII. Sow rye, for weak ones in cold weather, if you can.

V III. Separate all weak, or thin, or sick, from those strong, in the fall, and give them especial care.

IX. If any sheep is hurt, catch it at once and wash the wound with something healing.    If a limb is broken, bind it with splinters tightly, loosening as the limb swells.

X. Keep a number of good bells on the sheep.

XI. If one is lame, examine the foot, clean out between the hoofs, pare the hoof if unsound, and apply tobacco with blue vitriol boiled in water.

XII. Shear at once any sheep commencing to shed its wool, unless the weather is too severe.

*Remarks.*—These are excellent rules for the care of sheep, but as they do not give the strength of the vitriol wash for the foot, in rule XI, it will be well to use the recipe for foot wash, in cases needing such treatment.

**Sheep, Their Value for Fertilizing and Improving Worn Out Soil.**—A correspondent of the *American Farmer* writes on the subject of the capacity of sheep to improve soil, and to renovate and bring up worn out land. He says: "From many years' experience and observation I am fully convinced that plowing in green crops with lime—such as clover and others—is the most economical and speediest means that a farmer can use for bringing up worn soil. Yet it can be very profitably done by the use of sheep—in pasturing even. More than once and on more than one farm, I have seen dry, barren spots, such as gravel knolls and side-hills made fertile and productive in a single season, simply by salting a small flock of sheep on those barren spots twice a week during the summer; the sheep would be sure to resort there several times a day to lick up the salt, and thus leave their droppings, both liquid and solid, which are very rich fertilizers; then the next season the most rank and luxuriant growths of grass and grain would be produced on those 'galled spots' of any other portion of the whole field; thus the best kind of manure was applied and spread just where most wanted without any hard labor. Weight for weight, sheep manure is more fertilizing than either horse or cow manure, and next in value to hen or hog droppings. Sheep are valuable fertilizers I am very sure."

*Remarks.*—The author trusts that what has been said about sheep will induce all who have not got them upon the farm, to begin with them as soon as they can; and that those who have them will make use of them to clean up brier patches, weeds, etc., and also to make use of their fertilizing power to renovate worn out soils, gravel knolls, side-hills, etc.

**Sheep, Care of in Winter.**—The weak ones should be separated from the strong, and wethers from the ewes; and especial care should be given to ewes that are to drop their lambs early. The springing of the udder is an unfailing sign of approaching parturition. The ewe should then be removed to a separate pen and kept quiet, but should be visited at least every 3 hours, and the last thing at night. It is rarely that any help is needed, except in very cold weather, to wrap a piece of soft blanket about the lamb, and to help it, as soon as possible, to get its first meal from the mother, when it will be all right; and the ewe may be left for a few hours.

If apples are abundant in winter, a feed, once or twice a week, may be given to sheep; or, in their absence, a feed of turnips, or other roots, cabbage, etc., may be given them as often as necessary to avoid costiveness, or stretches, says a writer, an ailment common to sheep in this country, but unknown in Great Britain, where turnips are fed daily. Sheep feel the change from the green pastures to the dry feed of winter, as quickly, if not more so, than any other of our domestic animals, hence the importance of some of these juicy foods, in winter; and salt is of the same importance in winter as in summer; in fact it is better for any and all animals if they have daily access to salt.

But I doubt the efficiency of General Marshall's plan, of New York, in forcing sheep to eat the orts or coarse butts of poor hay left in the racks by other animals, simply to get what salt they need. He places these orts in box-racks under cover for the sheep, which he says they eat readily after they have been well sprinkled with salt water. But my plan would be, if I had poor hay, to cut it in a suitable cutter and sprinkle it with sweetened water if necessary (see "Fattening Cattle, Use of Molasses in"); then mixing in a little meal to make up for the poor hay, and so there should be no orts left, and give to all animals daily access to salt; but I should not force my sheep to eat the poorest parts of the poor hay, left by the other stock, to obtain what little salt they needed. Sheep should be fed with the best of hay if you expect them to do well.

**Sheep, Sulphur and Salt Valuable for.**—There are those among sheep breeders who consider, especially in winter, that sulphur, 4 ozs., to salt, 2 qts., mixed and put where sheep can have access to it, under shelter, is valuable in helping to ward off diseases, as foot rot, scab, mange, etc. It is undoubtedly valuable, occasionally, for all stock, as well as for persons, who by the "grandmother plan," which was a good one, mix it with cream of tartar and molasses every spring and take a tea-spoonful every morning for 3 mornings, and skip 3, for the whole family, till 9 doses had been taken. Sheep, however, will eat it mixed with salt without the molasses.

**Breeding Ewes, Care of, for Profit.**—Have good winter shelter, good clover hay, a few roots, a little grain daily, and water handy—water is more necessary in winter than in summer. Have no fears of their becoming too fat. If, occasionally, one gets too fat and drops her lamb out of season, she will be in season for the butcher, at a good price, after shearing. Sheep are cheap in the fall, when all are fat. Feed thus from the time they come into winter quarters, or earlier, if pasture is short, and until it is good in the spring; and your wool will be better and more of it, the ewes will be better supplied with milk, especially those raising twins; the lambs will be in better condition for the butcher; so will any of the flock, which from age or general failure to raise a lamb or two, it will be best to dispose of. If not cared for through the winter, but allowed to become poor, you can not sell till fall, when everybody else has them also for sale.

**Sheep, Peas, and Pea Straw, a Valuable Winter Food For.**— There are so many useful things in the following item, which every sensible man can see, who reads it, I am constrained to give them a place, although I do not know who the writer was. If I did know I should take great pleasure in giving him credit; still, I know so well that it contains too much good common sense to throw it away, and from what I know of raising peas for hogs, as given under that head, I know great benefit will arise to all who have suitable land for peas, if they raise them and use them as this writer directs for sheep. He says:

I. "I have made peas one of my principal crops for several years, and find these advantages: Peas are as sure a crop as any other, and one which leaves the ground in the best order for wheat. The yield will vary with the soil, 40 bush. being a large yield. In preparing the land I aim to fall plow and fit with cultivator in the spring; although the best corn I ever raised was on corn stubble, spring plowed. Peas are better if drilled, but can be sown broadcast on the furrow if rolled afterward. Peas like a fine, dry loam or sandy soil best, but will thrive well on a clayey soil, if well fitted. I never have threshed peas with a machine, as it splits them badly, and sheep will not relish the straw as well as if threshed with the flail. If the vines are very luxuriant, sheep will not eat them very closely, but if cut before all the top pods have grown white, sheep will not only eat, but relish the straw exceedingly well. If the straw is fed at night sheep will eat more than if fed in the morning or at noon.

II. *"Bugs in Peas, to Avoid.*—We have been troubled with bugs which sting the peas while yet soft, leaving the small eggs, which are hatched, the worm feeding upon the pea, leaving but a thin shell by the following spring. This is obviated by the early sowing so as to have the majority of the pods so hard by the time the fly arrives at maturity that it is impossible to pierce them. If the season be backward and this cannot be done, very late sowing will secure the same result. Good crops have been raised when sown as late as the 15th or 20th of May. The quantity of seed will depend on the soil. If very fine and rich, 1½ bus. to the acre; on ordinary soil, 2, and on very poor, 3, or better not sow any."

*Remarks.*—There is not an inconsistent statement in this gentleman's remarks. Never let no one fear to venture upon raising peas for this purpose. Beans have been considered especially the food for sheep, but peas are easier raised, and will, no doubt, do just as well as beans fed in like quantity, about a gill, I believe, for each sheep, once daily. I must say here, however, that I am of the opinion it would be a decided advantage in raising peas to sow sufficient oats with them to hold them up, as suggested in relation to raising them for hogs, which see. Oats are then fed also to sheep; then, as they are a great help in supporting pea vines, which are to be allowed to ripen for sheep, why not sow them together and feed them together? Whoever tries them both ways, I have not a doubt but what he will afterwards always sow them together.

## Sheep vs. Dogs—How to Give the Advantage to the Sheep.—

A remedy for sheep-killing dogs is given by a correspondent of the *Prairie Farmer*, which is better than legal enactments, as the case is settled without complaints, without lawyers, judge or jury. He says: "I have kept a flock of sheep for several years, varying from 100 to over 2,000 head, and for the last 8 years have not lost a sheep killed by dogs. I keep my sheep yarded nights, and occasionally, varying from once in two weeks to once a month, I go out at bedtime and place around the outside of the pen bits of meat containing strychnine, which I take up again early in the morning if not eaten during the night. Result, immunity from dogs, and an old well on the farm has received a layer of dogs and a layer of dirt until it is about full. I have never killed a man's dog through malice, or anywhere except on my own premises and in protection of my own property, and have not, to my knowledge, received any injury in retaliation for the death of any dog. The plan is just and right, and every fair-minded man must acknowledge it."

*Remarks.*—The author can see only one point in this plan which may be wrong. It is in that he put out his strychnined meat only once or twice a month, whereas I should think twice a week would be better if there were many dogs about.

**Fattening Sheep.**—An Ohio sheep-raiser, writing to the *Rural New Yorker*, says: "Sheep picked out for the butcher should be fed generously and regularly, and upon this point too much stress cannot be laid. Care should be taken, however, to give the sheep only just enough for one meal at each feeding time. My own experience agrees with that of most successful sheep owners, that fattening cattle should be fed three times a day, though some of my neighbors think twice often enough. It is also very important that the sheep should not be allowed to suffer from want of water; neither should they lack a supply of salt; for although salt is not so necessary to them in the winter as in summer, still they will thrive better if it is fed to them at least once a week at all seasons."

*Remarks.*—The author would say here that sheep as well as cattle should have daily access to salt and also to pure water. If fed salt only once a week they will eat so much of it as to make them over-dry, and consequently to overdrink, which is a bad thing to do. I have never seen an account of any animals over-eating salt when it is kept where they can have access to it whenever they like; and I believe they will eat only what is good for them if it is so placed.

**Pea and Oatmeal for Fattening Sheep.**—As nothing was said above as to what kind of food should be used for fattening sheep, the author would suggest peas and oats, which may have been grown together, or, better still, to grind them together; then cut nice hay and properly wet it with sweetened water if you like (see "Fattening Cattle, Molasses for," etc.); then mix in this mixed meal, and I will guarantee the fattening to be quickly and satisfactorily done. See also peas for sheep, above.

**Foot Rot in Sheep, Successful Remedy.**—Sulphuric acid, 2 ozs., water, 1 oz.; and put into the mixture 2 old copper cents (I say old, because the old ones are purer copper than the new ones), and when the cents are dissolved it is ready for use. DIRECTIONS—Remove all the rotten and decaying parts of the hoof with a knife or any convenient instrument—a knife like the blacksmiths use in horseshoeing, have the end bent up or around a little, is best— the knife being sharp to cut off if need be any projecting bits of the decaying hoof, avoiding if possible, any bleeding; then apply the mixture thoroughly to every part which was diseased. If thoroughly applied, once will generally be sufficient; but if there is any of the disease between the hoofs, besides cleaning out all that can be with the knife, a piece of soft cord or string must be wet with the mixture and drawn through to make thorough work of it and prevent its spreading again from this part.

*Remarks.*—Some persons have recommended tar a sa cure for the disease, but in my estimation there is nothing curative in it; but if the disease is first killed by the use of this acid mixture, or some of those below, then immediately apply tar over the affected part, it will protect the foot from the dampness of the ground and help to hold the acid mixture in place to make a more certain and positive cure. This acid mixture I am much in favor of, as it is very much like the celebrated Longworth cure of scrofula in persons. He puts 2 coppers into 1 oz. of nitric acid on a plate, and when effervescence ceases, *i. e.*, after it ceases to eat the copper any more, he then adds 2 ozs. of pure vinegar; then, with a swab, wash the scrofulous sores twice daily; and if it causes too much pain, reduce, so it can be borne, with a little rainwater. One man is reported in my "Second Receipt Book" as using this mixture upon his ankle for four-teen months, which effected a perfect cure, after years of suffering. The cop-per not only neutralizes much of the strength of either of the acids, but it adds to their power of destroying or killing the disease in sheep's feet, or on the scrofulous sores of persons, as above indicated. The difference, it will be seen, is, that for the foot-rot 2 ozs. of the acid is used to 1 of water, while for the scrofula 1 oz. only of the acid is used to 2 of vinegar, and this to be still reduced with water if need be, although the stronger it can be borne upon the scrofulous sore, the sooner will be the cure. There are those who think foot-rot in sheep, like scrofula, is a disease of the blood; but I think not, but that it is contagious and wholly external; while in treating scrofula internal altera-tives should be taken to make the quicker cure, still there can be no objection to the mixture of sulphur and salt, as given above, being placed where the sheep can have daily access to it. Persons should also take the sulphur mixture as given under the head of scrofula, which see.

### Sheep, Foot-Rot in—A Flockmaster's Sure Cure for.—A corre-

spondent signing himself "Flockmaster," writing to the *Post and Tribune*, says: "I have seen for the last year, inquiries for what will cure foot-root in sheep, and for the sake of the valuable animal I will give to the readers of the *Post and Tribune* a sure cure for the disease in all its stages: Muriatic acid, 3 ozs.; butter of antimony and corrosive sublimate; each, 1 oz. Mix in an open-mouthed bottle. Take the sheep and cut the decaying hoof away to the quick of the foot, as long as any opening can be found penetrating deeply into the hoof, but avoid making it bleed. [He don't tell us why, but blood neutralizes the butter of antimony.] Then with a smooth, sharp stick dip in the bottle and thoroughly rub the foot all over. It is a harsh treatment, but I will warrant a cure every time, if it is thoroughly applied."

*Remarks.*—He gives us no address, still I have no doubt of its efficacy. He says to "rub the foot all over," by which I suppose he means only the diseased part or parts, as it is no object to put it on the sound parts of the hoof; but a soft cord or string wet with it may be drawn between the hoofs, if there is any disease there. Care should always be used not to apply too freely, nor to get any of these mixtures upon your person, eyes, etc.; and don't let them lay around loose for children to get at, as they are poisonous as well as corrosive and destructive to healthy parts as well as to the diseased part.

**Another Remedy—Never Known to Fail.**—A writer in the *Ohio Farmer* says: "For foot-rot, here is a cure I have never known to fail: Take carbolic acid and pour it on a piece of copper—an old-fashioned penny will do —let it stand until the acid ceases to act on it. Be sure not to apply till the acid ceases to eat the copper. Keep the copper in all the time. Clean the hoof and apply with a swab. One or two applications will be sufficient."

*Remarks.*—He does not say how much acid. Carbolic acid is obtained by druggists in the form of crystals, but is generally kept dissolved in the least amount of water that will dissolve it. This is the kind he refers to, and 1 oz. may be put upon 1 cent, and if it eats it all up put in another, so there is some copper still left undissolved is the way to use it; otherwise, as in the above cases, to cleanse off decaying parts of the hoof before applying. But now we come to a

**Preventive of Foot-Rot in Sheep.**—A Mr. Karkeek, who is claimed to be good authority, writes to one of the agricultural papers that when the prevalence of wet weather makes it probable that foot-rot may set in, "it is easily prevented by carting a quantity of earth and throwing it up in the form of a mound in the center of the yard attached to the shed, and upon this mound strew small quantities of freshly slacked lime."

*Remarks.*—This confirms the general idea that foot-rot is brought on by external causes rather than internal, and hence the idea given in one of the "Short Rules for the Care of Sheep," and that is: "Keep sheep dry under foot with litter," etc. Sheep dearly love rolling, or even hilly, land, and cannot be well kept on low, wet grounds, and especially so if there are no knolls nor elevated dry grounds upon which they can gather themselves to rest and sleep, and hence the advantage of the mound in the yard or litter to keep their feet dry in winter.

**Sheep Ticks, Dip and Other Remedies for.**—It is important, soon after shearing sheep, to see that the lambs, especially, are freed from these pests; for after shearing, to get away from the light, and the exposures of the cold, when the old sheep have parted with their covering, the ticks will escape to the lambs, often to such an extent as to stunt their growth, reduce them in flesh, and seriously weaken them by the loss of blood; when, otherwise, they would be in their best condition. The *Hearth and Home* gives us the usual strength of the dip necessary to free them when numerous, as follows: "Cheap plug tobacco, 5 lbs., broken up and boiled in 2 pails of water; then 30 gals. added, will make dip enough for 100 lambs, or 50 sheep. After dipping keep them dry a day or two."

To dip them have a water-tight box large enough to hold a lamb, or a sheep, if any are to be dipped, so as to entirely cover them with the dip. Arrange a sloping table at the side of the box which will allow all the liquid to run back into it. Then take a lamb by the forelegs with one hand, with the other cover up the mouth and nostrils, let an assistant take the hind legs, and immerse the lamb entirely, long enough to allow the dip to penetrate the wool, lay the lamb on the sloping table and squeeze out the surplus liquid, and the operation is complete. If this is done every year, it is claimed that ticks will soon disappear altogether; but it strikes the author that ticks are as natural to sheep as lice are to hairy animals, and that they must be thus destroyed whenever they appear. If fowls are permitted access to the sheep yards they will eagerly search for ticks and pick them out of the wool, but we would rather trust to the more effectual process of dipping. Not long after this process of dipping, a careful examination of the lambs should be made, and if there is only occasionally a tick seen, every one of them must be snipped with a pair of small scissors; but if very many are left from a want of proper penetration of the dip into the wool, it must be repeated, to make a thorough destruction of them, to eradicate them from the flock, before cold weather sets in.

**Scab in Sheep, Successful Remedy.**—Quick silver, 1 lb.; Venice turpentine, ½ lb.; spirits of turpentine, 2 ozs.; melted lard, 4½ lbs. Directions—Work the first articles together thoroughly in a mortar; then mix into the warm lard and stir until cold. Apply to all scabs, and all places indicating the disease—at shearing, or whenever any indications appear—use a swab, or sponge, in applying, rubbing carefully when the skin demands it.

*Remarks.*—A farmer of Olney, Oregon, who had used it 10 years says: "It saves wool and sheep." There is not a doubt of the success of this ointment for scab in sheep, and I have not a doubt, either, but what it will cure all eruptive skin diseases of persons. If less in amount is needed, keep the same proportions. Let it be applied in fine weather, else keep the sheep under sheds for a few days; lest cold drenching rains might cause irritation from the quick silver, which is mercury. (See Scab Remedies also for other animals. See Sulphur and Salt, Valuable for Sheep, above.) It is also claimed that sulphur, moistened with Spirits of turpentine, and rubbed into the sores, will cure it. I am, then, of the opinion that it is caused by an itch mite, the same as itch, on persons, which sulphur will kill; then why not cure scab, which is an itch, on sheep, dogs, and all other animals.

**Sheep Marking Ink.**—Take linseed oil, 1 pt.; litharge, 2 ozs.; lampblack, 1 oz. Boil together, and it is ready to use; and it will not crisp or injure the wool.

**Sheep, Wash to Prevent Them from Barking Fruit Trees.**— The following wash is recommended as a sure preventive of sheep barking fruit trees: "Take soap, the dirtier and stronger the better, and make a very strong suds; dissolve ¼ lb. whale oil soap in every 6 gals., and into this stir, with brush or old stub of broom, sheep manure until it is as thick as good whitewash, and with this mixture wash the trees as high as the sheep can reach. It will be found that no sheep will come near enough to rub against them for at least two months, the time depending much on the amount of rain. Keep the mixture handy, and repeat the application as often as necessary—twice in a summer will often suffice. Sheep running among fruit trees should have plenty of good fresh water; it is thirst that first induces them to gnaw the bark, but, after they have once got a taste, they eat because they like it. The above mixture will effectually keep them away, and, besides it is a very good application for the health of the trees, keeping the bark smooth and fine, and killing any insects that may come in contact with it."

# HOGS.

**The Best Kind for Profitable Raising, etc.**—No matter how much the doctors may say against eating pork, it will always be eaten, and I am among the number who like my pork and beans, as well as ham and eggs, the ham part being nice and tender to begin with, and has been nicely cured, smoked, etc. I always expect to eat some of them as long as I may live, and it being the same with many, very many others, I will try to give a few ideas that shall benefit the others, to obtain the best breeds, how to prevent or cure their diseases, manner of feeding, etc., to the best possible profit. And as I desire to be as short as possible, I can not cover the point as to the difference in breeds, and as to their value in the markets, easier than to quote from the *Western Rural* upon these questions. It says:

**Raising Hogs.—Which the Most Profitable.**—"Did our farmer readers ever take a slate and pencil in an evening and estimate the difference between a good and poor breed of hogs? The increasing demand for ham and lard in all parts of the world shows that hogs that yield largely of these profitable parts are in demand. The consequence is there is a range in the market at this time at St. Louis, from $4.50 to $7.50, and at Chicago, from $4 to $7, showing a difference of three per cent. in favor of the good hog. Nor is this all. While the improved breeds of hogs can be made as easily and with equal food to average at 15 months old 350 pounds, as the 'greaser' hog will 175 pounds, or a little better hog will 225 pounds. If a farmer has 50 head of the latter class to sell now, he will get, at $4 per cwt., $1,125. If he has 50 'greasers,' which are too numerous in this country yet, he will get $700. But if he has 50 of the best Poland-China, Suffolk, Berkshire, etc., which have cost no more, and which have rendered a large amount of satisfaction, he will receive $2,450. These are figures that can-not be disputed, and are within the reach of every farmer who has 160 acres of land in cultivation. The number, weight, or price is not overestimated."

*Remarks.*—Remarks are almost absolutely out of the question, for figures don't lie, and there are too many whose experience have given them the $700, instead of the $1,125, or the $2,450. Don't do it again, is all that is neces-sary to add. As to feeding, etc., see that head. On the question of the best breeds, I will quote from a writer in the *Rural World*, of St. Louis, Mo., who gives the following reasons for his preference of the Berkshires, over all others. He says:

**Berkshires the Best.**—"While at St. Louis, I took a good deal of pains to study the tastes of the packers as the breed of hogs. I could

740

plainly see that they preferred those that had a strong dash of the Berkshire blood  Mine were all half, and some of them nearly full Berkshire, and they suited the buyers.  The Poland-Chinas that were young, and not of the coarser strains of that breed, were also in demand, and pleased the packers very much. Both breeds furnish good hams and shoulders, as well as side meat, and have but little offal.

"From a long experience, I am satisfied that I can fatten the Berkshire in one-half the time, and with one-half the corn required by the scrub breeds. I wish that accurate experiments for farm purposes could be made with this breed in comparison with the Chester White, Poland-China, Essex, or any other breed.    I feel certain that the Berkshire would bear off the palm. Was there ever a hardier, healthier breed?    Mine have never had an hour of sickness, nor mange, nor any skin disease.    Do you see any comparing with them as breeders?    Other breeds may have as many pigs, but will they raise as many nice, salable ones?    The Berkshires are so thoroughly established that they reproduce themselves in their offspring.    All their pigs are fine. They require no weeding out.  They are nicely turned, square built, plump fellows that please the eyes of all.  The color is good.  They are sufficiently active and industrious, and are good gleaners and grazers, are just the right size for the packers, and furnish the finest hams to be found anywhere. They have less offal, are not coarse, have small bones and are perfect."

*Remarks.*—Although it seems that the Berkshires have a clear track, yet I will give one more item in their favor, it being short, and right to the point, as follows:

**Berkshire Swine—Points of Superiority Over all Others.—** Mr. S. A. Knapp, an Iowa swine breeder, thus states his very high opinion of the Berkshires:

"The Berkshire hogs are superior to all others for the following reasons:

"1st.   They possess greater vitality, and hence are less liable to disease.

"2d.   They are more prolific.   Mature sows seldom raise less than 8 or 9 pigs.

"3d.   Being strictly a thoroughbred hog, the pigs are uniform—all choice.

"4th.   Their flesh is firmer than that of any other hog.  They furnish superior ham, shoulder, and bacon.  They bring a higher price for the English market."

*Remarks.*—Simply, "none others need apply."  By all means give them a trial.  Still, for family use, I prefer a smaller hog, which makes its best at about 150 to, at most, 200 lbs.  My stomach is not strong enough for the very large and very fat kind, but I know their great value for the market, and consequently to the farmer's profits.  There is another advantage claimed by many writers in favor of the Berkshire, and that is, that they are less liable to have hog cholera than most other breeds.

**A Small, Quick-Growing Hog Desirable.**—Another writer makes the following statement of the value of a small hog, as compared with the larger ones.  He says:

"A small, early maturing hog is much more valuable than a large one, as no more food will be required to raise two good, quick-growing ones than for a large but slow, all-lard-hog."

*Remarks.*—Some of both would be my plan ; let others suit themselves.

1. **Hog Cholera.—Its Cause and Best Known Remedies.— Cause.**—A writer for the *Country Gentleman,* of Bronson, Mich., speaking of the cause of cholera in hogs says: "I have never known an instance of cholera among hogs that had clean quarters and were fed regularly, kept warm and dry, although fed exclusively on corn, if they had also pure drink. The disease is not caused by any one thing alone, but by a combination of many unfavorable circumstances. To put a hog into a cold, wet, muddy place, exposed to hot days and chilling nights, compelled to pick its food out of the dirt and filth and drink from a filthy trough or hole, are enough to make the best of the swine race sick. All such abuses invite a sure penalty, and the wonder is that more do not get cholera, or something else, and die."

*Remarks.*—All writers upon this subject agree upon the same things, but none of them put it in such terse, or plain language. Some have written half a column, and some more, and not said half as much as this writer, with his few notes. Then give hogs clean quarters, feed them regularly, keep them warm and dry, feed corn, or any other suitable feed, and see that they have plenty of pure water, if you would avoid cholera. If you allow the other conditions of cold, wet and mud, and only a dirty hole to drink out of, it seems pretty certain that, generally, you will pay the penalty by losing your hogs. You see the difference, "you takes your choice."

**"Ringing" Hogs Claimed to be a Cause of Cholera.**—Quite a good many writing upon this subject of hog cholera, claim that the unhealthful habit of "ringing" hogs is a prominent cause of this disease ; together with the habit of always keeping hogs in the same pasture from year to year. A writer in the *Cincinnati Gazette* put it in the following shape:

"Another cause," he says, "is found in hogs occupying one field or pen from year to year, *without cleansing, or plowing under, the accumulated filth,* the hog constantly "rung," denying him a taste or smell of fresh earth, or the use of an instinct that teaches him in bilious derangements to search for bugs, worms, or vegetable roots, the natural excitants of stomach, liver and bowels, Another cause is scanty feeding, muddy, stagnant and filthy water, obliging them to allay their thirst often from the draining of their own discharges.

"When the disease first made its appearance a few years ago, it was characterized by many symptoms resembling cholera in the human being, even watery discharges, emaciation and rapid waste. Its most usual form now is loss of vitality, emaciation and drying up, with occasional paralysis, or an entire suspension of secretions; no discharges; with an inflammatory state of the liver, sympathetically affecting head, throat and lungs."

*Remarks.*—This last idea cannot be doubted, and hence should never be allowed. A "change of pasture" for hogs is of as much importance, and will give them as much pleasure and benefit as for other stock. The following receipt is this writer's plan of preventing, as well as curing the disease :

**3. Hog Cholera—Preventive and Cure**—"Madder, sulphur, resin, saltpetre and black antimony, each 1 lb., assafœtida, 3 oz.

*Directions.*—" Pulverize and mix well ; then feed three table-spoonfuls to each five hogs, three times a week, with a little salt, more bran, and ashes. [I take it this would be stirred into moistened bran, or bran-slop, from what he says below.] Commence feeding before the cholera gets into your neighborhood, and continue until it ceases from the same ; and if, during the time and before your hogs are properly medicated, one should take the disease, immediately remove it to a dry pen. Give one table-spoonful of this mixture in 1 gal. of water or table-slops once per day; and in order to make the cure doubly sure, take one-half pint soft soap, 1 table-spoonful pine (common) tar, 1 table-spoonful of lard ; warm and mix well, and drench the hog ; and my word for it, it will cure ninety-nine out of the hundred.

"If you will treat the first one or two in this manner, the disease will spread no further. And you must remember that as fast as the disease spreads, or in a ratio to the number infected, its malignancy increases, until it will almost defy control.

*Caution.*—" If the season should'be wet, keep your hogs on short timothy pasture ; if dry, on the best growth clover you have, and these are valuable helps. Sweet milk alone is said also to be good."

*Remarks.*—It is considered very important, if a hog is attacked with the disease, gets dumpish, lies around, or tries to get into the litter, or straw, of the pen, to remove him at once from the others, lest the disease spread, although quite a good many writers claim the disease is not contagious. Although it may not be contagious, yet perhaps it will spread in a herd if the sick ones are not separated from the others. See the last paragraph before the Caution above, as to its greater "malignancy," according to the number infected.

Everything that will throw even the least light on the subject of hog cholera is of such great importance that I cannot refrain from giving an Iowa man's opinion upon the origin of this disease. It is from the *Patron's Helper*, of Iowa. It is based upon close confinement, *i. e.*, always in the same pasture, and also upon ringing, to prevent their rooting up the soil. His argument is strong, and his theory undoubtedly correct. Then let piggy's nose go free to root as it pleases, as indicated below ; and also pay as much attention as possible to the plan of nice clover if the season is dry; and short timothy if the season is wet, as given in the last paragraph, or Caution, above, if you hope for success. The following are his ideas and argument :

**4. Hog Cholera—its Origin.**—"Let us watch our hogs in their ample pasture. Some are browsing the herbage, some are destroying it by extracting the roots. Others—what are they doing ? They are rooting into that woody hillside; into that hard, calcareous soil. The crackling sound indicates that they are *eating the clay with its limestone pebbles.* What can this be for ? Well, we cannot tell. We know it is a fact. It may effect something chemically; but we sometimes doubt that, it being too crude to enter into the animal economy. Perhaps its effect is mainly mechanical.

"The poor pig has no rights that man or dog are bound to respect, outside of his pen, so it is furnished a pen; may be one or two acres; frequently much less. In 'Mrs. Piggy' goes with her numerous progeny. Everything goes well for a while. They eat the grass and turn over the soil and thrive. The owner improves his herd by an infusion of Chester White, Poland-China or Berkshire blood. He is well satisfied with the profits of the investments.

"Anon! a change has come in the condition of things. The surface soil is now all rooted over. The desirable properties are exhausted or befouled with droppings. The pigs endeavor to dig deeper, but the filthy mass falls to the bottom; and soon it is said the pigs are not doing well.

"The owner changes their food, gives them sulphur and antimony and what not. He concludes they look a little better, but they don't do well yet. In fact, he sighs for the 'good old Elm Peelers and Prairie Rooters.' It does not stop here. The pigs are constipated, dyspeptic and mangy. Their blood is out of order, and ulcers are found on some so as to cause portions of the flesh to slough off. In fact, they have got the cholera. No wonder. Had the proprietor made a vegetable garden or a corn field of his hog lot a year or two ago, and furnished his hogs with another pasture, his improved hogs would have improved the strength and vigor of his herd, and also the condition of his finances."

*Remarks.*—If the result is liked, let every one go and do likewise; if not liked, take the sensible course that is sure to prevent the disease. Let their noses alone, and give them a large pasture, a woody one if possible. (See II in Reports below).

**5. Hog Cholera—Its General Symptoms and Treatment, by Prof. Cressey.**—The following was given through the *Scientific American.* The symptoms are given very full, and the treatment is a common-sense plan, and will undoubtedly be found very satisfactory, if taken before the diarrhœa sets in. The larger amount given, of course, will be understood for a large hog, and the smaller amount for a small one. He says:

"Hog Cholera is known as 'Blue Disease,' 'Red Soldier,' 'Distemper in Pigs,' etc. This is undoubtedly a blood disease, and belongs to the anthrax malignant type of fevers.

*Symptoms—First Stage.*—"The disease sets in and usually secures a firm hold upon the animal before its presence is suspected. The one affected will isolate himself from the rest and burrow in the litter, often remaining thus till death, though sometimes they will run about as if wild, grunting and squealing as if in great pain. Dullness, drooping head and ears, and loss of appetite are the symptoms observed, if at all, in the first stage. Now is the time to remove him from the herd.

*Second Stage.*—"In what may be called the Second Stage, the abdominal pains are indicated by lying on the belly, with fore-feet outstretched, and, when caused to move, uttering shrieks. The skin takes on a purple color, particularly upon the back and ears, along the abdomen and inside the thighs. The pulse is rapid, but feeble.

*Third Stage.*—"Diarrhœa sets in and becomes profuse in the Third Stage. The dejections are black and offensive. The pulse weakens and finally becomes imperceptible. Breathing is difficult and spasmodic, owing to the condition of the lungs, and an irritating cough comes on. General weakness is now apparent; the animal can scarcely stand, his legs get entangled like a tipsy man's, and complete paralysis soon results. Eruptions on the skin may have followed the first discoloration, which now are succeeded by sloughing and ulceration. Insensibility precedes death from three to six hours. The malady sometimes appears in less fatal forms, accompanied by colored skin and loss of appetite for a few days, when recovery follows; but this is uncommon. On *post mortem* (after death) examination the appearance of rapid decomposition is manifest, and all the tissues seemed transfused with blood.

*Treatment.*—" After diarrhœa sets in death is almost certain. Before that event, administer quickly—by means of a drenching-horn or long-necked bottle, and, if the pig is large, tying him to a post with a rope around his upper jaw—Epsom salts, 2 to 4 oz.; sulphur, 2 to 6 drs.; gentian and ginger (powdered), 1 to 2 drs.; molasses, 2 to 3 table-spoonfuls; gin, ½ pt. Clean bedding and comfortable pens, with light diet of vegetable food, are required. A free run in a bare pasture or lane is a great help. In this, as in all other sickness, when possible, prevention is the best treatment, and simply consists in careful feeding, plenty of vegetable food, cleanliness and exercise."

*Remarks.*—Of course, the "exercise" he refers to can only mean a large run—plenty of room; still I do not see that he will move about much in this condition. The room, or "exercise" should have been provided before this.

**6. Hog Cholera—Reports to the State Board of Agriculture of Illinois, with Preventive.**—The State Board of Agriculture, of Illinois, a short time since, sent out to the various swine-breeders of the State a series of questions to obtain all possible knowledge as to the cause and the best known remedies. The answers were in accordance, or agreeing generally with the ideas as given above. No positive cure was claimed to be known. Preventives, by care, removing sick ones from the herd, etc., were the leading recommendations. I will quote from only two or three of them; the first, because he claims exemption of his Berkshires; the second, because he gives a preventive in the line of medicines; and the last, because his herd escaped the disease by "good feeding and keeping, and giving plenty of salt."

I. The first was from George M. Caldwell, a breeder of Berkshires, of Carlinville. He says:

" I am satisfied that the Cholera is owing to the sudden transition from a laborious, half-starved condition to one of high feed ; and so convinced am I that, while I have a pig, I intend to feed him liberally until sold. During the last three years my best Berkshires were running by the side of the diseased stock, and some of the older sows with them nearly all the time. I have always fed my young Berkshires, and have lost none of them. I do not consider the disease contagious. My hogs died in the Branch, and some of my neighbors' hogs, just below, on the same stream, were healthy, and all the water they got was from the Branch. These hogs, however, were on clover, and fed some corn all the season."

*Remarks.*—Here you see strong reasons why this gentleman does not think the disease is contagious. The other two believe it is contagious.

II. The second is from Lemuel Milk, of Kankakee, who keeps on an average 1,000 head of hogs. He reports:

" My experience is, that the fat hogs are more liable to be attacked. I think that hogs having range of fields and woods are not so liable to be affected. I believe the disease is contagious—have no doubt of it from my experience and observation. I have used as a

**"Preventive of Hog Cholera.**—Copperas, black antimony and fenugreek seed, each 5 lbs.; sulphur, 4 lbs., and saltpetre, 2 lbs."

He does not tell us, but, of course, all should be pulverized and evenly mixed; and for dose and manner of giving, see "Hog Cholera Preventive and Cure," where quite a similar mixture is given—except less antimony, and the author would not use more than 2 lbs. of the antimony here given. He closed as follows:

"I have used as a remedy, with good result, carbolic acid, given in slop and sprinkled on the bedding of the sick hogs. Several weeks after, the diseased hogs recovered; they became strong and healthy, after every hair had come off. The hogs opened, that had died with cholera, generally had their stomachs full of worms."

III. The third is from O. B. Nichols, of Carlyle, Clinton county, also an extensive breeder. He says:

"I believe the disease contagious, because one-half to three-fourths of the herd die, as a general thing, when allowed to run and sleep together." And closed by saying: "While last year my neighbors suffered heavy losses, mine escaped the cholera, as I believe, by good feeding and good keeping, and by giving them plenty of salt.—*Springfield (Ill.) Correspondent of Chicago Tribune.*

**Hog Cholera—Two Well-Tried Cures for.**—The Greenville (Ill.) *Advocate* published these cures: "The first is from a correspondent at Mill Grove, who says the receipt was first published in the *Prairie Farmer* some years since. The quantity given is for 100 hogs and is mixed with slop to have enough for a few doses, say one pint of the slop to the hog, each time. The following is the receipt:

I. "Sulphur, 2 lbs.; black antimony, ¼ lb.; arsenic, 2 oz.

"Our correspondent says he has tried it on a lot of fifty hogs, and cured all that were able to walk to the trough to eat the slop.

"*The Second.*—Prof. J. B. Turner published the following preventives in the same paper (*Prairie Farmer*), which our correspondent says he has seen used with perfect satisfaction:

II. "Wood ashes, 1 pk.; salt, 4 lbs.; black antimony, copperas and sulphur, each, 1 lb.; saltpetre, ¼ lb. Pulverize and mix, moisten and put in a trough under a shed, where the hogs can have free access to it.

**8. Hog Cholera, Preventive and Cure.**—*Moore's Rural New Yorker* publishes the following: "We have recently published reports of a new and dangerous hog disease now prevailing in the western states. Hon. T. C. Jones, of Ohio, publishes in the Delaware, O., *Gazette* the following preventive treatment with directions what to do in case of an attack:

"'A mixture of ashes (wood), 1 pk.; salt, 4 lbs.; copperas, 7 lbs.; sulphur, 1 lb.; kept constantly in a trough, is of great service. If predisposed to cholera, hogs will eat it more freely than when free from all symptoms. If a hog gets down, try to get into him a gill (4 oz.) of coal oil in slops; it has sometimes been effective when other remedies have failed.'"

*Remarks.*—If 1 lb. of black antimony, pulverized, was added to the above I think it would be all the better for it. "Coal oil," of course, means "kerosene," which is getting to be used by some physicians for persons giving a few drops internally and rubbing it on freely, for throat diseases, rheumatism, etc.

**9. Calomel as a Cure for Hog Cholera.**—A Mr. Benj. J. Kemp, of Marion county, Ind., says he has cured all cases of hog cholera on his farm by giving sixty grains of calomel to each grown hog, mixing it with flour dough.

*Remarks.*—Although I am not much of a calomel man, yet I should have no fears of trying this ; but I should think better of Mr. K. if he had given his post-office address. I suppose, however, he wanted to avoid correspondence, like many others do now-a-days. The following is also from an Indiana man :

**10. Hog Cholera, Preventive and Cure.**—Madder, saltpetre and sulphur, each, 1 lb.; black antimony, $\frac{1}{4}$ lb.; assafœtida, 2 oz.

*Directions.*—All the articles to be pulverized and mixed thoroughly.

*Dose.*—In case they are sick, give four table-spoonfuls to five hogs once daily, in slop. Twice a week in the same proportion, as a preventive. *Tested.*—*Correspondence of the Indiana Farmer.*

*Remarks.*—This is much like No. 3, but I like this better, as it has only half the antimony in it as No. 3, and this man's mode of giving I also prefer. The severity of the disease and the great losses from it, is my excuse for giving all the information I have upon the subject of hog cholera. One more, and I am done.

**11. Soap Believed to Exempt Hogs from Cholera.**—A writer says :

"The exemption of hogs fed from the slops of hotels and private families from attacks of cholera is attributed to the fact that such slops contain a considerable amount of soapy water. The effect of potash is to cleanse the hog's intestines of worms, making them more vigorous and healthy, and a little soap fed with corn is therefore recommended both for economy and as a safeguard against disease.

*Remarks.*—Soap enters into the formation of many pills for its carminative properties, why should it be thought singular, or no account for hogs ? But so far as the alterative properties are concerned, the ashes in the above preventives would have the same effect. There is not a doubt but what hogs should have salt as regularly as cattle, or other domestic animals ; and a little ashes with it would be a benefit occasionally for all stock.

**12. Hog Cholera, Positive Remedy from "Navin on the Hog"; Valuable also for Chicken Cholera, and as a Condition Powder for Horses, Cattle, etc.**—After the foregoing matter had all been written I found the following from "Navin on the Hog," and which he so highly extols, I must give it a place, for I know it will prove valuable for *all* the conditions for which he recommends it. He says:

**1. For Hogs.**—Ginger and sulphate of iron (copperas), each 4 ozs.; black antimony, sulphur and nitre (saltpetre), each 2 ozs. All pulverized and mixed.

Dose, for a large hog, 1 tea-spoonful 3 times a day. For a hog less than 150 lbs., a level tea-spoonful only; smaller according to size.

*Remarks.*—He does not say how to give it, but like the others, I should give it in a little slops; or if the hog is too dumpish to eat, drench it in a little slop or gruel. He claims to have used it successfully in *every* case, from the commencement of the disease in his neighborhood. It being his condition powder, in use by him for ten years for horses. If diarrhœa in the hogs has set in, he takes alum, 2 ozs., and white-oak inner bark, 2 ozs., steeping the bark, mixing in the alum, and gives; and if it continues obstinate he gives lard, 1 lb. melted with spirits of turpentine, 1 table-spoonful; continuing the powder till the hair is bright, and the skin clean and healthy. He says it never failed him in ten years use of it, even in the last stages of the disease.

**For Chickens.**—He says, also, it is good for chicken cholera, 1 tea-spoonful in 1 pint of dough for 1 dozen chickens.

We shall have something now to say upon the subject of feeding and fattening hogs, and also upon the question as to the value of charcoal or carbon in some form as *preventive* as well as *curative* of other diseases, as diarrhœa or scours of hogs, arising from over-feeding while fattening, etc. The importance of charcoal for hogs while fattening is so generally believed we can scarcely open an agricultural paper which does not have something in its columns upon it. I will give the opinions of a few papers and persons, whose experience enables them to write what they know, and what the author feels assured he can recommend to his readers, to go and do likewise, expecting to receive the same satisfaction. Under the head of

**Carbon for Hogs,** the *Western Rural* says:

"There is no doubt in our mind of the benefit from feeding crude carbonaceous matter to swine when they are kept in close pens. The avidity with which hogs eat rotten wood is well known. Charcoal is but another form of carbon. Bituminous (having a kind of mineral filth in it, over soft mineral coal,) is still another form. The utility of feeding wood and coal has long been recognized. We, some years since, substituted the ordinary Western stone coal with the best results, where from two to five hundred hogs were kept in close pens and fed on the refuse of the city hotels. Something of the kind seems as necessary to them as salt to strictly herbivorous (herb-eating) animals. We have known them to consume a pound in the course of a day, and again they would not seek the coal for some time. Just what particular use the coal is in the animal economy is not so easy to answer. Swine are especially liable to scrofulous and inflammatory diseases. Carbon, in the shape of coal, is an antiseptic, and the probability is that it acts in this way in purifying the blood.'

**Charcoal, or Burnt Corn for Hogs.**—Under this head the *New England Farmer* says:

"We have but little doubt that charcoal is one of the best known remedies for the disordered state into which hogs drift; usually having disordered bowels, all the time giving off the worst kinds of evacuation. Probably the best form in which charcoal can be given is in the form of burnt corn—perhaps, because when given in other forms the hogs do not get enough. A distillery was burnt in Illinois, about which a large number of hogs were kept. Cholera prevailed among these hogs somewhat extensively. In the burning of the buildings a large amount of corn was consumed. To this burnt and partially burnt corn the hogs had access at will, and the sick commenced recovering at once, and a large proportion of them got well. Many farmers have practiced feeding scorched corn, putting it into a stove, or building a fire upon the ground, placing the ears upon it, leaving them till pretty well charred. Hogs fed on still-slops are liable to be attacked by irritation of the stomach and bowels, coming from too free generation of acid, from fermentation of food after eaten. Charcoal, whether it be produced by burning corn or wood, will neutralize the acid, in this way removing the irritating cause. The charcoal will be relished to the extent of getting rid of the acid, and beyond that it may not be. Hence it is well to let the wants of the hog be settled by the hog himself."

**Mineral Coal for Hogs.**—The following is from Judge Katon, in *Prairie Farmer,* He says:

"The hog seems to crave carbon in a concentrated form, and hence we may conclude it is necessary to his well-being. He will eat charcoal freely, which is tasteless and not nutritious. From the same natural prompting we see them eat wood when so decayed that they can do so.

"For myself I have for many years been in the habit of feeding my hogs with an abundance of our common bituminous (soft) coal, preferring the poorest, or that which contains a large amount of sulphur and iron, and, I think, with the happiest results. [Where iron is needed see those recipes containing copperas, which is the sulphate of iron — a good remedy for me.] Let a farmer who has never tried it throw in a lump of coal as large as his fist, and he will be surprised to see the hog leave the corn and crunch the coal, as if it were the most luscious morsel. Sulphur has long been known as a valuable remedial agent for hogs, and iron is a well-known tonic, acting specifically upon the blood, thickening and strengthening it. Here, then the hog, by eating the coal, gets other important elements besides the carbon.

"I have never known a hog well supplied with this coal, to be sick, or off his feed for a single day, and although I cannot give figures showing actual results of careful experiments to prove it, I believe hogs thus supplied will eat more and assimilate their food better, will make appreciably more pork, with a given amount of corn, than those which are without it. At least, I am well satisfied with the way in which my hogs thrive—grow and fatten—under this treatment. Coal is cheap, and others, if they have not done so, may try it at little expense."

*Remarks.*—It can thus be seen not only how general the opinion is, that carbon—charcoal, soft, or bituminous—mineral—coal, or properly and thoroughly burned corn are carbon—is almost, if not absolutely necessary for hogs while fattening; and it is as well known. also, that when they are pretty well fattened is the time when their stomachs are the most likely to get out of order from the over-feeding, or perhaps, more properly speaking, long and constant feeding. They refuse their food, become dumpish, and perhaps scours or diarrhœa sets in, and all the labor of feeding, and the value of the hog is lost by neglect to see that charcoal, soft or mineral coal, with plenty of sulphur in it or the burnt corn has been fed, or kept where the hogs could have free access to them; and salt and wood ashes mixed and kept also where they can partake of them as they like, should be attended to early in the fattening if you would avoid loss in the end. These more simple remedies will be found all-sufficient when cholera is not prevailing; when it is, then prepare also some of the preventives against that disease, which see above, which always means given before in this book.

**Hogs, Preparing Food for—Peas claimed Better than Corn.—**
The *Fostoria Review* informs us that a writer in one of their exchanges states:

"The present practice in any country, I believe, is to prepare food for hogs either by steeping, steaming or boiling, under the belief that cooking in any shape is better than giving in the raw state. But I now assert, on the strongest possible grounds—by evidence indisputable, again and again proved by actual trials, in various temperatures, with a variety of the same animals, variously conducted—that for fast and cheap production of pork, raw peas are fifty per cent. better than cooked peas or Indian corn in any shape."

*Remarks.*—I am well aware that raw peas, when young, that is, growing, but being what we know as "full," *i. e.* got their full size and ready to use "at table," if cut up and fed to hogs thus, they thrive and grow upon them very fast. As it is from decided statements of this kind that others are induced to try the experiment for themselves, and establish or refute such statements, I have given it a place. I have not a doubt but what the writer is honest in his position, and if further test shall prove it true, generally, there may be considerable profit to those who can raise more peas than corn to the acre, which no doubt many can. Still, I must say that I believe more pork can be made in the same time from either peas or corn if they are ground and properly cooked, or boiling water, at least, poured upon the meal, and the meal stirred as it should be, as will be seen in fattening cattle, than if fed unground and uncooked. There can be no doubt upon this position of properly cooked food being better for fattening purposes than uncooked. See " Meal and Hay for Fattening Stock—Scalding the Meal a great Saving."

**Hog Feeding Experience of an Iowa Breeder and Packer.—**A hog breeder and pork packer of Iowa gives his experience in the business to one of the agricultural papers as follows: He has demonstrated to his entire satisfaction that after his spring pigs had reached about 300 lbs. they ceased to grow with any profit. His pigs on the first of January weighed nearly as much as they did on the first of February, notwithstanding he had kept up the feeding. He is a great advocate of taking good care of hogs. He would never shut up his hogs more than five weeks before he wants to market them. His food early in the fall was pumpkins, steamed and mixed with middlings, the proportion being about one-half a bu. of middlings to 40 gals. of steamed pumpkins. His object was to develop the bone and muscle of the hog without adding fat. This he continued three months, and then put them in a close pen and fed them meal and middlings steamed. After shutting them up for five weeks they gained two pounds a day until they reached 300 lbs., and then ceased to grow to any extent.

*Remarks.*—Where this man used middlings to thicken his steamed pumpkin, to give bone and muscle, or to make his pigs grow, would be just the place for pea and oat meal to come in, as oats are generally sowed with peas, to help hold them up, as peas fill better if they stand up than they do when fallen down, as they almost always do if sowed alone. Boiled or steamed potatoes, when they are plenty, when the pumpkins are all used up, or part pumpkins and a part potatoes do excellently well, thickening with the pea and oat meal, and would generally be considered cheaper than the middlings as above mentioned.

**Hogs—Corn Claimed to be the Best Food for, and Best when Cooked.**—I am well aware that there are some people who yet think that it is not at all necessary to cook food for hogs, or other stock. I do not propose to enter into the discussion of the subject. I will say that I think common sense tells us that it is better to cook food to fatten hogs; but I will give an item from the *American Rural Home*, which was given under the above heading, then let every one judge for himself as to whether it is best to grind and cook corn, or to let the hogs grind and cook it for themselves. The item is as follows:

" Corn is the best feed for hogs, and may be fed in the ear, while soft, but when hard, should be ground fine and wet with hot water, or otherwise cooked, for it has been proved, by repeated experiments, that corn thus fed will make from one-third to one-half more pork than when fed unground and uncooked; and a bushel should make from ten to twelve pounds of meat when thus fed to good feeding stock."

*Remark.*—See above, Preparing Food for Hogs, Peas Claimed Better than Corn, etc.

**Fattening Hogs, Roots Valuable for.**—The *Dublin Farmers' Gazette* gives the following as to the value of roots for fattening pigs. "Pigs" is quite often used while speaking of these animals, when hogs would be the proper word. It says:

" Parsnips, carrots, Swedish turnips, and especially mangel-wurzel, will all fatten pigs. These roots ought not to be given in a raw state, but always cooked and mixed with beans, peas, Indian corn, oats or barley, all of which must be ground into meal. When pigs are fed on such cooked food as we have stated, the pork acquires a peculiarly rich flavor, and is much esteemed, especially for family use.

**Store Pigs, Value of Roots for.**—The following Item from the *American Agriculturist* will strengthen the above idea from the *Gazette*, and add another root to the list, as this item, no doubt, refers to the common field turnip, which is not enumerated in the other. I must add, however, what the *Agriculturist* does not mention, and that is, I think the turnips should be cooked. It says:

" Store pigs will thrive well on roots with a slop of bran, sour milk and water. A supply of roots on hand will greatly reduce the cost of feeding store pigs. Turnips that cannot well be fed to cows may be given to the pigs. Give your pigs a warm, dry bed."

*Remarks.*—It will be seen by referring to the Cattle Department that if the rootlets are trimmed off of the turnips, they can be fed to milch cows, without flavoring the milk.

**Store Pigs and Breeding Sows, Corn and Oats Ground Together for, Better than Either Alone.**—A writer upon this subject says:

" A bushel of corn weighs nearly twice as much as a bushel of oats, but if ground together the mixture makes a better feed for growing pigs and breeding sows than either grain alone."

*Remarks.*—There is not a doubt but what this is a fact—oats too light, alone, and corn heavier and more heating ; but when ground together, they combine all the elements needed for making growth ; but there is not a doubt, either, if they have a good patch of the artichoke to run to, named in the next item, they will thrive equally well on much less of meal. Try them, if you want a good thing for hogs, or children, either. Most persons are fond of them raw, as they have a pleasant sweetish taste. It is claimed, also, that they are a good preventive against hog cholera.

**Growing Hogs and Breeding Sows, Artichokes Valuable for, Amount Raised to the Acre.**—Prof. Johnson, the farm superintendent of the Agricultural College of Michigan, has given a good deal of attention to the artichoke as food for hogs, and thinks they are not only healthful, but that they give a certain sweetness to the pork. For fattening purposes, he says, "corn will always be most valuable ; but for growing swine, and before the fattening process begins, the artichoke furnishes excellent food." He planted a patch near the pens, and turned the breeding sows into them early in the spring, allowing them to "root, hog, or die," as suited them best, but found that the artichoke furnished a succulent, juicy food for the sows, just when it was most needed, and most difficult to obtain from other sources.

**Artichokes.—Amount to the Acre, Labor of Raising, Getting Rid of them when desired, and Preventive of Cholera, etc.**—I. It is but very little labor to raise artichokes. Plant on good soil, properly plowed and harrowed, then furrow it two or three feet apart as you choose, and an eye dropped every few inches, and properly covered, is about all the trouble; for they grow quickly and spread all over the ground so as to keep down weeds, especially after the first season. They yield from 300 to 800 or more bushels to the acre; the hogs dig them as wanted, and all they want, and it is said by plowing them up in June, when the tops are about a foot in height, they can be exterminated if desired. My father always used to have them growing along the garden fence for the pleasure of us children, but sixty years ago there was but little known of their value for swine, but many a one have I dug for eating raw, and for mother to pickle for table use, if the other pickles run out before spring. Of course the winter does not hurt them. A writer speaking of the danger of frost upon the ordinary roots for stock, says: "Beets endure but little frost, turnips improve with a little, carrots stand a good deal of it, but parsnips, salsify, and artichokes may be left out all winter with advantage."

II. **Preventive of Cholera.**—Another writer says: "Where the artichoke is planted largely in districts as food for hogs, the cholera has prevailed only to a very limited extent."

**Apples Good for Hogs, and Hogs Running in the Orchard Destroy the Codling Moth.**—Fallen apples may be gathered and fed, profitably to hogs, horses or cattle in moderation; but where one has enough hogs to consume all as they fall, it is probably the best thing to do to turn them into the orchard; as those that fall early, especially, contain the moth, whose sting, or eating into its heart, has caused it to fall thus early. The word codlin, as Shakespeare has it, means "almost an apple," hence we get the "codlin," or "codling moth"—a moth that makes codlins, or early falling apples, which, if not eaten or picked up soon and carried out of the orchard, the moth will return to the tree for further depredation and its own increase. "The destruction of the early fallen apples also destroys the moths and saves the remainder left upon the trees."

Sows Eating their Pigs, to Prevent, and Cure the Habit.—I. To prevent it, keep a trough of the following mixture where all the hogs can have access to it: Wood ashes, salt, sulphur and powdered charcoal, in about equal bulk, mixed, and see especially that sows partake of it about this period; then if they commence the eating of their young, give them in small pieces one pound of salt pork; and ten or twelve hours later give them half as much more as long as they will eat it, and see also that they have frequent tastes of this preventive mixture.

II. To Cure the Habit.—A little salt daily and a handful of charcoal to each hog once a week, it is claimed, will prevent cholera and other diseases; then, if the above mixture is kept where all hogs can eat of it at their pleasure, the author will guarantee it preferable to the salt and charcoal alone. Still, if cholera was prevailing in a neighborhood, he would advise some of the preventives found under that head, having antimony, saltpeter, etc., with the salt and charcoal. Keep on the safe side is a good motto to go by. And it is by thus satisfying the natural desire for what their systems need, that a ravenous taste is prevented, that of eating their pigs.

Scurvy Pigs, Simple Remedy.—Wash the scurvy hair and all parts troubled with the scurf thoroughly every day for a few times with buttermilk. A farmer who has tried this so many times as to be sure of his position, says: "It will entirely and speedily remove the scurf."

Lice on Hogs, Easy Remedy.—"Carbolic acid 1 oz. to water, 10 ozs., makes a wash that destroys the lice without injury to the hog." Then it would on other animals, as cattle, cats, dogs, fowls, etc.

Kidney-Worm in Hogs and "Fluke" in Sheep, Remedy for. —The *Rural Alabamian* asserts that kidney-worms in hogs, and the fluke-worms that infest the livers of sheep are identically the same. A parasitic insect—an insect drawing its whole support from another animal, as lice upon an animal, or worms in them—and the editor claims also "that lye made from hard-wood ashes, if given daily, will work a cure; also rubbing turpentine upon the loins."

*Remarks.*—There is nothing said as to the amount to be given, but we should say, if the lye is pretty strong, two or three table-spoonfuls in a small amount of slop, two or three times daily, would be plenty. Of course it could not be given without diluting, else it would destroy the mucous membrane of the mouth, throat, etc., as cows have been killed by drinking lye left where they could get at it. But why not salt and ashes mixed, in place of the salt and charcoal mentioned just above? If they will take enough of it, it will do as well without a doubt, and I have no doubt of their value in such cases.

**Corn and Pork, How to Get the Most from, by the Way of Feeding.**—The Chicago *Herald* informs its readers that "an Ohio pork grower has learned by experimenting that a bushel of corn fed on the cob will produce only nine pounds of pork, while an equal quantity, ground, and the meal fed raw, gives twelve pounds; but a bushel of corn boiled gives thirteen pounds, while if ground and the meal cooked, makes about $16\frac{1}{2}$ pounds."

*Remark.*—Now farmers, continue the old plan and get the nine pounds, or take the common sense plan, that is, do the best you know and obtain the $16\frac{1}{2}$, as you like best. Although every experiment might not exactly meet these figures, yet there is not a doubt but what they will come very near them.

# POULTRY.

**HENS, CHICKENS, TURKEYS, DUCKS AND GEESE.—** Winter Care of, upon a Large Scale—House For—Best Breeds, Etc.—As it has been thoroughly taught through the newspapers for several years passed that poultry raising upon a larger scale than about fifty hens could not be done safely, I propose to give a different idea, by quoting the report of a committee of the New York Farmers' Club, made through the *Hearth and Home*. All that is needed to carry on the business upon a large scale is to know how, and that is learned from this report, from one who has proved, by several years' experience, that it has been done and therefore can be done again. The committee was appointed by the Club to visit poultry yards and ascertain the best mode of carrying feathered stock through cold weather, which was as follows:

"On Wednesday last we spent the day at the farm of Warren Leland, 25 miles north of this city (New York), at Rye Station, and have derived, from a careful survey of his yards, ideas which we consider important. We find him carrying 150 turkeys, about 300 hens, a large drove of ducks, and several dozen of geese through the winter without the loss of any of his poultry by disease of any sort, and without the freezing of their feet or their legs. We learn that he never has maladies among his poultry, that he will allow the greater part of his hens to set in the spring, and each of them will yield an average brood of 10 chicks; so that he will raise about 3,000 chickens from his present flock, and his losses be very few. How does he do it? 1. His hens, ducks and geese have the best winter quarters we have ever seen provided for any of the feathered tribes. Their main barrack or hennery is a stone house 75 feet long and 20 feet wide, and faces south. The openings on the north side are small and filled with window-glass, and in some cases with double sash. Those on the south side are much larger, consisting of double doors, which are opened on sunny days. In the middle of the north side is a wide, old-fashioned fire-place, with crane and a big camp-kettle. Nearly every day in winter a fire is lit and fed with chunks, knots and old logs that would otherwise be knocked about the wood-yard. The walls are of stone, and the floor of rock or earth, so the fire can be left without the least danger. On cold days, and especially in cold rains, the hens gather before this fire and warm themselves and trim their feathers. The chimney can easily be closed, or the logs rolled out into the middle of the building, and feathers or sulphur used to make a fumigation. This is done whenever hen-lice appear; and the openings of the house can be closed so as to hold the fumigation till it penetrates to every crack. Smoke he finds better than carbolic acid, or kerosene, or whitewash to drive vermin.

"The roosts are oak slats 1 inch thick by 2½ inches wide, fastened to the rafters near the ridge. They are nailed at different heights and at proper intervals. About 2 feet below the perches is a scaffold of boards that fit quite closely. This is from time to time covered with plaster and ashes. About once a month the accumulations are shoveled down and piled up for the corn-field. He calculates that 50 hens yield in the course of a year as much com-

755

post as would be worth $50 in bone-meal; that is to say, if he threw away his hen-droppings, and had to buy the same amount of fertilizing salts in bone-dust, it would cost him $50. He has paid special attention to the comfort of his hens on the perch. They sit on a slat 2½ inches wide; their breast-feathers come down and cover their feet, and protect them from freezing in the coldest nights. Of course, there is no lack of dry ashes in their house, and he finds that after the fire goes out the hens use the hearth as a place to nestle and shake ashes through their feathers. They enjoy it, and it keeps them sound and comfortable.

"The offal of the farm, as entrails, feathers, heads, scraps from lard, and all the odds and ends from the kitchen are thrown into this house, and the hens pick it over, eating all they want. Then, as soon as spring opens, all this trash is shoveled and scraped out, composted and taken to the corn-field. Besides this refuse, his poultry eat about 1 bushel of corn a day in winter, and ½ a bushel in summer. He raises large crops of corn because he has strong manure to feed his crops with. In spring, after a hen has hatched, her nest is taken out, the straw burned, and the box whitewashed inside and out, then filled with fresh straw and put back for another family party.

**Best Breed.** — "After many trials of breeds he has settled upon the White Brahmas. They lay more uniformly the year through, make the best mothers, and the chicks grow the fastest. During summer his poultry have a wide range, and scour the fields for half a mile or more consuming grasshoppers. His turkeys nearly make their weight on grasshoppers and beetles, with a handful of corn night and morning. One man has little to do in spring and summer but to take care of chickens and young turkeys. In winter they require but little attention, and this man then attends to the calves and lambs."

"The cost of his poultry-meat—and he often kills in a season 300 turkeys and 3,000 chickens—he considers to be about 250 bushels of corn, and the wages of his hen-wife for half the time. His gains he cannot give exactly, for the poultry is eaten very freely by a large family and sent to the Metropolitan when prices are high, or the supply in market defective in quality. He does not keep exact account of his eggs, for, as a rule, he says the best thing to do with an egg is to let a good motherly hen make a chicken of it. Your committee conclude their report by an expression of opinion that the common ideas on the subject of poultry-raising on a large scale are erroneous. It has been said again and again in this Club and in farm journals that there is no use in trying to keep more than about 50 hens; if one goes deeper into the poultry business there is backset from lice and roup and gapes and cholera and the sudden death of hens and chicks from causes unknown. This is a fallacy. In the manner above described, by the wise use of smoke and lime and ashes and a fire, by cleanliness and a wide range in mild weather, we find Mr. Leland taking about 4,000 feathered animals through the season, for year after year, without calamity or loss, and on an expense that is very trifling and unfelt on a large farm."

*Remarks.*—I wish to speak here of two points particularly, which I believe to be worthy of absolute confidence. First, the perches being made of 2½ by 1 inch slats, fastened so they sit upon the flat or broad side of the perch, making it not only easier for the hen to sit upon it, but she does not have to cling her toes around a pole to be able to keep her position, which strains the cords and makes them more liable to freeze in winter. And second, these slats will not crack open by shrinking, as everybody knows poles do; thus preventing a harbor for lice, right under the hen, which amounts to more, as I know it must, than one would suppose by a mere thought upon the subject.

Another thought or two are worthy of consideration. Mr. Leland considers fumigation, smoke from feathers, or sulphur, better than kerosene, or carbolic acid washes. There is not a doubt of it, as the smoke will reach every crack and crevice, while many will be missed with the washes. And the idea of a chimney and a pretty large fire-place in the hen house, is really the grandest idea of all, by it he secures warmth, life, and health, to his poultry in damp, as well as cold winter weather. Let the size of the house be in proportion only to the number of poultry you wish to keep.

Now, all that is necessary to consider before engaging in the poultry business is, what does the market demand in my neighborhood, or within points I can quickly reach by rail?

Still, as some people will neglect their duties towards their poultry, and some will get cholera, gapes, roup, etc., I will give a few of the best remedies for them, manner of feeding, kinds of food considered best generally, their need of pure water, dust baths, etc. I will reverse the order of naming them and begin with

**Dust Baths, Necessary for Poultry to Keep them Free from Lice.**—Unless you have a fire-place in your poultry house, as in the case reported above, take dry, fine sand, or dry dust from the road, twenty measures (the size of the measure to be governed by the number of hens to be provided for); wood ashes, five measures; and "flowers" (fine) sulphur, one measure, and mix well together and place in large, shallow boxes, or in a corner of the poultry house; at all events, sheltered from rain and snow. They delight to bathe and dust themselves in this, as much as boys delight to bathe and frolic in the creeks of a warm summer day; besides it keeps the lice from troubling the poultry if the house and perches are kept free of them by washes or fumigation. The following is considered one of the best washes for a poultry house, perches, etc.

**Lice in Poultry Houses, the Best Wash to Destroy Them.**—Take 1 lb. of hard soap, sliced thin, and put into an iron kettle with water, 2 qts.; or soft soap and water, each 1 qt., and heat till it boils ; then remove from the fire and stir in kerosene, 1 qt., continuing the stirring until the kerosene is all absorbed into the mixture. This may be poured into a common pail of hot water, stirred well and immediately applied to the perches and every possible crevice about the house where the perches are fastened ; and if enough is made in these proportions, to wash the whole inside of the house and every nest-box (the nest being first taken out and burned, new straw being afterwards put in), it will be all the more certain to make a "clear riddance" of the lice. The composition I take from the *N. Y. Rural* of August 30, 1884, so it may be considered the latest thing out for this purpose ; and it may be noticed, it is much like Prof. Beal's remedy to kill bark lice on fruit trees. I know it will prove "too much" for all lice which it can be made to reach.

2. The following is from the *American Agriculturist*, is quite different from the above, is very thorough in its plan of work, and may therefore suit some people better by the removal of every cleat and everything else from the

poultry house before applying the wash. The carbolic acid is, no doubt, as effectual as the soap and kerosene, and may be used, if preferred, instead of the first above. The item was given in answer to an inquiry by O. Kellogg, of Bradford Co., Pa., whose poultry was infested with lice, and wanted to know how to get rid of them. The editor says :

"Take out of the house every perch, nest-box, or movable thing; remove all battens, cleats, or anything whereby a crevice is made, so that the inside is smooth. Then make a whitewash of fresh lime, into which put one ounce of carbolic acid to a pailful. Wash the house thoroughly with this. Then wash the outside. Then smear the perches with a mixture of lard and kerosene, putting it on thick, so that when the fowls roost they will get some of it on their feathers. Also, put some of it on each fowl, under the wings. This will clear the house, and the hens will clear themselves, if no recruits are furnished from the house.

"In a month, or less, if there is occasion, wash the house again, and grease the roosts ; take care to fill all holes and cracks in the poles. It would be well to pass the poles through a fire made of straw, exposing them to the flame, before greasing them."

**3. Lice on the Poultry, an Ointment or Grease for.**—If there are any lice on the poultry themselves, besides making a clean job of the house by one of the above plans, annoint the necks and heads, if any are to be seen there, and under the wings, around the "vent," and inside the thighs, legs, etc., every place where the feathers are not thick, with lard pretty well thickened with "flowers" (fine) sulphur, one ounce at least to one pound of lard. Sulphur is considered, with grease, to be death to lice, but be this as it may, the lice cannot crawl on the poles nor slats, if they are used as freely as they ought to be, if a good coat of the ointment is smeared over them ; and I can see no reason why some kerosene, say two table-spoonfuls to each pound of lard, may not be added, with the sulphur ointment for the poultry, as well as for the roosts, etc.

If poultry is badly covered with lice, some insect powder may be dusted among the feathers, not much will be needed, using the bellows as used for "bugs" about the bedsteads. At all events, keep the poultry free from lice, else do not keep poultry. If no insect powder is at hand, dust sulphur among the feathers, it will do equally well, at least many claim this to be "all-sufficient." It is recommended in the next item below by the *Iowa State Register.*

**I. To Prevent Lice Upon Setting Hens.**—Which says that two or three leaves of tobacco placed in the nest of a setting hen, then placing the eggs upon them, will kill or drive off any lice which may be upon the hen, and prevent them from getting upon them, which they frequently do while setting, even if not upon them at the commencement ; and

**II.** Sulphur sprinkled among the feathers, when the tobacco cannot be obtained, is good to destroy lice on the fowls, and to keep them at a distance.

**III.** Again, another writer says, to put a table-spoonful of sulphur in the nest of a hen or turkey to be "set," will destroy all lice upon the fowls, and also prevent them from getting into the nest and thus infesting the "setter." This should not be used too freely, lest it may injure the young chicks when they are hatched. Simply greasing the heads of very young chickens will prevent lice from getting upon them. The old nest should always be taken out and burned, and new straw used for each setting. The nest-box should also be always re-whitewashed at each setting.

IV. It is also claimed that hog's hair, used in place of straw for the nest, is never infested with lice. A writer says: "Hen lice won't stay in hog hair." Some writers claim that nine out of every ten hens that die, die from the effects of lice. Then "for heaven's sake," as we often hear said, keep your hens free from lice, else, as we have suggested, do not keep poultry. Whenever you see a hen drooping around, refusing to eat, and the comb looking blue or dark at the points or end, pick her up and look for lice, which, if found, "go for them" at once, as I have directed; clean the house, renew the dust bath, and put all things again in "tip top" order, And remember!

**Water, Clean and Pure—Its Importance Daily for Poultry.—A** writer in the *Fancier's Journal* believes that cholera will seldom trouble poultry if they have a daily supply of pure water, and " that the omission to furnish it is one of the worst forms of cruelty to animals." Another writer says: "Poultry should be as regularly watered as horses, cattle or any of the domestic animals." These statements from those in the business should be taken as the "word for the wise," which "is sufficient." The tonic given below can be occasionally used by putting into their drinking water, as there directed. It is believed to be more needed in winter than summer, unless disease is prevalent among them in the neighborhood. A few words now as to food for poultry, necessity for variety, etc.

I. Food—Several Kinds Necessary for Poultry to do Well.— It has been the custom to feed poultry almost wholly upon corn, summer and winter. But, as in other things, great improvement has been made, and it has been found as necessary to give a variety of food to fowls as it is to persons or other domestic animals if you want them to do their best. Corn, buckwheat, wheat, oats, cooked vegetables of all kinds, meats, cooked and raw, fruit, refuse from the table, raw cabbage in winter, as a substitute for the tender grasses they obtain in summer; and some think it important to cut fine and give them rowen or second growth hay, or dried grass, more correctly speaking in the winter; but the cabbage or other vegetables cooked, as aboved named, may take its place very satisfactorily; but one or the other, or both, at different times for variety's sake, would be better, and sour milk is also claimed to be "one of the best feeds for poultry, especially for young chickens, that can be given them," says the *New York Herald,* "as they thrive wonderfully upon a diet of sour milk, and it may be given them in place of water to great advantage."

II. Corn at night in winter time is especially valuable, from the increased heat or warmth it gives them during the cold months; while the other grains are better in summer for general feeding, sometimes mixed, at other times a feed of one, then the other.

III. **Buckwheat** is especially valuable as a fattener, and is also particularly an egg producer, besides it is well liked by poultry generally.

IV. **Oats** are not a favorite with poultry unless ground and made into dough, no doubt for the reason of its length of kernel, in the sharpness of the ends, making it difficult to swallow.

V. **Fine Gravel,** unless they have easy and near access to it, should always be kept where the poultry can scratch and pick it over, as they will do daily, and eat it in considerable quantities as an aid in cutting their food in the gizzard.

VI. **Charcoal,** broken finely, should also always be given them once or twice a week at all times of the year.

**Raising Chickens, by a City Woman, with Great Success.—** The following was reported through the *Country Gentleman.* The lady says: "I have brought up chickens by hand; had 103 at one time, and never had an insect (lice) on them. I put sulphur under their wings and on the backs of their heads, and once or twice put a pinch in their food, and they were perfectly free from these exhausting pests. Speaking of chickens, I would like to say for the benefit of novices (beginners) in chicken raising, I am one who never had a case of gapes among my chickens; never saw a chicken with the gapes. I think the reason was I never let them run in the damp, and if I saw any tendency to looseness of the bowels, I always put a stiff dose of cayenne pepper in the food every day until they were cured, and out of 109 chickens hatched I only lost four, and those died from accidents—boards fell on them. I never let my young chickens run unheeded in the grass. I fixed up what I called "my yard," with boards propped against sticks driven into the grass; and then I covered over the whole place with mosquito netting to keep the little ones in, and to prevent the old fowls from stealing the young chicken's food. Chickens must be fed every three or four hours at first. [Allow me to say here, not the first day, but after that.] I never feared hawks, for we kept Guinea hens, and never lost a chicken. Many country people have expressed astonishment that I, a city woman, should bring up chickens that never had the gapes. Great care did it. Never let a chicken get its feet wet, and it will never have the gapes. I always had plenty of coal ashes for the little things to roll and pick in; ashes, not cinders. If a number of chickens are in one place (I had about thirty in each place,) the ashes must be changed once a week while they are very young, and every other day as they grow older."

I will mention, for the good of others, I visited a family during the past summer (1884), in a village in Ohio, where the woman was raising about 100 chickens in a space not two rods square. I remarked to her, "you have four times as many chickens in that yard as you ought to have," etc. The cholera got amongst them and she lost a large number of them, not long after.

Many persons in different sections of the country are using some of the incubators, such as we see at the fairs, for hatching and raising chickens. Some use heat from lamps to keep the eggs at about 102 degrees F., and some use the heat produced by fermenting horse manure, for the same purpose ; but before any one goes into either plan extensively, they had better be certain they have not been humbugged or deceived in the information they received about the undertaking. To give proper instructions would require much more space than I can give it, hence this caution. There is no patent on the use of horse manure, nor that I am aware of on the use of lamps, still on some forms of apparatus connected with them, there are patents, I believe.

*Remarks.*—Observe here, care with sulphur prevented lice. Putting a little cayenne in the food if looseness appeared, saved them. Keeping out of wet grass saved from gapes, and cholera too, no doubt. The coal ashes made the dust-bath, and her care in changing the ashes often and keeping only about thirty in one place or yard, as she calls her different enclosures, kept them in a thriving and healthy condition. Notice, too, that Guinea hens are the specific, positive thing against hawks, (see their value also below in gardens, as devourers of bugs and all insects therein.

**Chicken Cholera, Successful Remedies.**—It has become a well-settled fact that if chickens have warm and dry, but well-ventilated houses, of a size to correspond with the number kept, with their dust-baths, are properly fed, and have free access to pure water daily, with ordinary care, they will hardly ever have cholera, or other diseases. Then if it begins, see in which of these points you have failed, and correct it at once. And

I. It has also been found that onions chopped and put into the food once a day for several days, then once a week, and also ground ginger, a little (I should say as freely as they would eat it) in their meal at their next feeding, every day or two will cure cholera; then I claim they will prevent it, if fed occasionally, when it is known to be prevalent in a neighborhood. A writer says: "Raw onions and a very little ginger against the world for curing cholera, if the disease has not been allowed to run too far," and adds, "too much whole corn we have found injurious; it should be in meal, and only given once in three or four days in hot weather

II. Common red pepper, or Cayenne, one tea-spoonful in a quart of milk, or a quart of meal, says Mrs. J. E. Duvall, of Jamestown, Pa., "is the way I cured mine." I know the Cayenne and the ginger are both valuable in cholera, or looseness of the bowels, of persons, why not with these smaller animals? It must so prove. A poultry fancier (one who has a special liking for raising poultry) "cures chicken cholera by feeding, every other day, for two weeks, bran mash, in which he puts a liberal dose of common red pepper. One old biddy," he says, "was determined to die, crouched in an out-of-the-way spot. But I sought her out, gave her a whole pepper, in doses, one hour apart, kept her in a warm place, and she, in a few days, gave me notice she could take care of herself."

III. "Hog's lard," another one claims, "cold, in doses of one level table-spoonful to a fowl, and if not better, repeated in twenty-four hours, is a tried and true remedy, and will cure if anything in creation will cure."

IV. Alum and copperas is also claimed to be a well-tested remedy for chicken cholera, given in the following manner: "At the first symptoms," (drooping and looseness) "dissolve, for each gallon of drinking water, one tea-spoonful of each, and put in; and at the same time give daily, in the soft feed, a little sharp sand at the rate of one tea-spoonful to each fowl. In severe cases, give at once, by hand, mixed in a little dough, a piece of alum and copperas, each the size of a pea, and also mix a tea-spoonful of sand with a little meal and water, for the fowl. Continue the medicated water, and sanded feed, until all signs of the disease disappear."

2. **Chicken Cholera, an "Infallible Remedy."**—A correspondent of the *Blade,* I believe, says:

"I have found a mixture of two ounces, each, of red pepper, alum, resin, and sulphur to be an infallible remedy for this scourge. Last summer I lost more than fifty common fowls from cholera, my Buff Cochins not being affected. I chanced to see the above mixture recommended, and tried it, mixing one table-spoonful in three pints of scalded corn meal, and, though several fowls were in the last stages of the disease, they recovered, and I have not lost a chicken since. In severe cases I would advise giving one-third of a tea-spoonful in a meal-pellet to each fowl every day till well. Put a small lump of alum, say the size of a hickory nut, in their drinking water."

*Remarks.*—This receipt calls for resin (rosin) as one of the ingredients; but from my knowledge of the nature of rosin and copperas, I should much prefer copperas in the place of the rosin, and with the copperas I should have no fears at all. The writer says: "Alum the size of a hickory nut, in their drinking water." This amount, or one tea-spoonful powdered, would be the right quantity for one quart, or enough for one dozen fowls, and then I'd also put in the same of copperas, or, preferably the tonic below, as there directed. If "Cochins" do not take this disease, they are correspondingly more valuable than other breeds.

**VI. Rue for Cholera.**—From the New York *Sun.* It says:

"Get a few cents' worth of garden rue at your nearest druggist's and break up fine and mix with chopped vegetables, meat, and cooked corn meal. Put a pinch of the rue leaves in the food every day, until there are no further signs of the cholera. Every poultry keeper should have a bed of rue in his garden to use whenever it is needed. Five cents' worth of rue seed will produce plants enough for a neighborhood, and they will grow almost anywhere."

*Remarks.*—With this disease, as with every other, in animals, as well as in persons, begin with the remedy you determine upon as the best, or the one you will try, "with the first symptoms," and you will have but little trouble, and less loss.

**Tonic for Poultry.**—The sulphate of iron, copperas, has often been recommended by poultry men as a valuable tonic for fowls of all kinds, especially valuable in the "moulting season," besides occasionally in summer, but more often in cold winter weather. Many formulas, or receipts, have been given for it, but I like the one best given by the *Southern Farmer,* being always ready to use when needed, as it is all given in ones, and will, therefore, be easily remembered, as follows:

"In one one gallon of warm water dissolve one pound of sulphate of iron (copperas) and then add one ounce of sulphuric acid. Put the mixture into a jug, from which it may be used as needed. To one quart of drinking water add one tea-spoonful of the solution It gives the water a rusty appearance and a pungent taste "

*Remarks.*—It is a disinfectant, keeping the drinking vessels free from living bacteria or mites, of living animals, from which it has been recently claimed, that cholera of persons arises. Once a week, or so, then, let more of it be put into the drinking vessels, and scrubbed around with an old broom, then nicely rinsed and turned up to the sun and dried, after the fowls have had their morning drink and gone upon their daily excursion for grasshoppers and other pickings.

1. **Gapes in Poultry.—Cause and Successful Remedies.—** I. **Cause.**—Although this disease is believed to be contagious and epidemic, *i. e.* one catches it from another, and is liable to affect a whole neighborhood, yet it is claimed to originate from foul water, exposures to wet, and a want of nourishing food. Then look out that none of these are allowed, and avoid gapes. The gapes are caused by the presence of worms or maggots in the heart, and trachea, or windpipe, which makes them gape, or, perhaps, more correctly speaking, to gasp for breath.

II. **Remedies.**—Camphor spirits, 1 or 2 tea-spoonfuls to 1 qt. of their drinking water at the commencement may prove all that is needed; but if any become bad, a bit of camphor gum the size of a grain of wheat, for a chick, and of a small pea for an older fowl, put into the throat and retained there until swallowed, is claimed to be a "sure cure." But a tea-spoonful of camphor spirits should also be put into each quart of their drinking water.

III. **Tobacco.**—Smoking them by putting the lot into a box, or boxes, with a pan of live coals in it, upon which sprinkle fine cut tobacco, covering up the box and smoking them till drunk. Says B. L. Scott in the *Blade*, "I will warrant every chicken."

IV. **Salt Butter** has cured bad cases, giving in the morning while they are hungry they will eat it readily. If too sick to eat put some down, the first time, the next morning they will eat it of themselves. Giving two or three times will generally be, sufficient. This, with pepper, is recommended below.

V. **Black Pepper.**— A Mrs. M. D. Bush, of Saline, Mich., informs the Detroit *Post and Tribune:* "Obtaining the grain pepper and grinding it, one tea-spoonful is mixed in a half tea-spoonful of Indian meal with a little water. Open the chicken's mouth, drop in one pill of it per day till cured. One dose will usually cure them, if given when first taken. Have seen no lice at all."

*Remarks.*—Seeing "no lice at all," shows she took good care of her chickens.

Another writer says that two or three grains of ground black pepper in a little fresh butter (it may be fresh made, but I prefer it salted as for table), two or three times a day for a week cures gapes. I have no doubt they will eat it readily, as I know they are fond of the stimulating taste of cayenne; why not then of the black? I believe the cayenne to be the better of the two for this disease. Many writers speak very highly of giving the camphor pills and putting it in their drinking water, one next below of brimstone as a preventive; why should not the use of the tonic, given in cholera above, be also a

preventive of gapes?  I believe it will be if given twice a week in the water
with other proper care.

2.  Gapes in Chickens.—Certain Preventive.—A correspondent
of the Germantown *Telegraph*, who lost 70 chickens the year before now says :
"That fresh water daily with a lump of roll brimstone kept in it will be found
a certain preventive."

*Remarks.*—From my knowledge of the value of sulphur in diphtheria, I
I have great faith in it as a preventive in gapes, as both diseases are supposed
to arise from living parasites in the throat, *and sulphur is death to them.*  I
should prefer, however, to sprinkle in flour of sulphur along the drinking
trough, to ensure a better distribution of it in all the water.   A tea-spoonful
to a quart would be sufficient, and the water stirred before the chickens come
to it.   And if allowed free access to it, I have no doubt, they would pick at
the sulphur and eat considerable of it.   Why not, by the way, mix this
amount of sulphur in a quart of their food, made by wetting up corn and oatmeal ground together, whenever there is gapes about, especially in wet
weather, if they have to be allowed to run out.   I know, from the nature of
it, it will pay.   (See also sulphur in roup, below.)   And this mixed feed twice
a week, is all the corn, or corn-meal poultry ought to have in summer, as corn
or corn-meal alone is too heating a food for warm weather.   Other grains
named previously, with scraps of meat, cooked vegetables, etc., should make
the summer food.   Boiled carrots are especially valuable.

1.  Roup in Poultry—Description of Successful Treatment,
Roup Pills, etc.—I will first give an item from the *London* (Ont.) *Free Press*,
because it gives the description of it, its cause, treatment. and the roup pills,
which can be used in the powder form if preferred, by mixing it in the feed of
corn and oat-meal mash, saving the trouble of catching each fowl and forcing
a pill down its throat.   It says:

"Whenever you have a northeast storm, with damp, chilly, disagreeable
weather, look out for the roup.   Roup is to the fowls what heavy colds are to
human individuals, and as we may have cold in the head, cold in the bowels,
sore throat, and other disturbances from cold, the term ' roup ' covers them all.
Roup in some forms is contagious, while in other shapes it may exist in a flock
without affecting any but those of weak constitutions.   The first thing to do
with the affected fowl is to clean out the nostrils, and every breeder should
have on hand a small syringe, which should be put to use early.   Roup, when
malignant, makes known its presence by a peculiar, disagreeable odor.   The
sick fowl looks dropsy, and a slight pressure on the nostrils causes a discharge,
which is very offensive in smell."

I.  Of Roup Treatment:  "Make a solution of copperas water, and with
the syringe inject some of it into the nostrils, and also down the throat.   [I
would use the tonic, of full strength, for this purpose; having the acid in it
makes it better than without.]   If the bird is no better in a few hours, try a
severer remedy, which is the injection of a mixture of coal oil and carbolic
acid.   Add 10 drops of carbolic acid to 1 table-spoonful of coal oil, and force a
small quantity into each nostril.   This will cure when all other remedies fail.
Night and morning give the roup pills or powder, either in the food or by
forcing it down the throat.   Add some, also, to the food of those that are
well."

II.   Roup Pills—"How to make Roup Pills," the *Free Press* continues, " is what most persons desire to know.   The basis of all roup pills or powders is asafetida.   This is combined with tonics and cathartics.   Here is the method, and by which a large quantity may be made at a small cost.   Take 1 tea-spoonful each of tincture of muriate of iron, red pepper, ginger, saffron, chlorate of potash, salt, and powdered rhubarb ; mix them intimately.   After thoroughly mixing add 3 table-spoonfuls of hypo-sulphate of soda, and mix together well.   Then incorporate this with 1 oz. of asafetida, working it together until the whole is completely mingled, occasionally softening it, when-ever necessary, with castor-oil.   This can be made into pills or dry powder. It is of the same composition as many of the roup pills, which are sold at 50 cents a box."

*Remarks.*—Unless fowls are bad, mixing this in the powder form into the feed will be the least trouble, mixing in enough so each fowl would get what would make a common sized pill.   If the tonic is used to inject a little into the nostrils, as in No. I. above, only a little, say ¼ tea-spoonful would be enough to inject into the throats at one time ; and it might do if reduced half with water.   The mouth, throat, eyes and nostrils, if much stuck up with the dis-charge, should be washed out clean with warm water, then sponged with the reduced tonic water, just above named, and for the eyes it might be reduced with two or three times as much water as of the tonic.   I should prefer this to the carbolic acid and kerosene, or coal oil.   The following with sulphur, or the next one after, with aconite, may be preferred.

**2.   Cure for Roup, with Sulphur.**—An agricultural writer says : "Last fall I had two roosters affected; the first one was almost choked to death when I found him, a hard, cheesy substance having formed in the wind-pipe.   I had saved the lives of others by taking it out with the point of a scissors.   In this case I took a piece of writing paper, made a funnel the size of a child's finger, opened the beak and another person blew a half tea-spoonful of sulphur down his throat.   We put him out, I supposed, to die, but he did not, and after the third dose he could crow as loudly as ever."

*Remarks.*—Sulphur has cured hundreds of cases of diphtheria of children, why not cure roup in fowls?   It undoubtedly did, and will, again.

**3.   Roup—Cure with Aconite, from the Canada Poultry Chronicle.**   The *Chronicle* says:

"When the fowl is attacked with the characteristic cough of this malady, or has tenacious mucus about the beak with difficulty of breathing, I place it in a wicker coop, in a quiet shed, and put before it a drinking fountain con-taining about a gill (4 ozs.) of water, with which I have mixed one drop of tincture of aconite.   In every instance during three years, this treatment has had an effect almost marvelous; for upon visiting the patient an hour or two afterwards, I have found that the symptoms have vanished.   The attack for a day or two is liable to return, yet each time in a lighter form, but, continuing the aconite water has in no instance with us failed completely to remove the ailment in about forty-eight hours."

*Remarks.*—If so bad when found, that they will not drink, pour a tea-spoon-ful of the aconite water down the throat, occasionally, once in an hour or two, until they can drink it.

**Scabby Legs of Poultry.**—Mix equal parts of lard and kerosene oil into a paste, with sulphur, and rub upon the legs daily until the scabs come off ; then rub on a little sweet oil, or a little lard or fresh butter will do as well.

**Egg-Eating Hens—Simple, but Certain Remedy For.**—Make an opening into the large end of an egg and let out the contents, beat it up and mix into it enough strong mustard to re-fill it, and paste on a bit of cloth to keep it in : then place it where the egg-eaters can see and get at it. They will " go for it " at once, and as quickly go away. It is too much for them. And as they take it for granted that all eggs are alike, they give up the habit. I cannot see why it would not be as good for egg-eating dogs as for hens.

**POULTRY.—The Average of Different Breeds as Layers.— Table, with Remarks upon Best Setters and Mothers, Winter Layers, etc.**—Experiments have shown the following to be about the average laying capacity of the different breeds, yearly, and the weight of eggs to the pound :

| BREEDS. | No. Eggs per lb. | No. Per Year. | BREEDS. | No. Eggs per lb. | No. Per Year. |
|---|---|---|---|---|---|
| Light Brahmas and Partridge Cochins. | 7 | 130 | Creve Cœurs | 8 | 140 |
| | | | Black Spanish | 7 | 140 |
| Dark Brahmas | 8 | 130 | Leghorns | 8 | 160 |
| Black, White and Buff Cochins | 7 | 115 | Hamburghs | 9 | 150 |
| | | | Polish | 9 | 125 |
| Plymouth Rocks | 8 | 150 | Dominiques | 9 | 135 |
| Houdans | 8 | 150 | Games | 9 | 130 |
| La Fleche | 7 | 150 | Bantams | 16 | 90 |

*Remarks.*—Thus it is seen that the Leghorns average more eggs generally than any other breed, but in our cold northern winters their combs and wattles freeze unless they have a warm house and good care. They sometimes do better than the above average given—remember than the table refers only to a general average. But I see a report in the *Blade*, from J. Bechtol, Polk City, Iowa, stating that he had bought a " rooster and a pullet of the Leghorns, she beginning to lay February 28, 1882, and up to July 30—153 days—he had 146 eggs, kept in a yard twenty by forty feet only."

Next to them come the Plymouth Rocks, Houdans, and the Hamburgs. While I was stopping in Eaton Rapids, Mich., for some weeks, two or three years ago, I saw a gentleman receiving at the express office, a number of Speckled Hamburgs, and in talking with him I found he had proved them excellent layers. They are quite a hardy breed, too. One writer speaks of the old " Bolton Grays" as being much like the Silver Pencilled Hamburgs, but beating them as layers, quite often producing 200 eggs a year. Thus, aside from the old Bolton Grays, which may not now be obtainable, this writer, J. G. McKeon, of Acworth, N. H., to the Boston *Cultivator*, says that " in his experience no variety of fowls equal the Hamburgs as layers, being small eaters, and wonderfully prolific, but on account of their small size, not

recommended for their flesh." The Plymouth Rocks and Brahmas are especially recommended as winter layers ; but it is also claimed that well-lighted
and warm quarters, with a variety of food, corn at night, a hot or warm mush
made of the mixed meal, or best ground feed for hens, with cooked potatoes
and cooked carrots in the morning, are especially valuable as egg-producing
food, with chopped meat at least once a week, and vegetables mixed with the
mixed meal, or oatmeal, made up as the "boarding-house hash," the noon feed
to be of mixed grains, is excellent as a winter plan of feeding when eggs in
large quantities are expected. I would add to the "hash" once or twice a
week, a tea-spoonful of powdered Cayenne to every quart of the mixture,
when, with all this care, I guarantee a "fair show" of eggs all winter. It
will be noted in the first item given under the head of poultry that of the large
breeds Mr. Leland considers, for general purposes, none will be found superior
to the Brahmas. The Buff Cochins, it is thought, make the best setters and
mothers, of all the others. Let people, then, supply themselves with the
breed that is best for what they wish to do—for eggs, the best layers ; for
chickens to sell, some of the large breeds that mature the quickest, etc., and
give care accordingly.

I will give, however, the following item from the *New England Farmer*,
upon the question of the best breed for farmers and families of the villages
who only desire to keep one kind, for home use, home sales, etc.; although I
think them equally valuable for shipping, if any one should desire at any time
to do so. This item will also confirm, in its statements, several observations
made in other places upon this subject.

**Best Breed of Fowls for Farmers and Families in Towns.—**
One breed is enough for the farm, or for villagers, keeping only for home use.
What is wanted is a good sized hen, a good layer, a good mother, a non-setter,
(not inclined or determined to set,) and a fine table fowl, which the Plymouth
Rocks are conceded to combine in a greater degree than any others. The
White Leghorns will beat them in the number of eggs ; and the Cochins and
Brahmas as a table fowl exclusively; but the last named being great consum-
ers of food, lose their prestige, or superiority. But let it be remembered,
whether on the farm, or in the village, it is care and attention to cleanliness,
food, and all other details of management which give their proper returns in
eggs and merit.

**Best Ground Feed for Hens.**—Cornmeal, oatmeal and middlings,
each 50 lbs., bran, 10 lbs., bone meal, 3 ozs., cayenne, 1 oz.; mix evenly
together for use,

*Directions.*—If you can afford it, put milk on the fire till it wheys, and is
scalding hot, if no milk, water, the same; add 1 tea-spoonful of salt for a
dozen fowls, and stir in of the mixed meal, to make a stiff batter, and bake
four hours. Crumble to feed. This meal can be fed dry, or as any other meal,
for much feeding; and if you have no milk to spare, it makes a feed nearly
equal, to boil meat scraps to a soup, adding potato parings and other vegetables, as for a common soup, then thickening with the meal and baking as
mentioned, for at least one feed daily.—*Poultry Journal.*

**Poultry Maxims, or Short Statements of Important Facts.—**

1.　Give hens constant access to lime, of which to make shells, and always give them access to gravel.

2.　A fresh egg has a lime-like surface, old ones become glossy and smooth.

3.　Charcoal in pieces the size of a pea, or burned corn once a week is valuable for all poultry.

4.　If eggs are expected, give a warm feed every morning of mashed vegetables so moist as to allow thickening with middlings, or corn, oats, wheat, and buckwheat ground together in equal quantities; buckwheat alone, or the mixed small grains, buckwheat being one of them, for the noon feed, and cracked corn, or whole kernels at night.　Once a week putting a tea-spoonful of cayenne into the morning feed, for 1 dozen fowls, and once a week, black pepper, twice as much, in its place, which not only increases the production of eggs, but wards off disease.

5.　Meat, chopped, and fed once a week induces laying, and poultry, young or old, are very fond of warm dish-water in winter, with a little corn meal, or mixed meal in it; and are also very fond of oatmeal gruel; and all the better if it can be made of milk, or at least half milk. It promotes warmth and makes flesh; but better with water only, than none.

6.　Wheat, oats, and barley boiled together, promotes laying, or either two of them; buckwheat is good with them, but does not want boiling more than half as long.

7.　Feed only what will be eaten up clean and at once, else they become too fat and quit laying; while in summer, any of the mixed or mashed feeds not eaten up, soon sours, and invites disease.

8.　Fine gravel, or coarse sawdust are as essential to the thriving of poultry as good and varied food.　They will not keep healthy without them.

9.　Early chickens must be fed by lamp-light at night, if expected to mature quickly.　They will soon learn to enjoy it; and four times by daylight, the last of these at early dark, the final at bed-time, if for an early market.

10.　Pullets generally begin to lay eggs in about eight months from hatching; then those hatched in March or April, if properly cared for, will be the more certain to make excellent winter layers.

11.　Gather eggs twice daily in summer, and three times in winter.

**Young Chickens—Best Food For—How Often to Feed, Etc.—** The following well-written and sensible instructions are from "Fanny Field," in the *Ohio Farmer*. She says:

"The first meal, which should not be given until the chicks are at least twelve hours old, is hard-boiled egg, crumbled fine, or stale wheat bread crumbs, moistened with milk.　We make it a rule to feed nothing the first week except the egg, bread crumbs and curds.　When a week old we begin on cooked oat meal, boiled potatoes, cooked rice, etc.　Cooked corn meal may be fed the second week, but we think they do better without any corn meal until the third or fourth week; then we give almost any cooked food, adding a little cooked meat when the egg is dropped from the bill of fare, unless insects are plenty. As soon as they are old enough to swallow the grains, give cracked corn, cracked oats, wheat, etc., at night. Two or three times a week mix a little bone meal with the feed—a table-spoonful to 1 pt. of feed. Season the food slightly with salt and pepper. Give milk to drink if you can get it. Feed often—five or six times a day. Feed all they will eat up clean, but do not leave any food around to sour. Sour, sloppy food is responsible for a good deal of mortality among the infant chicken population."

*Remarks.*—The "bone meal" referred to here is undoubtedly good; and if it cannot be obtained at the stores, which has been finely ground and put up for sale, the best substitute is to burn bones till white, then pound and pulverize them in an iron mortar as finely as practicable, will do very well, and is especially important until the chickens are allowed to take the range of the fields.

### Fattening Poultry for Market—Best Food for, Etc.—American, French and English Plans, Etc.

—"No fowl," says the *American Agriculturist,* "over two years old, should be kept in the poultry yard, except it be an extra good mother or a finely-feathered bird, desirable for breeding—such may be kept till 10 years old, or as long as useful. All other hens or roosters should be fattened for market at the end of the second year." They should be confined in a room or shed that can be closed and made quite dark, if you wish the greatest speed in fattening; the floor to be covered with two or three inches of sifted coal ashes, dry sand, dry earth, or dry straw; best in the order named. The food should be given four times a day, and pure water always before them.

1. The Americans think buckwheat meal, mixed with skimmed milk into a thick mush, with a tea-spoonful of salt to enough for 1 doz. fowls, is the best food for fattening; and that two weeks should do it, if the room is dark and cool. Then ship at once to market.

2. The French claim that no meal for fattening should be made from grain less than one year old, and that the water used in mixing should have suet added to it, at the rate of ¾ oz. to each 2 qts. of meal; and a small quantity of coarse gravel also added to aid the digestion; and no food to be given within twelve hours of the time the fowl is to be killed. They also feed largely of the Belgian yellow carrot, boiled or stewed, and mashed, claiming a very rich and peculiar flavor is imparted to the flesh by its use. All carrots that I ever saw are yellow, but the Belgian may be peculiarly so, and may be richer in flavor than our common kinds, still I think they will "fill the bill."

3. The English have a great liking for the flesh of the Dorking fowls, and prepare them for the London market by shutting up in a dark room, the same as the Americans and French do; but they feed a mixture of suet, 1 lb., chopped fine; sugar, ½ lb. with each 4 lbs. of meal; and give milk as their drink five or six times daily, and claim a gain of 2 lbs. a week; and with young turkeys, that even 3 lbs. a week is often gained. Thus turkeys might be brought up to about 40 lbs. for the New York market, where, of this weight at Christmas time, I see some of the papers claim they are worth $1 a pound. Bear in mind, however, that in all cases their droppings must be often removed

and the floor covering also renewed if the same room is continuously used. Best to rake over the floor covering daily.

**Dressing Poultry for the Market, the Best Way.**—There are two ways of dressing poultry for market—dry picked and scalded. Fowls dressed in the former way in all cases bring the highest prices. It should be the aim of every farmer, in disposing of his poultry, to ship it in as good condition as possible, in order to catch the eye of the butcher or grocer, and secure a ready sale. Greater skill is required to dry-pick than most people imagine, in order that the "bird" may look plump and handsome. To do this work properly, or with any degree of satisfaction, the fowls should be plucked when warm—that is, immediately after they are killed—as, if allowed to get cold before stripping, you are apt to tear the flesh. Commence by plucking the wing and tail feathers, then the back, from head to tail. Pluck the feathers from the "craw" crossways; stomach and breast feathers should be plucked downward—that is, from the legs to the head. In dressing poultry by this method you get a double advantage of those dressed by the hot-water process, as you can save all the feathers, being careful to keep separate all the tail and wing feathers; and where many are dressed, the sale of feathers amounts to quite an item of profit. Dressing poultry by the scalding process is by no means a good and profitable one, as it depreciates the value of the birds, they looking anything but dainty, and do what you will, they will never look enticing to the buyer; moreover, you lose the value of the feathers.

*Remarks.*—Allow me to say here, I think it best to wait long enough after killing, to allow the fowl to become a little cooled, as if the feathers are plucked too soon, as anyone can tell by trying, there will be a little blood settle into the orifices, from which the feathers are pulled, and thus make them a little spotted, if done too soon. This is of importance to observe. If they are killed as the French do it, they having a knife much like a screw-driver, the end being the sharpest, the legs held by another person, the mouth opened, the fowl being on its back, the knife is put just back of the "roof of the mouth," and pressed in to separate the vertebræ, or bones of the neck, which kills them quickly; and then hang up by the legs till done bleeding, the feathers may then be removed at once; and this hanging up by the legs, to bleed, should be done, if the head is cut off in the old way. The fowl keep better for being hung up to bleed; but, if the head is cut off, the skin must be pulled over the bone of the neck and tied, and all blood carefully removed from every part of the fowl, before packing. The entrails are never to be removed, unless so understood before shipping.

**Packing Poultry for Market.**—If poultry is killed in cold weather, for market, it ought to hang twenty-four hours before packing, to allow all animal heat to pass off, and thus prevent its spoiling; then pack in clean rye straw, if obtainable, but any straw, free from chaff and powdery dust, will do. First an inch of straw, at least, and the fowls placed in with straw between each, so they do not touch each other, then straw again; the top of the box, or barrel, so filled with straw that there shall be no shaking or jostling about. Mark plainly, to whom addressed, the number of chickens, and the weight of them; and also your own name on the package, to show you are not ashamed of your work, and to help the commission man to keep each lot by themselves, for they will soon learn who does his work the best.

**Guinea Fowl, Their Value to Keep Away Hawks, and Bugs from Garden Vines.**—Although the noise of these pretty animals is quite annoying to most people, yet, as this very noise scares off the hawks, they should be kept by all who raise many chickens; and also for the reason that they do not scratch the garden like our common chickens, but "go for the bugs," on all garden vines, without injuring the most delicate plants; hence it would be well to keep a few on every farm.

# AGRICULTURAL.

**The Successful Farmer.—What he Does, and What he Does Not,—Applicable to all Business Men.**—The successful farmer does nothing but farm. He invests his money as fast as made in a way to improve the farm. He informs himself by magazines, farm journals and books, as to his business, so he can do his work intelligently. Upon such farms no weeds are allowed to mature their seeds after the wheat or other crop is off; and no weeds in fence corners, nor other places, stand as high as a man's head; nor are fences, nor buildings neglected or dilapidated; no implements are left exposed to the weather, nor stock unsheltered and uncared for; but everything is attended to at the right time; and the consequences are natural and sure. Enterprise and thrift show themselves in everything.

*Remarks.*—A whole volume in but few words. Let every business man adopt the same rules, and he will be alike sure of success.

**Hay, Time to Cut.**—There is scarcely a subject of greater importance to the agriculturalist, than the proper time to cut hay, so it shall contain to the fullest extent its nourishing, or flesh-making, properties; and experiments in the United States, as well as in England, France and Germany go to show, most decidedly, that that time is: As soon as possible after the blossoming and setting of the seed, whether it be timothy or clover.

A writer in the *Prairie Farmer* says: "Do not wait for the grass, or the clover to get ripe before you cut it for hay. Any of the meadow grasses are in their prime for hay, so far as nourishment is concerned, just as soon as they are out of bloom."

Dr. Sturtevant, in the *Country Gentleman*, says: "According to the talk of Wolff, red clover hay, cut in full blossom, contains 13.4 per cent. of albuminoids (nourishment), and when ripe, only 9.4, or a loss of 80 pounds to each ton," and this he goes on to show amounts, in the New England States alone, to 5,000,000 tons difference in its nourishment.

Dr. Arnold says: "Dried grass is worth as much as cornmeal, pound for pound, while after grass has blossomed and is made into what is called hay, it is not worth half as much as cornmeal to feed out."

*Remarks.*—As these points are considered by most writers upon this subject to be the facts, nothing further need be said to induce sensible farmers to do this when possible considering other work; I will, however, give a word from a writer in the Germantown *Telegraph*, who says: "The greatest losses of farmers come from late cut hay, cold stables, and, consequently, poor stock." A word to the wise is sufficient.

# AGRICULTURAL. 773

**Manuring—Its Advantages Shown in the John Johnston Farm.**—The editor of the *Country Gentleman* gives the following account of a visit to this farm at Geneva, N. Y. And as I believe it to be applicable, generally, in all sections of our country, and of such great importance, I give it a place. He says:

"Mr. Johnston came to Geneva from Scotland, fifty-two years ago, with little capital, comparatively; but having much of the economy, energy and thrift necessary to enable any one to succeed in a comparatively new country. He is now, at the age of eighty-four, a hearty, vigorous farmer, able to oversee his farm and farm hands, and apparently as capable of directing and conducting all the operations necessary to make a farm pay, as at any time during his long life.

"On being asked where lay the secret of his success, replied, 'manure, sir, manure, and plenty of it.' The main object in his farming has always been to make all the yard manure possible; and by its free use he brought his wheat, which was then the staple crop in western New York, from 12 or 15 bushels per acre to 30, and became celebrated as a farmer who would be sure to have a crop sufficient to meet all obligations.

"After some years he purchased fifty acres adjoining his original farm, the owner of which said that manure would do no good on the land. In the barnyard there was three years' manure accumulated, which Mr. Johnston obtained with the farm. He paid $1,500 for the fifty acres, most of which he borrowed, 'but,' said he, 'that manure paid every cent for the farm.'"

*Remarks.*—If Mr. Johnston could double, or more than double, his crop, by the use of manure, other farmers can do the same. The object of this report is to induce them to do it. And until sufficient "yard manure" can be made by keeping more stock, a judicious use of some of the " fertilizers," or "phosphates," as the manufactured articles are called, or lime, or a mixture of lime, ashes, plaster, salt, and hen manure will be used. These were not known in Mr. Johnston's days as they are of later years.

**Salt, Its Uses as a Manure.**—A correspondent of the *Country Gentleman* says his experience in the use of salt in agriculture leads him to the following conclusions:

"It keeps the land cool and moist. It neutralizes drouth. It exterminates all soil vermin. It prevents potato rot. It glazes and stiffens straw, preventing crinkling and rust. It keeps the ground in such condition that the berry of many kinds of grain fills plumply, however long-continued the hot and dry weather may be."

*Remarks.*—Unleached ashes, probably " stiffens straw" more than salt does, especially if grain falls from over-manuring with stable manure.

2. **Salt as a Manure, Amount per Acre for Different Crops.** —The French and German agriculturists recommend, salt per acre, for clover, 150 lbs.; for wheat or flax, 250 ; and for barley and potatoes, 300 lbs., to be sown broadcast early in the season.

3. **Ashes, Lime, and Salt for Wheat.**—A Wisconsin wheat grower makes an important point on the use of ashes and lime and salt as a manure for wheat. He plowed up sod and sowed twelve bushels of unleached ashes, mixed with ten bushels of air-slacked lime, to three acres, before the wheat was sown, and when the wheat was up a little, he sowed on also one barrel of

salt, which gave him twenty bushels to the acre of plump, fine berry, weighing 62 lbs. to the bushel, while another acre of the same field, without these gave him only ten to the acre. Such facts as these tell the whole story. Go and do the same.

**Wheat-Growing Maxims, or, "Much in Little."**—A maxim being a condensation of a well-established fact, somebody has taken the labor of condensing several facts into short maxims upon the subject of raising wheat, and although they have got "into print" without credit to the originator, still as they contain so much of real value in so few words, I deem it best to give them a place :

I.   The best soil for wheat is a rich clay loam.

II.   Wheat likes a good, deep, soft bed.

III.   Clover turned under makes just such a bed.

IV.   The best seed is plump, heavy, oily and clean.

V.   About two inches is the best depth for sowing the seed.

VI.   The drill puts in the seed better and cheaper than broadcasting.

VII.   From the middle of September to the last of October is the best time for sowing.

VIII.   If drilled, one bush. of seed per acre ; if broadcasted, two bush.

IX.   One heavy rolling after sowing does much good.

X.   For flour, cut when the grain begins to harden ; for seed, not until it is hardened.

**Corn. Raising for Soiling, Winter and Spring Feeding.**—In answer to inquiries in the Detroit *Tribune* as to raising corn-fodder, J. E. Estes, of Commerce, Mich., gave his plan from ten years' experience. He says :

"I plow my ground early in spring ; keep it well cultivated until the first or middle of June, then I mark out with a marker thirty inches wide, sow with a one-horse drill four bushels per acre, keep well cultivated. It will soon cover the ground. Cut when the juice is sweet in the joints, with a common corn knife ; put in large stocks and let it stand until cold weather, then draw as you want it to use. In this way it will cure green and nice. I have raised from three to five acres for the last twelve years with good success."

*Remarks.*—All, so far as I know, agree that drilling is the best plan, especially so if it is probable that weeds will be troublesome ; then, by frequent cultivation they will be kept down ; but all do not agree as to the amount of seed per acre. In Western New York one claims that two bushels produce stalks nearer the right size than any other amount of seed—the thicker it stands the smaller the stalk. Ten acres of corn, no doubt, are now sown for fodder where one was ten years ago.

**2. Corn For Summer, Fall, and Winter Feeding—Time to Sow, Etc.**—For soiling in early summer, sow as early as the middle of May, in fair seasons. For later summer and fall feeding sow every two or three weeks after the first. For winter, sowing from the middle to the last of June is considered the best time for sowing. In all cases of drilling, keeping well cultivated is of the utmost importance ; and as soon as the ends of the leaves begin to get dry it is thought to be the best time to cut it, the juices then being just fully matured, the fodder gives the greatest amount of animal heat when fed. If drilled, cut with a common corn-cutter; if broadcast, cut with a cradle or self-raking reaper. Let lay until wilted and a little dry; then bind into moderate sized bundles and put about a dozen into a "stock" or "shock," binding the top securely to shed the rain and to keep standing until perfectly dry. And if drawn in at all, unless it is perfectly dry, it must not be stored too thick, as it gathers dampness and molds without these precautions, except in cold winter weather. The soil for this purpose, if not rich in itself, ought to be made so, as well as for rye.

**3. Corn Cut in the Blossom Better than Hay for Milch Cows.**—An Illinois dairyman, name not given, claims that "corn cut when in blossom, bound and set up till cured, is better for milch cows than the best hay." Certainly several tons of it can be raised where one of hay can be—then "go for it."

**4. Rye—Its Value for Fall and Spring—Green Feeding.**—Those who need fall and spring green feed for stock should not fail to take a piece of their best land, and if not naturally rich, make it so with barn-yard manure or good fertilizers, then plow and make fine with the harrow, and have it ready by the last of August or early in September, and sow to rye. This will give fall feed; and what is not cut till spring will grow up again, and give two or three more cuttings, according to the season. It is strange that more rye is not sown for this purpose, for it is wonderful what an amount of feed it will furnish upon good, rich soil.

**1. Sweet Potatoes, Fruits, Seed Corn, Etc., to Keep for Months, Even in the South.**—A correspondent of the *Southern Cultivator* writes that after testing every plan given for preventing decay in fruits without success, had adopted the following with entire success He says:

"Take good, perfect sand, free it from trash, etc., by sieving it. Put it in a large metallic vessel—I use large syrup boilers—mixing flour of sulphur through the whole, enough to fumigate it well, then heat to a temperature that will volatilize the sulphur. After maintaining this heat till the sand is dry, let the mass cool to a moderate warmth, and putting your sweet corn—or other grain difficult to keep—into barrels or boxes, pour the sand in, filling the same well, and packing down closely. In heating the sand, the vessel should be covered to retain as much as possible the sulphurous fumes. I put in the corn, stripped of the shuck, and thus the sand sieves well through the barrel. This certainly balks the wevils, and even rats do not burrow in it. It is applicable to any grain--even seed wheat, so difficult to preserve in this latitude. This sand keeps perfectly all such fruits as oranges, apples and lemons, putting them away in shallow boxes in a cool place. I've kept these fruits for months, perfect and plump, when if exposed to atmospheric heat and moisture they would have decayed in a few days."

*Remarks.*—This gentleman does not speak of sweet potatoes, but I know the dry sulphurous sand will do it, as well as other kinds of fruit, hence I have named them in my heading. I think, however, that apples should pass through what is called "a sweating," by laying two or three weeks about three feet thick on a barn floor before putting up for the next season's use, or before shipping on sea voyages. The same with sweet potatoes before putting into the sulphured sand. I have not a doubt, either, but what with a little extra care in packing and getting the sand well among them, and covering the boxes nicely, grapes may be kept in the same way for spring use. In our northern country, what he calls a "cool place," must not be such as to freeze in winter. Still,

2. **The True Secret of Keeping Fruit** over winter is, to keep it as near the freezing point as possible, not to freeze; say at 34° or 35°, which is 2 or 3 above freezing. But a few degrees above this, never above 50°, and always below 40°, is better; but to do this ice house arrangements must be made to suit one's conveniences, and amounts to be put up; the best plans for which all are now supposed to understand. With ice-houses the sand packing is not necessary; and for small amounts the "poor woman's", plan, next below, will be all sufficient.

3. **Keeping Sweet Potatoes over Winter in the Living Room.** —"A poor woman," says one of the editors of a northern paper, "just told us how she keeps her sweet potatoes over winter, as follows : When dug and properly dry for packing, she obtains dry sand, with which the bottoms of kegs or boxes are covered. Then a layer of sweet potatoes is put in, not touching each other; then sand, and so on. They are kept in the living room, raised two inches from the floor."

*Remarks.*—The only secrets seem to be dry sand and raising the boxes from the floor by means of strips of plank, to allow air under, as well as around them. Then, why not in any room or cellar that does not freeze ? They will do as well, at the same time being more out of the way. There is not a doubt, however, that the sulphur heated among the sand, in drying as above, is a very valuable addition.

4. **Sweet Potatoes. How to Grow and to Keep.**—It has been considered heretofore that sweet potatoes could only be grown upon sandy soil and in ridges ; but the *Ohio Farmer* informs its readers that they have grown 160 bushels to the acre of good, merchantable sweet potatoes upon thin clay soil, by a shallow cultivation, applying only ten good two-horse loads of manure, worked in with a cultivator after the shallow ploughing, and then planting in hills made on the ridges—the ridges three feet apart and the hills three feet from each other. He cultivated several times after plowing before planting, and made the hills high, so as to brush off three or four inches at the planting, to set the plants in fresh earth—only one plant to each hill. The hills are made small, to allow the sun to keep the hill warmer than if made large, and the shallow cultivation is to keep the potatoes nearer the surface than if ploughed deep. The idea of only one plant in a hill is to obtain larger potatoes than if two or more were allowed, on the same principle that not more than two stalks should be allowed to stand in a hill of common or "Irish" potatoes, as recommended below

**To Keep Well,** he dried them by spreading upon boards a few days in the sun as you would apples. [The great apple raiser, Pell, on the Hudson, who ships largely to England, "sweats" his apples two or three days, in his apple house, three feet thick, then takes to an upper room and spreads out to dry before packing.] Whether this would do as well for sweet potatoes I am not certain. Test, only, can settle that. There must be no bruising of either, if expected to keep long.

I. **POTATO CULTIVATION.—Soil Needed, Seed to Select, etc.—**I. SOIL NEEDED.—Perhaps no plant appreciates a good, rich soil more nor pays for it better, than the "Irish," or common potato. Then take your best soil and make it as rich as you can, if not already so.

II. SELECTING THE SEED.—Although in the United States it is generally understood that the "crown," or seed end eyes, are the best, yet there has been a controversy in England upon the subject of seed, some claiming for a number of years, that the stem end only should be planted ; and that these furnished a larger, and consequently a better potato. I think I can explain this difference of opinion readily, although I have but little experience in raising them. It is well known that the eyes on the seed end are much more numerous than on the stem end. It has been the custom generally, until recently, and is still the custom except by a few, to cut off the seed end and to put two or even three of these pieces to each hill. This, of course, gives a large number of stalks to each hill, while the stem end, having not half as many eyes, has only had two or three pieces to the hill, the stalk, of course, being equally less in number. And now, of late years, a few persons have found out that the hill of potatoes with only two or three stalks gives a larger, and consequently a better potato than the hills having many stalks. Therefore, the stem end men have got the largest and best potatoes, because they have less stalks in the hills, as they have less eyes. The author is willing to stand or fall by a fair test of this opinion.

III. **Potatoes. How Many to the Hill, Etc.—**It is claimed, of late years, by those who have tested it, that large potatoes only, should be selected for seed, and that only one eye should be kept on each piece, and only two pieces for a hill, if you want large marketable potatoes. Henry Ives, of Genesee Co., N. Y., says : "That cut seed from large potatoes yield 8 to 10 per cent. better than small ones planted whole." Another writer says : "You always find your largest potatoes when there is only one large vine." A writer in the *American Cultivator* reports he has thinned his potato vines, when they exceed this number, to two in a hill, and that his father did the same for fifty years before him. Pulling up the weaker ones as he would weeds from the hill." A writer in the *Indiana Farmer* says : "One great secret in potato cultivation, is, not to have too many eyes in one piece, and cut large ones for seed."

*Remarks.*—DIFFERENCES OF OPINION BALANCED BY COMMON SENSE.— The author has observed for over fifty years, being at this writing November 1884, nearly 68 years old, that in almost every attempted improvement, the experimenters go from one extreme to the other; then, as it used to be the custom to put 2 or 3 pieces of the seed-end of potatoes into a hill which would have from, perhaps, 4 to 6 eyes to a piece, they now come down to two pieces only, with only one eye to a piece. Now let common sense come in and make it 3 to 5 eyes, or stalks, to stand in each hill, and I will guarantee, all things being equal, as to richness of soil, proper cultivation, etc., the best results will be obtained. I have seen the statement of a writer, that one stalk of corn only to a hill, would give more corn to the acre than a larger number; but I say that soil that will not nourish three or four stalks to the hill is not as rich as it ought to be, and can be made. The same will hold good also, with potatoes.

2. "Hilling," or Level Cultivation, Which?—It is equally a conceded fact, of late years, that land which is fit for potatoes, at all, that is, dry, rich soil, it is best to cultivate without hilling, which allows the rainfall to settle about the roots and ensures also, larger and better potatoes than when "hilled up," which certainly turns the water away; as water has always run down hill, and no doubt, will still continue to do the same.

*Remarks.*—The "successful farmer" that we started this department with, only needs to see a point, when his common sense at once adopts it. The foregoing condensed facts are all he needs upon the subject referred to.

1. Potato Bugs Beaten.—A farmer of Goguac Prairie, near Battle Creek, Mich., gives to the *Inter-Ocean*, his plan of not only beating the potato bugs, but also getting remarkably fine and large potatoes, 1st by harrowing his ground to make the surface very loose and fine, then 2d, marking off, and dropping his potatoes on the surface, putting no dirt over them, but covering with straw, to the depth of a foot, which retains the moisture in the soil, and so far beats the bugs, that what few may get on to them above the straw, have never injured them, and the next best thing is, he gets large and clean potatoes by simply pitching over the straw and picking up the crop, besides saving the time otherwise spent in cultivation. Those having straw will do well to try it.

2. Bugs Kept Entirely from Potatoes. Another man, of Janesville, Wis., who had ten years' experience in Colorado, from which the "bug" started, claims entire success over them, by simply planting two or three flaxseeds in each hill, the bugs not attacking his potatoes at all, while his neighbors without the flax, were overrun with them. If as simple a thing as this will "beat the bugs," 'tis better than Paris green or hand-gathering. Certainly ten years was long enough to test it.

Seed Corn, Melons, Cucumbers, etc.—Selecting and Saving to Have the Best Results.—To have the best seed corn, go through the field and select and mark with red chalk the long, well-filled ears, and as soon as the husks begin to turn, gather them, and braid into traces and hang in a dry cool place. When to be planted break off the tip one-fourth the length of the ear, and throw among the corn for feed; the same with two or three rows of the ill-shaped kernels at the butt; for it is a well established fact that the corn from the butt ripens earlier than from the tip-end of the ear. What has been many times proved need not be done again, unless it be for one's own satisfaction. Take all the advantage possible in selecting wheat, or other grain, to use the plumpest and heaviest berries; and it would also be well to save that for seed from parts of the field that ripen the earliest, to get the best results.

II. Melon, Squashes, Cucumbers, Beans, Peas, and all seeds possible, should be kept in the pulp or shell till wanted for sowing, whenever possible. Select the earliest, full, medium sized melons, cucumbers, etc., growing three or four feet from the hill, and put stakes by them before you begin to pick for use or market. Let them ripen and rot down upon the vines; then put a piece of board under each one, mashing down to break the rind, so the juice will dry out; and when dry, cut off from the vine, and also cut off one-fourth of the blow-end and throw it away. When properly dry, put away in the pulp till wanted for planting. Seed thus kept sprouts quicker and is more vigorous in growth, and using only the stem-end seeds, insures an earlier ripening, the same as with corn, which has been well-proved many times. Even garden seeds are better when the stalks are nicely dry to put paper around them, to save scattering seeds and allow them to remain in the plant till wanted to sow or plant, as above. Of course all seeds must be secured from the ravages of their lovers, rats and mice.

**Weight, Pounds per Bushel of Grain, and Most Articles in Common Use.**—Shelled corn, 56 lbs.; corn in the ear, 70; wheat, 60; buckwheat, 52; rye, 56; oats, 32; barley, 48; onions, 57; potatoes, Irish, 60; sweet, 55; turnips, 55; beans, white, 60; castor, 46; clover seed, 60; timothy seed, 45; flax seed, 56; hemp seed, 44; dried peaches, 33; dried apples, 24 ; salt, coarse, 50; fine, 55; corn meal, 48; bran, 20; plastering hair, dry, 8; lime, "quick," *i. e.* unslacked, 80; stone coal, 80.

**Fruit Trees, Right Soil For, How to Plant.**—I. THE SOIL.— If the soil where an orchard is designed to be set out is not rich, it should be made so before setting out, by deep culture and plenty of barn-yard manure, well worked in with the previous crops.

II. HOW TO PLANT A TREE.—Dig the hole two or three inches deeper than needed; loosen up the bottom by pick, if needed, a few inches; then put in soil, the last inch or two actual surface soil, and place the tree upon it, spreading out the roots level with their starting point at the tree, and work the fine surface soil in among them, to leave no vacancies, keeping the fine fibres all in their natural directions and completely covered with the soil, packing the dirt as tightly as you can with the hand only, setting so that about four inches of dirt shall be above the roots; and this is to be sprinkled on in a fine state, being very careful that no one steps upon this loose soil, nor even to pat it, or pack it with the shovel; then it will settle naturally and evenly, not incline the tree more to one side than the other; and the first rain will have a chance to fill any possible crevices under the roots, in the settling of the loose soil. After a rain or two, mulch if you have suitable coarse manure for the purpose.—*Condensed from F. B. Elliott in the Cleveland Herald.*

**2. Fruit Trees.—Trimming, Best Time, etc.—**The best time to trim any fruit, or other trees, or vines, is to pinch off the buds or sprouts when you see one is growing where you don't want it; if too large to rub or pinch off, use the pocket knife; and although in July or August is considered the best time for trimming, yet branches not exceeding half an inch in diameter may be trimmed off at any time when the sap is not frozen. Still R. N. Handy, in *Green's Fruit-Grower*, says:

"That the best time to trim apple trees is from June to August, as the wounds then heal over much quicker and better than in the winter months." Good authority or corroboration. And the time to trim apple trees, is the time for all fruit trees.

**But Large Branches,** if they ever have to be removed, but will not have to be if properly trimmed from the beginning, should be trimmed off in February or March, so the wound will become dry before spring growth commences; and I would always cover a large wound with tallow, well rubbed in, or a coat of grafting-wax, no matter what time of year the trimming was done.

T. T. Lyon, of Coldwater, in the *Michigan Farmer*, tells his brother farmers that "in case of very thrifty, non-bearing trees," a thorough trimming in July or August will check wood-growth and encourage fruiting the next season.

**1. Manuring and Care of Orchards.—**If the soil was, or has been made rich before putting out an orchard, and mulching was done properly after setting out, whether it was fall or spring planting, and the mulch, coarse manure or litter was put on to extend beyond the extremities of the roots, as it always should, no further manuring will be needed for two or three years only as may be needed for such crops as are raised upon the ground; after that a good, thorough manuring again over the whole surface. It is deemed of more importance to mulch well soon after spring planting than fall, to prevent drying out the moisture from the loose dirt by the heat of summer, while in the north, snow generally protects over winter; but 'tis best to do it within two or three weeks after planting, if no mice are in the field, and if mice, the snow must be kept well tramped down around the trees, and if the tramping extends out over the mulching, 'tis likely to kill any mice nesting therein. See next receipt also against mice, rabbits, etc.

**I. Fruit Trees—To Protect From Mice and Borers.—**"M," a correspondent of the *Maine Farmer*, in answer to an inquiry of one signing himself "Novice," (one new in any business) says he has for ten years protected his trees from mice by binding a piece of birch bark around the base of the tree with twine, which lasts two or three years, or until the growth bursts the twine, then a new string is to be tied on again.

**II. Bores—To Protect Against Borers.—**Cover the lower end of the bark an inch or more with dirt. Where birch bark is not plenty, other barks, or why not tarred building-paper, as neither mice nor rabbits like the tar.

Again, he says, he has "never known mice to attack trees which received a coat of whitewash made of quick lime (unslacked lime), and applied in the fall of the year." Put in some soap, too, as in next.

III. **Fruit Trees—To Protect Against Rabbits.**—Dr. Hassby, in the *Western Planter*, protects his trees from rabbits by a wash "made from air-slacked lime and soft soap, brought to the consistency of common paint, with common flour paste added to make it adhere.

IV. **Again,** it is claimed that axle-grease and lard, equal parts, well mixed and rubbed upon young trees, protect from rabbits. The rosin in it, no doubt, is offensive to them, as I know the tarred paper is.

V. **Mice and Rabbits—Late Toledo Remedy Against Girdling Trees, Improved.**—A few days after I had prepared these items upon the care of fruit trees, I saw a report in the *Blade* of a meeting of the Horticultural Society, of this city, horticulture having more especial reference to garden culture, the word coming from the Latin *hortus*, a garden, and *cultor*, a cultivator, as Webster's "unabridged" informs us, wherein the secretary advised washing the lower part of the tree with the following mixture, as a protection against mice and rabbits girdling them: "Carbolic acid, 1 oz., mixed with strong soap-suds, 1 gal.; then diluted with 2 or 3 gals. of water."

**The Improvement.**—In place of the "strong soap suds," the author says, take one gallon of good soft soap and water, not more than one gallon, mixed with the carbolic acid, one ounce. This will give the strength of acid that Mr. Saunders, of the Washington public grounds, uses on his trees, which is not too strong, (see in pear blight); and it also gives a mixture more like Prof. Cook's, of Lansing, or Michigan Agricultural College, against bark lice, borers, and other pests, given below, insuring according to my best judgment, not only an improvement, but really one of the best, if not the best application which can be made against mice and rabbits, against the borers, and all other pests of the trees, as it makes a wash sufficiently thick to adhere well to the bark, leaving such a body of the mixture, too, upon the tree, that neither mice nor rabbits will like as food, for it is for this purpose they seek. This, of course, should be applied late in the fall, before these depredators begin their winter's work. See also among the receipts for sheep, a Wash to Prevent them from Barking Trees. It will be as good against rabbits and mice as sheep.

**Knowledge vs. Ignorance. Their Different Results.**—At the same meeting above named, Capt. Nixon said:

"As a general rule, success was the result of knowledge, failure the result of ignorance," which agrees well with our starting point in this department. The Successful Farmers which see. Then. as the wise man says, "Get knowledge, and with all thy getting, get understanding," for these things eradicate ignorance upon any and all subjects.

**Girdled Trees by Mice or Rabbits, to Restore the Bark.**—If a tree is not girdled entirely around, make a clay mortar, and apply a good thickness by means of cloths, and you are safe. A loamy soil will do, but if neither, then apply grafting-wax spread on cloth in the same way, melting to spread, covered with common mud from the road. Says a correspondent of the *Rural New Yorker*, "The bark will grow again without a scar."

**1. Fruit Trees, to Secure Against Bark Lice Borers, etc.—** Prof. A. J. Cook, of the Agricultural College, Lansing, Mich., informs the readers of the Detroit *Tribune*, that an application of soft soap to the trees the first week in June, and at the same time in July, will ensure safety against the borers ; and it also exterminates the bark lice, if the rough bark is scraped off to ensure the soap reaching them all.

**I. For the Lice**, the scraping may be done earlier, and the soap, diluted only enough to apply readily as a wash, but to extend to all large branches, and the trees will start into new life and more active growth from its application ; and, if done from the setting out of an orchard, there will be little or no trouble from these pests.

**II. The Borer** makes its appearance about the first of June and deposits its eggs upon the bark, near the ground, and another writer says, referring more particularly to the peach borer, "These pests can be entirely exterminated by removing a small portion of the earth from the body of the tree near the roots, and filling its place with a quart of soft soap. If the borer has attacked the tree this will kill him, and if not the soap will not injure the trees and the borer will not get at them through the soap."

If it is good for peach trees, it is as good for apple trees, or any other. Bands of cloth should be put around trees by the middle or last of June, to prevent the ascending of the pest that stings the fruit, and care taken to kill all that take "lodging" under the bands.

**III. Fruit Trees, Plants, etc.; Chloride of Lime Ensures Against Grubs, Vermin, etc., on Trees and Plants.—***Le Cultivateur*, a French journal, says:

"If chloride of lime be spread on the soil, or near plants, insects and vermin will not be found near them," and adds : "By its means plants will easily be protected from insect plagues by simply brushing over their stems with a solu- tion of it, or sprinkling upon. It has often been noticed that a patch of land which has been treated in this way remains religiously respected by grubs, while the unprotected beds around are literally devastated. Fruit trees may be guarded from the attacks of grubs by attaching to their trunks pieces of tow smeared with a mixture of hog's lard and chloride of lime, and ants and grubs already in possession will rapidly vacate their position. Butterflies, again, will avoid all plants whose leaves have been sprinkled over with this chloride of lime water."

*Remarks and Directions.*—This journal does not give the strength of the above mixture, but one ounce of the chloride to eight of lard would be plenty, no doubt, and one-half pound of the chloride to a pail of water, enough for the "solution."

**IV. Examination of the Trees for the Borer, and Remedy, if They Have Entered the Wood.**—Prof. Cook advises "a thorough examination of the trees in September, to ascertain whether the borer has gone

Into the wood. If he has he must be followed closely with a small wire, or he must be dug out with a sharp knife, making as small a cut as possible."

*Remarks.*—It will be remembered that the borer enters the wood a little under the soil, or very near it ; and if holes are cut to get them out, as above spoken of, you should apply the soap after it, and also cover the wounds with dirt, or with the clay mud bound on, if much above the ground, as for girdled trees, above.

**Fruit Trees, Old, Mossy, and Diseased Bark to Renew.**— The old plan for mossy and diseased bark, was, to sprinkle on thoroughly of wood ashes, but except there is moss to catch and hold the ashes, or many crevices in the bark, the ashes would amount to but little—the later plan of scraping and applying soft soap, reduced only to allow applying with a brush, as a wash, is quicker and better, and more destructive to caterpillars and other destructive insects which infest the trees ; but, lest the soap nor the ashes may prove sufficient in all cases, especially in pear blight, I will give the wash as used by Wm. Saunders, of Washington, D. C., who has, or has had, charge there, of the public grounds, as follows :

**Pear Blight, Diseased Bark, etc., Wash for.**—Put stone lime, ½ bu.; sulphur, 4 lbs. into a tight barrel, slacking the lime with hot water, to the consistency of common white-wash, keeping the barrel covered with an old piece of carpet ; and when to be applied, add carbolic acid ¼ oz. to each gal. of the wash. He applies it early in spring to the body and large branches; but thinks it would be better if applied later, or about the first of June, when borers, caterpillars, etc., appear. And if any diseased bark, he scrapes off or cuts off all that can be done readily.

*Remarks.*—This was reported to the Norfolk, Va., Horticultural Society, and spoken of highly for pear blight by G. B. Leighton, and it has also been recommended by others in the same favorable manner.

The *Germantown Telegraph*, however, speaks very highly of the ashes process to clean off old scaly and deadened bark, and also as being destructive to all insects infesting pear or apple trees. So let each person please himself. But if I was going to use the ashes I should make a wash of them, and put on, and not wait for rains to do the work, after having sprinkled them on dry, as recommended.

**Barren Trees, Remedy for.**—Let it be remembered that barren soil makes barren fruit trees. As it is not possible to grow fruit from the same soil every year unless a supply of manure, ashes, lime, bone-dust, and stable manure, is properly composted, and applied every other year in sufficient quantities at least 2 to 4 bush. to each tree, according to the size, and therefore the distance the roots extend, the larger share being out over the extremities of the roots, where the smaller fibres or suckers are. I do not mean growing sprouts called suckers, but the fibers of the roots which suck up the nourishment and thus help to make the fruit as well as add to the growth of the tree, foliage, etc. These roots and fibres often extend 8 to 10 feet from the tree, and at this outer point is the place for the largest portion of the fertilizers to be spread. Feed your fruit trees where the fibers of the roots are.

**Swamp Muck, Lime and Ashes, a Valuable Manure for Fruit Trees.**—"Lucky is he," says a writer, who owns a reclaimed swamp of muck, for he goes on to say, "If this is thrown out in a heap and mixed with lime it forms a stimulant to fruit trees which cannot harm, but never fails to invigorate in a wonderful manner, etc., to which I would say, use ashes also with the lime, in about equal proportions, and as freely as you can afford it, to be mixed between layers of the muck, in filling up. In the end, to be finely mixed before applying.

**Ashes—Their Value in Orchards and Garden.**— A gardener realized the value of ashes to be so great in the garden and orchard that he recently recommended, through the *Rural New Yorker,* that even the trimmings from apple trees, as soon as dry enough, with all weeds and other rubbish, be burned "for the fertilizing matter they contain." He gives a case where the trimmings of an orchard and the rubbish about had been burned, and the ashes put upon the outer roots of the trees to their great advantage, and squashes grew in great abundance on the ground where they were burned; and for experiment "a hill was planted ten feet off, manured with a small quantity of the ashes, and another with horse manure. The hill with the ashes grew three times as great as the other, and was twice as productive." Certainly a fair test.

*Remarks.*—The immortal Liebig, many years ago, pointed out the importance of potash to the soil for grain, tobacco, hemp, etc., and from this time on, the enterprising farmer has been using it more or less, according to his convenience of obtaining it, and means to purchase with, etc., until now, lime, ashes, and the nitrate of soda from South America, plaster, phosphates, etc., all come in to give a full supply. So fully was the editor of the *Scientific American* long ago satisfied of the importance of potash, lime, etc., for renewing the growth of old fruit trees, he gives us an experiment of his as follows. He says:

"Some twenty-five years ago, we treated an old hollow pippin apple tree as follows: The hollow, to the height of 8 feet, was filled and rammed with a compost of wood ashes, garden mould and a little waste lime. The filling was securely fastened in by boards. The next year the crop of sound fruit was 16 bushels from an old shell of a tree that had borne nothing of any account for some time. But the strangest part was what followed. For seventeen years after filling, the old tree continued to flourish and bear well."

*Remarks.*—Thus it appears, it makes no difference whether the potash in the ashes, with the lime, reach the tree through its roots or by absorption from the hollow of the old, rotting and decaying body. It has also been abundantly proved that even by putting a mixture of wood and coal ashes alone around the stems or trunks and roots of fruit trees, vines, currant and other fruit bushes, in early spring, has generally greatly benefited apples, peaches, grapes, etc., both in quality and quantity, and the trees, shrubs, vines, etc., last and bear much longer for it. Then, as it pays, in all points let it be done properly, and at the right time—"early spring."

**Potash—Its Value as a Manure for Fruit Trees, Crops, Etc., and in What it is Found.**—The foregoing has sufficiently shown the value of potash as a manure for orchards, so I need only say it is equally valuable for all crops; and now it remains only to show in what it is found. The fact is, nothing grows in the line of fruits nor crops, which does not contain it, and need its return, to keep up a supply. The potash of commerce is made from wood ashes; and grass, grain crops, and consequently all straw and weeds, leaves, barn-yard manure, roots, and fruits of all kinds, contain it; so any one can see that all these things which have passed the point of usefulness as food, etc., should find their way into the compost heap or manure pile, so that at the proper time, they, with the potash they contain, may be returned to the soil.

**Pear Culture—Great Success in—Applicable to All Other Fruit.**—A Mr. Quinn, at Newark, N. J., has a large pear orchard, in which he had been so successful, the editor of the *Horticulturist* paid him a visit the last of August, recently, to ascertain by what means he had been more successful than others. He found " the 'standards' were full to overflowing, and the 'dwarfs' so over-abundant as to need support," and continues: "Mr. Quinn's success in pear culture has been due to three points only:

I. " He cultivates his orchard constantly, permits no other crop to grow between, and allows no grass nor weeds to be seen, and mulches heavily in time of fruiting.

II. "He prunes in early summer and winter, carefully, and has thus built up an orchard of splendid shape, healthy limbs, and able to bear any reasonable amount of fruit without strain.

III. " He takes especial pains with packing, always using clean, new half-barrels, assorts into even grades, and packs solidly and handsomely."

*Remarks.*—The foregoing points are all of the utmost importance, in the cultivation of any fruit crop whatever, except perhaps, as apple trees are planted considerably farther apart than pears or plums for a few years at least other suitable crop may be cultivated between the rows, but never to the injury of the roots, and especially never galling the trees with the whiffletrees. Attention to all the above points and the various items previously given, no one need fail of being a successful horticulturist, where the market justifies its undertaking.

**Plum Trees. The Well-known Remedies Against the Curculios, Insuring a Full Crop of Fruit.**—Ever since 1832, when an old man by the name of David Thomas told his neighbors to "jar their plum trees and curculios on sheets, and destroy them," a few persons have practiced this plan and have had good crops of plums ; still, very many people will not take this trouble; let all such put their chicken coops under their plum trees like Daniel Billig does, and get crops that require propping up from their heavy loads ; or like Peter Myers, make a pen of one length of boards under each plum tree, and put two pigs in each pen, who also had to prop his trees to prevent their breaking down with plums. These were Illinois men, and their names got into the papers by a report of J. D. Piper to the Horticultural Society of that State.

II. **A French** gentleman, not many years since, had large orchards surrounding his mansion, among them about three acres in plums, from which although blossoming finely, he got no fruit ; he therefore fenced it up for a chicken yard, leaving the trees for shade ; but the very next year he was profoundly astonished by having a very large and abundant yield of plums, actually breaking down many branches.

III. **An Old** and successful fruit grower reports that to "plant tansy at the roots of the plum trees, or by hanging branches of the plant on the limbs of trees, you will not be annoyed with the curculio." And claims it is the most successful curculio preventive he has ever tried. Then why not good about other fruit trees ? Still I do not see that it can be grown about the roots and allow cultivation. I can, however, see that it would be quite a mulch in itself, as it grows abundant on good soil, and will mat down considerably. Then let no one further doubt, but follow one of these plans best suited to his convenience and, like these men, have a full yield of fruit. That it may be so, is the reason I have given these short accounts of past successes.

**Quinces. Their Successful Cultivation.**—Many persons put their quince trees, or "bushes," as more generally called, in the dryest and most out-of-the-way place they can find, then let them take care of themselves, *i. e.*, they receive no cultivation at all, grass and weeds reigning supreme. But the quince is a native of the sea shore, and although it does not need a wet soil, yet it does require a moist but porous, else a well-drained soil ; and to keep up its natural demand for a saline, or salt-loaded atmosphere of its sea-coast nativity, must not only be as well cultivated as Mr. Quinn's pear orchard above, but must also have a supply of salt, broadcast, as far as the roots extend. To a full-grown tree or bush three or four quarts will not be too much. The principal points above are from Dr. Sylvester, of Lyons, N. Y., through the *Prairie Farmer*, but my own knowledge and observation tells me the same things.

**Shade Trees, Where to Plant.**—Shade trees are usually planted too near the house, and also too near each other, making the rooms dark and damp, especially so if evergreens; nothing more out of place than large evergreens on the sunny sides of a house, but a few rows of them and other suitable timber groves on the north side make excellent wind-breaking protection for house, barn, sheds for stock, etc. It is well to have plenty of shade trees about, but set the more open topped on the east and south, the dark evergreens on the west and north, where none, or not enough, are yet provided.

**Forest Trees, Planting in the West, a Success.**—I see it stated in the *American Messenger*, for January, 1885, that Messrs. Douglas & Son, near Ft. Scott, Kansas, finding that 600 acres they planted with forest trees are a complete success, are planting 500 acres more. Before next April they will have 1,360,000 trees planted.

*Remarks.*—Others can do it as well as they; and if they do not wish to put out as many, can put out enough to break the winds from their houses, barns, sheds, etc., and soon have enough for their home use, for fence posts, fuel, etc. And as anyone who desires to put out trees would be likely to inquire, " what shall I put out ?" I will name a few kinds that have done well in the west, and show also what may be expected to be their growth in 10 to 20 years.

**Hardy Trees, Rapidity of Growth, etc.**—The following varieties, all things considered, are the best for general cultivation in the North-west:

Cottonwood, soft maple, silver poplar, black cherry, ash-leaved maple, catalpa, black walnut, and white walnut. H. C. Raymond, of Council Bluffs, Iowa, states that the following named varieties, planted when one foot in height, attained the following diameters and heights when ten years of age :

| | | | |
|---|---|---|---|
| Cottonwood,..................... | Diameter, 9 inches. | Height, 35 feet. |
| Soft Maple. ..... ................ | " 8 " | " 30 " |
| Silver Poplar.................... | " 9 " | " 30 " |
| Black Cherry ................... | " 6 " | " 28 " |
| Ash-leaved Maple.............. | " 5½ " | " 27 " |
| Catalpa ......................... | " 6 " | " 25 " |
| Black Walnut.................. | " 5 " | " 20 " |
| Butternut...................... | " 5 " | " 20 " |

Hon. Suel Foster, of Muscatine, Iowa, reports the following as the growth of the varieties named twenty years, after transplanting :

| | | | |
|---|---|---|---|
| Soft Maple.................... | Diameter, 16 inches. | Height, 35 feet. |
| Hard Maple.................. | " 14¼ " | " 20 " |
| Black Cherry................ | " 11 " | " 40 " |

The chestnut, twenty-four years from seed grew to be 10 to 16½ inches in diameter and 30 to 39 feet in height. The European larch, ten years, transplanted, attained a diameter of 4 to 7½ inches, and were 20 to 30 feet in height.

The Osage orange south of the north line of Missouri, the *Prairie Farmer* thinks is the quickest to give fence posts, and that they are more durable than any other, easily cut and split when green, but very hard when dry. Grapevine posts of this timber, perfectly sound after 14 years' use, and some poles of it of 4 to 5 inches in diameter lay the same length of time under the ledge and yet perfectly sound. They think it admirably adapted for farm timber and farm fuel all over the west and southwest, not too far north, of any other. For felloes of wheels it outsets 4 to 1 the best white oak, and valuable for all purposes that hard wood can be put to. Probably no timber is equal to the black walnut when large enough for sawing; and the hard maple for making one's own sugar, as they may be tapped by boring when 6 to 10 inches in diameter. The chestnut makes splendid rails, and furnishes a salable nut, if the children can spare them. Now let each one judge for himself according to his situation and his wants.

**Labels for Trees, Wood Very Durable.**—Make nice smooth strips of thin board, with a hole in one end for copper wire; then soak the strips in strong copperas water and dry them; then soak again in lime water, after which, write the name upon them and attach to branches with wire, loosely. Soaking in the two mixtures forms a gypsum, which is almost insoluble, and therefore very durable.—*Report of Horticultural Society, of Berlin.*

*Remarks.*—The report claims that the same processes of soaking twine, or netting would make them very durable, but as the proportions were not given, experiment would have to settle that, not to get the solution so strong as to rot the goods. For the wooden labels, it matters not how strong, if a pound to a bucket of water, so much the better, but one-fourth these amounts would be as "strong" as I should try them on netting, or twine for netting.

**Zinc Labels for Marking Trees, Plants, etc., to Write Name with Pencil or Ink.**—The *Horticulturist* says : "The best labels for trees or plants may be made by writing with a lead pencil when moist upon slips of zinc, and attaching with a copper wire." Although the *Country Gentleman* claims "this writing will last for years," yet I think it cannot show very plainly, and hence give the following :

**Ink for Zinc Labels, for Trees, Plants, etc.**—Take by weight, verdigris, 2 parts, say drs.; sal ammoniac, 1 dr.; water, 80 drs.

DIRECTIONS.—Rub the powders in a mortar with a little of the water at first. Then adding all, bottle and keep corked up to prevent the ammonia from escaping. Write upon the strips of zinc with a quill pen, shaking often while writing. Some attach the zinc labels by cutting one end narrow, then bend it around a limb. Others with copper wire. This ink makes a black mark that will show plainly, and also be durable.

**Fall Planting Best for Raspberries, Blackberries, Currants Gooseberries, Grapes, etc.**—The *Fruit Recorder* tells its readers that all of the above-named fruit "set out in the fall, even in October, before the leaf drops, will make double the growth and double the fruit the next year than if planted in the spring." I recommend its early setting, that the fall rains may settle the dirt nicely about the roots so they begin their growth with the opening of spring, "even throwing out rootlets in the fall," mulching before freezing with litter of any kind, manure, tan bark, sawdust, inverted sods, hay or straw,—over each hill—and they will come out all right in the spring, and begin to grow as soon as frost is out, scarcely a plant failing.

*Remarks.*—There isn't a doubt about it. And it is believed by the author that fall planting of fruit trees must be found equally advantageous, in being more likely to live and also to thrive better generally. And now, as we began this department with "The Successful Farmer, What he Does Not and What he Does, Applicable to All Business Men," we will close it with :

**The Happy Farmer, How He Does His Work, Equally Applicable to All Laborers, and to Everybody.**—The following thoughts have more reference to the spirit in which work is best done, than to the way, physically, of doing it. Carlyle says :

"Give us, O, give us the man who sings as his work! He will do more in the same time—he will do it better—he will persevere longer."

Another writer makes short work of it in the following couplet :

" Whistle and hoe, sing as you go ;
Shorten the row by the songs that you know."

Another thinks it important to "push things" "in life's earnest battle," as well as in war ; and also shows us that those "only prevail," or come off final victors, who " never say fail," by the following stanza :

" Keep pushing! 'tis wiser than sitting aside,
And sighing and watching and waiting the tide ;
In life's earnest battle, they only prevail,
Who daily march onward and never say fail."

No matter how distasteful any particular kind of work may be, in the beginning, if it is taken up with a feeling that one has got to " Hoe his own row," and that although there may be some other kind of work that would suit better ; yet, as this is all that offers for the present, I am going at it as I would if I loved it. Of such, a writer says :

" Who loves his work and knows how to spare,
May live and flourish anywhere."

Then all I have further to say is, go at whatever you have to do with cheerfulness, "sing," or " whistle," as suits you best ; but be cheerful, any-how ; "push things" whenever they need pushing ; never allow a thought of "giving up the ship," and you will soon love your work, and must " flourish" —succeed—almost " anywhere," and at almost anything, because entered upon with a "determination to conquer " be you farmer, laborer, or business man, boy or girl, man or woman, in the nature of things you must succeed.

# MECHANICAL.

**1. BRASS, TO CLEAN.**—Nitric acid, 1 part; sulphuric acid, ½ part; (half as much) in a stone jar. DIRECTIONS.—"Have ready a pail of fresh water, and a box of sawdust. Dip into the acid (or swab on), then into the water (or swab on), and rub with the sawdust. A brilliant color is immediate. If things are greasy, first dip into a strong solution of potash or soda (or swab on), to cut the grease. It is used at the U. S. arsenals, and considered the best in the world.

**2. How to Clean Brass, Copper, Tin, etc.**—The following mixture will be found the best thing for cleaning brass, copper, tin, stair-rods, taps, and even windows, and it is quite worth the trouble of making: Whiting, pulverized rotten stone, and soft soap, each 1 lb.; vinegar, 1 cup, and as much water as makes it a thick paste; spirits of turpentine ½ pint. DIRECTIONS.—Let it boil fully 10 minutes, and when nearly cold, add the turpentine, and store in wide-mouthed pickle jars of glass or stoneware. When to be used, put a very little of it on a rag, and rub the article until it becomes bright. Polish with a soft leather dipped in powdered bath-brick. Unless bath-brick is used, it soon tarnishes.

**3. Brass, the Dirtiest, to Clean Very Quickly.**—Finely rubbed bichromate of potassa, mixed with twice its bulk of sulphuric acid, and an equal quantity of water, will clean the dirtiest brass very quickly.

**4. Another.**—Clean brass with a paste made of oxalic acid, 1 oz.; rotten stone, 6 oz.; and enough whale oil and spirits of turpentine, in equal quantities to mix.

**5. Stained Brass, Silver, etc., to Clean.**—Whiting wet with aqua ammonia will clean stains from brass and silver, and is excellent for polishing door knobs, of brass, or silver, faucets, fenders, rods, etc.

*Remarks.*—All the foregoing are good, so take your choice of such as you can obtain the handiest.

**1. Steam Pipes to Cover, to Prevent Loss of Heat.**—Coal ashes 4 parts (qts. or bushels, no matter what the measure), sifted through a riddle 4 meshes to the inch; calcined plaster (of Paris), wheat flour, and fine dry clay, each 1 part (1 measure of each of these are used to 4 of ashes.)

DIRECTIONS—Mix ashes and fine clay together (with water), to the thickness of thin mortar, in a mortar-trough; mix the calcined plaster and flour together dry, and add to the ashes and clay mortar, as you want to use it; put it on the pipes in two coats, according to the size of the pipe. For a 6-inch pipe, 1st coat 1¼ inches thick, the 2d coat about ½ inch. Afterwards finish with a hard finish, same as for a room. About 2½ hours will be required to set, on a hot pipe.

**2. Steam Pipes, Protection Efficient and Cheap.**—A mechanic reports through the Detroit *Post and Tribune*, a little different from the above, you will see, using hair and leaving out the flour. He says: "One hundred lbs. of clay are mixed with water, and 100 lbs. of fine ashes added and well kneaded, then mix with 1 lb. of hair. This mixture is well incorporated and allowed to stand until needed to use. Just before using, 10 lbs. of ground plaster of Paris are mixed with it. The mixture, of course, soon sets, and cannot be kept over 12 hours after the plaster is added."

*Remarks.*—The clay should, no doubt, be dry, then made fine, else allowance made for the moisture in it; and this latter make no distinction as to ashes, whether wood or coal. I think cleanly sifted coal ashes preferable. The plaster of Paris, it will be seen too, is not calcined (dried in a hot kettle.) If so done, it sets quicker, which is its only advantage, and it may be an advantage, sometimes, not to have it set too quick. The hair, I think, a decided advantage, but it should be thoroughly whipped. If good for pipes, it must be equally good for boilers.

**"Zincing Iron"—Without a Battery.**—"The following" is an excellent and cheap method for preventing iron articles, exposed to the air, from rust. They are to be first cleaned by placing them in open wooden vessels, in water, containing ¾ to 1 per cent. ("¾ to 1 per cent.," means ¾ to to 1 pt., or part, to 100 pts. or parts, in the "wooden vessel" of water), of common sulphuric acid, and allow them to remain in it until the surface appears clean, (bright) or may be rendered so by scouring with a rag or wet sand. [This may be done in a revolving cylinder by machinery.] According to the amount of acid, they may require to remain in from 6 to 24 hours. [Then, if time is of any account, use more acid, up 5 or 6 per cent.] Fresh acid must be added according to the extent of use, and the amount of liquid; and when this is saturated with the sulphate of iron (the rust of iron from the articles being cleaned) it must be renewed. After removal from this bath ("wooden vessels,") the articles are rinsed in fresh water and scoured until they acquire a clean metallic surface (become "bright," as above remarked); and then they are to be placed in water, in which a little slacked lime has been stirred, and kept there until the next afternoon. When thus freed from rust, they are to be coated with a thin film of zinc, while cold, by means of chloride (more commonly called muriate) of zinc, which is made by filling three-fourths full a glazed earthen vessel with muriatic acid, then adding zinc clippings (little pieces of zinc) until effervescence ceases.

[Effervescence is shown by the rising of bubbles; when these stop rising, it has dissolved all the zinc it will cut, is saturated, as chemists say, and is then called muriate of zinc, and is the same as tinners use upon their seams before applying solder.]

"This liquid (muriate of zinc) is now to be turned off from the undissolved zinc and preserved in glass vessels.

"For use, it is poured into a sheet zinc vessel, of suitable size and shape for the objects or articles to be zineed, and about 1-30th part of its weight of finely powdered sal-ammoniac is to be added. The articles are to be immersed in this ("cold," as above mentioned), and a scum of fine bubbles forming on their surface in from one to two minutes, indicates the completion of this part of the operation. The articles are next drained so the excess may flow back into the vessel. The iron articles are thus coated with a thin film of zinc, and are to be placed on clean sheet-iron plates, heated from beneath, until perfectly dry, and then dipped piece by piece, with tongs, or other means, into very hot, though not glowing molten zinc, for a short time, until they acquire the temperature of the melted zinc, into which they are being dipped. They are then removed and beaten, or tapped lightly, to cause any excess of zinc to fall off, while yet hot."

**Nickel Plating, Without Battery.**—"To a dilute solution of the chloride of zinc—5 to 10 per cent.—(5 to 10 lbs. to 100 lbs. of water)—enough sulphate of nickel is to be added to give the solution a decidedly green color, and it is then to be heated to boiling in a porcelain vessel. The heating makes the solution cloudy, but does not injure it. The articles to be nickel plated are to be carefully cleaned of rust or grease, (see 1st receipt above for cleaning brass), and then suspended in the solution from 30 to 60 minutes, the bath being kept at a boiling temperature. When the articles are observed to be uniformly coated, they may be removed, washed in water, in which a little chalk is suspended, dried, and finally polished with chalk, or other suitable material."

*Remarks.*—This discovery is credited to a Prof. Slatba, and will be found valuable. Precipitated chalk is very fine, but rotten stone, as in some of the above receipts for polishing brass may be found preferable. Zincing is done mostly on small cast-iron articles, while this nickel-plating is used on a finer class of goods.

**Silver Plating, With a Battery.**—1. Dissolve 1 oz. of pure silver (like old coin) in nitric acid, by pouring the acid upon the silver until all is dissolved—perhaps 4 ozs. of acid to cut 1 of silver—then dissolve salt in soft water until very strong; now pour of this salt water into the acid and silver until all the silver sinks to the bottom, scientists say, until all is "thrown down;" then fill the jar or bottle with soft water, shake up, and let settle; then pour off carefully, and fill again and again, for three times, shaking well each time, or until there is no acid or taste of acid left. This, if carefully done, without waste, gives you 1 oz. of silver in fine powder.

2. In a suitable jar or dish, dissolve cyanide of potassium, 6 ozs. in soft rain water, 2 qts., into which put the silver powder, which will be dissolved therein, and this constitutes the plating solution.

3. In this solution the articles to be plated are to be suspended upon a silver hook. And in this solution must also be suspended a plate (generally in sheet form) or piece of pure silver, with about as much surface as there is surface to the articles to be plated, as it is necessary to keep the strength of

the solution up to this standard—the silver, therefore, that is deposited upon the articles being plated, dissolved off of the "plate, sheet, or piece of pure silver," as it is deposited upon the articles—the solution remaining full strength and ready for continued use. Of course the "battery" is connected with this "plating solution."

*Remarks.*—The battery used is the same as used by telegraphers, who will instruct one how to prepare and "connect" it. All articles to be plated must be freed from grease with a solution of potash or soda, as in the above processes. This is from a friend in Ann Arbor, whom I know to be reliable from over 25 years acquaintance.

**Steel—To Temper Very Hard.**—"Take water, 2 measures—no matter what size—wheat flour, ½ measure, and 1 of common salt.

DIRECTIONS.—Mix into a paste; heat the steel to be hardened enough to coat with the paste—by immersing it in the composition—after which heat it to a cherry red and plunge it in cold, soft water. If properly done, the steel will come out with a beautiful white surface, and very hard."

*Remarks.*—It is said this is the process by which Stubbs' files are tempered, which are recommended below, for drilling glass.

**1. Steel and Iron Machinery—To Keep From Rusting.**—Powdered camphor gum, ½ oz.; lard, 1 lb.; a little black lead.

DIRECTIONS.—Dissolve the gum in the lard by heat; remove the scum, stir in just black lead enough to give an iron shade. Rub this over cleaned steel or iron machinery of any kind, and leave on 24 hours; then rub with a soft linen cloth, and it is safe from rust for a long time.

**Iron or Steel Varnish—To Prevent Rust.**—Rosin, 120 parts (drs., ozs. or lbs.); gum sandarach, 180; gum lac (shellac), 60; spirits of turpentine, 120; and alcohol, 180 parts.

DIRECTIONS.—Pulverize the three first articles and melt together; and gradually (and carefully, to avoid taking fire), add the turpentine, continuing the heat until all are again dissolved (if they harden) in the turpentine; then add the alcohol, and filter through a fine cloth (muslin) or thick filtering paper, bottle and cork for use.—*Manufacturer and Builder.*

*Remarks.*—The straining or filtering indicates its intention for fine articles; without it, it would do for outside railings, or ornamentation; and if desired black, for iron balustrades, fence, etc., add a little fine lamp-black, which will adapt it to such work, and look very nicely. See also Black Paint. How to Make for Iron Work.

**3. Steel—Rust Upon—To Remove.**—Cover the steel for a couple of days with sweet oil; then with finely powdered unslacked lime (known as "quick" lime), rub the steel until all the rust is removed; re-oil to prevent further rust.—*Indian Domestic Economy.*

**2. Another** plan, is, to place the rusty article in a bowl of kerosene, else to wrap the steel in a cloth well wet with kerosene, and let it remain 24 hours, or more; then scour the rusty spots with brick dust.

*Remarks.*—If brick-dust is used, bath or bristol brick would be best, but the powdered unslacked lime would be better than either, as it has an active power in itself of removing rust, and if time cannot be given, this powdered quick-lime, and the sweet oil or the kerosene, will remove it in a few minutes, by thorough rubbing; so will it with ammonia. Always apply oil, or some of the oily mixtures, at the last, to prevent the rust from deeper penetration.

**4. Steel Dinner Knives, Rust to Remove.**—Cover the steel with sweet oil, well rubbed in; let them remain 48 hours, and then using unslacked lime, finely powdered, rub the knife till all the rust has disappeared.

*Remarks.*—I should not like to go without my meals while this process was going on; hence I should let them lie over night only, and risk the job at that.

**5. Steel Apparatus, and Fine Instruments, to Preserve Their Polish, by Preventing Rust**—Prof. Olmsford, of Yale College, says: "This is done effectually, by melting slowly together, lard, 6 or 8 oz., and rosin, 1 oz.; and stirring till cool. It can be wiped off nearly clean, if desired as in a case of knife blades, or it can be thinned with coal oil, or benzine. The surface should be bright and dry, when applied, as it does not prevent oxidation (rusting) already commenced."

*Remarks.*—If any spots of rust, remove first with the sweet oil and piece of quick lime, as below. And remember there must be no salt in the lard.

**6. Steel, or Iron Buckles, Jewelry, etc., to Clean.**—Take a piece of unslacked lime, free from grit, or hard specks, and touch it to sweet oil, then rub them with it, and finish with chamois or buckskin. For ornamental jewelry, see next below.

**1. Jewelry, Ornaments, Gold Chains, etc., to Clean.**—Wash in soap suds; rinse in dilute alcohol (half water, half alcohol), and lay in a box of dry sawdust to dry; then rubbing with the sawdust, is a nice way to clean such goods.

**2. Gilded Washed, or Plated Jewelry, to Clean.**—Henry M. M. Morrison, of Wis., says: "The work of cleansing gilt articles is a delicate task, but they may be cleaned by rubbing them very gently with a soft sponge or brush, dipped in a solution of borax, 1/2 oz., to water, 1 lb., (a pt. is a lb. the world around); then rinsing in pure water and drying with a soft linen rag."

**3. Another.**—To clean gilt jewelry, put cyanide of potassium, 1 oz. to boiling water 1/2 pt., and when cold, add aqua ammonia, 1/2 oz., and alcohol, 1 oz., brush gently the articles with this compound. Rinse and dry with a cloth, chamois, buckskin, or sawdust as in No. 1, above.

*Remarks.*—Cyanide of potash is poison, so don't let children drink it nor get it into a sore spot in using it.

**4. Silverware, to Keep it's Original Luster.**—The proprietor of one of the oldest silverware houses in Philadelphia says: "Housekeepers

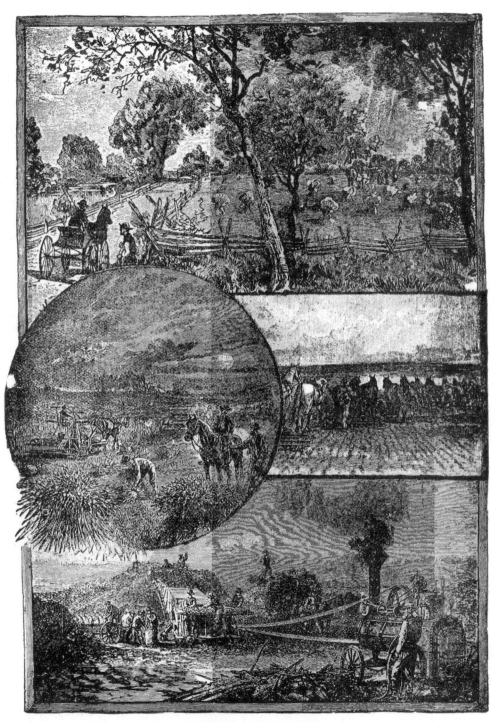

SUCCESSFUL FARMING.

ruin their silverware by washing it in soapsuds, which destroys the original luster, and makes it look like pewter. When it needs polishing, he says: take a piece of soft leather (chamois) and whiting and rub hard.

*Remarks.*—When, of course, never use soap in cleaning it, but take the following:

**5. Silverware, to Wash.**—"Put aqua ammonia, 1 tea-spoonful to very hot water, 1 pt., and wash quickly with a small soft brush, kept for the purpose only, and dry with a clean linen towel; then rub very dry with chamois. Washed in this manner silverware becomes again brilliant, and requires no polishing with any of the powders, or whiting usually employed, and lasts much longer.

*Remarks.*—Nothing could be more sensible, still the following is also sensible:

**6. Silverware, Knives and Forks, Tin, etc., to Brighten after Cleaning.**—Put the finishing touch to them by rubbing with old, dry newspaper. It is a fine polisher. Some of these receipts are quite domestic, but still they are equally mechanical.

**Silvering Powder.**—Chloride of silver, 1 dr.; potassa alum, 2 drs.; common salt and cream of tartar, each, 1 oz.

DIRECTIONS.—First dip the article to be silvered into a strong solution of salt in water, then rub with the powder; wash and dry with a soft cloth, and polish with any of the above plans.

*Remarks.*—Druggists in small places may say there is no "potassa alum," but there is, and also "ammonia alum."

**Zinc, to Clean.**—Take sulphuric acid, 1 oz.; water, 2 ozs.

DIRECTIONS.—Wash quickly with the mixture, rinse immediately with warm water, wipe dry with a cloth, and polish with whiting, brightens it nearly equal to new.

**Soldering German Silver.**—To solder German silver, pour out some spirits of salt into an earthen dish, and put a piece of zinc in it. Then scrape the parts clean that are to be soldered, and paint over with the spirits of salt. Next put a piece of pewter solder on the joint and apply the blow-pipe to it. Melt five parts of German silver and four parts of zinc into thin cakes, then powder it for solder.—*Rural New Yorker.*

*Remarks.*—The phrase, "spirits of salt," is the old name for muriatic acid, as now called; and all the zinc should be put in that the acid will dissolve; then it is called "muriate of zinc," which is what is to be put on. Where he says, "Then scrape the parts clean that are to be soldered, and paint over with the spirits of salt." This "muriate of zinc" is the proper "flux," or solution for all soldering. See Soldering Cast Iron, next below, calling for the "muriatic acid." It should be kept corked and away from children, as it is poisonous—eats or destroys clothing, as well as flesh, hence apply with a swab.

**2. Soldering Cast Iron.** A paper called the *Engineer* says that Soldering cast iron is generally considered to be very difficult, but it is only a question of thoroughly making bright the surface to be soldered, and using good solder and a clean swab, with muriatic acid.

*Remarks.*—The muriate of zinc is the article to use in this, as in all other solderings.

**Glass Globes, to Clean.**—If the globes are much stained by smoke, soak them in tolerably hot water with a little washing soda dissolved in it, then put a tea-spoonful of powdered carbonate of ammonia into a pan of lukewarm water, and with a tolerably hard brush wash the globes till the smoke stain disappears; rinse in clean, cold water, and let them drain till dry. They will be quite white and clear.

*Remarks.*—Aqua ammonia, which is more likely to be in the house, will do as well, but a tea-spoonful of either is not enough for a " pan of water," but only for a pint of water or one quart at most.

**1. White Paint, to Clean.**—Take a small quantity of fine whiting on a damp piece of flannel; rub gently over the soiled surface and the effect will almost equal the original purity.

*Remarks.*—See the next receipt for washing off, if needed.

**2. Oil-Painted Surfaces, to Clean.**—Take a piece of soft flannel, put it in warm water, and squeeze it till it feels dry; next dip gently on to some very finely pulverized French chalk, and rub the painted surface with the flannel; the effect will be the removal of all dust, greasy matter, and dirt; the surface is next washed with a clean sponge and water, and dried with a piece of wash-leather. This method does not injure the paint like soap, and produces a very good result.

*Remarks*—Wash-leather is split sheepskin, prepared as chamois, and used for the same purposes, very properly, too, because much cheaper.

**Tracing Paper, to Make.**—To wet common drawing paper, or any other kind, with benzine, it becomes transparent immediately, and can be placed over a drawing, or picture, to be transferred, by tracing with a pencil, ink, or water-colors, which will not spread nor run upon its surface. This is condensed from the *Engineering and Mining Journal,* and may be relied upon. If the work is not completed before the paper loses its transparency by evaporation of the benzine, you can dampen that part again, to complete it. This is a new discovery, and valuable.

**I. Glass, to Break as You Like.**—File a little notch in the edge, at the point you wish to break from; then put a suitably shaped red-hot iron upon the notch, and draw, slowly, in the direction you wish. A crack will follow the iron, caused by the heat, if not drawn too fast.

**2. Glass, to Drill.**—To drill glass, use a file drill, and keep it wet with a mixture of camphene and spirits of turpentine. Heretofore turpentine has been used alone. The camphene helps to give the drill a better bite.— *Scientific American.*

*Remarks.*—It is claimed that a Stubb's triangular, or 3-square file, ground to proper shape, makes the best drill for glass, and some have claimed that water only or turpentine, do equally well to keep the glass wet with. Again turpentine with garlic juice in it, is claimed to be the best. The file must be ground so that the edge is sharp, and the width that the hole is to be. The file perhaps, had best not be heated, as the temper can seldom be made equal to that of the maker, (if Stubbs tempers his files as given on page 793, why can not any good blacksmith do it?) but if heated, while hot shape it to suit, then re-temper as Stubbs is said to do? A man in Jackson, Mich., claimed, in writing to the *Scientific American*, that he had drilled 4 holes through ¼ inch plate glass in 15 minutes, and that water was equally as good as turpentine to keep wet with.

1. **Furniture, Black Walnut Stain.**—Take 1 pt. of very thin glue, its adhesiveness being just perceptible between the thumb and fingers. Put into it 1 tea-spoonful of raw umber, stir it well, and put on warm with a sponge or brush. When dry, brush off and varnish, or,

2. Take 1 tea-spoonful of Venetian red and ½ tea-spoonful of lampblack, mix into a paste and then dilute with 1 pt of glue-water, as before.—*Journal of Chemistry.*

3. **Ebony, or Black Stain Upon Pine, or Other Soft Woods.**—Make a strong decoction of logwood by boiling, and apply boiling hot, 3 or 4 times according to the shade desired, allowing it to dry between applications; then apply a solution of acetate of iron. This is made by putting iron filings into good vinegar. These penetrate the wood deeply, and are very black, or less deep, according to the number of applications.

4. **Polish, Fine For Furniture.**—Linseed oil, and old ale, each ½ pt.; the white of 1 egg, beaten; alcohol, and muriatic acid, each 1 oz., mix.

DIRECTIONS.—Dust the furniture, shake the polish, and apply with a wad of batting or cotton flannel, and finish with an old silk handkerchief.

*Remarks.*—This, and any of the others, will keep any length of time, if corked.

5. **Polish to Brighten Old Furniture, Pianos, etc.**—Dissolve orange shade, gum shellac, 4 oz. in 95 per cent. alcohol, 1 qt.; then add linseed oil, 1 qt.; spirits of turpentine, 1 pt.; shake and also add sulphuric ether, and aqua ammonia, each 4 oz. Shake well when used, rubbing until a polish appears.—*Good Cheer.*

6. **To Take Bruises Out of Furniture.**—Wet the part with warm water; double a piece of brown paper 5 or 6 times, soak it in warm water, and lay it on the place; apply on that a warm, but not hot, flat iron, till the moisture is evaporated. If the bruise be not gone, repeat the process. After two or three applications, the dent or bruise will be raised to the surface. If the bruise be small, merely soak it with warm water and hold a red-hot iron near the surface, keeping the surface continually wet. The bruise will soon disappear.

(NOTE—This valuable receipt was obtained from New Zealand.)

*Remarks.*—For the sweet-oil plan, see the next receipt.

7. **Polish, Excellent and Good.**—To make a good polish for furniture, take alcohol, good vinegar and sweet-oil, equal parts of each, or a little more of the last. Shake the bottle well, daily, for three weeks, when it is fit for use, but the longer it stands, the better it is. The furniture must be rubbed till the polish is dry. Apply every 2 or 3 months; and rub the furniture with

a dry cloth every time it is dusted. For dining-room tables and sideboards, use the polish every week, as it makes them beautifully bright.

*Remarks.*—White-wine vinegar, when it can be got, is considered the best.

8. **Polish for Pianos, etc.**—Raw linseed oil (raw, which is unboiled oil, the kind intended in all, except the last one given), 1 qt.; spirits of turpentine, ½ pt.; alcohol, benzine, and aqua ammonia, each, 4 oz. Shake when applied, and rub well.

9. **Polish, Cheap and Good.**—Gum shellac and rosin, each 2 oz.; alcohol, 1 pt.; mix and let stand 24 hours, or until dissolved, shaking occasionally; then add spi. 'ts of turpentine, 3 pts.; boiled linseed oil, 2 qts.; red analine, 15 grs.; oil of citronella, ½ oz. Shake well when used. Apply with cotton flannel.

*Remarks.*—This is given in large quantities, as it has been made and sold extensively. The analine is only to color, and the citronella to flavor.

**Furniture, Upholstered. Carpets, Furs, Fannels, Etc.—The Trade Secret for Ridding of Moths.**—A trade secret among upholsterers for ridding furniture, etc., of moths, is the following: " A set of furniture that seemed to be alive with the larvæ, and from which hundreds of these pests had been picked and brushed, was set into a room by itself. Three gallons of benzine was purchased, at 30 cents a gallon, retail. Using a small watering pot, with a fine rose-sprinkler, the whole upholstery was saturated through and through with the benzine. Result: Every moth, larvæ and egg was killed. The benzine dried out in a few hours, and its entire odor disappeared in 3 or 4 days. Not the slightest harm happened to the varnish, or wood, or fabric. or hair-stuffing. That was months ago, and not a sign of a moth has since appeared. The carpets were also sprinkled all around the sides of the room, with equally good effect. For furs, flannels—indeed, all woolen articles containing moths,—benzine is most valuable. Put them in a box, sprinkle them with benzine, close the box tightly, and in a day or two the pests will be exterminated, and the benzine will all evaporate on opening. In using benzine great care should be taken that no fire is near by, as it is very inflammable.—*Tecumseh* (Mich.) *Herald.*

*Remarks.*—There is not a doubt of this fact, for I know that benzine is "death to bed-bugs," and so is gasoline, which may be equally good for moths, and being much cheaper, is worthy of trial. It will evaporate, too, as quickly as the benzine.

1. **Paint—Cheap, as Used at Iowa College. Suitable for Fences, Cheap Buildings, Tenement Houses, Etc.**—Crude petroleum, 3 parts—qts. or gals.—boiled linseed oil, 1 part, with " mineral paint," for body.

*Remarks.*—A report having got into some of the papers, that such a paint had been used on some of the college buildings, an inquiry about its value led Prof. S. A. Knapp to make the following explanation. He says:

"Five buildings and considerable fence upon the Iowa Agricultural College Farm, have been painted with this preparation. Upon some of them it has been one year, and thus far it has appeared to be fully equal to more expensive paints, in body, durability and in retention of color. It is especially adapted to cheap outbuildings, covered with rough boards. If 25 lbs. of white lead be added to each 100 lbs. of mineral paint, the mixture answers a very excellent purpose for tenement houses. [I see another writer claims that 1 lb. of lead to 4 lbs. of mineral paint, is sufficient.] Many experienced painters have examined the buildings covered with this paint, and affirmed that it made a better covering than pure lead and oil. This is doubtless an extreme view. It may, however, fairly be considered as a reliable paint for protection of the fences and cheaper farm buildings."

2. **Black Paint—How to Make for Iron Fences, Balustrades, Farm Implements, Etc.**—Coal-tar, 2 qts.; benzine, or benzole, 1 pt., or a little more, to thin it, to lay on nicely with a brush. As the benzine is very evaporative, make no more than is to be used at the time.—*Industrial Monthly.*

*Remarks.*—This is claimed to be more durable than oil and lamp-black paints, even where that was varnished, having been in use three years when the report was made.

3. **Paint for Floors.**—A writer claims there "is but one paint suitable for floors, and this is French ochre. And, 1st, if the boards have shrunk, clean out the cracks, and, with a small brush, give them a heavy coat of boiled linseed oil, then putty them solid and smooth. 2d. Paint the whole floor with a mixture of much boiled oil and little ochre for the first coat; then after it is well dried, give two more coats of much ochre and little oil; and finally finish with a coat of first-rate copal varnish. It is extremely durable for floors, windows, or outside, such as verandas, porticoes and the like. A floor stain, he continues, is best mixed in oil, and finally varnished."

*Remarks.*—If "a floor stain is best mixed in oil and varnished," take the following:

4. **Floor Stain.**—"Boiled linseed oil, 1 gal.; 5 cts. worth, or 2 heaping table-spoonfuls of burnt umber; heat the oil hot in an iron kettle—soap will clean it easily—then stir in the finely powdered umber, and with an old paint brush apply it as hot as you can; then, says a lady in the *Blade,* farewell scrubbing. A mop, wrung out of warm water, will clean it nicely."

*Remarks.*—This amount was given for a floor of 14 to 16 feet square; but it is about twice as much as needed if only one coat is to be given. The following receipt may be liked better, as it has spirits of turpentine in it, which causes it to penetrate the wood more deeply; and it has some "dryer" also, which makes it dry quicker than without it. It was given in the Detroit *Post and Tribune,* coming from a painter, as follows.

5. **Stain Black Walnut for a Pine Floor, Light Shade.**—"For an ordinary sized room, boiled oil and spirits of turpentine, each 1 qt.; dryer, 1 gill (4 ozs.); burnt umber, ¼ lb. Mix thoroughly and thin, or your floor

will be black as your shoe nearly. [Then put in only sufficient of the umber to give the shade desired.] If the floor is not to be varnished, use turpentine, 1 pt. only, and boiled oil, 3 pts., to make it more glossy."

6. **Paint, Flexible, for Canvas.**—Yellow soap, thinly sliced, 2½ ozs.; boiling water, 1¼ gals. Dissolve the soap by more heat, if necessary, and grind the whole solution, while hot, with 125 lbs. of good oil-paint. Keep same proportions for any amount needed.

7. **Paint, Old, to Remove.**—Stone lime, 3 ozs.; pearlash, or saleratus, 1 oz.

DIRECTIONS.—Slack the lime with water, and mix in the pearlash, or saleratus, using only water enough to make a paste. Spread this upon the paint to be removed, and let it remain over night, or until soft, when it can all be scraped off.—*Scientific American.*

*Remarks.*—Where pearlash or saleratus cannot be obtained, sal soda may take their place.

**Fire-Proof Wash for Shingle Roofs.**—Freshly slacked lime, salt and fine sand, or wood ashes, equal parts, made into a wash and put on freely as any ordinary whitewash is done, is said to render shingles fifty-fold more safe against taking fire from falling cinders, or otherwise, in case of a fire in the vicinity.—*Fireman's Journal.*

1. **Cement, Crystal, or Liquid Glue for General Purposes.** —"Hard water, 3 qts.; white glue, 3 lbs.; dry white lead, ½ lb.; aqua ammonia, 1 oz.; spirits of camphor, 2 ozs.; salt, 1 heaping table-spoonful; alcohol, 1 qt.; gum shellac, ¼ lb.

DIRECTIONS.—Put the shellac into the alcohol until dissolved. Dissolve the glue in the water by putting into a tin dish and setting into a pan of hot water to prevent burning the glue, till dissolved; then put the glue water and shellac, dissolved in the alcohol, together in a pan or kettle, to allow all to be brought to a boiling heat, stir in the powdered white lead; then the ammonia and spirits of camphor, and lastly the salt; stir and boil a few minutes, and bottle while hot.

*Remarks.*—This receipt was sent to me by Albert Stockwell, of Flint, Mich., who, in canvassing for my receipt books, always carried this cement with him, for sale, to help in his expenses. He spoke very highly of its great strength as a cement.

2. **Cement for Iron Works.**—It is sometimes advisable to fix two pieces of iron, as pipes for water or steam, firmly together as a permanency. A rust cement is frequently used, and the materials are sal-ammoniac, sulphur and iron borings. If the cement is desired to act quickly, the proportions should be: Sal-ammoniac, 1 part by weight; sulphur, 2 parts; iron borings, 200 parts. The sal-ammoniac and sulphur should be pulverized, and the borings of iron tolerably fine and free from oil. The mixture should be made with water to a conveniently handled paste. The theory of its action is simply union by oxidation.

**3. Cement for Leather.**—Sulphide of carbon, 10 parts; spirits of turpentine, 1 part; into which, in a suitable bottle, put finely cut shreds of pure gutta percha, to make a thickly-flowing liquid. To remove grease from the belts or leather to be joined, put a cloth upon it, and apply a hot iron for a while; then apply the cement to both surfaces, put together and apply pressure until dry.

**4. Cement for Rubber, and to Fasten Rubber to Metal, Glass and Other Smooth Surfaces.**—"Powdered shellac is softened to ten times its weight of strong wat'r of ammonia, whereby a transparent mass is obtained, which becomes fluid after keeping some little time, without the use of hot water. In three or four weeks the mixture is perfectly liquid, and when applied it will be found to soften the rubber. As soon as the ammonia evaporates the rubber hardens again—it is said quite firmly—and thus becomes impervious both to gases and to liquids. For cementing sheet rubber or rubber material in any shape to metal, glass or other smooth surfaces the cement is highly recommended."

**II. Cement for Rubber Goods, Fastening Rubber Soles, Leather Patches, Straps, etc.**—Fill a bottle one-tenth full of native Indian rubber (gutta-percha) cut in minute shreds; pour in benzole till the bottle is three-quarters full; shake every few days until the mixture is as thick as honey. This dries quickly. It is useful to mend rubber shoes o. any other rubber goods, as a water and air-tight cement for bottles—simply dipping the corks into it, and for a hundred other purposes. Three coats of this will unite leather straps, patches and rubber soles with firmness. To make a patch invisible, shave the edge of the leather quite thin.

**5. Cement, Similar to that upon Postage Stamps, Gummed Labels, etc., Good for Scrap Books, Labeling on Tin, Glass, etc.**—Dextrine, 2 ozs.; acetic acid and alcohol, each, $\frac{1}{2}$ oz.; water, $2\frac{1}{2}$ ozs.

DIRECTIONS.—Mix the dextrine, acetic acid and water, stirring until thoroughly mixed; then add the alcohol. For attaching labels to tin, first rub the surface with a mixture of equal parts of muriatic acid and alcohol; then apply the label gummed with a very thin coating of the cement, and it will adhere almost as well as on glass. A thin coat only is needed on "scraps," for scrap books.

*Remarks.*—Knowing the value of a paste, or cement, somewhat similar to this, where the adhesion depended upon the dextrine, I have every confidence in this for all the purposes named.

**6. Cement for Small Leaks in Steam Boilers.**—Experiments have shown the following to be effectual for stopping small leaks from the seams of boilers, pipes, etc. Mix equal parts of air-slacked lime and fine sand; and finely powdered litharge equal to both the first. Keep the powder dry, in a bottle, or a covered box. When wanted to apply, mix, as much as needed, to a paste, with boiled linseed oil, and apply quickly, as it soon hardens.

II. **Cement, Steam-Tight, and Water-Tight for Joints.—** Pure white, and red leads, equal parts mixed with boiled linseed oil, to the consistency required, has been extensively used for this purpose.

**Steam Boilers, to Prevent Incrustation from Becoming Hard.** —A bar of zinc having accidentally been left in a steam boiler, when under repairs, it was afterwards found to have disappeared, or dissolved, by which the incrustations, instead of becoming hard, were muddy and soft, and hence easily removed. This proves that the zinc, and iron of the boiler, forms a battery, the zinc being consumed, while the iron is protected, which is claimed to be a valuable discovery in engineering. The size of the bar of zinc would necessarily depend upon the size of the boiler, and how long the run was to be between cleanings.

**Nails, to Drive Into Hard Seasoned Timber.—** The editor of the *New Genesee Farmer* gives the following account of witnessing an experiment of driving nails into hard seasoned timber, fairly dried. "The first two nails, after passing through a pine board, entered about an inch, only, into the hard wood, then doubled down under the hammer; but on dipping the points of six or eight nails into lard, every one was driven home without the least difficulty."

*Remarks.*—Carpenters who are engaged in repairing old buildings sometimes carry a small lump of tallow for the purpose on one of their boots or shoes.

**Calcimining.—** Take four lbs. of Paris white, put it in a pail, cover it with cold water and let it stand over night. Put into a kettle 4 oz. of glue, and cover it also with cold water. In the morning set the glue on the stove, and add enough warm water to make 1 qt.; stir it until dissolved. Add the glue to the Paris white, and pour in warm water till the pail is three-quarters full. Then add bluing, a little at a time, stirring it well until the mixture is slightly bluish. Use a good brush, and go over one spot on the wall till it is thoroughly wet. If your brush dries quickly, add more warm water, as the mixture is too thick. The brush must be kept wet. This mixture costs thirty-eight cents.—*Scientific American.*

**Sewing Machine Oil, to Make, and How to Use.—** Take the best paraffine oil, and the best sperm oil, equal parts. Mix.

**To Use.—** Clean off the old oil with benzine, or kerosene, then apply. This I obtained from a sewing-machine agent who said he had manufactured and sold much of this oil, having been in the business over 14 years. Machines should be cleaned and re-oiled as often as they become the least gummy.

# BEE-KEEPING.

[In order that I might give the people the benefits of experience in Bee-Keeping, I engaged Dr. A. B. Mason, one of the most successful bee-growers in the country, to write this chapter for this work.]

Motto: Keep all colonies strong, and don't put off till to-morrow what should be done to-day.

In order that those interested in the science of Bee-keeping, who may read the following on the subject, may understand the meaning of the terms I shall use, I will say that the home or receptacle for the bees is called a "hive," not a "skip," "skep stand," or "gum," etc., and the bees when in a hive make a "colony," not a "swarm," and when part of a colony leaves a hive by what is known as swarming, it is a swarm, but the moment it is put in a hive it is a colony.

The suggestions that follow are not intended for those largely engaged in bee-keeping, or those who understand the subject, but for those who wish to keep only enough colonies to furnish their tables with pure, healthful and most delicious sweet honey.

Any one wishing to be informed in regard to the natural history of the honey-bee, and for more elaborate instructions in regard to Bee-Keeping, should procure some standard work on the subject, such as "Langstroth on the Honey-Bee," which is a thoroughly scientific work; or, "Cook's Manual of the Apiary," or, "Quinby's Mysteries of Bee-Keeping," both of which are thoroughly practical, and up with the times.

Any good supply dealers can furnish any of the articles used in Bee-keeping. All references and directions are given for those of the Langstroth hive.

## HOW TO COMMENCE BEE-KEEPING.

The first thing to procure, if such is not already on hand, will be one or more colonies of bees, which, in its natural condition, during the honey season, will be composed of a fertile queen (the only perfect female in the colony), more or less drones (or males), and from 20,000 to 40,000 workers. Some speak of a "king-bee" also, but there is no king in a colony of bees.

## WHAT HIVE TO USE.

It is claimed by many that the hive known as the Langstroth is the one most in use. After having used different styles, for several years I adopted the Langstroth, and would rather pay for such than use any other, if furnished me for nothing. Whatever style may be adopted, let it by all means be one with movable frames, and have but one sized frame in the apiary.

In using the Langstroth hive, many prefer having it so narrow that it will hold but eight frames, claiming that number of frames is enough to raise the

803

necessary amount of brood, and obliging the bees to put the surplus honey in the sections or upper stories.

When referring to the Langstroth hive, reference is usually had to the size of frame, as it is immaterial what the external appearance of the hive may be, that being left to the taste or fancy of the bee-keeper.

Before commencing any operation with bees, it will generally be better to be provided with a bee-vail and a smoker, and if you don't want to be stung at all, get a pair of rubber gloves. The vail can be bought ready made for about fifty cents, or it can be made from bobinett. Brussel's net is much better but more expensive. Get 1½ yds., that is about ⅔ of a yard wide. Sew the ends together and hem one edge, and put a rubber cord in the hem of such length as will hold the vail close around the crown of the hat you wear, or use a hat as a bee-hat, and sew the vail, without the cord or hemming, to the edge of the rim. A smoker may be had for from 50 cents to $2.00, in which rotton wood or cotton rags may be burned. The rubber gloves will cost from $1.75 to $2.00.

## HOW TO PROCURE THE FIRST COLONIES, ETC.

If not already supplied with bees, it will be best to get them as near home as possible.

Italians are undoubtedly the best, and our motto demands that only strong colonies be purchased, and if purchased in the fall not more than two-thirds as much should be paid for them as they would be worth in the spring.

Prepare a place on the ground for the hives, and if it is where the hens will not scratch, remove the grass and cover so thickly with sawdust where the hives are to set, and for several inches beyond on all sides, that neither grass nor weeds will grow through it. Place the hives six or more feet apart each way, and have them face south or east. The reason for placing them so far apart will be given under the head of swarming. Put a stick two inches square and as long as the hive is wide under the front end of the hive, and a like piece, under the back end.

If the bees are not in the kind of hive that it is intended to be used, they may be readily transferred in either of the following ways.

## TRANSFERRING.

The best time for this method is early in the season, when there is but little honey and brood in the hive, and always on a warm day, if possible, when the bees are busily engaged in gathering honey. When fruit trees are in bloom is as good a time as any, although I have transferred in October with splendid success, but don't attempt it late in the season unless you understand the business.

Before commencing this operation, as many hives should be provided as there are colonies to be transferred. Get everything ready that may be needed. If the colony is in a box hive, the following will be needed: A hand-saw, a hammer, a chisel to cut nails, a sharp, thin knife (a pointed shoe or case knife is good), a board a few inches larger each way than the frame to be used, with one side covered with one or more thicknesses of flannel, a wing or a small brush broom, a small box without a top, a dish of water and a towel. In addition to these, something will be needed to hold the combs in place when fitted in the frames. The best things for this purpose can readily be made. Get some wire, about No. 14 is best, cut into pieces 11¼ inches long for the Langstroth frame. At ¼ inch from one end bend to a right angle, at ⅞ of an inch from this angle bend the same way as the first to a right angle. At 9¼ inches from this second angle bend the same way to a right angle. The first two bends form a hook that is to be placed over the top bar of the frame, and the last bend makes an end that is to be pushed under the bottom of the frame after it is filled with comb. Prepare 6 or more for each frame that is to be filled.

If the bees are at all disposed to rob, place what is to be used in some building or room where the bees can not enter. Now go to the hive to be transferred from and blow a little smoke in at the entrance. The object in smoking the bees is to frighten them, when they will fill themselves with honey, which puts them in the same condition a cross, hungry person is after a good dinner—good natured. It is said that a bee full of honey will not sting unless pinched in some way. Then move the hive to one side and set the new one without the frames in its place, and carry the old hive, bees and all, to where you have placed the things you are to use in transferring, and turn it bottom side up if it is a box hive. Place one edge of the small box, before spoken of, on one edge of the now turned-over hive. Either prop or hold up the opposite edge of the box and drum lightly on the hive with the hammer or a small stick, and you will soon see the bees going up into the box. In this way drive out all the bees that will readily leave, keeping them subdued with smoke. When all or nearly all the bees are in the box, empty them out on the ground or sawdust in front of the new hive. Now run the saw down one or two sides of the hive on the inside, cutting the combs and cross sticks loose from the sides, choosing the sides from which the flat sides of the comb can be most readily got at. Then, with the chisel, cut off the nails and remove the two sides of the hive. Remove one or more of the combs, or as much as will fill one of the frames and lay on the cloth that has been fastened to the board as already directed. The cloth prevents injuring the sealed brood as the uncovered board would do. Place one of the frames on this comb in such a way as to save as much of the brood as possible, and with a sharp, thin knife cut the comb to the size of the inside of the frame so it will fit snugly. Put on as many of the previously prepared wires as may be needed for the upper side. Then raise the board, comb and frame up edgewise, and turn the frame and its contents and lay the wire side down on the cloth and put wires on the now upper side, and it is ready to place in the new hive where the bees are. Proceed in the same manner till all the worker comb has been transferred, rejecting all drone comb, if there are other bees within two or three miles, and let your less careful neighbors raise the drones. Brush the remaining bees, if any, down in front of the new hive. The honey from the remaining pieces of comb can be extracted or fed back to the bees and the comb made into wax.

## GIVE FRAMES, OR STARTERS OF FOUNDATION.

If there is not enough suitable comb to fill all the frames, it will be best to fill the empty ones with comb foundation. Cut the foundation so as it will reach within one-eighth of an inch of the ends of the frame and about three-eighths of an inch narrower than the inside of the frame. If you cannot afford so much foundation, put a strip of any width (called starters) from half an inch to wider along the center of the under side of the top bar of the frames, so as to give the bees a guide by which to build their combs straight in the frames, and to make sure that they will be straight, place each frame with these guide pieces in them, between frames of comb if possible, but do not separate the combs that have brood in them till settled warm weather, or the brood may get chilled.

As soon as the bees have fastened the combs securely in the frames, which will be in from one to three days, the wires should be removed.

Another method of transferring is called the Heddon plan, in which the combs are not transferred, and is as follows:

Prepare a hive and have the frames filled with comb, if possible; if not, put in full sheets of foundation, or strips, as already directed, and place it where the one stands that is to be transferred.

If one or more combs of brood can be procured from some other hive and put in this the bees will be more apt to be contented with their new home. If neither combs or foundation can be had, proceed as directed under the heading "How to get straight combs."

This method of transferring should not be attempted except in warm weather and when there is a good flow of honey. About swarming time is the best.

Now drive out nearly all of the bees, as before directed, making sure that the queen is driven out with them, and empty them down in front of the new hive, and see that all enter. Then place the old hive a few feet back of its old location with entrance in the opposite direction from what it was before. After two or three days, move the old hive a few inches towards its old location and also turn the entrance a little towards its former direction, and so continue to do every day or two till it stands by the side of the new hive with the entrance the same way, which should be accomplished in at least three weeks from the time the transfer was made.

In twenty-one days from the time of the transfer all the young bees will be hatched in the old hive, when all the bees should be driven from it and united with the colony in the new hive, first destroying the queen that is with the bees just driven out. The old hive may now be taken apart, the honey be extracted from the combs, and then melt them into wax. If the surplus arrangements have not been added to the new hive it may now be done. This method of transferring saves much work and perhaps many stings.

The future methods of procedure will depend on what kind of honey it is intended to secure, comb or extracted, not strained, as some call it.

## COMB HONEY.

It will generally be best for those keeping but a few colonies to buy the hives already prepared with the needed fixtures. I would advise the use of sections holding not more than 2 pounds, one lb. is better and not over 1¾ inches wide. The comb is more apt to be built straight in the narrow sections than in the wider ones.

Fill each section with a very thin comb foundation, fastening it firmly at the top, letting it come within ⅛ of an inch of each end and ¼ of an inch of the bottom of the section. If it is not desirable to use so much foundation, cut it into triangular pieces, long enough up and down to reach within ¼ of an inch of the bottom of the section. If foundation is not used, it will hasten and aid the bees in starting in the sections to procure some nice white pieces of comb and cut and use as directed for foundation.

Be sure and have everything in readiness for immediate use, for a few days after makes the difference between a good supply of honey and none at all.

If the colony is strong, (and none other should be kept), and it is gathering honey, the sections may be put on as soon as the wires are removed from the transferred combs. The honey secured from fruit bloom is dark colored and usually bitter, and may be extracted and kept to be fed back to the bees if at any time they should need feeding, or it can be used in making honey vinegar. When the sections are nearly filled with honey, and the bees are still gathering, they should be raised up and another tier prepared like the first placed under it on the hive. The bees will usually commence at once to work in the new and also finish the old ones. As soon as the old ones are finished they should be removed, for the longer they are left on the hive the darker they will become, for the bees do not always have clean feet. When the second tier of sections is nearly finished, remove the under tier, and should the honey flow continue, they should be raised and another tier put under as at first, and the operation should be repeated as often as necessary. After being removed from the hive, comb honey should be kept in a warm dry room, never in a cellar, unless warm and dry, and never allowed to freeze.

## EXTRACTED HONEY.

In addition to the appliances already on hand as before spoken of, a honey extractor and a honey knife will be needed if extracted honey is to be secured. An extractor can be had from $6 to $25, the price depending upon the size and style. A good one can be bought for from $8 to $14, and a knife for from 50 cents to $1.50.

Procure a hive the same as for comb honey, but in place of the sections, etc., get one or more extra stories with frames, to put on the lower hive. Some of the most successful producers of extracted honey use upper stories only 6 inches deep. Fill the frames with foundation, or put in starters, as directed under transferring. If the colony is strong and gathering honey rapidly, the second story may be put on as soon as the wires are removed from the transferred combs, otherwise not till a surplus is being gathered. If the colony is not strong enough to occupy the whole of the second story, 2 or 3 frames and a division board may be put in and the remainder of the lower story be kept covered so as to retain the heat of the bees. When the second story is nearly filled with honey it may be extracted, or it may be raised up and another prepared as before directed, be put under it, and so continue to do till the honey season closes and the extracting can all be done at once. But the better plan is to do the extracting as soon as the honey flow from each kind of flowers ceases, for the mixing of different kinds of honey destroys their distinctive flavors. The better way is to extract the yield from fruit bloom as soon as white clover begins to yield honey, and then again after white clover and before basswood, and after basswood and before the yield of dark honey from fall flowers. As different localities often yield different kinds of honey, each one must judge for himself when to extract.

Another method is to have hives of only one story in which the bees raise brood, this is called the brood nest. If honey is coming in rapidly it may be be necessary to extract 2 or 3 times a week, so as to give the queen room to deposit eggs. If this is neglected the cells will be filled with honey and brood rearing will necessarily have to cease, and as the amount of honey gathered depends upon the number of bees, it is desirable to raise as many as possible, that is, keep all colonies strong.

When ready to extract, blow a little smoke in at the entrance of the hive. If the honey is to be extracted from the brood nest move the hive just back of where it now stands and place an empty one, without any covering, in its place. Remove the cover and quilt off the hive to be extracted from, and if the bees are cross smoke them enough to make them quiet. Have ready another empty hive or comb holder in which to place the combs to be extracted. Remove one of the combs and shake the adhering bees into the empty hive on the old stand. Such bees as have not been shaken off should be brushed off with a wing or brush. Then place this comb in the empty hive or comb holder. Proceed in like manner with the remaining combs. If any of them do not need extracting place them in the hive where the bees have been shaken. Take the combs to the honey extractor and with the uncapping knife remove the cappings from as many of the combs as the comb basket will contain. Then by revolving the comb basket the honey will be thrown out of one side of the combs, which should then be reversed and the honey thrown, or extracted, from the other side. Proceed in this manner till all have been extracted, when the combs should be placed in the hive where the bees are and the hive closed up. Proceed in like manner with all the colonies that need extracting. If the combs contain unsealed brood be careful not to revolve them so rapidly as to throw it out. A little practice will soon enable one to do it properly. Should there be upper stories to extract from, and not from the brood nest, the hive need not be moved, and the bees may be shaken on the ground in front of the hive.

## SWARMING.

Swarming is the natural method of obtaining increase, and usually occurs during the latter part of May or in June when the colony has become populous and the bees are actively engaged in breeding and gathering honey. Usually about 10 o'clock, or between 10 and 2, on a bright, warm day, the greater portion of the workers not engaged in gathering stores, having their honey sacks filled with honey, rush from the hive as though a ghost were after them. After flying about for a short time, the swarm usually lights on some convenient tree or bush. During an experience of twenty years I have known but one swarm to leave for parts unknown without first lighting.

To prevent constant watching and anxiety in swarming time, I clip off two-thirds or more of one of the wings of the queen as soon as she commences to deposit eggs.

A swarm will not "run away" unless a queen accompanies it, and she can not go if one of her wings is nearly gone. Be sure and remove enough of the wing, or the queen will still be able to fly, although it will be apt to be quite slowly, if too little has been taken off.

A swarm may light without a queen being with it, the same as if the queen accompanied it, but it will finally return to its old home.

If two or more swarms issue at the same time they are very apt to light together, if they light at all. When they miss their queens and return they are pretty sure to divide up and go to their own hives.

I have previously given directions for placing the hives at least 6 feet apart, and on or near the ground. The reason of this can now be readily seen. If a swarm issues when no one sees it the queen will not be likely to crawl 6 feet and enter the wrong hive and be killed, and the hive being on the ground, she can crawl back and enter her own hive. It will not do to let them swarm and go back many times, or they may become disgusted with their queen and destroy her, and while the swarming fever lasts it interferes materially with honey gathering and brood rearing.

## HIVING A SWARM.

If the queen's wing has not been clipped, a good way to proceed is to place the hive where it is to stand permanently. Have the frames filled with foundation, or with starters in them as before directed. If there is a supply of extra combs use them in place of foundation.

As soon as the swarm issues take one or more combs from the hive the swarm has come from, at least one of the combs to have young brood in (but *be sure* there is no queen cell on either of them) and place in the center of the hive prepared for the swarm. Place the frames left in the old hive in the center and fill the empty places thus made with frames that have been prepared for the new hive. Have ready a box or basket that will hold 6 or 8 quarts, without top, and as soon as the swarm has lighted shake or brush the bees into it, and as soon as the bees have settled on it carry them to the hive prepared for them and gradually shake or brush out a few at the entrance of the hive, and as soon as they begin to enter, the remaining bees may be poured out in front of the hive.  All should be made to enter, so as to be sure that the queen is in, or they might swarm out.  The hive should also be shaded during the hottest part of the day, and it would be better if every hive could be shaded in the same way during warm weather.

## MY METHOD.

I clip a wing of every one of my queens, and when a swarm issues proceed as follows :  As soon as a swarm is seen coming out, go with a queen cage or glass tumbler to the hive and watch for the queen, which, being clipped, will soon be seen crawling on the ground, making vain attempts to fly.  Place her in the cage or tumbler.  Be careful in going to the hive that you do not step on her.

As soon as the swarm is all out move the hive it has just left two or more rods away, and put a new hive, prepared as before directed, in its place.  As before stated, the swarm will usually return without lighting, and as soon as they begin to enter let the queen loose at the entrance, and be sure she enters the hive.  If the swarm should light the same as if the queen were with it, it can be hived as already directed, letting the queen run in with the first that enter.

As soon as the other bees have all entered move the hive to where it is to remain and place the old one in its former location and the work is done.  Sometimes the swarm while circling around in the air finds the old hive, even when moved some distance away, and will enter unless prevented by again moving it, or covering it up.

Hives in which swarms are to be put should be kept in the shade for if left in the sun they will sometimes become so warm that the newly hived swarms will not stay in them.

## AFTER SWARMS.

If it is not desirable to have more than one swarm from each colony, it may be prevented in either of the following ways :

If extra queens are in readiness all the queen cells should be destroyed as soon as the colony has swarmed and a new queen be given to it.  This will save the old colony from being without a laying queen for over two weeks.  Care must be taken to remove every queen cell before attempting to introduce the queen.

Another method is to remove all the queen cells but one as soon as the colony has swarmed, and at the farthest not later than six or seven days after the swarm has issued.  If all the queen cells but one are destroyed as soon as the swarm has issued other cells will sometimes be started, so it will be better to to wait, or examine again for queen cells in three or four days.

Occasionally the colony will swarm without having started any queen cells, in which case it will be twenty-four or more days before it will have a laying queen unless one is furnished it.

## HOW TO CLIP A QUEEN'S WING.

As soon as the queen has commenced to deposit eggs, usually about eight or ten days after being hatched, take hold of the left wing with the left thumb and whichever finger comes most handy, (or if left handed use the right hand), being careful not to grasp or squeeze the abdomen, raise her from the comb, and let her stand on another finger or on the knee, and with a small pair of sharp scissors, one blade of which is carefully passed under the right wing, clip off at least ⅔ of it, being very careful not to injure either of her legs, then replace her on the comb among the bees.

## HOW TO GET STRAIGHT COMBS.

If no foundation is to be used, and the bees are to make their own combs, and it is desired to have them straight in the frames, it may be easily accomplished in the following manner:

Have the lower side of the top bar of the frames made V shaped. Raise the back end of the hive about 6 inches, and as the bees always begin comb building at the highest point, they will begin at the back end of the frames. When they have started comb nearly half the length of the frames they are at work on, reverse every other one, putting the front end of the frames at the back end of the hive, and if the combs already built are straight, the filling out of the other ends of the frames will necessarily be straight. It will be well to look at the combs occasionally while they are being built, and if they are being started wrong, or are being made crooked, they can readily be bent and fixed straight. A little attention to this will easily secure that much to be desired object, straight combs. When the combs are started the full length of the top bar, the back end of the hive should be lowered to the right position.

## ROBBING.

When the flow of honey ceases, bees are very much inclined to rob. To prevent this, keep the entrance to the hive closed to the size necessary for the use of the colony. If robbing has already begun, close the entrance so that but one or two bees can pass at a time. If this does not stop it, cover the entrance with some loose, wet hay or straw. Bees do not like to crawl through this, and the colony will generally be able to repel the attack.

## WINTERING.

It is well known that to winter bees successfully is the most difficult part of bee-keeping, and this one thing may be put down as an axiom: Extremes of heat or cold are detrimental to bees. If the temperature becomes extremely low, the bees take more food to keep up the animal heat; they become uneasy and throw off much moisture which may condense and freeze around the cluster encasing them in a solid wall of ice, thus preventing them reaching the honey, and they actually starve with plenty of honey in the hive. The remark is often made in the spring by those that had a few colonies and lost them in the winter. "My bees all died with lots of honey in the hive; I wonder what was the reason?"

If the temperature becomes too high they will also become restless and eat more than is for their good, become diseased, foul their combs and hive, and die with plenty of honey in the combs.

## CELLAR WINTERING.

It will readily be seen that it is desirable to avoid either of these extremes, heat and cold. To do this, as soon as there is settled cold weather, which in this locality is usually about the middle of November, place the bees in a dark, quiet cellar that will keep vegetables well, and maintain an even temperature of about 45°. Of course the bees should have plenty of honey to eat, and 25 lbs. will be none too much to last them till they can gather a supply in the spring. To prepare them for the cellar remove everything above the frames and put three or four sticks, ½ inch square, and nearly as long as the hive is wide inside, crosswise on the frames, and put on a new honey quilt. This will give the needed ventilation, retain the heat, and give the bees a chance to move over the tops of the frames. This should be done before cold weather, so when it is time to put the bees in winter quarters all it will be necessary to do will be to remove the cap and carefully place the colony in the cellar.

## OUTDOOR WINTERING.

If the bees are to be wintered out doors 35 lbs. of honey will be none too much for each colony. A new quilt and sticks should take the place of the old quilt the same as for cellar wintering. Corn fodder or straw may be placed about each hive to aid in keeping off the cold, but the entrance should be left partially open and shaded from the sun.

A better method of outdoor protection is to take a box without top or bottom and 8 or 10 inches larger each way than the outside of the hive and as high as may be needed. Place this box over the hive and fix the entrance so that the bees can get out and in, and fill the space between the box and hive with chaff, cut straw or dry leaves, well pressed down, and cover the top of the hive in the same way, and finish by covering the box with a flat, or slanting, roof that is water tight.

The best outdoor wintering arrangement I have ever seen is that used by H. D. Cutting, of Clinton, Mich., now and for several years past, Secretary of the Michigan State Bee-keepers' Association. It is simple, cheap and durable. I don't know that he ever made one to sell. It is very easily made and can be taken apart and put away (in the flat) in a moment and will last for years. It is made of lumber ⅜ or ½ inch thick, dressed on one or both sides, or it need not be dressed at all. Cut it so it will be 8 or 10 inches longer than the hive for the sides, and 8 or 10 inches longer than the hive is wide for the ends. For each hive make 8 pieces or cleats, about 1 inch square and 4 inches longer than the hive is high, unless the cover is high.

To make the sides place 1 of the inch square pieces ½ an inch from the end of the board cut for the sides, if ½ inch stuff is used, or ⅜ of an inch if ⅜ stuff is used, and nail fast; making as wide as the cleats are long, and put another cleat at the other end in the same way. For the end pieces place the cleats 1 inch from the ends of the boards that have been cut for the ends; make as many of these as may be needed. The sides and ends may be fastened at the corners with two hooks at each corner, or screws may be used if more convenient. The cover may be made like a house roof, or in any way that may suit ones fancy or convenience, always making sure that it is water tight. Set the hive to be prepared for winter on a board that is as wide as the inside of the above described box, and some longer than its length so as to furnish an alighting place for the bees. Fix an entrance for the bees and place the box in position, and pack as already directed. The ends of the cleats will stand on the edges of the bottom board so that rains will not wet the packing.

Whatever method of protection is adopted, whether it be corn fodder, straw, or packing in a box, it should not be removed till settled warm weather in the spring.

## MY METHOD OF WINTERING.

As soon as possible after the frost has killed the flowers so that the bees can gather little or no bee-bread, I examine each colony and select such combs as have little or no bee-bread in them, and place as many in one side of the hive as the bees may need to cluster on, and put in a division board. If there is not honey enough in the selected combs for the bees to winter on, I uncap the honey in some or all of the others, and place them on the other side of the division board so the bees will carry it over into the combs they are to winter on. If there is still a lack of winter stores, I feed more honey or syrup made of either granulated, or coffee A sugar. Don't feed poor sugar if you wish to save the bees.

The empty or extra combs are put away to be used again in the spring. At this time put on the sticks and new honey quilt as before directed, and when it becomes settled cold weather, place all in the cellar.

The object in taking away the bee-bread is to prevent the loss of bees from diarrhea. I have wintered in this way with perfect success for the last seven winters, not losing a colony from disease.

During cold weather all the bees need to eat is food which will produce heat, and that is furnished by the honey or sugar syrup, which, when pure, is fully digested, leaving nothing to be discharged as feces, consequently there can be no diarrhea, unless it be induced by extremes of heat or cold.

I believe that colonies wintered in the cellar are more apt to become weak from the loss of bees in the spring than those that are wintered outdoors if properly protected; but those wintered in the cellar consume much less honey.

The same protection may be given them when they are brought from the cellar in the spring, as has been recommended for outdoor wintering, and will largely, if not wholly prevent spring dwindling.

Whatever method of wintering may be adopted, the secret of doing it successfully is, to keep the bees in an even temperature, and with little, or no nitrogenous food. Pollen, called also bee-bread, is nitrogenous food.

If the bees are wintered in the cellar, place them on their summer stands as early in the spring as they can gather pollen from willow and soft maple blossoms. If convenient place each hive where it stood the previous season.

With the division board keep the bees crowded on as few combs as they may choose to occupy, moving it and giving new combs from those removed when preparing for winter, as often as they may need them.

If it is desired to keep the honey quilt clean for future winter use it may be removed and the one taken off in the fall replaced; but it will be well to put the wintering quilt on top of the other to help retain the heat 'till settled warm weather.

## HONEY VINEGAR.

All waste honey, and that with a bitter and unpleasant taste may be made into vinegar that is better flavored than that made from cider.

When extracting honey, the dishes used will have honey adhering to them which should be rinsed off with as little water as possible, and the sweetened water thus obtained should be put in a keg, barrel or crock and placed where it will be kept warm. During warm weather it may be placed in the sun, and so covered that air may readily enter, and dirt and flies be excluded. The cappings removed from the combs with the uncapping knife, after the honey has drained from them, may be washed with water, and will add materially to the amount of sweetened water. The sweeter the water the stronger the vinegar will be; but it will not sour as rapidly if made too sweet at first.

## ENEMIES OF BEES.

Bees have many enemies, but I shall notice but two, the toad and the moth-miller. The only objection that I know of to the hive resting on the ground is, that it makes it convenient for Mr. or Mrs. Toad to readily reach the bees, where they will quietly sit and make a square meal of bees. Although they are good in the garden and on the farm, they are bad around the bee-hives. Be sure and keep them away, even if you are obliged to kill them.

The moth-miller is sometimes very troublesome, but seldom does any harm if all colonies are kept strong. Don't invest in moth-proof hives, or moth traps, but keep all the colonies strong and the moth-miller will not trouble.

## FOUL BROOD.

Among the diseases of bees, foul brood takes first rank. The success of the most convenient method of curing it (and the one I shall give) would indicate that the cause of the disease is in the honey; but the disease itself is developed in the young brood, causing it to die, usually before it is sealed over. It may also lurk in and about the hive, and a hive that has contained a diseased colony should not be again used for any purpose till thoroughly disinfected by boiling.

When a colony is badly diseased it may frequently be known by the odor without opening the hive. To me it is very much like that given off by the melting of bad glue.

It may be quite readily known on examination of the combs, especially if badly diseased. If but few cells of brood are affected it may not be detected by one not acquainted with it, and if extracted honey is taken may readily be communicated to every colony, for it is very contagious.

When the brood first dies it usually has the appearance of pus, or "matter," and settles down in the lower back corner of the cell, and is light colored; but the longer it is dead the darker it becomes, sometimes getting almost black.

If the disease is suspected, take a pin and with the head slowly attempt to remove the putrid mass from one of the cells. If it clings to the pin and also to the cell, and stretches out like a thread of rubber, and finally lets go the pin and draws back into the cell, it is quite safe to call it foul brood.

Being so contagious, it, by many, is considered difficult to cure; so much so that it is directed to burn a good log or brush-heap, and when well on fire throw the hive, bees and all, into the fire. But this is a useless waste, the bees, hive, and frames may be saved and the combs melted into wax. Probably the best way is to have a starving box to hold about a peck, with one side off, or an empty hive may be used. Shake and brush all the bees of the diseased colony into the starving box and cover the open side with wire cloth, so that not a bee can escape, and do not let a single bee from the colony being treated go to any other colony, for it will be pretty sure to carry the disease with it. Set this box in a cool, dark place, where no bees can reach it, placing the box so that the wire cloth will be on the side, not on the top or bottom.

Now melt the combs into wax, and thoroughly boil the hive and frames and everything connected with it, in water, and it is again ready for use. Do not use the old location again unless it has been thoroughly scalded, ground and all, with boiling water, or covered one or more inches deep with salt, which is to be left to be dissolved by the rains and dews.

After the bees have been in the box two or more days some of the bees will be seen falling to the bottom, having consumed all the honey taken with them, and are actually starving. If they were well filled with honey when put in the box it may be six or more days before the honey is all used up. When a few bees fall to the bottom, say 100, more or less, and are crawling slowly about, they may be placed in the boiled or some other hive that has been prepared with foundation or starters.

I would not use any comb for a few days, for if any of the bees should still have any foul honey it would be deposited in the cells and so continue the disease.

The bees in the starving-box must be very closely watched, for when their honey is all consumed they soon die. Look at them several times a day after the second day.

To cleanse the hands or anything else that it will not do to put into boiling water, prepare a solution of salycilic acid as follows:

Salycilic acid, 16 grs.; borax, 16 grs.; water, 1 oz. Put in a bottle and shake often till the acid and borax are dissolved.

Thoroughly moisten the hands, etc., with this preparation and no fears need be entertained of spreading the disease by handling some other bees or hive.

# GLOSSARY,

OR

# DICTIONARY OF MEDICAL TERMS

## USED IN THIS WORK.

**Ab-do-men.** The belly, or the lower front part of the body.

**Ab-lu-tion.** Washing of the body externally; cleansing by water.

**Ab-nor-mal.** Unnatural; irregular; not according to rule.

**Ab-or-tion.** Childbirth before the proper time.

**Ab-ra-sion.** A superficial wound caused by bruising the skin.

**Ab-sorb-ent.** Glands and vessels which absorb or suck up substances; medicines which absorb, or combine with acid matter in the stomach or bowels.

**Ac-couch-eur.** A man who attends mothers in childbirth.

**Ac-e-tab-u-lum.** The socket that receives the head of the thigh bone.

**A-cho-li-a.** Not sufficient of bile.

**A-cid.** Sour, sharp, pungent, bitter or biting to the taste.

**Ac-tual Cau-te-ry.** Used in surgery; burning or searing with a hot iron.

**Ac-u-punc-ture.** Pricking with needles; one of the operations of surgery.

**Ac-ute.** Diseases attended with violent symptons; the reverse of chronic.

**Ad-he-sive.** Tenacious, sticky; apt or tending to adhere.

**Ad-he-sive Plaster.** Sticking plaster.

**Ad-i-pose.** Membrane or tissue; fat.

**A-dult Age.** Manhood or womanhood; a person who has attained full size and age.

**Af-fec-tion.** Disorder, disease, malady.

**Al-bu-men.** An element found in both animal and vegetable substances. The white of an egg.

**Al-bu-mi-nose.** A substance produced in the stomach during digestion.

**Al-i-ment.** Nourishment, nutrition; anything necessary for the support of life.

**Al-i-ment-a-ry Ca-nal.** The entire passage through the whole intestines from the mouth; the passage for the aliments.

**Al-ka-li.** A substance which, when united to acids, neutralizes them.

**Al-ter-a-tive.** A remedy which gradually restores healthy action.

**Al-ve-o-lar.** Relating to the sockets of the teeth.

**Al-vine.** Relating to the intestines.

**Am-au-ro-sis.** A loss or decay of sight, produced by various causes.

817

**Am-en-or-rhe-a.** An obstruction of the menstrual discharges; absence of the menses.

**Am-ni-ot-ic Liquid.** The fluid surrounding the fœtus of the womb.

**Am-pu-ta-tion.** The act of cutting off a limb or other part of the body.

**A-na-sar-ca.** A dropsy of the whole body; a general dropsy.

**A-nas-to-mose.** To communicate with each other; applied to arteries and veins.

**A-nat-o-my.** Study of the body.

**An-em-i-a.** Lack of blood; a comparatively bloodless state.

**An-es-the-sia.** Numbness or paralysis of sensation.

**An-eu-rism.** A soft tumor, caused by the rupture of the coats of an artery.

**An-i-mal-cules.** Animals so minute as to be visible only with a microscope.

**An-o-dyne.** Any medicine which will allay pain and induce sleep.

**Ant-a-cid.** A substance which neutralizes acids; alkalies are antacids.

**An-thel-min-tic.** A medicine that destroys worms.

**An-thrax.** A dusky red or purplish kind of tumor, occurring in the neck.

**An-ti-bil-ious.** An opposing medicine counteractive of bilious complaints.

**An-ti-dote.** A preventive, or remedy for, poison or any disease.

**An-ti-dys-en-ter-ic.** A cure for dysentery.

**An-ti-e-met-ic.** A remedy to check vomiting.

**An-ti-lith-ic.** A medicine to prevent or remove urinary calculi or gravel.

**An-ti-mor-bif-ic.** Anything to prevent or remove disease.

**An-ti-pe-ri-o-dic.** That which cures periodic diseases, such as ague, intermittent fever, etc.

**An-ti-scor-bu-tic.** A remedy used for the scurvy; blood purifiers.

**An-ti-sep-tic.** Whatever resists or removes putrefaction or mortification.

**An-ti-spas-mod-ic.** Remedy for cramps, spasms, and convulsions.

**A-nus.** The external opening of the rectum, lower intestines.

**A-or-ta.** The great artery from the heart.

**Ap-a-thy.** Insensibility to pain.

**A-pe-ri-ent.** A mild purgative or laxative.

**Ap-pe-tite.** A desire for food or drink.

**Ar-o-ma.** The agreeable odor of plants and other perfumed substances.

**Ar-o-mat-ic.** Spicy and fragrant drugs.

**Ar-te-ry.** A vessel that conveys the blood from the heart to the organs.

**Ar-thro-di-a.** A joint movable in any direction.

**Ar-tic-u-la-tion.** The union of bones with each other, as at the joints.

**Ar-tic-u-la-ted.** Having joints.

**As-car-i-des.** Pinworms found in the lower portion of the bowels.

**As-ci-tes.** Dropsy of the abdomen.

**As-phyx-ia.** Apparent death, as from drowning.

**As-sim-i-la-tion.** The process by which food is changed into tissue.

**As-then-ic.** Debilitated.

**As-trin-gent.** A medicine which contracts or puckers up surfaces with which they come in contact; used in flooding, diarrhea, etc.

**At-o-ny.** Debility; defect of muscular power.

**At-ro-phy.** A loss of strength and wasting of flesh without any sensible cause.

**At-ten-u-ants.** Medicines for reducing the weight of the body.

**Au-ri-cle.** A cavity of the heart.

**Aus-cul-ta-tion.** The art of detecting disease by listening to the sounds of lungs, heart, etc.

**Ax-il-la.** The armpit; hence axillary, pertaining to the armpit.

**Ax-il-la-ry Glands.** Situated in the armpit, secreting a fluid of peculiar odor.

**Bal-sam-ics.** Medicines possessing healing properties.

**Bile** or **Gall.** A secretion from the liver which aids digestion.

**Blis-ter.** A thin watery bladder on the skin.

**Bou-gie.** A taper body introduced into a passage or sinus to keep it open or enlarge it.

**Bright's Disease.** A dangerous disease of the kidneys.

**Bron-chi-tis.** Inflammation of the bronchial tubes; the branches of the windpipe in the lungs.

**Ca-chex-y.** A bad state of the body. It may be caused by blood poisons.

**Cal-cu-lus.** Stone or gravel found in the kidneys and bladder.

**Cal-lous.** Hard or firm.

**Ca-lor-ic.** Heat.

**Cap-il-la-ry.** Fine, hair-like.

**Cap-si-cum.** Cayenne pepper.

**Cap-sule.** A dry, hollow vessel containing the seed or fruit.

**Car-bon-ic Acid Gas.** A gas of two parts of oxygen and one part of carbon.

**Ca-ri-es.** Ulceration of a bone.

**Car-min-a-tives.** Medicines which allay pain by expelling wind from the stomach and bowels; an aromatic medicine.

**Ca-rot-id Artery.** The great arteries of the neck that convey blood to the heart.

**Car-ti-lage.** A hard elastic substance of the body; gristle.

**Ca-ta-me-ni-a.** The monthly discharges of women.

**Cat-a-plasm.** A poultice.

**Ca-tarrh.** A discharge from the head or throat; a flow of mucus.

**Ca-thar-tic.** An active purgative.

**Cath-e-ter.** A curved instrument introduced into the bladder, for drawing off the urine.

**Caus-tic.** Burning; a corroding or destroying substance which burns or corrodes living tissues, as nitrate of silver, potash, etc.

**Cau-ter-y.** A burning or searing any part of the body.

**Cell.** A small elementary form found in vegetable and animal tissue.

**Cer-e-bel-lum.** The lower and back part of the brain.

**Cer-e-bral.** Pertaining to the brain.

**Cer-e-brum.** The upper and front part of the brain.

**Cer-e-bro-Spinal.** Pertaining to the spinal cord and brain.

**Ce-ru-men.** The wax of the ear.

**Cha-lyb-e-ate.** Containing iron in solution, as found in mineral springs.

**Chan-cre.** A venereal or syphilitic sore.

**Chol-a-gogues.** Medicines that cause an increased flow of bile, such as calomel and podophyllin.

**Chol-er-ic.** Easily irritated; irritable.

**Chor-dee.** A painful drawing of the chords of the penus. It occurs in gonorrhea.

**Chron-ic.** To continue for a long time, and becoming a fixed condition of the system.

**Chyle.** A milky fluid, mixing with and forming the blood.

**Chyme.** The pulp formed by the food after it has been for some time in the stomach, mixed with the gastric secretions.

**Cir-cu-la-tion.** The motion of the blood, which is propelled by the heart through the body.

**Clav-i-cle.** Collar-bone.

**Co-ag-u-la-tion.** A change from a fluid to a solid condition, as in the coagulation of the blood.

**Co-ag-u-lum.** A clot of blood.

**Co-a-lesce.** To grow together; to unite.

**Col-lapse.** Sudden failure or prostration of the vital functions.

**Col-liq-ua-tive.** Excessive discharges from the body which weaken the system.

**Co-lon.** A portion of the large intestine.

**Co-ma, Com-a-tose.** Stupor; disposed to sleep.

**Com-press.** A bandage, made with several folds of linen.

**Con-cus-sion.** A violent shock.

**Con-flu-ent.** Running together.

**Con-ges-tion.** An accumulation of blood.

**Con-junc-ti-va.** The membrane that lines the eyelid and covers the eye.

**Con-sti-pa-tion.** Costiveness.

**Con-ta-gious.** Catching, or that which may be communicated by contact.

**Con-tu-sion.** A bruise.

**Con-va-les-cence.** An improvement in health after sickness.

**Con-vul-sions.** Involuntary and violent movements of the body.

**Cor-dial.** A medicine that stimulates and raises the spirits.

**Cor-ne-a.** The transparent membrane in the fore part of the eye.

**Cor-rob-o-rants.** Tonics or strengthening medicines.

**Cor-ro-sive.** Substances that consume or eat away.

**Coun-ter-ir-ri-ta-tion.** Driving disease from one part by irritating another part.

**Cra-ni-um.** The skull.

**Cri-sis.** The turning point of a disease.

**Cu-ta-ne-ous.** Pertaining to the skin.

**Cu-ti-cle.** The outer skin.

**Cyst.** A bag or sac containing matter or other fluid.

**De-bil-ity.** Weakness.

**De-coc-tions.** Medicines that are prepared by boiling.

**Deg-lu-ti-tion.** The act of swallowing.

**De-liq-ui-um.** The act of fainting.

**De-lir-i-um.** Wildness, temporary loss of the mind.

**De-mul-cents.** A mucilaginous medicine, as flaxseed or gum Arabic.

**Den-ti-tion.** The act or process of cutting teeth.

**Den-tri-frice.** A preparation for cleaning the teeth.

**De-ob-stru-ent.** A mild laxative.

**De-ple-tion.** To diminish the quantity of blood by blood-letting or other process.

**Dep-u-ra-tion.** Cleansing from impure matter.

**De-ter-gent.** Cleansing medicines as laxatives and purgatives.

**Di-ag-no-sis.** The act of determining diseases by symptoms.

**Di-a-pho-ret-ics.** Medicines which aid or produce perspiration or sweating.

**Di-a-phragm.** Midriff; the muscular division between the chest and the abdomen.

**Di-ath-e-sis.** Tendency of the body to any form of disease, as scrofulous diathesis.

**Di-e-te-tic.** Relating to diet.

**Dil-a-ta-tion.** Act of spreading in all directions.

**Di-lu-ted.** Reducing the strength of liquids with water.

**Di-lu-ting.** Weakening.

**Dis-cu-tient.** Medicines which scatter or drive away tumors.

**Dis-in-fec-tants.** Articles which purify infected places.

**Dis-lo-ca-tion.** A bone out of its socket.

**Di-u-ret-ic.** A medicine that increases the amount of urine.

**Dor-sal.** Having reference to the back.

**Dras-tics.** Active or strong purgatives.

**Du-o-de-num.** The first of the small intestines.

**Dys-cra-sia.** A bad habit, producing generally a diseased condition of the system.

**Dys-pep-sia.** Difficult of digestion.

**Dys-pha-gi-a.** Difficulty of swallowing.

**Dysp-nœ-a.** Obstructing the breath.

**Dys-u-ri-a.** Difficulty and pain in discharging urine.

**Eb-ul-li-tion.** The motion of a liquid by which it gives off bubbles of vapor.

**Ef-fer-vesce.** To foam as in soda-water.

**Ef-flor-es-cence.** Redness of the surface, as in measles, etc.

**Ef-flu-vi-a.** Exhalations from substances, as from flowers or decaying matter.

**Ef-fu-sion.** An escape of fluids from their natural position into the tissues or cavities of the body.

**E-lec-tri-za-tion.** Medical use of electricity.

**E-lec-tu-ary.** Medicines prepared with honey.

**E-lim-i-na-tion.** To escape from the body, as by the pores of the skin.

**E-mac-i-ate.** To waste away; to grow thin.

**Em-bry-o.** The early stage of the fœtus.

**Em-e-sis.** The act of vomiting.

**Emet-ics.** Medicines which produce vomiting.

**Em-men-a-gogue.** A medicine which will aid the menstrual discharge.

**E-mol-li-ent.** A softening medicine, flaxseed, etc.

**E-mul-sion.** A mucilage from the emollients.

**E-nam-el.** The outside covering of the teeth.

**En-ceph-a-lon.** The whole brain.

**En-cys-ted.** Enclosed in a cyst or sac.

**En-dem-ic.** A disease peculiar to certain localities.

**E-ne-ma.** An injection by the rectum.

**En-er-va-tion.** A reduction of strength.

**En-te-ri-tis.** Inflammation of the bowels.

**E-phem-e-ral.** Of short duration.

**Ep-i-dem-ic.** A disease that prevails in a certain district.

**Ep-i-derm-is.** The outer skin; the cuticle.

**Ep-i-gas-tric.** Pertaining to the upper part of the abdomen.

**Ep-i-glot-tis.** Trap-door cartilage at the root of the tongue, preventing food or drink from entering the wind-pipe.

**Ep-i-lep-tic.** Subject to epilepsy, convulsions, or the falling sickness.

**E-piph-o-ra.** A surplus secretion of tears, causing what is termed a watery eye.

**Ep-i-spas-tic.** Blistering.

**Ep-is-tax-is.** Nose bleed.

**Er-e-thism.** Morbid energetic action of irritability.

**E-ro-sion.** Eating away; corrosion.

**Er-rhine.** A medicine to promote the discharge of mucus from the nose.

**E-ruc-ta-tion.** Raising wind from the stomach; belching.

**E-rup-tion.** Pimples or blotches on the skin.

**Es-char.** The dead part, which falls off from the surface.

**Es-cha-rot-ic.** An application which sears or destroys the flesh.

**Eu-sta-chi-an Tube.** A narrow canal leading from the side of the throat to the internal ear.

**E-vac-u-a-tion.** The discharge by stool or passing of urine from the bladder.

**Ex-ac-er-ba-tion.** Violent increase in a disease.

**Ex-an-the-ma.** An eruptive disease, as small-pox, scarlet fever, measles.

**Ex-ci-sion.** The act of cutting out or off.

**Ex-cit-ant.** A stimulant; a nerve remedy.

**Ex-cor-i-ate.** To wear off the skin in any way.

**Ex-cres-cence.** An unnatural growth of a part, as a wart or tumor.

**Ex-cre-tion.** That which is thrown off.

**Ex-fo-li-ate.** Scaling or peeling off.

**Ex-ha-la-tion.** Throwing off of vapor, air, gas, etc.

**Ex-os-to-sis.** An unnatural growth from a bone; a bony tumor.

**Ex-pec-to-rant.** A medicine which produces or aids the discharge of mucus from the bronchial tubes or lungs.

**Ex-pec-to-rate.** To discharge mucus or saliva from the mouth.

**Ex-pi-ra-tion.** The act of expiring; breathing out the air from the lungs.

**Ex-trav-a-sa-tion.** A collection of blood into a cavity, or under the skin, a blood blister.

**Fæ-cal.** Relating to the fæces.

**Fæ-ces.** The natural discharges of the bowels.

**Fa-ci-al.** Having reference to the face.

**Far-i-na-ceous.** Containing starch, as farinaceous food, meal or flour from vegetables.

**Fau-ces.** The pharynx and back part of the mouth.

**Feb-ri-fuge.** A medicine to drive away fever, producing perspiration.

**Fe-brile.** Having reference to fever; feverish.

**Fe-mur.** The thigh bone.

**Fet-id.** Having a disagreeable odor.

**Fi-brine.** Animal matter found in blood.

**Fi-brous.** Composed of small threads or fibres of animal or vegetable matter.

**Fil-ter.** To strain through a paper made for that purpose.

**Fil-tra-tion.** Straining.

**Fist-u-la.** An ulcer.

**Flac-cid.** Flabby, soft, relaxed; as a flaccid muscle.

**Flat-u-len-cy, Fla-tus.** To inflate the stomach with gas.

**Flood-ing.** Uterine hemorrhage.

**Flush.** A flow of blood to the face.

**Flux.** An unusual discharge from the bowels, diarrhea.

**Fœ-tus.** The child in the womb.

**Fo-men-ta-tion.** Bathing by means of flannels dipped in hot water or medicated liquid.

**For-mi-ca-tion.** An unpleasant sensation, like the creeping of ants.

**For-mu-la.** A medical prescription.

**Fract-ure.** A broken bone.

**Fric-tion.** Rubbing with the dry hand or coarse cloth.

**Fu-mi-ga-tion.** Smoking a room or anything to be cleansed.

**Func-tion.** The particular acting of an organ, as the function of the heart.

**Fun-da-ment.** The anus; the lower extremity of the rectum.

**Fun-gus.** A spongy flesh in wounds, as proud flesh, a soft cancer which bleeds when touched.

**Gal-van-i-za-tion.** Use of the galvanic current.

**Gan-gli-on.** A knot or lump on tendons; an enlargement in the course of a nerve.

**Gan-grene.** Partial death of a part, often ending in entire mortification.

**Gar-gle.** A wash for the mouth and throat.

**Gastric.** Belonging to the stomach.

**Gastric Juice.** Secretion of the stomach.

**Gas-tri-tis.** Inflammation of the stomach.

**Ges-ta-tion.** The period of pregnancy.

**Gland.** A soft body, the function of which is to secrete some fluid.

**Glot-tis.** The opening into the windpipe at the root of the tongue.

**Glu-te-us.** A name applied to the muscles of the hip.

**Gran-u-la-tion.** The healing of a wound or ulcer with healthy matter.

**Gru-mous.** Thick, clotted, concreted; as grumous blood.

**Gut-tur-al.** Relating to the throat.

**Hab-it.** A peculiar state or temperament of the body; pre-disposed to do some particular thing.

**Hec-tic.** A remitting fever.

**Hem-a-le-mes.** Hemorrhage from the stomach.

**Hem-a-tu-ra.** Hemorrhage from the bladder.

**Hem-a-to-sis.** An excessive or morbid quantity of blood.

**Hem-i-ple-gia.** Paralysis of one side of the body.

**He-mop-ty-sis.** A spitting of blood.

**Hem-or-rhage.** A flow of blood, as from the lungs, nose, etc.

**Hem-or-rhoids.** The piles; bleeding piles.

**He-pat-ic.** Relating to the liver.

**Her-ba-ceous.** Pertaining to herbs.

**Hereditary.** Inherited from a parent.

**Her-pes.** Disease of the skin, as tetter, ringworm, etc.

**Her-ni-a.** A rupture, and protrusion of some part of the bowels.

**Hu-mors.** The fluids of the body, excluding the blood.

**Hy-dra-gogue.** A medicine that produces a watery discharge from the bowels, used in dropsy.

**Hy-drar-gy-rum.** Metallic mercury, quicksilver; a physician's name for calomel.

**Hy-dro-gen.** One of the elementary principles, always existing in water, of which it composes the ninth part.

**Hy-dro-pho-bia.** The rabid qualities of a mad dog.

**Hy-gi-ene.** The art of preserving health by diet.

**Hyp-o-chon-dri-a-cal.** Melancholy; low-spirited.

**Hyp-not-ics.** Medicines which produce sleep.

**Hy-po-der-mic.** To insert under the skin.

**Hy-ster-ic-al.** Subject to hysteria; nervous.

**I-chor.** A biting, watery, and acrid discharge from ulcers.

**Id-i-op-a-thy.** An unhealthy condition not preceded by any other disease.

**Id-i-o-syn-cra-sies.** Peculiarity of constitution or temperament.

**Il-e-ous.** Colic in the small intestines.

**Il-i-ac Re-gion.** Region of the small intestines.

**Im-be-cil-i-ty.** Weakness of mind.

**Im-mer-se.** To plunge under water.

**In-a-ni-tion.** Emptiness; weakness; exhaustion.

**In-cor-po-rate.** To mix medicines.

**In-cu-ba tion.** To hatch eggs; slow development of disease.

**In-ci-sor.** A front tooth.

**In-di-gest-i-ble.** Not easily digested.

**In-dis-po-si-tion.** A poor state of health.

**In-fec-ti-ous.** Contagious.

**In-flam-ma-tion.** Attended with heat; a redness or swelling of any part.

**In-fu-sion.** Medicine prepared by steeping, not boiling.

**In-ges-tion.** Forcing into the stomach.

**In-jec-tion.** Any preparation sent into some part of the body by means of a syringe.

**In-oc-u-la-tion.** Communicating a disease to a healthy person by injecting contagious matter in the skin.

**Is-chu-ra.** Not able to pass the urine.

**In-spi-ra-tion.** Drawing air into the lungs.

**In-spis-sa-tion.** The act of thickening by boiling or evaporation.

**In-teg-u-ment.** A covering; the skin.

**In-ter-cos-tal.** Between the ribs.

**In-ter-mit-tent.** Ceasing at intervals; fevers which come on at regular intervals.

**In-tes-tines.** The bowels.

**Jug-u-lar.** Applied to the veins of the throat.

**Lac-er-a-ted.** Torn from.

**Lach-ry-mal.** Pertaining to the tears.

**Lac-ta-tion.** Act of nursing, or sucking.

**Lan-ci-na-ting.** Piercing, as with a sharp pointed instrument; hence lanci-nating pain.

**Lan-guor.** Feebleness; lassitude of body.

**Lar-ynx.** The upper part of the windpipe.

**Lax-a-tive.** A gentle cathartic; a medicine that loosens the bowels.

**Le-sion.** A flesh wound.

**Leth-ar-gy.** Excessive drowsiness.

**Leu-cor-rhe-a.** A whitish discharge from the womb.

**Lig-a-ture.** A thread for tying blood-vessels to prevent bleeding.

**Li-ga-tion.** The art of using a ligature.

**Lin-i-ment.** A fluid lotion or wash to be applied by friction.

**Lith-on-trip-tic.** A medicine to dissolve the stone or gravel in the bladder.

**Li-thot-o-my.** The operation of cutting to remove the stone in the bladder.

**Liv-id.** Black and blue spot on the surface.

**Lo-chi-al.** Pertaining to discharges from the womb after childbirth.

**Lum-ba-go.** Rheumatic pains in the loins and small of the back.

**Lum-bar.** Pertaining to the loins.

**Lymph.** A thin, colorless fluid in the lymphatic vessels.

**Lym-phat-ic.** Small vein-like vessels pervading the body; absorbents.

**Mac-er-a-tion.** Steeping or softening with water.

**Mac-u-lar.** Colored spots; blemishes.

**Mal-Bad.** Mal practice; not according to science.

**Ma-la-ri-a.** Bad air; air which tends to cause disease supposed to arise from decayed vegetable matter.

**Mal-for-ma-tion.** Irregular formation or structure of parts.

**Ma-lig-nant.** Violent; dangerous; liable to produce death.

**Mar-row.** A soft substance in the bones.

**Mas-ti-ca-tion.** The act of chewing.

**Mas-tur-ba-tion.** Self-abuse. The most injurious, self-destroying of all habits.

**Ma-te-ri-a Medica.** The science of medicine.

**Ma-trix.** The womb.

**Mat-u-ra-tion.** The formation of pus or matter in any part of the body.

**Me-dul-la Oblongata.** A nervous mass in the lower part of the brain.

**Men-ses, Menstruation.** The monthly sickness of women.

**Men-stru-um.** A liquid used to dissolve solid substances.

**Me-phit-ic.** Suffocating; noxious; pestilential.

**Met-a-car-pus,** That portion of the hand between the wrist and fingers.

**Me-tas-ta-sis.** A change of disease from one location to another.

**Met-a-tar-sus.** The part of the foot between the ankle and the toes.

**Mi-as-ma, Miasmata.** Malaria; exhalations from swamps, lowlands and decaying matter.

**Mor-bid.** Unhealthy; deseased; corrupt.

**Mor-bif-ic.** Producing disease.

**Mor-bus.** A disease of the bowels; cholera morbus.

**Mu-ci-lage.** A glutinous, watery solution of gum.

**Mu-cus.** Animal mucilage secreted by the mucous membrane.

**Mus-cles.** A bundle of fibres; the organs of motion; they constitute the flesh.

**Nar-cot-ics.** Medicines that produce sleep, relieve pain, or stupefy.

**Nau-se-a.** Sickness at the stomach; may increase until vomiting takes place.

**Na-vel.** Center of the abdomen.

**Ne-gus.** A liquid made of wine, water, sugar, nutmeg, and lemon juice.

**Ne-phr-it-is.** Inflammation of the kidneys.

**Neph-ros.** The kidney.

**Ner-vine.** A medicine that soothes a nervous excitement.

**Neu-ral-gia.** Pain in the nerves.

**Neu-ras-the-nia.** Nervous exhaustion.

**Noc-tur-nal.** Occurring in the night.

**Nor-mal.** Natural and healthy condition.

**Nos-trum.** A patent medicine.

**Nu-tri-tious.** A substance possessing nourishment.

**Ob-tuse.** Dull, not acute.

**Œ-de-ma.** A watery swelling.

**Ol-fac-tory Nerves.** The nerves of smell.

**O-men-tum.** The covering of the bowels.

**Oph-thal-mi-a.** Disease of the eye. Inflammation of the eyes.

**O-pi-ates.** Medicines which promote sleep.

**Op-tic Nerve.** The nerve which enters the back part of the eye.

**Or-thop-nœ-a.** Asthma; great difficulty of breathing, caused by diseases of the heart or diaphragm.

**Os-si-fy.** To change flesh or other soft matter into a hard, bony substance; from osteo, a bone or like a bone.

**O-vum.** An egg.

**Ox-y-gen.** A gas that forms one-fifth of the atmosphere.

**Pal-ate.** The partition separating the cavity of the mouth from that of the nose.

**Pal-pi-ta-tion.** A fluttering or unnatural action of the heart, in which it beats too rapidly and strongly.

**Pan-a-ce-a.** A remedy for all diseases; a universal medicine.

**Pa-pil-la.** A red point upon the tongue or elsewhere.

**Par-a-cen-te-sis.** Puncturing of the chest or abdomen for the purpose of drawing off water.

**Pa-ral-y-sis.** Palsy; losing control of any part of the system.

**Par-a-lyt-ic.** One affected with paralysis.

**Par-a-ple-gi-a.** Paralysis of the lower portion of the body.

**Par-ox-ysm.** A fit of disease at certain periods.

**Pa-thol-o-gy.** Doctrine of disease.

**Par-tu-ri-tion.** Childbirth.

**Pec-tor-al.** Relating to the chest.

**Pel-vis.** A bony cavity forming the lower part of the trunk of the body.

**Pep-sin.** A peculiar substance in the stomach which aids digestion.

**Per-i-car-di-um.** The sac containing the heart.

**Per-i-car·dit-is.** Inflammation of the pericardium.

**Per-spi-ra-tion.** Sweat.

**Per-i-ne-um.** The part between the anus and organs of generation

**Per-i-os-te-um.** The membrane covering the bones.

**Per-i-to-ne-um.** The membrane which lines the abdomen and covers the bowels.

**Pe-te-chi-æ.** Purple spots which appear upon the skin in low fevers.

**Phag-e-den-ic.** Corroding, eating; applied to ulcers.

**Pha-lan-ges.** The bones which form the fingers and toes.

**Phleg-mat-ic.** Dull; sluggish; heavy.

**Phar-ynx.** The upper part of the throat.

**Phlo-gis-tic.** Tendency to inflammatory.

**Phthys-ic-al.** A condition of the system tending to pulmonary consumption.

**Phlegm.** A mucus from the bronchial tubes.

**Ple-thor-ic.** Of a full habit of body; corpulence.

**Pleu-ra.** A membrane that covers the lungs and folds upon the sides.

**Pleu-ri-sy.** Inflammation of the pleura.

**Pneu-mo-ni-a.** Inflammation of the lungs.

**Pol-y-pus.** A pear shaped tumor.

**Pre-scrip-tion.** A physician's formula for the preparation of medicines.

**Probe.** An instrument for examining the depth of a wound.

**Prog-no-sis.**  Guessing the termination of a disease.

**Pro-lap-sus Ani.**  Falling of the anus.

**Pro-lap-sus Uteri.**  Falling of the uterus.

**Pros-tra-tion.**  Loss of strength.

**Pro-phy-lac-tic.**  A medicine to prevent disease.

**Pty-a-lism.**  A copious flow of saliva; salivation.

**Pu-ber-ty.**  Full growth; perfection.

**Pu-er-pe-ral.**  Fever at or soon after childbirth.

**Plu-mon-a-ry.**  Pertaining to, or affecting the lungs.

**Pul-mon-i-tis.**  Inflammation of the lungs.

**Pulse.**  The beating of the heart or blood-vessels, especially of the arteries.

**Pulp.**  A soft mass.

**Pun-gent.**  Piercing, biting, stimulating.

**Pur-ga-tive.**  A gentle cathartic; a medicine acting on the bowels to loosen them.

**Pur-u-lent.**  Consisting of pus or matter.

**Pus.**  Unhealthy matter.

**Pus-tules.**  Elevations of the skin containing pus.

**Pu-tre-fac-tion.**  To decompose by fermentation.

**Pu-tres-cent.**  Pertaining to the process of putrefaction.

**Py-ro-sis.**  A peculiar disease of the stomach better known as water-brash.

**Rec-tum.**  The lower portion of the large intestine.

**Re-frig-er-ant.**  Medicines which lessen the heat of a body.

**Reg-i-men.**  The regulation of diet and habit in order to restore health or to cure disease.

**Res-o-lu-tion.**  To return to health; dispersion of an inflammation before pus has formed.

**Re-solv-ents.**  Applied to inflammations.

**Res-pi-ra-tion.**  The process of breathing.

**Re-sus-ci-ta-tion.**  Reviving from apparent death, as drowning.

**Ret-i-na.**  The internal nervous tissue of the eye.

**Ru-be-fa-cients.**  Medicines that causes redness of the skin, as mustard, radish leaves, etc.

**Ru-bif-ic.**  To make red.

**Sac-cha-rine.**  Having the properties of sugar.

**Sa-li-va.**  The spittle; the secretions of the mouth.

**Sal-i-va-tion.**  Increase of the secretion of saliva.

**San-a-tive.**  A curative medicine; to heal.

**San-guine.**  Abounding in blood, or having the color of blood.

**Sa-ni-es.**  A thin discharge from wounds or ulcers.

**Scab.**  A formation over a sore in healing.

**Scarf-skin.**  The outer skin of the body.

**Scir-rhous.**  Hard; knotty, generally of a cancerous nature.

**Scor-bu-tic.**  Partaking of the nature of scurvy.

**Scro-tum.**  The bag containing the testicles.

**Se-cre-tion.** The separation of any substance from the blood for a particular purpose.

**Sed-a-tive.** The opposite of stimulation. A quieting medicine which allays irritation and soothes pain.

**Sed-en-tary.** Sedentary habit; accustomed to, or requiring much sitting; inactive.

**Seid-litz.** A village in Bohemia, from which Seidlitz powders derived its name.

**Sem-i-nal.** Pertaining to or contained in seed.

**Se-rous.** Thin, watery substance, like whey.

**Serum.** The watery, or milky portions of the blood.

**Sin-a-pism.** A mustard plaster.

**Sin-ew.** That which unites flesh to a bone.

**Slough.** Death from a part; the part that separates from a wound.

**Slough-ing.** The act of separating the dead flesh from a sore.

**Sol-u-tion.** Composed of a liquid and a solid substance.

**Sol-vent.** Having the power to dissolve solid substances.

**Sor-des.** The dark matter deposited upon the lips and teeth in low fevers.

**Spasm.** A sudden contraction of the muscles; cramps, convulsions.

**Spe-cif-ic.** An infallible remedy.

**Spi-nal Col-umn.** The back-bone.

**Spi-nal Cord.** The nervous marrow in the backbone.

**Spleen.** The milt; it is situated in the abdomen and attached to the stomach.

**Squa-mous.** Having scales.

**Ster-num.** The breast-bone.

**Ster-tor.** Noisy breathing; snoring.

**Ster-to-rous.** The act of snoring.

**Stim-u-lants.** Medicines that are calculated to excite a healthy action.

**Sto-mach-ic.** A cordial for the stomach, exciting its action.

**Sto-mat-i-tis.** Inflammation of the mouth.

**Stool.** A discharge from the bowels.

**Stran-gu-ry.** Difficult and painful passage of urine.

**Strict-ure.** Unnatural contraction of any passage of the body.

**Stru-ma.** Scrofula.

**Stupor.** Insensibility; numbness.

**Styp-tic.** A medicine which stops bleeding.

**Sub-cu-ta-ne-ous.** Under the skin.

**Sudor.** Sweat.

**Su-dor-if-ics.** Medicines that cause sweating.

**Sup-pos-i-to-ries.** Medicinal substances introduced into the rectum to favor or restrain evacuations, or to ease pain.

**Sup-pu-ra-tion.** The act of forming pus.

**Sut-ure.** The peculiar saw-like joint uniting the bones of the skull.

**Symp-tom.** A sign or token of disease.

**Syn-co-pe.** To swoon; fainting.

**Syph-i-lis.**  A contagious disease from sexual intercourse with those who have venereal disease.

**Syph-i-li-tic.**  Pertaining to the venereal disease or pox.

**Syr-inge.**  An instrument for injecting liquids into the bowels, ear, throat, or other parts of the body.

**Tan-nic Acid.**  An astringent made from oak bark.

**Tem-per-a-ment.**  A peculiar habit of body.

**Ten-don.**  A fibrous cord attached to the extremity of a muscle.

**Te-nes-mus.**  Difficulty and pain at stool; a painful bearing down sensation in the lower bowels.

**Te-pid.**  Warm, but not hot.

**Ter-tian.**  Occurring every other day.

**Tes-tes.**  The testicles.

**Tes-ti-cles.**  Two glandular bodies situated in the scrotum, belonging to the male organs of generation.

**Tet-a-nus.**  Locked jaw.

**Tib-i-a.**  The large bone of the leg below the knee.

**Tinct-ure.**  Medicine dissolved in alcohol.

**Tho-rax.**  The chest.

**Tor-mi-na.**  Severe griping pains.

**Ton-ics.**  Remedies intended to strengthen the system.

**Ton-sil.**  Glands situated on each side of the throat.

**Tor-pid.**  Dull; stupid; lifeless.

**Tra-che-a.**  The windpipe.

**Tu-ber-cle.**  A pimple, swelling, or small tumor.

**Tu-me-fac-tion.**  The act of forming a tumor.

**Tu-mor.**  An enlargement of any part of the body; a swelling.

**Ty-phoid.**  Resembling typhus; weak; low.

**Ty-phus.**  A nervous fever, malignant, infectious, etc.

**Ul-cer.**  A sore which discharges pus.

**Um-bil-ic.**  Pertaining to the navel.

**U-rea.**  A substance found in the urine.

**U-re-ter.**  The duct leading from the kidneys to the bladder.

**U-re-thra.**  Duct leading out from the bladder; the canal of the penis through which the urine passes from the body.

**U-rine.**  Water from the bladder.

**U-ter-us.**  The womb.

**Vac-ci-nate.**  To inoculate with the cow-pox by inserting the vaccine in the skin.

**Vac-cine.**  Matter of the cow-pox.

**Va-gi-na.**  The passage from the womb to the vulva.

**Vag-in-is-mus.**  Spasm of the vagina, caused by morbid irritability.

**Val-e-tu-di-na-ri-an.**  A person of a weak, sickly constitution.

**Va-ri-o-lous.**  Pertaining to small pox.

**Ven-e-ry.**  Sexual indulgence.

**Ve-nous.**  Relating to the veins.

**Ven-ti-la-tion.** A free admission or motion of air.

**Ver-mi-fuge.** A medicine intended to destroy worms.

**Ver-ti-go.** Dizziness; swimming of the head.

**Ves-i-cle.** A little bladder of water formed under the skin.

**Vir-u-lent.** Extremely injurious; malignant; poisonous.

**Vi-rus.** Contagious poison.

**Vis-ce-ra.** The internal organ of the body.

**Vis-cid.** Sticky; tenacious.

**Vol-a-tile.** Easily evaporated; substances that evaporate on exposure to the atmosphere.

**Vul-ner-a-ry.** Pertaining to wounds.

**Vul-va.** The external opening of the female genitals.

**Whites.** Fluor Albus.

**Zy-mot-ic.** Contagious diseases, such as may be inoculated.

# Publisher's Notices.

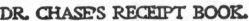

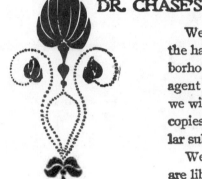

### DR. CHASE'S RECEIPT BOOK.

We desire to place a copy of this work in the hands of every family, and, if the neighborhood has been canvassed and there is no agent through whom it can be purchased, we will send by mail, free of postage, single copies to any address on receipt of the regular subscription price.

We at all times desire agents. The terms are liberal, and the agency to sell this work in any field will afford a good living to any man or woman of intelligence. Agents will be assigned territory in the order of their application. For name and address of the publishers, see title page.

### DR. CHASE'S FAMILY MEDICINES.

So great has become the demand for Dr. Chase's Family Medicines (many think we are the manufacturers because we publish Dr. Chase's book), owing to the fact that they possess great merit, that we are in almost daily receipt of letters of inquiry which not only make extra work for us in answering the correspondence, but inquirers do not receive as prompt attention as they would if they addressed the manufacturers direct. All inquiries for Dr. Chase's remedies should be addressed to

THE DR. A. W. CHASE MED. CO.,
No. 18 Ellicott St.,
BUFFALO, N. Y

832

# MEDICAL INDEX.

833

# GENERAL INDEX.